Dental RADIOGRAPHY

PRINCIPLES AND TECHNIQUES

SIXTH EDITION

Joen M. Iannucci, DDS, MS
Professor of Clinical Dentistry
The Ohio State University
College of Dentistry
Columbus, Ohio

Laura Jansen Howerton, RDH, MS
Retired Educator
The Ohio State University, Columbus, Ohio
The University of North Carolina, Chapel Hill, North Carolina
Wake Technical Community College
Raleigh, North Carolina

ELSEVIER

Elsevier
3251 Riverport Lane
St. Louis, Missouri 63043

DENTAL RADIOGRAPHY: PRINCIPLES AND TECHNIQUES, SIXTH EDITION ISBN: 978-0-323-69550-3

Library of Congress Control Number: 2021943199

Content Strategist: Joslyn Dumas/Kelly Skelton
Senior Content Development Manager: Luke Held
Senior Content Development Specialist: Maria Broeker
Publishing Services Manager: Deepthi Unni
Senior Project Manager: Manchu Mohan
Senior Design Direction: Amy L. Buxton

Printed in India.

Last digit is the print number: 9 8 7 6 5 4

To my son, Michael—
To my dad, Angelo—
To my mom, Dolores—

*Thank you for your everlasting love,
your encouragement, and a life filled with laughter.*

To all my students, past & present—
*Thank you for everything that you have taught me,
and for the sincere privilege of being a part of your lives.*

JMI

To my husband, Bruce, who inspires me every day of my life.

LJH

REVIEWERS

Deborah Bush-Munson, CDA, EFDA, MS
Associate Professor
Dental Technologies
St. Louis Community College at Forest Park
St. Louis, Missouri

Joanne Clare Gibbons-Smyth, CDA, BA, ID
Certified Dental Assistant Program Chairperson
Science Tech and Health CDA Department
Okanagan College
Kelowna, British Columbia

Tonya Hance, BAAS, CDA, RDA
Dental Assisting Program Director
Health Science
Grayson College
Denison, Texas

Linda Adams Hiter, RDH, BS, MDH
Dental Hygiene Instructor
Dental Hygiene Program
Mississippi Delta Community College
Moorhead, Mississippi

Dean Lefebvre, MAED, BS, RDH, CAET
Instructor in the Dental Hygiene Program
School of Health Sciences
Saskatchewan Polytechnic
Regina, Saskatchewan, Canada

Angie Maida, CDA, RDH, Med
Program Director, Associate Professor
Dental Hygiene Department
Chattanooga State Community College
Chattanooga, Tennessee

Tena A Phillips, DDS
Assistant Professor
Dental Assisting and Dental Hygiene Programs
Chattanooga State Community College
Chattanooga, Tennessee

Jennifer S Sherry, RDH, MSEd
Associate Professor
Dental Hygiene Program
Southern Illinois University
Carbondale, Illinois

Michelle Thibault, RDH
Manager, Dental Programs
Niagara College
Welland, Ontario, Canada

Laura J Webb, MSHSA, RDH, FAADH, CDA-Emeritus
Dental Hygiene Education Program Consultant & Continuing Education Provider
LFW Education Services
Fallon, Nevada

PREFACE

Welcome to the sixth edition of *Dental Radiography: Principles and Techniques*. The purpose of this text is to present the basic principles of dental imaging and provide detailed information about imaging techniques. This text offers a straightforward, reader-friendly format with a balance of theory and technical instruction to develop dental imaging skills. Our goal with this sixth edition, as with previous editions, is to facilitate teaching and learning.

ABOUT THIS EDITION

The simplicity and organization of this text makes it exceptionally easy to use. To facilitate learning, the sixth edition is divided into manageable parts for both the student and faculty:

- Radiation Basics
- Equipment and Digital Imaging Basics
- Film, Processing, and Film Mounting Basics
- Dental Radiographer Basics
- Technique Basics
- Extraoral and Three-Dimensional Imaging Basics
- Normal Anatomy Basics
- Image Interpretation Basics

Each chapter includes a variety of features to aid in learning. A list of **objectives** to focus the reader on the important aspects of the material is presented at the beginning of every chapter. **Key terms** are highlighted in blue and bold typeface as they are introduced in the text. A complete **glossary** of more than 600 terms is included at the end of the book. Detailed, easy-to-follow, step-by-step procedures are designed to guide the student for the various intraoral and extraoral techniques. The material is organized in an instructionally engaging way that ensures technique mastery and serves as a valuable reference tool. **Summary tables and boxes** are included throughout the text. These provide easy-to-read synopses of text discussions that support visual learners and serve as useful review and study tools. **Quiz questions** are included at the end of each chapter to immediately test knowledge. **Answers and rationales** to the quiz questions are provided to instructors on the Evolve website.

NEW TO THIS EDITION

The sixth edition recognizes the updates in radiation history, specifically the history of three-dimensional imaging and the recognition of oral and maxillofacial radiology as a specialty of dentistry. The changes in infection prevention protocols for imaging procedures are detailed, with a discussion of COVID-19, respiratory hygiene and cough etiquette, and updated CDC guidelines.

The latest classification system of periodontal and peri-implant diseases is presented with a detailed description of radiographic findings to aid in interpretation and diagnosis of periodontal disease.

Also new to this edition are a variety of exceptional technique videos. These videos are part of the Student Resources on Evolve that are included with each new textbook purchase and there are accompanying Interactive Video Questions and Answers.

This edition updates and expands the chapters on digital and three-dimensional imaging with the most current technology, ensuring students are prepared to practice in the modern dental office. Many images have been added that illustrate not only normal anatomic structures but common dental findings as well. The extraoral bite-wing image is introduced and presented as a valuable diagnostic aid.

Throughout the text, a **Helpful Hint** feature highlights important material and offers tips to aid student understanding. The hints help the student learn and recognize and prevent the most common technique pitfalls while providing a checklist to guide both the novice and the experienced dental radiographer.

Photographs have been updated throughout the text to depict the newest equipment, and revised art includes new illustrations of anatomy and technique. These enhancements help clearly delineate the various learning features and engage the student in the content. Enhanced line drawings are included to improve the clarity in this highly visual subject area.

ABOUT EVOLVE

A companion Evolve website is available to students and instructors. The site offers a wide variety of additional learning tools and greatly enhances the text for both students and instructors.

FOR THE STUDENT

Evolve Student Resources offers the following:

- **Self-Study Examination**. Over 250 multiple-choice questions are provided in an instant feedback format. This helps students prepare for class and reinforces what they've studied in the text.
- **Case Studies**. Scenarios similar to those found on the National Board Dental Hygiene Examination (NBDHE), as well as clinical and dental imaging patient findings, are presented with challenging self-assessment questions. There is also a case scenario in each chapter followed by three to five questions.
- **Additional Case Scenarios**. Case Studies are included for each chapter and accompanied by multiple choice questions.
- **Interactive Exercises**
    - **Labeling Exercises**. Drag-and-drop device assembly and labeling of equipment, along with positioning drawings and photographs.
    - **Dental Image Identification Exercises**. Drag-and-drop film mounting and digital imaging.
- **Technique Videos**. New to this edition.

FOR THE INSTRUCTOR

Evolve Instructor Resources offers the following:

- **TEACH Instructor Resource Manual**. Includes the following:
    - **TEACH Lesson Plans**. Detailed instruction by chapters and sections, with content mapping.
    - **TEACH PowerPoint Slides**. Slides of text and images separated by chapter.
    - **TEACH Student Handouts**. Exercises provide extra practice in the classroom.
    - **Test Bank in ExamView**. Approximately 1000 objective-style questions with accompanying rationales, CDA and NBDHE exam tags, and page/section references for textbook remediation.
- **Answers to Textbook Quiz Questions, Case Studies, and Case Scenarios**. A mixture of fill-in-the-blank and short-answer questions for each chapter, with self-submission and instant feedback and grading.

- **Answers to the Workbook and Laboratory Manual**.
- **Image Collection**. All the text's images available electronically for download into PowerPoint or other classroom lecture formats.

WORKBOOK AND LABORATORY MANUAL

Dental Radiography: A Workbook and Laboratory Manual is a companion to the textbook that seeks to provide a complete and comprehensive solution for dental assisting (DA) and dental hygiene (DH) educational programs. The first section of the Workbook contains written exercises and critical-thinking exercises organized into seven modules that follow the seven parts of the textbook, designed to offer students extra practice and reinforce the material. The second section is structured as a Laboratory Manual, presenting the material and instructions needed for students to perform each of the radiographic techniques, establishing competency in the radiography clinic through active learning.

FROM THE AUTHORS

Are there any tricks to learning dental imaging? Most definitely! Attend class. Stay awake. Pay attention. Ask questions. Read the book. Learn the material. Do not cram. Prepare for tests. Help your classmates. Do not give up.

We hope that you will find the textbook and Evolve website to be the most comprehensive learning package available for dental imaging.

Joen M. Iannucci, DDS, MS
Laura Jansen Howerton, RDH, MS

ACKNOWLEDGMENTS

We express our deepest appreciation to our families, friends, and colleagues for their unending support during preparation of this manuscript.

The sixth edition of this textbook would not have been possible without the incredible commitment and enthusiastic dedication of the team at Elsevier—which includes Joslyn Dumas, Senior Content Strategist; Kelly Skelton, Content Strategist; Luke Held, Senior Content Development Manager; Maria Broeker, Senior Content Development Specialist; Manchu Mohan, Senior Book Project Manager; Amy Buxton, Senior Book Designer; Balaji Dhandapani, Web Content Coordinator; and David Dipazo, Senior Producer, Video Specialist. This group of people has worked as a cohesive crew, giving 100% effort with an excellent work ethic.

We would also like to acknowledge the generosity and willingness of many dental manufacturing companies who gave their permissions to display imaging equipment. The authors would also like to thank the staff and dental offices of Dr. Timothy W. Godsey of Chapel Hill, North Carolina, Drs. Robert D. Elliott and Julie R. Molina of Cary, North Carolina, and Dr. W. Bruce Howerton, Jr., of Franklinton, North Carolina, for all their contributions of sample images. In addition, a note of thanks to Drs. Anthony Mecham and Kenneth Abramovitch for their enthusiasm in the education of dental radiology.

Joen M. Iannucci, DDS, MS
Laura Jansen Howerton, RDH, MS

CONTENTS

PART I Radiation Basics and Dental Image Characteristics

PART II Equipment and Digital Imaging Basics

PART III Film Imaging Basics

PART IV Dental Radiographer Basics

PART V Intraoral Technique Basics

PART VI Extraoral Imaging Basics

PART VII Normal Anatomy Basics

PART VIII Image Interpretation Basics

1

Radiation History

LEARNING OBJECTIVES

After completion of this chapter, the student will be able to do the following:

1. Define the key terms associated with dental radiation.
2. Summarize the importance of dental images.
3. List the uses of dental images.
4. Summarize the discovery of x-radiation.
5. Recognize the pioneers in dental x-radiation and their contributions and discoveries.
6. List the highlights in the history of x-ray equipment and film.
7. List the highlights in the history of dental radiographic techniques.
8. List the highlights in the history of digital imaging.

The dental radiographer cannot appreciate current x-ray technology without looking back to the discovery and history of x-radiation. A thorough knowledge of x-radiation begins with a study of its discovery, the pioneers in dental x-radiation, and the history of dental x-ray equipment, image receptors, and radiographic techniques. In addition, before the dental radiographer can begin to understand x-radiation and its role in dentistry, an introduction to basic dental imaging terms and a discussion of the importance of dental images are necessary. The purpose of this chapter is to introduce basic dental imaging terms, to detail the importance of dental images, and to review the history of x-radiation.

DENTISTRY AND X-RADIATION

Basic Terminology

Before studying the importance of dental images and the discovery and history of x-rays, the student must understand the following basic terms pertaining to dentistry and x-radiation:

Radiation: A form of energy carried by waves or a stream of particles

X-radiation: A high-energy radiation produced by the collision of a beam of electrons with a metal target in an x-ray tube

X-ray: A beam of energy that has the power to penetrate substances and record image shadows on receptors (photographic film or digital sensors)

Radiology: The science or study of radiation as used in medicine; a branch of medical science that deals with the therapeutic use of x-rays, radioactive substances, and other forms of radiant energy

Radiograph: An image or picture produced on a receptor (radiation-sensitive film, phosphor plate, or digital sensor) by exposure to ionizing radiation; a two-dimensional representation of a three-dimensional object

Dental radiograph: A photographic image produced on a receptor by the passage of x-rays through teeth and related structures

Radiography: The art and science of making radiographs by the exposure of a receptor to x-rays

Dental radiography: The production of radiographs of the teeth and adjacent structures by the exposure of an image receptor to x-rays

Dental radiographer: Any person who positions, exposes, and processes dental x-ray image receptors

Image: A picture or likeness of an object

Image receptor: A recording medium; examples include x-ray film, phosphor plate, or digital sensor

Imaging, dental: The creation of digital, print, or film representations of anatomic structures for the purpose of diagnosis

Importance of Dental Images

The dental radiographer must have a working knowledge of the value and uses of dental images. Dental images are a necessary component of comprehensive patient care. Dental images enable the dental professional to identify many conditions that may otherwise go undetected and to see conditions that cannot be identified clinically. An oral examination without dental images limits the dental practitioner to what is seen clinically—the teeth and soft tissue. With the use of dental images, the dental radiographer can obtain a wealth of information about the teeth and supporting bone.

Detection is one of the most important uses of dental images (Box 1-1). Through the use of dental images, the dental radiographer can detect disease. Many dental diseases and conditions produce no clinical signs or symptoms and are typically discovered only through the use of dental imaging.

DISCOVERY OF X-RADIATION

Roentgen and the Discovery of X-rays

The history of dental radiography begins with the discovery of the x-ray. Wilhelm Conrad Roentgen (pronounced "ren-ken"), a Bavarian

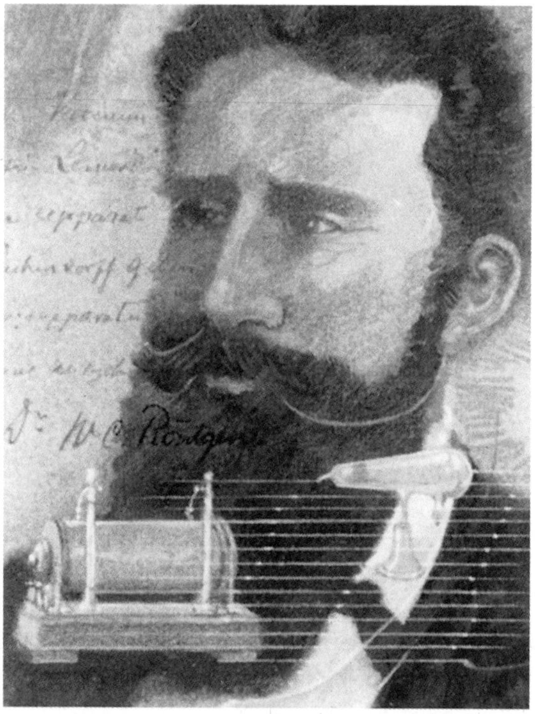

Fig 1-1 Roentgen, the father of x-rays, discovered the early potential of an x-ray beam in 1895. (Courtesy Carestream Health Inc., Rochester, NY.)

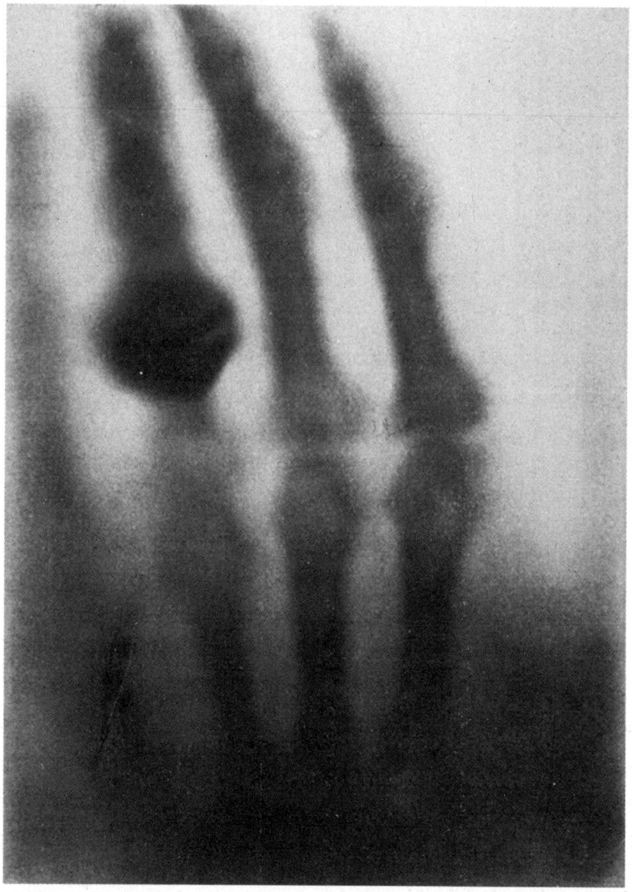

Fig 1-2 Hand mit Ringen (Hand with Rings): print of Wilhelm Roentgen's first "medical" x-ray, of his wife's hand, taken on December 22, 1895 and presented to Ludwig Zehnder of the Physik Institut, University of Freiburg, on January 1, 1896.

BOX 1-1 Uses of Dental Images

- To detect lesions, diseases, and conditions of the teeth and surrounding structures that cannot be identified clinically
- To confirm or classify suspected disease
- To localize lesions or foreign objects
- To provide information during dental procedures (e.g., root canal therapy, placement of dental implants)
- To evaluate growth and development
- To illustrate changes secondary to caries, periodontal disease, and trauma
- To document the condition of a patient at a specific point in time
- To aid in development of a clinical treatment plan

physicist, discovered the x-ray on November 8, 1895 (Figure 1-1). This monumental discovery revolutionized the diagnostic capabilities of the medical and dental professions and, as a result, forever changed the practice of medicine and dentistry.

Before the discovery of the x-ray, Roentgen had experimented with the production of cathode rays (streams of electrons). He used a vacuum tube, an electrical current, and special screens covered with a material that glowed (fluoresced) when exposed to radiation. He made the following observations about cathode rays:

- The rays appeared as streams of colored light passing from one end of the tube to the other.
- The rays did not travel far outside the tube.
- The rays caused fluorescent screens to glow.

While experimenting in a darkened laboratory with a vacuum tube, Roentgen noticed a faint green glow coming from a nearby table. He discovered that the mysterious glow, or "fluorescence," was coming from screens located several feet away from the tube. Roentgen observed that the distance between the tube and the screens was much greater than the distance cathode rays could travel. He realized that something from the tube was striking the screens and causing the glow. Roentgen concluded that the fluorescence must be the result of some powerful "unknown" ray.

In the following weeks, Roentgen continued experimenting with these unknown rays. He replaced the fluorescent screens with a photographic plate. He demonstrated that shadowed images could be permanently recorded on the photographic plates by placing objects between the tube and the plate. Roentgen proceeded to make the first radiograph of the human body; he placed his wife's hand on a photographic plate and exposed it to the unknown rays for 15 minutes. When Roentgen developed the photographic plate, the outline of the bones in her hand could be seen (Figure 1-2).

Roentgen named his discovery x-rays, the "x" referring to the unknown nature and properties of such rays. (The symbol *x* is used in mathematics to represent the unknown.) He published a total of three scientific papers detailing the discovery, properties, and characteristics of x-rays. During his lifetime, Roentgen was awarded many honors and distinctions, including the first Nobel Prize ever awarded in physics.

Following the publication of Roentgen's papers, scientists throughout the world duplicated his discovery and produced additional information on x-rays. For many years after his discovery, x-rays were referred to as "roentgen rays," radiology was referred to as "roentgenology," and radiographs were known as "roentgenographs."

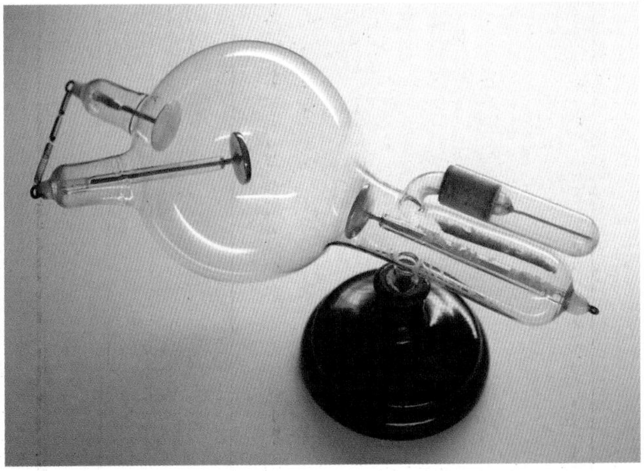

Fig 1-3 Early Crookes x-ray tube from the Museum of Wilhelm Conrad Roentgen in Würzburg, Germany. These first-generation "cold cathode" x-ray tubes were used from the 1890s until about 1920. Copyright User: Aida / Wikimedia Commons / CC-BY-SA-3.0 [http://creativecommons.org/licenses/by-sa/3.0] / GFDL [https://en.wikipedia.org/wiki/Wikipedia:Text_of_the_GNU_Free_Documentation_License] / https://commons.wikimedia.org/wiki/File:X-ray_tube_2.jpg

Earlier Experimentation

The primitive vacuum tube used by Roentgen in the discovery of x-rays represented the collective findings of many investigators. Before the discovery of x-rays in 1895, a number of European scientists had experimented with fluorescence in sealed glass tubes.

In 1838, a German glassblower named Heinrich Geissler built the first vacuum tube, a sealed glass tube from which most of the air had been evacuated. This original vacuum tube, known as the *Geissler tube*, was modified by a number of investigators and became known by their respective names (e.g., the *Hittorf-Crookes tube*, the *Lenard tube*).

Johann Wilhelm Hittorf, a German physicist, used the vacuum tube to study fluorescence (a glow that results when a fluorescent substance is struck by light, cathode rays, or x-rays). In 1870 he observed that the discharges emitted from the negative electrode of the tube traveled in straight lines, produced heat, and resulted in a greenish fluorescence. He called these discharges cathode rays. In the late 1870s, William Crookes, an English chemist, redesigned the vacuum tube and discovered that cathode rays were streams of charged particles. The tube used in Roentgen's experiments incorporated the best features of the Hittorf and Crookes designs and was known as the *Hittorf-Crookes tube* (Figure 1-3).

In 1894, Philip Lenard discovered that cathode rays could penetrate a thin window of aluminum foil built into the walls of the glass tubes and cause fluorescent screens to glow. He noticed that when the tube and screens were separated by at least 3.2 inches (8 cm), the screens would not fluoresce. It has been postulated that Lenard might have discovered the x-ray if he had used more sensitive fluorescent screens.

PIONEERS IN DENTAL X-RADIATION

After the discovery of x-rays in 1895, a number of pioneers helped shape the history of dental radiography. The development of dental radiography can be attributed to the research of hundreds of investigators and practitioners. Many of the early pioneers in dental radiography died from overexposure to radiation. At the time x-rays were discovered, nothing was known about the hidden dangers that resulted from using these penetrating rays.

Shortly after the announcement of the discovery of x-rays in 1895, a German dentist, Otto Walkhoff, made the first dental radiograph. He placed a glass photographic plate wrapped in black paper and rubber in his mouth and submitted himself to 25 minutes of x-ray exposure. In that same year, W. J. Morton, a New York physician, made the first dental radiograph in the United States using a skull. He also lectured on the usefulness of x-rays in dental practice and made the first whole-body radiograph using a 3 × 6 ft sheet of film.

C. Edmund Kells, a New Orleans dentist, is credited with the first practical use of radiographs in dentistry in 1896. Kells exposed the first dental radiograph in the United States using a living person. During his many experiments, Kells exposed his hands to numerous x-rays every day for years. This overexposure to x-radiation caused the development of numerous cancers in his hands. Kells' dedication to the development of x-rays in dentistry ultimately cost him his fingers, later his hands, and then his arms.

Other pioneers in dental radiography include William H. Rollins, a Boston dentist who developed the first dental x-ray unit. While experimenting with radiation, Rollins suffered a burn to his hand. This initiated an interest in radiation protection and later the publication of the first paper on the dangers associated with radiation. Frank Van Woert, a dentist from New York City, was the first to use film in intraoral radiography. Howard Riley Raper, an Indiana University professor, established the first college course in radiography for dental students.

Table 1-1 lists highlights in the history of dental radiography. The development of dental radiography has moved forward from these early discoveries and continues to improve even today as new technologies become available.

HISTORY OF DENTAL X-RAY EQUIPMENT

In 1913, William D. Coolidge, an electrical engineer, developed the first hot-cathode x-ray tube, a high-vacuum tube that contained a tungsten filament. Coolidge's x-ray tube became the prototype for all modern x-ray tubes and revolutionized the generation of x-rays.

In 1923, a miniature version of the x-ray tube was placed inside the head of an x-ray machine and immersed in oil. This served as the precursor for all modern dental x-ray machines and was manufactured by the Victor X-Ray Corporation of Chicago (Figure 1-4). Later, in 1933, General Electric introduced a new machine with improved features. From that time on, the dental x-ray machine changed very little until a variable kilovoltage machine was introduced in 1957. Later, in 1966, a recessed long-beam tubehead was introduced.

HISTORY OF DENTAL X-RAY FILM

From 1896 to 1913, dental x-ray packets consisted of glass photographic plates or film cut into small pieces and hand-wrapped in black paper and rubber. The hand wrapping of intraoral dental x-ray packets was a time-consuming procedure. In 1913 the Eastman Kodak Company manufactured the first prewrapped intraoral films and consequently increased the acceptance and use of x-rays in dentistry. The first machine-made periapical film packets became available in 1920.

The films currently used in dental radiography are greatly improved compared with the films of the past. At present, fast film requires a very short exposure time, less than 2% of the initial exposure times used in 1920, which, in turn, reduces the patient's exposure to radiation.

HISTORY OF DENTAL RADIOGRAPHIC TECHNIQUES

The intraoral techniques used in dentistry include the bisecting technique, the paralleling technique, and the bite-wing technique.

TABLE 1-1 Highlights in the History of Dental Imaging

Year	Event	Pioneer/ Manufacturer
1895	Discovery of x-rays	W. C. Roentgen
1896	First dental radiograph	O. Walkhoff
1896	First dental radiograph in United States (skull)	W. J. Morton
1896	First dental radiograph in United States (living patient)	C. E. Kells
1901	First paper on dangers of x-radiation	W. H. Rollins
1904	Introduction of bisecting technique	W. A. Price
1913	First dental text	H. R. Raper
1913	First prewrapped dental films	Eastman Kodak Company
1913	First x-ray tube	W. D. Coolidge
1920	First machine-made film packets	Eastman Kodak Company
1923	First dental x-ray machine	Victor X-Ray Corp, Chicago
1925	Introduction of bite-wing technique	H. R. Raper
1933	Concept of rotational panoramics proposed	
1947	Introduction of long-cone paralleling technique	F. G. Fitzgerald
1948	Introduction of panoramic radiography	
1955	Introduction of D-speed film (Kodak Ultra-speed)	
1957	First variable-kilovoltage dental x-ray machine	General Electric
1978	Introduction of dental xeroradiography	
1981	Introduction of E-speed film (Kodak Ektaspeed)	
1987	Introduction of intraoral digital imaging in France	
1989	Dental tomography scanners become available	
1994	Introduction of Kodak Ektaspeed Plus film	
1995	Introduction of digital sensor for panoramic unit	
1998	Introduction of cone-beam computed tomography (CBCT) for dental use	
1999	CBCT scanners available in Europe	
1999	Oral and maxillofacial radiology becomes a specialty in dentistry	
2000	Introduction of F-speed film (Kodak/ Carestream Dental INSIGHT)	
2001	CBCT scanners available in the United States	

The dental practitioners who developed these radiographic techniques include Weston Price, a Cleveland dentist, who introduced the bisecting technique in 1904, and Howard Riley Raper, who redefined the original bisecting technique and introduced the bite-wing technique in 1925. Raper also wrote one of the first dental radiography textbooks in 1913.

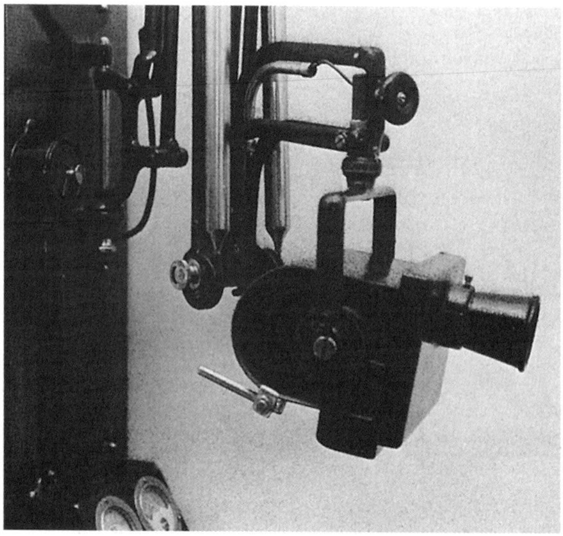

Fig 1-4 Victor CDX shockproof tube housing (1923). (Courtesy Goaz PW, White SC: *Oral radiology and principles of interpretation*, ed 2, St Louis, 1987, Mosby.)

The paralleling technique was introduced by C. Edmund Kells in 1896. Later, in 1920, Franklin W. McCormack used the technique in practical dental radiography. F. Gordon Fitzgerald, the "father of modern dental radiography," revived interest in the paralleling technique with the introduction of the long-cone paralleling technique in 1947.

The extraoral technique used most often in dentistry is panoramic radiography. In 1933 Hisatugu Numata of Japan was the first to expose a panoramic radiograph; however, the film was placed lingually to the teeth. Yrjo Paatero of Finland is considered to be the "father of panoramic radiography." He experimented with a slit beam of radiography, intensifying screens, and rotational techniques.

HISTORY OF DENTAL DIGITAL IMAGING

Radiographs have been produced using radiographic film for well over a century. Traditional radiography is being replaced by digital imaging in the dental office. Digital imaging is one of the most significant advances that have occurred in dentistry.

Digital imaging allows for instant and easy transmission of images and electronic storage. The capability to reduce patient exposure to radiation while increasing diagnostic potential has profound implications. In addition, chemical waste associated with traditional radiography is reduced, which benefits the environment.

In 1987, the technology that is used to support dental digital imaging was introduced in France when the first intraoral imaging sensor was introduced. In 1989 an article describing direct digital imaging technology was first published in U.S. dental literature. Since then, digital imaging technology has become widely accepted and has evolved with improvements in sensor design and supporting technology.

HISTORY OF THREE-DIMENSIONAL DIGITAL IMAGING

In 1999, cone-beam computed tomography was introduced to dentistry; this allows for viewing of the oral structures in three dimensions. Up to this point in time, imaging techniques allowed viewing of structures in two dimensions only; no magnification, distortion, or superimposition of structures is seen with three-dimensional digital imaging. This type of extraoral imaging allows for diagnosis of disease and image guidance of surgical procedures. Three-dimensional digital imaging will have a considerable effect on the field of dentistry.

HISTORY OF ORAL AND MAXILLOFACIAL RADIOLOGY EDUCATION

In 1999, the American Dental Association recognized its ninth specialty program: Oral and Maxillofacial Radiology (OMFR). This program provides advanced training in radiology of the oral and maxillofacial region, including the management of diseases and disorders. Persons interested in this program complete a 2- or 3-year residency term after completion of dental school, followed by an international board examination. OMFR joins the other specialty programs of dentistry including oral and maxillofacial surgery, orthodontics, endodontics, pediatric dentistry, periodontics, prosthodontics, dental public health, oral and maxillofacial pathology, dental anesthesiology, oral medicine, and orofacial pain.

SUMMARY

- An x-ray is a beam of energy that has the power to penetrate substances and record image shadows on an image receptor.
- A radiograph is a two-dimensional representation of a three-dimensional object.
- An image receptor is a recording medium; examples include x-ray film, phosphor plate, or digital sensor.
- Dental imaging is the creation of digital, print, or film representations of anatomic structures for the purpose of diagnosis.
- Disease detection is one of the most important uses for dental images.
- Wilhelm Conrad Roentgen discovered the x-ray in 1895.
- Following the discovery of the x-ray, numerous investigators contributed to advancements in dental radiography.
- Digital imaging, one of the most significant advances in dentistry, allows for instant review and transmission of images, reduces patient exposure, and improves the diagnostic potential.
- In 1999, cone-beam computed tomography was introduced, which allows for viewing of the oral and maxillofacial complex in three dimensions.
- Also in 1999, the American Dental Association recognized oral and maxillofacial radiology as a specialty field of dentistry.

BIBLIOGRAPHY

Frommer HH, Stabulas-Savage JJ: Ionizing radiation and basic principles of x-ray generation. In Radiology for the dental professional, ed 9, St Louis, 2011, Mosby.

Haring JI, Lind LJ: The importance of dental radiographs and interpretation. In Radiographic interpretation for the dental hygienist, Philadelphia, 1993, Saunders.

Johnson ON: History of dental radiography. In Essentials of dental radiography for dental assistants and hygienists, ed 9, Upper Saddle River, NJ, 2011, Prentice Hall.

Langlais RP: Exercises in oral radiology and interpretation, ed 4, St Louis, 2004, Saunders.

Langland OE, Langlais RP: Early pioneers of oral and maxillofacial radiology, Oral Surg Oral Med Oral Pathol 80(5):496, 1995.

Langland OE, Langlais RP, Preece JW: Production of x-rays. In Principles of dental imaging, ed 2, Baltimore, MD, 2002, Lippincott Williams & Wilkins.

Mallya SM, Lam EWN: Physics. In White and Pharoah's oral radiology: principles and interpretation, ed 8, St Louis, 2019, Elsevier.

Mallya SM, Lam EWN: Safety and protection. In White and Pharoah's oral radiology: principles and interpretation, ed 8, St Louis, 2019, Elsevier.

Miles DA, Van Dis ML, Williamson GF, et al: X-ray properties and the generation of x-rays. In Radiographic imaging for the dental team, ed 4, St Louis, 2009, Saunders.

Mosby's dental dictionary, ed 2, St Louis, 2008, Mosby.

WEBSITES

American Dental Association: Dental Specialties. https://www.ada.org/en/ncrdscb/dental-specialties

U.S. Food and Drug Administration: Dental Cone-Beam Computed Tomography. www.FDA.gov

QUIZ QUESTIONS

Matching

For questions 1 to 9, match each term (a to i) with its corresponding definition.

a. Radiation
b. Radiograph
c. Radiograph, dental
d. Radiographer, dental
e. Radiography
f. Radiography, dental
g. Radiology
h. X-radiation
i. X-ray

_____**1.** A photographic image produced on a receptor by the passage of x-rays through teeth and related structures.

_____**2.** A beam of energy that has the power to penetrate substances and record image shadows on photographic film.

_____**3.** A form of energy carried by waves or a stream of particles.

_____**4.** Any person who positions, exposes, and processes x-ray image receptors.

_____**5.** The production of radiographs by the exposure of a receptor to x-rays.

_____**6.** A high-energy radiation produced by the collision of a beam of electrons with a metal target in an x-ray tube.

_____**7.** The science or study of radiation as used in medicine.

_____**8.** The production of radiographs of the teeth and adjacent structures by the exposure of image receptors to x-rays.

_____**9.** A two-dimensional representation of a three-dimensional object.

For questions 10 to 19, match the dental pioneers with their contributions (a to j).

a. Used paralleling technique in practical dental radiography
b. Discovered x-rays
c. Developed first x-ray tube
d. Introduced bisecting technique
e. Exposed first dental radiograph
f. Wrote first paper on the danger of x-radiation
g. Exposed first dental radiograph in the United States (skull)
h. Introduced long-cone paralleling technique
i. Wrote first dental text; introduced bite-wing technique
j. Exposed first dental radiograph in the United States (living patient)

____**10.** Coolidge

____**11.** Fitzgerald

____**12.** Kells

_____13. McCormack
_____14. Morton
_____15. Price
_____16. Raper
_____17. Roentgen
_____18. Rollins
_____19. Walkhoff

Ordering

Arrange the following in order of discovery from earliest to latest:

_____20. Introduction of F-speed film
_____21. Introduction of D-speed film
_____22. Introduction of panoramic radiography
_____23. Cone-beam scanners available in the United States
_____24. Introduction of intraoral digital imaging
_____25. Introduction of cone-beam computed tomography

Essay

26. Discuss the importance of dental images.
27. Summarize the discovery of x-radiation.

2

Radiation Physics

LEARNING OBJECTIVES

After completion of this chapter, the student will be able to do the following:

1. Define the key terms associated with radiation physics.
2. Identify the structure of the atom.
3. Describe the process of ionization.
4. Discuss the difference between radiation and radioactivity.
5. List the two types of ionizing radiation and give examples of each.
6. List the characteristics of electromagnetic radiation.
7. List the properties of x-radiation.
8. Identify the component parts of the x-ray machine.
9. Label the parts of the dental x-ray tubehead and the dental x-ray tube.
10. Describe in detail how dental x-rays are produced.
11. List and describe the possible interactions of x-rays with matter.

To understand how x-rays are produced, the dental radiographer must understand the nature and interactions of atoms. A complete understanding of x-radiation includes an understanding of the fundamental concepts of atomic and molecular structure and a working knowledge of ionization, ionizing radiation, and the properties of x-rays. An understanding of the dental x-ray machine, x-ray tube, and circuitry is also necessary. The purpose of this chapter is to present the fundamental concepts of atomic and molecular structure, to define and characterize x-radiation, to provide an introduction to the x-ray machine, and to describe in detail how x-rays are produced. This chapter also includes a discussion of the interactions of x-radiation with matter.

FUNDAMENTAL CONCEPTS

Atomic and Molecular Structure

The world is composed of matter and energy. Matter is anything that occupies space and has mass; when matter is altered, energy results. The fundamental unit of matter is the atom. All matter is composed of atoms, or tiny invisible particles. An understanding of the structure of the atom is necessary before the dental radiographer can understand the production of x-rays.

Atomic Structure. The atom consists of two parts: (1) a central nucleus and (2) orbiting electrons (Figure 2-1). The identity of an atom is determined by the composition of its nucleus and the arrangement of its orbiting electrons. At present, 118 different atoms have been identified.

Nucleus. The nucleus, or dense core of the atom, is composed of particles known as *protons* and *neutrons* (also known as nucleons). Protons carry positive electrical charges, whereas neutrons carry no electrical charge. The nucleus of an atom occupies very little space; in fact, most of the atom is empty space. For example, if an atom were imagined to be the size of a football stadium, the nucleus would be the size of a football.

Atoms differ from one another on the basis of their nuclear composition. The number of protons and neutrons in the nucleus of an atom determines its mass number or atomic weight. The number of protons inside the nucleus equals the number of electrons outside the nucleus and determines the atomic number of the atom. Each atom has an atomic number, ranging from that of hydrogen, the simplest atom, which has an atomic number of 1, to that of ununoctium, the most complex atom known, which has an atomic number of 118. Atoms are arranged in the ascending order of atomic number on a chart known as the periodic table of the elements (Figure 2-2). Elements are substances made up of only one type of atom.

Electrons. Electrons are tiny, negatively charged particles that have very little mass; an electron weighs approximately 1/1800 as much as a proton or neutron. The arrangement of the electrons and neutrons in an atom resembles that of a miniature solar system. Just as the planets revolve around the sun, electrons travel around the nucleus in well-defined paths known as orbits or shells.

An atom contains a maximum of seven shells, each located at a specific distance from the nucleus and representing different energy levels. The shells are designated with the letters K, L, M, N, O, P, and Q; the K shell is located closest to the nucleus and has the highest energy level (Figure 2-3). Each shell has a maximum number of electrons it can hold (Figure 2-4).

Electrons are maintained in their orbits by the electrostatic force, or attraction, between the positive nucleus and the negative electrons. This is known as the binding energy, or binding force, of an electron. The binding energy is determined by the distance between the nucleus and the orbiting electron and is different for each shell. The strongest binding energy is found closest to the nucleus in the K shell, whereas electrons located in the outer shells have a weak binding energy. The binding energies of orbital electrons are measured in electron volts (eV) or kilo electron volts (keV). (One kilo electron volt equals 1000 electron volts.)

The energy required to remove an electron from its orbital shell must exceed the binding energy of the electron in that shell. A great amount of energy is required to remove an inner-shell electron, but electrons loosely held in the outer shells can be affected by lesser energies. For example, in the tungsten atom, the binding energies are as follows:

70 keV	K-shell electrons
12 keV	L-shell electrons
3 keV	M-shell electrons

Note that the binding energy is greatest in the shell closest to the nucleus. To remove a K-shell electron from a tungsten atom, 70 keV (70,000 eV) of energy would be required, whereas only 3 keV (3000 eV) of energy would be necessary to remove an electron from the M-shell.

Molecular Structure. Atoms are capable of combining with each other to form molecules. A molecule can be defined as two or more atoms joined by chemical bonds, or the smallest amount of a substance that possesses its characteristic properties. As with the atom, the molecule is also a tiny invisible particle. Molecules are formed in one of two ways: (1) by the transfer of electrons or (2) by the sharing of electrons between the outermost shells of atoms. An example of a simple molecule is water (H_2O); the symbol H_2 represents two atoms of hydrogen, and the symbol O represents one atom of oxygen (Figure 2-5).

Ionization, Radiation, and Radioactivity

The fundamental concepts of atomic and molecular structure just reviewed allow an understanding of ionization, radiation, and radioactivity. Before the dental radiographer can understand how x-rays are produced, a working knowledge of ionization and the difference between radiation and radioactivity is necessary.

Ionization. Atoms can exist in a neutral state or in an electrically unbalanced state. Normally, most atoms are neutral. A neutral atom contains an equal number of protons (positive charges) and electrons (negative charges). An atom with an incompletely filled outer shell is electrically unbalanced and attempts to capture an electron from an

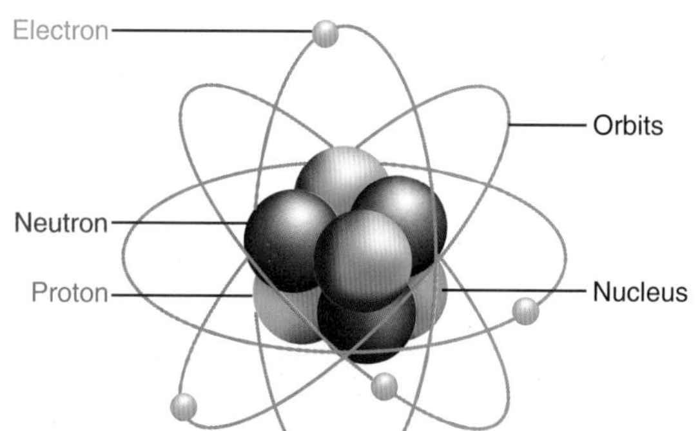

Fig 2-1 The atom consists of a central nucleus and orbiting electrons.

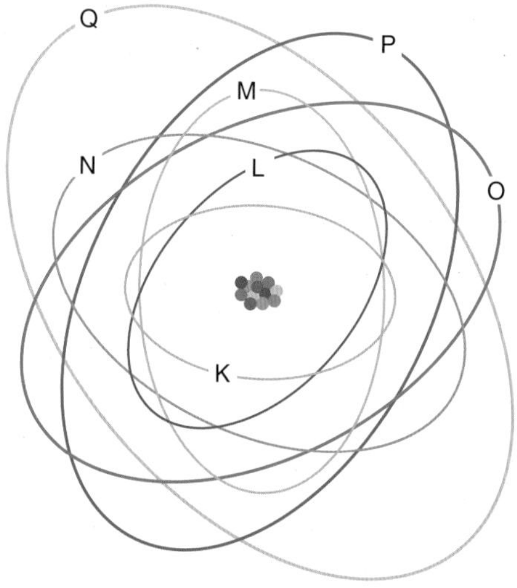

Fig 2-3 Orientation of electron orbits (shells) around the nucleus.

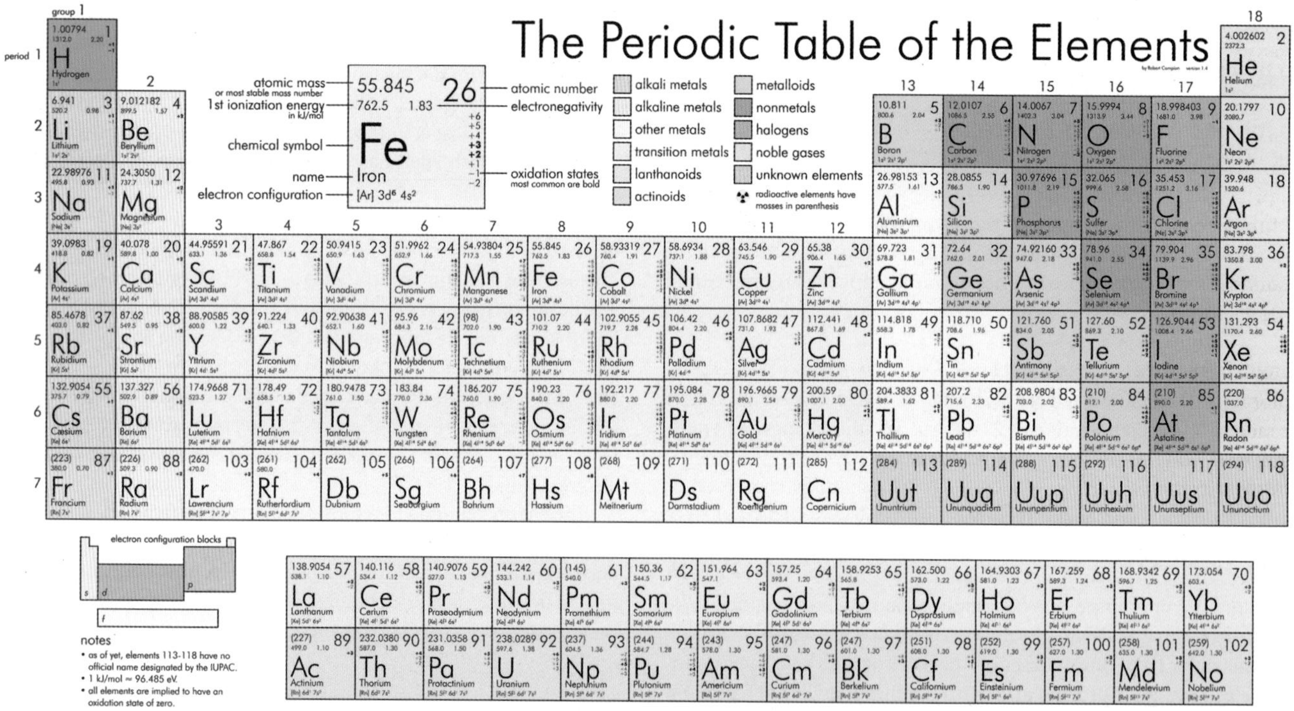

Fig 2-2 Periodic table of the elements. (User:2012rc / Wikimedia Commons / CC-BY-3.0 [https://creativecommons.org/licenses/by/3.0/legalcode] https://commons.wikimedia.org/wiki/File:Periodic_table_large.svg.)

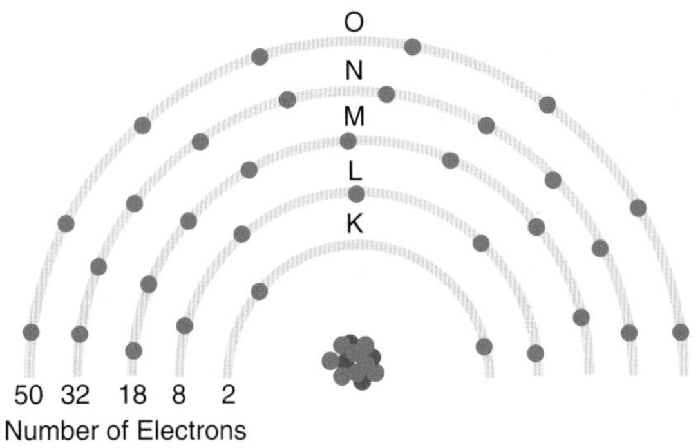

Fig 2-4 Maximum number of electrons that can exist in each shell of a tungsten atom. Redrawn from Langlais RP: *Exercises in oral radiology and interpretation*, ed 4, St. Louis, 2004, Saunders.

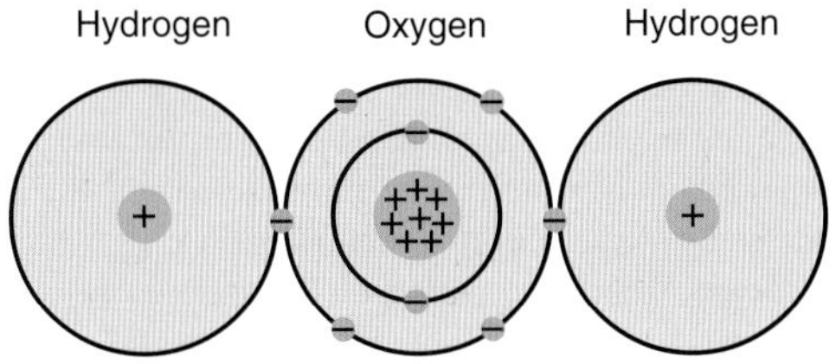

Fig 2-5 A molecule of water (H_2O) consists of two atoms of hydrogen connected to one atom of oxygen.

adjacent atom. If the atom gains an electron, it has more electrons than protons and neutrons, and therefore it has a negative charge. Similarly, the atom that loses an electron has more protons and neutrons and thus has a positive charge. An atom that gains or loses an electron and becomes electrically unbalanced is known as an ion.

Ionization is the production of ions, or the process of converting an atom into ions. Ionization deals only with electrons and requires sufficient energy to overcome the electrostatic force that binds the electron to the nucleus. When an electron is removed from an atom in the ionization process, an ion pair results. The atom becomes the positive ion, and the ejected electron becomes the negative ion (Figure 2-6). This ion pair reacts with other ions until electrically stable, neutral atoms are formed.

Radiation and Radioactivity. Radiation, as defined in Chapter 1, is the emission and propagation of energy through space or a substance in the form of waves or particles. The terms *radioactivity* and *radiation* are sometimes confused; it is important to note that they do not have the same meaning.

Radioactivity can be defined as the process by which certain unstable atoms or elements undergo spontaneous disintegration, or decay, in an effort to attain a more balanced nuclear state. A substance is considered radioactive if it gives off energy in the form of particles or rays as a result of the disintegration of atomic nuclei.

In dentistry, radiation (specifically x-radiation) is used, not radioactivity.

Ionizing Radiation

Ionizing radiation can be defined as radiation that is capable of producing ions by removing or adding an electron to an atom. Ionizing radiation can be classified into two groups: (1) particulate radiation and (2) electromagnetic radiation.

Particulate Radiation. Particulate radiations are tiny particles of matter that possess mass and travel in straight lines and at high

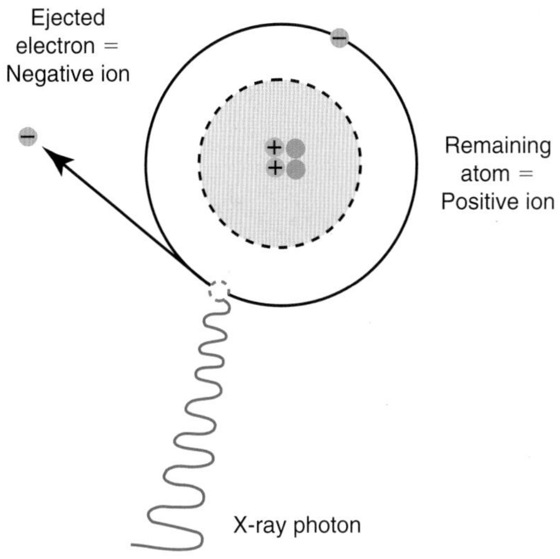

Fig 2-6 An ion pair is formed when an electron is removed from an atom; the atom is the positive ion, and the ejected electron is the negative ion.

TABLE 2-1 Particulate Radiations

Particle	Mass Units	Charge	Origin
Alpha particle	4.003000	+2	Nucleus
Electron			
• Beta particle	• 0.000548	• −1	• Nucleus
• Cathode rays	• 0.000548	• −1	• X-ray tube
Protons	1.007597	+1	Nucleus
Neutrons	1.008986	0	Nucleus

speeds. Particulate radiations transmit kinetic energy by means of their extremely fast-moving, small masses. Four types of particulate radiations are recognized (Table 2-1), as follows:

1. Electrons can be classified as beta particles or cathode rays. They differ in origin only.
   a. Beta particles are fast-moving electrons emitted from the nucleus of radioactive atoms.
   b. Cathode rays are streams of high-speed electrons that originate in an x-ray tube.
2. Alpha particles are emitted from the nuclei of heavy metals and exist as two protons and neutrons, without electrons.
3. Protons are accelerated particles, specifically hydrogen nuclei, with a mass of 1 and a charge of +1.
4. Neutrons are accelerated particles with a mass of 1 and no electrical charge.

Electromagnetic Radiation. Electromagnetic radiation can be defined as the propagation of wavelike energy (without mass) through spacc or matter. The energy propagated is accompanied by oscillating electric and magnetic fields positioned at right angles to one another, thus the term *electromagnetic* (Figure 2-7).

Electromagnetic radiations are man-made or occur naturally; examples include cosmic rays, gamma rays, x-rays, ultraviolet rays, visible light, infrared light, radar waves, microwaves, and radio waves. Electromagnetic radiations are arranged according to their energies in what is termed the electromagnetic spectrum (Figure 2-8). All energies of the electromagnetic spectrum share common characteristics.

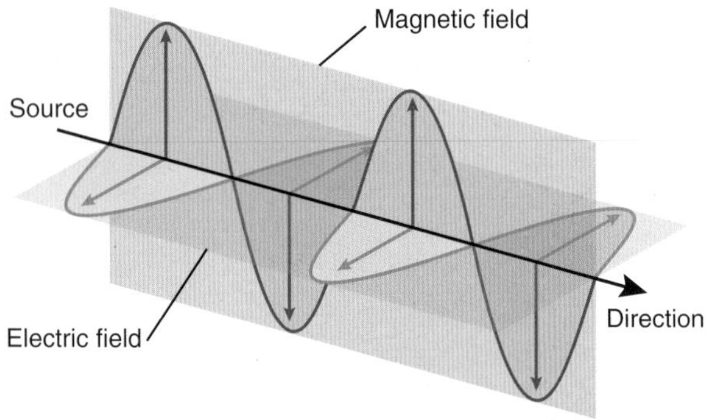

Fig 2-7 Oscillating electric and magnetic fields are characteristic of electromagnetic radiations.

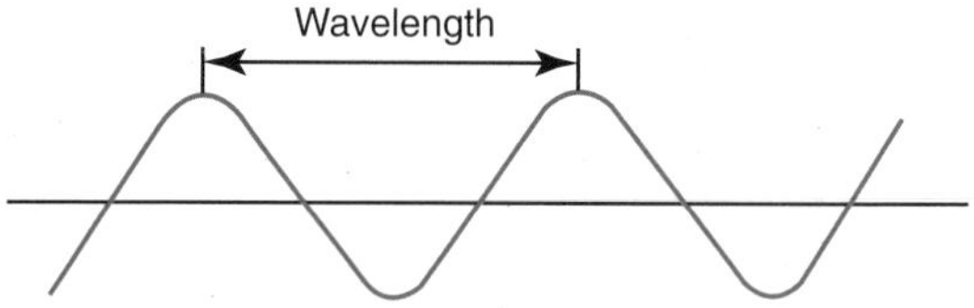

Fig 2-9 Wavelength is the distance between the crest (peak) of one wave and the crest of the next.

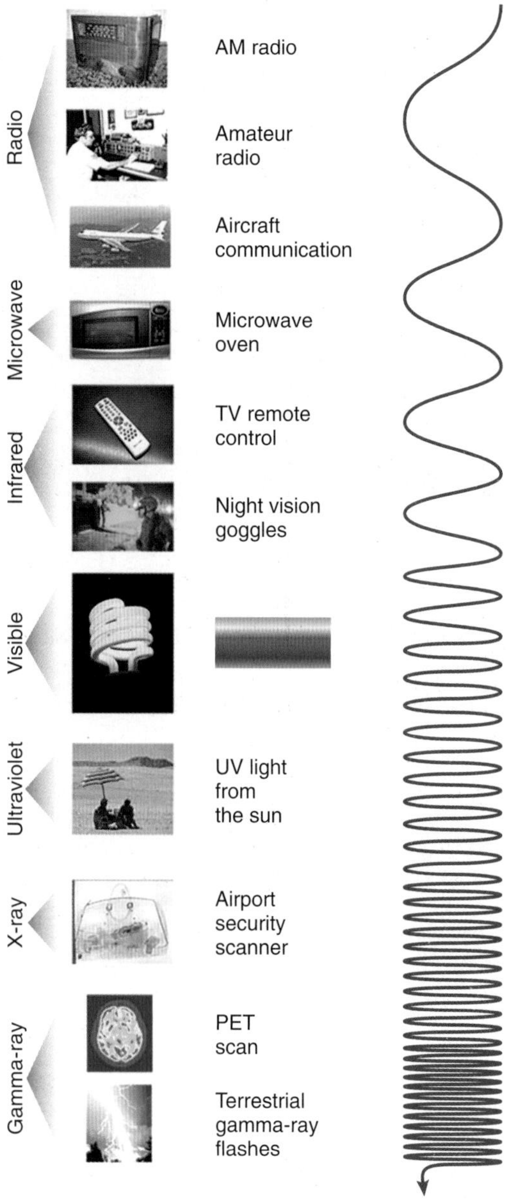

Fig 2-8 Electromagnetic energy spectrum. (Courtesy Imagine the Universe: The Electromagnetic Spectrum. NASA.gov. Last modified March, 2013. http://imagine.gsfc.nasa.gov/science/toolbox/emspectrum1.html)

Depending on their energy levels, electromagnetic radiations can be classified as ionizing or non-ionizing. In the electromagnetic spectrum, only high-energy radiations (cosmic rays, gamma rays, and x-rays) are capable of ionization.

Electromagnetic radiations are believed to move through space as both a particle and a wave; therefore two concepts, the particle concept and the wave concept, must be considered.

Particle concept. The particle concept characterizes electromagnetic radiations as discrete bundles of energy called photons or quanta. Photons are bundles of energy with no mass or weight that travel as waves at the speed of light and move through space in a straight line, "carrying the energy" of electromagnetic radiation.

Wave concept. The wave concept characterizes electromagnetic radiations as waves and focuses on the properties of velocity, wavelength, and frequency, as follows:

- Velocity refers to the speed of the wave. All electromagnetic radiations travel as waves or a continuous sequence of crests at the speed of light (3×10^8 meters per second [186,000 miles per second]) in a vacuum.
- Wavelength can be defined as the distance between the crest of one wave and the crest of the next (Figure 2-9). Wavelength determines the energy and penetrating power of the radiation; the shorter the distance between the crests, the shorter is the wavelength and the higher is the energy and ability to penetrate matter. Wavelength is measured in nanometers (nm; 1×10^{-9} meters, or one billionth of a meter) for short waves and in meters (m) for longer waves.
- Frequency refers to the number of wavelengths that pass a given point in a certain amount of time (Figure 2-10). Frequency and wavelength are inversely related; if the frequency of the wave is high, the wavelength will be short, and if the frequency is low, the wavelength will be long.

The amount of energy an electromagnetic radiation possesses depends on the wavelength and frequency. Low-frequency electromagnetic radiations have a long wavelength and less energy. Conversely, high-frequency electromagnetic radiations have a short wavelength and more energy.

For example, communications media use the low-frequency, longer waves of the electromagnetic spectrum; the wavelength of a radio wave can be as long as 100 m, whereas the wavelength of a television wave is approximately 1 m. In contrast, diagnostic radiography uses the high-frequency, shorter waves in the electromagnetic spectrum; x-rays used in dentistry have a wavelength of 0.1 nm, or 0.0000000001 m.

HELPFUL HINT

How to Remember Wavelengths

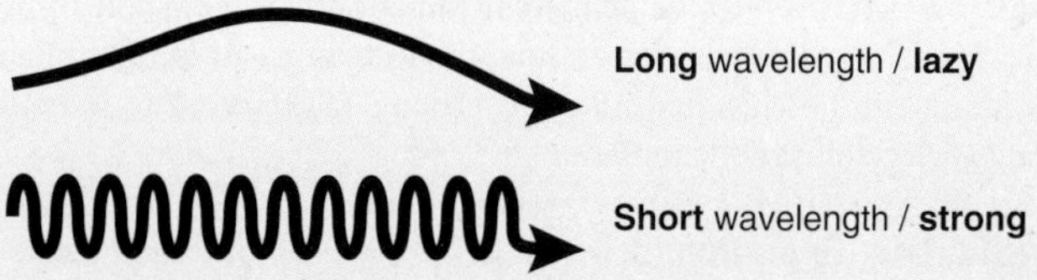

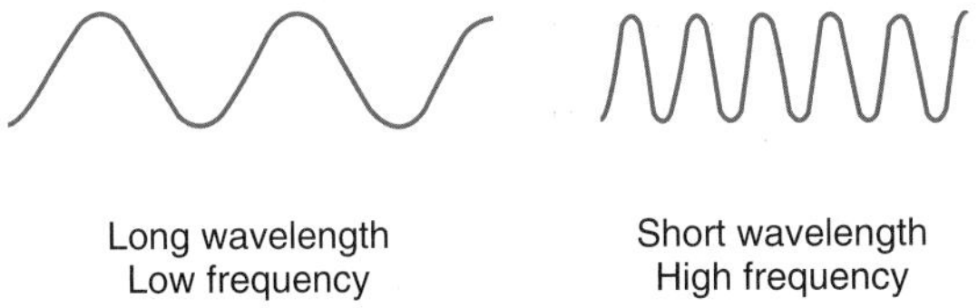

Fig 2-10 Frequency is the number of wavelengths that pass a given point in a certain amount of time. The shorter the wavelength, the higher the frequency will be, and vice versa.

BOX 2-1 Properties of X-Rays

- *Appearance:* X-rays are invisible.
- *Mass:* X-rays have no mass or weight.
- *Charge:* X-rays have no charge.
- *Speed:* X-rays travel at the speed of light.
- *Wavelength:* X-rays travel in waves and have short wavelengths with a high frequency.
- *Path of travel:* X-rays travel in straight lines and can be deflected, or scattered.
- *Focusing capability:* X-rays cannot be focused to a point and always diverge from a point.
- *Penetrating power:* X-rays can penetrate liquids, solids, and gases. The composition of the substance determines whether x-rays penetrate or pass through, or are absorbed.
- *Absorption:* X-rays are absorbed by matter; the absorption depends on the atomic structure of matter and the wavelength of the x-ray.
- *Ionization capability:* X-rays interact with materials they penetrate and cause ionization.
- *Fluorescence capability:* X-rays can cause certain substances to fluoresce or emit radiation in longer wavelengths (e.g., visible light and ultraviolet light).
- *Effect on receptor:* X-rays can produce an image on a receptor.
- *Effect on living tissues:* X-rays cause biologic changes in living cells.

X-RADIATION

X-radiation is a high-energy, ionizing electromagnetic radiation. As with all electromagnetic radiations, x-rays have the properties of both waves and particles. X-rays can be defined as weightless bundles of energy (photons) without an electrical charge that travel in waves with a specific frequency at the speed of light. X-ray photons interact with the materials they penetrate and cause ionization.

X-rays have certain unique properties or characteristics. It is important that the dental radiographer be familiar with the properties of x-rays (Box 2-1).

X-RAY MACHINE

X-rays are produced in the dental x-ray machine. For learning purposes, the dental x-ray machine can be divided into three study areas: (1) the component parts, (2) the x-ray tube, and (3) the x-ray generating apparatus.

Component Parts

The dental x-ray machine consists of three visible component parts: (1) control panel, (2) extension arm, and (3) tubehead (Figure 2-11).

Control Panel. The control panel of the dental x-ray machine contains an on-off switch and indicator light, an exposure button and indicator light, and control devices (time, kilovoltage, and milliamperage selectors) to regulate the x-ray beam. The control panel is plugged into an electrical outlet and appears as a panel or a cabinet mounted on the wall outside the dental operatory.

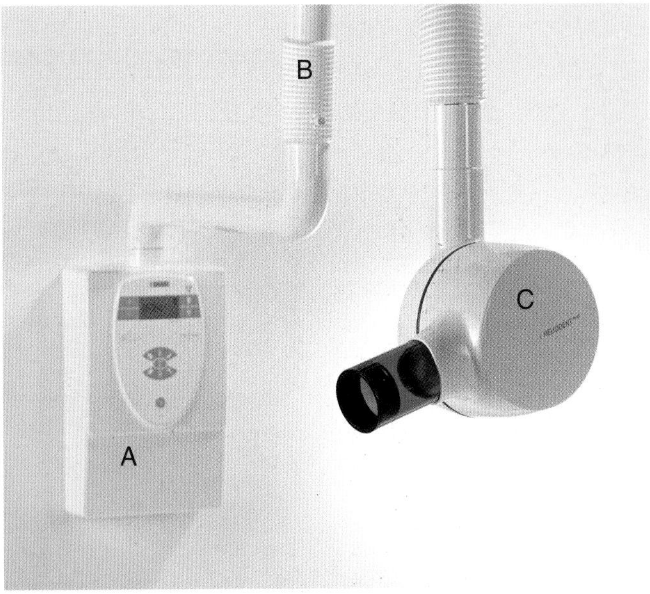

Fig 2-11 Three component parts of dental x-ray machine: **A,** control panel; **B,** extension arm; **C,** tubehead. (Courtesy Dentsply Sirona USA, Charlotte, NC.)

Extension Arm. The wall-mounted extension arm suspends the x-ray tubehead and houses the electrical wires that extend from the control panel to the tubehead. The extension arm allows for movement and positioning of the tubehead.

Tubehead. The x-ray tubehead is a tightly sealed, heavy metal housing that contains the x-ray tube that produces dental x-rays. The component parts of the tubehead include the following (Figure 2-12):

- Metal housing, or the metal body of the tubehead that surrounds the x-ray tube and transformers and is filled with oil—protects the x-ray tube and grounds the high-voltage components.
- Insulating oil, or the oil that surrounds the x-ray tube and transformers inside the tubehead—prevents overheating by absorbing the heat created by the production of x-rays.
- Tubehead seal, or the aluminum or leaded-glass covering of the tubehead that permits the exit of x-rays from the tubehead—seals the oil in the tubehead and acts as a filter to the x-ray beam.
- X-ray tube, or the heart of the x-ray generating system (discussed later) (Figure 2-13).
- Transformer, or a device that alters the voltage of incoming electricity (also discussed later).
- Aluminum disks, or sheets of 0.5-mm-thick aluminum placed in the path of the x-ray beam, filter out the nonpenetrating, longer-wavelength x-rays (Figure 2-14). Aluminum filtration is discussed in Chapter 4.
- Lead collimator, or a lead plate with a central hole that fits directly over the opening of the metal housing, where the x-rays exit—restricts the size of the x-ray beam (Figure 2-15). Collimation is also discussed in Chapter 4.
- Position-indicating device (PID), or open-ended, lead-lined cylinder that extends from the opening of the metal housing of the tubehead—aims and shapes the x-ray beam (Figure 2-16). The PID is sometimes referred to as the *cone.*

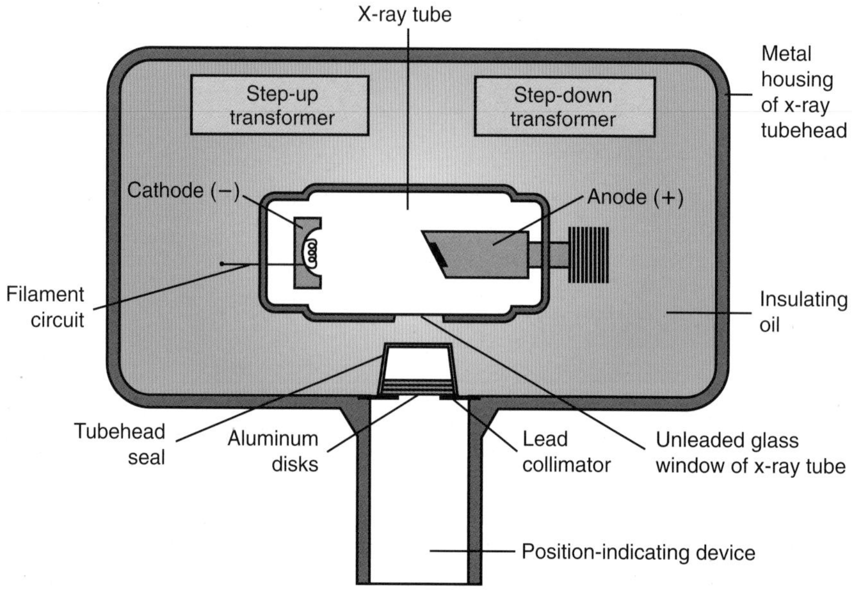

Fig 2-12 Diagram of dental x-ray tubehead.

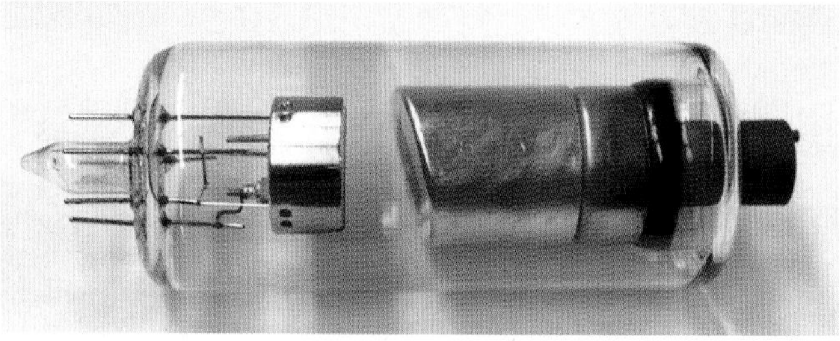

Fig 2-13 Actual dental x-ray tube. (Courtesy Mallya SM, Lam EWN: Physics. In *White and Pharoah's oral radiology: principles and interpretation*, ed 8, St. Louis, 2019, Elsevier.)

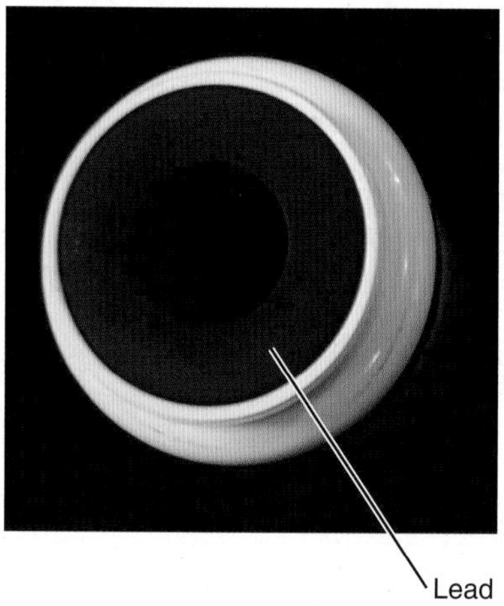

Fig 2-15 The lead collimator, or lead plate with a central opening, restricts the size of the x-ray beam.

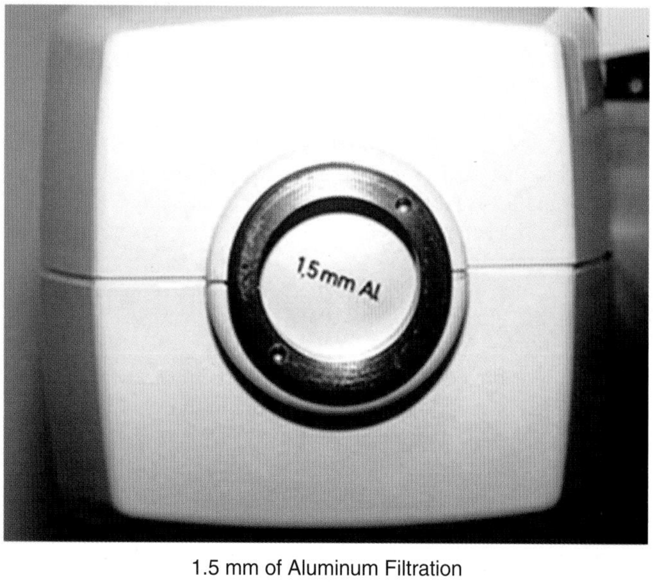

Fig 2-14 Aluminum filtration disk in x-ray tubehead. (© ADAA. Reprinted from the ADAA Continuing Education Course Radiation Biology, Safety and Protection for Today's Dental Team, <http://www.adaausa.org/>.)

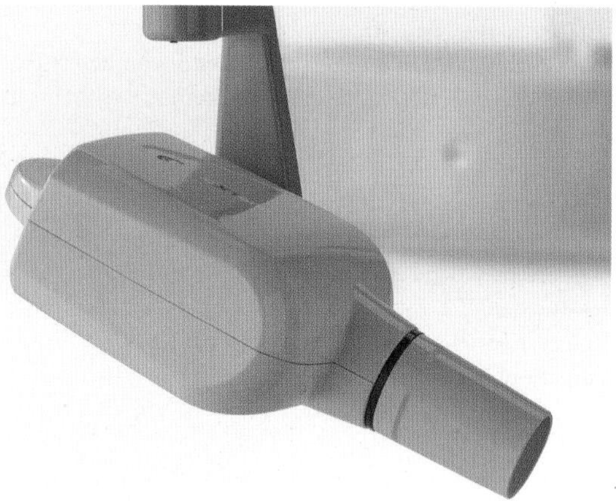

Fig 2-16 Position-indicating device (PID), or cone. (Courtesy Cefla North America, Inc., Charlotte, NC.)

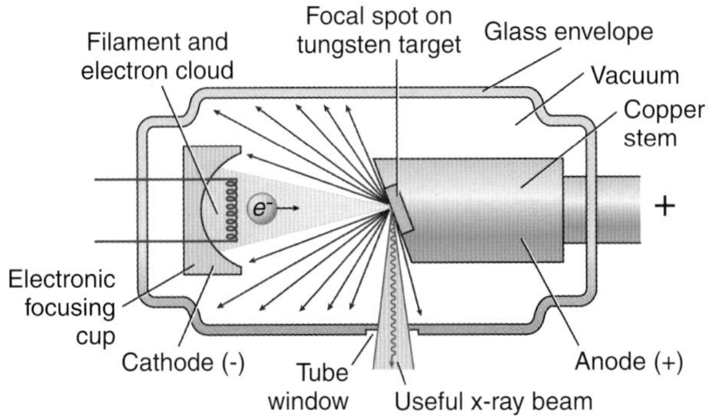

Fig 2-17 Diagram of x-ray tube.

X-Ray Tube

The x-ray tube is the heart of the x-ray generating system; it is critical to the production of x-rays and warrants a separate discussion from the rest of the x-ray machine. The x-ray tube is a glass vacuum tube from which all the air has been removed. The x-ray tube used in dentistry measures several inches long by 1 inch in diameter. The component parts of the x-ray tube include a leaded-glass housing, negative cathode, and positive anode (Figure 2-17).

Leaded-Glass Housing. The leaded-glass housing is a leaded-glass vacuum tube that prevents x-rays from escaping in all directions. One central area of the leaded-glass tube has a "window" that permits the x-ray beam to exit the tube and directs the x-ray beam toward the aluminum disks, lead collimator, and PID.

Cathode. The cathode, or negative electrode, consists of a tungsten wire filament in a cup-shaped holder made of molybdenum. The purpose of the cathode is to supply the electrons necessary to generate x-rays. In the x-ray tube, the electrons produced in the negative cathode are accelerated toward the positive anode. The cathode includes the following:

- The tungsten filament, or coiled wire made of tungsten, which produces electrons when heated.
- The molybdenum cup, which focuses the electrons into a narrow beam and directs the beam across the tube toward the tungsten target of the anode.

Anode. The anode, or positive electrode, consists of a wafer-thin tungsten plate embedded in a solid copper rod. The purpose of the anode is to convert electrons into x-ray photons. The anode includes the following:

- A tungsten target, or plate of tungsten, which serves as a focal spot and converts bombarding electrons into x-ray photons.
- The copper stem, which functions to dissipate the heat away from the tungsten target.

X-Ray Generating Apparatus

To understand how the x-ray tube functions and how x-rays are produced, the dental radiographer must understand electricity and electrical currents, electrical circuits, and transformers.

Electricity and Electrical Currents. Electricity is the energy that is used to make x-rays. Electrical energy consists of a flow of electrons through a conductor; this flow is known as the electrical current. The electrical current is termed direct current (DC) when the electrons flow in one direction through the conductor. The current is a steady constant electrical charge. The term alternating current (AC) describes an electrical current in which the electrons flow in two, opposite directions. The current alternates between positive and negative, resulting in a voltage waveform shaped like a sine wave. Rectification is the conversion of AC to DC. The dental x-ray tube acts as a self-rectifier in that it changes AC into DC while producing x-rays. This ensures that the current is always flowing in the same direction, more specifically, from cathode to anode.

Generators on older machines produced an x-ray beam with a wavelike pattern, whereas newer constant-potential (DC) x-ray machines produce a homogeneous beam of consistent wavelengths during radiation exposure. DC type x-ray machines create a steady supply of power, and consequently the x-rays that are produced are smooth and consistent. The smoothness of the DC x-rays reduces patient exposure to radiation, an important consideration for patient protection. Both AC

HELPFUL HINT

How to Remember Cathode and Anode

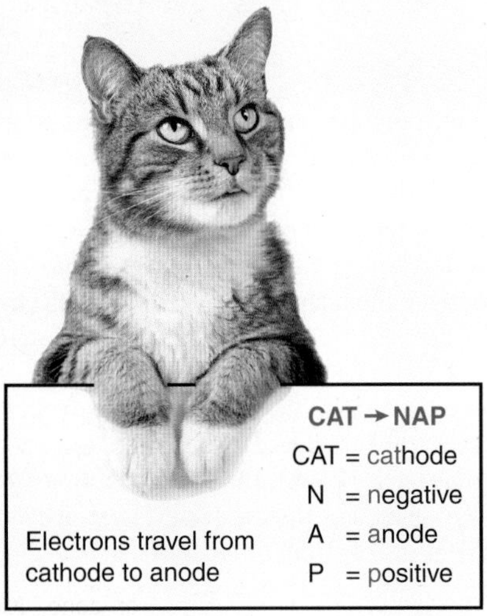

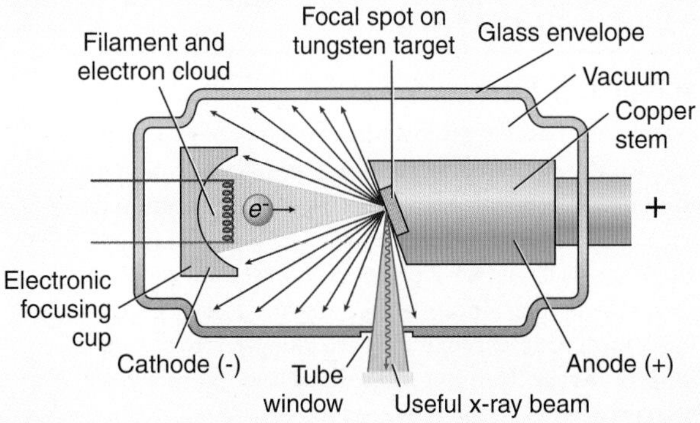

and DC units are capable of producing diagnostic images using conventional film or digital sensors. DC units operate at a slightly lower kilovoltage than AC units.

Amperage is the measurement of the number of electrons moving through a conductor. Current is measured in amperes (A) or milliamperes (mA). Voltage is the measurement of electrical force that causes electrons to move from a negative pole to a positive one. Voltage is measured in volts (V) or kilovolts (kV).

In the production of x-rays, both the amperage and the voltage can be adjusted. In the x-ray tube, the amperage, or number of electrons passing through the cathode filament, can be increased or decreased by the milliamperage (mA) adjustment on the control panel of the x-ray machine. The voltage of the x-ray tube current, or the current passing from the cathode to the anode, is controlled by the kilovoltage (kV) adjustment on the control panel.

Circuits. A circuit is a path of electrical current. Two electrical circuits are used in the production of x-rays: (1) a low-voltage, or filament, circuit and (2) a high-voltage circuit.

The filament circuit uses 3 to 5V, regulates the flow of electrical current to the filament of the x-ray tube, and is controlled by the milliampere settings. The high-voltage circuit uses 65,000 to 100,000V, provides the high voltage required to accelerate electrons and to generate x-rays in the x-ray tube, and is controlled by the kilovoltage settings.

Transformers. A transformer is a device that is used to either increase or decrease the voltage in an electrical circuit (Figure 2-18). Transformers alter the voltage of the incoming electrical current and then route the electrical energy to the x-ray tube. In the production of dental x-rays, three transformers are used to adjust the electrical circuits: (1) the step-down transformer, (2) the step-up transformer, and (3) the autotransformer.

A step-down transformer is used to decrease the voltage from the incoming 110- or 220-line voltage to the 3 to 5V used by the filament circuit. A step-down transformer has more wire coils in the primary coil than in the secondary coil (see Figure 2-18). The coil that receives the alternating electrical current is the primary, or input, coil; the secondary coil is the output coil. The electrical current that energizes the primary coil induces a current in the secondary coil. The high-voltage circuit uses both a step-up transformer and an autotransformer. A step-up transformer is used to increase the voltage from the incoming 110- or 220-line voltage to the 65,000 to 100,000 volts used by the high-voltage circuit. A step-up transformer has more wire coils in the secondary coil than in the primary coil (see Figure 2-18). An autotransformer serves as a voltage compensator that corrects for minor fluctuations in the current.

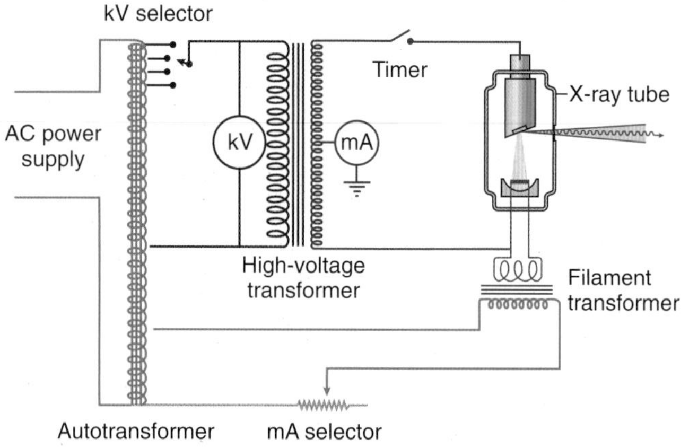

Fig 2-18 Three different transformers are used in the production of dental x-rays. Courtesy Mallya SM, Lam EWN: Physics. In *White and Pharoah's oral radiology: principles and interpretation*, ed 8, St. Louis, 2019, Elsevier.

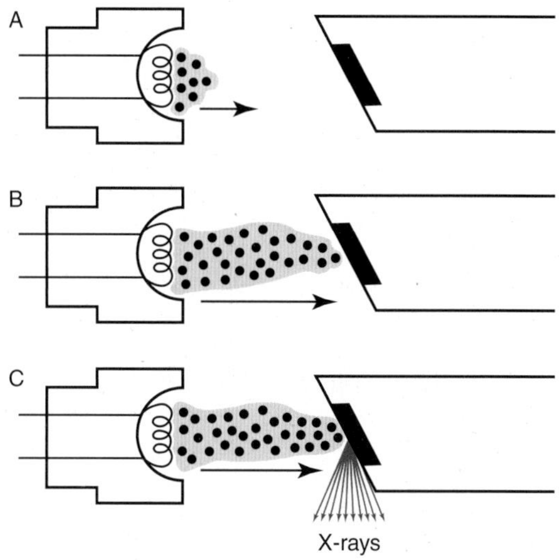

Fig 2-19 The production of dental x-rays occurs in the x-ray tube. **A,** When the filament circuit is activated, the filament heats up, and thermionic emission occurs. **B,** When the exposure button is activated, the electrons are accelerated from the cathode to the anode. **C,** The electrons strike the tungsten target, and their kinetic energy is converted to x-rays and heat.

PRODUCTION OF X-RADIATION

Production of Dental X-Rays

With the component parts of the x-ray machine, the x-ray tube, and the x-ray generating apparatus reviewed, a discussion of the production of dental x-rays is now possible. Following is a step-by-step explanation of x-ray production (Figure 2-19):

1. Electricity from the wall outlet supplies the power to generate x-rays. When the x-ray machine is turned on, the electrical current enters the control panel through the cord plugged into the wall outlet. The current travels from the control panel to the tubehead through the electrical wires in the extension arm.
2. The current is directed to the filament circuit and step-down transformer in the tubehead. The transformer reduces the 110 or 220 entering-line voltage to 3 to 5V.
3. The filament circuit uses the 3 to 5V to heat the tungsten filament in the cathode portion of the x-ray tube. Thermionic emission occurs, defined as the release of electrons from the tungsten filament when the electrical current passes through it and heats the filament. The outer-shell electrons of the tungsten atom acquire enough energy to move away from the filament surface, and an electron cloud forms around the filament. The electrons stay in an electron cloud until the high-voltage circuit is activated.
4. When the exposure button is pushed, the high-voltage circuit is activated. The electrons produced at the cathode are accelerated across the x-ray tube to the anode. The distance between the cathode and anode is very short, less than ½ inch. The molybdenum cup in the cathode directs the electrons to the tungsten target in the anode.
5. The electrons travel from the cathode to the anode. When the electrons strike the tungsten target, their energy of motion (kinetic energy)

is converted to x-ray energy and heat. Less than 1% of the energy is converted to x-rays; the remaining 99% is lost as heat.

6. The heat produced during the production of x-rays is carried away from the copper stem and absorbed by the insulating oil in the tubehead. The x-rays produced are emitted from the target in all directions; however, the leaded-glass housing prevents the x-rays from escaping from the x-ray tube. A small number of x-rays are able to exit from the x-ray tube through the unleaded glass window portion of the tube.
7. The x-rays travel through the unleaded glass window, the tubehead seal, and the aluminum disks. The aluminum disks remove or filter the longer wavelength x-rays from the beam.
8. Next, the lead collimator restricts the size of the x-ray beam. The x-ray beam then travels down the lead-lined PID and exits the tubehead at the opening of the PID.

Types of X-Rays Produced

Not all x-rays produced in the x-ray tube are the same; x-rays differ in energy and wavelength. The energy and wavelength of x-rays vary based on how the electrons interact with the tungsten atoms in the anode. The kinetic energy of the electrons is converted to x-ray photons through one of two mechanisms: (1) general (braking) radiation and (2) characteristic radiation.

General Radiation. Speeding electrons slow down because of their interactions with the tungsten target in the anode. Many electrons that interact with the tungsten atoms undergo not one but many interactions within the target. The radiation produced in this manner is known as **general radiation**, or **braking radiation (bremsstrahlung)**. The term *braking* refers to the sudden stopping of high-speed electrons when they hit the tungsten target in the anode. Most x-rays are produced in this manner; approximately 70% of the x-ray energy produced at the anode can be classified as general radiation.

General (braking) radiation is produced when an electron hits the nucleus of a tungsten atom or when an electron passes very close to the nucleus of a tungsten atom (Figure 2-20). An electron rarely hits the nucleus of the tungsten atom. When it does, however, all its kinetic energy is converted into a high-energy x-ray photon. Instead of hitting the nucleus, most electrons just miss the nucleus of the tungsten atom. When the electron comes close to the nucleus, it is attracted to the nucleus and slows down. Consequently, an x-ray photon of lower energy results. The electron that misses the nucleus continues to penetrate many atoms, producing lower energy x-rays before it imparts all of its kinetic energy. As a result, general radiation consists of x-rays of many different energies and wavelengths.

Characteristic Radiation. **Characteristic radiation** is produced when a high-speed electron dislodges an inner-shell electron from the tungsten atom and causes ionization of that atom (Figure 2-21). Once the electron is dislodged, the remaining orbiting electrons are rearranged to fill the vacancy. This rearrangement produces a loss of energy that results in the production of an x-ray photon. The x-rays produced by this interaction are known as *characteristic x-rays.*

Characteristic radiation accounts for a very small part of x-rays produced in the dental x-ray machine. It occurs only at 70 kV and above because the binding energy of the K-shell electron is approximately 70 keV.

Definitions of X-Radiation

Terms such as *primary, secondary,* and **scatter** are often used to describe x-radiation. Understanding the interactions of x-radiation with matter requires a working knowledge of these terms, as follows:

- **Primary radiation** refers to the penetrating x-ray beam that is produced at the target of the anode and that exits the tubehead. This x-ray beam is often referred to as the **primary beam**, or **useful beam**.
- **Secondary radiation** refers to x-radiation that is created when the primary beam interacts with matter. (In dental radiography, "matter" includes the soft tissues of the head, the bones of the skull, and the teeth.) Secondary radiation is less penetrating than primary radiation.
- **Scatter radiation** is a form of secondary radiation and is the result of an x-ray that has been deflected from its path by the interaction with matter. Scatter radiation is deflected in all directions by the patient's tissues and travels to all parts of the patient's body and to all areas of the dental operatory. Scatter radiation is detrimental to both the patient and the radiographer.

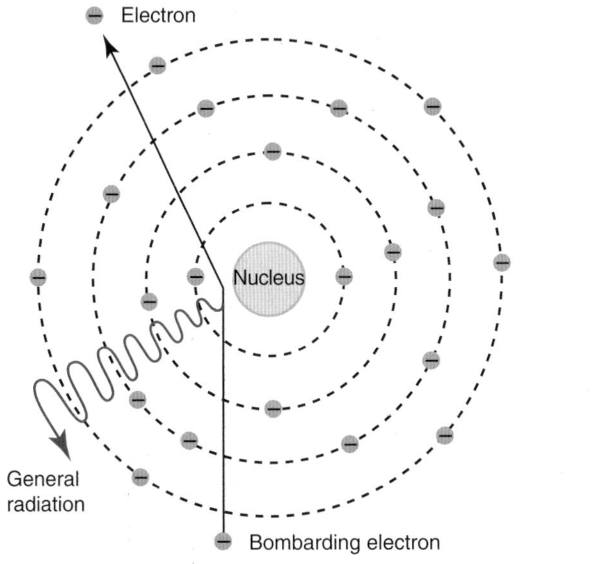

Fig 2-20 When an electron that passes close to the nucleus of a tungsten atom is slowed down, an x-ray photon of lower energy known as *general (braking) radiation* results.

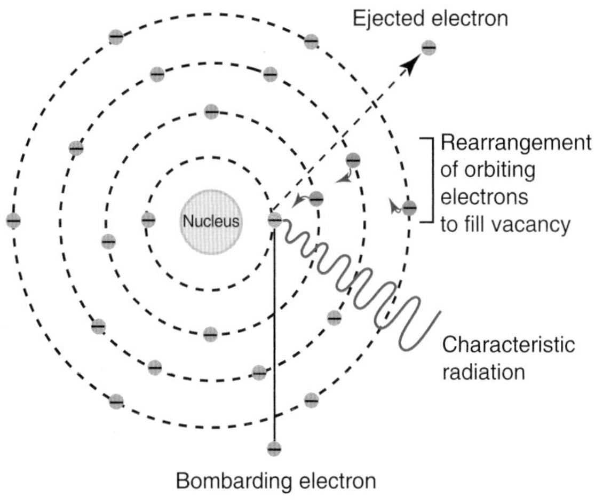

Fig 2-21 An electron that dislodges an inner-shell electron from the tungsten atom results in the rearrangement of the remaining orbiting electrons and the production of an x-ray photon known as *characteristic radiation.*

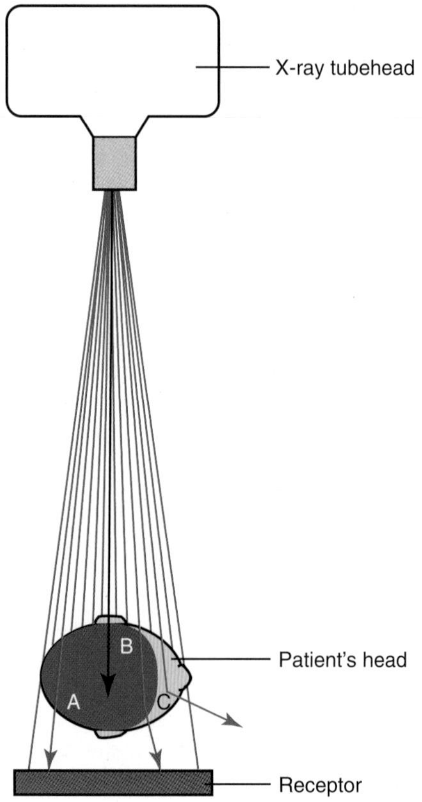

Fig 2-22 Three types of radiation interactions with the patient may occur. **A**, The x-ray photon may pass through the patient without interaction and reach the receptor. **B**, The x-ray photon may be absorbed by the patient. **C**, The x-ray photon may be scattered onto the receptor or away from the receptor.

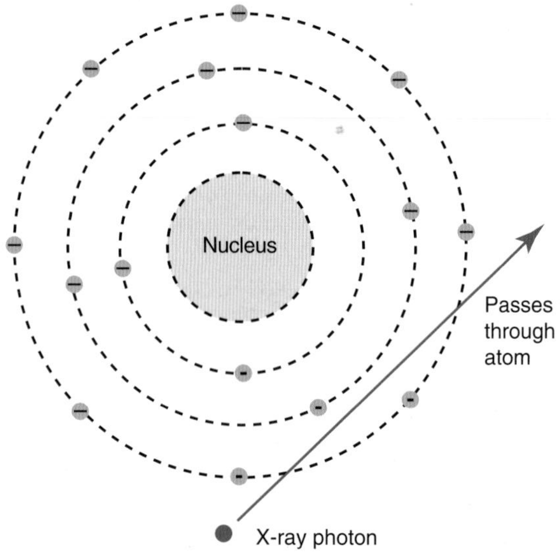

Fig 2-23 When an x-ray photon passes through an atom unchanged, no interaction has taken place.

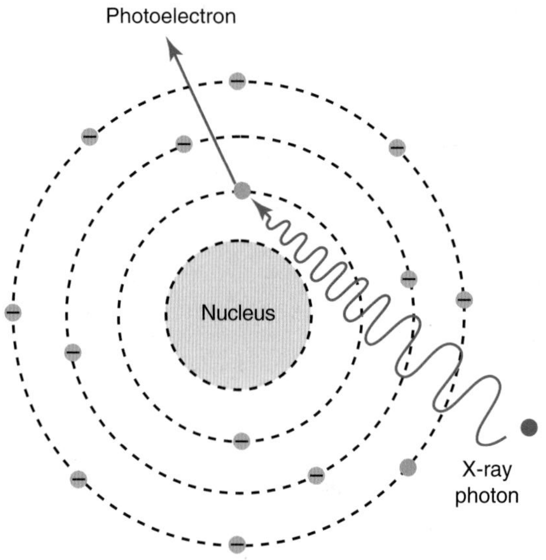

Fig 2-24 When an x-ray photon collides with an inner-shell electron, a photoelectric effect occurs: The photon is absorbed and ceases to exist, and a photoelectron with a negative charge is produced.

INTERACTIONS OF X-RADIATION

What happens after an x-ray exits the tubehead? When x-ray photons arrive at the patient with energies produced by the dental x-ray machine, one of the following events may occur:

- X-rays can pass through the patient without any interaction.
- X-ray photons can be completely absorbed by the patient.
- X-ray photons can be scattered (Figure 2-22).

Knowledge of atomic and molecular structures is required to understand such interactions and effects. At the atomic level, four possibilities can occur when an x-ray photon interacts with matter: (1) no interaction, (2) absorption or photoelectric effect, (3) Compton scatter, and (4) coherent scatter.

No Interaction

It is possible for an x-ray photon to pass through matter or the tissues of a patient without any interaction (Figure 2-23). The x-ray photon passes through the atom unchanged and leaves the atom unchanged. The x-ray photons that pass through a patient without interaction are responsible for producing densities and make dental radiography possible.

Absorption of Energy and Photoelectric Effect

It is possible for an x-ray photon to be completely absorbed within matter, or the tissues of a patient. **Absorption** refers to the total transfer of energy from the x-ray photon to the atoms of matter through which the x-ray beam passes. Absorption depends on the energy of the x-ray beam and the composition of the absorbing matter or tissues.

At the atomic level, absorption occurs as a result of the photoelectric effect. In the **photoelectric effect**, ionization takes place. An x-ray photon collides with a tightly bound, inner-shell electron and gives up all its energy to eject the electron from its orbit (Figure 2-24). The x-ray photon imparts all of its kinetic energy to the orbital electron, is absorbed, and ceases to exist. The ejected electron is termed a *photoelectron* and has a negative charge; it is readily absorbed by other atoms because it has very little penetrating power. The atom that remains has a positive charge. The photoelectric effect accounts for 30% of the interactions of the dental x-ray beam with matter.

Compton Scatter

It is possible for an x-ray photon to be deflected from its path during its passage through matter. The term *scatter* refers to this type of radiation. At the atomic level, the Compton effect accounts for most of the scatter radiation.

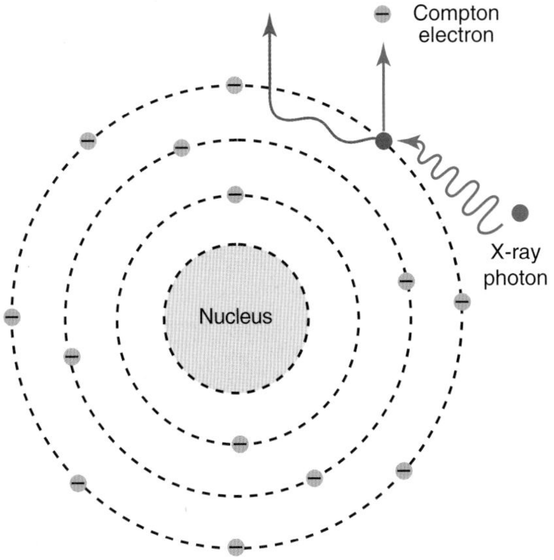

Fig 2-25 When an x-ray photon collides with an outer-shell electron and ejects the electron from its orbit, Compton scatter results: The photon is scattered in a different direction at a lower energy, and the ejected electron is referred to as a *Compton*, or *recoil, electron.*

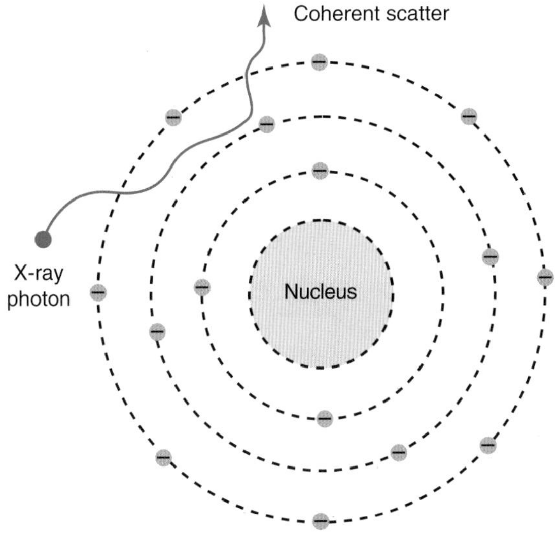

Fig 2-26 When an x-ray photon is scattered and no loss of energy occurs, the scatter is termed *coherent.*

In Compton scatter, ionization takes place. An x-ray photon collides with a loosely bound, outer-shell electron and gives up part of its energy to eject the electron from its orbit (Figure 2-25). The x-ray photon loses energy and continues in a different direction (scatters) at a lower energy level. The new, weaker x-ray photon interacts with other atoms until all its energy is gone. The ejected electron is termed a Compton electron, or recoil electron, and has a negative charge. The remaining atom is positively charged. Compton scatter accounts for 62% of the scatter that occurs in diagnostic radiography.

Coherent Scatter

Another type of scatter radiation that may take place when x-rays interact with matter is known as coherent scatter, or unmodified scatter. Coherent scatter involves an x-ray photon that has its path altered by matter (Figure 2-26). Coherent scatter occurs when a low-energy x-ray photon interacts with an outer-shell electron. No change in the atom occurs, and an x-ray photon of scattered radiation is produced. The x-ray photon is scattered in a different direction from that of the incident photon; no loss of energy and no ionization occur. Essentially, the x-ray photon is "unmodified" and simply undergoes a change in direction without a change in energy. Coherent scatter accounts for 8% of the interactions of the dental x-ray beam with matter.

SUMMARY

- An atom consists of a central nucleus composed of protons, neutrons, and orbiting electrons.
- Most atoms exist in a neutral state and contain equal numbers of protons and neutrons.
- When unequal numbers of protons and electrons exist, the atom is electrically unbalanced and is termed an *ion.*
- The production of ions is termed *ionization;* an ion pair (a positive ion and a negative ion) is produced. The atom is the positive ion, and the ejected electron is the negative ion.
- Ionizing radiation is capable of producing ions and can be classified as *particulate* or *electromagnetic.*
- Electromagnetic radiations (e.g., x-rays) exhibit characteristics of both particles and waves and are arranged according to their energies.
- The energy of an electromagnetic radiation depends on wavelength and frequency.
- A low-energy radiation has a low frequency and a long wavelength; a high-energy radiation has a high frequency and a short wavelength.
- X-rays are weightless, neutral bundles of energy (photons) that travel in waves with a specific frequency at the speed of light.
- X-rays are generated in an x-ray tube located in the x-ray tubehead.
- The x-ray tube consists of a leaded-glass housing, a negative cathode, and a positive anode. Electrons are produced in the cathode and accelerated toward the anode; the anode converts the electrons into x-rays.
- After x-rays exit the tubehead, several interactions are possible: The x-rays may pass through the patient (no interaction), may be completely absorbed by the patient (photoelectric effect), or may be scattered (Compton scatter and coherent scatter).

BIBLIOGRAPHY

Frommer HH, Stabulas-Savage JJ: Ionizing radiation and basic principles of x-ray generation. In Radiology for the dental professional, ed 9, St Louis, 2011, Mosby.

Johnson ON: Characteristics and measurement of radiation. In Essentials of dental radiography for dental assistants and hygienists, ed 9, Upper Saddle River, NJ, 2011, Prentice Hall.

Johnson ON: The dental x-ray machine: components and functions. In Essentials of dental radiography for dental assistants and hygienists, ed 9, Upper Saddle River, NJ, 2011, Prentice Hall.

Mallya SM, Lam EWN: Physics. In White and Pharoah's oral radiology: principles and interpretation, ed 8, St. Louis, 2019, Elsevier.

QUIZ QUESTIONS

Multiple Choice

____ 1. Which electrons have the greatest binding energy?
- a. N-shell
- b. M-shell
- c. L-shell
- d. K-shell

____ 2. What type of electrical charge does the electron carry?
- a. positive
- b. negative
- c. no charge
- d. positive or negative

____ 3. Which term describes two or more atoms that are joined by chemical bonds?
- a. ion
- b. ion pair
- c. molecule
- d. proton

____ 4. Which statement describes ionization?
- a. atom without a nucleus
- b. atom that loses an electron
- c. atom with equal numbers of protons and electrons
- d. none of the above

____ 5. Which term describes the process by which unstable atoms undergo spontaneous disintegration in an effort to attain a more balanced nuclear state?
- a. radiation
- b. radioactivity
- c. ionization
- d. ionizing radiation

____ 6. Which is *not* a type of particulate radiation?
- a. alpha particles
- b. beta particles
- c. protons
- d. nucleons

____ 7. Which is *not* a type of electromagnetic radiation?
- a. electrons
- b. radar waves
- c. microwaves
- d. x-rays

____ 8. Which statement is incorrect?
- a. Velocity is the speed of a wave.
- b. Wavelength is the distance between waves.
- c. Frequency is the number of wavelengths that pass a given point in a certain amount of time.
- d. Frequency and wavelength are inversely related.

____ 9. Which statement is incorrect?
- a. X-rays travel at the speed of sound.
- b. X-rays have no charge.
- c. X-rays cannot be focused to a point.
- d. X-rays cause ionization.

____ 10. Which statement is correct?
- a. X-rays are a form of electromagnetic radiation; visible light is not.
- b. X-rays have more energy than does visible light.
- c. X-rays have a longer wavelength than does visible light.
- d. X-rays travel more slowly than does visible light.

Identification

For questions 11 to 20, identify each of the labeled structures in Figure 2-27.

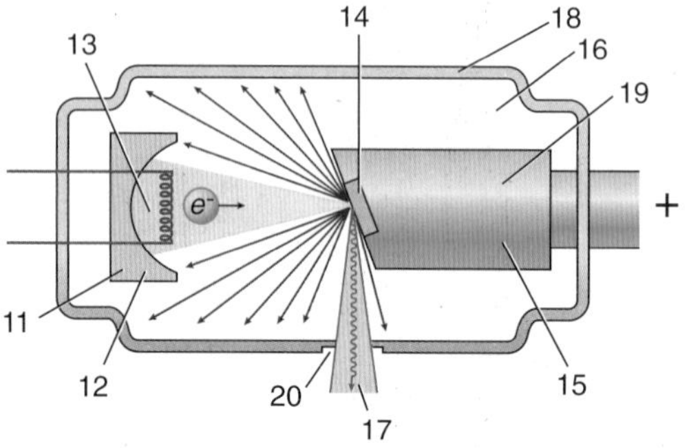

Fig 2-27 Dental x-ray tube.

For questions 21 to 28, identify each of the labeled structures in Figure 2-28.

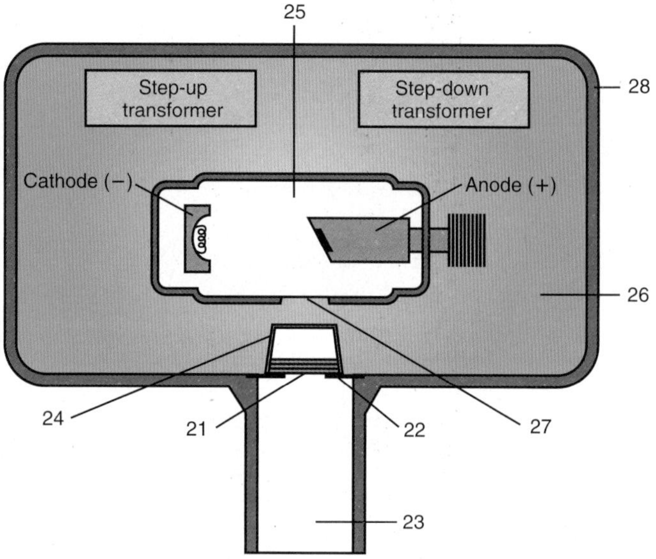

Fig 2-28 Dental x-ray tubehead.

Multiple Choice

____ 29. Which regulates the flow of electrical current to the filament of the x-ray tube?
- a. high-voltage circuit
- b. low-voltage circuit
- c. high-voltage transformer
- d. low-voltage transformer

____ 30. Which is used to increase the voltage in the high-voltage circuit?
- a. step-up transformer
- b. step-down transformer
- c. autotransformer
- d. step-up circuit

____ 31. Which does *not* occur when the high-voltage circuit is activated?
a. The unit produces an audible and visible signal.
b. Electrons produced at the cathode are accelerated across the tube to the anode.
c. X-rays travel from the filament to the target.
d. Heat is produced.

____ 32. Which is the location where x-rays are produced?
a. positive cathode
b. positive anode
c. negative cathode
d. negative anode

____ 33. Which is the location where thermionic emission occurs?
a. positive cathode
b. positive anode
c. negative cathode
d. negative anode

____ 34. Which accounts for 70% of all the x-ray energy produced at the anode?
a. general radiation
b. characteristic radiation
c. Compton scatter
d. coherent scatter

____ 35. Which occurs only at 70 kV or higher and accounts for a very small part of the x-rays produced in the dental x-ray machine?
a. general radiation
b. characteristic radiation
c. Compton scatter
d. coherent scatter

____ 36. Which describes primary radiation?
a. radiation that exits the tubehead
b. radiation that is created when x-rays come in contact with matter
c. radiation that has been deflected from its path by the interaction with matter
d. none of the above

____ 37. Which describes scatter radiation?
a. radiation that exits the tubehead
b. radiation that is more penetrating than primary radiation
c. radiation that has been deflected from its path by interaction with matter
d. none of the above

____ 38. Which type of scatter occurs most often with dental x-rays?
a. Compton
b. coherent
c. photoelectric
d. none of the above

Identification

For questions 37 to 40, identify the x-radiation interaction with matter in Figures 2-29, 2-30, 2-31, and 2-32.

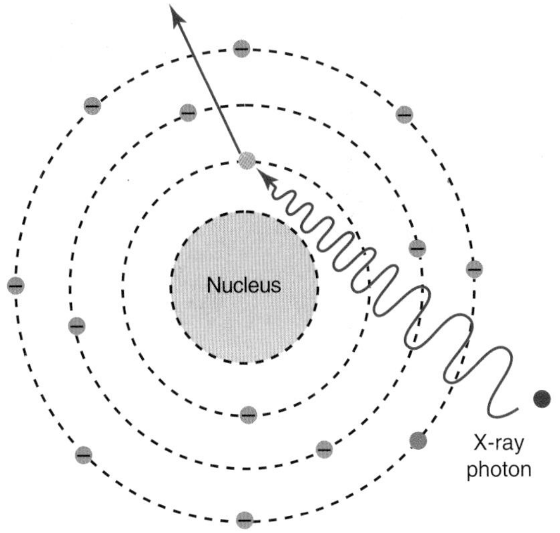

Fig 2-29

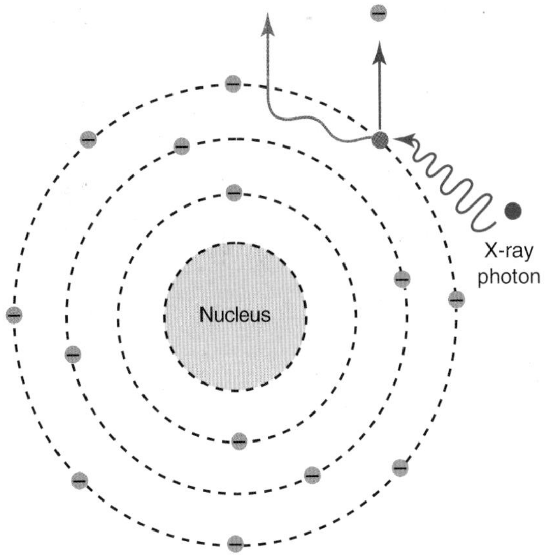

Fig 2-30

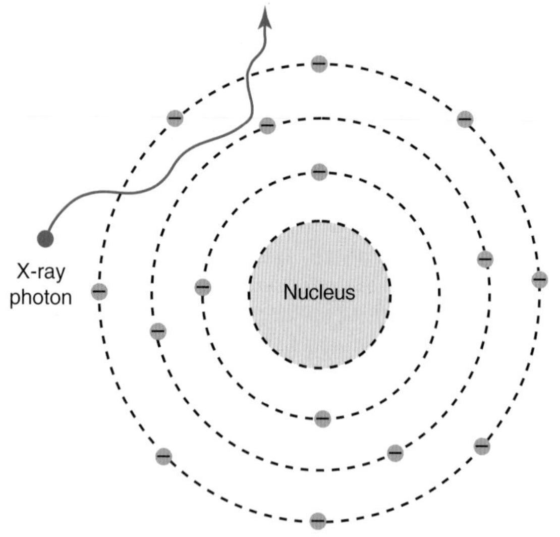

Fig 2-31

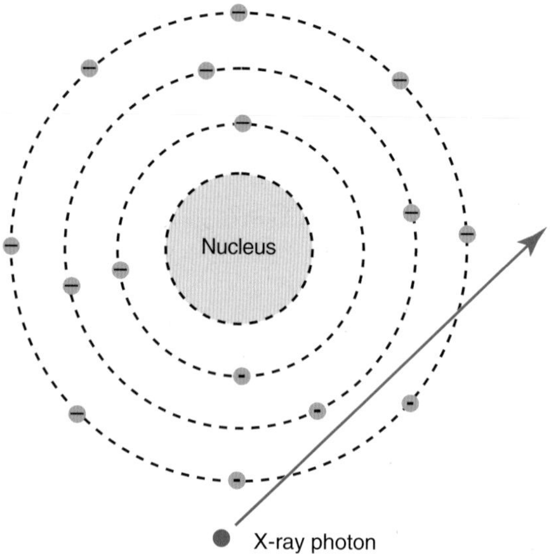

Fig 2-32

Multiple Choice

For questions 41 to 44, refer to Figures 2-29, 2-30, 2-31, and 2-32.

_____ **41.** The interaction of x-radiation with matter illustrated in Figure 2-29 demonstrates:
- **a.** no scatter; no ionization
- **b.** no scatter; ionization
- **c.** scatter; no ionization
- **d.** scatter; ionization

_____ **42.** The interaction of x-radiation with matter illustrated in Figure 2-30 demonstrates:
- **a.** no scatter; no ionization
- **b.** no scatter; ionization
- **c.** scatter; no ionization
- **d.** scatter; ionization

_____ **43.** The interaction of x-radiation with matter illustrated in Figure 2-31 demonstrates:
- **a.** no scatter; no ionization
- **b.** no scatter; ionization
- **c.** scatter; no ionization
- **d.** scatter; ionization

_____ **44.** The interaction of x-radiation with matter illustrated in Figure 2-32 demonstrates:
- **a.** no scatter; no ionization
- **b.** no scatter; ionization
- **c.** scatter; no ionization
- **d.** scatter; ionization

Identification

For questions 45 to 48, identify the wavelengths and frequency in Figure 2-33.

_____ **45.** Which has the shortest wavelength?

_____ **46.** Which has the longest wavelength?

_____ **47.** Which has the lowest frequency?

_____ **48.** Which has the highest frequency?

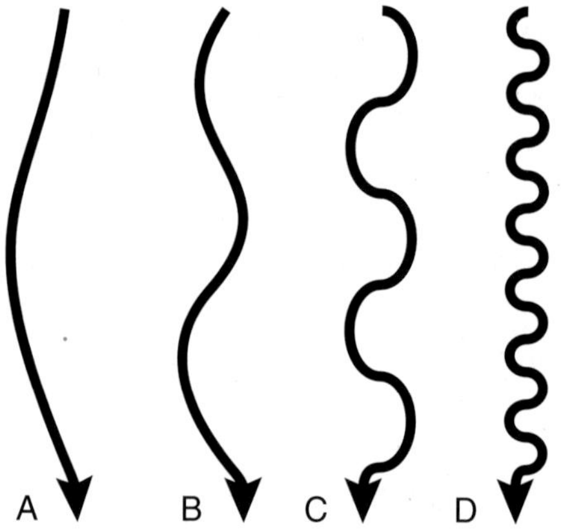

Fig 2-33

3

Radiation Biology

LEARNING OBJECTIVES

After completion of this chapter, the student will be able to do the following:

1. Define the terms associated with radiation injury.
2. Describe the mechanisms and theories of radiation injury.
3. Define and discuss the dose-response curve and radiation injury.
4. Describe the sequence of radiation injury and list the determining factors for radiation injury.
5. Discuss the short-term and long-term effects and the somatic and genetic effects of radiation exposure.
6. Describe the effects of radiation exposure on cells, tissues, and organs and identify the relative sensitivity of a given tissue to x-radiation.
7. Define the units of measurement used in radiation exposure.
8. List common sources of radiation exposure.
9. Discuss risk and risk estimates for radiation exposure.
10. Discuss dental radiation and exposure risks.
11. Discuss the risk versus benefit of dental images.

All ionizing radiations are harmful and produce biologic changes in living tissues. The damaging biologic effects of x-radiation were first documented shortly after the discovery of x-rays. Since that time, information about the harmful effects of high-level exposure to x-radiation has increased based on studies of atomic bomb survivors, workers exposed to radioactive materials, and patients undergoing radiation therapy. Although the amount of x-radiation used in dental imaging is small, biologic damage does occur.

The dental radiographer must have a working knowledge of radiation biology, the study of the effects of ionizing radiation on living tissue, to understand the harmful effects of x-radiation. The subject of radiation biology is a common discussion point from patients who question the need and frequency of radiographic exams; therefore it is essential to comprehend and appreciate these concepts. The purpose of this chapter is to describe the mechanisms and theories of radiation injury, to define the basic concepts and effects of radiation exposure, to detail radiation measurements, and to discuss the risks of radiation exposure.

RADIATION INJURY

Mechanisms of Injury

In diagnostic imaging, not all x-rays pass through the patient and reach the dental x-ray receptor; some are absorbed by the patient's tissues. *Absorption*, as defined in Chapter 2, refers to the total transfer of energy from the x-ray photon to patient tissues. What happens when x-ray energy is absorbed by patient tissues? Chemical changes occur that result in biologic damage. Two specific mechanisms of radiation injury are possible: (1) ionization and (2) free radical formation.

Ionization. X-rays are a form of ionizing radiation; when x-rays strike patient tissues, ionization results. As described in Chapter 2, ionization is produced through the photoelectric effect or Compton scatter and results in the formation of a positive atom and a dislodged negative electron. The ejected high-speed electron is set into motion and interacts with other atoms within the absorbing tissues. The kinetic energy of such electrons results in further ionization, excitation, or breaking of molecular bonds, all of which cause chemical changes within the cell that result in biologic damage (Figure 3-1). Ionization may have little effect on cells if the chemical changes do not alter sensitive molecules, or such changes may have a profound effect on structures of great importance to cell function (e.g., DNA).

Free Radical Formation. X-radiation causes cell damage primarily through the formation of free radicals.* Free radical formation occurs when an x-ray photon ionizes water, the primary component of living cells. Ionization of water results in the production of hydrogen and hydroxyl free radicals (Figure 3-2). A free radical is an uncharged (neutral) atom or molecule that exists with a single, unpaired electron in its outermost shell. It is highly reactive and unstable; the lifetime of a free radical is approximately 10^{-10} seconds. To achieve stability, free radicals may (1) recombine without causing changes in the molecule, (2) combine with other free radicals and cause changes, or (3) combine with ordinary molecules to form a toxin (e.g., hydrogen peroxide [H_2O_2]) capable of producing widespread cellular changes (Figure 3-3).

Theories of Radiation Injury. Damage to living tissues caused by exposure to ionizing radiation may result from a direct hit and absorption of an x-ray photon within a cell or from the absorption of an x-ray photon by the water within a cell accompanied by free radical formation. Two theories are used to describe how radiation damages biologic tissues: (1) the direct theory and (2) the indirect theory.

Direct Theory. The direct theory of radiation injury suggests that cell damage results when ionizing radiation directly hits critical areas, or targets, within the cell. For example, if x-ray photons directly strike the DNA of a cell, critical damage occurs, causing injury to the irradiated organism. Direct injuries from exposure to ionizing radiation occur infrequently; most x-ray photons pass through the cell and cause little or no damage.

Indirect Theory. The indirect theory of radiation injury suggests that x-ray photons are absorbed within the cell and cause the formation of

*A free radical with no charge is denoted by a dot following the chemical symbol (e.g., H•). A free radical with a charge is an ion.

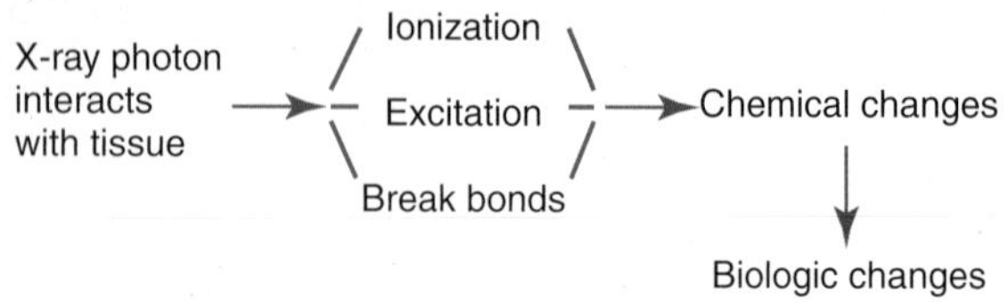

Fig 3-1 The x-ray photon interacts with tissues and results in ionization, excitation, or breaking of molecular bonds, all of which cause chemical changes that result in biologic damage.

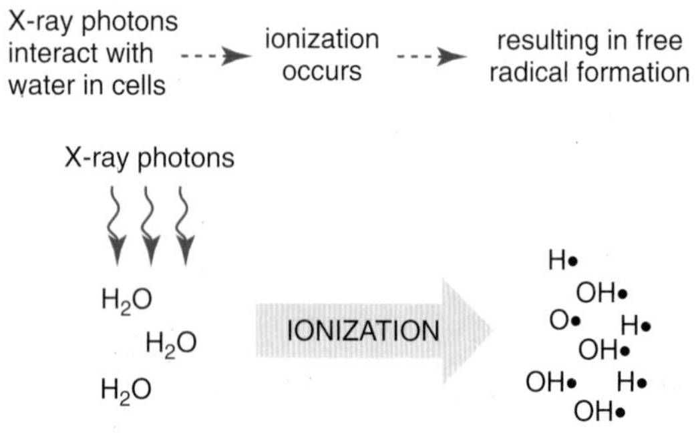

Fig 3-2 Examples of free radicals created when water is irradiated.

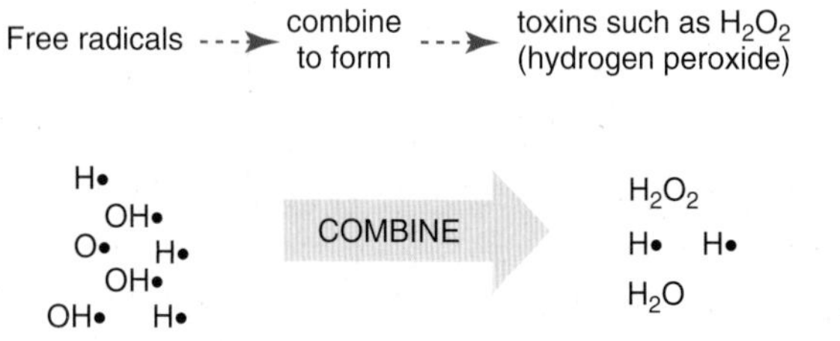

Fig 3-3 Free radicals can combine with each other to form toxins such as hydrogen peroxide.

toxins, which in turn damage the cell. For example, when x-ray photons are absorbed by the water within a cell, free radicals are formed. The free radicals combine to form toxins (e.g., H_2O_2), which cause cellular dysfunction and biologic damage. An indirect injury results because the free radicals combine and form toxins, not because of a direct hit by x-ray photons. Indirect injuries from exposure to ionizing radiation occur frequently because of the high water content of cells. The chances of free radical formation and indirect injury are great because cells are 70% to 80% water.

HELPFUL HINT

X-Rays Are Harmful

- All ionizing radiations are **harmful**.
- All ionizing radiations produce **biologic changes** in tissues.
- It is discouraged to use the term "safe" x-rays.

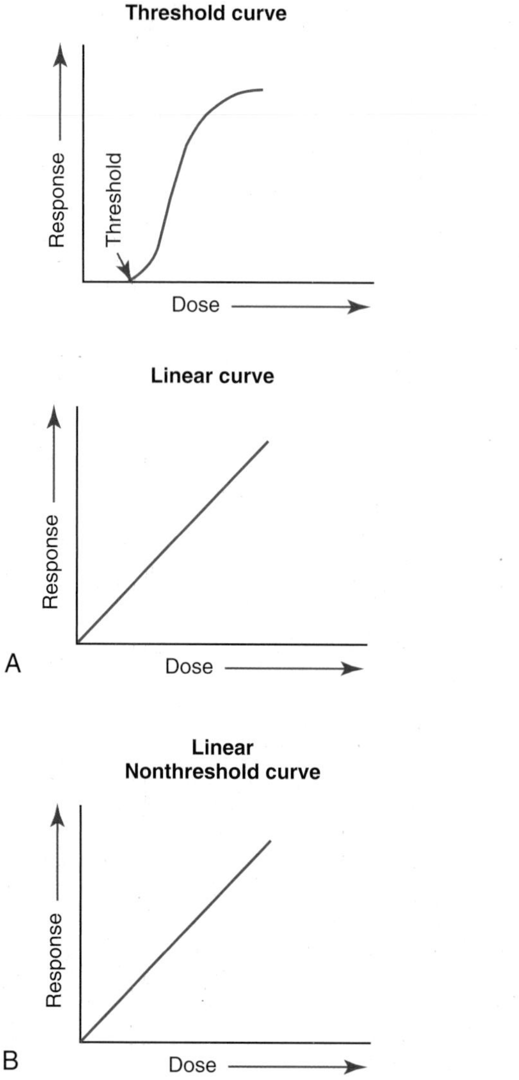

Fig 3-4 A, *Threshold curve:* This curve indicates that below a certain level (threshold), no response is seen. B, *Linear curve:* This curve indicates that response is proportional to dose. C, *Linear nonthreshold curve:* This dose-response curve indicates that a response is seen at any dose. It is essentially the same as the linear curve.

Dose-Response Curve

If all ionizing radiations are harmful and produce biologic damage, what level of exposure is considered acceptable? To establish acceptable levels of radiation exposure, it is useful to plot the dose administered and the damage produced. With radiation exposure, a **dose-response curve** can be used to correlate the "response," or damage, of tissues with the "dose," or amount, of radiation received.

When dose and damage are plotted on a graph, a linear, nonthreshold relationship is seen. A linear relationship indicates that the response of the tissues is directly proportional to the dose. A nonthreshold relationship indicates that a threshold dose level for damage does not exist. A nonthreshold dose-response curve suggests that no matter how small the amount of radiation received, some biologic damage does occur (Figure 3-4). Consequently, no safe amount of radiation exposure exists. In dental imaging, as mentioned earlier, although the doses received by patients are low, damage does occur.

Most of the information used to produce dose-response curves for radiation exposure comes from studying the effects of large doses of radiation on populations—for example, atomic bomb survivors. In the low-dose range, however, minimal information has been documented; instead, the curve has been extrapolated from animal and cellular experiments.

TABLE 3-1 **A Comparison of Non-Stochastic and Stochastic Effects of Radiation**

	Non-Stochastic Effects (deterministic effects)	Stochastic Effects
Example	**Mucositis** resulting from radiation therapy to oral cavity	**Radiation-induced cancer**
Caused by	Killing of many cells	Sub-lethal damage to DNA
Threshold dose?	**Yes:** Sufficient cell killing required to cause a clinical response	**No:** Even one photon could cause a change in DNA that leads to a cancer
Severity of clinical effects & dose	**Proportional to dose;** the greater the dose, the greater the effect	**Independent of dose; all-or-none response-** an individual either has effect or does not
Probability of having effect & dose	**Probability of effect independent of dose;** all individuals show effect when dose is above threshold	**Probability of effect proportional to dose;** the greater the dose, the greater the chance of having the effect

TABLE 3-2 **Tissue and Radiation Effect**

Tissue or Organ	Radiation Effect
Bone marrow	Leukemia
Reproductive cells (ova, sperm)	Genetic mutations
Salivary gland	Carcinoma
Thyroid	Carcinoma
Skin	Carcinoma
Lens of eye	Cataracts

Stochastic and Nonstochastic Radiation Effects

The deleterious effects of ionizing radiation on human tissue can be divided into two types: stochastic and nonstochastic. Stochastic effects occur as a direct function of dose. The probability of occurrence increases with increasing absorbed dose; however, the severity of effects does not depend on the magnitude of the absorbed dose. As in the case of nonthreshold radiation effects, stochastic effects do not have a dose threshold. Stochastic effects occur as a result of the effect of ionizing radiation on chromosomes that result in genetic mutations. Examples of stochastic effects include induction of leukemia and other cancers (i.e., tumors).

Nonstochastic effects (deterministic effects) have a threshold and increase in severity with increased absorbed dose. Nonstochastic effects occur only after a threshold of exposure has been exceeded. The severity of deterministic effects increases as the dose of exposure increases. Because of an identifiable threshold level, appropriate radiation protection mechanisms and occupational exposure dose limits can be put in place to reduce the likelihood of these effects occurring. Nonstochastic effects are caused by significant cell damage (lethal DNA damage) or cell death. The physical effects occur when the cell death burden is large enough to cause obvious functional impairment of a tissue or organ.

Examples of nonstochastic effects include skin erythema, loss of hair, cataract formation, decreased fertility, radiation sickness, teratogenesis, and fetal death. Compared with stochastic effects, nonstochastic effects require larger radiation doses to cause serious impairment of health. Table 3-1 compares stochastic and nonstochastic effects of radiation.

Sequence of Radiation Injury

Chemical reactions (e.g., ionization, free radical formation) that follow the absorption of radiation occur rapidly at the molecular level. However, varying amounts of time are required for these changes to alter cells and cellular functions. As a result, the observable effects of radiation are not visible immediately after exposure. Instead, after exposure, a latent period occurs. A latent period can be defined as the time that elapses between exposure to ionizing radiation and the appearance of observable clinical signs. The latent period may be short or long, depending on the total dose of radiation received and the amount of time, or rate, it took to receive the dose. The more radiation received and the faster the dose rate, the shorter the latent period.

After the latent period, a period of injury occurs. A variety of cellular injuries may result, including cell death, changes in cell function, breaking or clumping of chromosomes, formation of giant cells, cessation of mitotic activity, and abnormal mitotic activity.

The last event in the sequence of radiation injury is the recovery period. Not all cellular radiation injuries are permanent. With each radiation exposure, cellular damage is followed by repair. Depending on a number of factors, cells can repair the damage caused by radiation. Most of the damage caused by low-level radiation is repaired within the cells of the body.

The effects of radiation exposure are additive, and unrepaired damage accumulates in the tissues. The cumulative effects of repeated radiation exposure can lead to health problems (e.g., cancer, cataract formation, or birth defects). Table 3-2 lists disorders that may result from the cumulative effects of repeated radiation exposure on tissues and organs.

Determining Factors for Radiation Injury

In addition to understanding the mechanisms, theories, and sequence of radiation injury, it is important to recognize the factors that influence radiation injury. The factors used to determine the degree of radiation injury include the following:

- Total dose: Quantity of radiation received, or the total amount of radiation energy absorbed. More damage occurs when tissues absorb large quantities of radiation.
- Dose rate: Rate at which exposure to radiation occurs and absorption takes place (dose rate=dose/time). More radiation damage takes place with high dose rates because a rapid delivery of radiation does not allow time for the cellular damage to be repaired.
- *Amount of tissue irradiated:* Areas of the body exposed to radiation. Total-body irradiation produces more adverse systemic effects than if small, localized areas of the body are exposed. An example of total-body irradiation is the exposure of a person to a nuclear energy disaster. Extensive radiation injury occurs when large areas of the body are exposed because of the damage to the blood-forming tissues.
- *Cell sensitivity:* More damage occurs in cells that are most sensitive to radiation, such as rapidly dividing cells and young cells (see later discussion).
- *Age:* Children are more susceptible to radiation damage than are adults.

HELPFUL HINT

Determining Factors

Total Dose
More damage with *more* dose

Dose Rate
More damage with *fast* rate

Amount of Tissue
More damage with *more* tissue exposed

Cell Sensitivity
More damage with *sensitive* cells

Age
More damage in *children*

RADIATION EFFECTS

Short-Term and Long-Term Effects

Radiation effects can be classified as either short-term or long-term effects. After the latent period, effects that are seen within minutes, days, or weeks are termed short-term effects. Short-term effects are associated with large amounts of radiation absorbed in a short time (e.g., exposure to a nuclear accident or the atomic bomb). Acute radiation syndrome (ARS) is a short-term effect and includes nausea, vomiting, diarrhea, hair loss, and hemorrhage. Short-term effects are not applicable to dentistry.

Effects that appear after years, decades, or generations are termed long-term effects. Long-term effects are associated with small amounts of radiation absorbed repeatedly over a long period. Repeated low levels of radiation exposure are linked to the induction of cancer, birth abnormalities, and genetic defects.

Somatic and Genetic Effects

All the cells in the body can be classified as either somatic or genetic. Somatic cells are all the cells in the body except the reproductive cells. The reproductive cells (e.g., ova, sperm) are termed genetic cells. Depending on the type of cell injured by radiation, the biologic effects of radiation can be classified as somatic or genetic.

Somatic effects are seen in a person who has been irradiated. Radiation injuries that produce changes in somatic cells produce poor health in the irradiated individual. Major somatic effects of radiation exposure include the induction of cataracts and cancer, including leukemia. These changes, however, are not transmitted to future generations (Figure 3-5).

Genetic effects are not seen in the irradiated person but are passed on to future generations. Radiation injuries that produce changes in genetic cells do not affect the health of the exposed individual. Instead, the radiation-induced mutations affect the health of the offspring (see Figure 3-5). Genetic damage cannot be repaired.

Radiation Effects on Cells

The cell, or basic structural unit of all living organisms, is composed of a central nucleus and surrounding cytoplasm. Ionizing radiation may affect the nucleus, the cytoplasm, or the entire cell. The cell nucleus is more sensitive to radiation than is the cytoplasm. Damage to the nucleus affects the chromosomes containing DNA and results in disruption of cell division, which, in turn, may lead to disruption of cell function or cell death.

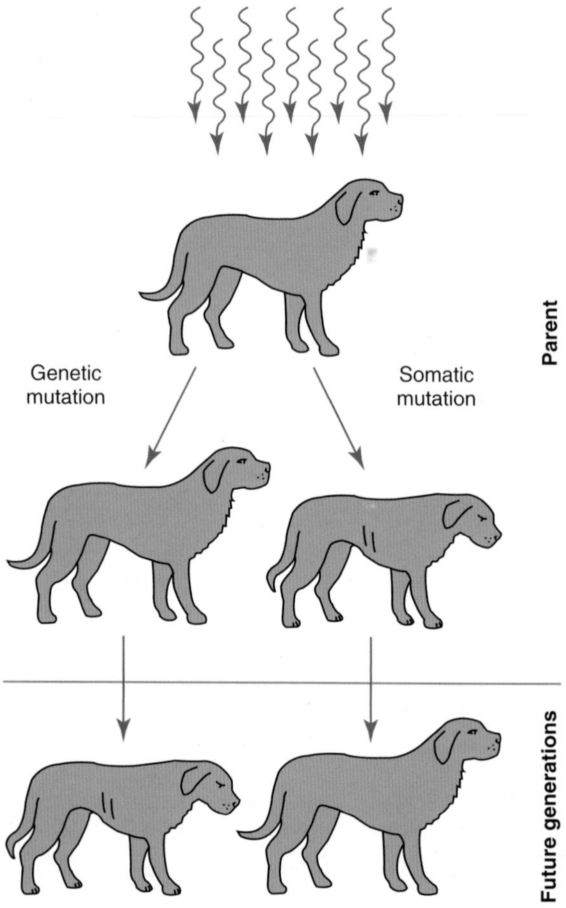

Fig 3-5 A somatic mutation produces poor health in the exposed animal but does not produce mutations in subsequent generations. In contrast, a genetic mutation does not affect the exposed animal but produces mutations in future generations.

Not all cells respond to radiation in the same manner. A cell that is sensitive to radiation is termed radiosensitive; one that is resistant is termed radioresistant. The response of a cell to radiation exposure is determined by the following:

- Mitotic activity: Cells that divide frequently or undergo many divisions over time are more sensitive to radiation.
- Cell differentiation: Cells that are immature or are not highly specialized are more sensitive to radiation.
- Cell metabolism: Cells that have a higher metabolism are more sensitive to radiation.

Cells that are radiosensitive include blood cells, immature reproductive cells, and young bone cells. The cell that is most sensitive to radiation is the small lymphocyte. Radioresistant cells include cells of bone, muscle, and nerve (Table 3-3).

Radiation Effects on Tissues and Organs

Cells are organized into the larger functioning units of tissues and organs. As with cells, tissues and organs vary in their sensitivity to radiation. Radiosensitive organs are composed of radiosensitive cells and include the lymphoid tissues, bone marrow, testes, and intestines. Examples of radioresistant tissues include the salivary glands, kidney, and liver.

In dentistry, some tissues and organs are designated as "critical" because they are exposed to more radiation than are others during

TABLE 3-3 Tissue and Organ Sensitivity to Radiation

Tissue or Organ	Sensitivity to Radiation	Tissue or Organ	Sensitivity to Radiation
Radiosensitive Tissues		**Radioresistant Tissues or Organs**	
Small lymphocyte 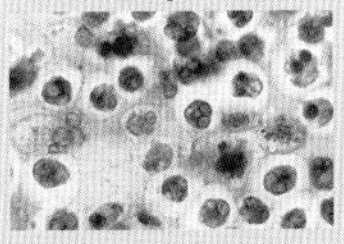 From the CDC Public Health Image Library (PHIL 10614). http://phil.cdc.gov/.	**High**	**Muscle tissue** 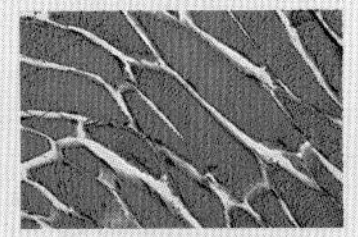 Copyright Bildpoet/iStock.com	**Low**
Bone marrow 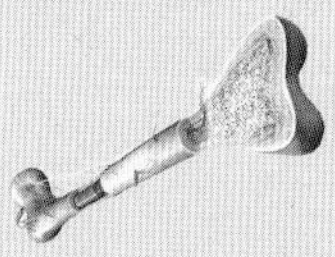 Copyright Sciencepics/Shutterstock.com	**High**	**Nerve tissue** 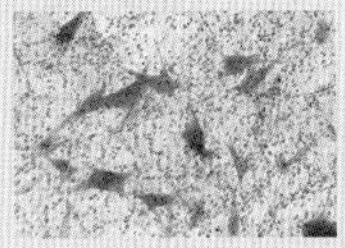 Copyright BeholdingEye/iStock.com	**Low**
Reproductive cells 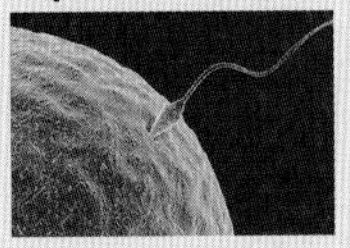 Copyright cornishman/iStock.com	**High**	**Mature bone and cartilage** 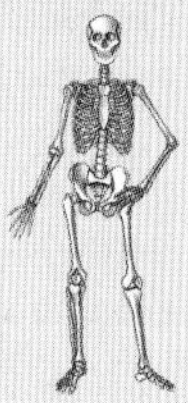 From Herlihy: *The Human Body in Health and Illness*, ed 5, St. Louis, 2014, Saunders.	**Fairly low**
Intestinal mucosa 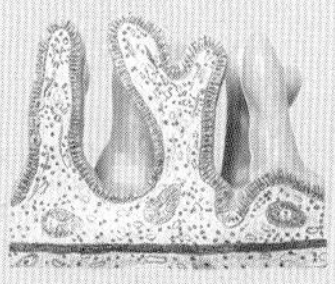 Copyright Ericsphotography/iStock.com	**High**	**Salivary gland** 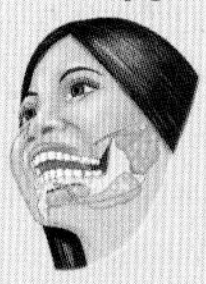 From Patton & Thibodeau: *Essentials of Anatomy and Physiology*, ed 1, St. Louis, 2012, Mosby.	**Fairly low**
Skin 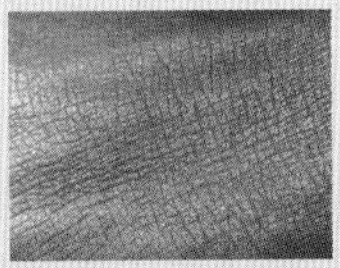 Copyright Nico_blue/iStock.com	**Fairly high**	**Thyroid gland** 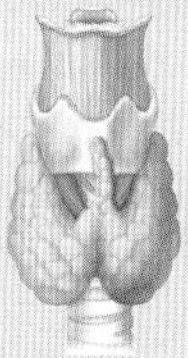 From Patton & Thibodeau: *Anatomy and Physiology*, ed 8, St. Louis, 2013, Mosby.	**Fairly low**
Lens of eye 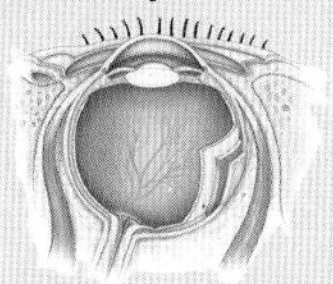 From Patton & Thibodeau: *The Human Body in Health and Disease*, ed 6, St. Louis, 2014, Mosby.	**Fairly high**	**Kidney** 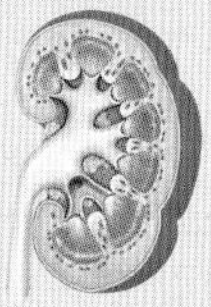 From Patton & Thibodeau: *Anatomy and Physiology*, ed 8, St. Louis, 2013, Mosby.	**Fairly low**
Oral mucosa 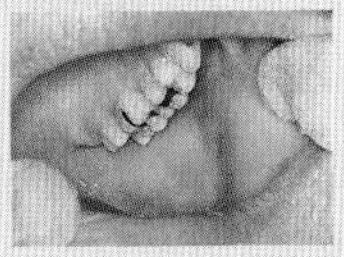 From Robinson and Bird: *Essentials of Dental Assisting*, ed 5, St. Louis, 2013, Mosby.	**Fairly high**	**Liver** 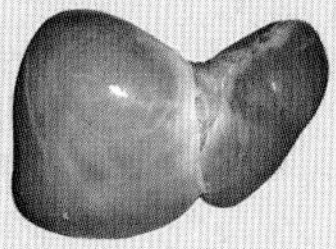	**Fairly low**

imaging procedures. A critical organ is an organ that, if damaged, diminishes the quality of a person's life. Critical organs exposed during dental imaging procedures in the head and neck region include the following:

- Thyroid gland
- Bone marrow
- Skin
- Lens of the eye

RADIATION MEASUREMENTS

Units of Measurement

Radiation can be measured in the same manner as other physical concepts such as time, distance, and weight. Just as the unit of measurement for time is minutes, for distance miles or kilometers, and for weight pounds or kilograms, the International Commission on Radiation Units and Measurements (ICRU) has established special units for the measurement of radiation. Such units are used to define three quantities of radiation: (1) exposure, (2) dose, and (3) dose equivalent. The dental radiographer must know radiation measurements to discuss exposure and dose concepts with the dental patient.

At present, two systems are used to define radiation measurements: (1) The older system is referred to as the *traditional system*, or *standard system;* and (2) the newer system is the metric equivalent known as the *SI system*, or *Système International d'Unités (International System of Units)*.

The traditional units of radiation measurement include the following:

- Roentgen (R)
- Radiation absorbed dose (rad)
- Roentgen equivalent (in) man (rem)

The SI units of radiation measurement include the following:

- Coulombs/kilogram (C/kg)
- Gray (Gy)
- Sievert (Sv)

This text uses both traditional and SI units of measurement; the dental radiographer should be familiar with both systems and know how to convert measurements from one system to the other (Table 3-4). In addition, the dental radiographer must be familiar with a number of physics terms used in the definitions of both traditional and SI units of radiation measurement (Table 3-5).

TABLE 3-4 Units of Radiation Measurement

Unit	Definition	Conversion
Traditional System		
Roentgen (R)	1 R = 87 erg/g	1 R = 2.58×10^{-4} C/kg
Radiation absorbed dose (rad)	1 rad = 100 erg/g	1 rad = 0.01 Gy
Roentgen equivalent (in) man (rem)	1 rem = rad × QF	1 rem = 0.01 Sv
SI System		
Coulombs per kilogram (C/kg)	—	1 C/kg = 3880 R
Gray (Gy)	1 Gy = 0.01 J/kg	1 Gy = 100 rad
Sievert (Sv)	1 Sv = Gy × QF	1 Sv = 100 rem

J, Joule; *QF*, quality factor; *SI*, International System of Units.

TABLE 3-5 Radiation Measurement Terms

Term	Definition
Coulomb (C)	Unit of electrical charge; the quantity of electrical charge transferred by 1 ampere in 1 second.
Ampere (A)	Unit of electrical current strength; current yielded by 1 volt against 1 ohm of resistance.
Erg (erg)	Unit of energy equivalent to 1.0×10^{-7} joules or to 2.4×10^{-8} calories.
Joule (J)	SI unit of energy equivalent to the work done by the force of 1 newton acting over the distance of 1 meter.
Newton (N)	SI unit of force; the force that, when acting continuously on a mass of 1 kilogram, will impart to it an acceleration of 1 meter per second squared (m/sec^2).
Kilogram (kg)	Unit of mass equivalent to 1000 grams or 2.205 pounds.

Exposure Measurement

The term exposure refers to the measurement of ionization in air produced by x-rays. The traditional unit of exposure for x-rays is the roentgen (R). The roentgen is a way of measuring radiation exposure by determining the amount of ionization that occurs in air. A definition follows:

> *Roentgen: The quantity of x-radiation or gamma radiation that produces an electrical charge of 2.58×10^{-4} coulombs in a kilogram of air at standard temperature and pressure (STP) conditions.*

In measuring the roentgen, a known volume of air is irradiated. The interaction of x-ray photons with air molecules results in ionization, or the formation of ions. The ions (electrical charges) that are produced are collected and measured. One roentgen is equal to the amount of radiation that produces approximately 2 billion, or 2.08×10^9, ion pairs in one cubic centimeter (cm^3) of air.

The roentgen has limitations as a unit of measure. It measures the amount of energy that reaches the surface of an organism but does not describe the amount of radiation absorbed. The roentgen is essentially limited to measurements in air only; it does not measure radiation absorbed by the body. By definition, it is used only for x-rays and gamma rays and does not include other types of radiation.

No SI unit for exposure that is equivalent to the roentgen exists. Instead, exposure is simply stated in coulombs per kilograms (C/kg). The coulomb (C) is a unit of electrical charge. The unit C/kg measures the number of electrical charges, or the number of ion pairs, in 1 kg of air. The conversions for roentgen and coulombs per kilogram can be expressed as follows:

$$1\text{R} = 2.58 \times 10^{-4}\ \text{C} / \text{kg}$$

$$1\text{C} / \text{kg} = 3.88 \times 10^{3}\ \text{R}$$

Dose Measurement

Dose can be defined as the amount of energy absorbed by a tissue. The radiation absorbed dose, or rad, is the traditional unit of dose. Unlike the roentgen, the rad is not restricted to air and can be applied to all forms of radiation. The rad measures radiation absorbed by the body but does not take into account the radiosensitivity of different tissues. A definition follows:

Rad: A special unit of absorbed dose that is equal to the deposition of 100 ergs of energy per gram of tissue (100 erg/g).

Using SI units, 1 rad is equivalent to 0.01 joule per kilogram (0.01 J/kg). The SI unit equivalent to the rad is the gray (Gy), or 1 J/kg. The conversions for rad and Gy can be expressed as follows:

1 rad = 0.01 Gy

1 Gy = 100 rad

Dose Equivalent Measurement

Different types of radiation have different effects on tissues. The dose equivalent measurement is used to compare the biologic effects of different types of radiation. The traditional unit of the dose equivalent is the roentgen equivalent (in) man, or rem. A definition follows:

Rem: The product of absorbed dose (rad) and a quality factor specific for the type of radiation.

To place the exposure effects of different types of radiation on a common scale, a quality factor (QF), or dimensionless multiplier, is used. Each type of radiation has a specific QF based on different types of radiation producing different types of biologic damage. For example, the QF for x-rays is equal to 1.

The SI unit equivalent of the rem is the sievert (Sv). Conversions for the rem and sievert can be expressed as follows:

1 rem = 0.01 Sv

1 Sv = 100 rem

The sievert is the preferred unit of measurement of absorbed radiation dose currently used in dentistry. The sievert not only accounts for absorbed dose in soft tissues, but also takes into consideration the radiosensitivity of certain tissues.

Measurements Used in Dental Imaging

In dental imaging, the gray and sievert are equal, and the roentgen, rad, and rem are considered approximately equal. Smaller multiples of these radiation units are typically used in dentistry because of the small quantities of radiation used during imaging procedures. The prefixes "milli-," meaning 1/1000, and "micro-," meaning 1/1,000,000, allow the dental radiographer to express small quantities of exposure, dose, and dose equivalent. For example, 1 millisievert (mSv) = 0.001 Sv and 1 microsievert (μSv) = 0.000001 Sv.

HELPFUL HINT

Sievert Conversion Chart

1.000000 Sv	=	1000.000 mSv	=	1,000,000 μSv
0.010000 Sv	=	10.000 mSv	=	10000 μSv
0.001000 Sv	=	1.000 mSv	=	1000 μSv
0.000010 Sv	=	0.010 mSv	=	10 μSv
0.000001 Sv	=	0.001 mSv	=	1 μSv

RADIATION RISKS

Sources of Radiation Exposure

To understand radiation risks, the dental radiographer must be familiar with the potential sources of radiation exposure. This knowledge can then be used to better understand the radiation risks associated with dentistry.

Humans are exposed daily to radiation from both natural and synthetic sources. Natural, or background, radiation sources include radon in the air; uranium, radium, and thorium in the earth; cosmic rays from outer space and the sun; radioactive potassium in food and water; and radioactive material found within the human body. Radon gas arising from the soil is the single greatest source of exposure to background radiation in the United States.

Exposure to background radiation varies depending on where a person lives. The cosmic exposure depends on the elevation above sea level; the higher the altitude, the more exposure to cosmic rays. Terrestrial exposure comes from the ground; an example includes naturally occurring uranium-enriched soil. Type of home construction also effects exposure; a brick home has a higher natural radiation level than a home made of wood. Internal radiation exposure depends on the food and water that a person ingests. Foods such as bananas and Brazil nuts naturally contain higher levels of radiation than other foods, and most water supplies naturally contain radon. In the United States the average person is exposed to approximately 3.1 mSv of background radiation per year.

In addition to naturally occurring background radiation, modern technology has created artificial, or human-made, sources of radiation. The average person is exposed to approximately 3.1 mSv of human-made radiation per year. Consumer products (e.g., luminous wristwatches, televisions, computer screens), fallout from atomic weapons, weapons production, and the nuclear fuel cycle are all sources of human-made radiation exposure.

Medical radiation is the greatest contributor to human-made radiation exposure. Medical radiation includes medical imaging procedures, dental imaging, fluoroscopy, radiation therapy, nuclear medicine, and computed tomography (CT) imaging. Medical radiation exposure accounts for nearly half of the annual total exposure received. In the United States the average person is exposed to a total of 6.2 mSv of radiation per year (3.1 mSv from natural sources + 3.1 mSv from human-made sources=6.2 mSv total). See Figure 3-6.

To estimate personal annual radiation dose, visit the American Nuclear Society (ANS) website and use the interactive dose chart (http://www.ans.org/pi/resources/dosechart/).

Table 3-6 summarizes radiation sources and exposure.

Risk and Risk Estimates

A risk can be defined as the likelihood of adverse effects or death resulting from exposure to a hazard. In dental imaging, risk is the likelihood of an adverse effect, specifically cancer induction, occurring from exposure to ionizing radiation.

The potential risk of dental imaging inducing a fatal cancer in an individual has been estimated to be approximately 3 in 1 million. The risk of a person developing cancer spontaneously is much higher, or 3300 in 1 million. To keep the concept of risk in perspective, the risk of incurring a fatal cancer from dental imaging procedures should be compared with commonplace risks. For example, a 1-in-1-million risk of a fatal outcome is associated with each of the following activities: riding 10 miles on a bike, 300 miles in a car, or 1000 miles in an airplane; or smoking 1.4 cigarettes per day. These risk estimates suggest that death is more likely to occur from common activities than from

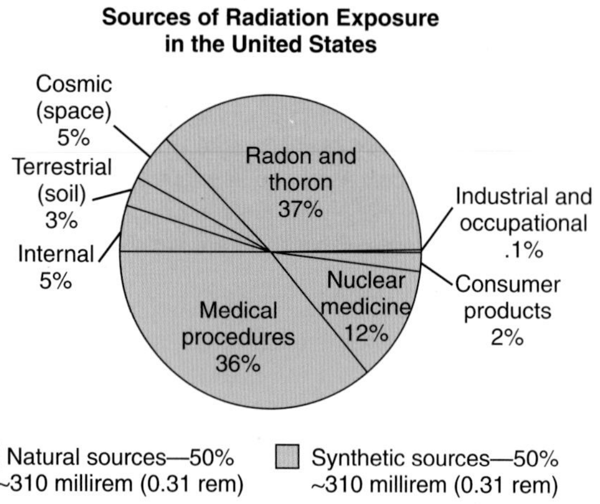

Fig 3-6 Radiation sources that contribute to the average annual U.S. radiation dose of 6.2 mSv. Approximately 75% of this dose is split between radon/thoron gas and diagnostic medical procedures. (Data from National Council on Radiation Protection and Measurements. Report No. 160—Ionizing radiation exposure of the population of the United States, Bethesda, MD, 2009.)

TABLE 3-6 Radiation Sources and Exposure

Radiation Source	Whole Body (mrem/year)	Whole Body (mSv/year)
Natural/Background		
Radon	200.00	2.00
Cosmic	27.00	0.27
Terrestrial	28.00	0.28
Internal	39.00	0.39
Artificial/Human-Made		
Medical or dental	53.00	0.53
Consumer products	9.00	0.09
Other		
Occupational	<1.00	<0.001
Nuclear fuel cycle	<1.00	<0.001
Fallout	<1.00	<0.001

mrem, millirem; *mSv*, millisievert.

dental imaging procedures and that cancer is much more likely to be unrelated to radiation exposure. In other words, the risks from dental imaging are not significantly greater than the risks of other everyday activities in modern life.

Dental Radiation and Exposure Risks

To calculate the risk from dental imaging procedures, doses to critical organs must be measured. As previously defined, damage to a critical organ diminishes the quality of an individual's life. With dental imaging procedures, the critical organs at risk include the thyroid gland and active bone marrow. The skin and eyes may also be considered critical organs.

Risk Elements.

Thyroid gland. Although the primary beam does not irradiate the thyroid gland in dental imaging procedures, thyroid radiation exposure does occur. An estimated dose of 6000 mrad (0.06 Gy) is necessary to produce cancer in the thyroid gland; such a large dose does not occur in dental imaging.

Bone marrow. The areas of the maxilla and mandible exposed during dental imaging account for a very small percentage of active bone marrow. The risk of cancer induction (leukemia) is directly associated with the amount of blood-producing tissues irradiated and the dose. Leukemia is induced most likely at doses of 5000 mrad (0.05 Gy) or more; a dose of such magnitude does not occur in dental imaging.

Skin. A total of 250 rad (2.5 Gy) in a 14-day period causes erythema, or reddening, of the skin. To produce such changes, more than 500 dental films (F-speed film, exposure rate 0.7 R/second) in a 14-day period would have to be exposed. This scenario does not occur in dental imaging.

Eyes. More than 200,000 mrad (2 Gy) are necessary to induce cataract formation (cloudiness of lens) in the eyes. Again, such high doses are not a consideration in dental imaging.

Patient Exposure and Dose

Dental patients must be protected from excess exposure to radiation. (Chapter 4 discusses patient protection in detail.) How much radiation exposure results from dental imaging? The amount of exposure varies, depending on the following:

- *Receptor choice:* Using digital sensors reduces radiation exposure. The use of sensors can reduce exposure time by 50% to 90% compared with conventional radiography. Radiation exposure can be limited by using the fastest film available. The use of F-speed film instead of D-speed reduces the absorbed dose by 60%.
- *Collimation:* Radiation exposure can be limited by using rectangular collimation. The use of rectangular collimation instead of round collimation reduces the absorbed dose by 60% to 70%.
- *Technique:* Radiation exposure can be limited by increasing the target-receptor distance. The use of the paralleling technique and increased target-receptor distance reduces the skin dose.

Risk Versus Benefit of Dental Images

X-radiation is harmful to living tissues. Because biologic damage results from x-ray exposure, dental images should be prescribed for a patient only when the benefit of disease detection outweighs the risk of biologic damage. When dental images are properly prescribed and exposed, the benefit of disease detection far outweighs the risk of damage from x-radiation (see Chapter 4).

TABLE 3-7 Doses and Risks Associated with Dental Radiographic Examinations

Technique	Effective Dose in Microsieverts	Days of per Capita Background	Probability of *x* in a Million Fatal Cancer
Intraoral Techniques			
Single PA or PBW image with digital receptor and rectangular collimation	2	5 hours	0.1
Single PA or PBW image with digital receptor and round collimation	9	1	0.5
FMX with digital receptors and rectangular collimation	35	4	2
4 BWs with digital receptors and rectangular collimation	5	14 hours	0.3
FMX with digital receptors and round cone	171	20	9
Not recommended by ADA FMX with D film speed and round cone	388	46	21
Extraoral Plane Projections			
Panoramic—digital	16	2	1
Cephalometric—digital	5	14 hours	0.3
Cone Beam CT			
Large field of view	68	8	4
Adult exposure (42-mA setting)	91	11	5
Pediatric exposure (14-mA default setting)	57	7	3
Average field of view (varies from 5 mA to 38 mA)	21	2	1

From Ludlow JB: The risks of radiographic imaging, *Dimens Dent Hyg* 10(6):56, 2012.
ADA, American Dental Association; *BW*, bite-wing; *CT*, computed tomography; *FMX*, full mouth x-ray; *PA*, periapical; *PBW*, posterior bite-wing.

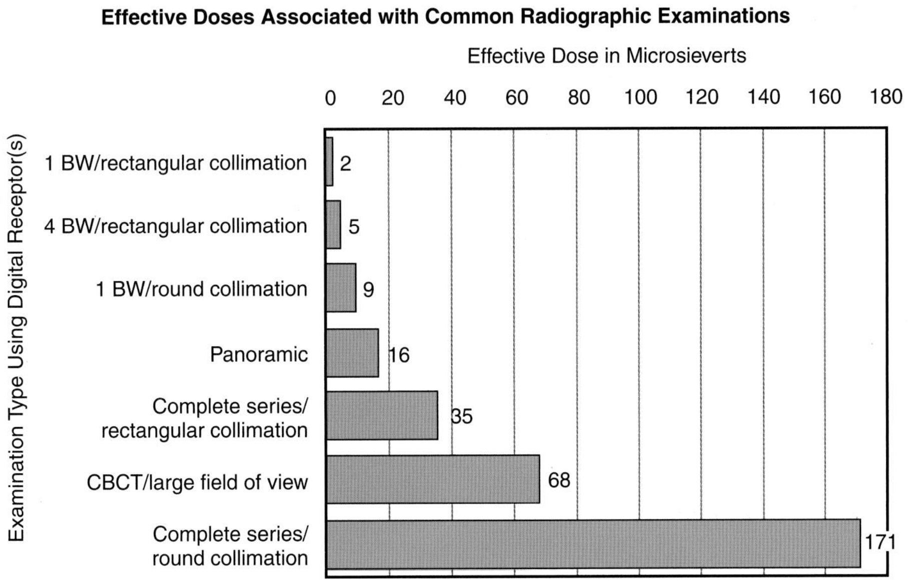

Fig 3-7 Effective doses associated with common radiographic examinations. Data from Ludlow JB: The risks of radiographic imaging, *Dimens Dent Hyg* 10(6):56, 2012.

SUMMARY

- All ionizing radiation is harmful and produces biologic changes in living tissue.
- Radiation injury results from ionization or free radical formation.
- A dose-response curve is used to demonstrate the response (damage) of tissues to the dose (amount) of radiation received.
- A threshold dose for damage does not exist, and the response of tissues is directly proportional to the dose received.
- Radiation injury follows a sequence of events: latent period, period of injury, and period of recovery.
- Radiation injury is affected by total dose, dose rate, amount of tissue irradiated, cell sensitivity, and patient's age.
- Short-term radiation effects occur when large amounts of radiation are absorbed in a short period; long-term radiation effects occur when small amounts of radiation are absorbed over a long time.
- Radiation effects are classified as somatic (seen in the irradiated person) or genetic (passed on to future generations).
- Cellular response to radiation depends on mitotic activity, cell differentiation, and cell metabolism.
- Radiosensitive cells include blood cells, immature reproductive cells, young bone cells, and epithelial cells.
- Radioresistant cells include the cells of bones, muscle, and nerve.
- Exposure is the measurement of ionization in air produced by x-rays; the units for exposure are the roentgen (R) and coulombs per kilogram (C/kg).
- Dose is the amount of energy absorbed by a tissue; the units for dose are the radiation absorbed dose (rad) and the gray (Gy).
- Dose equivalent measurement is used to compare the biologic effects of different types of radiation; the units for dose equivalent are the roentgen equivalent (in) man (rem) and the sievert (Sv).
- The risks of radiation exposure involved in dental imaging are not significantly greater than other everyday risks in life.
- The amount of exposure a patient receives from dental imaging depends on the receptor, collimation, and technique used.
- Dental images should be prescribed for a patient only when the benefit of disease detection outweighs the risk of damage from x-radiation.

BIBLIOGRAPHY

Bernstein DI, Clark SJ, Scheetz JP, et al: Perceived quality of radiographic images after rapid processing of D- and F-speed direct-exposure intraoral x-ray films, Oral Surg Oral Med Oral Pathol Oral Radiol Endod 96(4):486, 2003.

Frommer HH, Stabulas-Savage JJ: Biologic effects of radiation. In Radiology for the dental professional, ed 9, St Louis, 2011, Mosby.

Johnson ON: Effects of radiation exposure. In Essentials of dental radiography for dental assistants and hygienists, ed 9, Upper Saddle River, NJ, 2011, Prentice Hall.

Ludlow JB: The risks of radiographic imaging, Dimens Dent Hyg 10(6):56, 2012.

Mallya SM, Lam EWN: Safety and protection. In White and Pharoah's oral radiology: principles and interpretation, ed 8, St. Louis, 2019, Elsevier.

Mallya SM, Lam EWN: Biologic effects of ionizing radiation. In White and Pharoah's oral radiology: principles and interpretation, ed 8, St. Louis, 2019, Elsevier.

Miles DA, Van Dis ML, Williamson GF, et al: Radiation biology and protection. In Radiographic imaging for the dental team, ed 4, St Louis, 2009, Saunders.

National Council on Radiation Protection and Measurements: Report No. 160—Ionizing radiation exposure of the population of the United States, Bethesda, MD, 2009.

QUIZ QUESTIONS

Multiple Choice

____ **1.** The latent period in radiation biology is the time between:

a. initial injury and repair
b. subsequent doses of radiation
c. cell rest and cell mitosis
d. exposure to x-radiation and clinical symptoms
e. none of the above

____ **2.** A free radical:

a. is an uncharged molecule
b. has an unpaired electron in the outer shell
c. is highly reactive and unstable
d. combines with molecules to form toxins
e. all of the above

____ **3.** Direct radiation injury occurs when:

a. x-ray photons hit critical targets within a cell
b. x-ray photons pass through the cell
c. x-ray photons are absorbed and form toxins
d. free radicals combine to form toxins
e. none of the above

____ **4.** Indirect radiation injury occurs when:

a. x-ray photons hit critical targets within a cell
b. x-ray photons pass through the cell
c. x-ray photons are absorbed and form toxins
d. x-ray photons hit the DNA of a cell
e. none of the above

____ **5.** Which relationship describes the response of tissues to radiation?

a. linear
b. linear, threshold
c. linear, nonthreshold
d. nonlinear, nonthreshold
e. none of the above

____ **6.** Which factor(s) contribute(s) to radiation injury?

a. total dose
b. dose rate
c. cell sensitivity
d. age
e. all of the above

____ **7.** Which statement is correct?

a. Short-term effects are seen with small amounts of radiation absorbed in a short period.
b. Short-term effects are seen with small amounts of radiation absorbed in a long period.
c. Long-term effects are seen with small amounts of radiation absorbed in a short period.

d. Long-term effects are seen with small amounts of radiation absorbed in a long period.
e. None of the above.

____ 8. Radiation injuries that are not seen in the person irradiated but that occur in future generations are termed:
a. somatic effects
b. genetic effects
c. cumulative effects
d. short-term effects
e. long-term effects

____ 9. Which is most susceptible to ionizing radiation?
a. bone tissue
b. small lymphocyte
c. muscle tissue
d. nerve tissue
e. epithelial tissue

____ 10. The sensitivity of tissues to radiation is determined by:
a. mitotic activity
b. cell differentiation
c. cell metabolism
d. all of the above
e. none of the above

____ 11. Which is considered radioresistant?
a. immature reproductive cells
b. young bone cells
c. mature bone cells
d. epithelial cells
e. none of the above

____ 12. An organ that, if damaged, diminishes the quality of an individual's life is termed:
a. critical
b. somatic
c. cumulative
d. radioresistant
e. none of the above

____ 13. The traditional unit for measuring x-ray exposure in air is termed:
a. gray
b. coulombs per kilogram
c. rem
d. rad
e. roentgen

____ 14. Which radiation unit is determined by the quality factor (QF)?
a. roentgen
b. rad
c. rem
d. gray
e. coulombs per kilogram

____ 15. The unit for measuring the absorption of x-rays is termed:
a. roentgen
b. rad
c. rem
d. quality factor
e. sievert

____ 16. Which conversion is correct?
a. $1\,R = 2.58 \times 10^{-4}\,C/kg$
b. $1\,rad = 0.1\,Gy$
c. $1\,rem = 0.1\,Sv$
d. $1\,Gy = 10\,rad$
e. $1\,Sv = 10\,rem$

____ 17. Which traditional unit does not have an SI equivalent?
a. roentgen
b. rad
c. rem
d. quality factor
e. none of the above

____ 18. Which measurement is used only for x-rays?
a. sievert
b. gray
c. rem
d. rad
e. roentgen

____ 19. Which conversion is correct?
a. $1\,R = 2.58 \times 10^{-4}\,C/kg$
b. $1\,Gy = 100\,rad$
c. $1\,Sv = 100\,rem$
d. $1\,rem = rad \times QF$
e. all of the above

____ 20. What is the approximate average dose of **background radiation** received by an individual in the United States?
a. 100 mrem/0.01 mSv
b. 100 mrem/1.0 mSv
c. 300 mrem/3.0 mSv
d. 500 mrem/5.0 mSv
e. 1000 mrem/10.0 mSv

____ 21. What is the greatest contributor to **artificial radiation** exposure?
a. radioactive materials
b. medical radiation
c. consumer products
d. weapons production
e. nuclear fuel cycle

____ 22. The amount of radiation exposure an individual receives varies depending on:
a. receptor type
b. collimation
c. technique
d. both a and b
e. all of the above

____ 23. A single intraoral image using a digital sensor results in an effective exposure dose of:
a. 0.002 mSv
b. 0.020 mSv
c. 0.200 mSv
d. 2.000 mSv
e. 20.00 mSv

____ 24. What is the dose at which leukemia induction is most likely to occur?
a. 500 mrad (0.005 Gy)
b. 1000 mrad (0.01 Gy)
c. 2000 mrad (0.02 Gy)
d. 5000 mrad (0.05 Gy)
e. none of the above

____ 25. Which statement is incorrect?
a. X-radiation is not harmful to living tissues.
b. Dental images benefit the patient.
c. In dental imaging, the benefit of disease detection outweighs the risk of damage from radiation.
d. Dental images should be prescribed only when the benefit outweighs the risk.
e. Biologic damage results from x-ray exposure.

Ordering

Arrange the following examination types using digital receptors in order of effective dose, from smallest (A) to largest (E).

_____ **26.** panoramic
_____ **27.** single periapical/rectangular collimation
_____ **28.** complete series/round collimation
_____ **29.** complete series/rectangular collimation
_____ **30.** single bite-wing/round collimation

Arrange the annual sources of radiation exposure in the United States from smallest (A) to largest (E).

_____ **31.** medical procedures
_____ **32.** cosmic (space)
_____ **33.** radon and thoron
_____ **34.** terrestrial (soil)
_____ **35.** consumer products

4

Radiation Protection

LEARNING OBJECTIVES

After completion of this chapter, the student will be able to do the following:

1. Define the key terms associated with radiation protection.
2. Describe in detail the basics of patient protection before x-ray exposure.
3. Discuss the different types of filtration, and state the recommended total filtration for dental x-ray machines operating above and below 70 kV.
4. Describe the collimator used in dental x-ray machines and state the recommended diameter of the useful beam at the patient's skin.
5. List six ways to protect the patient from excessive radiation during x-ray exposure.
6. Describe the importance of receptor handling and processing after patient exposure to x-radiation.
7. Discuss operator protection in terms of adequate distance, shielding, and avoidance of the useful beam.
8. Describe personnel and equipment monitoring devices used to detect radiation.
9. Discuss radiation exposure guidelines, including radiation safety legislation, maximum permissible dose (MPD), and the ALARA concept.
10. Discuss with the dental patient radiation protection steps used before, during, and after exposure to x-radiation.

Many of the early pioneers in dental radiography suffered from the adverse effects of radiation. As discussed in Chapter 1, some of these pioneers lost their fingers, limbs, and, ultimately, lives to excessive doses of radiation. The hazards of radiation are now well documented, and radiation protection measures can be used to minimize radiation exposure for both the dental patient and the dental radiographer. The purpose of this chapter is to discuss patient protection before, during, and after exposure to x-rays; to detail operator protection methods; and to present radiation exposure and safety guidelines. In addition, this chapter includes a discussion of patient education about radiation protection.

PATIENT PROTECTION

X-radiation causes biologic changes in living cells and adversely affects all living tissues. With the use of proper patient protection techniques, the amount of x-radiation received by a dental patient can be minimized. Patient protection techniques can be used before, during, and after exposure to x-radiation.

Before Exposure

Patient protection measures can be used before any x-radiation exposure. Proper prescribing of dental images and the use of equipment that complies with state and federal radiation guidelines can minimize the amount of x-radiation that a dental patient receives.

Prescribing Dental Images. The first important step in limiting the amount of x-radiation received by a dental patient is the proper prescribing, or ordering, of dental images. The person responsible for prescribing dental images is the dentist. The dentist uses professional judgment to make decisions about the number, type, and frequency of dental images. Depending on the clinical examination of the patient, the images prescribed may include one survey (e.g., periapical) or a combination of surveys, such as bite-wing, panoramic, and cone-beam computed tomography (CBCT). The assessment of the patient's imaging history, the availability of alternate diagnostic tools, and the anatomic features of the patient are also important considerations when ordering dental images.

Every patient's dental condition is different, and, consequently, every patient should be evaluated for dental images on an individual basis. Examination should never include a predetermined number of images, nor should images be exposed at predetermined time intervals. For example, the dentist who prescribes a set number of images (e.g., four bite-wings) at a set interval (e.g., every 6 months) for every patient is not taking the individual needs of the patient into consideration.

The American Dental Association (ADA) Council on Scientific Affairs, in conjunction with the U.S. Department of Health and Human Services, Public Health Service, Food and Drug Administration (FDA), has adopted guidelines for prescribing the number, type, and frequency of dental images. These guidelines, titled *Dental Radiographic Examinations: Recommendations for Patient Selection and Limiting Radiation Exposure*, revised in 2012, summarize the recommendations that promote patient protection in diagnostic dental imaging (Table 4-1). For the most recent information and update on prescribing dental images, visit *www.ADA.org* and *www.FDA.gov*.

Proper Equipment. Another important step in limiting the amount of x-radiation a dental patient receives is the use of proper equipment. The dental x-ray tubehead must be equipped with appropriate aluminum filters, lead collimator, and position-indicating device.

Filtration. Two types of **filtration** are used in the dental x-ray tubehead: inherent filtration and added filtration.

Inherent filtration. **Inherent filtration** takes place when the primary beam passes through the glass window of the x-ray tube, the insulating oil, and the tubehead seal. The inherent filtration of the dental x-ray machine is equivalent to approximately 0.5 to 1.0 millimeter (mm) of aluminum. Inherent filtration alone does not meet the standards regulated by state and federal laws. Therefore added filtration is required.

Added filtration. **Added filtration** refers to the placement of aluminum disks in the path of the x-ray beam between the collimator and

TABLE 4-1 Recommendations for Prescribing Dental Radiographs (2012)

	PATIENT AGE AND DENTAL DEVELOPMENTAL STAGE				
Type of Encounter	**Child with Primary Dentition (prior to eruption of first permanent tooth)**	**Child with Transitional Dentition (after eruption of first permanent tooth)**	**Adolescent with Permanent Dentition (prior to eruption of third molars)**	**Adult, Dentate or Partially Edentulous**	**Adult, Edentulous**
New patient* being evaluated for oral diseases	Individualized radiographic exam consisting of selected periapical/occlusal views and/or posterior bite-wing images if proximal surfaces cannot be visualized or probed.	Individualized radiographic exam consisting of posterior bite-wing images with panoramic bite-wings and selected periapical images.	Individualized radiographic exam consisting of posterior bite-wings with panoramic exam or posterior bite-wings and selected periapical images.		Individualized radiographic exam, based on clinical signs and symptoms.
	Patients without evidence of disease and with open proximal contacts may not require radiographic exam at this time.		A full-mouth intraoral radiographic exam is preferred when patient has clinical evidence of generalized oral disease or a history of extensive dental treatment.		
Recall patient* with clinical caries or at increased risk for caries[†]	Posterior bite-wing exam at 6- to 12-month intervals if proximal surfaces cannot be examined visually or with probe			Posterior bite-wing exam at 6- to 18-month intervals	Not applicable
Recall patient* with no clinical caries and not at increased risk for caries[†]	Posterior bite-wing exam at 12- to 24-month intervals if proximal surfaces cannot be examined visually or with probe		Posterior bite-wing exam at 18- to 36-month intervals	Posterior bite-wing exam at 24- to 36-month intervals	Not applicable
Recall patient* with periodontal disease	Clinical judgment as to the need for and type of radiographic images for the evaluation of periodontal disease. Imaging may consist of, but is not limited to, select bite-wing and/or periapical images of areas where periodontal disease (other than nonspecific gingivitis) can be demonstrated clinically.				Not applicable
Patients (New and Recall) for monitoring of dentofacial growth and development, and/or assessment of dental/skeletal relationships	Clinical judgment as to need for and type of radiographic images for evaluation and/or monitoring of dentofacial growth and development or assessment of dental and skeletal relationships.		Clinical judgment as to need for and type of radiographic images for evaluation and/or monitoring of dentofacial growth and development, or assessment of dental and skeletal relationships. Panoramic or periapical exam to assess developing third molars.	Usually not indicated for monitoring of growth and development. Clinical judgment as to the need for and type of radiographic image for evaluation of dental and skeletal relationships.	
Patient with other circumstances including, but not limited to, proposed or existing implants, other dental craniofacial pathoses, restorative/endodontic needs, treated periodontal disease and caries remineralization	Clinical judgment as to need for and type of radiographic images for evaluation and/or monitoring in these conditions.				

CLINICAL SITUATIONS FOR WHICH RADIOGRAPHS MAY BE INDICATED INCLUDE, BUT ARE NOT LIMITED TO
Positive Historical Findings 1. Previous periodontal or endodontic treatment 2. History of pain or trauma 3. Familial history of dental anomalies 4. Postoperative evaluation of healing 5. Remineralization monitoring 6. Presence of implants, previous implant-related pathosis or evaluation for implant placement
Positive Clinical Signs/Symptoms 1. Clinical evidence of periodontal disease 2. Large or deep restorations 3. Deep carious lesions 4. Malposed or clinically impacted teeth 5. Swelling 6. Evidence of dental/facial trauma 7. Mobility of teeth 8. Sinus tract ("fistula") 9. Clinically suspected sinus pathosis 10. Growth abnormalities 11. Oral involvement in known or suspected systemic disease 12. Positive neurologic findings in the head and neck 13. Evidence of foreign objects 14. Pain and/or dysfunction of the temporomandibular joint 15. Facial asymmetry 16. Abutment teeth for fixed or removable partial prosthesis 17. Unexplained bleeding 18. Unexplained sensitivity of teeth 19. Unusual eruption, spacing, or migration of teeth 20. Unusual tooth morphology, calcification, or color 21. Unexplained absence of teeth 22. Clinical tooth erosion 23. Peri-implantitis

*Modified from American Denta Association, US Food and Drug Administration: Dental radiographic examinations: recommendations for patient selection and limiting radiation exposure. http://www.ada.org/~/media/ADA/Member%20Center/FIles/Dental_Radiographic_Examinations_2012.ashx. Accessed November 17, 2015.

These recommendations are subject to clinical judgment and may not apply to every patient. They are to be used by dentists only after reviewing the patient's health history and completing a clinical examination. Even though radiation exposure from dental radiograph is low, once a decision to obtain radiographs is made it is the dentist's responsibility to follow the ALARA Principle (As Low as Reasonably Achievable) to minimize the patient's exposure.

†Factors increasing risk for caries may be assessed using the ADA Caries Risk Assessment forms (0-6 years of age and over 6 years of age).

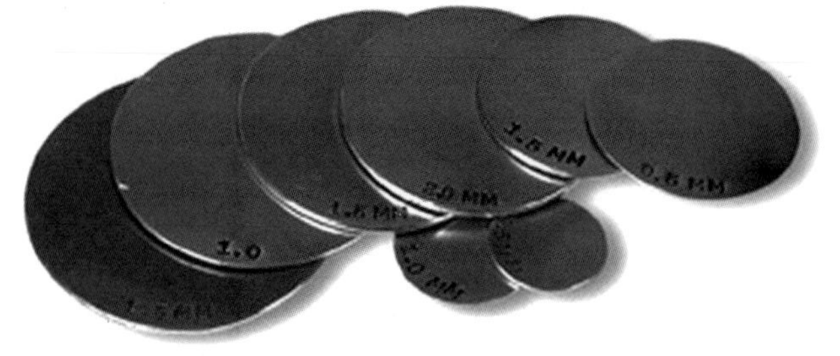

Fig 4-1 Aluminum disks range in thickness from 0.5 mm to 2.0 mm and are available in a variety of diameters. (Courtesy Margraf Corporation, Jenkintown, PA.)

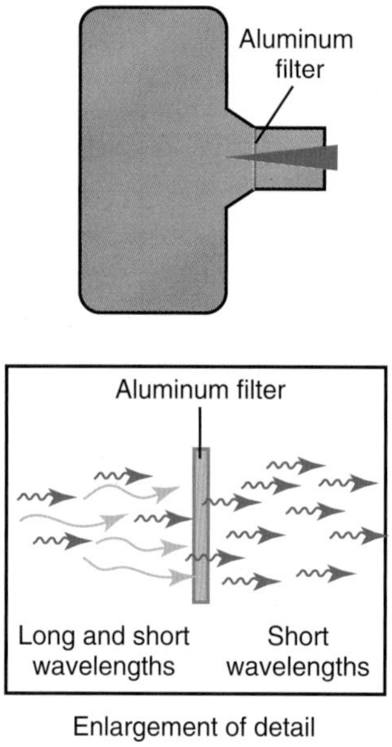

Fig 4-2 Aluminum disks are placed in the path of the beam to filter out the low-energy, longer-wavelength x-rays that are harmful to the patient.

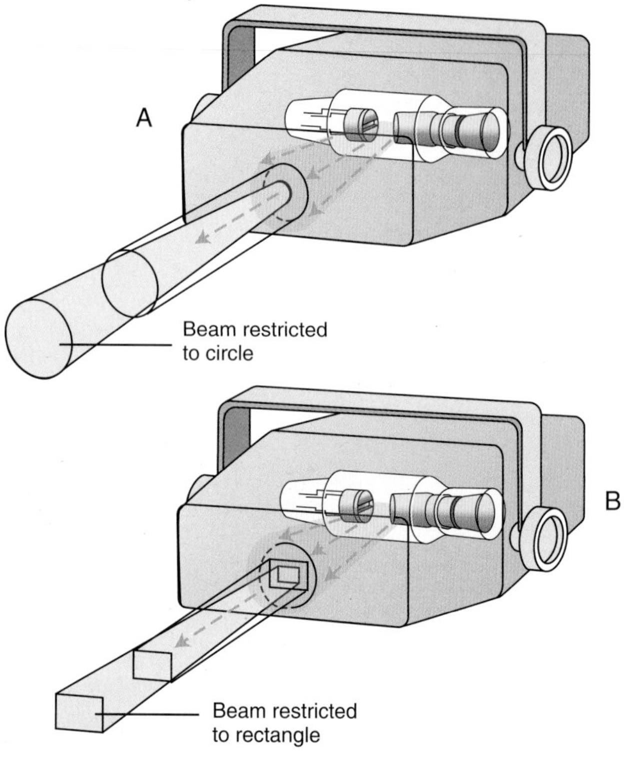

Fig 4-3 Collimation of an x-ray beam (*blue*) is achieved by restricting its useful size. A, Circular collimator. B, Rectangular collimator restricts area of exposure to just larger than the detector size and thereby reduces unnecessary patient exposure. (Courtesy White SC, Pharaoh MJ: Oral radiology: principles and interpretation, ed 7, St Louis, 2014, Mosby.)

the tubehead seal in the dental x-ray machine (Figure 4-1). Aluminum disks can be added to the tubehead in 0.5-mm increments. The purpose of the aluminum disks is to filter out the longer-wavelength, low-energy x-rays from the x-ray beam (Figure 4-2). The low-energy, longer-wavelength x-rays are harmful to the patient and are not useful in diagnostic radiography. Filtration of the x-ray beam results in a higher energy and more penetrating useful beam.

Total filtration. State and federal laws regulate the required thickness of total filtration (inherent plus added filtration). Dental x-ray machines operating at or below 70 kilovoltage (kV) require a minimum total of 1.5 mm aluminum filtration, and machines operating above 70 kV require a minimum total of 2.5 mm aluminum filtration.

Collimation. Collimation is used to restrict the size and shape of the x-ray beam and to reduce patient exposure. A collimator, or lead plate with a hole in the middle, is fitted directly over the opening of the machine housing where the x-ray beam exits the tubehead (Figure 4-3).

A collimator may have either a circular (round) or rectangular opening (Figure 4-4). A *rectangular* collimator restricts the size of the x-ray beam to an area slightly larger than a size 2 intraoral receptor and significantly reduces patient exposure. A rectangular collimator exposes 60% less tissue than a circular collimator.

A *circular* collimator produces a cone-shaped beam that is 2.75 inches in diameter, considerably larger than a size 2 intraoral receptor (Figure 4-5, A). Rectangular collimators may also be added to the open end of a circular position-indicating device (PID) to reduce the amount of tissue being radiated (see Figure 4-5, B). When using a circular collimator, federal regulations require that the x-ray beam be collimated to a diameter of no more than 2.75 inches as it exits from the position-indicating device and reaches the skin of the patient (Figure 4-6).

Position-indicating device. The position-indicating device (PID) appears as an extension of the x-ray tubehead and is used to direct the x-ray beam. The PID may also be referred to as the *cone*. On early dental x-ray machines, the PID was a closed, pointed plastic cone. When the x-rays exited the pointed cone, the beam penetrated the plastic and produced excess scatter radiation (Figure 4-7). To eliminate this cone-produced scatter radiation, the conical PID is no longer used in dentistry. The term *cone*, however, may still be used to refer to the PID.

Two types of PIDs are currently used: rectangular and round (cylindrical). Open-ended, lead-lined rectangular or round PIDs limit the production of scatter radiation (Figure 4-8). Both rectangular and circular PIDs are typically available in two lengths: short (8-inch) and long (16-inch). The long PID is preferred because less divergence of the x-ray beam occurs (Figure 4-9). Like the rectangular collimator, the rectangular PID is most effective in reducing patient exposure.

During Exposure

Patient protection measures are used before and during x-ray exposure. A thyroid collar, lead apron, digital sensors or fast film, and beam alignment devices are all used during x-ray exposure to limit the amount of radiation received by the patient. Proper selection of exposure factors and good technique further protect the patient from excessive exposure to x-radiation.

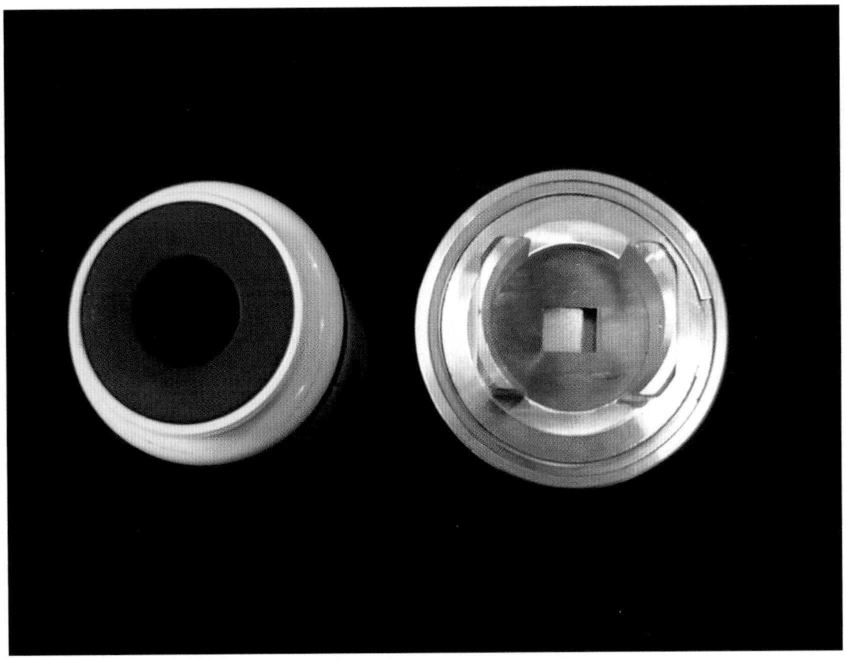

Fig 4-4 The hole in the collimator may be either circular or rectangular in shape.

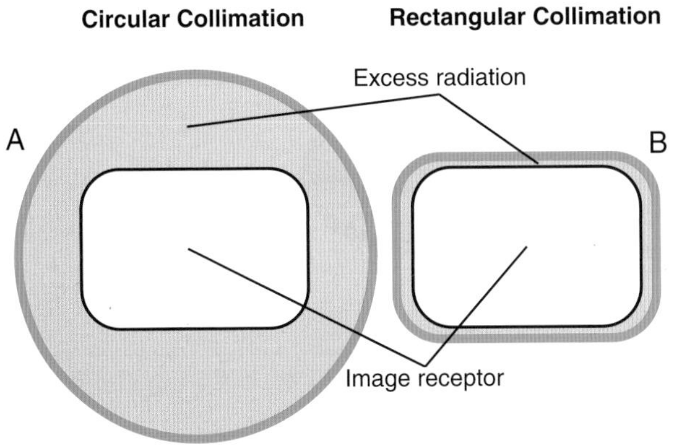

Fig 4-5 Comparison of excess radiation area using circular (**A**) and rectangular collimator (**B**). (Courtesy Castellanos S, Jain RK: Reduce radiation with rectangular collimation, Dimensions of Dental Hygiene. February 2013; 11(2): 46, 48–50.)

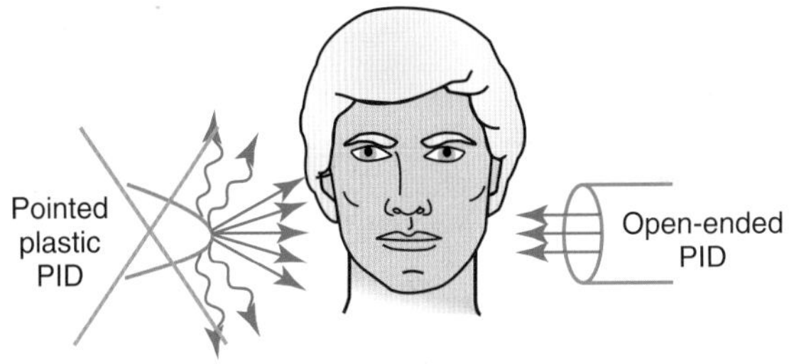

Fig 4-7 A plastic, pointed position-indicating device (*PID*) produces scatter radiation and is no longer used in dentistry.

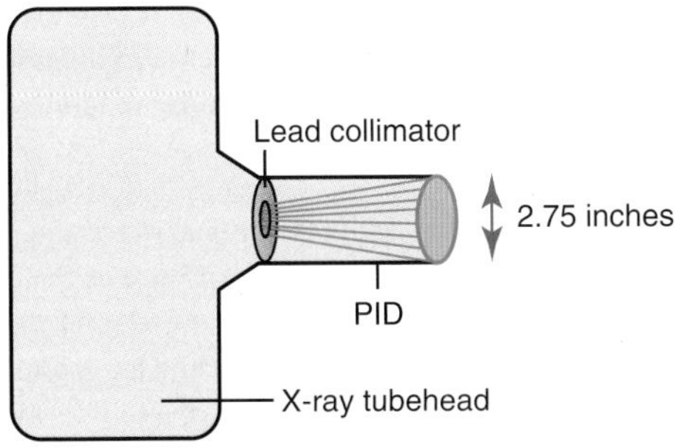

Fig 4-6 Federal regulations require that the diameter of a collimated x-ray beam be restricted to 2.75 inches at the patient's skin. *PID*, Position-indicating device.

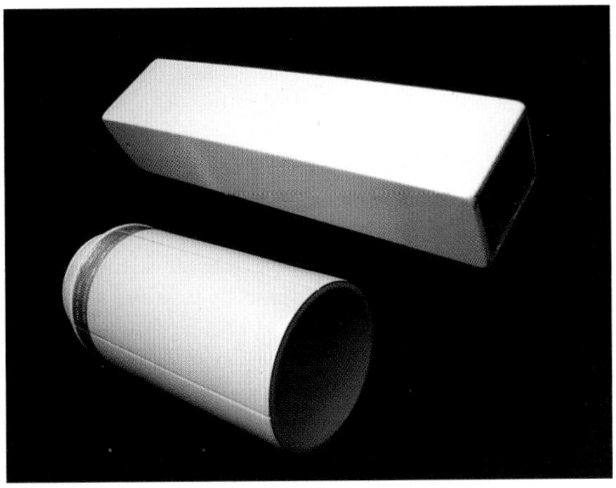

Fig 4-8 Open-ended, lead-lined circular and rectangular position-indicating devices (PIDs).

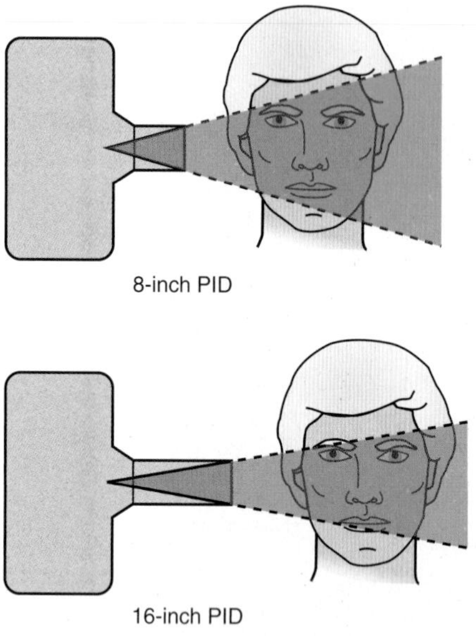

Fig 4-9 Compared with a short (8-inch) position-indicating device (*PID*), the longer (16-inch) PID is preferred because it produces less divergence of the x-ray beam.

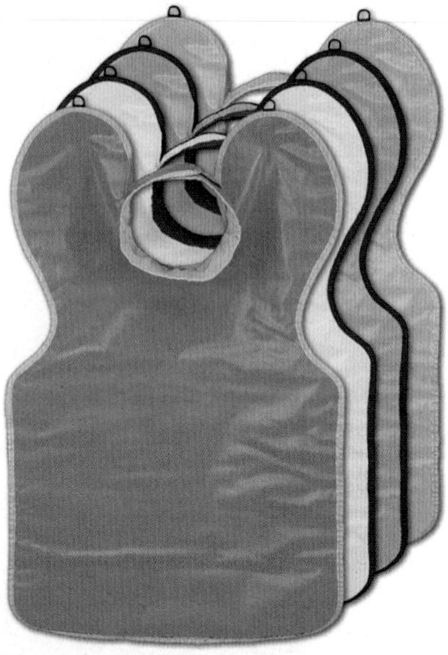

Fig 4-11 The thyroid collar may be attached to the lead apron or may be used as a separate shield. (Courtesy DUX Dental, Oxnard, CA.)

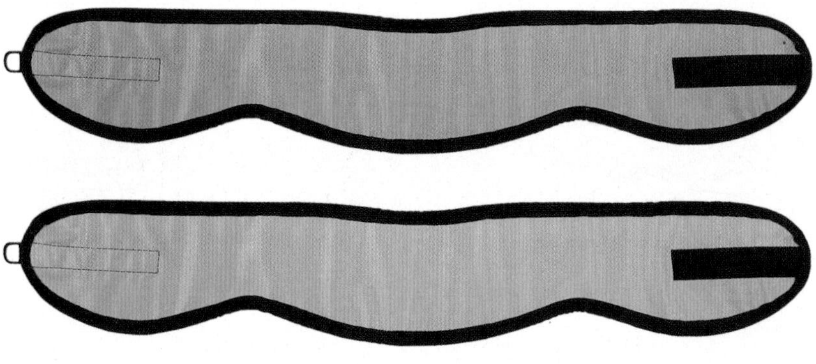

Fig 4-10 A thyroid collar provides important radiation protection. (Courtesy DUX Dental, Oxnard, CA.)

Thyroid Collar. The thyroid collar is a flexible lead shield that is placed securely around the patient's neck to protect the thyroid gland from scatter radiation (Figure 4-10). The lead prevents radiation from reaching the gland and protects the highly radiosensitive tissues of the thyroid. The thyroid collar may exist as a separate shield or as part of the lead apron.

Because of its location, the thyroid gland is exposed to x-radiation during oral imaging procedures. The use of the thyroid collar is recommended for all intraoral exposures. However, its use is not recommended with extraoral exposures because it obscures information and results in a nondiagnostic image.

Lead Apron. The lead apron is a flexible shield placed over the patient's chest and lap to protect the reproductive and blood-forming tissues from scatter radiation; the lead prevents the radiation from reaching these radiosensitive organs (Figure 4-11). Use of a lead apron is recommended for both intraoral and extraoral exposures. To be effective, lead shields should have at least 0.25 mm of lead or lead equivalent. Many state laws mandate the use of a lead apron on all patients. Lead-free aprons made of alloy sheeting are also available for use during intraoral or panoramic radiography. Without the weight of lead, these aprons weigh 30% less and are comfortable and easy to handle while providing the same protection as does the traditional lead apron.

Much discussion has emerged over the use and necessity of the lead apron, and differing opinions exist. According to some, the lead apron is now considered outdated and unnecessary equipment. Well-designed modern x-ray equipment and low doses of radiation for common imaging procedures may make the routine use of lead aprons unnecessary. However, in keeping with the ALARA Principle (see later discussion), the lead apron is an important part of radiation protection and should be used for *all* patients. If a difference in opinion still exists in determining whether a lead apron should be used, it is advised to check with the state dental board.

Image Receptors. Compared with traditional film radiography, digital image receptors require less radiation exposure of the patient. Use of a digital receptor is the most effective method of reducing a patient's radiation exposure. The lowered absorbed dose is significant with regard to patient protection from excessive radiation. Digital imaging is discussed in detail in Chapter 8.

When digital sensors are not used, fast film is the most effective method of reducing a patient's exposure to x-radiation. Currently, F-speed film, or *InSight*, is the fastest intraoral film available and is recommended by the ADA. F-speed film provides an additional 20% reduction in exposure over E-speed films (and 60% reduction in exposure from earlier D-speed film, or *Ultra-Speed*).

Beam Alignment Devices. Beam alignment devices are also effective in reducing a patient's exposure to x-radiation. A beam alignment device helps stabilize the receptor in the mouth and reduces the chances of movement (Figure 4-12). Beam alignment devices align the receptor precisely with the beam and are recommended for periapical and bite-wing images.

Exposure Factor Selection. Chapter 5 discusses the selection of exposure factors (kilovoltage, millamperage, and time) which influences the quality of dental images. Consequently, proper exposure factor selection can limit the amount of radiation that a patient receives. To limit patient exposure, operators should use an optimal kilovoltage setting of 60 to 80 kV, a milliamperage setting of 6 to 8 mA, and the shortest exposure time possible to create a diagnostic image.

Proper Technique. Proper technique helps create a diagnostic image and reduce the amount of exposure a patient receives. Images that are nondiagnostic must be retaken; this results in additional exposure of the patient to radiation. The reexposure of an image, or *retake, must be avoided at all times.*

To produce diagnostic images, the radiographer must have a thorough knowledge of the techniques used in dental imaging. Common techniques include the paralleling technique, bisecting technique, and bite-wing technique (see Chapters 19, 20, and 21, respectively). In addition to knowing exactly how each receptor is exposed, an organized exposure sequence routine is important for the effective application of a technique.

After Exposure

The radiographer's role in limiting the amount of x-radiation received by a patient does not end during exposure. After the receptors have been exposed, meticulous handling, proper processing techniques, and image retrieval are critical for the production of high-quality diagnostic images.

Proper Receptor Handling. Proper receptor handling is necessary to produce diagnostic images and to limit patient exposure to x-radiation. From the time the receptors are exposed until they are processed or retrieved, careful handling is crucial. Artifacts caused by improper handling result in nondiagnostic images (see Chapters 10, 22). A nondiagnostic image must be retaken, which exposes the patient to excessive radiation.

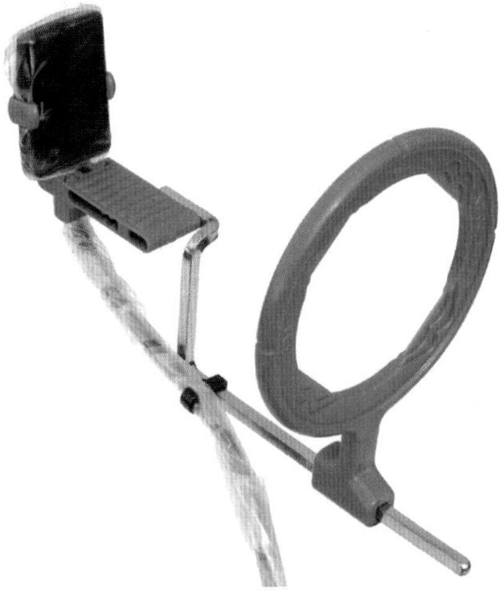

Fig 4-12 Beam alignment devices reduce the patient's exposure to radiation by stabilizing the receptor in the mouth. (Courtesy Dentsply Rinn Corporation, York, PA.)

Proper Film Processing/Image Retrieval. Proper film processing (developing) and proper retrieval of digital images are also necessary to produce diagnostic images and to limit patient exposure to x-radiation. Improper film processing or image retrieval can render images nondiagnostic, thereby requiring retakes and needlessly exposing the patient to excessive x-radiation.

OPERATOR PROTECTION

The dental radiographer must use proper protection measures to avoid occupational exposure to x-radiation (e.g., primary radiation, leakage radiation, scatter radiation). The use of proper operator protection techniques can minimize the amount of radiation that a dental radiographer receives. Operator protection measures include following protection guidelines and using radiation-monitoring devices.

Protection Guidelines

The purpose of operator protection guidelines is to provide the dental radiographer with the basic safety information needed when working with x-radiation. Such guidelines are based on the following rule: *The dental radiographer must avoid the primary beam.* Operator protection guidelines include recommendations on distance, position, and shielding.

Distance and Position Recommendations. Ideally, the radiographer should either leave the room or take a position behind a suitable barrier or wall during exposures. If leaving the room is not possible or if no barrier is available, the radiographer must adhere to distance and position recommendations. One of the most effective ways for the operator to avoid the primary beam and limit x-radiation exposure is to maintain an adequate distance during exposure. The dental radiographer must stand at least 6 feet (2 meters) away from the x-ray tubehead during x-ray exposure. When maintaining this distance is not possible, a protective barrier must be used. This recommendation is based on the inverse square law, which states that the intensity of the beam diminishes as the distance from the source increases. The further the radiographer is from the x-ray tubehead, the less intense the x-ray beam, causing less potential for occupational exposure. Another important way for the operator to avoid the primary beam is to maintain proper positioning during x-ray exposure.

To avoid the primary beam, which travels in a straight line, the dental radiographer must position himself or herself perpendicular to the primary beam, or at a 90-degree to 135-degree angle to the beam (Figure 4-13). To avoid the primary beam, proper operator position during exposure includes the following:

- The dental radiographer must never hold a receptor in place for a patient.
- The dental radiographer must never hold or stabilize the x-ray tubehead.

Shielding Recommendations. Adequate shielding can greatly reduce the occupational exposure of the dental radiographer. Protective barriers that absorb the primary beam can be incorporated into the office design, thus protecting the operator from primary and scatter radiation. Whenever possible, the dental radiographer should stand behind a protective barrier, such as a wall, during x-ray exposure. Most

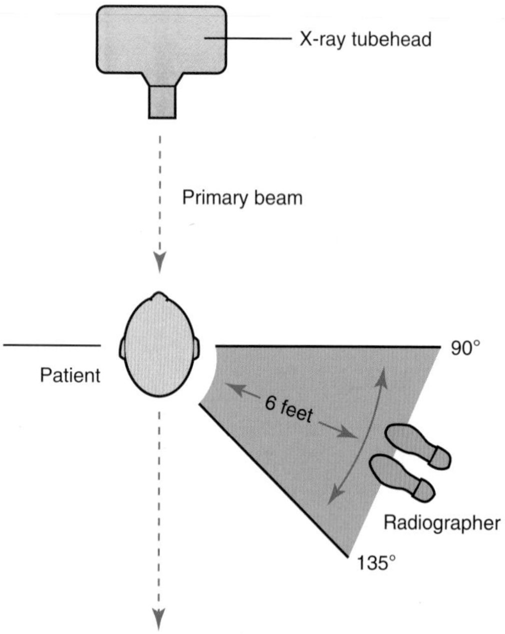

Fig 4-13 Operator protection guidelines suggest that the dental radiographer stand at an angle of 90 to 135 degrees to the primary beam.

dental offices incorporate adequate shielding in walls through the use of several thicknesses of common construction materials such as drywall. A leaded glass window or the use of a mirror is beneficial to monitor the patient during exposure.

Radiation Monitoring

Radiation monitoring can also be used to protect the dental radiographer and includes the monitoring of both equipment and personnel. The use of radiation monitoring can identify excessive occupational exposure.

Equipment Monitoring. Dental x-ray machines must be monitored for leakage radiation. **Leakage radiation** is any radiation, with the exception of the primary beam, that is emitted from the dental tubehead. For example, if a dental x-ray tubehead has a faulty tubehead seal, leakage radiation results. Dental x-ray equipment can be monitored for leakage radiation using a device that can be obtained through the state health department or from the manufacturers of dental x-ray equipment.

Personnel Monitoring. The amount of x-radiation that reaches the body of the dental radiographer can be measured through the use of a personnel-monitoring device known as a **radiation monitoring badge** (film badge dosimeter or film badge). A radiation monitoring badge can be obtained from a badge service company.

The radiation monitoring badge consists of a piece of radiographic film in a plastic holder (Figure 4-14). Each radiographer should have his or her own badge; the badge should be worn at waist level whenever the dental radiographer is exposing images with either film or digital sensors. When not being worn, badges should be stored in a radiation-safe area. A radiation monitoring badge should *never* be worn when the radiographer is undergoing x-ray exposure.

After the dental radiographer has worn the badge for a specified interval (e.g., 1 month), the badge is returned to the service company. The company processes and evaluates the badge for exposure and then provides the dental office with an exposure report for each radiographer. Often the service company may provide an additional badge to keep in a radiation-safe area during the specified interval to use as a reference monitor for each individual office.

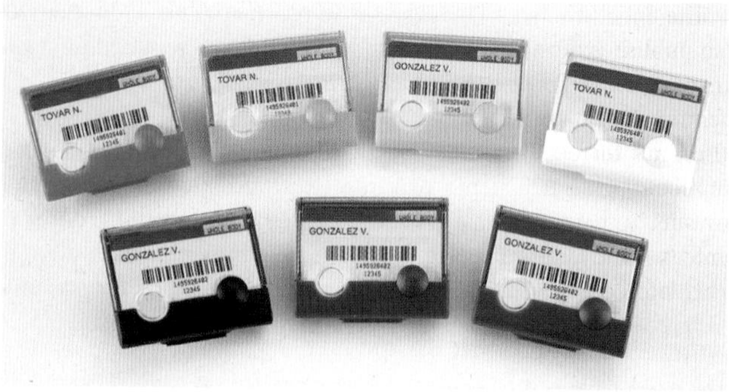

Fig 4-14 A radiation monitoring badge is used to measure the radiation exposure received by the dental radiographer. (Courtesy ICCARE, Irvine, CA.)

RADIATION EXPOSURE GUIDELINES

All x-radiation is harmful. Radiation exposure guidelines have therefore been established to protect the patient and operator from excessive exposure. These guidelines include radiation safety legislation and exposure limits for the general public and for persons who are occupationally exposed to radiation. Strict adherence to radiation exposure guidelines is mandatory for all dental radiographers.

Radiation Safety Legislation

Radiation safety legislation has been established at both state and federal levels to protect the patient, the operator, and the general public from radiation hazards. At the federal level, the Radiation Control for Health and Safety Act was enacted in 1968 to standardize the operation of x-ray equipment. Also, in 1981 the federal Consumer-Patient Radiation Health and Safety Act was enacted to address the issues of educating and certifying operators of radiographic equipment.

Radiation legislation in the United States varies greatly from state to state; the dental radiographer must be familiar with the laws that apply to his or her workplace. For example, in some states, before a dental radiographer can expose patients to radiation, he or she must successfully complete a radiation safety examination. Continuing education hours dedicated to dental imaging may also be required.

Maximum Permissible Dose

Radiation protection standards dictate the maximum dose of radiation that an individual can receive. The **maximum permissible dose (MPD)** is defined by the National Council on Radiation Protection and Measurements (NCRP) as the maximum dose equivalent that a body is permitted to receive within a specific period. The MPD is the maximum dose of radiation that the body can endure with little or no injury.

The NCRP published the complete set of basic recommendations specifying dose limits for exposure to ionizing radiation. The most recent NCRP report states that the current MPD for occupationally exposed persons, or those who work with radiation (e.g., dental radiographers), is 50 mSv/year (0.05 Sv/year or 5.0 rem/year). It is recommended that dental radiographers not exceed a maximum dose of 50 mSv in any 1 year. For pregnant dental personnel, the radiation exposure limit is 0.5 mSv per month during the pregnancy months. For nonoccupationally exposed persons (i.e., the general public), the current MPD is approximately 1 mSv/year (0.1 rem/year).

The International Commission on Radiologic Protection (ICRP) also publishes recommendations for radiation protection. It is important to note that the NCRP and ICRP do not always agree on recommended dose limits. The current ICRP Publication 103 recommended dose limit for occupational exposure is 20 mSv/year averaged over 5 consecutive years (100 mSv in 5 years) with no more than 50 mSv in any single year. The ICRP recommended dose limit for the public is 1 mSv/year, with a higher value being allowed in special circumstances provided that the average over 5 years does not exceed 1 mSv/year.

Cumulative Occupational Dose

Occupationally exposed workers must not exceed an accumulated lifetime radiation dose. This is referred to as the cumulative occupational dose. In the publication titled *Limitation of Exposure to Ionizing Radiation NCRP Report 116*, the NCRP has recommended that an individual's cumulative occupational effective dose not exceed the worker's age multiplied by 10 mSv. Thus for a 50-year-old worker, the NCRP would recommend a cumulative occupational dose of no more than 50 × 10 mSv = 500 mSv (0.5 Sv).

ALARA Concept

The ALARA ("as low as reasonably achievable") concept states that all exposure to radiation must be kept to a minimum. To protect both patients and operators, every possible method of reducing exposure to radiation should be employed to minimize risk. The radiation protection measures detailed in this chapter can be used to minimize patient and operator exposure, thus keeping radiation exposure "as low as reasonably achievable."

RADIATION PROTECTION AND PATIENT EDUCATION

Patients often have questions about radiation exposure. The dental radiographer must be prepared to answer such questions and to educate the dental patient about radiation protection topics. Patient education about radiation protection may take the form of an informal conversation or printed literature.

The dental radiographer must be prepared to explain exactly how patients are protected before, during, and after x-ray exposure. An informal discussion can take place as the dental radiographer prepares the patient for x-ray exposure. For example, while placing the lead apron and thyroid collar on the patient, the dental radiographer can make the following comments:

- "Before we get started, let me tell you just how our office does all that is possible to protect you from unnecessary radiation."
- "Before we expose you to any radiation, the dentist custom-orders your x-rays based on your individual needs. The x-ray equipment we use is tested to ensure that state and federal radiation safety guidelines are met."
- "During x-ray exposure, we use a thyroid collar and a lead apron to protect your body from excessive radiation. We use a digital sensor or the fastest film available and a device to hold the receptor so that your fingers are not exposed to radiation. We also use proper technique so that we can avoid making mistakes that require further exposure."
- If using digital imaging: "Our office uses digital imaging procedures that reduce your exposure to radiation significantly compared with traditional, film-based radiography."
- "Even after your dental images have been exposed, we take steps to process and handle the receptors carefully so that we don't have to repeat any procedures."
- "Hopefully, this quick review of radiation protection techniques has answered some of the questions you may have about dental x-rays. What questions do you have before we begin?"

In addition to such an informal discussion, the patient can be given printed handouts or pamphlets outlining the steps used to protect patients from excessive radiation. This information can be placed in the reception area or in the room where dental images are exposed.

SUMMARY

- Before x-ray exposure, proper prescribing of dental images and proper use of radiographic equipment can minimize the amount of radiation that a patient receives.
- The dentist must prescribe images based on the individual needs of patients.
- In the x-ray tubehead, aluminum disks are used to filter out the longer-wavelength, low-energy x-rays from the x-ray beam.
- In the x-ray tubehead, a collimator (lead plate with a hole in the middle) is used to restrict the size and shape of the x-ray beam.
- A position-indicating device (PID) is used to direct the x-ray beam; the rectangular PID is preferred and is most effective in reducing patient exposure to x-rays.
- A thyroid collar, a lead apron, fast film, digital imaging, and a beam alignment device can be used during x-ray exposure to protect the patient from excessive exposure to radiation. Proper selection of exposure factors and good technique can also be used to protect the patient.
- After x-ray exposure, careful handling of the receptors (film or sensor), film-processing techniques, and accurate image retrieval are critical for the production of diagnostic images.
- During x-ray exposure, the dental radiographer must always follow operator protection guidelines and always avoid the primary beam by maintaining adequate distance and using proper positioning and shielding.
- The dental radiographer must never hold a receptor or the tubehead in place for a patient during x-ray exposure.
- Radiation monitoring may include the monitoring of both equipment and personnel.
- Federal and state laws protect the patient, the operator, and the general public from radiation hazards.
- Exposure limits have been established for the general public and persons who work with radiation. The maximum permissible dose (MPD) for persons who work with radiation (e.g., dental radiographers) is 50 mSv/year (0.05 Sv/year or 5.0 rem/year). The MPD for the general public is 1 mSv/year (0.1 rem/year).
- The ALARA (as low as reasonably achievable) concept states that all exposure to radiation must be kept to a minimum.
- The dental radiographer must be prepared to explain to patients the steps taken to provide protection before, during, and after x-ray exposure.

TECHNIQUE VIDEOS

View the Technique Videos and complete the accompanying Interactive Exercises that are available as part of the Student Resources on the companion Evolve website for this textbook.

BIBLIOGRAPHY

Bernstein DI, et al: Perceived quality of radiographic images after rapid processing of D- and F-speed direct-exposure intraoral x-ray films, Oral Surg Oral Med Oral Pathol Oral Radiol Endod 96(4):486, 2003.

Frommer HH, Stabulas-Savage JJ: Operator protection. In Radiology for the dental professional, ed 9, St Louis, 2011, Mosby.

Frommer HH, Stabulas-Savage JJ: Patient protection. In Radiology for the dental professional, ed 9, St Louis, 2011, Mosby.

Haring JI, Lind LJ: The importance of dental radiographs and interpretation. In Radiographic interpretation for the dental hygienist, Philadelphia, 1993, Saunders.

ICRP: The 2007 Recommendations of the International Commission on Radiological Protection. ICRP Publication 103, Ann ICRP 37:2, 2007.

Johnson ON: Patient relations and education. In Essentials of dental radiography for dental assistants and hygienists, ed 9, Upper Saddle River, NJ, 2011, Prentice Hall.
Johnson ON: Radiation protection. In Essentials of dental radiography for dental assistants and hygienists, ed 9, Upper Saddle River, NJ, 2011, Prentice Hall.
Langland OE, Langlais RP, Preece JW: Radiologic health and protection. In Principles of dental imaging, ed 2, Baltimore, 2002, Lippincott Williams & Wilkins.
Mallya SM, Lam EWN: Physics. In White and Pharoah's oral radiology: principles and interpretation, ed 8, St. Louis, 2019, Elsevier.
Mallya SM, Lam EWN: Safety and protection. In White and Pharoah's oral radiology: principles and interpretation, ed 8, St. Louis, 2019, Elsevier.
Miles DA, Van Dis ML, Jensen CW, et al: Intraoral radiographic technique. In Radiographic imaging for the dental team, ed 4, St Louis, 2009, Saunders.
Miles DA, Van Dis ML, Jensen CW, et al: Radiation biology and protection. In Radiographic imaging for the dental team, ed 4, St Louis, 2009, Saunders.
National Council on Radiation Protection and Measurements (NCRP): Limitation of exposure to ionizing radiation, NCRP Report No. 116, 1993, NCRP.
National Council on Radiation Protection and Measurements: Ionizing radiation exposure of the population of the United States, NCRP Report No. 160, 2009, NCRP.

USEFUL WEBSITES

American Dental Association (ADA): www.ada.org/en/member-center/oral-health-topics/x-rays
International Atomic Energy Agency (IAEA): www.iaea.org/resources/rpop/health-professionals/dentistry/patients
U.S. Food and Drug Administration (FDA): www.fda.gov/Radiation-Emitting-Products/RadiationEmittingProductsandProcedures

QUIZ QUESTIONS

True or False

_____ 1. Every patient should be evaluated individually prior to prescribing dental images.
_____ 2. The 8-inch PID is more effective than the 16-inch PID in reducing radiation exposure of the patient.
_____ 3. Pointed cones should not be used because of increased scatter radiation.
_____ 4. The thyroid collar must be worn for both intraoral and extraoral exposures.
_____ 5. If necessary, the dental radiographer may hold a receptor in the patient's mouth to ensure a diagnostic image.

Multiple Choice

_____ 6. Which statement describes the function of a filter in a dental x-ray tubehead?
- **a.** It reduces the size and shape of the beam.
- **b.** It removes low-energy x-rays.
- **c.** It removes the dose of radiation to the thyroid gland.
- **d.** It decreases the mean energy of the beam.

_____ 7. Which is *not* a component of inherent filtration?
- **a.** oil
- **b.** unleaded glass window
- **c.** a leaded PID
- **d.** tubehead seal

_____ 8. Which is the most effective method of reducing patient exposure to radiation?
- **a.** lead apron
- **b.** fast films
- **c.** circular PID
- **d.** film-holding devices

_____ 9. Which position-indicating device is most effective in reducing patient exposure?
- **a.** conical
- **b.** rectangular
- **c.** circular
- **d.** all are equally effective in reducing patient exposure

_____ 10. Which device restricts the size and shape of the x-ray beam?
- **a.** filter
- **b.** collimator
- **c.** barrier
- **d.** film badge

_____ 11. Which material is used as a collimator?
- **a.** lead
- **b.** aluminum
- **c.** copper
- **d.** all of the above

_____ 12. Which describes the function of filtration?
- **a.** increases scatter radiation
- **b.** increases divergent rays
- **c.** increases long wavelengths
- **d.** reduces low-energy waves

_____ 13. Which is the recommended size of the beam at the patient's face?
- **a.** 2.75 inches
- **b.** 3.25 inches
- **c.** 3.50 inches
- **d.** 4.00 inches

_____ 14. Which term describes the dose of radiation that the body can endure with little or no chance of injury?
- **a.** radiation limit
- **b.** maximum permissible dose
- **c.** occupationally exposed dose
- **d.** ALARA

_____ 15. Which statement is true of a radiation monitoring badge?
- **a.** It should be worn when the radiographer is undergoing x-ray exposure.
- **b.** It can be shared between employees.
- **c.** It should be worn at waist level when exposing x-ray receptors.
- **d.** All of the above are true.

Fill in the Blank

16. Provide the requirements for proper filtration:
Machines operating at 70 kV or lower require __________ mm aluminum.
Machines operating above 70 kV require __________ mm aluminum.
17. State the angle at which the dental radiographer should stand in relationship to the primary beam:__________ degrees.
18. State the formula for the cumulative occupation dose:
____
__________________________.
19. State the maximum permissible dose for occupationally exposed persons: __________ mSv/year (__________ rem/year).

5

Radiation Characteristics

LEARNING OBJECTIVES

After completion of this chapter, the student will be able to do the following:

1. Define the key terms associated with radiation characteristics.
2. Describe the effect that the kilovoltage has on the quality of the x-ray beam and identify the range of kilovoltage required for dental imaging.
3. Describe how kilovoltage affects the density and contrast of the image.
4. Describe how milliamperage influences the quantity of the x-ray beam and identify the range of milliamperage required for dental imaging.
5. Describe how milliamperage affects the density of the image and how exposure time and milliamperage are related.
6. Describe how kilovoltage, milliamperage, exposure time, and source-to-receptor distance influence the intensity of the x-ray beam.
7. Calculate an example of radiation intensity using the inverse square law.
8. Explain how the half-value layer determines the penetrating quality of the x-ray beam.

Radiation characteristics include x-ray beam quality, quantity, and intensity. Variations in the character of the x-ray beam influence the quality of the resulting images.

The dental radiographer must have a working knowledge of radiation characteristics and exposure factors. The purpose of this chapter is to detail the concepts of x-ray beam quality and quantity, define the concept of beam intensity, and discuss how exposure factors influence these characteristics.

Current dental x-ray units have control panels with preset, predetermined exposure factors (kV, mA, time) for the various anatomic areas of the maxilla and mandible, so no manual operator adjustment choices are needed (Figure 5-1). On older x-ray units, the exposure factors could be manually adjusted by the operator. Whereas all current dental x-ray units allow for the adjustment of time, the ability to adjust kilovoltage and milliamperage varies from model to model. On many current dental x-ray units, manual adjustments of kilovoltage and milliamperage are not an option. Although today's x-ray units allow only for limited operator adjustments, the dental radiographer still needs a working knowledge of how changing exposure factors affects the appearance of resultant images.

X-RAY BEAM QUALITY

Wavelength determines the energy and penetrating power of radiation. X-rays with shorter wavelengths have more penetrating power, whereas those with longer wavelengths are less penetrating and more likely to be absorbed by matter. In dental imaging, the term *quality* is used to describe the mean energy or penetrating ability of the x-ray beam. The quality, or wavelength and energy, of the x-ray beam is controlled by kilovoltage.

Voltage and Kilovoltage

Voltage is a measurement of force that refers to the potential difference between two electrical charges. Inside the dental x-ray tubehead, voltage is the measurement of electrical force that causes electrons to move from the negative cathode to the positive anode. Voltage determines the speed with which they move. When voltage is increased, the speed of the electrons is increased. The electrons strike the target with greater force and energy, resulting in a penetrating x-ray beam with a short wavelength.

Voltage is measured in volts or kilovolts. The **volt (V)** is the unit of measurement used to describe the potential that drives an electrical current through a circuit. Dental x-ray equipment requires the use of high voltages. Most radiographic units operate using kilovolts; 1 **kilovolt (kV)** is equal to 1000 volts. It is common to refer to tube voltage as "kilovoltage," which is abbreviated as kV, the same as its unit, the kilovolt. The term **kilovoltage (kV)** is the maximum voltage, or peak voltage of an alternating current (AC) (Figure 5-2). In older units, the kilovoltage fluctuated depending on the voltage waveform applied to the tube. In current dental x-ray units, this fluctuation is so very small that the kilovoltage can be considered as a fixed value during exposure.

In the past, dental x-ray units were available with adjustable settings ranging from 65 to 100 kV. With these units, the kilovoltage could be adjusted according to the individual diagnostic needs of patients. For example, a higher kilovoltage setting was used when the area to be examined was dense or thick. The use of higher kV produces more penetrating dental x-rays with greater energy, whereas the use of lower kV produces less penetrating dental x-rays with less energy. Current intraoral x-ray units include adjustable settings that range from 60 to 70 kV, or else a fixed setting of 70 kV. If the unit has a fixed kV, that kV number is found imprinted on the face of the control panel. On units that allow for the adjustment of kilovoltage, a kV button is found on the control panel.

The **quality**, or wavelength and energy, of the x-ray beam is controlled by the kilovoltage. The kilovoltage regulates the speed and energy of the electrons and determines the penetrating ability of the x-ray beam. Increasing the kilovoltage results in a higher energy x-ray beam with increased penetrating ability.

Density and Kilovoltage

Density is the overall darkness or blackness of an image. An adjustment in kilovoltage results in a change in the density of a dental

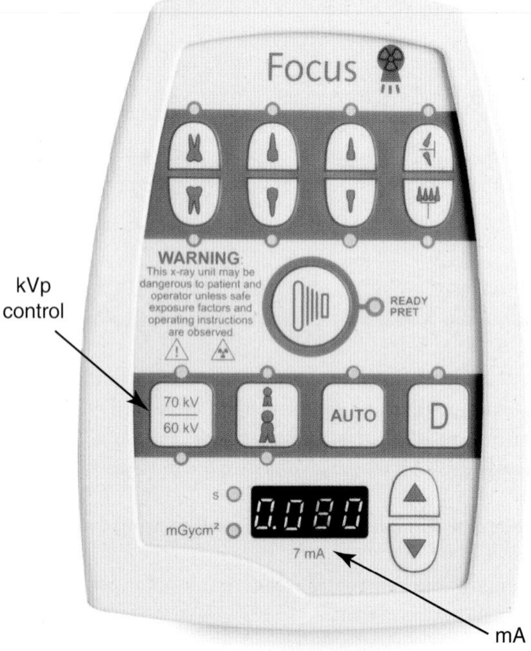

Fig 5-1 Kilovoltage (kV) control and milliamperage (mA) of the unit are located on the dental x-ray machine. (Courtesy KaVo Imaging, Brea, CA.)

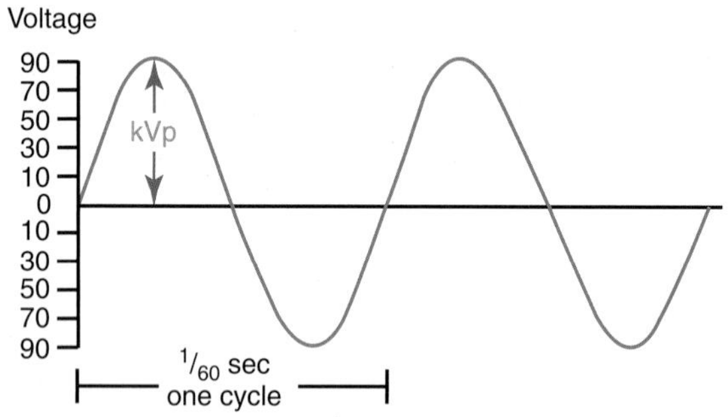

Fig 5-2 Kilovoltage (kV) controls the quality of the x-ray beam and measures the peak voltage of the current.

image. If the kilovoltage is increased while other exposure factors (milliamperage, exposure time) remain constant, the resultant image exhibits an increased density and appears darker (Figure 5-3). If the kilovoltage is decreased, the resultant image exhibits a decreased density and appears lighter (Figure 5-4). Table 5-1 summarizes the effect of kilovoltage on density (also see Chapter 6). With digital imaging, special image enhancement software can be used to change the density by adjusting the brightness. For example, if a digital image is too dark or too light, the brightness can be adjusted so that the image is readable. In comparison, if film is used and the density is nondiagnostic, the image must be retaken with adjusted exposure factors.

Contrast and Kilovoltage

Contrast refers to how sharply dark and light areas are differentiated or separated on an image. An adjustment in kilovoltage results in a change in the contrast of a dental image. When lower kilovoltage settings are used, a high-contrast image will result. An image with "high" contrast has many black areas, many white areas, and few shades of gray

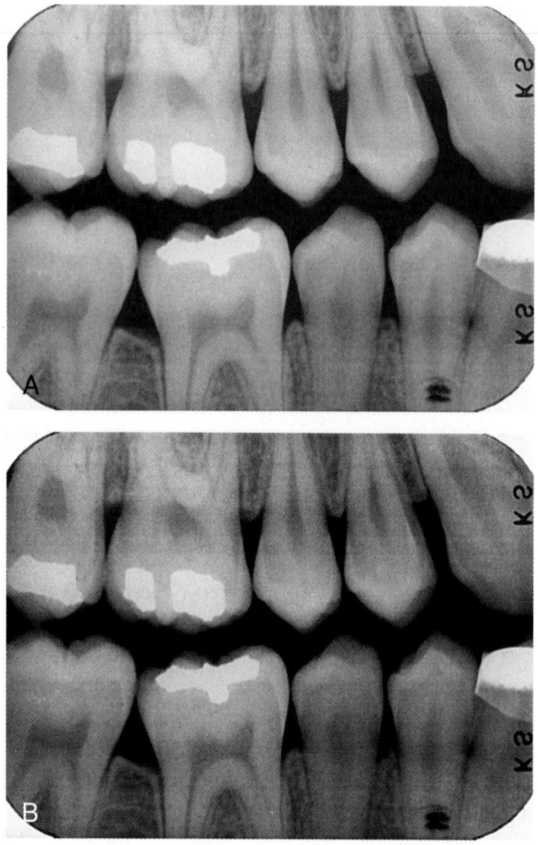

Fig 5-3 **A,** Diagnostic radiograph. **B,** Increase in kilovoltage results in an image that exhibits increased density; the image appears darker.

(Figure 5-5). An image with high contrast is useful for detecting and determining the progression of dental caries.

With higher kilovoltage settings, low contrast results. An image with "low" contrast has many shades of gray instead of areas that are predominantly black and white (Figure 5-6). An image with low contrast is useful for the detection of periodontal or periapical disease. In dental imaging, a compromise between high and low contrast is desirable. See Table 5-1 for a summary of the effect of kilovoltage on contrast (also see Chapter 6).

With digital imaging, special image enhancement software can be used to change the contrast by altering the distribution of the gray levels seen in the image. A digital image can be adjusted so that the contrast is higher, which is desirable in caries interpretation, or so that the contrast is lower, which is desirable in evaluating periodontal disease. In comparison, if film is used and the contrast is incorrect, the image must be retaken with adjusted exposure factors.

Exposure Time and Kilovoltage

Exposure time refers to the interval of time during which x-rays are produced. The timer controls the length of exposure time and determines how long the x-rays will be emitted from the machine. The longer the exposure time, the more x-rays are delivered, and a darker image results. Every x-ray machine has a timer. The timer is the exposure factor that is recommended to adjust in order to lighten or darken an image. For example, to get the same end result, a larger patient may require more x-ray exposure time, whereas a smaller patient may require less x-ray exposure time. The timer may be calibrated in either seconds or impulses, depending on when the unit was manufactured.

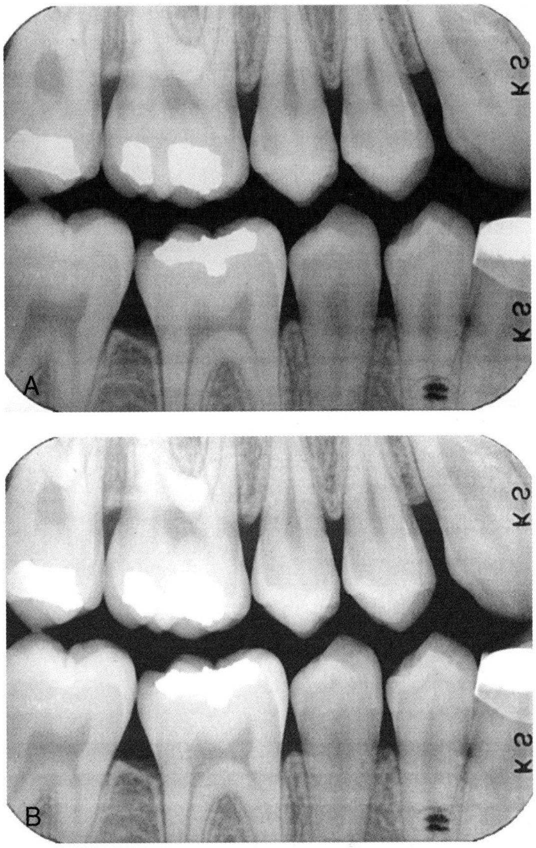

Fig 5-4 **A,** Diagnostic radiograph. **B,** Decrease in kilovoltage results in an image that exhibits decreased density; the image appears lighter.

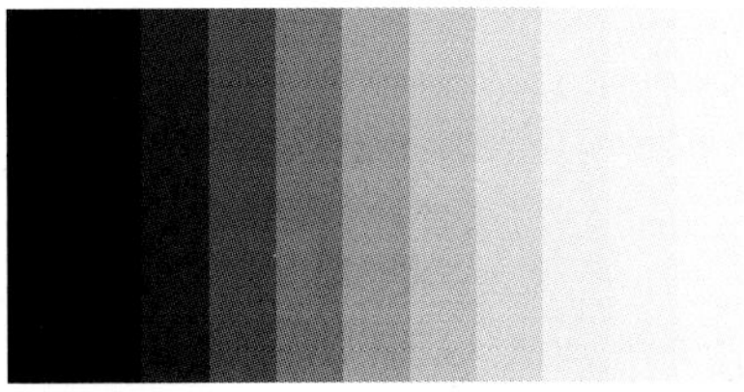

Fig 5-5 Image produced with lower kilovoltage exhibits high contrast; many light and dark areas are seen, as demonstrated by the use of the stepwedge.

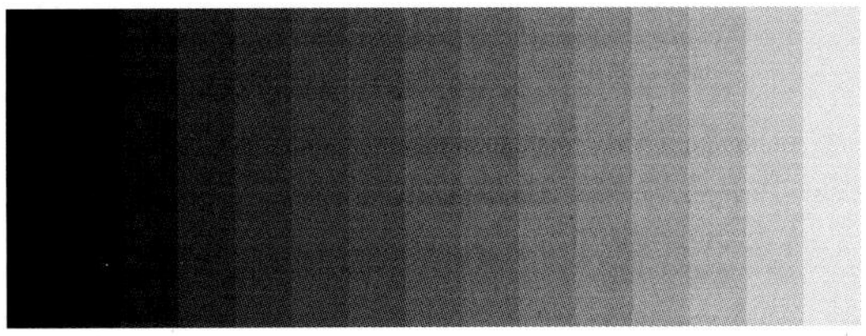

Fig 5-6 Image produced with higher kilovoltage exhibits low contrast; many shades of gray are seen instead of black and white.

TABLE 5-1 Effect of Kilovoltage (kV) on Image Density and Contrast

Adjustment	Density	Contrast
↑ kV	↑ (Darker)	Low
↓ kV	↓ (Lighter)	High

↑, Increase; ↓, decrease.

On older units, exposure time may be indicated as "pulses" or "impulses." An impulse is a term of measurement that refers to the fact that x-rays are created in a series of bursts or pulses rather than in a continuous stream. One impulse occurs every 1/60 of a second; therefore 60 impulses occur in 1 second. Newer x-ray units designed to be used with digital imaging use exposure times measured in hundredths of a second, instead of impulses of 1/60 of a second.

Kilovoltage and exposure time are inversely related. On older x-ray units, if the kilovoltage was changed, the exposure time needed to be adjusted in order to maintain the diagnostic density of an image. When kilovoltage was increased, the exposure time was decreased in order to compensate for the penetrating power of the x-ray beam. When kilovoltage was decreased, the exposure time was increased.

X-RAY BEAM QUANTITY

Quantity of the x-ray beam refers to the number of x-rays produced in the dental x-ray unit.

Amperage and Milliamperage

Amperage determines the amount of electrons passing through the cathode filament. An increase in the number of electrons available to travel from the cathode to the anode results in production of an increased number of x-rays. The quantity of the x-rays produced is controlled by milliamperage.

The ampere (A) is the unit of measure used to describe the number of electrons, or current, flowing through the cathode filament. The number of amperes needed to operate a dental x-ray unit is small; therefore amperage is measured in milliamperes. One milliampere (mA) is equal to 1/1000 of an ampere. It is common to abbreviate milliamperage as mA, the same as its unit, the milliampere. Some dental x-ray units have a fixed milliamperage setting, whereas others have a milliamperage adjustment on the control panel (see Figure 5-1). In the past, dental x-ray units were available with adjustable setting choices of 7 mA or 15 mA. With these units, the mA setting could be chosen according to the individual diagnostic needs of patients. For example, the higher mA setting was used when the area to be examined was dense or thick. The use of 15 mA produced more dental x-rays, whereas the use of 7 mA produced fewer dental x-rays. Current intraoral x-ray units may include adjustable settings that range from 6 to 8 mA, or else a fixed setting of 7 mA. If the unit has a fixed mA, that mA number is found imprinted on the face of the control panel.

Milliamperage regulates the temperature of the cathode filament. A higher milliampere setting increases the temperature of the cathode filament and consequently increases the number of electrons produced. An increase in the number of electrons that strike the anode increases the number of x-rays emitted from the tube.

The quantity, or number of x-rays emitted from the tubehead, is controlled by milliamperage. Milliamperage controls the amperage of the filament current and the amount of electrons that pass through the filament. As the milliamperage is increased, more electrons pass through the filament, and more x-rays are produced. For example, if the milliamperage is increased from 7 to 15 mA, approximately twice as many electrons travel from the cathode to the anode, and approximately twice as many x-rays are produced.

TABLE 5-2 Effect of Milliamperage (mA) on Image Density

Adjustment	Density
↑ mA	↑ (Darker)
↓ mA	↓ (Lighter)

↑, Increase; ↓, decrease.

TABLE 5-3 Guidelines for Adjusting Kilovoltage (kV), Milliamperage (mA), and Exposure Time

Adjustment	Exposure*
↑ kV	↓ Exposure time
↓ kV	↑ Exposure time
↑ mA	↓ Exposure time
↓ mA	↑ Exposure time

↑, Increase; ↓, decrease.
*Adjustment in exposure time needed to maintain diagnostic density of image.

Density and Milliamperage

Milliamperage, as with kilovoltage, has an effect on the density of a dental image. An increase in milliamperage increases the overall density and results in a darker image. Conversely, a decrease in milliamperage decreases the overall density and results in a lighter image. Table 5-2 summarizes the effect of milliamperage on density.

As previously described, with digital imaging, special image enhancement software can be used to change the density by adjusting the brightness. In comparison, if film is used and the density is nondiagnostic, the image will need to be retaken with adjusted exposure factors.

Exposure Time and Milliamperage

Milliamperage and exposure time are inversely related. On older units, if the milliamperage was changed, the exposure time also needed adjustment in order to maintain the diagnostic density of an image. When milliamperage was increased, the exposure time was decreased. When milliamperage was decreased, the exposure time was increased.

Table 5-3 lists guidelines for adjusting kilovoltage, milliamperage, and exposure time.

HELPFUL HINT

How to Remember Quality and Quantity

kV = quality

mA = quantity

k – l – m – n

Modified from istock.com/stevanovicigor

EXPOSURE FACTOR TIPS

All dental x-ray machines have three exposure factor settings: kV, mA, and time. As described in this chapter, changing any one of these three exposure factors changes the appearance of the resultant image.

On dental x-ray units, only the exposure time setting is always adjustable. Most manufacturers recommend that once an x-ray unit has been installed, calibrated, and inspected, it is best **not** to adjust the kV and mA. Instead, adjust only the exposure time to make any needed changes. There is less potential for confusion, errors, and retakes when only the exposure time is adjusted. The exposure time adjustment is based on patient size; it should be decreased with small children and increased with adults with large jaws.

X-RAY BEAM INTENSITY

Quality refers to the energy or penetrating ability of the x-ray beam; *quantity* refers to the number of x-ray photons in the beam. Quality and quantity are described together in a concept known as *intensity*. Intensity is defined as the product of the quantity (number of x-ray photons) and quality (energy of each photon) per unit of area per unit of time of exposure, as follows:

$$\text{Intensity} = \frac{(\text{No. of photons}) \times (\text{Energy of each photon})}{(\text{Area}) \times (\text{Exposure rate})}$$

Intensity of the x-ray beam is affected by a number of factors, including kilovoltage, milliamperage, exposure time, and distance.

Kilovoltage

Kilovoltage regulates the penetrating power of the x-ray beam by controlling the speed of the electrons traveling between the cathode and the anode. Higher kilovoltage settings produce an x-ray beam with more energy and shorter wavelengths; higher kilovoltage levels increase the intensity of the x-ray beam.

Milliamperage

Milliamperage controls the penetrating power of the x-ray beam by controlling the number of electrons produced in the x-ray tube and the number of x-rays produced. Higher milliampere settings produce a beam with more energy, increasing the intensity of the x-ray beam.

Exposure Time

Exposure time, as with milliamperage, affects the number of x-rays produced. A longer exposure time produces more x-rays. An increase in exposure time produces a more intense x-ray beam.

Distance

The distance traveled by the x-ray beam affects the intensity of the beam. Distances that must be considered when exposing a dental image include the following (Figure 5-7):

- Target-surface distance: The distance from the source of radiation (tungsten target in anode) to the patient's skin
- Target-object distance: The distance from the source of radiation (tungsten target in anode) to the tooth
- Target-receptor distance: The distance from the source of radiation (tungsten target in anode) to the receptor

The distance between the source of radiation and the receptor has a marked effect on the intensity of the x-ray beam. As x-rays travel from their point of origin or away from the target anode, they diverge like waves of light and spread out to cover a larger surface area.

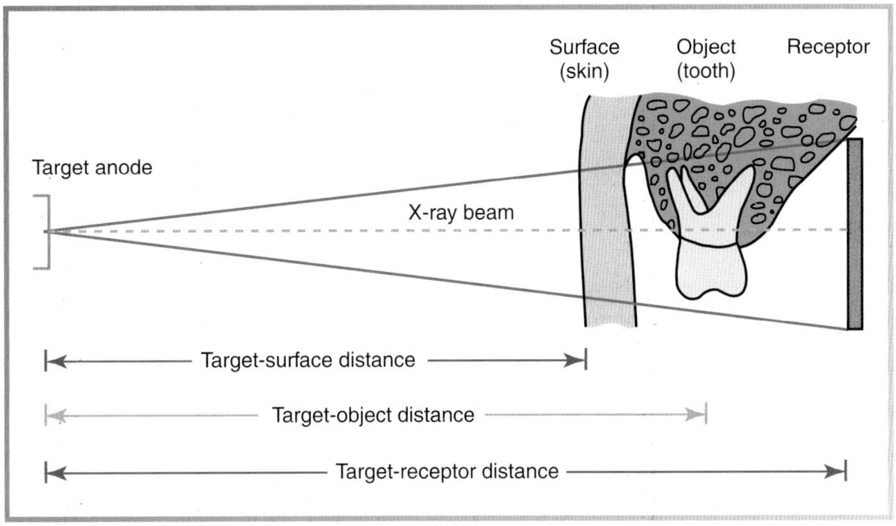

Fig 5-7 Distances to consider when exposing dental radiographs: target-surface, target-object, and target-receptor distance.

HELPFUL HINT

How to Remember Distance and Intensity

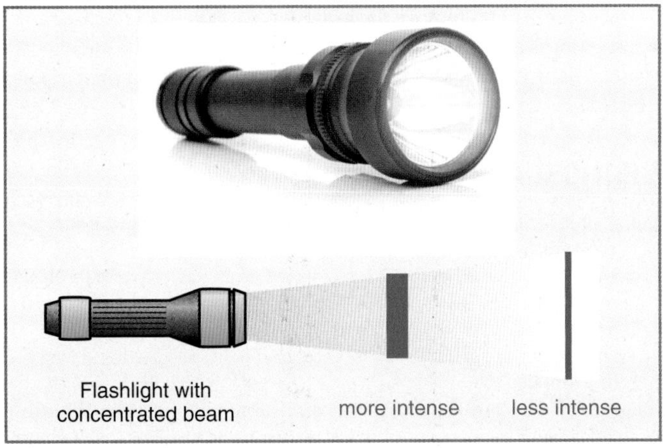

Modified from istock.com/connect11

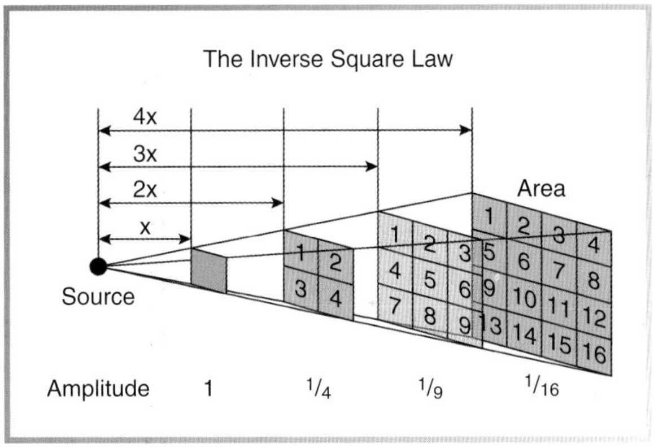

Fig 5-8 The inverse square law states that the intensity of radiation is inversely proportional to the square of the distance from the source. Note that as the source-to-receptor distance is doubled, the radiation is one fourth as intense.

As x-rays travel away from their source of origin, the intensity of the beam lessens. Unless a corresponding change is made in one of the other exposure factors (kilovoltage), the intensity of the x-ray beam is reduced as the distance increases. The inverse square law is used to explain how distance affects the intensity of the x-ray beam.

Inverse Square Law

The inverse square law is stated as follows:

The intensity of radiation is inversely proportional to the square of the distance from the source of radiation.

"Inversely proportional" means that as one variable increases, the other decreases. When the source-to-receptor distance is increased, the intensity of the beam is decreased.

According to the inverse square law, when the target-receptor distance is doubled, the resultant beam is one-fourth as intense (Figure 5-8). When the target-receptor distance is reduced by half, the resultant beam is four times as intense.

The following mathematical formula is used to calculate the inverse square law.

$$\frac{\text{Original intensity}}{\text{New intensity}} = \frac{\text{New distance}^2}{\text{Original distance}^2}$$

Example

If the target-receptor distance is changed from 8 inches to 16 inches, how does this increase in source-to-receptor distance affect the intensity of the beam?

$$\frac{1}{x} = \frac{16^2}{8^2}$$

$$\frac{1}{x} = \frac{256}{64}$$

$$\frac{1}{x} = \frac{4}{1}$$

$$x = \frac{1}{4}$$

This mathematical formula reveals that the beam will be one-fourth as intense if the target-receptor distance is changed from 8 to 16 inches (assuming that kilovoltage and milliamperage remain constant). In this example, the inverse square law reveals that doubling the distance from the source of radiation to the receptor results in a beam that is one-fourth as intense.

HELPFUL HINT

How to Remember Inverse Square Numbers

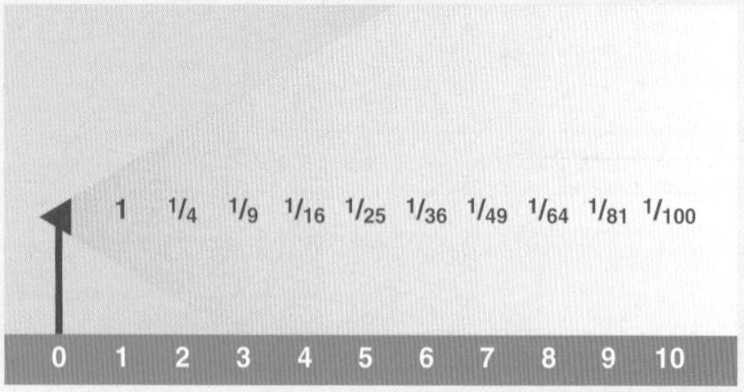

If distance is doubled = 1/4 as intense (inverse of 2^2)

If distance is tripled = 1/9 as intense (inverse of 3^2)

If distance is quadrupled = 1/16 as intense (inverse of 4^2)

Remember: The intensity of the radiation is inversely proportional to the square of the distance. This is also true for lighting used in professional photography.

Half-Value Layer

To reduce the intensity of the x-ray beam, aluminum filters are placed in the path of the beam inside the dental x-ray tubehead. Aluminum filters are used to remove the low-energy, less penetrating, longer-wavelength x-rays. Aluminum filters increase the mean penetrating capability of the x-ray beam while reducing the intensity. When placed in the path of the x-ray beam, the thickness of a specified material (e.g., aluminum) that reduces the intensity by half is termed the **half-value layer (HVL)**.

For example, if an x-ray beam has an HVL of 4 mm, a thickness of 4 mm of aluminum would be necessary to decrease its intensity by half. Measuring the HVL determines the penetrating quality of the beam. The higher the half-value layer, the more penetrating the beam. (Filtration of the x-ray beam was discussed in Chapter 4.)

SUMMARY

- Radiation characteristics include x-ray beam quality, quantity, and intensity.
- X-ray units may or may not have adjustable dials or buttons for kilovoltage, milliamperage, and time.
- *Quality* refers to the mean (average) energy or penetrating ability of the x-ray beam and is controlled by the kilovoltage.
- Increased kilovoltage produces x-rays with increased energy, shorter wavelength, and increased penetrating power; kilovoltage affects density and contrast.
- *Quantity* refers to the number of x-rays produced and is controlled by the milliamperage.
- Increased milliamperage produces an increased number of x-rays; milliamperage affects density.
- Exposure time also influences the number of x-rays produced.
- Exposure factors include kV, mA, and time.
- All current dental x-ray units allow for the adjustment of exposure time, whereas the ability to adjust kV and mA varies from model to model.
- Once an x-ray unit has been installed, calibrated, and inspected, it is best *not* to adjust the kV and mA. Instead, adjust only the exposure time to make any needed changes.
- With digital imaging, special image enhancement software can be used to change the density and contrast. In comparison, if film is used and the density and/or contrast is nondiagnostic, the image must be retaken with adjusted exposure factors.
- *Intensity* is the total energy contained in the x-ray beam in a specific area at a given time; intensity is affected by kilovoltage, milliamperage, exposure time, and distance.
- Increased kilovoltage, milliamperage, or exposure time results in increased intensity of the x-ray beam.
- Intensity of the x-ray beam is reduced with increased distance. The *inverse square law* is used to explain how distance affects the intensity of the x-ray beam.
- An aluminum filter is placed in the path of the x-ray beam to reduce the intensity and remove the low-energy x-rays from the beam.
- The thickness of aluminum placed in the path of the x-ray beam that reduces the intensity by half is termed the *half-value layer (HVL)*.

BIBILIOGRAPHY

Frommer HH, Stabulas-Savage JJ: Image formation. In Radiology for the dental professional, ed 9, St Louis, 2011, Mosby.

Frommer HH, Stabulas-Savage JJ: Image receptors. In Radiology for the dental professional, ed 9, St Louis, 2011, Mosby.

Frommer HH, Stabulas-Savage JJ: Ionizing radiation and basic principles of x-ray generation. In Radiology for the dental professional, ed 9, St Louis, 2011, Mosby.

Johnson ON: The dental x-ray machine: components and functions. In Essentials of dental radiography for dental assistants and hygienists, ed 9, Upper Saddle River, NJ, 2011, Prentice Hall.

Johnson ON: Producing quality radiographs. In Essentials of dental radiography for dental assistants and hygienists, ed 9, Upper Saddle River, NJ, 2011, Prentice Hall.

Mallya SM, Lam EWN: Physics. In White and Pharoah's oral radiology: principles and interpretation, ed 8, St. Louis, 2019, Elsevier.

Miles DA, Van Dis ML, Williamson GF, et al: Image characteristics. In Radiographic imaging for the dental team, ed 4, St Louis, 2009, Saunders.

Miles DA, Van Dis ML, Williamson GF, et al: X-ray properties and the generation of x-rays. In Radiographic imaging for the dental team, ed 4, St Louis, 2009, Saunders.

QUIZ QUESTIONS

Multiple Choice

____ 1. In dental imaging, the quality of the x-ray beam is controlled by:
   a. kilovoltage
   b. milliamperage
   c. exposure time
   d. source-to-receptor distance

____ 2. Identify the kilovoltage range for current dental x-ray machines:
   a. 50 to 60 kV
   b. 60 to 70 kV
   c. 70 to 100 kV
   d. greater than 100 kV

____ 3. A higher kilovoltage produces x-rays with:
   a. greater energy levels
   b. shorter wavelengths
   c. more penetrating ability
   d. all of the above

____ 4. Identify the unit of measurement used to describe the amount of electric current flowing through the x-ray tube:
   a. volt
   b. ampere
   c. kilovoltage
   d. force

____ 5. Radiation produced with high kilovoltage results in:
   a. short wavelengths
   b. long wavelengths
   c. less penetrating radiation
   d. lower energy levels

____ 6. In dental imaging, the quantity of radiation produced is controlled by:
   a. kilovoltage
   b. milliamperage
   c. exposure time
   d. both b and c

____ 7. Increasing milliamperage results in an increase in:
   a. temperature of the filament
   b. mean energy of the beam
   c. number of x-rays produced
   d. both a and c

____ 8. Identify the milliamperage range used for current dental x-ray machines:
   a. 1 to 5 mA
   b. 6 to 8 mA
   c. 9 to 15 mA
   d. greater than 15 mA

____ 9. The overall blackness or darkness of an image is termed:
   a. contrast
   b. density
   c. overexposure
   d. polychromatic

____ 10. If kilovoltage is decreased with no other variations in exposure factors, the resultant image will:
   a. appear lighter
   b. appear darker
   c. remain the same
   d. either a or b

____ 11. Identify the term that describes how dark and light areas are differentiated on an image:
   a. contrast
   b. density
   c. intensity
   d. polychromatic

____ 12. An image that has many light and dark areas with few shades of gray is said to have:
   a. high density
   b. low density
   c. high contrast
   d. low contrast

____ 13. The image described in question 12 was produced with:
   a. low kilovoltage
   b. high kilovoltage
   c. low milliamperage
   d. high milliamperage

____ 14. Increasing milliamperage alone results in an image with:
   a. high contrast
   b. low contrast
   c. increased density
   d. decreased density

____ 15. The total energy contained in the x-ray beam in a specific area at a given time is termed:
   a. kilovoltage
   b. beam quality
   c. intensity
   d. milliampere-second

____ 16. Increasing which of these four exposure controls will increase the intensity of the x-ray beam: (1) kilovoltage, (2) milliamperage, (3) exposure time, (4) source-to-receptor distance?
   a. 1 and 2
   b. 2 and 3
   c. 1, 2, and 3
   d. 1, 2, 3, and 4

____ 17. If the target-receptor distance is doubled, the resultant beam will be:
   a. four times as intense
   b. twice as intense
   c. half as intense
   d. one-fourth as intense

____ 18. If the target-receptor distance is tripled, the resultant beam will be:
   a. one-half as intense
   b. one-fourth as intense
   c. one-ninth as intense
   d. one-sixteenth as intense

____ 19. The half-value layer is the amount of:
   a. lead that restricts the diameter of the beam by half
   b. copper needed to cool the anode
   c. aluminum needed to reduce scatter radiation by half
   d. aluminum needed to reduce x-ray beam intensity by half

____ 20. If the half-value layer is 3 mm, what thickness of aluminum is necessary to decrease the intensity by half?
   a. 1.5 mm
   b. 3 mm
   c. 6 mm
   d. 9 mm

6

Dental X-Ray Image Characteristics

LEARNING OBJECTIVES

After completion of this chapter, the student will be able to do the following:

1. Define the key terms associated with image characteristics.
2. Differentiate between radiolucent and radiopaque areas on a dental image.
3. Describe a diagnostic dental image.
4. List the two visual characteristics of the radiographic image.
5. List the factors that influence density and contrast.
6. Discuss the difference between high contrast and low contrast.
7. Describe film contrast and subject contrast.
8. Describe the difference between short-scale contrast and long-scale contrast.
9. Identify images of high contrast, low contrast, no contrast, short-scale contrast, and long-scale contrast.
10. Describe a stepwedge and explain its function.
11. List the three geometric characteristics of the radiographic image.
12. List the factors that influence sharpness, magnification, and distortion.

Dental x-ray image features include both visual characteristics and geometric characteristics. A variety of factors affect the visual image characteristics of density and contrast, as well as the geometric image characteristics of sharpness, magnification, and distortion.

The dental radiographer must have a working knowledge of the characteristics that apply to dental imaging. The purpose of this chapter is to describe in detail the visual image characteristics of density and contrast; to define the geometric image characteristics of sharpness, magnification, and distortion; and to discuss how influencing factors affect these image characteristics. Terms that apply to both digital and film-based imaging are identified in this chapter. Additional information concerning digital imaging characteristics is discussed in Chapter 8.

DENTAL X-RAY IMAGE CHARACTERISTICS

A dental image appears black and white with varying shades of gray. When viewed on a light source or computer monitor, the darkest area of the image appears black, and the lightest area appears white. Two terms are used to describe the black areas and the white areas on a dental image: *radiolucent* and *radiopaque*, respectively. These terms are used in both digital and film-based imaging.

- **Radiolucent** refers to that portion of an image that is dark or black. A structure that appears radiolucent lacks density and permits the passage of the x-ray beam with little or no resistance. For example, air space freely permits the passage of dental x-rays and appears radiolucent on a dental image (Figure 6-1).
- **Radiopaque** refers to that portion of an image that appears light or white. Radiopaque structures are dense and absorb or resist the passage of the x-ray beam. For example, structures that resist the passage of the x-ray beam include enamel, dentin, and bone and appear radiopaque on a dental image (Figure 6-2).

In both digital and film-based imaging, the ideal dental image is not too light and not too dark. The quality of a dental image is determined by its characteristics. These image characteristics include the visual characteristics of density and contrast, as well as the geometric characteristics of sharpness, magnification, and distortion. The ideal dental image is a diagnostic one. A **diagnostic image** provides a great deal of information; the images exhibit proper density and contrast, are of the same shape and size as the object exposed, and have sharp outlines.

VISUAL CHARACTERISTICS

Two visual characteristics—density and contrast—directly influence the diagnostic quality of a dental image.

Density

The overall blackness or darkness of a dental image is termed **density**.

Description. When a processed dental film is viewed against a light source, the relative transparency of areas on the image depends on the distribution of black silver particles in the emulsion. Darker areas represent heavier deposits of black silver particles. Density is this degree of silver blackening.

Images of teeth and supporting structures must have enough density to be viewed on a light source; however, if the density of an image appears too light or too dark, the image is considered nondiagnostic. An image with the correct density allows the radiographer to view black areas (such as air spaces), white areas (including enamel, dentin, and bone), and gray areas (for example, soft tissue) (Figure 6-3).

Influencing Factors. A number of factors have a direct influence on the density of a dental image. As discussed in Chapter 5, three **exposure factors** control the density of a dental image, as follows:

- Kilovoltage (kV)
- Milliamperage (mA)
- Exposure time

Any increase in such exposure factors, separately or combined, increases the density of a dental image. In addition, the subject thickness influences density (Table 6-1).

Kilovoltage. As presented in Chapter 5, many of today's dental x-ray machines do not allow for the adjustment of **kilovoltage** (kV). On units that do allow for adjustment, an increase in kV increases density by producing x-rays of higher energy. If the kilovoltage is increased, the

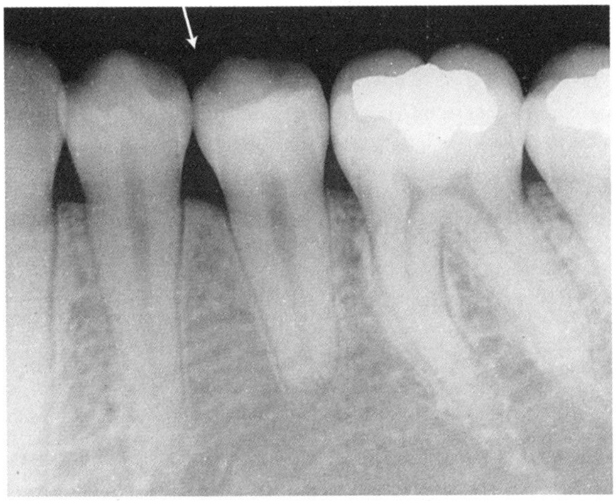

Fig 6-1 Air space (*arrow*) appears radiolucent, or dark, because the dental x-rays pass through freely.

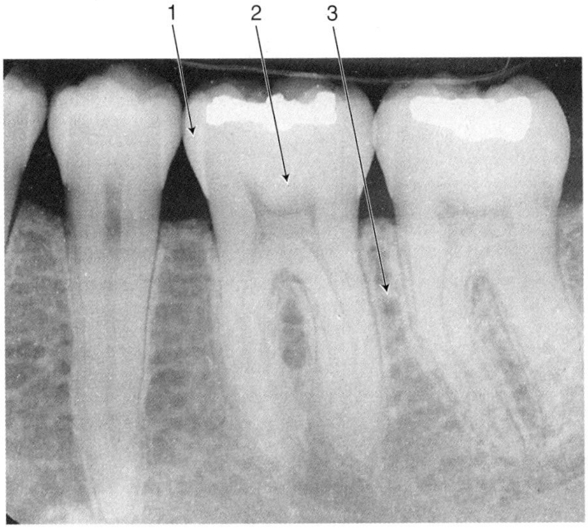

Fig 6-2 Dense structures, such as enamel (1), dentin (2), and bone (3), resist the passage of x-rays and appear radiopaque, or white.

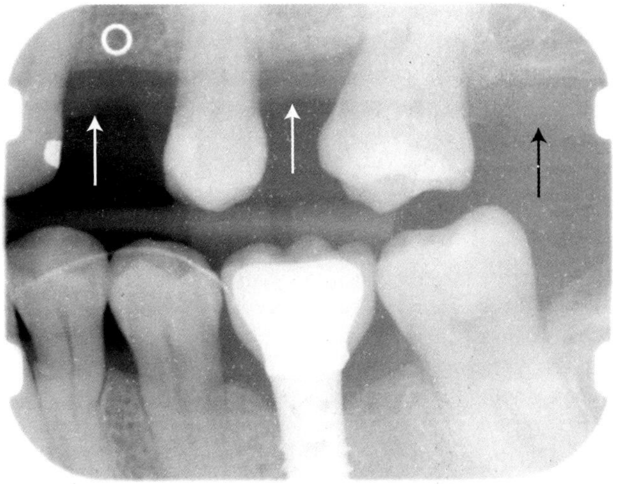

Fig 6-3 Note the grayish area in the upper arch (*arrows*); this represents the gingival tissues.

TABLE 6-1 Visual Characteristics and Influencing Factors

Visual Characteristic	Influencing Factors	Effect of Influencing Factors
Density	mA	↑ mA=↑ density
		↓ mA=↓ density
	kV	↑ kV=↑ density
		↓ kV=↓ density
	Time	↑ Time=↑ density
		↓ Time=↓ density
	Subject thickness	↑ Thickness=↓ density
		↓ Thickness=↑ density
Contrast	kV	↑ kV=long-scale contrast; low contrast
		↓ kV=short-scale contrast; high contrast

mA, milliamperage; *kV*, kilovoltage; ↑, increased; ↓, decreased.

density increases, and the image appears darker. Conversely, if kilovoltage is decreased, the density decreases, and the image appears lighter.

The adjustment of kilovoltage has been compared with adjusting a spray nozzle on a garden hose. Like the spray nozzle, the kilovoltage controls the force of the emerging x-rays. Using a low kilovoltage setting is similar to "opening up" the nozzle on a hose to create a fine mist. The x-rays have less power and do not penetrate well. As a result, the image is mostly black and white. Using a high kilovoltage setting is similar to "closing down" the spray nozzle on a hose to create a single, powerful stream of water. The beam is highly

HELPFUL HINT

Adjusting Kilovoltage

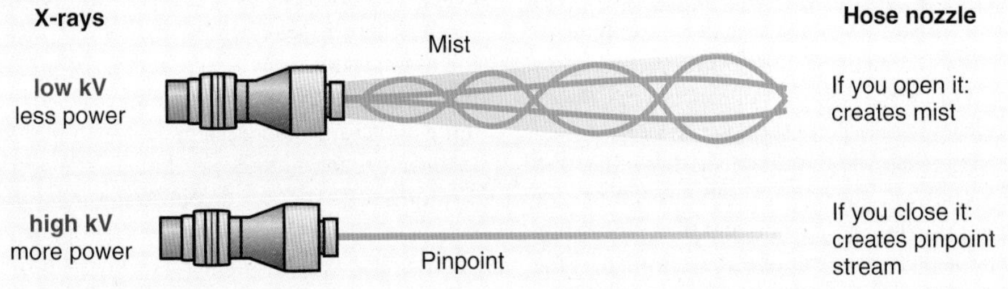

penetrating and has high energy. As a result, many shades of gray are seen in the resultant image.

Milliamperage. In dental x-ray machines that allow for adjustment of milliamperage (mA), an increase in mA produces more x-rays that the receptor is exposed to and, as a result, increases density. If the milliamperage is increased, the density increases, and the image appears darker. Conversely, if the milliamperage is decreased, the density decreases, and the image appears lighter.

Exposure time. Density is directly related to exposure time. An increase in exposure time increases density by increasing the total number of x-rays that reach the receptor surface. If the exposure time is increased, more x-rays reach the receptor, the density increases, and the image appears dark. Conversely, if the exposure time is decreased, the density decreases, and the image appears lighter.

The x-ray timer controls the exposure time by turning the flow of x-rays on or off. It has been compared with a water faucet. For example, if the faucet is open for a certain period, a specific amount of water will flow. If the faucet is opened for twice that amount of time, twice the amount of water will flow. The same is true with exposure time. If a receptor is exposed to x-radiation for a specific period, a specific amount of x-rays are produced. If the time is doubled, the amount of x-rays produced is doubled. The longer the exposure time, the more x-ray photons reach the receptor and continue to darken the image.

Subject thickness. Fewer x-rays reach the receptor in a patient with an increased amount of soft tissue, muscle, or thick, dense bones. As a result, the image has less density and appears lighter. Adjustments in kV, mA, or exposure time can be made to compensate for the subject thickness that varies with the size of the patient.

HELPFUL HINT

Density and Size of Patient

- Subject thickness=small patient
  ↓ thickness=↑ density/**darker**
  If patient is **small**, need to ↓ **kV, mA**, or **time**
- Subject thickness=large patient
  ↑ thickness=↓ density/**lighter**
  If patient is **large**, need to ↑ **kV, mA**, or **time**

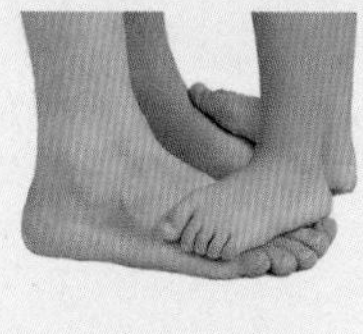

Contrast

The difference in the degrees of blackness (densities) between adjacent areas on a dental image is termed contrast.

Description. The differences in the amount of light transmitted through adjacent areas of a dental image can also be described as contrast. When viewed on a light source, a dental image that has very dark areas and very light areas demonstrates high contrast; the dark and light areas are strikingly different. An image that does not have very dark and very light areas but instead has many shades of gray demonstrates low contrast. In dental imaging, a compromise between low contrast and high contrast is preferred. The overall contrast of a dental image is determined by the film contrast and the subject contrast.

Film contrast. Film contrast refers to the characteristics of the film that influence radiographic contrast. The characteristics that influence contrast include the inherent qualities of the film and film processing. The inherent qualities of the film are determined and controlled by the film manufacturer and cannot be changed. Film processing, however, is under the control of the dental radiographer. Development time or the temperature of the developer solution affects the contrast of a dental radiograph. For example, an increase in development time or developer temperature results in a film with high contrast.

Subject contrast. Subject contrast refers to the characteristics of the subject (the dental patient) that influence radiographic contrast. Subject contrast is determined by the size and thickness of patient tissues. Increasing or decreasing the kilovoltage can alter subject contrast. When a high kilovoltage is used, low subject contrast results, and many shades of gray are seen on the dental radiograph. Conversely, when a low kilovoltage is used, high subject contrast results, and areas of black and white are seen on the image.

Influencing Factors. Only one exposure factor has a direct influence on the contrast of a dental image. As discussed in Chapter 5, the kilovoltage affects contrast.

Kilovoltage. Increasing the kilovoltage produces higher energy x-rays and affects contrast by increasing the overall energy of the x-ray beam. X-rays with higher energy are better able to penetrate tissue. As a result, more variations in tissue density are recorded on the receptor and appear as varying shades of gray. A higher kilovoltage setting produces an image with decreased or low contrast; the radiograph exhibits many shades of gray. Conversely, a lower kilovoltage setting produces an image with increased or high contrast; the radiograph has many black-and-white areas.

Table 6-1 summarizes the effects of kilovoltage on contrast. Figure 6-4 provides a series of dental radiographs showing the influence of kilovoltage on both density and contrast.

Scales of Contrast. The range of useful densities seen on a dental image is termed the scale of contrast. In dental radiography, the terms short-scale contrast and long-scale contrast may be used to describe the appearance of an image.

Short-scale contrast. A dental image that shows only two densities, areas of black and areas of white, has a short contrast scale. A lower kilovoltage range results in an image with a short-scale contrast; many areas of black and white, rather than shades of gray, are seen. An image that exhibits a short contrast scale can also be described as having high contrast, in which the black-and-white areas are easily distinguished from each other (Table 6-2).

Long-scale contrast. A dental image that exhibits many densities, or many shades of gray, has a long contrast scale. A higher kilovoltage range results in an image with a long-scale contrast; many shades of gray, rather than areas of black and white, are present. An image that exhibits a long contrast scale can also be described as having low contrast, in which areas of gray are not easily distinguished from each other (see Table 6-2).

Short-scale vs. long-scale contrast. So, which type of contrast is preferred in dental images? If the operator is suspicious of finding dental caries on the patient's images, decreasing the kilovoltage to produce short-scale contrast may be beneficial. The carious lesion appears radiolucent as a result of the demineralization of the hard tooth structure (see Chapter 33). A short-scale contrast may help allow the radiolucent caries "stand out" more on the image because it demonstrates more black and white areas (Figure 6-5). On the other hand, if the operator is treating a patient with periodontal issues, an increase in the kilovoltage may be recommended to produce long-scale contrast. The long-scale contrast demonstrates many shades of gray; this may be beneficial to see the subtle changes in bone loss associated with periodontal disease (see Chapter 34) (Figure 6-6).

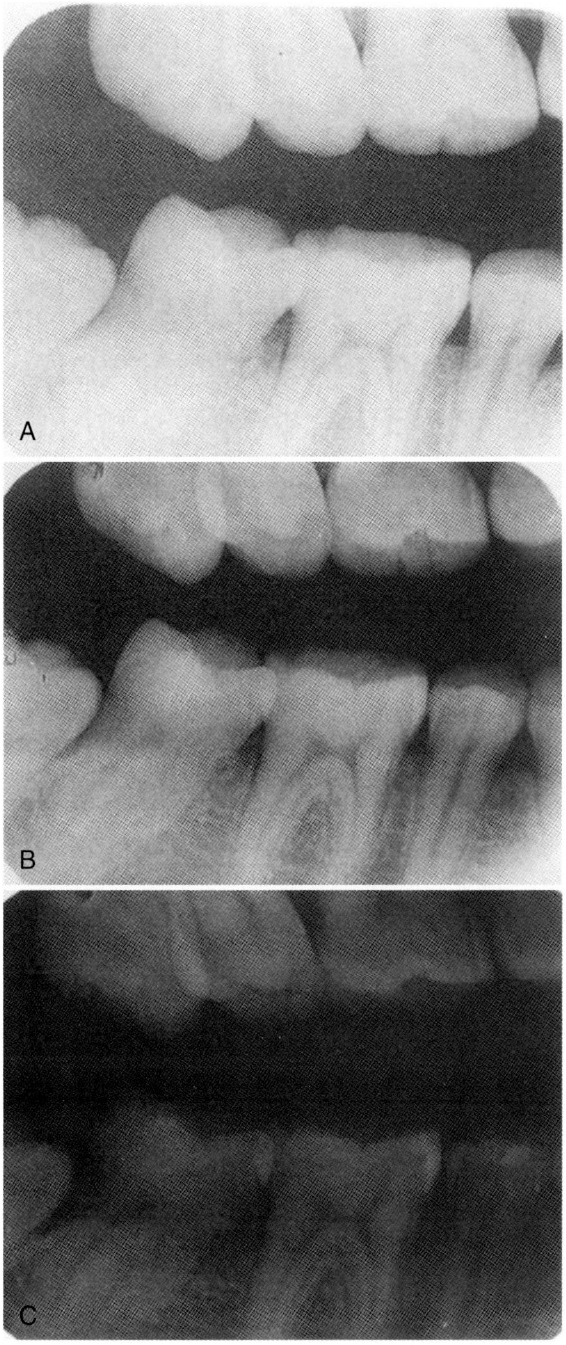

Fig 6-4 Exposure series showing the influence of kilovoltage (kV). **A,** When kV is low, the result is low density and high contrast. **B,** The optimal image is created when a proper balance between kV and milliamperage (mA) is obtained. This image is considered optimal because it provides a full range of tones from white to black. **C,** When kV is high, the result is very high density with very low contrast. (Courtesy Carestream Health, Inc., Rochester, NY.)

TABLE 6-2 The Effect of Kilovoltage on Contrast

Kilovoltage	Contrast	Scale of Contrast	Example
High	Low	Long-scale	See Figure 6-16.
Low	High	Short-scale	See Figure 6-16.

kV, kilovoltage.

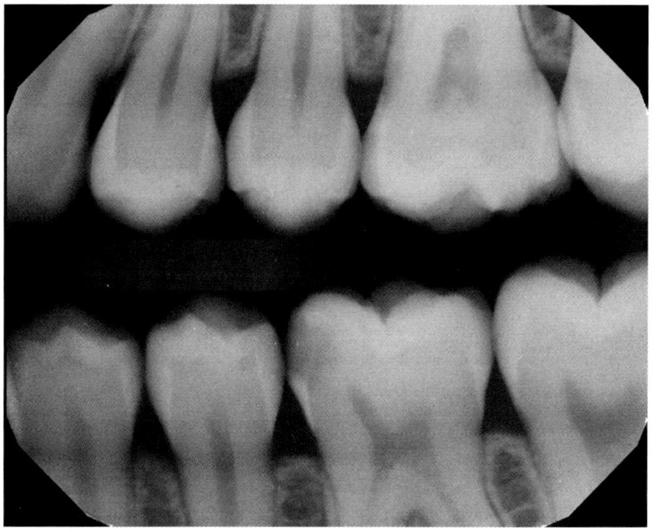

Fig 6-5 A premolar bite-wing reveals carious lesions in both the maxillary and mandibular teeth. The lower kVp setting produces more areas of black and white, allowing the caries to be better viewed.

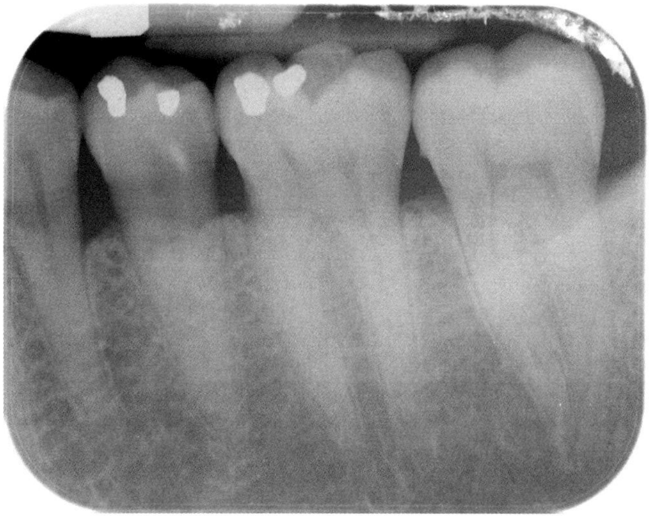

Fig 6-6 A periapical image reveals horizontal bone loss and calculus deposits. The higher kVp setting produces many shades of gray, allowing for subtle bony changes to be seen.

Stepwedge. A device known as a stepwedge can be used to demonstrate short-scale contrast and long-scale contrast. A stepwedge consists of uniform-layered thicknesses of an x-ray-absorbing material, usually aluminum. The typical stepwedge is constructed of aluminum steps in 2-mm increments (Figure 6-7). When a stepwedge is placed on top of an image receptor and exposed to x-rays, the different steps absorb varying amounts of x-rays. As a result, different densities appear on the dental image.

The use of a stepwedge to demonstrate corresponding densities and contrast scales is illustrated in Figure 6-8. The stepwedge can be used to monitor the qualities of the film, the film processing, and the digital sensor, as well as calibration of the x-ray machine. Quality control tests using the stepwedge are discussed in Chapter 17.

HELPFUL HINT

Contrast

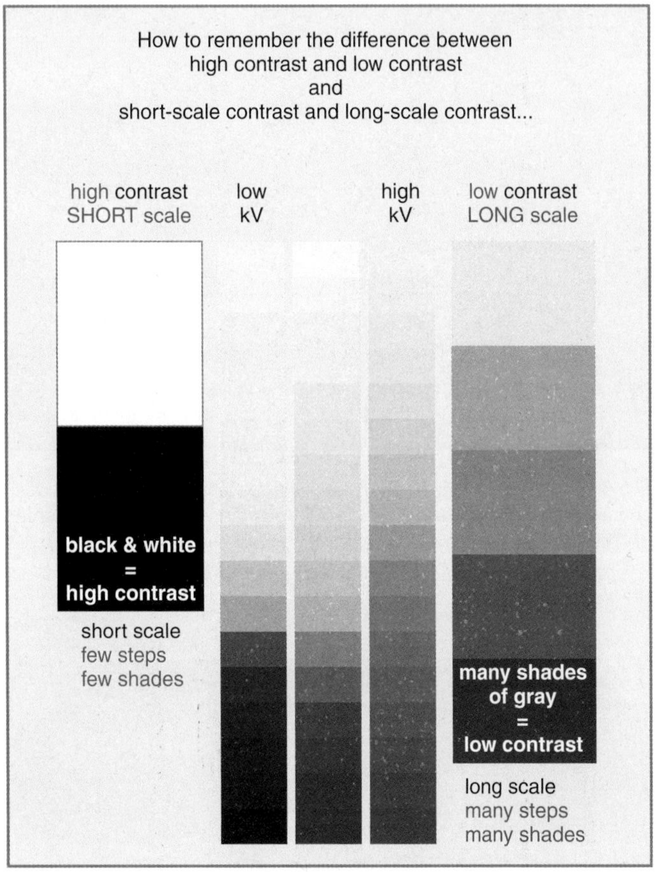

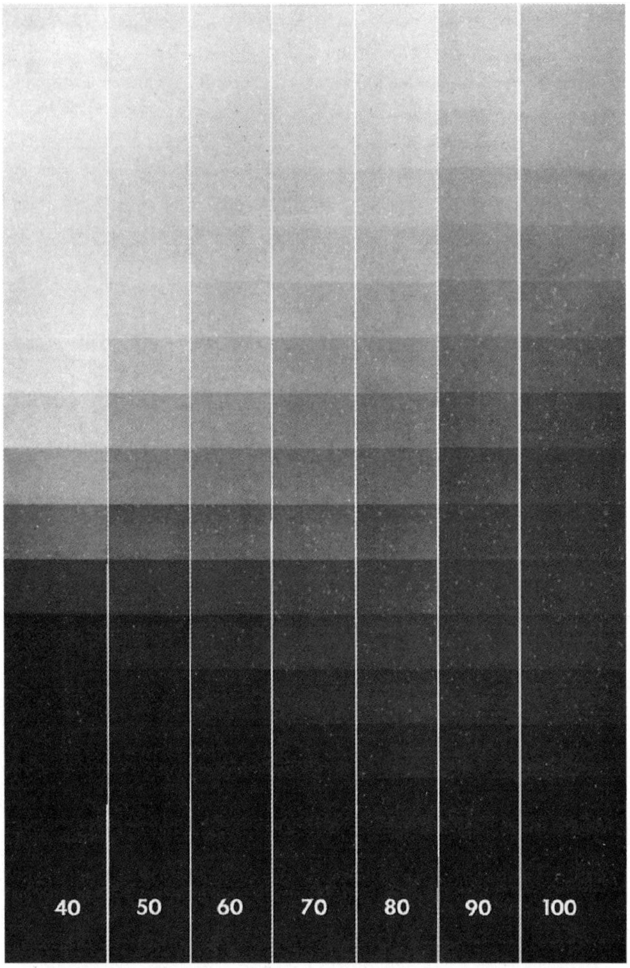

Fig 6-8 Seven radiographs of a stepwedge made at 40 to 100 kV shown side by side. As the kV was increased, the mA was reduced to maintain a roughly uniform middle-step density. Note the long grayscale (low-contrast) image with high kV and the short grayscale (high-contrast) image when using low kV. (Courtesy Carestream Dental, a division of Carestream Health Inc.)

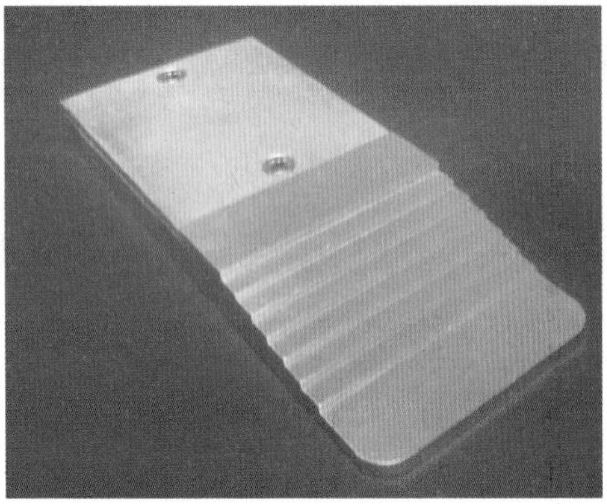

Fig 6-7 A stepwedge is made of uniform-layered thicknesses. (Courtesy Harry B. Rusk Co., Wichita, KS., www.harrybrusk.com.)

GEOMETRIC CHARACTERISTICS

Three geometric characteristics—sharpness, magnification, and distortion—influence the diagnostic quality of a dental image. These geometric characteristics must be controlled to produce an accurate radiographic image. Although sharpness is preferred on all images, magnification and distortion must be minimized to produce an accurate radiographic image of the tooth and surrounding structures.

Sharpness

Sharpness (also known as *detail, resolution*, or *definition*) refers to the capability of the receptor to reproduce the distinct outlines of an object—in other words, how well the smallest details of an object are reproduced on a dental image.

Description. A certain lack of image sharpness, or unsharpness, is present in every dental image. The fuzzy, unclear area that surrounds a structure (e.g., a tooth) on an image is termed the *penumbra* (from the Latin *pene*, meaning "almost," and *umbra*, meaning "shadow"). **Penumbra** can be defined as the unsharpness, or blurring, of the edges.

Influencing Factors. The sharpness of an image is influenced by the following three factors (Table 6-3):

- Focal spot size
- Film composition
- Movement

Focal spot size. The focal spot size influences sharpness. As described in Chapter 2, the tungsten target of the anode serves as a **focal spot**; this small area converts bombarding electrons into x-ray

TABLE 6-3 Geometric Characteristics and Influencing Factors

Geometric Characteristic	Influencing Factors	Effects of Influencing Factors
Sharpness	Focal spot size	↓ Focal spot size = ↑ sharpness
		↑ Focal spot size = ↓ sharpness
	Film composition	↓ Crystal size = ↑ sharpness
		↑ Crystal size = ↓ sharpness
	Movement	↓ Movement = ↑ sharpness
		↑ Movement = ↓ sharpness
Magnification	Target-receptor distance	↑ Target-receptor distance = ↓ magnification
		↓ Target-receptor distance = ↑ magnification
	Object-receptor distance	↑ Object-receptor distance = ↑ magnification
		↓ Object-receptor distance = ↓ magnification
Distortion	Object-receptor alignment	Object and receptor parallel = ↓ distortion
		Object and receptor not parallel = ↑ distortion
	X-ray beam angulation	Beam perpendicular to object and receptor = ↓ distortion
		Beam not perpendicular to object and receptor = ↑ distortion

↓, decreased; ↑, increased.

photons. The focal spot concentrates the electrons and creates an enormous amount of heat. To limit the amount of heat produced and to prevent damage to the x-ray tube, the size of the focal spot is limited. The size of the focal spot ranges from 0.6 to 1.0 mm^2 and is determined by the manufacturer of the x-ray equipment; most manufacturers use the smallest focal spot area possible based on heat production restrictions.

The smaller the focal spot area, the sharper the image; the larger the focal spot area, the greater the loss of image sharpness (Figure 6-9). If x-rays were produced from one spot or a single "point source," no unsharpness would be present (Figure 6-10). However, a single point source of x-ray production is impossible because of the limited capacity of the x-ray tube.

Film composition. The composition of the film emulsion influences sharpness. Sharpness is relative to the size of the crystals found in the film emulsion. The emulsion of faster film contains larger crystals that produce less image sharpness, whereas slower film contains smaller crystals that produce more image sharpness. Unsharpness occurs because the larger crystals do not produce object outlines as well as smaller crystals do.

Movement. Movement influences image sharpness. A loss of image sharpness occurs if the tubehead, the receptor, or the patient moves during x-ray exposure (Figure 6-11). Even slight amounts of movement result in unsharpness, which may cause the image to be nondiagnostic (Figure 6-12).

Magnification

Image magnification refers to a radiographic image that appears larger than the actual size of the object it represents.

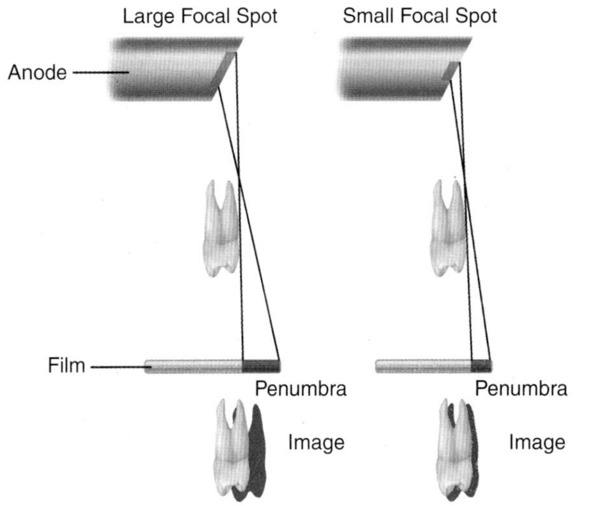

Fig 6-9 The smaller the focal spot area, the sharper the image; the larger the focal spot area, the greater the amount of penumbra, and the greater the loss of image sharpness.

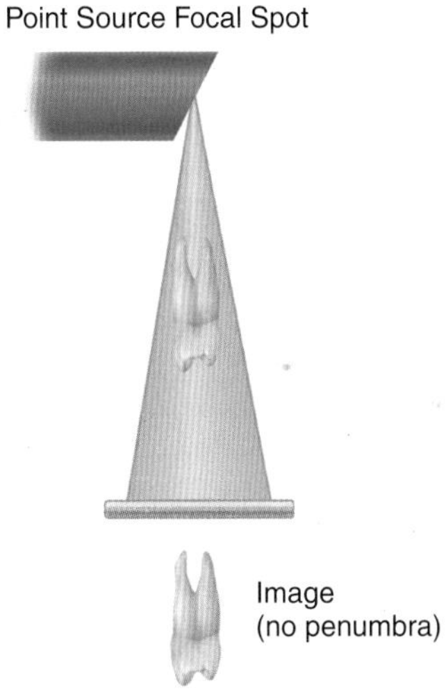

Fig 6-10 Theoretical "point source" of x-rays would produce a sharp image without penumbra.

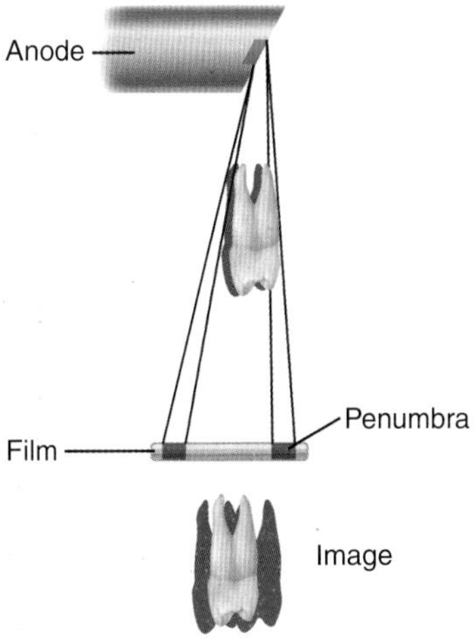

Fig 6-11 Diagram illustrating the influence of motion on image sharpness. Note that the image outline is blurred because of penumbra.

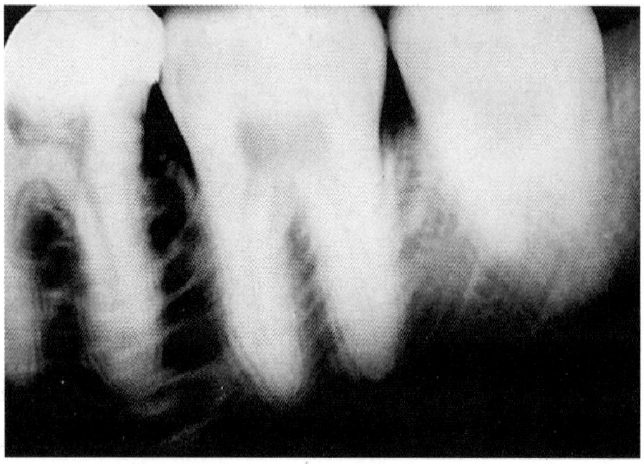

Fig 6-12 Image of a patient who moved during x-ray exposure. Note the blurred image outline.

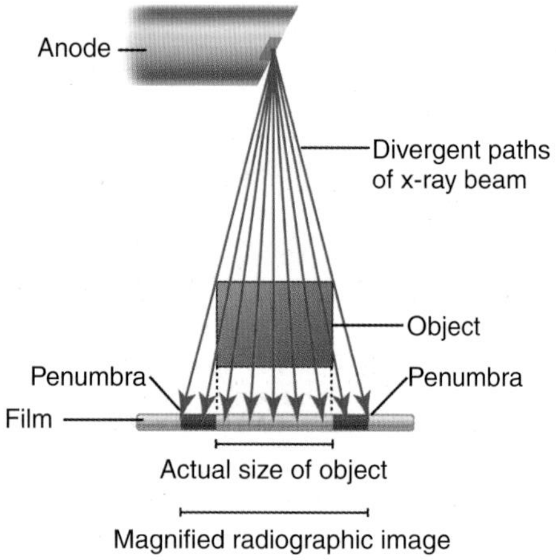

Fig 6-13 Diagram illustrating magnification as a result of the divergent paths of the x-ray beam.

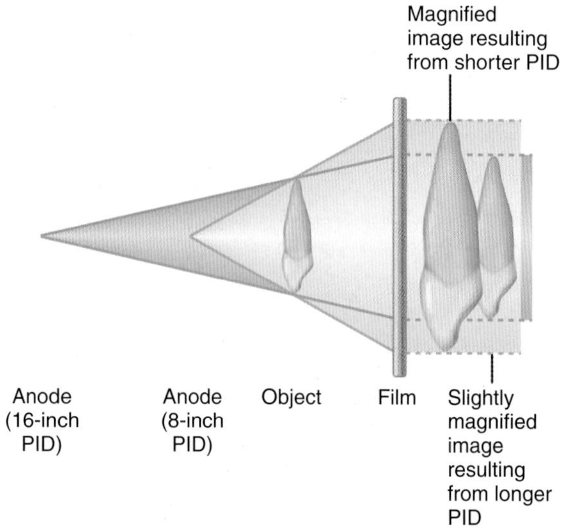

Fig 6-14 A longer position-indicating device (PID) (16 inches) and target-receptor distance results in less image magnification.

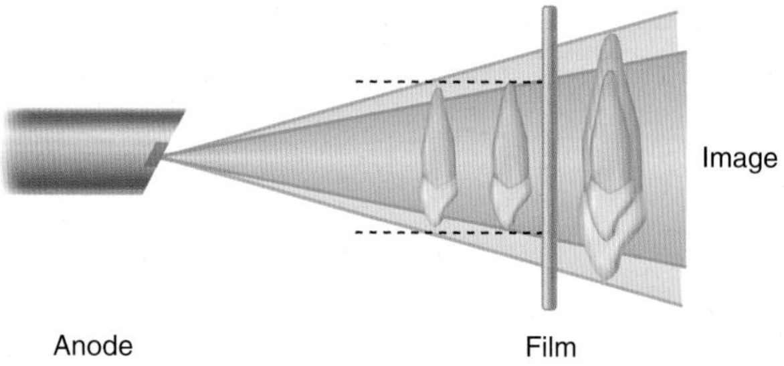

Fig 6-15 Object-receptor distance. Note that the closer the tooth is to the receptor, the less magnification is seen on the image.

Description. Magnification, or enlargement of a radiographic image, results from the diverging x-ray beam. As detailed in Chapter 2, x-rays travel in diverging straight lines, radiating from the focal spot. Because of these diverging paths, some degree of image magnification is present in every dental image (Figure 6-13).

Influencing Factors. The magnification on a dental image is influenced by the following (see Table 6-3):

- Target-receptor distance
- Object-receptor distance

Target-receptor distance. As defined in Chapter 5, the target-receptor distance (also known as the *source-to-receptor distance*) is the distance between the source of x-rays (focal spot on the tungsten target) and the image receptor. The target-receptor distance is determined by the length of the position-indicating device (PID). When a longer PID is used, more parallel rays from the middle of the x-ray beam strike the object rather than the diverging x-rays from the periphery of the beam. As a result, a longer PID and target-receptor distance result in less image magnification, and a shorter PID and target-receptor distance result in more image magnification (Figure 6-14). Although the longer PID is preferred because it limits magnification, the long (16-inch) cone may be bulky or difficult to maneuver around the patient. Current x-ray machines are manufactured with a recessed focal spot, meaning that the dental x-ray tube is recessed, or placed in the rear section of the tubehead. This allows for the use of a shorter PID while still maintaining the extended target-receptor distance.

Object-receptor distance. The object-receptor distance is the distance between the object being radiographed (the tooth) and the image receptor. The tooth and the receptor should always be placed as close together as possible. The closer the tooth is to the receptor, the less the image is enlarged. A decrease in object-receptor distance results in a decrease in magnification, and an increase in object-receptor distance results in an increase in image magnification (Figure 6-15).

Distortion

Dimensional distortion of a radiographic image is a variation in the true size and shape of the object being radiographed. A distorted image does not have the same size and shape as the object being radiographed.

Description. A distorted image results from the unequal magnification of different parts of the same object. Distortion results from improper receptor alignment or beam angulation. Foreshortened and elongated images are examples of distortion.

Influencing Factors. The dimensional distortion of a radiographic image is influenced by the following (see Table 6-3):

- Object-receptor alignment
- X-ray beam angulation

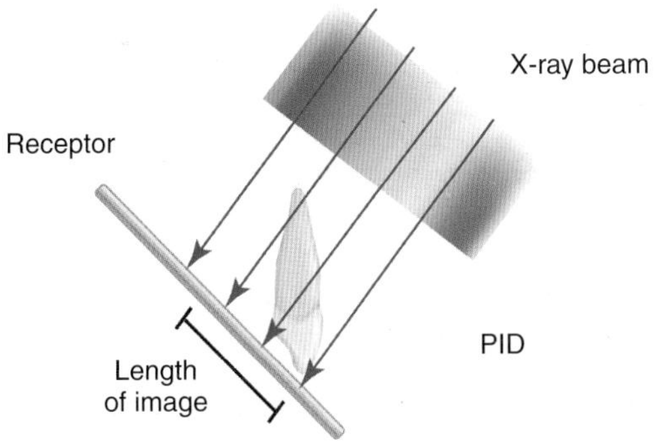

Fig 6-16 If the tooth and receptor are not parallel, an angular relationship is formed, and a distorted image results. In this example, the length of the tooth that appears on the image is shorter than the actual tooth.

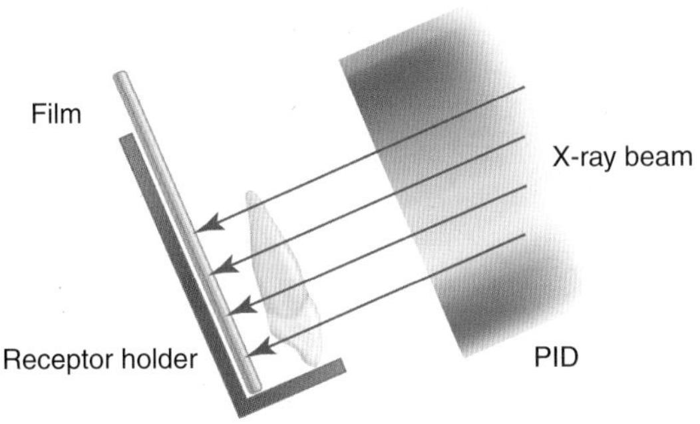

Fig 6-17 To limit distortion, the central ray of the x-ray beam must be perpendicular to the tooth and the receptor.

Object-receptor alignment. To minimize dimensional distortion, the object and receptor must be parallel to each other. If the object (tooth) and receptor are not parallel, an angular relationship results. An angular relationship produces a variation of distances between the tooth and the receptor that results in a distorted image. A distorted image may appear too long or too short (Figure 6-16). Such distortions are discussed in the chapters on technique basics.

X-ray beam angulation. To minimize dimensional distortion, the x-ray beam must be directed perpendicular to the tooth and the receptor. The central ray of the x-ray beam must be as nearly perpendicular to the tooth and receptor as possible to record the adjacent structures in their true spatial relationships (Figure 6-17).

SUMMARY

- A number of factors influence the visual image characteristics of density and contrast as well as the geometric characteristics of sharpness, magnification, and distortion.
- Milliamperage, kilovoltage, and exposure time can be used to adjust the density of a dental radiograph. Subject thickness also influences the density of an image.
- Of the three exposure factors, only the kilovoltage has a direct influence on contrast.
- An image that exhibits areas of black and white is termed *high contrast* and is said to have a short contrast scale.
- An image that exhibits many shades of gray is termed *low contrast* and is said to have a long contrast scale.
- A stepwedge can be used to demonstrate short-scale and long-scale contrast patterns.
- The factors that influence the visual characteristics of density and contrast are reviewed in Table 6-1.
- The factors that influence the geometric characteristics of sharpness, magnification, and distortion are reviewed in Table 6-3.
- To create a sharp image using film, choose an x-ray unit with the smallest focal spot possible, use a film with small crystals in the emulsion, and limit patient, tubehead, and image receptor movements.
- To limit image magnification, use the longest target-receptor distance and the shortest object-receptor distance.
- To limit image distortion, position the receptor and the tooth parallel to each other, and direct the x-ray beam perpendicular to the receptor and the tooth.

BIBLIOGRAPHY

Frommer HH, Stabulas-Savage JJ: Image formation. In Radiology for the dental professional, ed 9, St Louis, 2011, Mosby.

Frommer HH, Stabulas-Savage JJ: Image receptors. In Radiology for the dental professional, ed 9, St Louis, 2011, Mosby.

Johnson ON: Producing quality radiographs. In Essentials of dental radiography for dental assistants and hygienists, ed 9, Upper Saddle River, NJ, 2011, Prentice Hall.

Mallya SM, Lam EWN: Film imaging. In White and Pharoah's oral radiology: principles and interpretation, ed 8, St. Louis, 2019, Elsevier.

Miles DA, Van Dis ML, Jensen CW, et al: Image characteristics. In Radiographic imaging for the dental team, ed 4, St Louis, 2009, Saunders.

QUIZ QUESTIONS

Multiple Choice

____ 1. The portion of a dental image that appears dark or black is termed:
   a. dense
   b. radiolucent
   c. radiopaque
   d. transparent

____ 2. The portion of a dental image that appears light or white is termed:
   a. radiolucent
   b. radiopaque
   c. dense
   d. high density

____ 3. Which appears most radiolucent on a dental image?
   a. bone
   b. enamel
   c. dentin
   d. air space

____ 4. Which appears most radiopaque on a dental image?
   a. bone
   b. enamel
   c. dentin
   d. all of the above

____ 5. The overall blackness or darkness of a dental image is termed:
   a. density
   b. contrast

c. subject thickness
d. diagnostic quality

_____ 6. Increasing the milliamperage (mA) will cause:
a. an increase in density; the image appears darker
b. an increase in density; the image appears lighter
c. a decrease in density; the image appears darker
d. a decrease in density; the image appears lighter

_____ 7. Increasing the operating kilovoltage (kV) will cause:
a. an increase in density; the image appears darker
b. an increase in density; the image appears lighter
c. a decrease in density; the image appears darker
d. a decrease in density; the image appears lighter

_____ 8. Increasing the exposure time will cause:
a. an increase in density; the image appears darker
b. an increase in density; the image appears lighter
c. a decrease in density; the image appears darker
d. a decrease in density; the image appears lighter

_____ 9. A dental patient has thick soft tissues and dense bones. To compensate for this increase in subject thickness and to provide an image of diagnostic density, the dental radiographer may:
a. increase the exposure time
b. increase the milliamperage
c. increase the kilovoltage
d. any of the above

_____ 10. The difference in the degrees of densities between adjacent areas on a dental image is termed:
a. film contrast
b. contrast
c. subject thickness
d. diagnostic quality

_____ 11. A dental image that demonstrates many shades of gray is said to have:
a. high contrast
b. low contrast
c. high density
d. low density

_____ 12. A dental image that demonstrates very dark areas and very light areas is said to have:
a. high contrast
b. low contrast
c. high density
d. low density

For questions 13 to 17, refer to Figure 6-18.

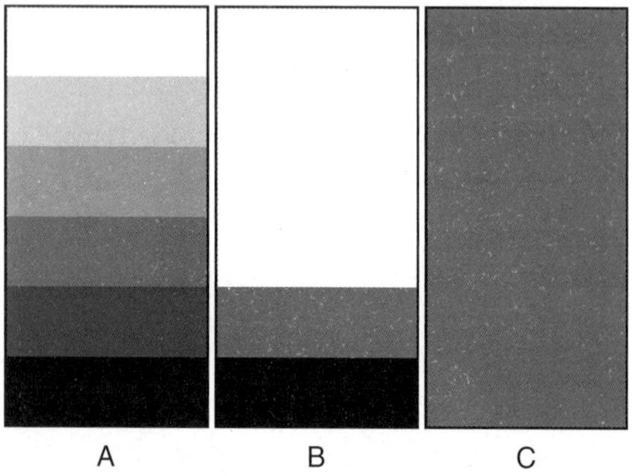

Fig 6-18

_____ 13. In Figure 6-18, which exhibits high contrast?
a. A
b. B
c. C

_____ 14. In Figure 6-18, which exhibits low contrast?
a. A
b. B
c. C

_____ 15. In Figure 6-18, which exhibits long-scale contrast?
a. A
b. B
c. C

_____ 16. In Figure 6-18, which exhibits short-scale contrast?
a. A
b. B
c. C

_____ 17. In Figure 6-18, which exhibits no contrast?
a. A
b. B
c. C

_____ 18. The one exposure factor that has a direct influence on the contrast of a dental image is:
a. kilovoltage
b. milliamperage
c. exposure time
d. subject thickness

_____ 19. The type of contrast preferred in dental imaging is:
a. low contrast
b. long-scale contrast only
c. short-scale contrast only
d. a compromise between short-scale contrast and long-scale contrast

_____ 20. The stepwedge is used for all of the following except:
a. to demonstrate short-scale and long-scale contrast
b. to monitor quality control of film processing
c. to increase the penetrating quality of the x-ray beam
d. to demonstrate densities

_____ 21. The capability of the receptor to reproduce distinct outlines of an object is termed:
a. sharpness
b. magnification
c. distortion
d. diagnostic quality

_____ 22. The unsharp or blurred edges seen on an image are termed:
a. distortion
b. umbra
c. penumbra
d. contrast

_____ 23. The geometric characteristic that refers to an image that appears larger than its actual size is termed:
a. distortion
b. detail
c. definition
d. magnification

_____ 24. A variation in the true size and shape of the object being imaged is termed:
a. magnification
b. distortion
c. sharpness
d. resolution

Fill in the Blank

For questions 25 to 35, fill in the blank with the words *increase* or *decrease*.

_____ 25. Decrease focal spot size = ___________ sharpness.

_____ 26. Increase crystal size = ___________ sharpness.

_____ 27. Decrease crystal size = ___________ sharpness.

_____ 28. Decrease movement = ___________ sharpness.

_____ 29. Increase movement = ___________ sharpness.

_____ 30. Increase target-receptor distance = ___________ magnification.

_____ 31. Increase object-receptor distance = ___________ magnification.

_____ 32. Decrease object-receptor distance = ___________ magnification.

_____ 33. Object and receptor are parallel = ___________ distortion.

_____ 34. Beam perpendicular to object and receptor = ___________ distortion.

_____ 35. Beam not perpendicular to object and receptor = ___________ distortion.

7

Dental X-Ray Equipment

LEARNING OBJECTIVES

After completion of this chapter, the student will be able to do the following:

1. Define the key terms associated with dental x-ray equipment.
2. Discuss the regulation of dental x-ray machines at the federal, state, and local levels.
3. Recognize dental x-ray machines used for intraoral and extraoral exposures.
4. Describe a portable dental x-ray unit and how operator exposure is limited during use.
5. Identify the component parts of the dental x-ray machine.
6. Describe the purpose and use of dental x-ray receptor holders, beam alignment devices, and collimating devices.
7. Identify commonly used dental x-ray receptor holders, beam alignment devices, and collimating devices.

The dental radiographer must be familiar with dental x-ray equipment, receptor holders and beam alignment devices used in digital and film-based imaging. The purpose of this chapter is to introduce the dental radiographer to a variety of intraoral and extraoral dental x-ray machines, to detail the component parts of x-ray machines, and to describe the more common dental x-ray receptor holders, beam alignment devices, and collimating devices.

DENTAL X-RAY MACHINES

A variety of intraoral and extraoral dental x-ray machines is available for diagnostic purposes. Dental x-ray machines vary in both design and operation. The dental radiographer must have a clear understanding of the operating procedures for the specific equipment that is used in the dental office to avoid improper exposure of patients and dental personnel.

Performance Standards

Before 1974, no federal standards existed for the manufacture of dental x-ray machines. All dental x-ray machines manufactured after 1974 must, however, meet specific federal guidelines regulating diagnostic equipment performance standards. The federal government regulates the manufacture and installation of dental x-ray equipment. State and local governments regulate how dental x-ray equipment is used and dictate codes that pertain to the use of x-radiation. Depending on state and local radiation safety codes, dental x-ray equipment must be registered, inspected, and monitored periodically. A fee is typically charged for such services.

Types of Machines

Dental x-ray machines may be used to expose intraoral or extraoral receptors. Some machines are used only for intraoral exposures (Figure 7-1), whereas others are limited to extraoral exposures (Figure 7-2). State-of-the-art x-ray machines produce a wide variety of imaging types (Figure 7-3).

Some intraoral units are portable and allow for exposures outside of the dental office in sites such as nursing homes and mobile clinics (Figure 7-4). These lightweight, handheld units are battery powered and have been recently approved for use in dentistry by the U.S. Food and Drug Administration. Scientific studies have shown that these units can be held stable during exposure and produce high-quality diagnostic images. Operator exposure is limited by the use of a lead acrylic disk shield that surrounds the PID and minimizes backscatter from the patient. Handheld x-ray units are approved in many, but not all, states. Each individual state radiation control board determines the use and protection requirements for such units.

Component Parts: Intraoral X-Ray Machine

As detailed in Chapter 2, the typical intraoral dental x-ray machine features three component parts: (1) tubehead, (2) extension arm, and (3) control panel.

Tubehead. The tubehead, or tube housing, contains the x-ray tube that produces dental x-rays (Figure 7-5). Extending from the tubehead opening is the position-indicating device (PID), or cone. The PID may be round or rectangular in shape and restricts the size of the x-ray beam.

Extension Arm. The extension arm suspends the x-ray tubehead, houses the electrical wires, and allows for movement and positioning of the tubehead.

Control Panel. The control panel, which allows the dental radiographer to regulate the x-ray beam, is plugged into an electrical outlet and appears as a console or cabinet. A control panel may be mounted on a floor pedestal, a wall support, or a remote wall location outside the dental operatory. A single control panel may be used to operate more than one x-ray unit located in adjacent rooms. The control panel consists of (1) an on-off switch and indicator light, (2) an exposure button

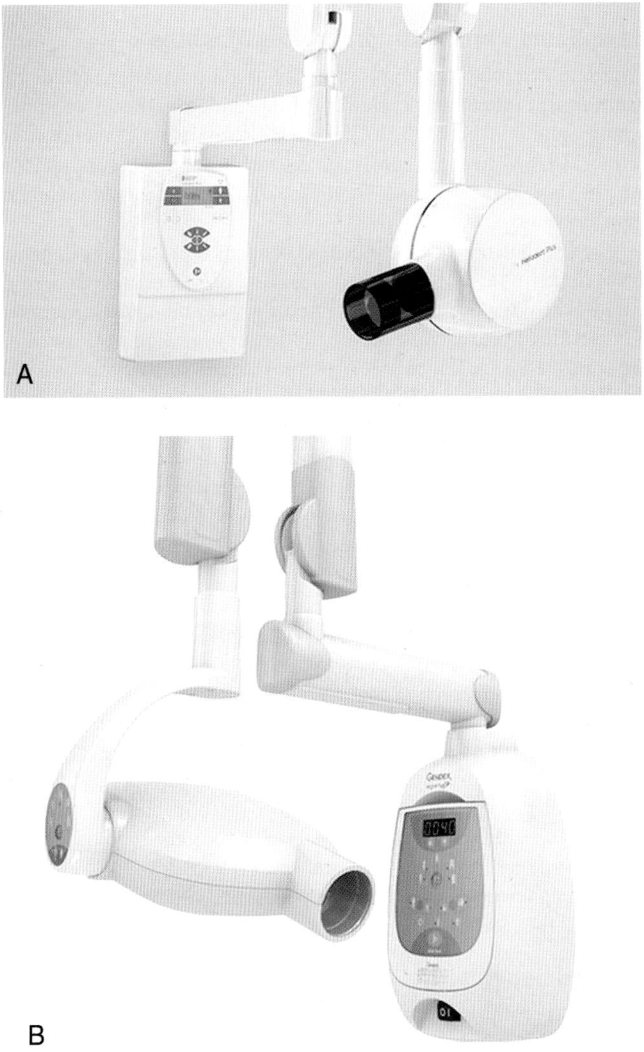

Fig 7-1 **A,** Heliodent Plus intraoral x-ray machine. (Courtesy Dentsply Sirona USA, Charlotte, NC.) **B,** KaVo Focus intraoral x-ray machine. (Courtesy KaVo Imaging, Brea, CA.)

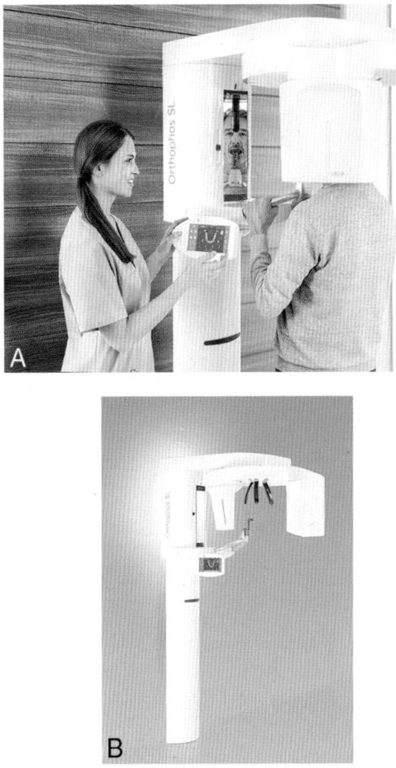

Fig 7-2 **A,** Orthophos E extraoral x-ray machine. **B,** Orthophos SL 2D/3D extraoral x-ray machine. (Courtesy Dentsply Sirona USA, Charlotte, NC.)

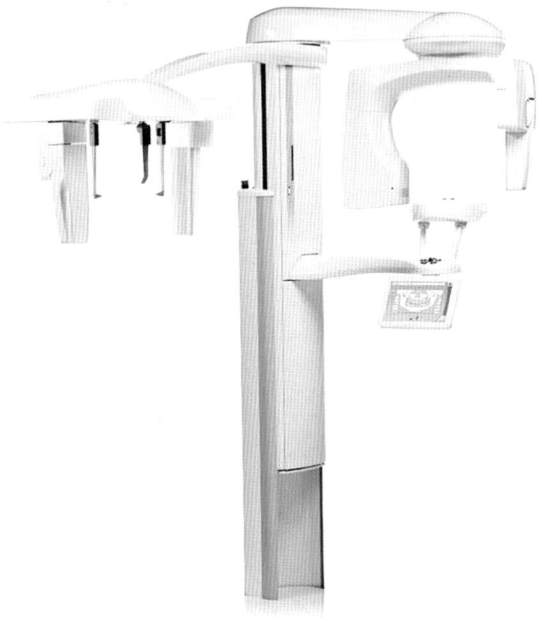

Fig 7-3 The Planmeca Promax 2D S3 offers a complete maxillofacial imaging system, including panoramic, sinus and TMJ imaging, as well as extraoral bite-wings. (Courtesy Planmeca USA Inc., Hoffman Estate, IL.)

and exposure light, (3) a control device for time, and (4) with some units, control devices for kilovoltage and milliamperage (Figure 7-6).

On-off switch. The on-off switch must be placed in the "on" position to operate the dental x-ray equipment. An indicator light is illuminated when the equipment is turned on.

Exposure button. The exposure button activates the machine to produce x-rays. The dental radiographer must firmly depress the exposure button until the preset exposure time is completed. As a visible sign that x-rays are being produced, an exposure light on the control panel is illuminated during x-ray exposure. In addition, a beep sounds during x-ray exposure as an audible signal that x-rays are being produced. The exposure light turns off and the beep stops when the x-ray exposure is completed.

Control devices. The control devices that regulate the x-ray beam include the timer and the kilovoltage (kV) and milliamperage (mA) selectors. The timer determines the length of exposure time in seconds. The kV and mA selectors permit the dental radiographer to adjust and set the correct kilovoltage and milliamperage. Some dental x-ray units have preset programmable settings for the various anatomic areas of the maxilla and the mandible or for different sizes of patients, thus eliminating the need to set the individual controls of kV, mA, and time.

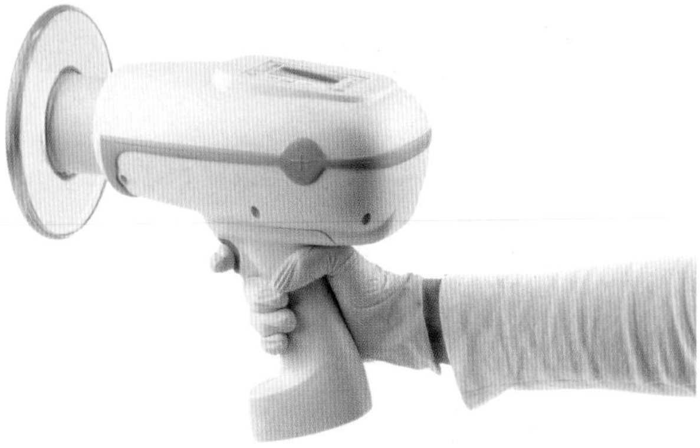

Fig 7-4 NOMAD Pro 2 Handheld X-Ray. (Courtesy Aribex, Charlotte, NC.)

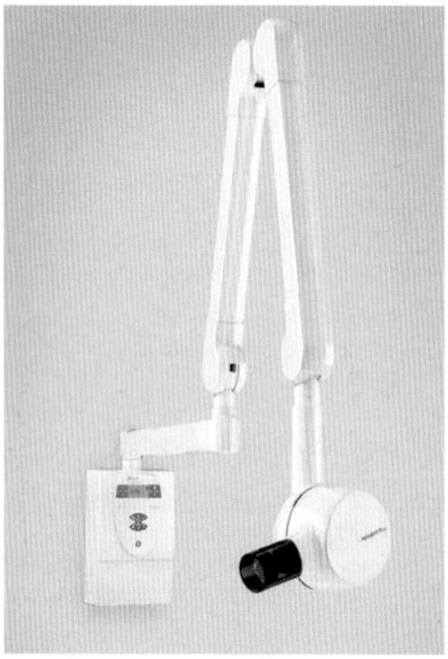

Fig 7-5 The tubehead of the Heliodent Plus contains the x-ray tube. (Courtesy Dentsply Sirona USA, Charlotte, NC.)

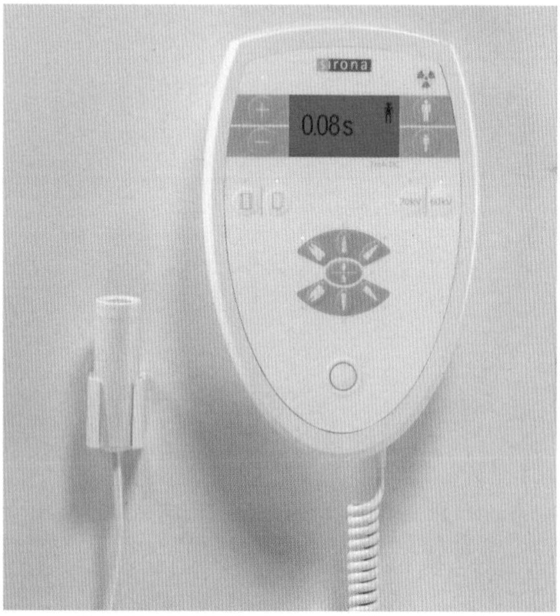

Fig 7-6 Heliodent control panel. (Courtesy Sirona Dental Inc. USA, Charlotte, NC.)

Component Parts: Extraoral X-Ray Machine

Common extraoral imaging techniques used in dentistry include the panoramic, cephalometric, skull imaging, and cone-beam computer tomography (Chapters 25, 26, and 27). The main components of an extraoral x-ray machine consist of the tubehead; positioning devices for the lateral head, chin, forehead, and anterior teeth; and an exposure control panel.

As mentioned earlier, the tubehead contains the x-ray tube that produces dental x-rays. The PID may be round or rectangular, as seen in intraoral imaging machines. Most often, the x-ray tubehead is mounted on one side of the machine, where the sensor or detector is located on the opposite side. Stabilizing devices for the head, chin, and sides of the face are not only important in positioning the patient correctly, but also aid in keeping the patient still during exposure time. Exposure times may range from a few moments up to 20–30 seconds. A bite-block may also be required to keep the anterior teeth separated for ease of viewing anatomic structures. Manufacturers of extraoral machines program the exposure settings to accommodate a wide variety of patients.

DENTAL X-RAY RECEPTOR HOLDERS AND BEAM ALIGNMENT DEVICES

A receptor holder is a device used to hold and align intraoral dental x-ray receptors in the mouth. Receptor holders eliminate the need for the patient to stabilize the receptor. With certain intraoral techniques (e.g., paralleling technique), the use of a receptor-holding device is required. Specific intraoral techniques and receptor-holding devices are discussed in Chapters 19, 20, and 21. A beam alignment device is used to help the dental radiographer position the PID in relation to the tooth and the receptor.

Types of Receptor Holders

Intraoral receptor holders are commercially available from a number of manufacturers. The simplest holder is a disposable Styrofoam bite-block with a backing plate and a slot for receptor retention; examples include XCP Bite-Block and Stabe Bite-Block (Rinn Corporation) (Figure 7-7). Molded-plastic devices that can be sterilized are also available, including the Snap-A-Ray, formerly named EEZEE-Grip, which is a double-ended instrument that holds the receptor between two serrated plastic grips that can be locked in place (Figure 7-8). Other receptor-holding products include EndoRay and Uni-bite (Figure 7-9).

In digital radiography, a sensor is held in place by a bite-block attachment or by devices that aim the beam and sensor accurately. Beam alignment devices must be used to stabilize and secure the sensor (Figure 7-10).

Types of Beam Alignment Devices

Beam alignment devices, which are available from a number of manufacturers, are used to indicate the PID position in relation to the tooth and receptor. The XCP and BAI beam alignment devices (Rinn) feature plastic bite-blocks, plastic aiming rings, and metal indicator arms (Figure 7-11). These devices are available with bite-blocks designed to hold traditional film or digital sensors. For use in conjunction with a beam alignment device, a collimating device may be retrofitted onto the end of a standard PID to restrict the size of the x-ray beam and limit radiation exposure. Examples of such devices include the IDI Tru-Image™ x-ray positioning system (Figure 7-12) and the Rinn Universal collimator (Figure 7-13).

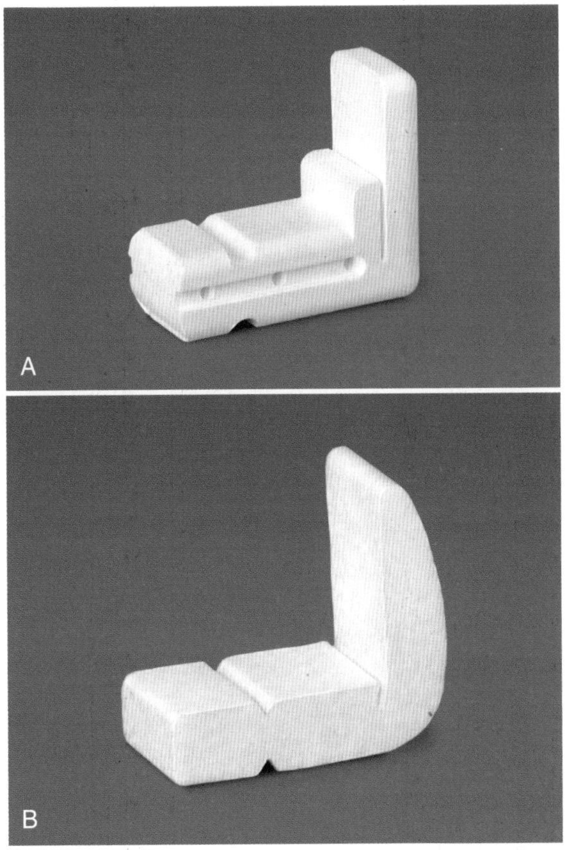

Fig 7-7 A, XCP Bite-Block. B, Stabe Bite-Block. (Courtesy Dentsply Rinn Corporation, York, PA.)

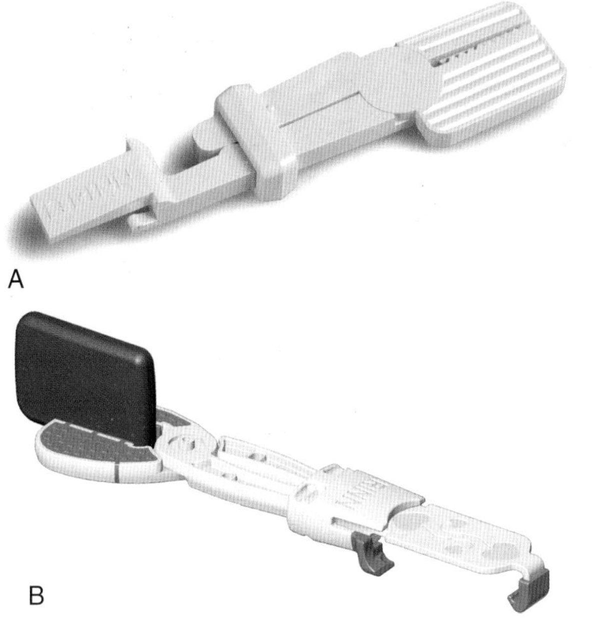

Fig 7-8 A, Snap-A-Ray film holder. The film can be positioned for anterior areas and most posterior areas. B, Snap-A-Ray holder for use with a digital sensor. (Courtesy Dentsply Rinn Corporation, York, PA.)

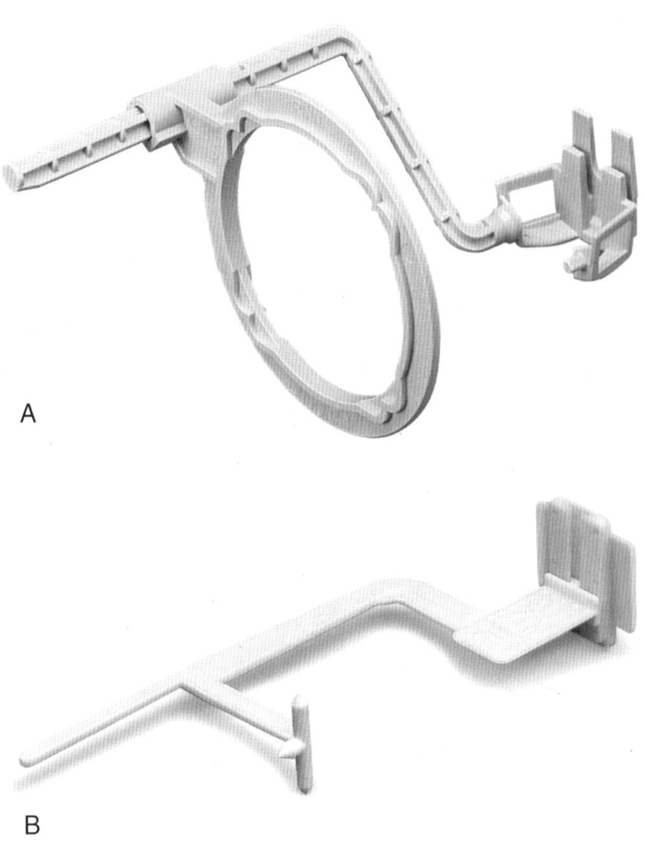

Fig 7-9 A, The EndoRay film holder is used during root canal procedures. It fits around rubber dam clamps and allows space for files to protrude from the tooth. B, The Uni-bite is a universal film holder that can be used with the bite-wing technique or the long-cone paralleling technique for exposure. (Courtesy Dentsply Rinn Corporation, York, PA.)

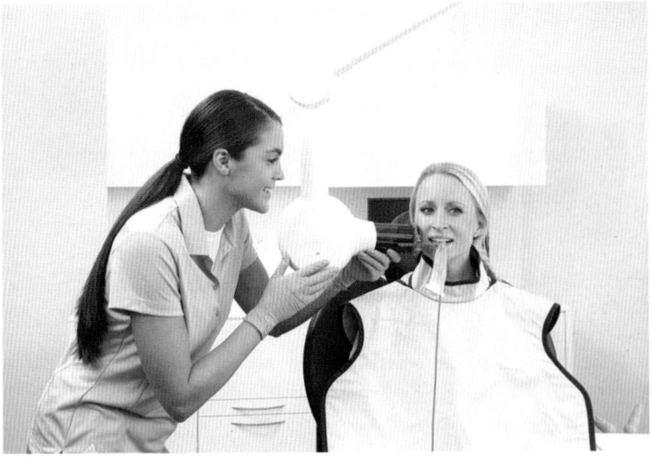

Fig 7-10 A beam alignment device is used to stabilize and secure the digital sensor. (Courtesy Dentsply Sirona USA, Charlotte, NC.)

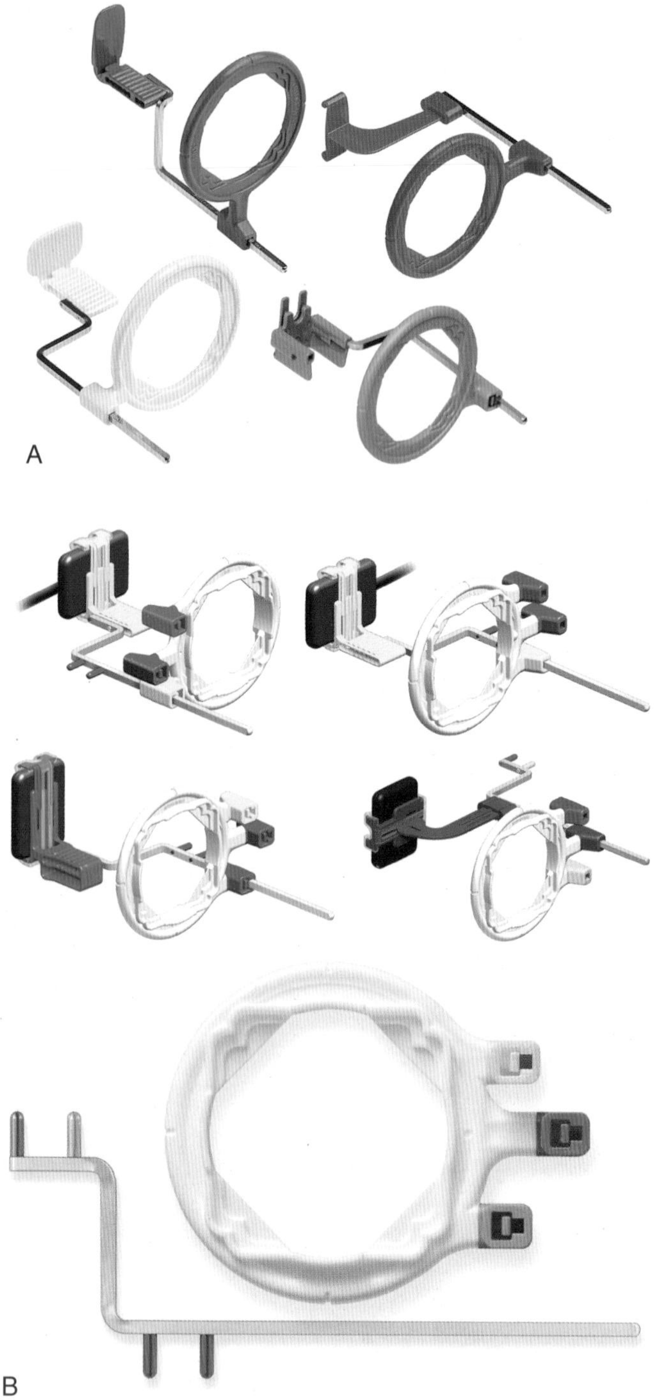

Fig 7-11 A, XCP instruments. The blue instruments are used in the anterior region, the yellow instruments in the posterior region, and the red instruments with the bite-wing technique. The turquoise instruments are used for endodontic procedures. B, XCP-ORA instruments include one ring and one arm. (Courtesy Dentsply Rinn Corporation, York, PA.)

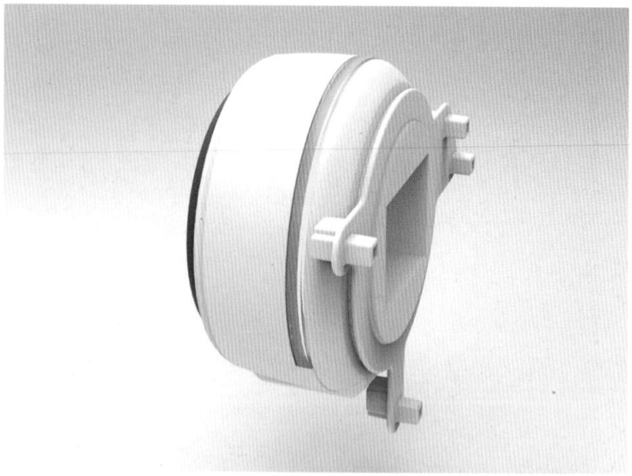

Fig 7-12 Tru-Image™ x-ray positioning system. (Courtesy Interactive Diagnostic Imaging LLC, Marietta, GA.)

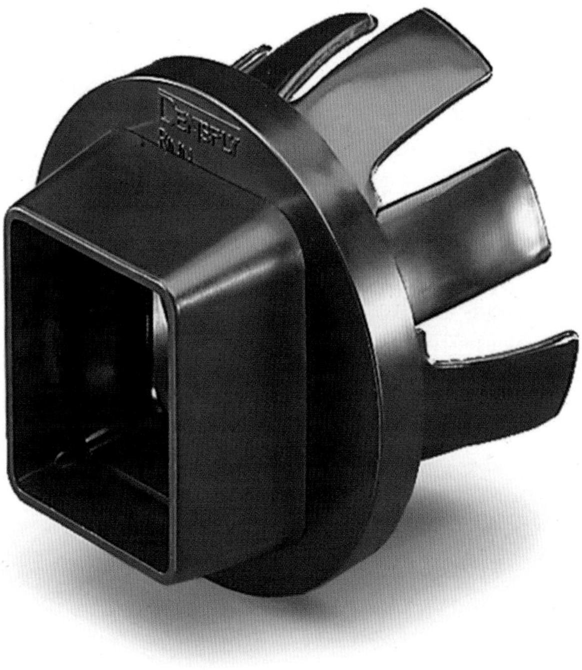

Fig 7-13 Rinn XCP Universal Collimator. (Courtesy Dentsply Rinn Corporation, York, PA.)

SUMMARY

- The dental radiographer must be familiar with how x-ray equipment, receptor holders, beam alignment devices, and collimating devices are used in dentistry.
- State and local governments regulate how dental x-ray equipment is used. Depending on state and local radiation safety codes, dental x-ray equipment must be registered, inspected, and monitored periodically. Dental x-ray units may be used to expose intraoral or extraoral receptors.
- Portable dental x-ray units allow for exposures at sites outside of the dental office.
- The typical intraoral dental x-ray machine consists of three component parts: (1) tubehead, (2) extension arm, and (3) control panel.
- The typical extraoral dental x-ray machine consists of three component parts: (1) tubehead, (2) positioning devices, and (3) control panel.
- A receptor holder is used to stabilize an intraoral receptor, either a film or a sensor.

- A beam alignment device helps the dental radiographer position the PID in relation to the tooth and the receptor.
- A collimating device may be used to further restrict the size of the x-ray beam and reduce patient exposure.

BIBLIOGRAPHY

Frommer HH, Stabulas-Savage JJ: Operator protection. In Radiology for the dental professional, ed 9, St Louis, 2011, Mosby.

Frommer HH, Stabulas-Savage JJ: Patient protection. In Radiology for the dental professional, ed 9, St Louis, 2011, Mosby.

Johnson ON: The periapical examination. In Essentials of dental radiography for dental assistants and hygienists, ed 9, Upper Saddle River, NJ, 2011, Prentice Hall.

Mallya SM, Lam EWN: Intraoral projections. In White and Pharoah's oral radiology: principles and interpretation, ed 8, St. Louis, 2019, Elsevier.

QUIZ QUESTIONS

Multiple Choice

____ 1. No federal standards existed for dental x-ray machines manufactured before the year:
a. 1954
b. 1964
c. 1974
d. 1984

____ 2. Dental receptors placed inside the mouth are termed:
a. intraoral
b. extraoral
c. occlusal
d. all of the above

____ 3. The component part of the dental x-ray machine that contains the x-ray tube is termed the:
a. control panel
b. tubehead
c. extension arm
d. console

____ 4. The component part of the dental x-ray machine that allows movement and positioning of the tubehead is termed the:
a. control panel
b. extension arm
c. console
d. position-indicating device (PID)

____ 5. The dental radiographer can regulate the x-ray beam (kilovoltage, milliamperage, time) through the use of the:
a. control panel
b. extension arm
c. tubehead
d. PID

____ 6. An instrument that is used to help the dental radiographer position the PID in relation to the tooth and receptor is the:
a. receptor holder
b. beam alignment device
c. collimating device
d. none of the above

____ 7. A device that is used to stabilize an intraoral receptor is termed:
a. beam alignment
b. collimator
c. receptor holder
d. none of the above

____ 8. Which of the following is used to restrict the size of the x-ray beam to the size of an intraoral receptor?
a. collimating device
b. receptor holder
c. beam alignment device
d. none of the above

True or False

____ 9. The federal government dictates how dental x-ray equipment is used.

____ 10. State and local governments dictate codes that pertain to the use of dental x-ray equipment.

____ 11. Portable dental x-ray units are approved in all states.

____ 12. Studies have shown that a portable dental x-ray unit can be used to produce high-quality diagnostic images.

____ 13. With a portable dental x-ray unit, operator exposure is limited by using a lead acrylic disk shield around the PID.

____ 14. An example of a collimating device is the Tru-Align Aiming Device.

____ 15. An example of a beam alignment device is the Snap-A-Ray.

8

Digital Imaging

LEARNING OBJECTIVES

After completion of this chapter, the student will be able to do the following:

1. Define the key terms associated with digital imaging.
2. Describe the purpose and use of digital imaging.
3. Discuss the fundamentals of digital imaging.
4. Describe radiation exposure in digital imaging.
5. List and describe the equipment used in digital imaging.
6. List and describe the two types of digital imaging.
7. Describe the patient and equipment preparations required for digital imaging.
8. List and discuss the advantages and disadvantages of digital imaging.

Advances in technology have produced a significant effect in the profession of dentistry and in dental imaging. For more than a century, film was the only medium and recording device for dental imaging. Today, digital imaging is commonplace along with all of the other computerized aspects of a dental practice, including electronic patient records, appointment scheduling, insurance claim processing, and accounts receivable. Patient treatment rooms may feature additional technology such as intraoral digital cameras, digital blood pressure equipment, and electronic charting and treatment planning.

In dental imaging, advances in technology have resulted in a unique "filmless" system known as digital imaging. Since its introduction to dentistry in 1987, digital imaging has influenced not only how dental disease is *recognized* but also how it is *diagnosed*. Digital imaging is a dependable and versatile technique that provides clear, detailed images and enhances interpretation and diagnosis. Before the dental radiographer can use this very specialized technology, an understanding of the basic concepts, which includes terminology, purpose, use, and fundamentals, is necessary. In addition, the dental radiographer must have a working knowledge of the equipment used in digital imaging.

The purpose of this chapter is to present the basic concepts of digital imaging, to introduce the various types, and to discuss the advantages and disadvantages of this form of imaging. Throughout this chapter, numerous references are made to film for comparison purposes. Please refer to Chapter 9 for a complete discussion of film-based imaging.

BASIC CONCEPTS

Digital imaging is a technique used to record dental images. Unlike conventional dental radiography techniques discussed in Chapter 9, no film or processing chemistry is used. Instead, digital imaging uses an electronic sensor and specialized computer software that produces images almost instantly on a computer monitor. Before the dental radiographer can use this technique competently, a thorough understanding of the terminology and fundamentals of digital imaging is necessary. Knowledge of related radiation exposure, equipment, and types of digital imaging is also required.

Terminology

Analog image: Radiographic image produced by conventional film.

Analog-to-digital converter: Method used to convert data elements acquired by the sensor are communicated to the computer in analog form and then converted into digital form.

Bit-depth image: Number of possible gray-scale combinations for each pixel (e.g., 8 bit-depth image has gray-scale combination of 2^8, which equals 256 shades of gray).

Charge-coupled device (CCD): Solid-state silicon chip detector that converts light or x-ray photons into an electrical charge or signal; in digital imaging, CCD is found in the sensor.

Digital imaging: Filmless imaging system; a method of capturing an image using a sensor, breaking it into electronic pieces, and presenting and storing the image using a computer and related imaging software.

Digital image: An image composed of pixels that can be stored in a computer.

Digital subtraction: One feature of digital imaging; a method of reversing the gray scale as an image is viewed; radiolucent images (normally black) appear white, and radiopaque images (normally white) appear black.

Digitize: In digital imaging, to convert an image into a digital form that, in turn, can be processed by a computer.

Direct digital imaging: Method of obtaining a digital image, in which an intraoral sensor is exposed to x-radiation to capture a dental image that can be viewed on a computer monitor.

Indirect digital imaging: Method of obtaining a digital image, in which a sensor is scanned after exposure to x-radiation and then converted into a digital form that can be viewed on a computer monitor.

Line pairs/millimeter (lp/mm): Measurement used to evaluate the ability of the computer to capture the resolution (or detail) of an image.

Pixel: A discrete unit of information. In digital electronic images, digital information is contained in, and presented as, discrete units of information; also termed *picture element*.

Sensor: In digital imaging, a receptor that is used to capture an intraoral or extraoral image.

Storage phosphor imaging: Method of obtaining a digital image in which the image is recorded on a phosphor-coated plate and then placed into an electronic processor, where a laser scans the plate and produces an image on a computer monitor.

Purpose and Use

The purpose of digital imaging is to generate images that can be used in the diagnosis and assessment of dental disease. The images produced are diagnostically equivalent or better compared with film-based imaging, thus enabling the dental radiographer to see conditions that cannot be identified clinically and to identify many conditions that may otherwise go undetected. Digital imaging allows the radiographer to obtain a wealth of information about teeth and supporting structures. Uses of digital imaging include the following:

- To detect lesions, diseases, and conditions of teeth and surrounding structures that cannot be detected clinically
- To confirm or classify suspected disease
- To localize lesions or foreign objects
- To provide information during dental procedures (e.g., root canal therapy instrumentation and surgical placement of implants)
- To evaluate growth and development
- To illustrate changes secondary to caries, periodontal disease, or trauma
- To document the condition of a patient at a specific point in time
- To aid in the development of a clinical treatment plan

Fundamentals

The term *digital imaging* refers to a method of capturing an image using a sensor, breaking the image into electronic pieces, and presenting and storing the image using a computer and imaging software. Film-based images are produced when x-ray photons strike an intraoral film; the information recorded on the film is known as an analog image. Analog images are depicted by a continuous spectrum of gray shades between the extremes of white and black. It might be helpful to visualize a painting done entirely in black, grays, and white; these shades flow together on a canvas, and it is difficult to see where one shade ends and another begins. In digital imaging, the sensor receives the analog information and converts it to a digital image in the computer processing unit. The digital image is an array of picture elements, called *pixels*, with discrete gray values for each pixel. Imagine the same black, gray, and white painting just described, but in a mosaic pattern instead of the shades flowing together. Each tiny square of the mosaic is similar to an individual pixel.

Traditional film-based imaging consists of x-radiation interacting with the silver halide crystals of the film emulsion, production of a latent image, and chemical processing to convert the latent image into a visible image. In digital imaging, a sensor is used as the receptor to capture the dental images. The sensor is used in place of dental film. As in film-based imaging, the x-ray beam is directed at the receptor. An electronic charge is produced on the surface of the sensor; this electronic signal is digitized, or converted into digital form. The sensor, in turn, transmits this information to a computer, and the computer stores the incoming electronic signal. Data elements acquired by the sensor are communicated to the computer in analog form and then converted into digital form by the use of an *analog-to-digital converter (ADC)*. Software is used to store the image electronically. The image is displayed within seconds to minutes and may be readily manipulated to enhance its appearance for interpretation and diagnosis.

In dental imaging, the term digital image (*not* radiograph or x-ray film) is used to describe the pictures that are produced (Figure 8-1). Digital imaging systems are not limited to intraoral images; panoramic, cephalometric, cone-beam computer tomography, and other extraoral images may also be obtained (Figure 8-2). For example, if the extraoral film traditionally used in panoramic radiography is replaced with an electronic sensor, that sensor delivers the image information to a computer for storage in digital format. As with intraoral digital imaging, the extraoral images are displayed using imaging software on a computer monitor and may be stored for future use.

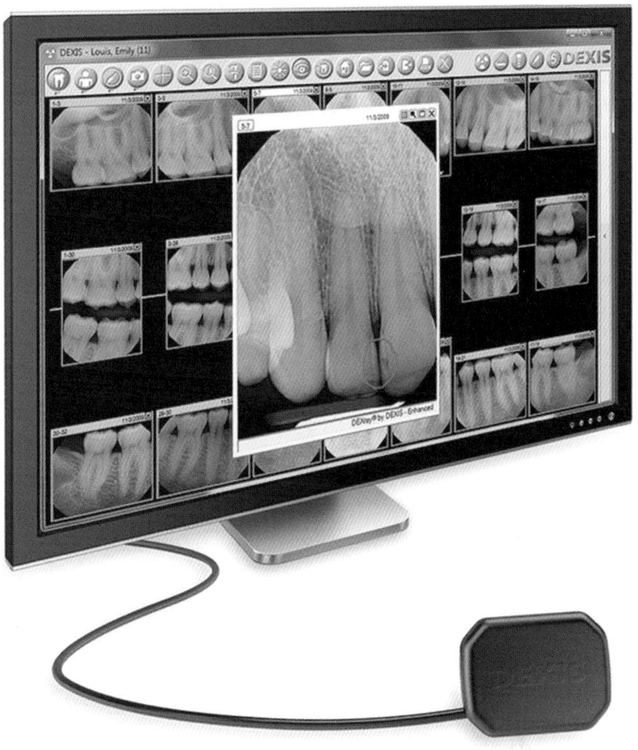

Fig 8-1 A full mouth series of digital images displayed on a computer monitor. (Courtesy KaVo Imaging, Brea, CA.)

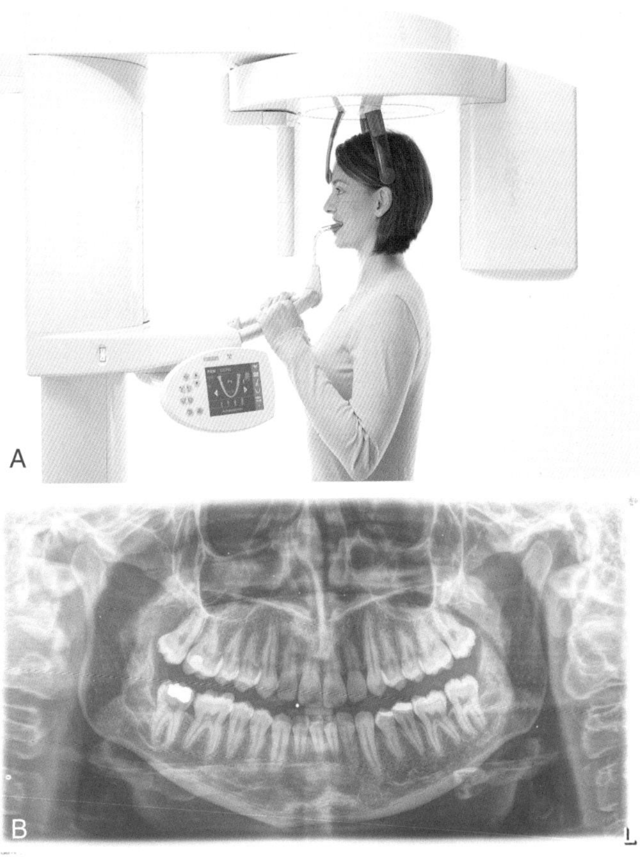

Fig 8-2 **A,** A panoramic machine used with digital imaging. **B,** An example of a panoramic digital image. (Courtesy Sirona USA, Charlotte, NC.)

Radiation Exposure

Digital imaging requires less x-radiation exposure than film-based imaging. Less x-radiation is necessary to form a digital image on the sensor because the sensor is more sensitive to x-radiation than is conventional film. Depending on the speed of film that is being used, exposure times for digital imaging are 50% to 90% less than those required for conventional radiography. For example, the typical exposure time required to produce an image for digital imaging is 0.05 seconds. This exposure time is much less than the 0.2 seconds required for intraoral film used in conventional radiography. With less radiation exposure, the absorbed dose to the patient is significantly reduced. Less radiation exposure supports the ALARA principle, and therefore the use of digital imaging is highly recommended.

Equipment

Digital imaging requires the use of specialized equipment. The essential components of a digital imaging system include an intraoral dental x-ray unit, a sensor, and a computer with imaging software.

X-Ray Unit. A conventional intraoral dental x-ray unit may be used in both film-based and digital imaging. If the dental x-ray unit has a timer that uses impulses (allowing for 1/60 of a second), the timer must be adapted to allow for exposures in 1/100 of a second. If the timer cannot be adapted, the unit will need to be replaced. A standard dental x-ray unit that is adapted for digital imaging is still functional for film-based imaging (Figure 8-3). Dental x-ray units that are designed for digital imaging are modern in appearance and feature adjustments for shorter exposure times, better image quality, and reduced patient radiation.

Sensor. In digital imaging, the receptor that is used is a sensor. As previously defined, the sensor is a detector that is used to capture the dental image (Figure 8-4). Intraoral sensors vary in size, thickness, and stiffness; some are thick and rigid, whereas others mimic conventional film in size and flexibility (Figure 8-5). Manufacturers produce intraoral sensors similar in dimension to sizes 0, 1, 2, and 4 of films, as well as extraoral sensors for panoramic and cephalometric projections (Figure 8-6). Intraoral sensors used in digital imaging systems may be wired or wireless. The term *wired* refers to the fact that the imaging sensor is physically linked by a fiber optic cable to a computer that records the generated signal (Figure 8-7). In wired systems, the common cable length varies from 3 to 9 feet; the shorter the cable, the more limited the range of motion (Figure 8-8). The term *wireless* refers to an imaging sensor that is *not* linked by a cable; the wireless sensor sends data to the computer via wi-fi, a wireless networking technology that uses radio waves. Wireless sensors are thicker than wired sensors and are battery powered. The image quality is not affected by the wireless transmission. Wireless sensors are more expensive than their wired counterparts.

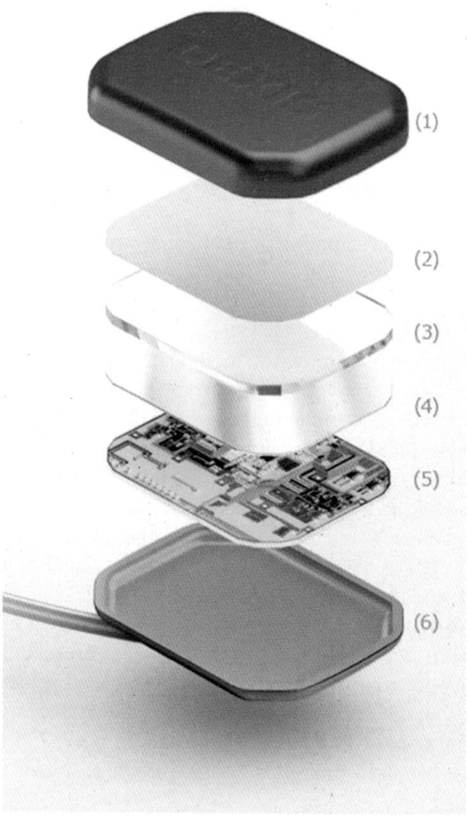

Fig 8-4 Component parts of a sensor. Dexis Platinum Sensor (1) front casing—forms watertight and light-tight barrier, (2) scintillator screen—converts x-ray beam into visible light, (3) fiber optic face plate—transmits light to sensor surface, (4) CMOS imaging chip—captures light from screen and creates a charge in each pixel, (5) sensor electronics—reads the charge in each pixel and transmits to computer, and (6) back casing /protective shield & cable—forms watertight and light-tight barrier and prevents backscatter. (Courtesy KaVo Imaging, Brea, CA.)

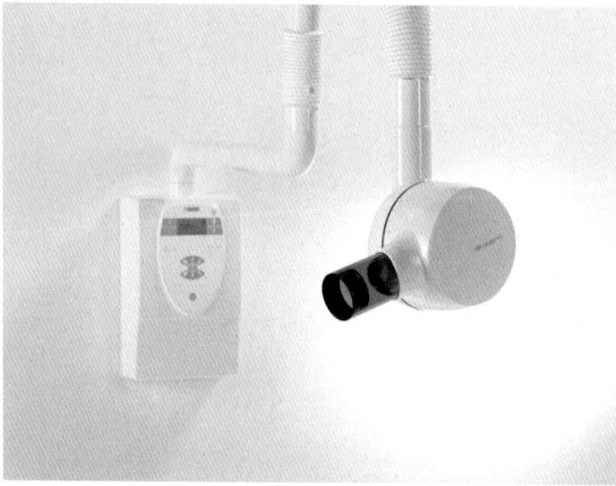

Fig 8-3 A conventional source of x-radiation is used with digital imaging. (Courtesy Sirona USA, Charlotte, NC.)

Fig 8-5 Wired sensor, intraoral film, and digital phosphor plate. (Courtesy Gail F. Williamson, Indianapolis, IN.)

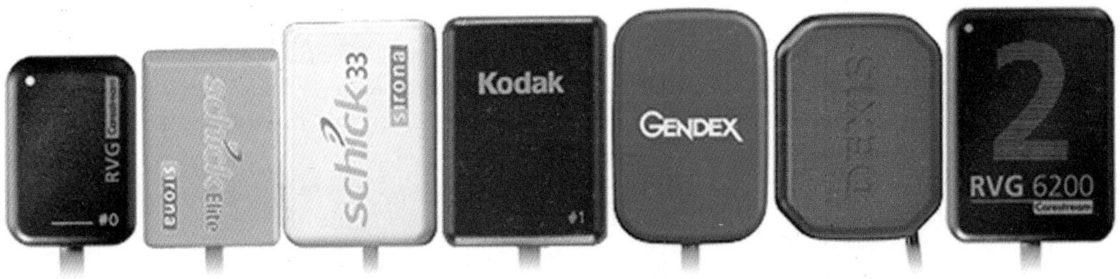

Fig 8-6 Examples of wired sensors. (Courtesy repairdds.com.)

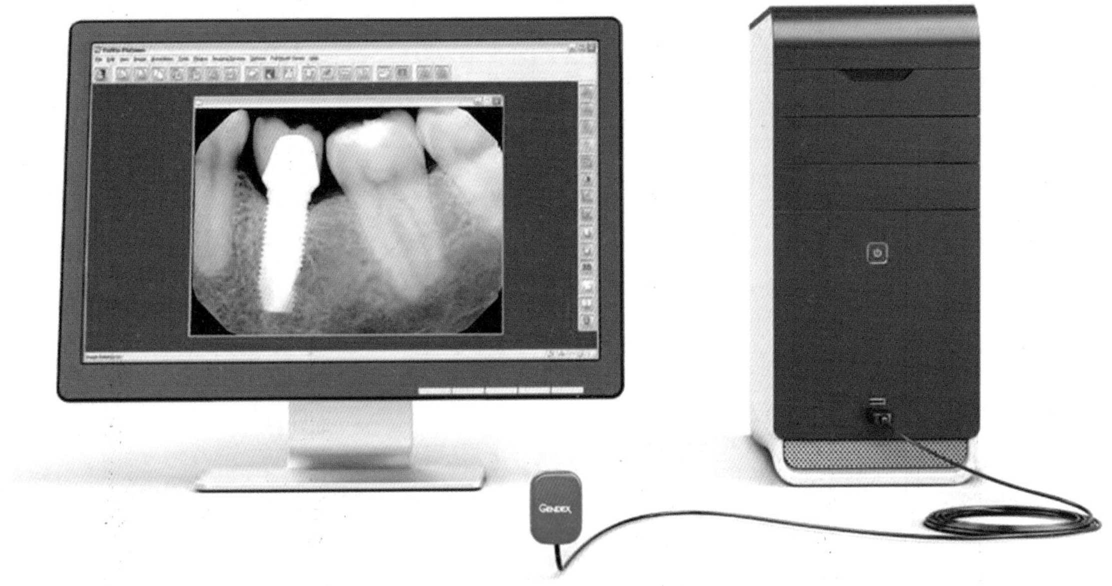

Fig 8-7 A wired sensor used with digital imaging showing the intraoral sensor at one end and the link to the computer at the other end. (Courtesy KaVo Imaging, Brea, CA.)

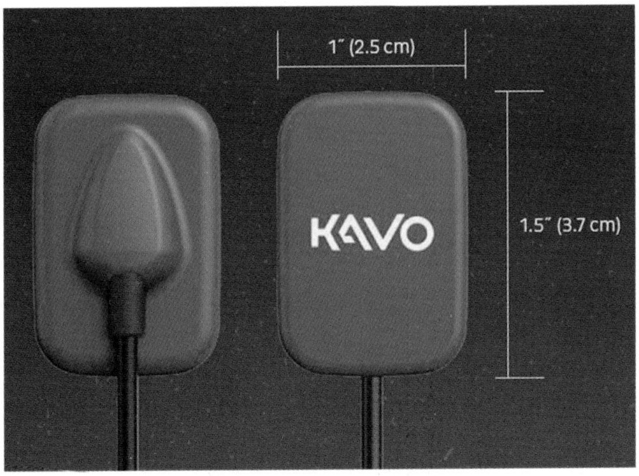

Fig 8-8 Intraoral sensor, front and back views. (Courtesy KaVo Imaging, Brea, CA.)

The most popular types of direct digital sensor technology include the charge-coupled device and the complementary metal oxide semiconductor. Both are rigid, solid-state detectors made of silicon that are arranged in an array of x-ray sensitive pixels.

Charge-coupled device. The charge-coupled device (CCD) is a common receptor used in dental digital imaging. The CCD technology used in digital imaging relies on a specialized and costly fabrication process. The CCD is a solid-state detector that contains a silicon chip with an electronic circuit embedded in it. This silicon chip is sensitive to x-radiation or light. The CCD is not a new technology; it was initially developed in the 1960s and has been used in many devices, including fax machines, home video cameras, microscopes, and telescopes. The electrons that compose the silicon chip in the CCD can be visualized as being divided into an arrangement of blocks or picture elements known as *pixels*. A pixel is a small box, or "well," into which the electrons produced by the x-ray exposure are deposited. A pixel is the digital equivalent of a silver crystal used in conventional radiography. As opposed to a film emulsion that contains a *random* arrangement of silver crystals, a pixel is structured in an *ordered* arrangement. The CCD functions to sense transmitted light and translate it into an electronic message. Each pixel is approximately 40 μm to 20 μm in size and is configured into rows arranged in a matrix of 512 × 512 pixels. The pixel size varies depending on the digital receptor, and the size of the pixel has an influence on the image resolution.

The x-ray photons that come into contact with the CCD cause electrons to be released from the silicon and produce a corresponding electronic charge. Consequently, each pixel arrangement, or *electron potential well*, contains an electronic charge proportional to the number of electrons that reacted within the well. Furthermore, each electronic well corresponds to a specific area on the linked computer screen. When x-radiation activates electrons and produces such electronic charges, an electronic latent image is produced. The latent image is then transmitted and stored in a computer and can be converted to a visible image on screen or printed on paper.

Complementary metal oxide semiconductor—active pixel sensor. The complementary metal oxide semiconductor (CMOS) is a solid-state detector similar to the CCD that has built-in control functions, smaller pixel size, and lower power requirements. The CMOS detector is silicon based and differs from the CCD detector in the way that the pixels are read. Although the CMOS process is the standard in the making of chips, it was not until the active pixel sensor (APS) was developed that CMOS became useful as a sensor in dental digital imaging. This sensor technology is termed the complementary metal oxide semiconductor—active pixel sensor (CMOS-APS). The CMOS-APS is a CMOS detector with active amplifying transistors integrated into each pixel to improve signal output. The advantages of the CMOS-APS technology are that the individual pixels can be made smaller, the power requirements are less, and the production cost of the chip is lower. CMOS sensors can be connected to a computer using a low-power external connection such as a USB.

Computer. In digital imaging, a computer with imaging software is used to store the incoming electronic signal. The imaging software is responsible for converting the electronic signal from the sensor into a shade of gray that is viewed on the computer monitor. Each pixel is represented numerically in the computer by location and the color level of the gray. The range of numbers for a pixel varies from 0 (black) to 255 (white), which creates 256 shades of gray, referred to as a pixel's *gray-scale resolution*. In comparison, the human eye can perceive only 32 shades of gray.

The number of possible gray-scale combinations per pixel is known as the bit-depth image. The computer software for the digital system determines the bit-depth image. For each pixel, the number of possible gray-scale combinations is 2^N; for example, an 8 bit-depth image has a gray-scale combination of 2^8, which equals 256 shades of gray. The software also allows for manipulation of the pixels, enhancing contrast and density without additional x-ray exposure of the patient.

The imaging software digitizes, processes, and stores information received from the sensor. The exposure can be viewed immediately on the computer monitor. An image is recorded on a computer monitor in 0.5 to 120 seconds, far less time than required for conventional film processing (Figure 8-9). This speed of image recording is extremely useful during certain dental procedures, such as the placement of surgical implants or during endodontic instrumentation. The image may be stored permanently in the computer, printed out as a hard copy for the patient record, or transmitted electronically to insurance companies or referring dental specialists.

Various computer-viewing features are available with digital imaging software systems. Digital systems feature split-screen technology, which allows the operator to view and compare multiple images on the same screen (Figure 8-10). This feature is helpful for comparison and to

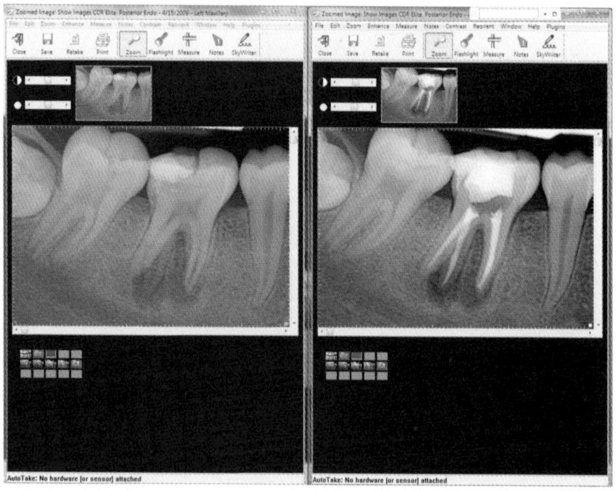

Fig 8-10 Split-screen technology that assists the dental professional to view several images of tooth #30 simultaneously. (Courtesy Sirona USA, Charlotte, NC.)

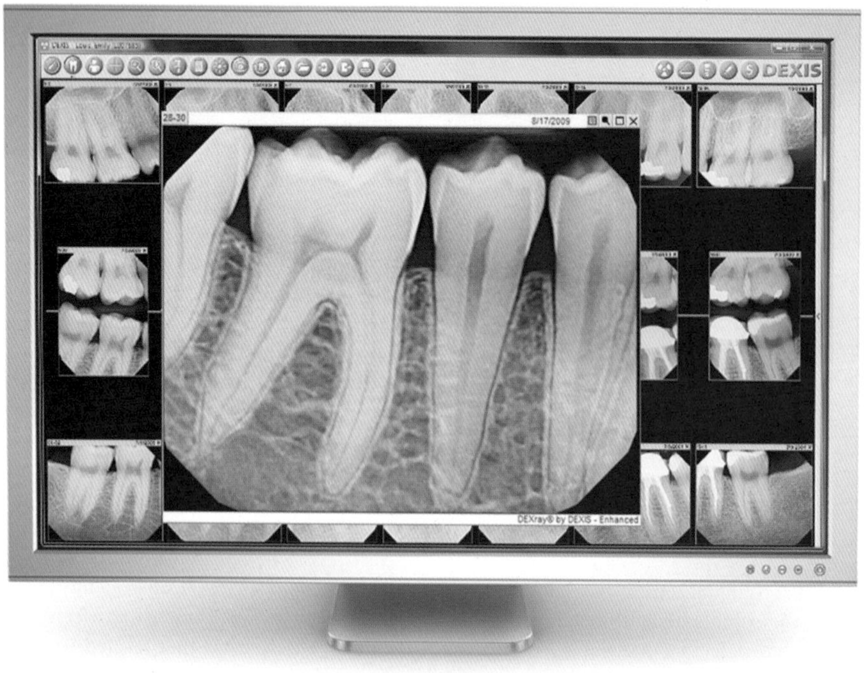

Fig 8-9 A digital image of the mandibular right periapical region as seen on a computer monitor. (Courtesy KaVo Imaging, Brea, CA.)

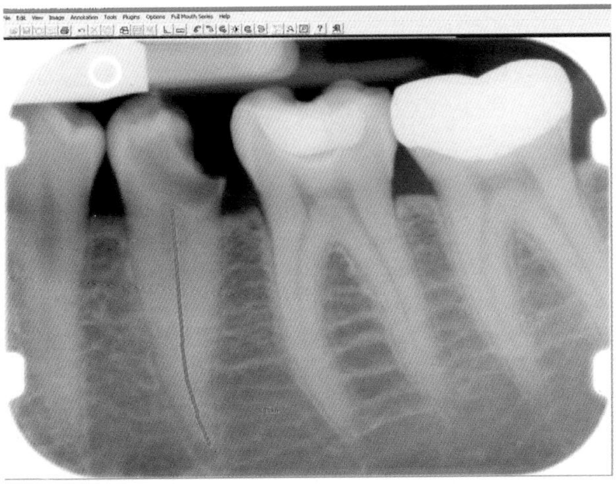

Fig 8-11 An example of a measurement tool as part of the imaging software. (Courtesy Dr. Donald Tyndall, The University of North Carolina School of Dentistry, Chapel Hill, NC.)

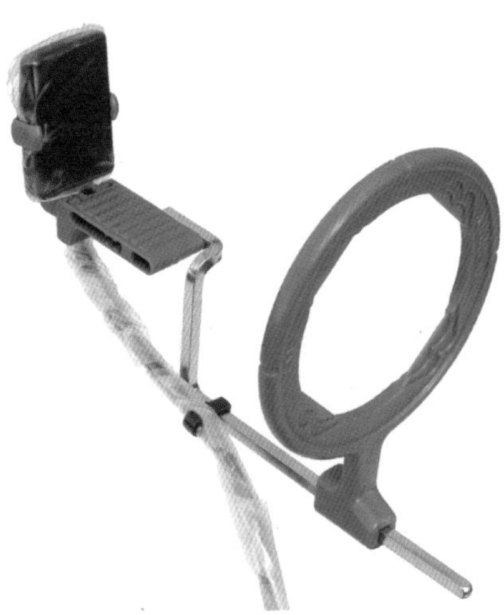

Fig 8-12 A beam alignment device assembled for the anterior region holds the digital sensor and secures the wire attachment. (Courtesy Dentsply Rinn Corporation, York, PA.)

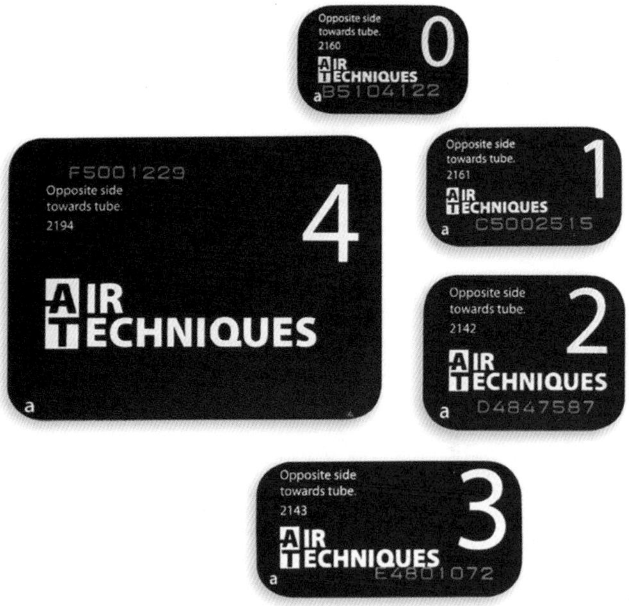

Fig 8-13 Examples of intraoral phosphor sensor sizes. (Courtesy Air Techniques, Melville, NY.)

evaluate the progression of caries or periodontal disease—for example, by comparing previous to current bite-wing images.

Digital systems also provide a feature that allows specific images to be magnified up to four times the original size. This feature is helpful when evaluating the apical area of a tooth. Many digital systems include a measurement tool as part of the imaging software. Measurement tools are valuable in therapies such as endodontic procedures or in implant treatment planning. Linear and angular measurements must be made with the proper projection geometry, avoiding such errors as elongation or foreshortening, which may distort the measurements (Figure 8-11).

TYPES OF DIGITAL IMAGING

Two methods of obtaining a digital image currently exist: (1) direct digital imaging and (2) indirect digital imaging.

Direct Digital Imaging

Direct digital imaging is a method of obtaining a digital image using an intraoral sensor that is exposed to x-radiation to transfer information *directly* to a computer with imaging software. The essential components of a direct digital imaging system include an intraoral dental x-ray unit, a sensor, and a computer with imaging software. An intraoral sensor with a fiber optic cable linked to the computer, or a wireless sensor, is placed into the mouth of the patient and exposed to x-radiation (Figure 8-12). The sensor captures the dental image and then transmits the image directly to a computer monitor. Within seconds of exposing the sensor to radiation, an image appears on the computer screen. Software is then used to enhance and store the image. Extraoral imaging machines also use direct digital sensors with either CCD or CMOS detectors.

Indirect Digital Imaging

Indirect digital imaging is a method of obtaining a digital image from a sensor after exposure to x-radiation by using a scanner to convert information into a digital form so that it can then be viewed on a computer monitor. Unlike direct digital imaging, there is an extra step—the scanning. The essential components of an indirect digital imaging system include an intraoral dental x-ray unit, a PSP plate, a scanner, and a computer with imaging software. A common type of indirect digital imaging is storage phosphor imaging. Storage phosphor imaging is also referred to as *photo-stimulable phosphor imaging* (PSP). PSP imaging has been in use since 1981 and has been the basis of hospital digital imaging systems. The use of a PSP receptor or "plate" is considered indirect digital imaging because a scanning process in needed to digitize the image and transmit the image to a computer.

In this system, a reusable imaging plate coated with phosphors known as a *PSP plate* is used. This PSP plate is flexible like film and similar in size, shape, and thickness (Figure 8-13). The intraoral PSP plate is reusable and is placed into the mouth in the same way as an intraoral film is positioned. PSP plates are manufactured for both intraoral and extraoral imaging. A PSP plate functions similarly to the intensifying screen that is used to expose an extraoral film—after exposure, it converts x-ray energy into light. This image remains on the reusable plate until it is erased after the scanning process. In past years, images were

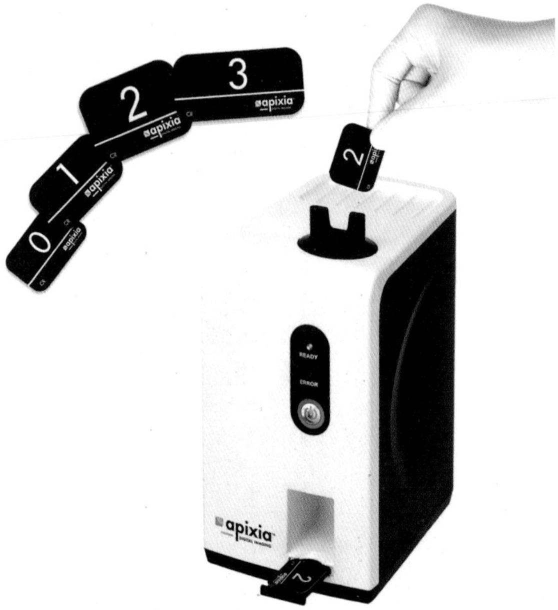

Fig 8-14 A storage phosphor imaging system, illustrating the laser scanning device and the intraoral and extraoral PSP digital sensors. (Courtesy Apixia Digital Imaging, Industry, CA.)

erased or cleared from the PSP plates by exposure to viewbox light for several minutes. Currently, manufacturers use technology that scans and retrieves the digital image, followed by a clearing step for reuse of the PSP plate (Figure 8-14). Once the image is erased, the plate may be disinfected and then inserted into a disposable barrier envelope for reuse. Extreme care must be taken when exposing, handling, and wrapping these receptors because bending or scratching can damage PSP plates. With careful handling, the typical PSP plate is designed to be reused 50 or more times.

When exposed to x-rays, a PSP plate records diagnostic data. A high-speed scanner is then used to convert the information into electronic files. The plate is placed into an electronic "scanner" or processor, and a laser then scans the plate and produces an image that is transferred to computer imaging software. Because of this step involving laser scanning, which can take 30 seconds to several minutes, this type of digital imaging is less rapid than direct digital. The dental radiographer must make certain to orient the PSP plate in the patient's mouth so that the correct side faces the beam. To aid in placement, *"opposite side toward tube"* is printed on the PSP plate. Currently, some PSP systems do not distinguish images that have been exposed backward (similar to placing a film in the mouth with the colored side facing the tubehead). Therefore it is recommended that the dental radiographer review the mounted digital images and confirm the images with the clinical findings while the patient is present in the dental chair. Table 8-1 summarizes the comparisons between direct and indirect digital imaging.

STEP-BY-STEP PROCEDURES

Step-by-step procedures for the use of digital imaging systems vary from manufacturer to manufacturer. It is critical to refer to the manufacturer's instruction booklet for information on the operation of the system, equipment preparation, patient preparation, and exposure. Only general guidelines concerning intraoral sensor preparation and placement are provided here.

TABLE 8-1 Comparison of Digital Imaging Receptors

	DIRECT	INDIRECT
description	• sensor exposed to x-radiation • DIRECTLY transmits information to computer with imaging software for viewing	• PSP plate exposed to x-radiation • INDIRECTLY transmits information first to a scanner to produce an image then to a computer for viewing
sensor	• SOLID STATE SENSOR (CCD, CMOS)	• PSP PLATES (photostimulable phosphor plates)
light sensitive	• no	• yes • semidark environment needed for plate handling • darkroom red safelights cannot be used
required equipment	• computer / software / monitor • cable or wireless connection to computer	• computer / software / monitor • plate is not connected to computer • laser scanning device • light-tight polyvinyl envelopes for each plate
viewing time	• almost instantaneous, within seconds • no processing or scanning needed	• lag time from exposure to viewing • requires time for scanning • 30 seconds to several minutes
workflow	• improved workflow • increased efficiency	• no improvement in workflow • time needed to place plate in envelope, prepare separate plate needed for each exposure, scanning, and erasing after use
required number	• one sensor used for multiple exposures	• one plate used for each individual exposure, similar to film*
sizes	• 0, 1, 2	• 0, 1, 2, 3, 4
thickness	• bulkier and thicker than film*	• same thickness of film*
receptor active area	• smaller than total surface area of film*	• similar to film*
infection prevention	• disposable protective plastic sleeve	• disposable barrier envelope
strength	• durable • most damage occurs at cable connection • requires careful handling	• subject to wear and tear and prone to artifacts • easily damaged by bending or scratching • requires careful handling
reusable	• yes	• yes, after scanning and erasing • may be reused > 50 times
life span	• unlimited, unless damaged	• limited

*Refer to Chapter 9, Dental X-Ray Film.

Intraoral Sensor Preparation

Digital imaging involves the placement of the intraoral sensor in the mouth of the patient, using the same technique as in film-based imaging. Whether using indirect or direct digital imaging, it is important that the individual sensors be protected from oral fluids. A PSP plate is placed in a disposable barrier sleeve that is waterproof (Figure 8-15). Rigid digital sensors, wired or wireless, must be covered with a disposable barrier sleeve (Figure 8-16). Digital sensors cannot withstand heat sterilization. A rubber finger cot may be placed underneath the disposable barrier sleeve to further protect the wired or wireless sensor and to prevent cross-contamination between patients.

Intraoral Sensor Placement

Beam alignment devices designed to accommodate the thickness of the intraoral digital sensor must be used to stabilize the receptor in the mouth. The beam alignment device aims the beam and positions the sensor accurately. The *paralleling technique* is the preferred placement method because of the dimensional accuracy of images produced and the ease of standardizing such images. As with conventional intraoral film, the sensor is centered over the area of interest. Various manufacturers have produced beam alignment devices that can be used with both wired and wireless digital sensors, as well as PSP plates (Figure 8-17).

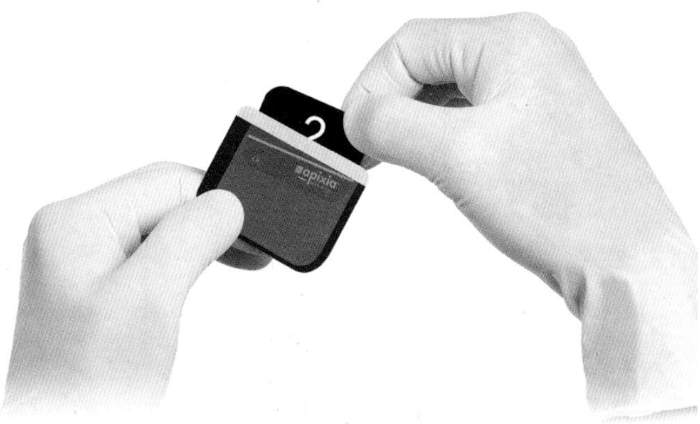

Fig 8-15 A barrier envelope is used to seal and protect the PSP sensors from contamination. (Courtesy Apixia Digital Imaging, Industry, CA.)

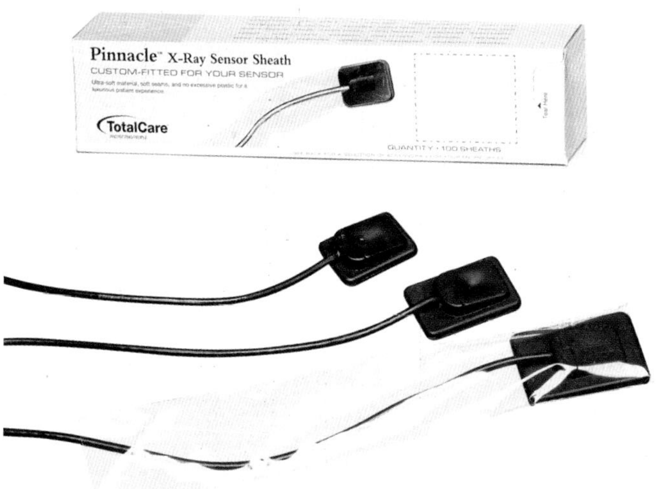

Fig 8-16 A wired digital sensor wrapped in a protective plastic sleeve. (Courtesy Kerr TotalCare, Orange, CA.)

ADVANTAGES AND DISADVANTAGES

As with film-based imaging, digital imaging has both advantages and disadvantages. Box 8-1 summarizes the advantages and disadvantages of digital imaging compared with the use of film-based imaging (Chapter 9).

Advantages of Digital Imaging

Superior gray-scale resolution. A primary advantage of digital imaging is the superior gray-scale resolution that results. Digital imaging

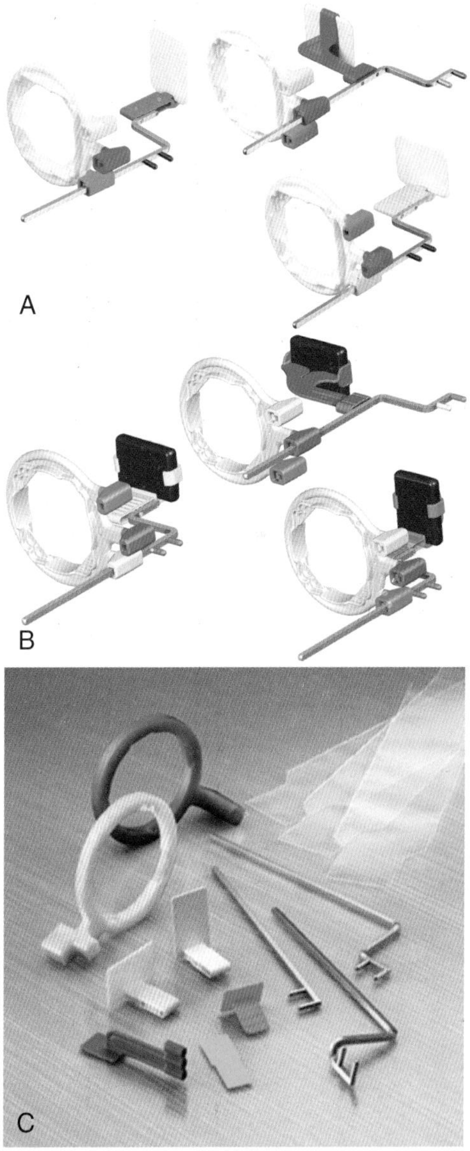

Fig 8-17 **A,** Beam alignment devices holding film for anterior, posterior, and bite-wing exposures. **B,** The same beam alignment devices updated with digital sensors for anterior, posterior, and bite-wing exposures. **C,** Beam alignment devices manufactured with adhesive backing to hold digital sensors in place. (Courtesy Dentsply Rinn Corporation, York, PA.)

uses up to 256 shades of gray compared with the 16 to 25 shades of gray differentiated on conventional film. This advantage is critical because diagnosis is often based on contrast discrimination. The ability to manipulate the density and contrast of the digital image without additional exposure of the patient to x-radiation is also an important advantage (Figure 8-18). In addition, studies have investigated the diagnostic capability of the intraoral sensor used in digital imaging.

Digital imaging enables the dental professional to identify dental disease just as with traditional film methods. One of the ways to measure the diagnostic value of digital imaging is through its ability to capture detail, or resolution. Line pairs/millimeter (lp/mm) is a measurement of the ability of the digital system to capture the detail in an image. Most digital imaging manufacturers maintain a range of 6 to 22 lp/mm. The human eye can recognize only approximately 8 lp/mm. All the current digital systems produce a diagnostically acceptable image with high definition.

Reduced exposure to x-radiation. Another primary advantage of the digital imaging system is the reduction in patient exposure to x-radiation. Decreased exposure results from the sensitivity of the sensor. The radiation exposure for digital imaging systems is 50% to 90% less than that required for film used in conventional radiography.

Increased speed of image viewing. Dental professionals and patients are able to view the digital images instantaneously, which allows for immediate interpretation and evaluation. Chairside viewing of the digitized image on a computer monitor within moments after exposure continues to be a compelling reason for the growing popularity of this technology.

Lower equipment and film cost. Long-term digital imaging eliminates the need to purchase conventional film, costly processing equipment, and processing solutions. With digital imaging, darkroom and processing solutions and maintenance are unnecessary. Also, environmental costs are reduced because the disposal hazards of processing chemicals, silver salts in film emulsion, and lead foil sheets are avoided. The elimination of darkroom processing errors is also an advantage.

Increased efficiency. Dental professionals can be more productive because digital imaging does not interrupt routine patient treatment or care. Dental practices that also use electronic charting have the advantage that the operator can access both patient data and digital images simultaneously. Both image storage and communication are easier with digital networking. The digital image can be incorporated into the electronic record of the patient, and the image can be printed out whenever needed. Digital images can also be electronically transmitted to referring dentists and specialists, insurance companies, or consultants.

Enhancement of diagnostic image. Features such as colorization and zooming allow users to highlight conditions such as bone resorption caused by periodontal disease or to help detect small areas of decay. Additional features commonly available in image software include brightness, contrast, sharpness, image orientation, and pseudocolor alteration.

Another feature that can be used to enhance a diagnostic image is digital subtraction. With digital subtraction, the gray scale is reversed so that radiolucent images (normally black) appear white and radiopaque images (normally white) appear black (Figure 8-19). Digital subtraction also eliminates distracting background information. For example, this feature permits the operator to remove

BOX 8-1 Advantages and Disadvantages of Digital Imaging in Comparison to Film-based Imaging

ADVANTAGES

1 – superior image resolution
2 – reduced patient exposure
3 – increased speed of image viewing
4 – lower equipment & supply costs
5 – increased efficiency
6 – enhancement options for images

DISADVANTAGES

1 – initial set-up costs
2 – image quality
3 – sensor size & thickness
4 – infection control
5 – wear and tear
6 – legal issues

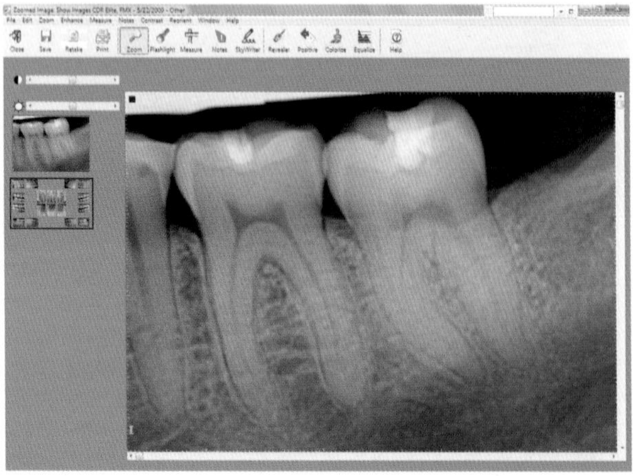

Fig 8-18 Magnification of a periapical image from a full mouth series, which allows the dental professional to take a closer look at teeth #18 and #19. (Courtesy Sirona USA, Charlotte, NC.)

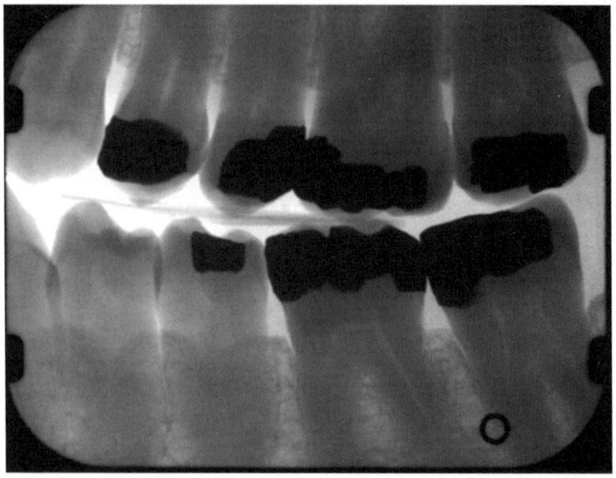

Fig 8-19 An example of digital subtraction of a bite-wing image. (Courtesy Dr. Donald Tyndall, The University of North Carolina School of Dentistry, Chapel Hill, NC.)

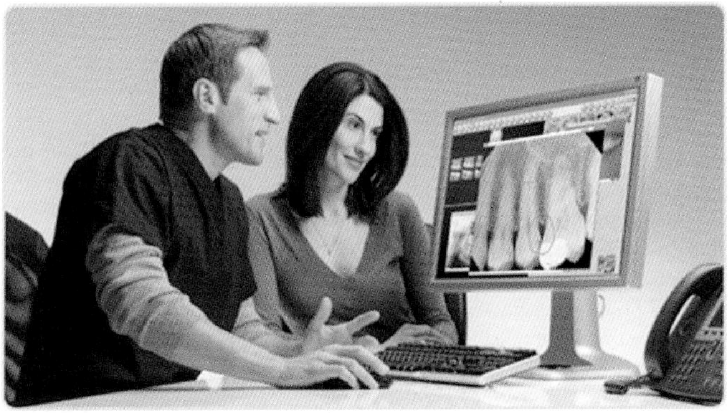

Fig 8-20 Patient education is made easier with larger dental images. (Courtesy KaVo Imaging, Brea, CA.)

all anatomic structures that have not changed between imaging examinations to facilitate identification of changes in diagnostic information.

Effective patient education tool. Digital images can be an effective tool in patient education and interaction. Patients can view digital images along with the operator, which facilitates dialogue and rapport and increases a patient's understanding of the disease process and acceptance of treatment modalities. In addition, the size of the digitized image on the 15-inch or 17-inch computer screen (compared with a 2-inch piece of film) makes the digital image an attractive patient education tool (Figure 8-20).

Eco-friendly alternative. Because digital imaging does not use any chemical processing or generate any hazardous waste materials, it is considered to be better for the environment by providing a "greener" alternative to traditional radiography.

Disadvantages of Digital Imaging

Initial setup costs. The initial cost of purchasing a digital imaging system is a disadvantage. The cost depends on the manufacturer, the level of computer equipment currently in the office, and auxiliary features such as the intraoral camera. Maintenance and repairs must also be considered.

Image quality. At one time, image quality was a source of debate. The spatial resolution of an image is defined as the number of line pairs per millimeter (lp/mm). Conventional dental x-ray film has a resolution of 12 to 20 lp/mm. A digital imaging system using a CCD sensor has a resolution closer to 10 lp/mm. Considering that the human eye can perceive only 8 to 10 lp/mm, a CCD system is significantly more effective in the recognition of dental disease. Many studies have reported on the ability of the digital image to capture early caries, bone loss, and periapical lesions. The majority of this research has shown that digital imaging performs at least as well as, and at times even better than, traditional radiography.

Sensor size and thickness. Some digital sensors are thicker and less flexible than intraoral film. Patients may complain about the bulkiness of the sensor, which may cause discomfort or elicit the gag reflex. However, with increasing experience and familiarity with the use of these rigid sensors, sensor placement becomes less of an issue. In addition, manufacturers have produced many varieties of sensor holders to stabilize sensor placement (Figure 8-21).

Infection prevention. Digital sensors cannot withstand heat sterilization. Therefore these sensors require complete coverage with disposable plastic barrier sleeves that must be changed between patients to prevent cross-contamination.

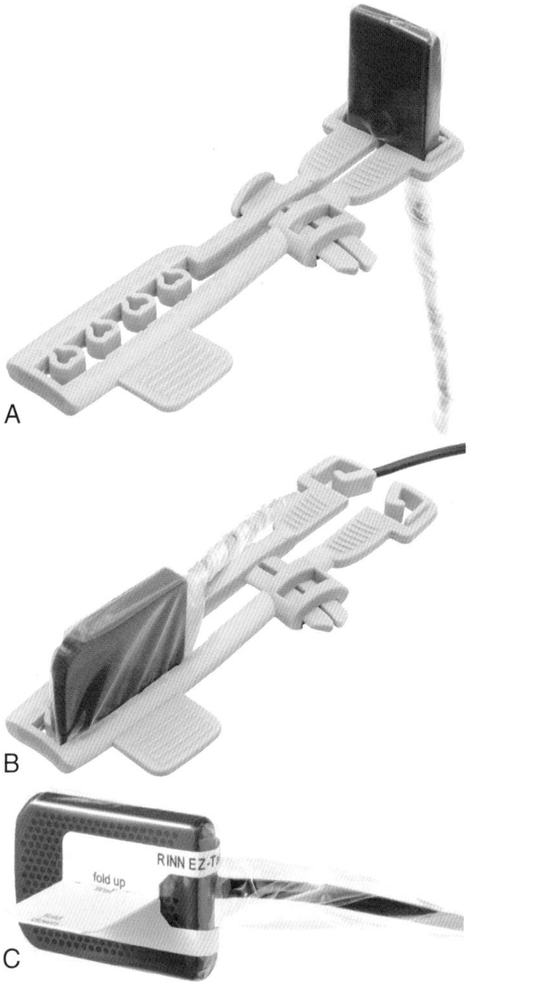

Fig 8-21 **A, B,** Anterior and posterior receptor holders are shown with direct digital sensors. **C,** A direct digital sensor fitted with an adhesive bite-wing tab. (Courtesy Dentsply Rinn Corporation, York, PA.)

Wear and tear. The receptors used in the PSP system are vulnerable to wear and tear and may have a limited lifespan. The PSP plates are not designed to have the edges bent or softened to accommodate individual patient anatomy. If bending or scratching of the plates occurs, permanent defects will appear on all images exposed, which may obscure diagnostic information.

Legal issues. Because the original digital image can be enhanced, it is questionable whether digital images can be used as evidence in lawsuits. To address this concern, manufacturers have included in the software a warning feature that appears if the image displayed on the monitor is not comparable with the original image. A file copy of the original image should always be saved and stored on the computer, even when characteristics such as density and contrast have been changed.

Box 8-1 summarizes the advantages and disadvantages of incorporating a digital imaging system into a dental practice.

SUMMARY

- Digital imaging is a method of capturing an image and displaying it on a computer monitor; no film or film processing chemicals are required.

- A conventional dental x-ray unit is used as the radiation source in digital imaging. An intraoral sensor is placed inside the patient's mouth and exposed to x-radiation. The electronic charge produced on the sensor is digitized (or converted into digital form) and is then viewed on a computer monitor. Sensors may also be used for extraoral imaging.
- Advantages of digital imaging include superior gray-scale resolution, reduced patient exposure to x-radiation, increased speed of image viewing, lower equipment and receptor costs, increased time efficiency, enhanced patient education, viewing options to enhance the diagnostic information of the image, and an eco-friendly alternative to processing chemical waste.
- Disadvantages of digital imaging include initial setup costs of the digital system, size of the intraoral sensor, wear and tear of sensors, legal issues, and the inability to heat-sterilize the sensor.

BIBLIOGRAPHY

Brennan J: An introduction to digital radiography in dentistry, J Orthod 29:66, 2002.

Frommer HH, Stabulas-Savage JJ: Digital imaging. In Radiology for the dental professional, ed 9, St. Louis, 2011, Mosby.

Levato C: Are you ready for digital radiography?, Dent Pract Finance 7:17, 1999.

Lusk LT: Comparison of film-based and digital radiography, J Pract Hygiene 7:45, 1998.

Mallya SM, Lam EWN: Digital imaging. In White and Pharoah's oral radiology: principles and interpretation, ed 8, St. Louis, 2019, Elsevier.

Miles DA, Van Dis ML, Jensen CW, et al: Digital imaging. In Radiographic imaging for the dental team, ed 4, St. Louis, 2009, Saunders.

Parks ET, Williamson GF: Digital radiography: an overview, J Contemp Dent Pract 3(4):23, 2002.

Razmus TF, Williamson GF: An overview of oral and maxillofacial imaging. In Current oral and maxillofacial imaging, Philadelphia, 1996, Saunders.

Tyndall DA, Ludlow JB, Platin E, et al: A comparison of Kodak Ektaspeed Plus film and the Siemens Sidexis digital imaging system for caries detection using receiver operating characteristic analysis, Oral Surg Oral Med Oral Pathol Oral Radiol Endod 85:113, 1998.

Van der Stelt PF: Filmless imaging: The uses of digital radiography in dental practice, J Am Dent Assoc 136(10):1379, 2005.

Van der Stelt PF: Better imaging: The advantages of digital radiography, J Am Dent Assoc 139(3):7S, 2008.

QUIZ QUESTIONS

Matching

For Questions 1 to 8, match each term with its corresponding definition.

a. charge-coupled device
b. digital radiography
c. digital subtraction
d. digitize
e. direct digital imaging
f. pixel
g. sensor
h. storage phosphor imaging

____ **1.** A detector that is used to capture the dental image.
____ **2.** An image receptor found in the intraoral sensor.
____ **3.** A form of indirect digital imaging in which the image is recorded on phosphor-coated plates and then placed into an electronic processor, where a laser scans the plate and produces an image on a computer screen.
____ **4.** To convert an image into digital form that, in turn, can be processed by a computer.
____ **5.** A method of obtaining a digital image in which an intraoral sensor is exposed to x-rays to capture an image that can be viewed on a computer monitor.
____ **6.** A discrete unit of information; a picture element.
____ **7.** A method of reversing the gray scale as a digital image is viewed.
____ **8.** A filmless imaging system; a method of capturing an image using a sensor, breaking the image into electronic pieces, and presenting and storing the image using a computer.

True or False

____ **9.** In digital imaging, the term used to describe the picture that is produced is *radiograph*.
____ **10.** Digital imaging requires more x-radiation than conventional radiography.
____ **11.** The x-radiation source used in most digital imaging systems is a conventional dental x-ray unit.
____ **12.** Compared with film emulsion, the pixels used in digital imaging are structured in an orderly arrangement.
____ **13.** All intraoral sensors can be heat-sterilized after use.
____ **14.** The preferred exposure method for intraoral digital imaging is the paralleling technique.
____ **15.** One advantage of a digital imaging system is the superior gray-scale resolution that results.
____ **16.** Digital subtraction is an advantage in digital imaging because distracting background information is eliminated from the image.
____ **17.** The manipulation of the original digital images can be considered a legal issue.

Multiple Choice

____ **18.** Digital imaging was introduced to dentistry in:
a. 1967
b. 1977
c. 1987
d. 1997

____ **19.** Digital imaging can be used for:
a. detecting conditions of teeth and surrounding structures
b. evaluating the growth and development of jaws
c. confirmation of suspected disease
d. all of the above

____ **20.** Digital imaging requires less radiation than does conventional radiography because:
a. the sensor is larger
b. the sensor is more sensitive to x-rays
c. the exposure time is increased
d. the pixels sense transmitted light quickly

_____ **21.** The image receptor found in the intraoral sensor is termed:
a. CCD
b. pixel
c. semiconductor chip
d. software

_____ **22.** Digital imaging systems can be used for which images?
a. bite-wing
b. panoramic
c. cephalometric
d. all of the above

_____ **23.** All of the following are advantages of digital imaging except:
a. digital subtraction
b. the ability to enhance the image
c. size of the intraoral sensor
d. patient education

9

Dental X-Ray Film

LEARNING OBJECTIVES

After completion of this chapter, the student will be able to do the following:

1. Define the terms associated with dental x-ray film.
2. Discuss why the radiographer should be familiar with dental x-ray film.
3. Describe film composition and latent image formation.
4. List the different types of x-ray film used in dentistry.
5. Define intraoral film and describe intraoral film packaging.
6. Identify the types and sizes of intraoral film available.
7. Discuss film speed.
8. Define extraoral film and describe extraoral film packaging.
9. Discuss the differences between intraoral film and extraoral film and identify the types of extraoral film available.
10. Describe the difference between screen and nonscreen films.
11. Describe the use of intensifying screens and cassettes.
12. Describe duplicating film.
13. Discuss proper film storage and protection.

Although an increasing number of dental practices are transitioning from film to digital imaging, traditional film continues to be used in dental practices. Consequently, the dental radiographer must be familiar with both film and digital imaging in order to be prepared to work in a variety of offices. A dental radiography text would not be complete without an overview of dental x-ray film.

The dental radiographer must have a working knowledge of dental x-ray film. The film used in dental radiography is a type of photographic film that has been adapted for dental use. An image is produced on dental x-ray film when it is exposed to radiation that has passed through teeth and adjacent structures. To avoid film-related errors that result in increased patient exposure to x-radiation, the dental radiographer must understand the composition of the x-ray film and latent image formation. In addition, the dental radiographer must be familiar with the types of film used in dental radiography, as well as with film storage and protection.

The purpose of this chapter is to provide an overview of dental x-ray film; to define film composition; to detail latent image formation; to describe the types of intraoral, extraoral, and duplicating film used in dental radiography; and to discuss film storage and protection.

DENTAL X-RAY FILM COMPOSITION AND LATENT IMAGE

In dental radiography, the x-ray beam passes through teeth and adjacent structures and reaches the x-ray film. The dental x-ray film serves as a recording medium, or **image receptor**; the term **image** refers to a picture or likeness of an object, and the term **receptor** refers to something that responds to a stimulus. Images are recorded on the dental x-ray film when the film is exposed to a stimulus—specifically, energy in the form of x-radiation or light. To understand how these images result, an understanding of film composition and latent image formation is necessary.

Film Composition

The x-ray film used in dentistry has four basic components: (1) a film base, (2) an adhesive layer, (3) film emulsion, and (4) a protective layer (Figure 9-1).

Film Base. The **film base** is a flexible piece of polyester plastic 0.2 mm (200 microns) in thickness that is constructed to withstand heat, moisture, and chemical exposure. The film base is transparent and exhibits a slight blue tint that is used to emphasize contrast and enhance image quality. The primary purpose of the film base is to provide a stable support for the delicate emulsion. The base also provides strength.

Adhesive Layer. The **adhesive layer** is a thin layer of adhesive material that covers both sides of the film base. The adhesive layer is added to the film base before the emulsion is applied and serves to attach the emulsion to the base.

Film Emulsion. The **film emulsion** is a coating attached to both sides of the film base by the adhesive layer to give the film greater sensitivity to x-radiation. The emulsion is a homogeneous mixture of gelatin and silver halide crystals.

Gelatin. The **gelatin** is used to suspend and evenly disperse millions of microscopic silver halide crystals over the film base. During film processing, the gelatin absorbs the processing solutions and allows the chemicals to react with the silver halide crystals.

Halide crystals. A **halide** is a chemical compound that is sensitive to radiation or light. The halides used in dental x-ray film are made up of the element silver plus a halogen (bromine or iodine). Silver bromide ($AgBr$) and silver iodide (AgI) are two types of **silver halide crystals** found in the film emulsion; the typical emulsion is 80% to 99% silver bromide and 1% to 10% silver iodide. The silver halide crystals absorb radiation during x-ray exposure and store energy from the radiation (Figure 9-2).

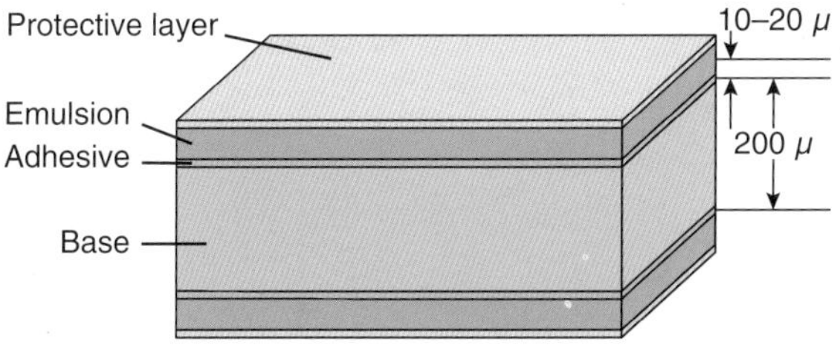

Fig 9-1 Components of dental x-ray film.

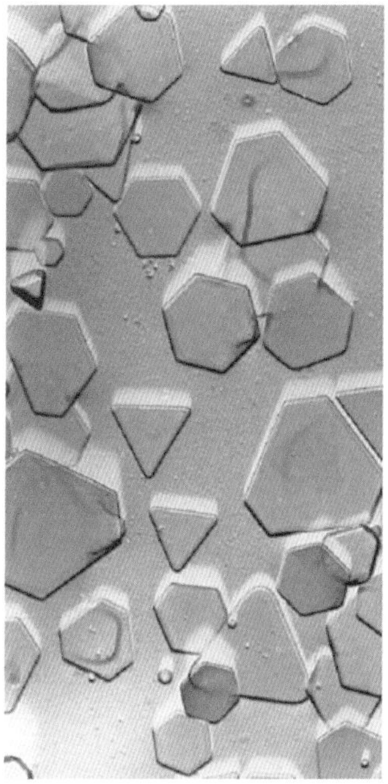

Fig 9-2 Scanning electron micrograph of emulsion of INSIGHT film showing flat tubular silver bromide crystals, which capture electrons. (Courtesy Carestream Health, Inc., Rochester, NY.)

Protective Layer. The **protective layer** is a thin, transparent coating placed over the emulsion. It serves to protect the emulsion surface from manipulation, as well as mechanical and processing damage.

Latent Image Formation

Silver halide crystals absorb x-radiation during x-ray exposure and store the energy from the radiation. Depending on the density of the objects in the area exposed, silver halide crystals contain various levels of stored energy. For example, the silver halide crystals on the film that are positioned behind an amalgam restoration receive almost no radiation. Amalgam is dense and absorbs the x-ray energy. As a result, the silver halide crystals are not energized. In contrast, the silver halide crystals that correspond to air space (no density) receive more radiation and are highly energized.

The stored energy within the silver halide crystals forms a pattern and creates an invisible image within the emulsion on the exposed film. This pattern of stored energy on the exposed film cannot be seen and is referred to as a **latent image**. The latent image remains invisible within the emulsion until it undergoes chemical processing procedures. When the exposed film with latent image is processed, a visible image results (see Chapter 10).

How does the stored energy of the silver halide crystals result in a latent image? When the x-ray photons hit the surface of the film emulsion, some silver bromide crystals are exposed and energized, while other crystals are not exposed. The silver bromide crystals exposed to x-ray photons are ionized, and the silver and bromine atoms are separated. Irregularities in the lattice structure of the exposed crystal, known as **sensitivity specks**, attract the silver atoms. These aggregates of neutral silver atoms are known as **latent image centers** (Figure 9-3). Collectively, the crystals with aggregates of silver at the latent image centers become the latent image on the film.

> **HELPFUL HINT**
>
> ***Definition of Latent***
>
> Existing but not yet developed; hidden; concealed
>
> ***late**nt* → comes ***late**r*
>
> Something latent is present but not visible.

TYPES OF DENTAL X-RAY FILM

Three types of x-ray film may be used in dental radiography: (1) intraoral film, (2) extraoral film, and (3) duplicating film.

Intraoral Film

An **intraoral film** is a film that is placed *inside* the mouth during x-ray exposure. An intraoral film is used to examine teeth and supporting structures.

Intraoral Film Packaging. Each intraoral film is packaged to protect it from light and moisture; the film and its surrounding packaging are referred to as a **film packet**. In dentistry, the terms "film packet" and "film" are often used interchangeably. Film packets are packaged in convenient plastic trays or cardboard boxes that can be recycled (Figure 9-4). Boxes of intraoral film are labeled with the type of film, film speed, film size, number of films per individual packet, total number of films enclosed, and the film expiration date.

An intraoral x-ray film packet is made up of four separate items: (1) x-ray film, (2) paper film wrapper, (3) lead foil sheet, and (4) outer film wrapping (Figure 9-5).

X-ray film. The intraoral **x-ray film** is a double-emulsion film (emulsion on both sides). Double-emulsion film is used instead of single-emulsion film (emulsion on one side) because it requires less radiation exposure to produce an image. A film packet may contain one film (**one-film packet**) or two films (**two-film packet**). A two-film packet produces two identical images with the same amount of exposure necessary to produce a single image. The two-film packet is used when a duplicate record of a radiographic examination is needed (e.g., for insurance claims, patient referrals, etc.).

A small, raised bump known as the **identification dot** is located in one corner of the intraoral x-ray film (Figure 9-6). The raised bump is used to determine film orientation. After the film is processed, the raised identification dot is used to distinguish between the left and right sides of the patient. The dot is significant in film mounting and interpretation (see Chapter 11).

Paper film wrapper. The **paper film wrapper** within the film packet is a protective sheet that covers the film and shields the film from light.

Lead foil sheet. The **lead foil sheet** is a single piece of lead foil within the film packet that is located behind the film wrapped in protective paper. The thin lead foil sheet is positioned behind the film to shield the film from backscattered (secondary) radiation that results in film fog.

The manufacturer-placed embossed pattern on the lead foil sheet is visible on a processed radiograph if the film packet is inadvertently positioned in the mouth backward and then exposed (Figure 9-7).

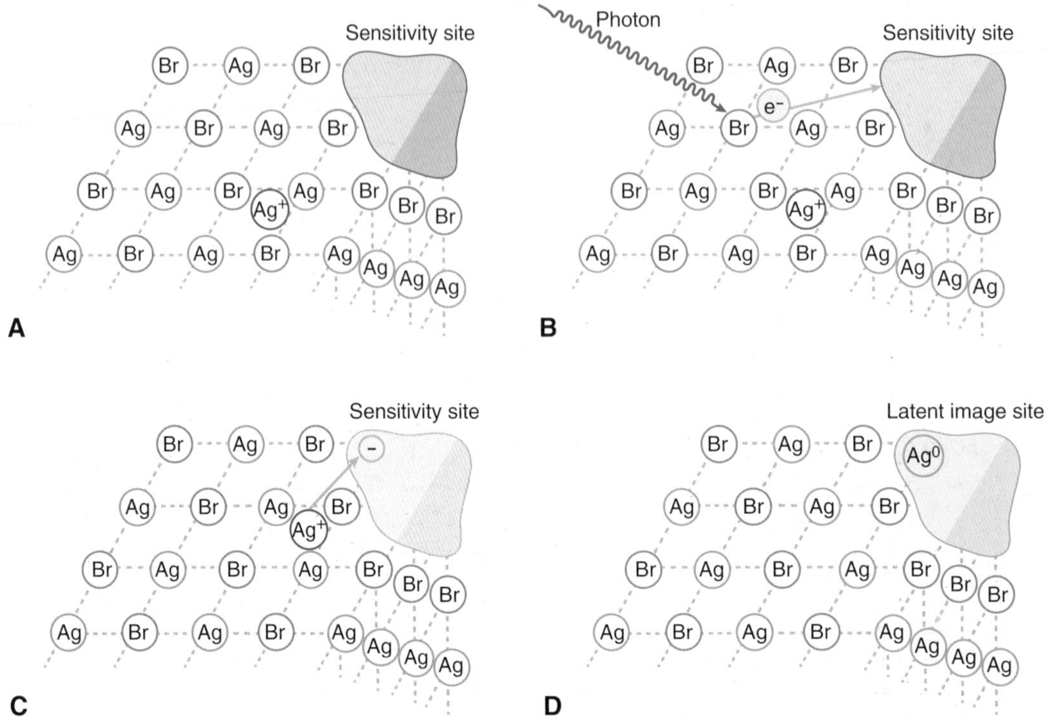

Fig 9-3 A, An x-ray film emulsion contains mostly silver and bromide ions in a crystal lattice. There are also free interstitial silver ions that form sensitivity sites. B, Exposure of the crystal to x-ray photons releases electrons. The electrons have sufficient kinetic energy to move within the crystal. When electrons reach a sensitivity site, they impart a negative charge to this region. C, Free interstitial silver ions (with a positive charge) are attracted to the negatively charged sensitivity site. D, When the silver ions reach the sensitivity site, they acquire an electron and become neutral silver atoms. These silver atoms now constitute a latent image site. The collection of latent image sites over the entire film constitutes the latent image. Developer causes the neutral silver atoms at the latent image sites to initiate the conversion of all the silver ions in the crystal into one large grain of metallic silver. The bromine dissolves in the developer.

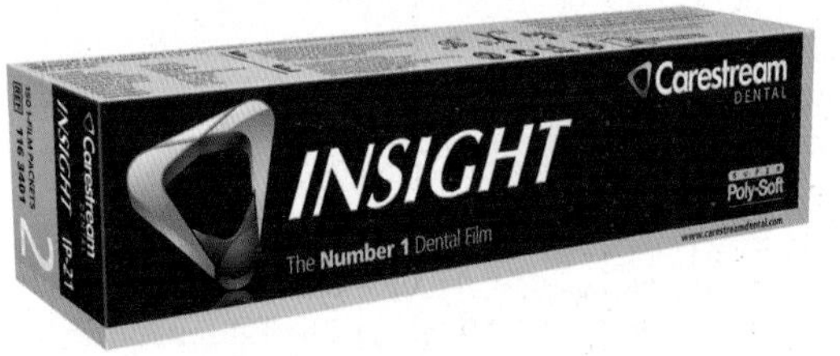

Fig 9-4 Intraoral film packets in a cardboard box that can be recycled. (Courtesy Carestream Health, Inc., Rochester, NY.)

This error may result in a retake if the resultant image is too light and nondiagnostic.

Outer package wrapping. The outer package wrapping is a soft-vinyl or paper wrapper that hermetically seals the film packet, protective paper, and lead foil sheet. This outer wrapper serves to protect the film from exposure to light and oral fluids.

The outer wrapper of the film packet has two sides: (1) the tube side and (2) the label side.

Tube side. The tube side is solid white and has a raised bump in one corner that corresponds to the identification dot on the x-ray film. When placed in the mouth, the white side (tube side) of the film packet must face the teeth and the tubehead. An easy way to remember this is "white in sight"—the white side of the film should be facing the operator when placed in the mouth. Another way to remember this is that "the white side of the film faces the white teeth."

Label side. The label side of the film packet has a flap used to open the film packet and remove the film before processing. The label side is color-coded to identify films outside of the plastic packaging container; the manufacturer uses color coding to distinguish one-film and two-film packets and film speeds (Table 9-1). When placed in the mouth, the color-coded side (label side) of the packet must face the tongue.

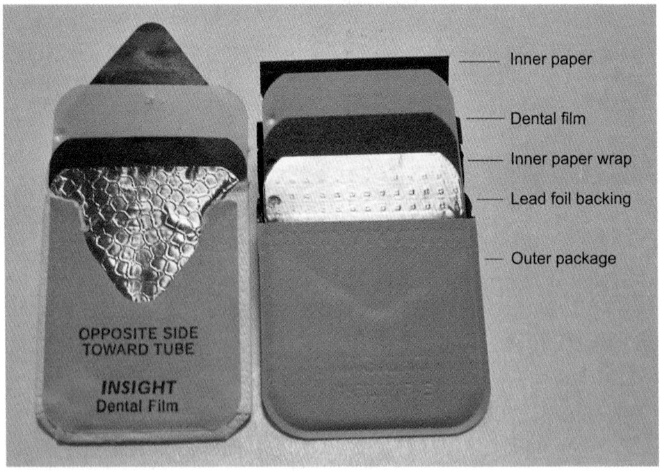

Fig 9-5 The four items that compose an intraoral film packet include the black paper film wrapper, the intraoral film, lead foil backing and the outer package wrapping. (Courtesy Carestream Health, Inc., Rochester, NY.)

The following information is printed on the label side of the film packet (Figure 9-8):

- A circle or dot that corresponds with the raised identification dot on the film
- The statement "opposite side toward tube"

HELPFUL HINT

Remembering the Tube Side of the Film Packet

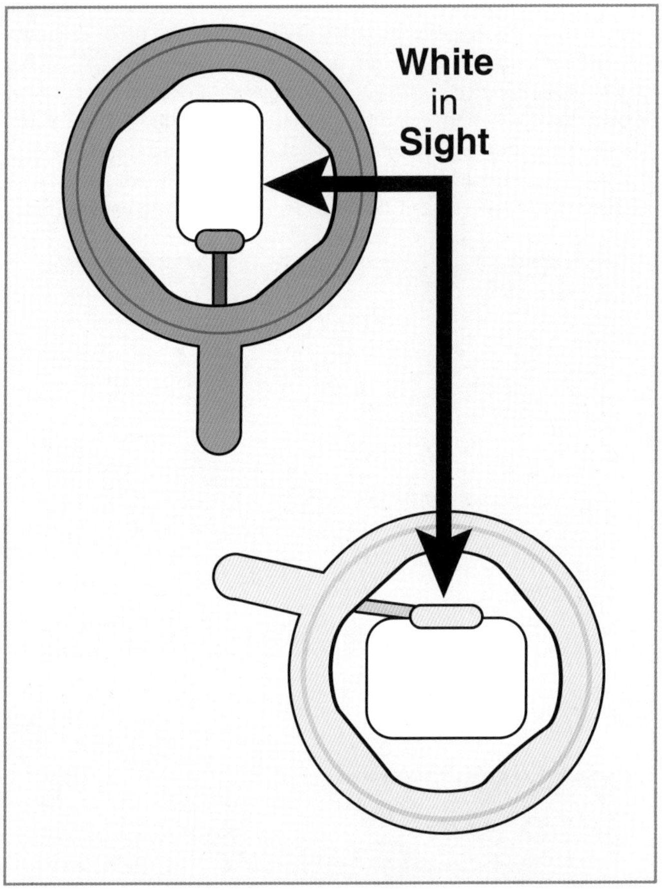

- The manufacturer's name (may or may not appear, depends on manufacturer)
- The film speed (example: INSIGHT)
- The number of films enclosed (example: one-Film or two-Film)

Intraoral Film Types. Three types of intraoral films are available: (1) periapical, (2) bite-wing, and (3) occlusal.

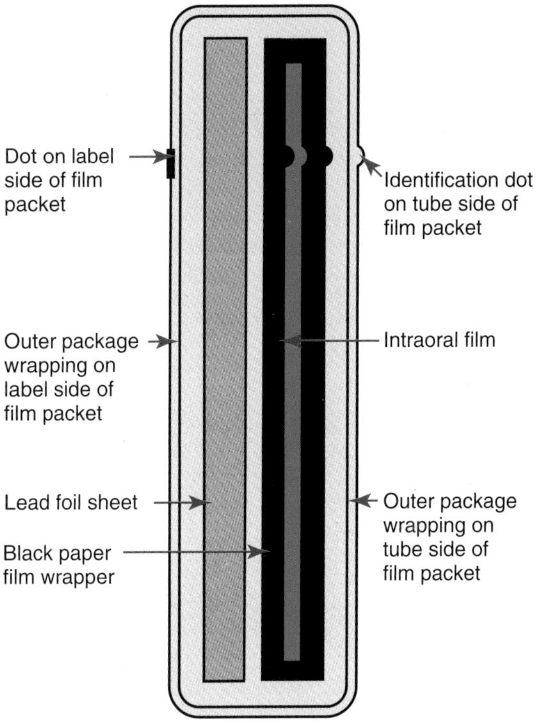

Fig 9-6 Labeled film packet.

HELPFUL HINT

Tube Side and Label Side of Film Packets

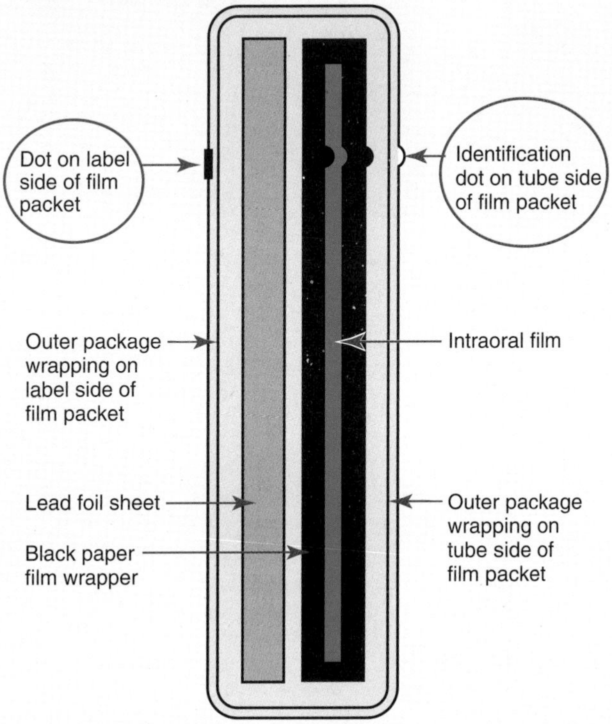

- **TUBE SIDE** is solid white
- Dot is a "**b**ump"

- **LABEL SIDE** has color
- Dot is f**la**t

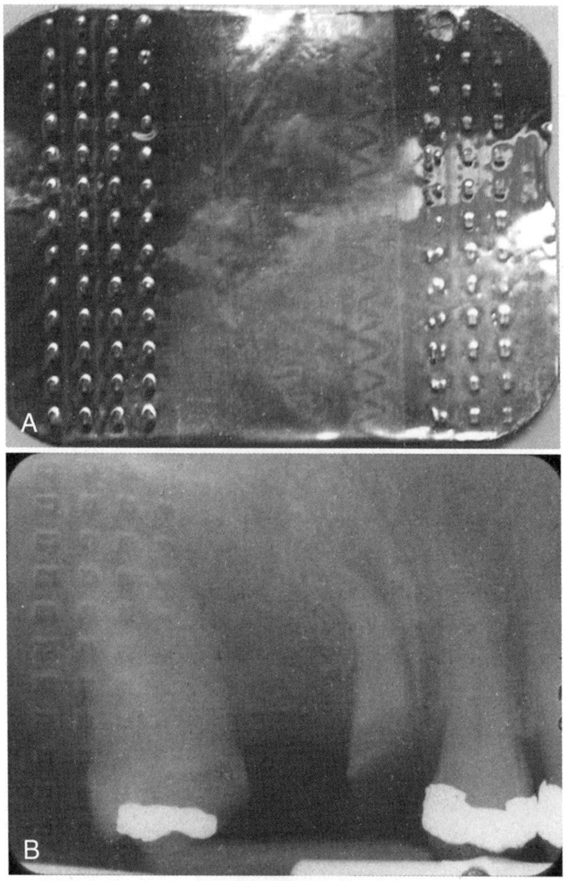

Fig 9-7 **A,** The lead foil insert in this packet has a raised diamond pattern across both ends. **B,** Radiograph showing the raised diamond pattern from the lead backing when the film is positioned backward in the mouth. (Courtesy Bird DL, Robinson DS: *Modern dental assisting,* ed 10, St Louis, 2012, Saunders.)

TABLE 9-1 Color Codes for Carestream Film Packets

	PACKETS	
Film Type	**One-Film**	**Two-Film**
Ultra-Speed (D-Speed)	Mint	Gray
Insight (F-Speed)	Violet	Tan

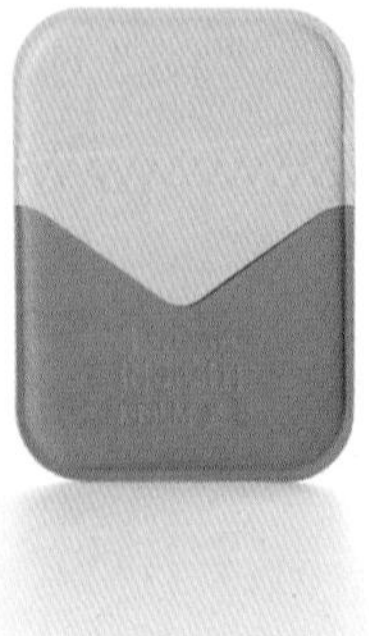

Fig 9-8 The label side of a film packet. (Courtesy Carestream Health, Inc., Rochester, NY.)

Periapical film. The periapical film is used to examine the entire tooth (crown and root) and supporting bone (Figure 9-9). The term *periapical* is derived from the Greek root *peri*, meaning "around," and the Latin cross reference *apex*, referring to the terminal end of a tooth root. As the term suggests, this type of film shows the tip of the tooth root and surrounding structures, as well as the crown.

Bite-wing film. The bite-wing film is used to examine the crowns of both maxillary and mandibular teeth on one film (Figure 9-10). The bite-wing film is particularly useful in examining interproximal, or adjacent, tooth surfaces. The bite-wing film has a "wing," or a tab, attached to the tube side of the film (Figure 9-11). The patient "bites"

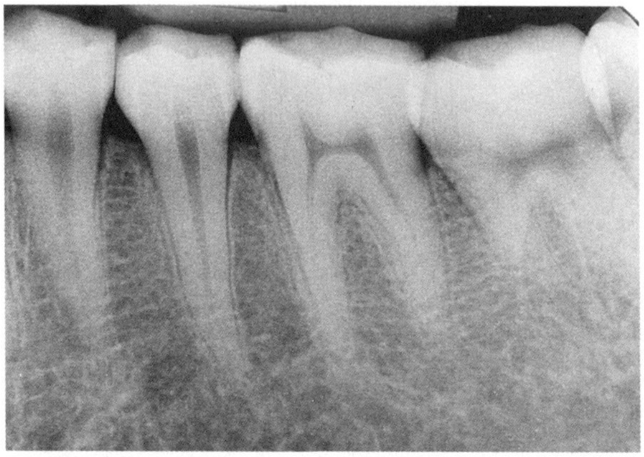

Fig 9-9 A periapical image. (Courtesy Carestream Health, Inc., Rochester, NY.)

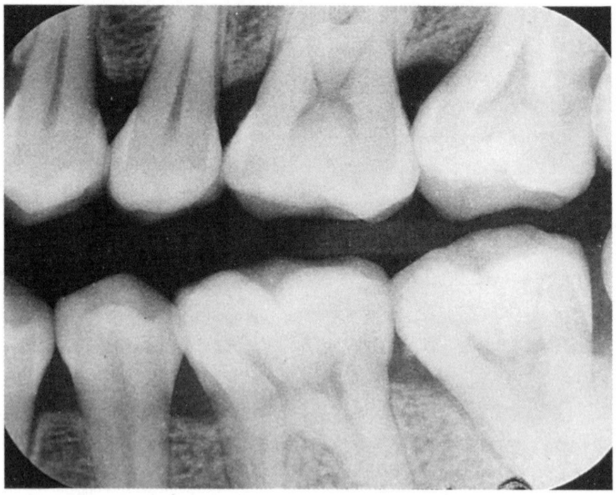

Fig 9-10 A bite-wing image. (Courtesy Carestream Health, Inc., Rochester, NY.)

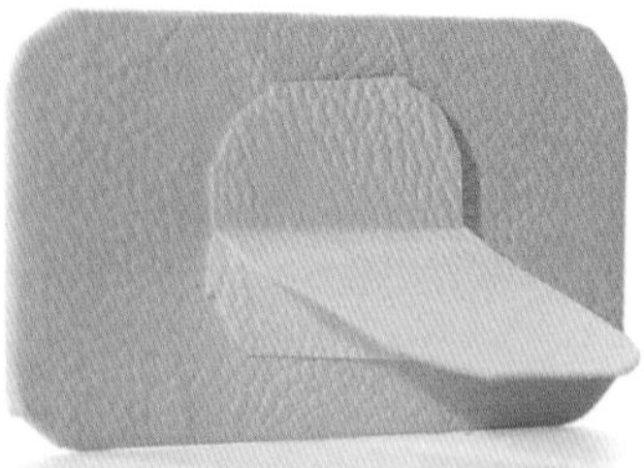

Fig 9-11 The bite-wing tab attached to the film. (Courtesy Carestream Health, Inc., Rochester, NY.)

on the wing to stabilize the film. Bite-wing films may be purchased with tabs attached to the film or may be constructed from a periapical film and bite-wing loop.

Occlusal film. The occlusal film is used for examination of large areas of the maxilla or the mandible (Figure 9-12). The occlusal film is so named because the patient "occludes," or bites on, the entire film. The occlusal film is larger than periapical or bite-wing films.

Intraoral Film Sizes. The intraoral film is manufactured in five sizes to accommodate the varying mouth sizes of children, adolescents, and adults; the larger the number, the larger is the size of the film. Different sizes of film are used with periapical, bite-wing, and occlusal exposures (Figure 9-13).

Periapical film. Three sizes (0, 1, and 2) of the periapical film are available.

- The *size 0* periapical film is the smallest intraoral film available and is used for very small children.
- The *size 1* periapical film is used primarily to examine the anterior teeth in adults, but may also be used with children.
- The *size 2* periapical film, also known as the standard film, is used to examine the anterior and posterior teeth in adults.

Bite-wing film. Three sizes (0, 2, and 3) of the bite-wing film are available. With the exception of the size 3 film, the size and shape of the bite-wing film are identical to the size and shape of the periapical film.

- The *size 0* bite-wing film is used to examine the posterior teeth in small children.
- The *size 2* bite-wing film is used to examine the posterior teeth in older children and adults. This is the most frequently used bite-wing film.
- The *size 3* film is longer and narrower than the standard size 2 film and is used only for bite-wing images. This bite-wing film shows all the posterior teeth on one side of the arch in one radiograph.

Occlusal film. The occlusal film is the largest intraoral film and is almost four times as large as a standard size 2 periapical film.

- The *size 4* occlusal film is used to show large areas of the maxilla or the mandible.

Intraoral Film Speed. Film speed refers to the amount of radiation required to produce a radiograph of standard density. Film speed, or *sensitivity*, is determined by the following:

1. Size of the silver halide crystals
2. Thickness of the emulsion
3. Presence of special radiosensitive dyes

Film speed determines how much radiation and how much exposure time are necessary to produce an image on a film. For example, a fast film requires less radiation exposure because the film responds more quickly; a fast film responds more quickly because the silver halide crystals in the emulsion are larger. The larger the crystals, the faster the film speed.

An alphabetical classification system is used to identify film speed. X-ray films are given speed ratings ranging from A speed (the slowest) to F speed (the fastest). Only D-speed, E-speed, E/F-speed, and F-speed film are used for intraoral radiography. The E/F-speed film is between the E- and F-speed categories. The American Dental Association (ADA) and the American Academy of Oral and Maxillofacial Radiology (AAOMR) currently recommend the use of F-speed film. The F-speed film requires 60% of the exposure time of the D-speed film and has comparable image contrast and resolution.

The use of F-speed film results in less radiation exposure of the patient. The F-speed film is a faster film than the D-speed film because of the larger crystals and the increased amount of silver bromide in the emulsion. Current F-speed films not only reduce the radiation dose to the patient but also provide stable contrast characteristics under various processing conditions.

The speed of a film is clearly indicated on the label side of the intraoral film packet and on the outside of the film box or container.

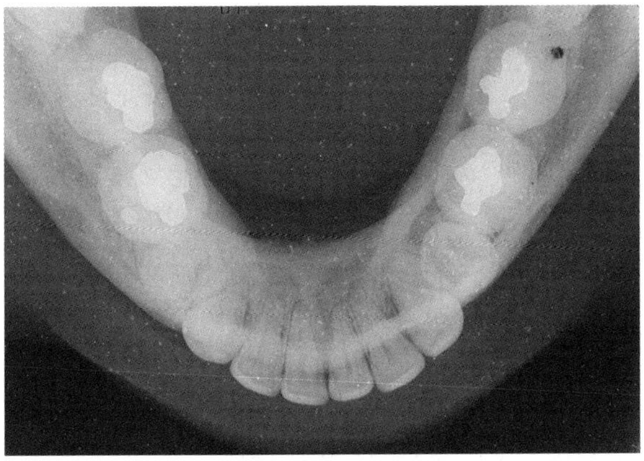

Fig 9-12 An occlusal image. (Courtesy Carestream Health, Inc., Rochester, NY.)

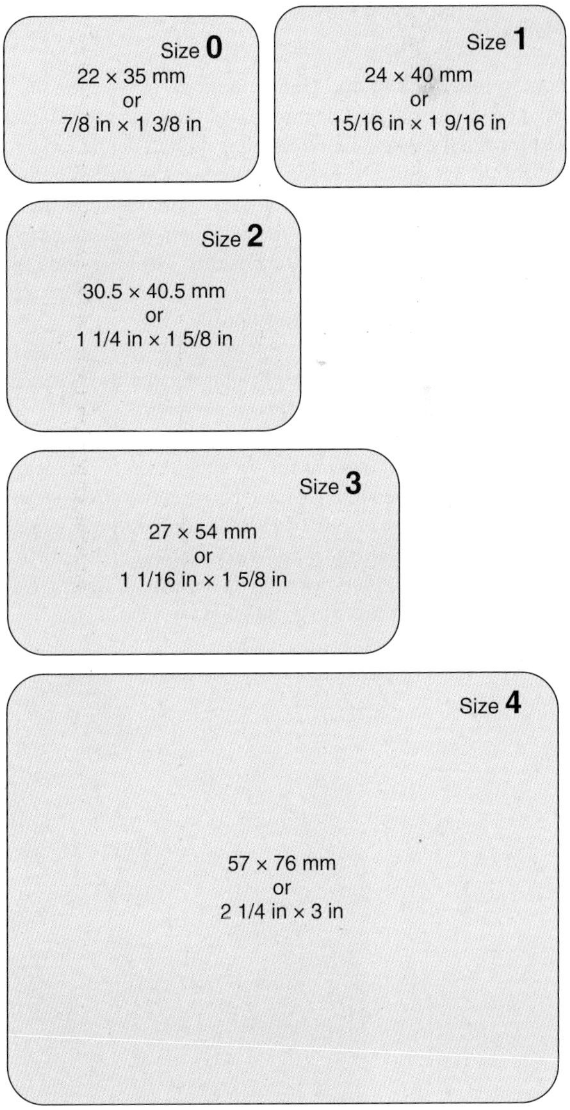

Fig 9-13 Films sizes 0, 1, 2, 3, 4 and measurements.

HELPFUL HINT

Film Speed

- **FASTER FILM** creates images that are <u>less</u> sharp due to **LARGE** crystal size
  - **FAST—LESS—LARGE**
- **SLOWER FILM** creates images that are <u>more</u> sharp due to **SMALL** crystal size
  - **SLOW—MORE—SMALL**

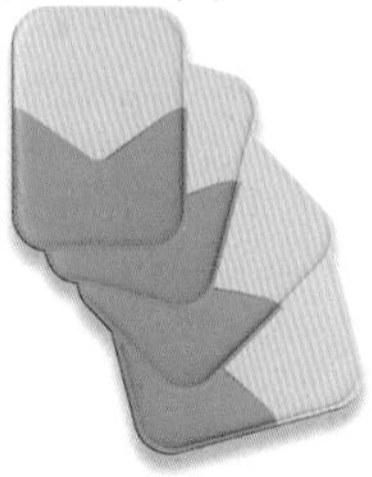

Extraoral Film

An **extraoral film** is placed *outside* the mouth during x-ray exposure. Extraoral images are used to examine large areas of the skull or jaws. Common extraoral images include panoramic and cephalometric. A **panoramic image** shows a panoramic (wide) view of the maxilla and the mandible and surrounding structures on a single image (Figure 9-14). A **cephalometric image** exhibits the bony and soft tissue areas of the facial profile (Figure 9-15).

Extraoral Film Packaging. Unlike intraoral films, extraoral films are designed for use outside the mouth and therefore are not enclosed in moisture-proof packets. Extraoral films used in dental radiography are available in 5 × 7-inch and 8 × 10-inch sizes, as well as in the panoramic 5 × 12-inch and 6 × 12-inch sizes. Extraoral films are boxed in quantities of 50 or 100. Some manufacturers separate each piece with protective paper. Labels on the boxes of extraoral films contain information including the type of film, film size, total number of films enclosed, and expiration date (Figure 9-16).

Extraoral Film Types. Two types of film may be used in extraoral radiography: (1) screen film and (2) nonscreen film.

Screen film. The majority of extraoral films are screen films. A **screen film** is a film that requires the use of a screen for exposure (see later discussion). A screen film is placed between two special intensifying screens in a cassette (Figure 9-17). When the cassette is exposed to x-rays, the screens convert the x-ray energy into light, which, in turn, exposes the screen film. The screen film is sensitive to fluorescent light rather than to direct exposure to x-radiation.

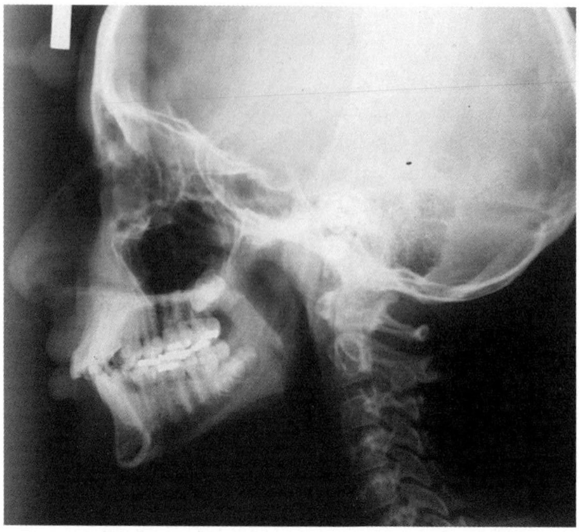

Fig 9-15 A cephalometric image. (Courtesy Bird DL, Robinson DS: *Modern dental assisting*, ed 10, St Louis, 2012, Saunders.)

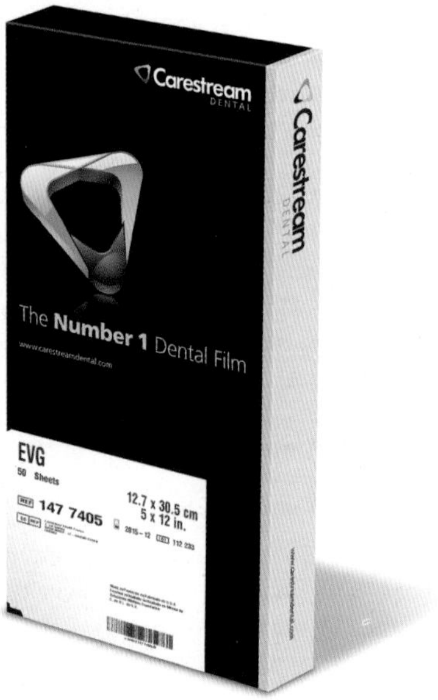

Fig 9-16 Extraoral film boxes are labeled with information on the type of film, film size, number of films enclosed, and expiration date. (Courtesy Carestream Health, Inc., Rochester, NY.)

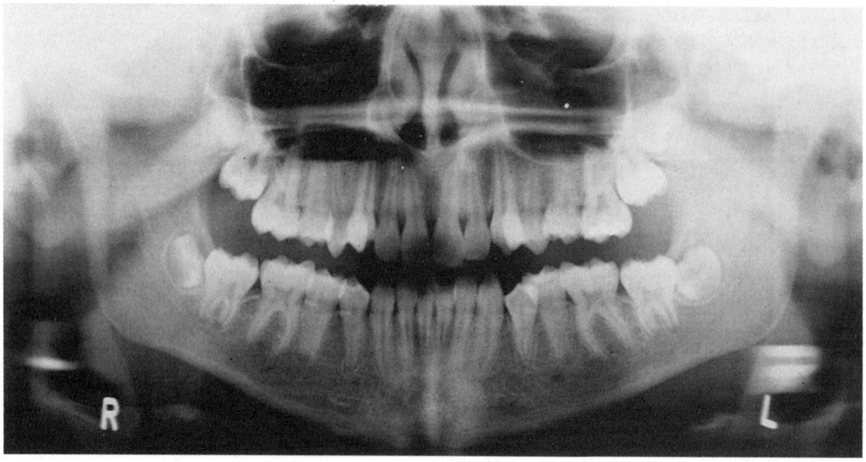

Fig 9-14 A panoramic image. (Courtesy Carestream Health, Inc., Rochester, NY.)

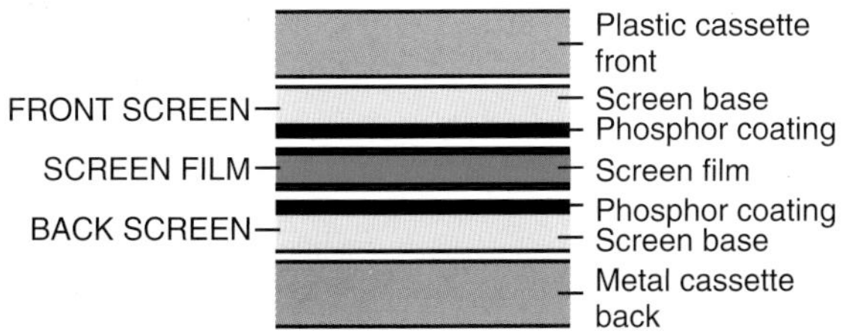

Fig 9-17 Inside cassette, the screen film is placed between two intensifying screens.

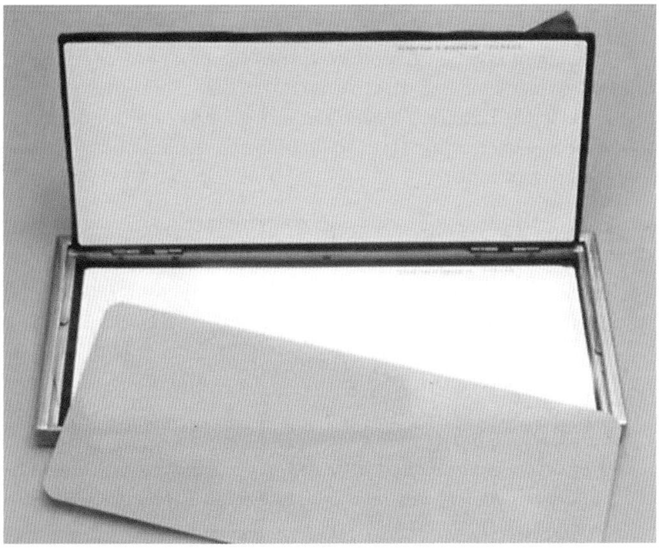

Fig 9-18 Cassette in open position, showing front and back intensifying screens and a piece of film. (Courtesy Mallya SM, Lam EWN: Film imaging. In *White and Pharoah's oral radiology: principles and interpretation*, ed 8, St. Louis, 2019, Elsevier.)

Films used in a screen-film combination are sensitive to specific colors of fluorescent light. Some screen films are sensitive to blue light (X-Omat DBF film), whereas others are sensitive to green light (T-Mat film). Blue-sensitive film must be paired with screens that produce blue light, and green-sensitive film must be paired with screens that produce green light. Properly matched film-screen combinations are imperative to obtain high-quality images and to minimize exposure of the patient.

Nonscreen film. A nonscreen film is an extraoral film that does not require the use of screens for exposure. A nonscreen extraoral film is exposed directly to x-rays; the emulsion is sensitive to direct x-ray exposure rather than to fluorescent light. A nonscreen extraoral film requires more exposure time than does a screen film and is not recommended for use in dental radiography.

Extraoral Film Equipment. In extraoral radiography, screen films are used in combination with two special equipment items: (1) intensifying screens and (2) cassettes.

Intensifying screens. An intensifying screen is a device that transfers x-ray energy into visible light; the visible light, in turn, exposes the screen film. These screens intensify the effect of x-rays on the film. With the use of intensifying screens, less radiation is required to expose a screen film, and the patient is exposed to less radiation.

In extraoral radiography, a screen film is sandwiched between two intensifying screens of matching size and is secured in a cassette (Figure 9-18). An intensifying screen is a smooth plastic sheet coated

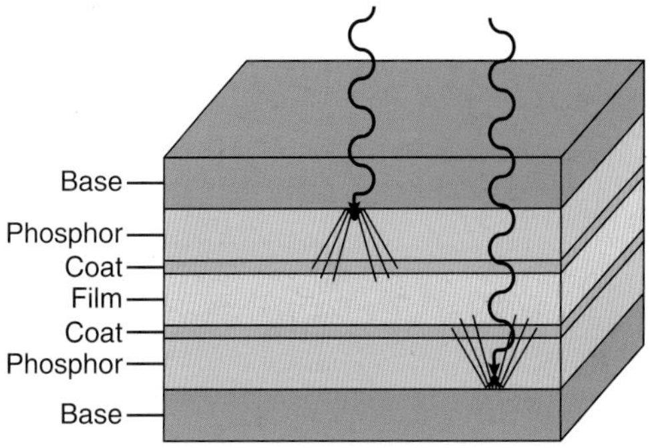

Fig 9-19 Phosphors in the intensifying screen emit visible light when hit by x-ray photons. Multiple visible light photons then strike and expose the film.

with minute fluorescent crystals known as phosphors. When exposed to x-rays, the phosphors fluoresce and emit visible light in the blue or green spectrum; the emitted light then exposes the film (Figure 9-19). As discussed in Chapter 2, one of the properties of electromagnetic radiation is that x-rays cause certain materials (e.g., phosphors) to fluoresce.

Conventional calcium tungstate screens have phosphors that emit blue light. The newer rare earth screens have phosphors that are not commonly found in the earth (thus "rare earth") and emit green light. Rare earth intensifying screens are more efficient at converting x-rays into light than are calcium tungstate intensifying screens. As a result, rare earth screens require less x-ray exposure than do calcium tungstate screens and are considered faster. The use of rare earth screens means less exposure of the patient to x-radiation. Rare earth intensifying screens (LANEX screens) are designed for use with green-sensitive film (T-Mat film), whereas conventional screens (X-Omatic screens) are used with blue-sensitive film (X-Omat DBF film).

Cassette. A cassette is a special device that is used to hold the extraoral film and the intensifying screens. Cassettes are available in a variety of sizes that correspond to film and screen sizes. A cassette may be flexible or rigid; most cassettes are rigid, although the panoramic cassette may be flexible (Figure 9-20).

A rigid cassette is more expensive but usually lasts longer than a flexible cassette does. A rigid cassette also better protects screens from damage. The film fits the rigid cassette exactly and cannot be loaded incorrectly. To load the flexible cassette properly, however, the film must be placed between the two screens and pushed to the end of the cassette.

Both rigid and flexible cassettes must be "light-tight" not only to protect the extraoral film from exposure but also to hold the intensifying screens in perfect contact with the extraoral film. Contact between the screen and the film is critical; lack of contact between screen and film results in loss of image sharpness.

A rigid cassette has a front cover and a back cover. The front cover is placed in such a way that it faces the tubehead and is usually constructed of plastic to permit the x-ray beam to pass through. The back cover is constructed of heavy metal and serves to reduce scatter radiation. Intensifying screens are installed inside the front and back covers of the cassette. The film is positioned between the two intensifying screens. Each screen exposes one side of the film.

The cassette must be marked to orient the finished radiograph; a metal letter "L" is attached to the front cover of the cassette to indicate the patient's left side, and a metal letter "R" indicates the patient's right side.

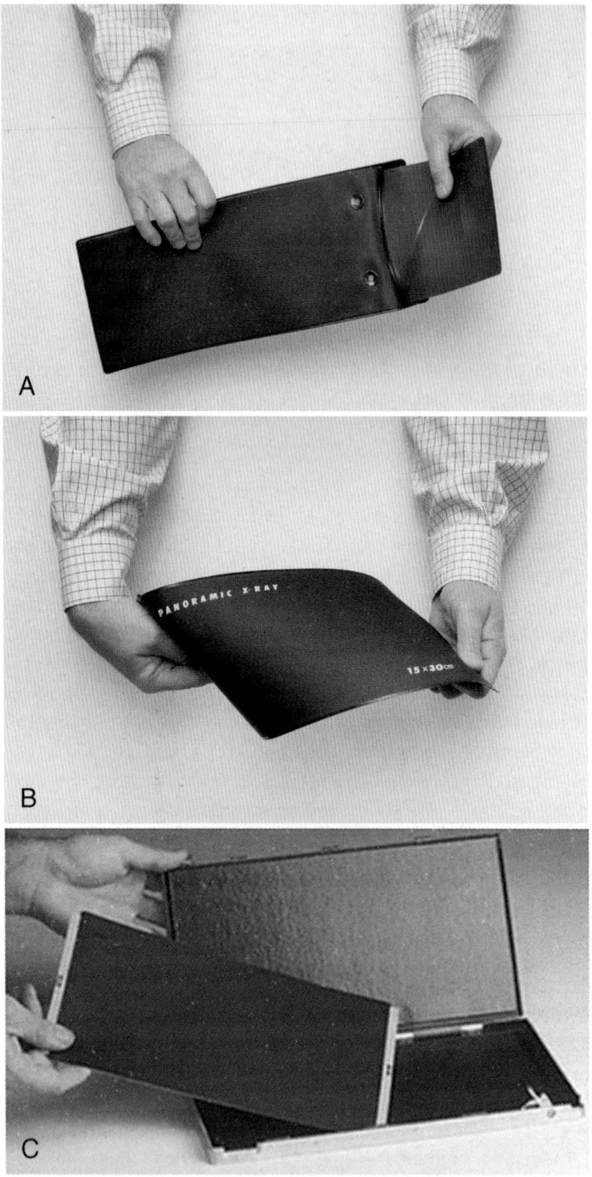

Fig 9-20 A and B, Close-up views of a flexible 5 × 12-inch panoramic cassette. (Courtesy KaVo Imaging, Brea, CA.) C, Rigid panoramic cassette.

Duplicating Film

A **duplicate radiograph** is one that is identical to the original x-ray film. In dentistry, duplicate radiographs are used for patient referrals to specialists, for insurance claims, and as teaching aids. A special film, or duplicating film, is required to make a duplicate radiograph.

Description. In dental radiography, a **duplicating film** is a type of photographic film used to make an identical copy of an intraoral or extraoral radiograph. Unlike intraoral and extraoral films, the duplicating film is used only in a darkroom setting and is not exposed to x-rays.

When examined in the darkroom under safe light conditions, duplicating film has an emulsion on one side only. The emulsion side of the film appears dull, whereas the side without the emulsion appears shiny. The emulsion side of the duplicating film must contact the original processed film during the duplication process. (Chapter 10 describes the equipment necessary for film duplication and the duplication process.)

Packaging. Duplicating films are boxed in sets of 50 sheets and are available in three sizes: 5 × 12-inch, 6 × 12-inch, and 8 × 10-inch.

FILM STORAGE AND PROTECTION

Films are adversely affected by heat, humidity, and radiation. To prevent film fog (see Chapter 10), unexposed, unprocessed films must be kept in a cool, dry place. The optimum temperature for film storage ranges from 50° F to 70° F, and the optimum relative humidity level ranges from 30% to 50%. Films must be stored in areas that are adequately shielded from sources of radiation and should not be stored in areas where patients are exposed to x-radiation. Lead-lined or radiation-resistant film dispensers and storage boxes are ideal to prevent film fog.

All dental x-ray films have limited shelf life. Each box or container of films is clearly labeled with an expiration date. Films must be used before the labeled expiration date. The "first-in, first-out" rule of thumb should be applied to film use; the oldest films in stock should always be used before new films.

SUMMARY

- The dental x-ray film is an image receptor that has four basic components: (1) a film base, (2) an adhesive layer, (3) film emulsion, and (4) a protective layer.
- An image is recorded on the dental x-ray film when the film is exposed to x-radiation.
- The silver halide crystals in the film emulsion absorb the x-radiation during x-ray exposure and store the energy from the radiation. The stored energy forms an invisible pattern on the emulsion and is known as the *latent image.*
- When the exposed film with the latent image undergoes chemical processing, a visible image results.
- Three types of film are used in dental radiography: (1) intraoral, (2) extraoral, and (3) duplicating.
- The intraoral film is placed inside the mouth and is then exposed; the extraoral film is placed outside the mouth and is then exposed; and the duplicating film is used to make a copy of an original radiograph and is not exposed to x-rays.
- An intraoral film packet is made up of four separate items: (1) x-ray film, (2) paper film wrapper, (3) lead foil sheet, and (4) outer package wrapping.
- Intraoral films are manufactured in five sizes (0, 1, 2, 3, 4); the larger the number, the larger the size of the film.
- Intraoral films are available in D-speed, E/F-speed, and F-speed. The F-speed film reduces patient exposure to radiation by 60% compared with the D-speed film, with no loss of image contrast or quality.
- Extraoral films are typically screen films and require the use of intensifying screens and a cassette for exposure.
- Intensifying screens transform x-ray energy into visible light, which in turn exposes the screen film.
- The use of intensifying screens requires less radiation to expose a screen film and results in less radiation exposure of the patient.
- The duplicating film is a special type of photographic film used to make an identical copy of an intraoral or extraoral radiograph.
- The duplicating film is used in a darkroom setting and is not exposed to x-radiation.
- Films are adversely affected by heat, humidity, and radiation. Film must be stored away from sources of radiation, at a temperature of 50° to 70° F, and with a relative humidity level of 30% to 50%.
- Dental films should always be used before the expiration date printed on the label.

BIBLIOGRAPHY

Frommer HH, Stabulas-Savage JJ: Image formation. In Radiology for the dental professional, ed 9, St Louis, 2011, Mosby.

Frommer HH, Stabulas-Savage JJ: Image receptors. In Radiology for the dental professional, ed 8, St Louis, 2005, Mosby.

Johnson ON: Dental x-ray films. In Essentials of dental radiography for dental assistants and hygienists, ed 9, Upper Saddle River, NJ, 2011, Prentice Hall.

Mallya SM, Lam EWN: Digital Imaging. In White and Pharoah's oral radiology: principles and interpretation, ed 8, St. Louis, 2019, Elsevier.

Miles DA, Van Dis ML, Jensen CW, et al: Film processing and quality assurance. In Radiographic imaging for the dental team, ed 4, St Louis, 2009, Saunders.

QUIZ QUESTIONS

Fill in the Blank

1. The component of the x-ray film described as "a thin transparent coating that is placed over the emulsion" is termed:

____

2. The component of the x-ray film described as "a flexible piece of plastic that withstands heat, moisture, and chemical heat" is termed:

____

3. The chemical compounds that change when exposed to radiation or light are termed:

____

4. The invisible pattern of stored energy on the exposed film is termed:

____

Identification

For questions 5 to 11, identify the items indicated on the intraoral film packet illustrated in Figure 9-21.

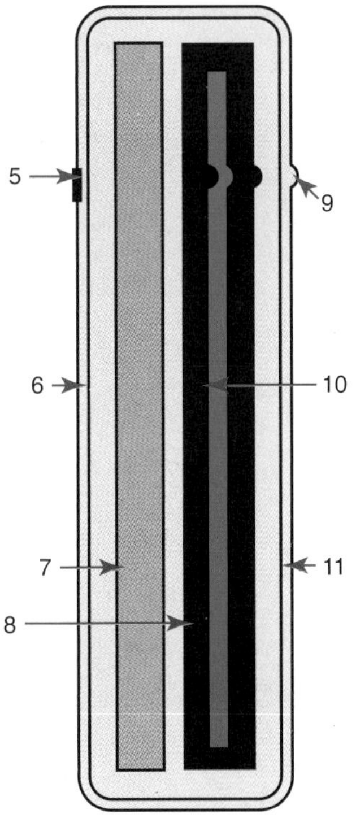

Fig 9-21

Multiple Choice

____ 12. Dental x-ray film that is placed inside the mouth and used to examine the teeth and supporting structures is termed:
- **a.** duplicating
- **b.** extraoral
- **c.** intraoral
- **d.** none of the above

____ 13. The identification dot on the intraoral film is significant because it:
- **a.** indicates the patient's right or left side
- **b.** determines film orientation
- **c.** is important in film mounting
- **d.** all of the above

____ 14. One advantage of a film with an emulsion coating on both sides (double-emulsion film) is that:
- **a.** the film requires less radiation exposure to make an image
- **b.** the image produced is less distorted
- **c.** the film has less sensitivity to radiation
- **d.** processing solutions are absorbed more easily

____ 15. The purpose of a lead foil sheet in the film packet is to:
- **a.** protect the film from primary radiation
- **b.** protect the film from saliva
- **c.** protect the film from backscattered radiation
- **d.** distinguish between the patient's right and left sides

____ 16. Which is not found on the label side of the film packet?
- **a.** film speed
- **b.** expiration date
- **c.** the phrase "opposite side toward tube"
- **d.** number of films enclosed

____ 17. Which film size is known as the *standard film*?
- **a.** 0
- **b.** 1
- **c.** 2
- **d.** 3

____ 18. Which is the largest intraoral film size?
- **a.** 4
- **b.** 3
- **c.** 2
- **d.** 1

____ 19. The film characteristic that is "the amount of radiation needed to produce a radiograph of standard density" is:
- **a.** contrast
- **b.** speed
- **c.** image resolution
- **d.** size

____ 20. The speed of a film is determined by the size of the silver halide crystals in the emulsion. Identify the true statement:
- **a.** The larger the crystals, the faster the film speed.
- **b.** The larger the crystals, the slower the film speed.
- **c.** The smaller the crystals, the faster the film speed.
- **d.** None of the above are correct.

_____ **21.** A film that is placed outside the mouth during x-ray exposure is termed:
- **a.** extraoral
- **b.** intraoral
- **c.** duplicating
- **d.** periapical

_____ **22.** A screen film is more sensitive to fluorescent light than to direct exposure to x-rays.
- **a.** True
- **b.** False

_____ **23.** Nonscreen extraoral film is commonly used in extraoral radiography.
- **a.** True
- **b.** False

_____ **24.** The device that transfers x-ray energy into visible light is termed a(n):
- **a.** cassette
- **b.** nonscreen film
- **c.** screen film
- **d.** intensifying screen

_____ **25.** The intensifying screen that emits green light and must be used with green-sensitive film is termed:
- **a.** calcium tungstate
- **b.** rare earth
- **c.** phosphor
- **d.** rare tungstate

_____ **26.** The device used to hold the extraoral film and intensifying screens is termed a:
- **a.** screen holder
- **b.** film holder
- **c.** cassette
- **d.** any of the above

_____ **27.** Which statement is true?
- **a.** Cassettes are available in sizes that correspond to film and screen sizes.
- **b.** A flexible cassette is more expensive than is a rigid cassette.
- **c.** Film can be loaded incorrectly in the rigid cassette.
- **d.** Film cannot be loaded incorrectly in the flexible cassette.

_____ **28.** What results if the intensifying screen is not in perfect contact with the screen film?
- **a.** The screen may be damaged.
- **b.** The film may be damaged.
- **c.** A loss of image sharpness occurs.
- **d.** None of the above.

_____ **29.** Which statement about the duplicating film is false?
- **a.** It is not exposed to x-rays.
- **b.** It is used in the darkroom.
- **c.** It may be placed intraorally or extraorally.
- **d.** It is used to make copies of radiographs.

_____ **30.** Identify the ideal temperature and humidity levels for film storage:
- **a.** 50° F to 70° F; 30% to 50%
- **b.** 60° F to 80° F; 50% to 60%
- **c.** 70° F to 90° F; 60% to 70%
- **d.** below 50° F; 0% to 30%

10

Film Processing

LEARNING OBJECTIVES

After completion of this chapter, the student will be able to do the following:

1. Define the key terms associated with processing of dental x-ray film.
2. Briefly describe how a latent image becomes a visible image.
3. Discuss the advantages of automatic film processing.
4. List and identify the component parts of the automatic film processor.
5. Describe the mechanism of automatic film processing.
6. List and discuss the four procedural steps for automatic film processing.
7. Describe the care and maintenance of the automatic film processor and automatic processing solutions.
8. List and discuss the five steps of manual film processing.
9. List the four basic ingredients of the developer solution.
10. List the four basic ingredients of the fixer solution.
11. Identify the parts of the processing tank: insert tanks, master tank, and lid.
12. Identify the equipment accessories needed for manual film processing.
13. List the procedural steps for manual film processing.
14. Describe the care and maintenance of the processing solutions, equipment, and equipment accessories used in manual film processing.
15. Discuss the primary function of the darkroom, as well as the location and size requirements necessary for the darkroom.
16. Discuss room lighting and safelighting.
17. Discuss miscellaneous requirements necessary in the darkroom.
18. Discuss waste management of items used in the darkroom.
19. Discuss the equipment requirements and procedural steps for film duplication.
20. Describe film processing problems that result from time and temperature errors.
21. Describe film processing problems that result from chemical contamination errors.
22. Describe film processing problems that result from film handling errors.
23. Describe film processing problems that result from lighting errors.

Traditional film continues to be used in dental practices. Although increasing numbers of dentists have transitioned from film-based to digital imaging, many offices still rely on film and processing. As long as film continues to be used, an understanding of film processing is needed. Film processing procedures directly affect the quality of a dental radiograph. The dental radiographer must have a working knowledge of film processing procedures, problems, and solutions.

The purpose of this chapter is to detail film processing procedures, to discuss automatic and manual film processing, to describe darkroom requirements, and to explain film duplication procedures. In addition, this chapter discusses common processing problems and provides solutions.

FILM PROCESSING

Film processing refers to a series of steps that produce a visible permanent image on a dental radiograph. The purpose of film processing is twofold:

- To convert the latent (invisible) image on the film into a visible image
- To preserve the visible image so that it is permanent and does not disappear from the dental radiograph

Film Processing Fundamentals

As detailed in Chapter 9, the silver halide crystals in the film emulsion absorb x-radiation during x-ray exposure and store the energy from the radiation. The stored energy within the silver halide crystals forms a pattern and creates an invisible image within the emulsion on the exposed film. This pattern of stored energy on the exposed film cannot be seen and is referred to as the **latent image**. The latent image remains invisible within the film emulsion until it undergoes chemical processing procedures.

From Latent Image to Visible Image. How does the latent image become a visible image? Under special darkroom conditions, a chemical reaction takes place when a film with a latent image is immersed in a series of special chemical solutions. During processing, a chemical reaction occurs, and the halide portion of the *exposed, energized* silver halide crystal is removed; chemically, this is referred to as a **reduction**. Reduction of the exposed silver halide crystals results in precipitated black metallic silver.

During film processing, selective reduction of the exposed silver halide crystals occurs. **Selective reduction** refers to the reduction of the energized, exposed silver halide crystals into black metallic silver, while the *unenergized, unexposed* silver halide crystals are removed from the film. The latent image is made visible through processing procedures (Figure 10-1), as follows:

- The film is placed in a chemical known as the **developer solution** for a specific amount of time and at a specific temperature. The developer distinguishes between the exposed and unexposed silver halide crystals. The developer initiates a chemical reaction that reduces the exposed silver halide crystals into black metallic silver and creates dark or black areas on a dental radiograph. At the same time, the unexposed silver halide crystals remain virtually unaffected by the developer.

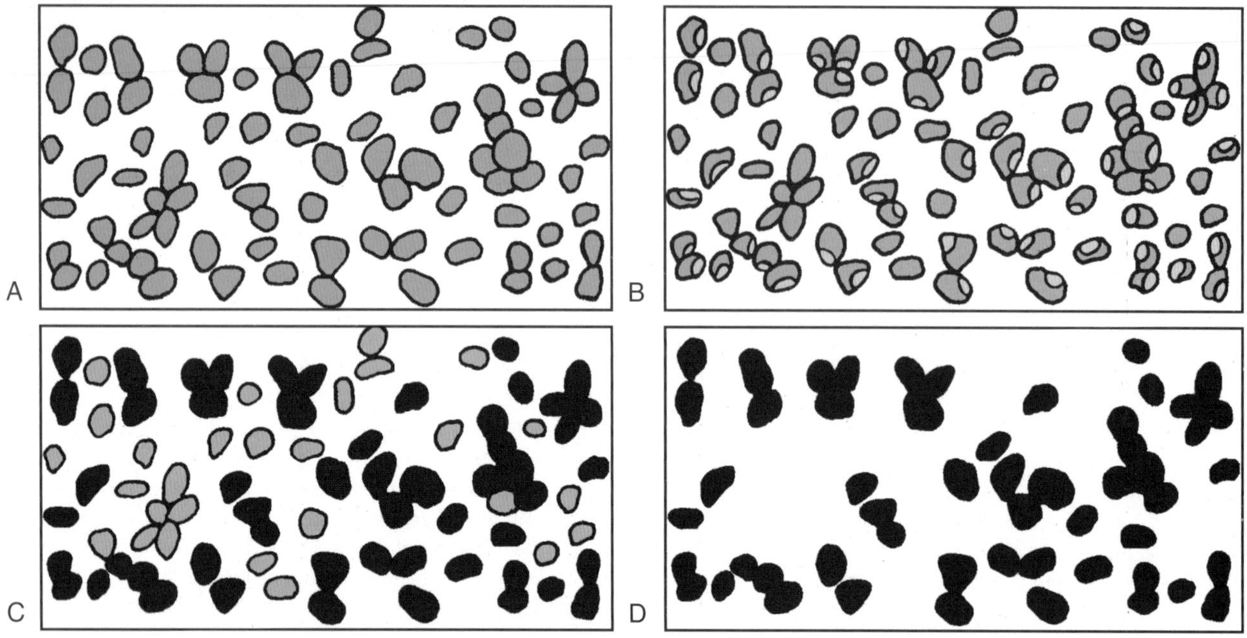

Fig 10-1 A, Schematic distribution of silver halide grains. The gray areas indicate a latent image produced by exposure. B, Partial development begins to produce metallic silver (*yellow*) in exposed grains. C, Development completed. D, Unexposed silver grains have been removed by fixing.

- The film is placed in a chemical known as the fixer solution for a specific amount of time. The fixer solution removes the unexposed silver halide crystals and creates white or clear areas on the dental radiograph. Meanwhile, the black metallic silver is not removed and remains on the film.

The Visible Image. The visible image that results on a dental radiograph is made up of black, white, and gray areas. Deposits of black metallic silver create the black areas seen on a dental radiograph. The amount of deposited black metallic silver seen on a dental radiograph varies depending on the structures being radiographed. The white areas on a dental radiograph result from the removal of the unexposed silver halide crystals. The amount of unexposed silver halide crystals removed depends on the structures being radiographed. As discussed in Chapter 6, structures that permit the passage of the x-ray beam appear black, or *radiolucent* (see Figure 6-1), as follows:

Radiolucent: A radiolucent structure is one that readily permits the passage of the x-ray beam and allows more x-rays to reach the film. If more x-rays reach the film, more silver halide crystals in the film emulsion are exposed and energized, thus resulting in increased deposits of black metallic silver. A radiograph with large deposits of black metallic silver appears black, or radiolucent.

As discussed in Chapter 6, structures that resist the passage of the x-ray beam appear white or *radiopaque* (see Figure 6-2), as follows:

Radiopaque: A radiopaque structure is one that resists the passage of the x-ray beam and restricts or limits the amount of x-rays that reach the film. If no x-rays reach the film, no silver halide crystals in the film emulsion are exposed, and no deposits of black metallic silver are seen. A radiograph with areas of unexposed silver halide crystals that have been removed during processing and with no black metallic silver deposits appears white, or radiopaque.

Film Processing Techniques

Two types of film processing techniques are discussed in this text: automatic and manual. Although automatic processing is used far more often than manual film processing, both are presented with step-by-step procedures to be used as a guide, if needed. Many dental practices using digital imaging choose to maintain automatic processing equipment as a backup option in the event of computer or software failures. In addition, some dental practices choose to maintain manual film processing capability in the event of automatic processor failure.

AUTOMATIC FILM PROCESSING

Automatic processing is a simple way of processing dental x-ray films.

Film Processing Steps

Automatic film processing consists of the following four steps:

1. Development
2. Fixing
3. Washing
4. Drying

The essential piece of equipment required for automatic processing is the automatic film processing machine, or automatic processor. A variety of automatic film processors are commercially available (Figure 10-2). Some automatic processors are limited to certain sizes of x-ray film, whereas others are capable of processing several different film sizes. Some automatic film processors are restricted to use under safelight conditions, whereas others, with daylight loaders, or light-shielded compartments, can be used in a room with white light (Figure 10-3). Automatic processors also vary in plumbing requirements and replenishment systems.

Many dental personnel prefer automatic processing as a method of film processing for the following reasons:

1. Less processing time is required.
2. Time and temperatures are automatically controlled.
3. Less equipment is used.
4. Less space is required.

Automatic film processing has a number of advantages. The major advantage is the time saved; an automatic processor requires only

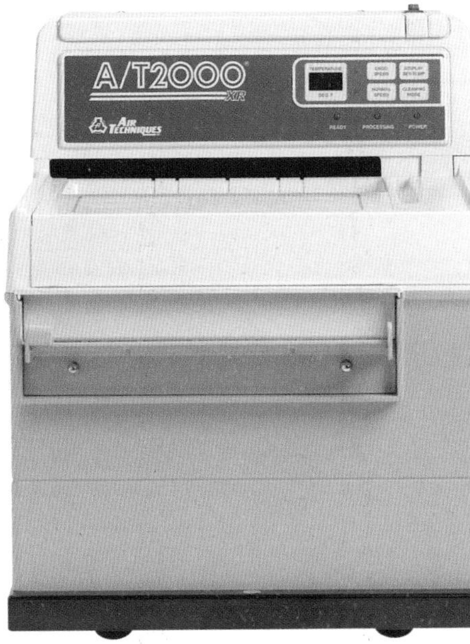

Fig 10-2 A typical automatic film processor used in the dental office. (Courtesy Air Techniques Inc., Melville, NY.)

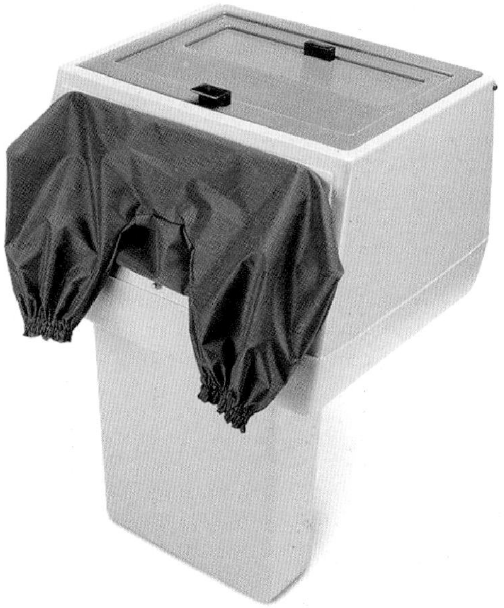

Fig 10-3 A daylight loader, which may be attached to the top of an automatic processor. (Courtesy Air Techniques Inc., Melville, NY.)

4 to 6 minutes to develop, fix, wash, and dry the film, whereas manual film processing techniques require up to 1 hour. Another advantage is the automatic control of time and temperature; the automatic processor maintains the correct temperature of solutions and controls the processing time, thus providing uniform film processing.

Equipment Requirements

When the automatic processor is properly maintained, this equipment produces high-quality radiographs. The automatic processor uses a roller transport system to move the unwrapped dental x-ray film through the developer, fixer, water, and drying compartments. Each component of the automatic processor contributes to the mechanism of automatic film processing and has a specific function (Figure 10-4), as follows:

- The **processor housing** encases all the component parts of the automatic processor.
- The **film feed slot** is an opening on the outside of the processor housing used to insert unwrapped films into the automatic processor.
- The **roller film transporter** is a system of rollers used to move the film rapidly through the developer, fixer, water, and drying compartments. Motor-driven gears or belts propel the rollers. The primary function of the rollers is to move the film through the automatic processor. In addition to moving the film, the rollers produce a wringing action that removes the excess solution from the emulsion as the film moves from compartment to compartment. This wringing action eliminates the need for an additional rinse step between the developer and fixer solutions (as seen in manual processing). The motion of the rollers also gently agitates the processing solutions, contributing to the uniformity of the processing.
- The **developer compartment** holds the developer solution. The developer solution used in an automatic processor is a specially formulated, highly concentrated chemical solution designed to react at temperatures between 80° F and 95° F. As a result of the high temperatures, development occurs rapidly. The developer solution used in manual film processing is not the same as the developer used in automatic film processing and should *never* be used in an automatic processor.
- The **fixer compartment** holds the fixer solution. The film is transported directly from the developer solution into the fixer *without* a rinsing step. The fixer solution used in an automatic processor is a specially formulated, highly concentrated chemical solution that contains additional hardening agents. In the fixer solution, the film is rapidly fixed or "cleared" and then hardened. The fixer solution used in manual film processing is not the same as the fixer used in automatic film processing and should *never* be used in an automatic processor.
- The **water compartment** holds circulating water. Water is used to wash the films after fixing. After washing, the wet film is transported from the water compartment to a drying chamber.
- The **drying chamber** holds heated air and is used to dry the wet film.
- A **replenisher pump** and **replenisher solutions** are used to maintain proper solution concentration and levels automatically in some automatic processors, whereas other processors require the operator to add the necessary replenishing solutions.
- The **film recovery slot** is an opening on the outside of the processor housing where the dry, processed radiograph emerges from the automatic processor.

Step-by-Step Procedures

Before processing, the exposed dental x-ray film and automatic processor (without daylight loader) must be present in the darkroom. Specific infection prevention procedures that pertain to automatic film processing are detailed in Chapter 16. For procedural steps, see Procedure 10-1.

Care and Maintenance

The automatic processor and automatic processing solutions must be carefully maintained. The manufacturer's recommendations for care and maintenance must be followed meticulously.

Automatic Processor. The automatic processor requires routine preventive maintenance. Without proper cleaning and replenishment,

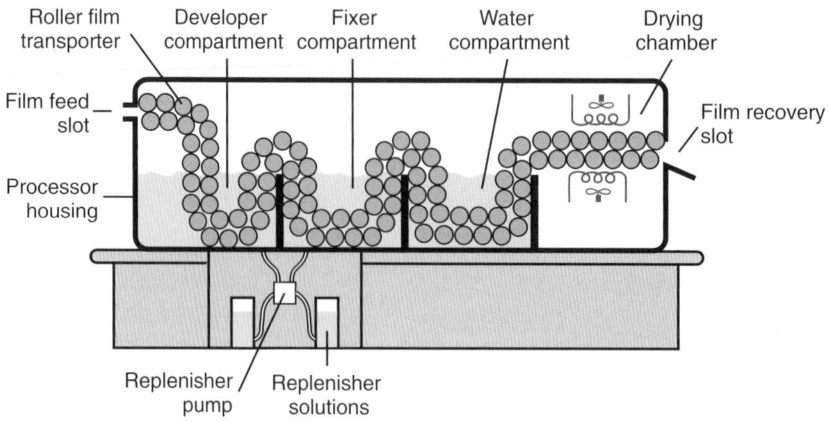

Fig 10-4 Component parts of the automatic processor.

PROCEDURE 10-1 Automatic Film Processing

1. Prepare the darkroom.
   - If a daylight loader is not part of the automatic processor, the films must be processed in the darkroom.
   - Close and lock the door of the darkroom, turn off the overhead white light, and turn on the safelights.
2. Prepare the films.
   - For intraoral films, carefully unwrap each exposed film over a clean work surface using proper infection prevention procedures (see Chapter 16).
   - Dispose of all film packet wrappings and recycle lead foil.
   - For extraoral films, carefully remove the film from the cassette.
   - Handle all films by the edges only.
3. Insert the films.
   - Insert each unwrapped film into the film feed slot of the processor, one at a time.
   - Allow at least 10 seconds between insertions of films.
   - Alternate sides or slots, whenever possible.
   - Make certain that films are straight when inserted. (When films are turned sideways or inserted too quickly, overlapping may occur during processing. Overlapped films result in nondiagnostic radiographs.)
4. Process and retrieve the films.
   - After the films have been inserted into the automatic processor, allow 4 to 6 minutes for automated processing to occur.
   - Retrieve the processed radiographs from the film recovery slot on the outside of the automatic processor.

the automatic processor will malfunction. A cleaning and replenishment schedule must be established and followed strictly to ensure optimum automatic processor performance.

Depending on the volume of films processed, the automatic processor requires daily or weekly cleaning. An extraoral-size cleaning film is used to clean the rollers of the automatic processor and is typically run through the processor at the beginning of each day. The cleaning film removes any residual gelatin or dirt from the rollers. Each week the rollers must be removed from the automatic processor, cleaned in warm running water, and then soaked for 10 to 20 minutes. The manufacturer's recommendations for daily and monthly cleaning of the automatic processor must be carefully followed.

Processing Solutions. If the automatic processor does not have automatic replenishment, the processing solution levels in the automatic processor must be checked at the beginning of each day and replenisher added as necessary. Failure to add replenisher results in exhausted solutions and nondiagnostic radiographs. Processing solutions in the automatic processor must be replaced every 2 to 6 weeks, depending on the number of films processed and the replenishment schedule. The manufacturer's recommendations for the changing of solutions must be carefully followed.

MANUAL FILM PROCESSING

The vast majority of dental practices that use film-based imaging use automatic processing. As manual film processing becomes less popular, there is limited need for detailed information. However, if the radiographer is employed in a dental practice that still uses this processing technique, the detailed information provided here can be used as a step-by-step guide. Instructors using this text may choose to spend limited time on the topic of manual film processing. Manual film processing (also known as *hand processing* or *tank processing*) is a simple method of developing, rinsing, fixing, and washing dental x-ray films. To process films manually, the dental radiographer must be knowledgeable about specific equipment requirements, step-by-step processing procedures, and care and maintenance of the equipment and supplies.

Film Processing Steps

Manual film processing consists of the following five steps:

1. Development
2. Rinsing
3. Fixing
4. Washing
5. Drying

Development. The first step in film processing is development. A chemical solution known as the *developer* is used in the development process. The purpose of the developer is to reduce the exposed, energized silver halide crystals chemically to black metallic silver. The developer solution softens the film emulsion during this process.

Rinsing. After development, a water bath is used to wash or rinse the film. Rinsing is necessary to remove the developer from the film and stop the development process.

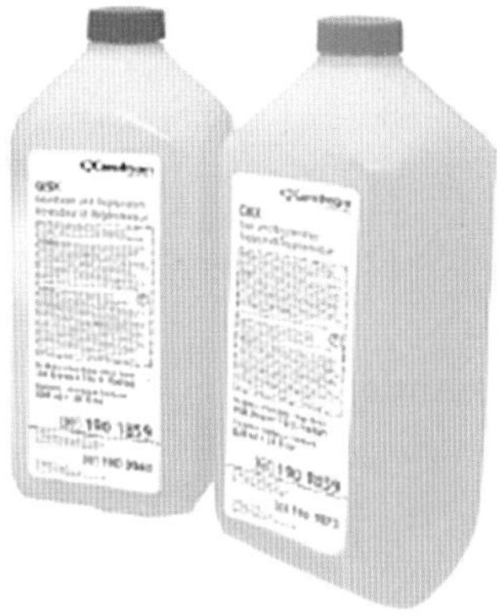

Fig 10-5 Liquid concentrates of developer and fixer. (Courtesy Carestream Health, Inc., Rochester, NY.)

Fixing. After rinsing, fixing takes place. A chemical solution known as the *fixer* is used in the fixing process. The purpose of the fixer is to remove the unexposed, unenergized silver halide crystals from the film emulsion. The fixer hardens the film emulsion during this process.

Washing. After fixing, a water bath is used to wash the film. A washing step is necessary to thoroughly remove all excess chemicals from the emulsion.

Drying. The final step in film processing is the drying of the films. Films may be air-dried at room temperature in a dust-free area or placed in a heated drying cabinet. Films must be completely dried before handling for mounting and viewing.

Film Processing Solutions

Film processing solutions may be obtained in the following forms:

- Powder
- Ready-to-use liquid
- Liquid concentrate

Both the powder and the liquid concentrate forms must be mixed with distilled water. The liquid concentrate form is popular and is used in most dental offices; it is easy to mix and occupies little storage space (Figure 10-5). It is important to follow the manufacturer's recommendations for the preparation of such solutions.

Fresh chemicals produce the best radiographs. To maintain freshness, film processing solutions must be replenished daily and changed every 3 to 4 weeks; more frequent changing of solutions may be necessary when large numbers of films are processed. "Normal" use is defined as 30 intraoral films per day.

As described under Film Processing Steps, two special chemical solutions are necessary for film processing: developer and fixer.

Developer Solution. The developer solution contains four basic ingredients: (1) developing agent, (2) preservative, (3) accelerator, and (4) restrainer (Table 10-1).

Developing agent. The developing agent (also known as the *reducing agent*) contains two chemicals, hydroquinone (paradihydroxybenzene) and elon (monomethyl-para-aminophenol sulfate). The purpose of the developing agent is to reduce the exposed silver halide crystals chemically to black metallic silver.

Hydroquinone generates the black tones and the sharp contrast of the radiographic image. Hydroquinone is temperature sensitive; it is inactive below 60° F and very active above 80° F. Because this chemical is sensitive to temperature, the temperature of the developing solution is critical. The optimal temperature for the developer solution is 68° F.

TABLE 10-1 Developer Composition

Ingredient	Chemical	Function
Developing agent	Hydroquinone	Converts the exposed silver halide crystals to black metallic silver
		Slowly generates the black tones and contrast in the image
	Elon	Converts the exposed silver halide crystals to black metallic silver
		Quickly generates the gray tones in the image
Preservative	Sodium sulfite	Prevents rapid oxidation of the developing agents
Accelerator	Sodium carbonate	Activates the developer agents
		Provides the necessary alkaline environment for the developing agents
		Softens the gelatin of the film emulsion
Restrainer	Potassium bromide	Prevents the developer from developing the unexposed silver halide crystals

Elon, also known as *metol*, acts quickly to produce a visible radiographic image. Elon generates the many shades of gray seen on a dental radiograph. This chemical is not temperature sensitive. If hydroquinone and Elon were used individually and not in combination, Elon would produce a film that appeared gray with indistinct contrast, whereas hydroquinone would produce a film that appeared black and white. Using a combination of these chemicals produces a film with black, white, and shades of gray.

Preservative. The antioxidant sodium sulfite is the preservative used in the developer solution. The purpose of the preservative is to prevent the developer solution from oxidizing in the presence of air. The reducing agents hydroquinone and Elon are not stable in the presence of oxygen and readily absorb oxygen from the air. If these agents react with oxygen, the action of the developer solution is weakened. The preservative helps to prevent this weakening and to extend the useful life of hydroquinone and Elon.

Accelerator. The alkali sodium carbonate is used in the developer solution as an accelerator. The purpose of the accelerator (also called the *activator*) is to activate the developing agents. The developing agents are active only in an alkaline (high-pH) environment. For example, hydroquinone and Elon do not develop when used alone; the presence of an alkaline accelerator is required. The accelerator not only provides the necessary alkaline environment for the developing agents but also softens the gelatin of the film emulsion so that the developing agents can reach the silver halide crystals more effectively.

Restrainer. The restrainer used in the developing solution is potassium bromide. The purpose of the restrainer is to control the developer and to prevent it from developing the exposed and unexposed silver halide crystals. Although the restrainer stops the development of both exposed and unexposed crystals, it is most effective in stopping development of the unexposed crystals. As a result, the restrainer prevents the radiographic image from appearing fogged; a fogged film appears dull gray, lacks contrast, and is nondiagnostic.

Fixer Solution. The fixer solution contains four basic ingredients: (1) fixing agent, (2) preservative, (3) hardening agent, and (4) acidifier (Table 10-2).

TABLE 10-2 Fixer Composition

Ingredient	Chemical	Function
Fixing agent	Sodium thiosulfate; ammonium thiosulfate	Removes all the unexposed undeveloped silver halide crystals from the emulsion
Preservative	Sodium sulfite	Prevents the deterioration of the fixing agent
Hardening agent	Potassium alum	Shrinks and hardens the gelatin in the emulsion
Acidifier	Acetic acid; sulfuric acid	Neutralizes the alkaline developer and stops further development

Fixing agent. The fixing agent (also known as the *clearing agent*) is made up of sodium thiosulfate or ammonium thiosulfate and is commonly called hypo. The purpose of the fixing agent is to remove or clear all unexposed and undeveloped silver halide crystals from the film emulsion. This chemical "clears" the film so that the black image produced by the developer becomes readily distinguished.

Preservative. The same preservative used in the developer solution, sodium sulfite, is also used in the fixer solution. The purpose of the preservative is to prevent the chemical deterioration of the fixing agent.

Hardening agent. The hardening agent used in the fixer solution is potassium alum. The purpose of the hardening agent is to harden and shrink the gelatin in the film emulsion after the accelerator in the developer solution has softened it.

Acidifier. The acidifier used in the fixer solution is acetic acid or sulfuric acid. The purpose of the acidifier is to neutralize the alkaline developer. Any unneutralized alkali may cause the unexposed crystals to continue to develop in the fixer. The acidifier also produces the necessary acidic environment required by the fixing agent.

Equipment Requirements

Like automatic film processing, manual film processing has specific equipment requirements. Manual film processing equipment includes a processing tank and related equipment accessories.

Processing. The essential piece of equipment required for manual processing is a processing tank. A processing tank is a container divided into compartments to hold the developer solution, water bath, and fixer solution. A processing tank has two insert tanks and one master tank (Figure 10-6), as follows:

- Insert tanks. Two removable 1-gallon insert tanks hold the developer and fixer solutions. The insert tanks are placed within the master tank in a floating position. The developer solution is typically placed in the insert tank on the left, and the fixer solution is placed in the insert tank on the right. The water in the master tank separates the two insert tanks.
- Master tank. The master tank suspends both insert tanks and is filled with circulating water. The water surrounds both floating insert tanks. An overflow pipe is used to control the water level in the master tank.

Ideally, the processing tank should be constructed of stainless steel, which does not react with processing solutions and is easy to clean. The processing tank should be equipped with a light-tight lid that is used to cover the solutions at all times. The cover protects the solutions from oxidation and evaporation, and during processing it protects the developing films from exposure to light.

The temperature of the circulating water in the master tank controls the temperatures of the developer and fixer solutions. A processing tank must be supplied with both hot and cold running water and a mixing valve. The water temperature is controlled through a mixing valve, which mixes the incoming hot and cold water (as in bathroom showers) to produce a water bath that maintains an optimum temperature of 68° F.

Equipment Accessories

In addition to a processing tank, a few accessory equipment items, including a thermometer, timer, and film hangers, are necessary for manual film processing.

Thermometer. A nonmercury thermometer is necessary for manual processing and is used to determine the temperature of the developer solution. A floating thermometer or one that is clipped to the side of the developer tank may be used (Figure 10-7). A thermometer containing metal or alcohol solution is recommended over one that contains mercury. Mercury is a toxic substance, and spills must be handled according to Environmental Protection Agency (EPA) standards.

A thermometer must be placed directly in the developer solution and not in the water bath. Why? As previously stated, the temperature of the water in the master tank controls the temperature of the developer and fixer solutions in the insert tanks. The water in the master tank reaches the desired temperature almost as soon as it is turned on. The water, however, must circulate in the master tank for some time to equalize the temperatures of the processing solutions. Depending on the size of the insert tanks and the temperature of the solutions, the developer and fixer solutions may take up to 1 hour to reach the temperature of the water bath.

Using a thermometer, the developer temperature must always be checked before processing. The optimum temperature for development is 68° F. Below 60° F, the chemicals work too slowly and result in underdevelopment. Over 80° F, the chemicals work too rapidly and produce film fog. The temperature of the developer determines development time. A time-temperature chart can be used to determine development time (Table 10-3). It is important to note that these temperatures refer to manual processing only.

HELPFUL HINT

Temperature for Manual Processing

68° F is the optimal temperature for the developer solution.

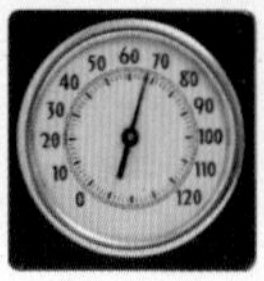

Timer. An accurate timer is also necessary for manual processing. X-ray film is processed in chemical solutions for specific intervals indicated by the manufacturer of the processing solutions. A timer is used to indicate such intervals (e.g., how long films have been placed in the developer solution, rinse water, fixer solution, and wash water). A timer is used to signal the radiographer that the films must be removed from the current processing solution. Development time depends on the temperature of the developer solution and must be adjusted based on time-temperature guidelines (see Table 10-3).

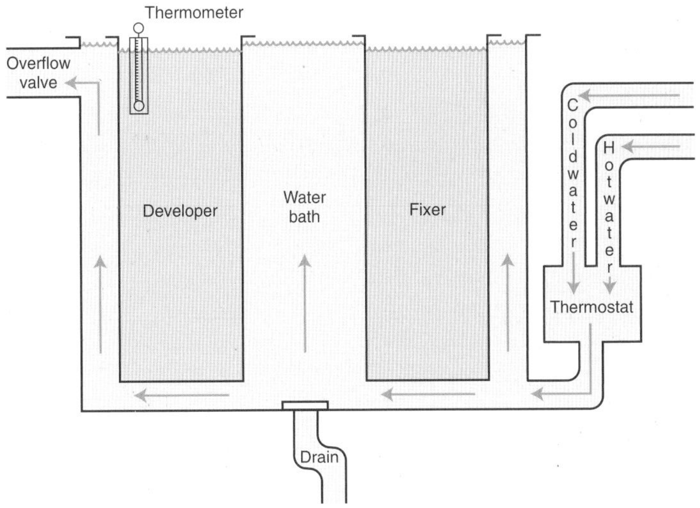

Fig 10-6 Processing tanks showing developing and fixing tank inserts in bath of running water with overflow drain. (Courtesy Frommer HH and Stabulas Savage, JJ: *Radiology for the Dental Professional*, ed 9, St. Louis, 2011, Mosby.)

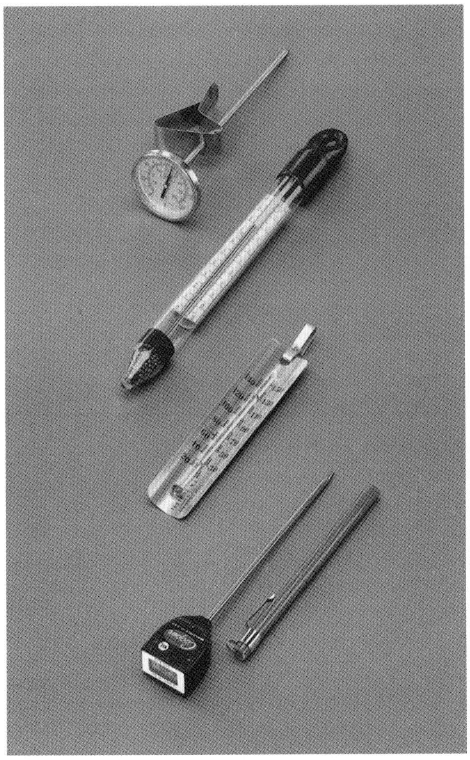

Fig 10-7 Examples of various thermometers used in manual film processing. (Courtesy Flow Dental, Deer Park, NY.)

Film Hangers. Film hangers (also known as *film racks* or *processing hangers*) are necessary for manual processing. A film hanger is a device equipped with clips used to hold films during processing (Figure 10-8). Film hangers are made of stainless steel and include an identification tab or label. Film hangers are available in various sizes and can hold up to 20 intraoral films.

Miscellaneous Equipment. A **stirring rod** or **stirring paddle** is a necessary piece of equipment for manual processing. A stirring rod is used to agitate the developer and fixer solutions before processing. The stirring action mixes the chemicals and equalizes the temperature of the solutions. The stirring rod or paddle may be plastic or glass. Another useful item for manual processing is a *plastic apron*, which is used to protect clothing during the processing of films and the mixing of chemicals.

Step-by-Step Procedures

Before processing the manual film, the exposed dental x-ray film and necessary equipment must be present in the darkroom. Specific infection prevention procedures that pertain to manual film processing are detailed in Chapter 16. For procedural steps, see Procedure 10-2.

Care and Maintenance

The processing solutions, equipment, and equipment accessories used in manual processing must be carefully maintained.

Processing Solutions. The manufacturer's instructions for the storage, mixing, and use of processing solutions must be carefully followed. Processing solutions deteriorate with exposure to air, continued use, and chemical contamination. Exhausted processing solutions result in nondiagnostic radiographs and therefore must be replaced. Processing solutions should be changed every 3 to 4 weeks; more frequent replacement of solutions may be necessary when large numbers of films are processed. It is suggested that both the developer and fixer solutions be changed at the same time. The processing solutions that require care and maintenance include the developer, fixer, and replenisher solutions.

Developer solution. The developer solution becomes depleted from evaporation and the removal of small amounts from the tank on the film hanger and films. With time and use, the developer solution decreases not only in volume but in strength as well. A weakened or exhausted developer solution does not fully develop the latent image and produces a nondiagnostic radiograph with reduced density and contrast.

TABLE 10-3 Manual Processing Temperatures and Times*

Developer Temperature		Time in Developer (minutes)	Rinse Time (minutes)	Time in Fixer (minutes)	Wash Time (minutes)
68° F	20.0° C	5.0	0.5	10	10
70° F	21.0° C	4.5	0.5	9-10	10
72° F	22.0° C	4.0	0.5	8-9	10
76° F	24.5° C	3.0	0.5	6-7	10
80° F	26.5° C	2.5	0.5	5-6	10

*Recommendations by Carestream Dental for INSIGHT film. Recommended water temperature for rinse, fixer, and wash is 60-85° F (15.5-29.5° C).

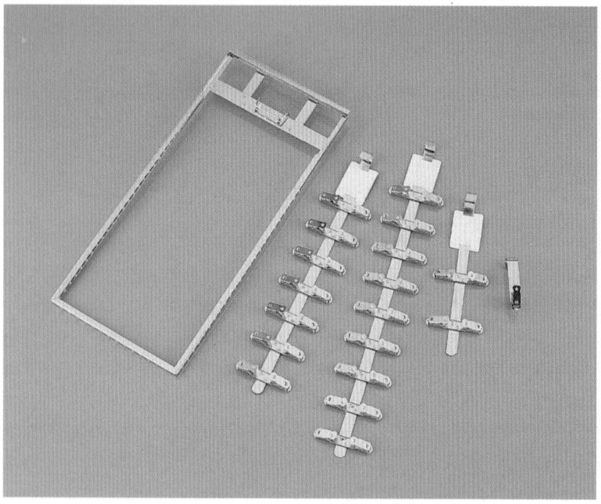

Fig 10-8 A variety of film hangers. (Courtesy Dentsply Rinn Corporation, York, PA.)

Six ounces of developer solution are typically added to the developer tank at the beginning of each day. When the tank is holding its maximum capacity (e.g., 1 gallon), 6 ounces must be removed before adding the replenisher.

Fixer solution. Fixer solution also decreases because of evaporation and the removal of small amounts from the tank on the film hanger and films. In addition, the fixer solution is diluted with water each time films are transferred from the rinse water to the fixer; this gradual dilution weakens the solution.

With time and use, the fixer solution decreases not only in volume but in strength as well. A full-strength fixer ensures adequate "clearing" of the film and hardening of the film emulsion. An exhausted or depleted fixer does not stop the chemical reaction sufficiently to maintain film clarity; the films will turn a yellow-brown color, transmit less light, and lose their diagnostic quality.

Three ounces of fixer solution are typically added to the fixer tank at the beginning of each day. When the tank is holding its maximum capacity (e.g., 1 gallon), 3 ounces must be removed before adding the replenisher.

Replenisher solution. To maintain adequate freshness, strength, and solution levels, both the developer and the fixer solution must be replenished daily. A replenisher is a superconcentrated solution that is added to the processing solutions to compensate for the loss of volume and strength that results from oxidation. Oxidation, or the process that occurs when developer and fixer solutions combine with oxygen and lose strength, takes place when the processing solutions are exposed to air. A breakdown of the chemicals in the processing solutions results, shortening the length of time the solutions can be used to produce diagnostic radiographs. Replenishment maintains adequate concentrations of chemicals, which ensures uniform results between solution changes.

Processing Tank. The interaction between the mineral salts in water and the carbonate in the processing solutions produces deposits on the inside walls of the insert tanks. Such deposits contaminate the processing solutions. To produce diagnostic radiographs, the processing tank must be kept clean.

The master and insert tanks are typically cleaned each time the solutions are changed. A commercial stainless steel tank cleaner or a solution of hydrochloric acid and water (1.5 ounces hydrochloric acid to 128 ounces of water) can be used to remove the mineral salts and carbonate deposits. Abrasive-type cleansers are not recommended for cleaning processing tanks; the cleansers may react unfavorably with the processing solutions. For procedural steps, see Procedure 10-3.

Miscellaneous Equipment. Cleanliness of manual processing equipment is essential. Film hangers and stirring paddles must be cleaned after each use. Both must be thoroughly cleaned, rinsed, and dried. The plastic apron used to protect clothing should also be wiped clean after each use.

THE DARKROOM

The primary function of a darkroom is to provide a completely darkened environment in which x-ray film can be handled and processed to produce diagnostic radiographs. The darkroom must be properly designed and well equipped.

Room Requirements

A well-planned darkroom makes processing easier. The ideal darkroom is the result of careful planning and must have the following characteristics:

1. Convenient location
2. Adequate size
3. Correct lighting equipment
4. Ample work space with adequate storage
5. Temperature and humidity control

Location and Size

The location of the darkroom must be convenient; ideally, it should be located near the area where x-ray units are installed. The darkroom must be large enough to accommodate film processing equipment and

PROCEDURE 10-2 Manual Film Processing

1. Identify the solutions.
   - Typically, the insert tank on the left is used for the developer, and the insert tank on the right is used for the fixer.
   - The fixer solution is easily identified by its vinegar-like odor.
2. Check the solution levels.
   - If the developer level is low, add fresh developer.
   - If the fixer level is low, add fresh fixer solution.
   - Never add water to raise the level of the solutions; it dilutes the strength of the chemicals.
3. Stir the solutions.
   - To avoid chemical contamination, use different paddles to stir the developer and the fixer.
   - Stirring the solutions mixes the chemicals and equalizes the temperature of the solutions.
4. Check the temperature.
   - Check the temperature of the developer solution.
   - The optimum temperature for the developer is between 68° F and 70° F; however, temperatures between 68° F and 80° F may be used.
   - Sufficient time must then be allowed for the developer to reach the correct temperature.
5. Label the hanger.
   - Label the film hanger with the name of the patient and the date of exposure.
6. Prepare the darkroom.
   - Close and lock the door of the darkroom.
   - Turn off the overhead white light, and turn on the safelights.
7. Unwrap the films.
   - For intraoral films, carefully unwrap each exposed film over a clean work surface using proper infection control procedures (see Chapter 16).
   - Dispose of all film packet wrappings and recycle lead foil.
   - For extraoral films, carefully remove the film from the cassette.
   - Handle all films holding them on the edges only.
8. Load the hanger.
   - Clip each unwrapped film to the labeled film hanger, one film to a clip.
   - Verify that each film is securely attached by running a finger along the film edge.
   - Reattach any loose films.
9. Set the timer.
   - On the basis of the temperature of the developer solution and the manufacturer's instructions, set the timer.
   - A time-temperature chart is used to determine such time intervals (see Table 10-3).
   - If the optimal temperature of 68° F is used, the recommended development time is 5 minutes.
10. Immerse the films, and activate the timer.
    - Immerse the film hanger with films into the developer solution.
    - Films must not contact other films or the side of the processing tank during development.
    - Gently agitate the film hanger up and down several times to prevent air bubbles from clinging to the film.
    - Hang the film rack on the edge of the insert tank and make certain that all films are immersed in the developer.
    - Activate the timer and cover the processing tank.
11. Remove the films from the developer, and rinse.
    - When the timer goes off, uncover the processing tank.
    - Remove the film hanger with films from the developer solution and place it in the circulating water of the master tank.
    - Agitate for 20 to 30 seconds.
    - Remove and drain excess water for several seconds.
12. Determine the fix time.
    - On the basis of the development time, determine the fixing time and set the timer. A time-temperature chart is used to determine such time intervals (see Table 10-3).
    - Fixing time is approximately double the development time.
13. Immerse the films, and activate the timer.
    - Immerse the film hanger with films in the fixer solution.
    - Gently agitate it up and down several times.
    - Hang the film rack on the edge of the insert tank and make certain that all films are immersed in the fixer.
    - Activate the timer and cover the processing tank.
14. Remove the films from the fixer solution and place into the water wash.
    - When the timer goes off, uncover the processing tank, remove the film hanger with films from the fixer, and allow the excess fixer to drain back into the fixer tank.
    - Place the film hanger with films in the circulating water.
    - Allow the films to wash for a minimum of 20 minutes.
15. Dry the films.
    - Remove the film hanger with films from the wash water and gently shake off excess water.
    - Cover the processing tank.
    - To air-dry the films, suspend the film hanger with films from a rod or drying rack in a dust-free area over a drip pan.
    - If a heated drying cabinet is used, the temperature should not exceed 120° F.
16. Remove the films from the rack.
    - Remove the dry radiographs from the film hanger and place them in an envelope labeled with the patient's name and date of exposure.
    - Outside the darkroom, use a viewbox to examine the processed films placed in a labeled film mount.
17. Clean up.
    - After manual processing procedures have been completed, clean all processing equipment and work surfaces.
    - Make certain to clean hangers and clips after each use.
    - A clean darkroom is essential for the production of diagnostic radiographs.

to allow ample work space. A darkroom should measure at least 16 to 20 square feet and provide enough space for one person to work comfortably. The size of the darkroom is determined by the following factors:

1. Volume of films processed
2. Number of persons using the room
3. Type of processing equipment used (processing tanks versus automatic processor)
4. Space required for duplication of films and storage

Lighting

As the term "darkroom" suggests, this room must be completely dark and must exclude all visible white light. The term **light-tight** is often used to describe the darkroom. To be considered light-tight, no light leaks can be present. Any white light that "leaks" into the darkroom (e.g., from around a door or through a vent) is termed a **light leak**. In a darkroom, when all the lights are turned off and the door is closed, no white light should be seen. Any white light coming around the door, through a vent or keyhole, or through a wall or ceiling seam is a light

PROCEDURE 10-3 Cleaning the Processing Tank

1. Drain the tanks.
   - Pull the drain plugs in the insert tanks and master tank.
   - Drain all liquid from each tank.
2. Clean and soak the tanks.
   - Pour cleaning solution into the master and insert tanks.
   - If the insert tanks are heavily coated with deposits, allow the tanks to soak for 30 minutes.
3. Scrub and rinse the tanks.
   - After soaking, use a brush to scrub all surfaces of the insert and master tanks and the tank cover.
   - Rinse thoroughly with water, wipe clean, and dry.
4. Add fresh solutions.
   - Pour fresh developer solution into the left insert tank and fresh fixer solution into the right insert tank.
   - Fill insert tanks until the solution level reaches the indicated fill line, about 1 inch from the top of the tank.
   - Fill the master tank with water.
5. Cover the tanks.
   - Place the lid on the processing tank.
   - The tank lid should be removed only when changing or adding solutions, when checking the developer temperature, or when processing films.

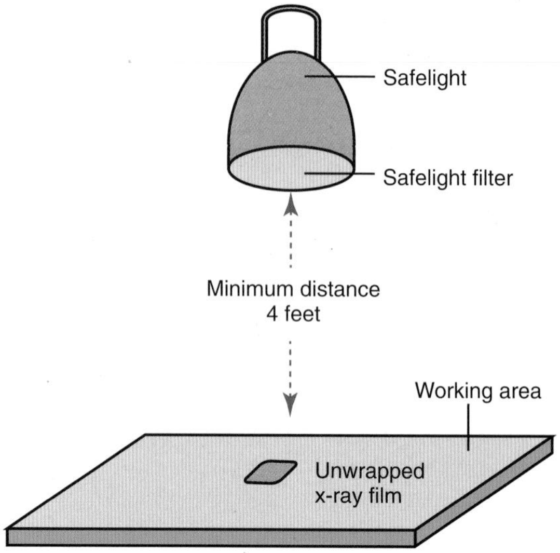

Fig 10-9 A minimum distance of 4 feet must exist between the safelight and the work area.

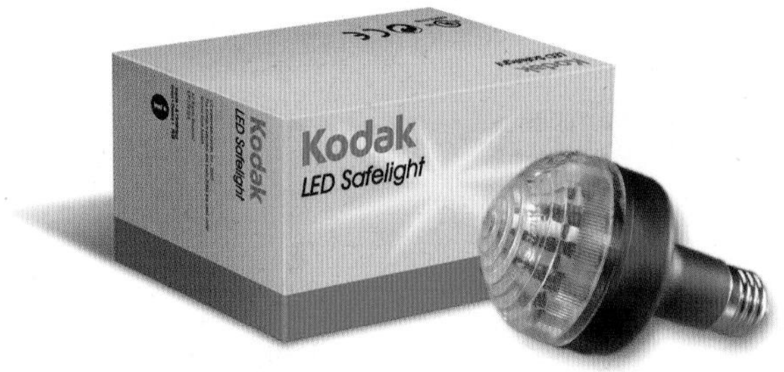

Fig 10-10 LED safelights are available for intraoral and extraoral films. (Courtesy Carestream Health, Inc., Rochester, NY.)

leak and must be immediately corrected with weather stripping or black tape. As previously discussed, x-ray film is extremely sensitive to visible white light. Any leaks of white light in the darkroom cause film "fogging." A fogged film appears dull gray, lacks contrast, and is nondiagnostic.

Two types of lighting are essential in a darkroom, as follows:

- **Room lighting**. Room lighting is required for procedures not associated with the act of processing films. An overhead white light that provides adequate illumination for the size of the room is necessary to perform tasks such as cleaning, stocking materials, and mixing chemicals.
- **Safelighting**. The special type of lighting used to provide illumination in the darkroom is termed *safelighting*. It is a low-intensity light composed of long wavelengths in the red-orange portion of the visible light spectrum. Safelighting provides sufficient illumination in the darkroom to carry out processing activities safely without exposing or damaging the film. Proper safelighting does not rapidly affect unwrapped x-ray film and does not cause film fogging.

A safelight typically consists of a lamp equipped with a frosted low-wattage bulb (15 watts or less) and a safelight filter. A **safelight filter** removes the short wavelengths in the blue-green portion of the visible light spectrum that are responsible for exposing and damaging x-ray film. At the same time, a safelight filter permits the passage of light in the red-orange range; consequently, the illumination in a darkroom is red. Most x-ray films have a reduced sensitivity to this red-orange range and are not affected by minimal exposure to the safelight. LED safelights are also available that emit light in the film-safe red spectrum. LED safelights provide twice as much visible light as conventional systems, do not require filters, and provide the most illumination without film damage.

Under safelight conditions, it is necessary to maintain an adequate safelight illumination distance and to keep film handling times to a minimum. Films that are unwrapped too close to the safelight or exposed to safelight illumination for more than 2 to 3 minutes appear fogged. A safelight must be placed a minimum of 4 feet (1.2 meters) away from the film and work area (Figure 10-9), and unwrapped films must be processed immediately under safelight conditions.

A number of safelights with different types of filters are available for use in the darkroom. Some safelights are used exclusively with intraoral films, some are used exclusively with extraoral films, and others are designed for use with both (Figure 10-10). For example, a universal safelight filter recommended for use in a darkroom in which both extraoral screen films and intraoral films are processed is the GBX-2 safelight filter by Carestream Health. Recommendations for specific safelights and filters depend on the type of film exposed (intraoral or extraoral) and are provided by the film manufacturer; such information is indicated on the outside of the film package.

Miscellaneous Requirements

The **darkroom work space** must include an adequate counter area where films can be unwrapped before processing. A clean, organized work area is essential; the work area must be kept absolutely clean, dry, and free of processing chemicals, water, dust, and debris. If an unwrapped film comes into contact with any such substance before processing, an "artifact" results, and the quality of the dental radiograph is compromised.

The **darkroom storage space** must include ample room for chemical processing solutions, film cassettes, and other miscellaneous radiographic supplies. Storage of unopened boxes of intraoral film in the darkroom is *not* recommended; a reaction between the fumes from chemical processing solutions and the film emulsion may occur that will result in film fogging. Boxes of opened extraoral film, however, must be stored in the darkroom. A light-tight storage drawer is necessary to protect opened boxes of unexposed extraoral film.

The temperature and humidity level of the darkroom must be controlled to prevent film damage. A room temperature of 70° F is recommended; if the room temperature exceeds 90° F, film fogging results. A relative humidity level of between 50% and 70% should be maintained. When humidity levels are too high, the film emulsion does not dry. When humidity levels are too low, static electricity becomes a problem and causes film artifacts.

A signal light on the outside of the darkroom door is helpful to indicate when a radiographer is inside performing processing procedures. It is helpful to electrically coordinate the outside signal light to turn on automatically when the safelight is turned on inside the darkroom. Unless the darkroom door can be locked from the inside, opening the darkroom door at an inappropriate time can ruin a series of developing films.

A utility sink with running water is useful in the darkroom. With manual processing, the darkroom plumbing must include both hot and cold running water along with mixing valves to adjust the water temperature in the processing tanks. Other miscellaneous items needed in the darkroom include boxed gloves and a wastebasket for the disposal of film wrappings and contaminated gloves.

Waste Management

Developer. Used developer is not typically a hazardous waste. It can be discharged to a sanitary sewer system. Unused developer may be hazardous because of a high pH. Check the material safety data sheet (MSDS) for the pH of the solution. If the solution pH is above 12.5, it is considered hazardous. It is important to remember that developer is caustic and should be handled with care. If any question remains, the local sewer authority should be contacted before discharging. *Never* discharge used or unused developer to a septic system.

Fixer. Fixer solutions and rinse waters following fixer baths generally contain silver at concentrations above 5.0 ppm, making them hazardous. Solutions should be run through a silver recovery unit to remove silver. After the silver is removed, the solutions may be discharged to the sanitary sewer system. Recovered silver must be disposed of via an approved waste carrier for recycling or disposal. If a silver recovery unit is not available, a company may be contacted to pick up the untreated fixer solutions. Store such solutions in labeled containers. *Never* discharge the fixer solution into a septic system.

HELPFUL HINT

Recycling

Processed film, unprocessed film, and lead foil must be recycled and not placed in the trash.

Film. Processed films should not be discarded with normal office trash. These processed films contain silver, with radiolucent areas containing the most silver. Safe disposal includes returning the films to the manufacturer for recycling or using a certified waste carrier. Undeveloped film packets contain unreacted silver and lead; such packets should be collected in an approved waste container. When the container is full, an approved waste carrier or supplier should be contacted for removal. Lead foils may be collected separately in recycling containers that are located in the darkroom. When full, the container should be sent for recycling.

FILM DUPLICATION

An identical copy of an intraoral or an extraoral radiograph is made through the process of film duplication. Duplicate radiographs may be used when referring patients to specialists, for insurance claims, and as teaching aids (see Chapter 9). The dental radiographer must be familiar with the equipment requirements and procedural steps for film duplication.

Equipment Requirements

The duplication of film requires the use of a film duplicator and duplicating film. A film duplicator is a light source that is commercially available from manufacturers, such as the Wolf X-Ray Corporation (Figure 10-11). A film duplicator provides a diffused light source that evenly exposes the special duplicating film.

Step-by-Step Procedures

Before duplication occurs, the films to be duplicated, the duplicating film, and the film duplicator must be present in the darkroom. Similar to film processing, film duplication must take place in a light-tight darkroom. For procedural steps, see Procedure 10-4.

PROCESSING PROBLEMS AND SOLUTIONS

Processing problems may result in nondiagnostic radiographs. As described in Chapter 6, a diagnostic radiograph provides a great deal of information. Diagnostic images exhibit proper density and contrast, have sharp outlines, and are of the same shape and size as the object being radiographed (Figure 10-13).

Processing problems may occur for a number of reasons, including the following:

- Time and temperature errors (Table 10-4)
- Chemical contamination errors (Table 10-5)
- Film handling errors (Table 10-6)
- Lighting errors (Table 10-7)

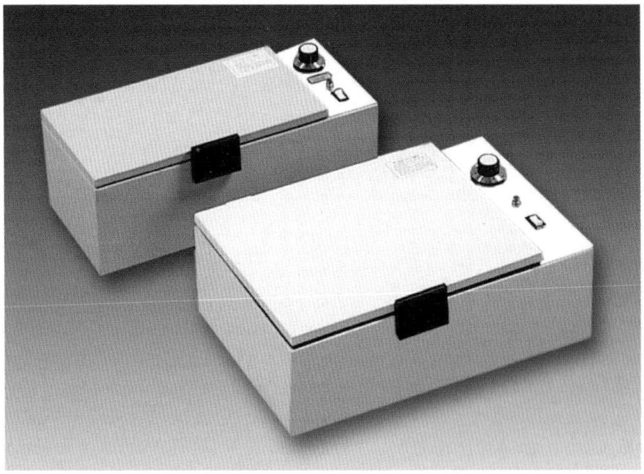

Fig 10-11 Examples of film duplicators. (Courtesy Wolf X-Ray Corporation, Deer Park, NY. www.wolfxray.com.)

PROCEDURE 10-4 Film Duplication

1. Arrange the original set of processed films in anatomic order.
   - Place the dental radiographs to be duplicated on the light screen of the film duplicator.
   - Use manufacturer-supplied film organizers to arrange the films and block out extraneous light (Figure 10-12).

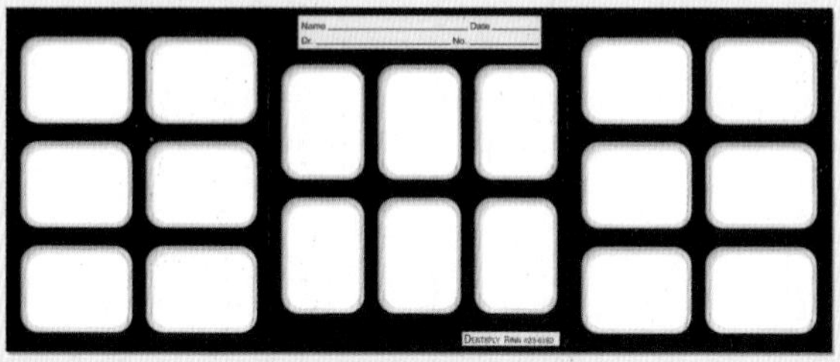

Fig 10-12 An x-ray "organizer," on which films are placed for duplication. (Courtesy Miles DA, Van Dis ML, Jensen CW et al: *Radiographic imaging for dental auxiliaries*, ed 3, Philadelphia, 1999, Saunders.)

2. Place the duplicating film.
   - Place the duplicating film on top of the arranged set of films.
   - Make certain the emulsion side is down on the duplicating film. *Note:* The emulsion side will appear dull and gray or lavender in color.
3. Secure the duplicator lid.
   - Close the lid of the film duplicator and fasten it securely to ensure adequate contact between the original films and the duplicating film. *Note:* To prevent blurring of the image, good contact must be maintained between the duplicating film and the films that are being duplicated.
   - Without good contact, the duplicate film appears fuzzy and shows less detail than the original film.
4. Set the timer.
   - Select the exposure time, set the adjustable timer, and activate the light source to expose the duplicating film. *Note:* An adjustable timer on the film duplicator controls the exposure time.
   - The adjustable timer controls the amount of light emitted from the film duplicator; the light passes through the original films and exposes the duplicating film. The longer the duplicating film is exposed to light, the lighter it appears. This is the opposite of x-ray film; x-ray film appears darker with longer exposure to light.
   - Exposure time depends on the type of duplicator used and the density of the original films being duplicated.
5. Process the duplicating film.
   - Process the duplicating film using manual processing techniques or the automatic processor.
6. Label the duplicate radiograph.
   - Label the processed duplicate radiographs with the patient's name and date of exposure.
   - Also, label the radiographs to indicate the patient's right (R) and left (L) sides.

A variety of processing errors may occur with manual and automatic film processing. Whereas some errors are unique to manual or automatic processing, others may occur with either technique. Processing errors may cause a partial or total absence of images or obscure images that are present. Films that appear light, dark, yellow-brown, or fogged are the result of processing errors. Films that appear scratched or contaminated with dirt, saliva, or fingerprints are the result of faulty film handling during processing. Reticulation and fingernail and static artifacts may also result from poor processing and film handling techniques.

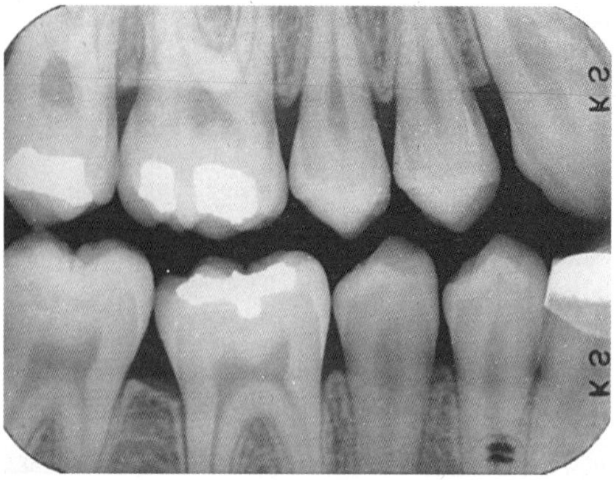

Fig 10-13 A diagnostic radiograph with images that exhibit proper density and contrast.

Many processing errors can be attributed to more than one cause. The dental radiographer must be able to recognize the appearance of common processing errors, identify potential causes of such errors, and know what steps are necessary to correct the problems.

Time and Temperature

Underdeveloped Film

Appearance. The film appears light (Figure 10-14).

Type of processing. Automatic or manual.

Problems. Underdeveloped films may result from the following:

- Inadequate development time
- Inaccurate timer
- Low developer temperature
- Inaccurate thermometer
- Depleted or contaminated developer solution

Solution. To prevent underdeveloped films, do the following:

- Check the temperature of the developer and the time the film must remain in the developer solution.
- Increase the time the film remains in the developer, as needed.
- Replace faulty and inaccurate thermometers and timers.
- When the developer solution is depleted or contaminated, replace it.

Overdeveloped Film

Appearance. The film appears dark (Figure 10-15).

Type of processing. Automatic or manual.

Problems. Overdeveloped films may result from the following:

- Excess development time
- Inaccurate timer
- High developer temperature
- Inaccurate thermometer
- Concentrated (overactive) developer solution

Solution. To prevent overdeveloped films, do the following:

- Check the temperature of the developer and the time that the film should remain in the developer solution.
- Decrease the time the film remains in the developer, as needed.
- Replace faulty and inaccurate thermometers and timers.
- If the developer solution is overactive, replace it.

Reticulation of Emulsion

Appearance. The film appears cracked (Figure 10-16).

Type of processing. Manual.

TABLE 10-4 Time and Temperature: Problems and Solutions

Example	Appearance	Problems	Solutions
Underdeveloped film 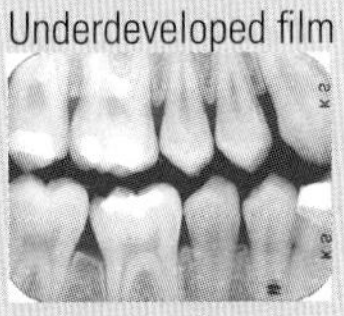	Light	Inadequate development time	Check development time.
		Developer solution too cool	Check developer temperature.
		Inaccurate timer or thermometer	Replace faulty timer or thermometer.
		Depleted or contaminated developer solution	Replenish developer with fresh solutions as needed.
Overdeveloped film 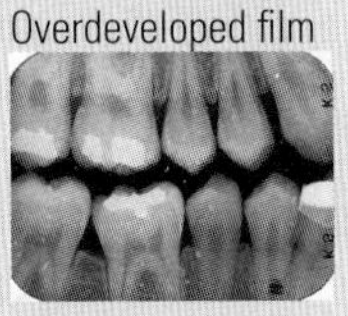	Dark	Excessive developing time	Check development time.
		Developer solution too hot	Check developer temperature.
		Inaccurate timer or thermometer	Replace faulty timer or thermometer.
		Concentrated developer solution	Replenish developer with fresh solutions, as needed.
Reticulation of emulsion 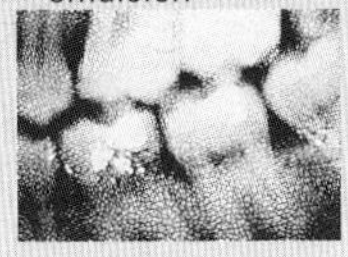	Cracked	Sudden temperature change between developer and water bath	Check temperature of processing solutions and water bath; avoid drastic temperature differences.

TABLE 10-5 Chemical Contamination: Problems and Solutions

Example	Appearance	Problems	Solutions
Developer spots 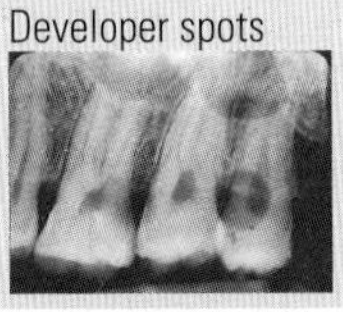	Dark or black spots	Developer comes in contact with film before processing	Use a clean work area in the darkroom.
Fixer spots 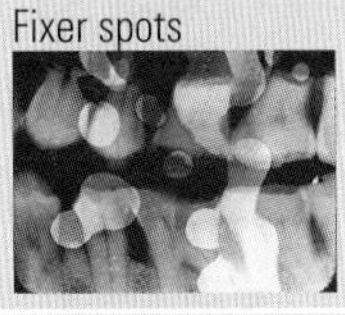	White or light spots	Fixer comes in contact with film before processing	Use a clean work area in the darkroom.
Yellow-brown stains 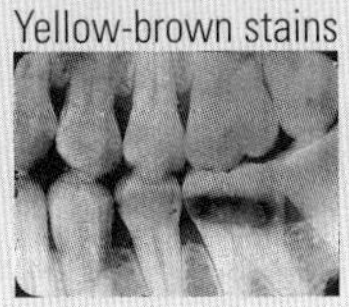	Yellow-brown color	Exhausted developer or fixer	Replenish chemicals with fresh solutions, as needed.
		Insufficient fixing time	Use adequate fixing time.
		Insufficient rinsing	Rinse for a minimum of 20 minutes.

Problem. Reticulation of emulsion results when a film is subjected to a sudden temperature change between the developer solution and the water bath.

Solution. To prevent reticulation of emulsion, do the following:

- Check the temperatures of the processing solutions and of the water bath.
- Avoid drastic temperature differences between the developer and the water bath.

Chemical Contamination

Developer Spots

Appearance. Dark spots appear on the film (Figure 10-17).

Type of processing. Manual.

Problem. Developer spots are seen when the developer solution comes in contact with the film before processing.

Solution. To avoid developer spots, do the following:

- Use a clean work area in the darkroom.
- To ensure a clean working surface, place a paper towel on the work area before unwrapping films.

Fixer Spots

Appearance. White spots appear on the film (Figure 10-18).

Type of processing. Manual.

Problem. Fixer spots are the result of fixer solution coming in contact with the film before processing.

Solution. To avoid fixer spots, do the following:

- Use a clean work area in the darkroom.
- To ensure a clean working surface, place a paper towel on the work area before unwrapping films.

TABLE 10-6 Film Handling: Problems and Solutions

Example	Appearance	Problems	Solutions
Developer cutoff 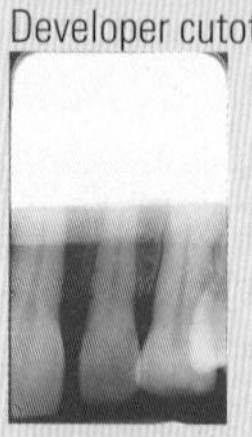	Straight white border	Undeveloped portion of film caused by low level of developer	Check developer level before processing; add solution if needed.
Fixer cutoff 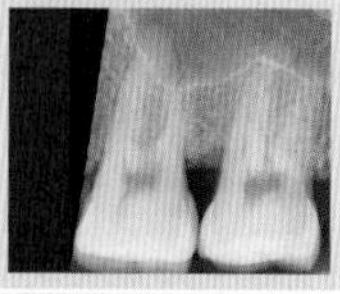	Straight black border	Unfixed portion of film caused by low level of fixer	Check fixer level before processing; add solution if needed.
Overlapped films 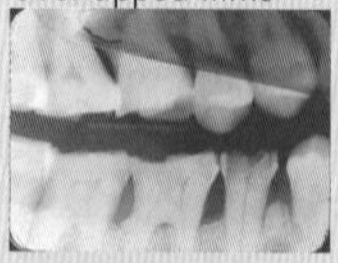	White or dark areas appear on film where overlapped	Two films contacting each other during processing	Separate films so that no contact takes place during processing.
Air bubbles* 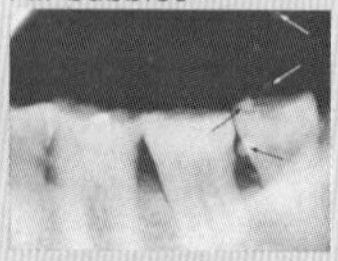	White spots	Air trapped on the film surface after being placed in the processing solutions	Gently agitate film racks after placing in processing solutions.
Fingernail artifact 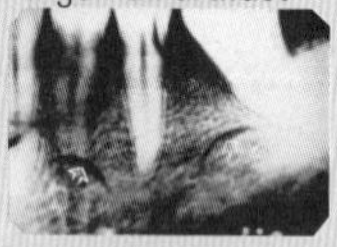	Black crescent-shaped marks	Film emulsion damaged by operator's fingernail during rough handling	Gently handle films, holding them on the edges only.
Fingerprint artifact 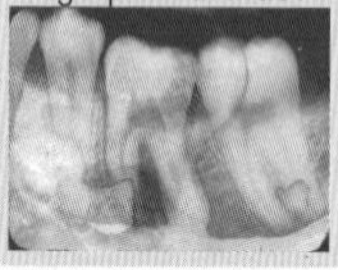	Black fingerprint	Film touched by fingers that are contaminated with fluoride or developer	Wash and dry hands thoroughly before processing films.
Static electricity 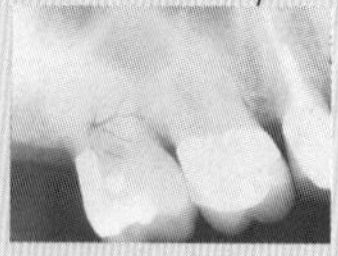	Thin, black, branching lines	Occurs when a film packet is opened quickly	Open film packets slowly.
		Occurs when a film pack is opened before radiographer touches a conductive object	Touch a conductive object before unwrapping films.
Scratched film 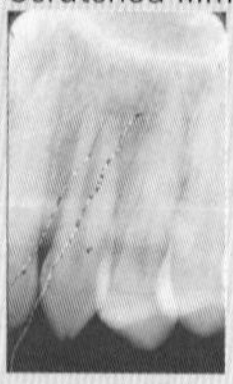	White lines	Soft emulsion removed from film by a sharp object	Use care when handling films and film racks.

*From Langlais RP: *Exercises in oral radiology and interpretation*, ed 4, St Louis, 2004, Saunders.

Yellow-Brown Color

Appearance. The film appears yellowish brown (Figure 10-19).

Type of processing. Manual.

Problems. Yellow-brown films result from the following:

- Use of exhausted developer or fixer
- Insufficient fixing time
- Insufficient rinsing

Solution. To prevent yellow-brown films, do the following:

- Replace the depleted developer and fixer solutions with fresh chemicals.
- Make certain that films have adequate fixing time and adequate rinse time.
- Rinse processed films for a minimum of 20 minutes in circulating cool water.

TABLE 10-7 Lighting: Problems and Solutions

Example	Appearance	Problems	Solutions
Light leak 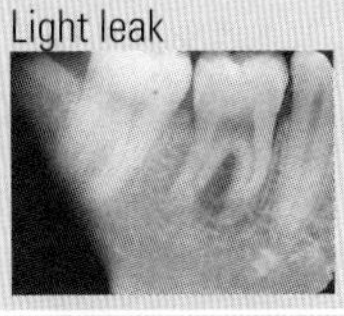	Exposed area appears black	Accidental exposure of film to white light	Examine film packets for defects before using.
			Never unwrap films in the presence of white light.
Fogged film 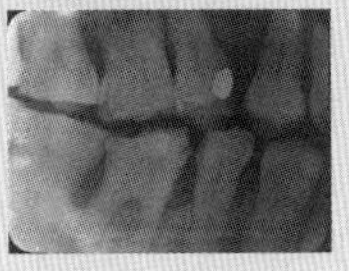	Gray; lack of detail and contrast	Improper safelighting	Check filter and bulb wattage of safelight.
		Light leaks in darkroom	Check darkroom for light leaks.
		Outdated films	Check the expiration date on film packages.
		Improper film storage	Store films in a cool, dry, protected area.
		Contaminated solutions	Avoid contaminated solutions by covering tanks after each use.
		Developer solution too hot	Check temperatures of developer.

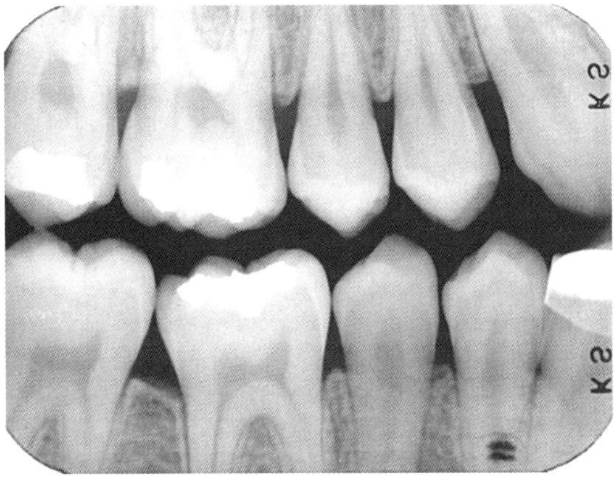

Fig 10-14 An underdeveloped film appears light.

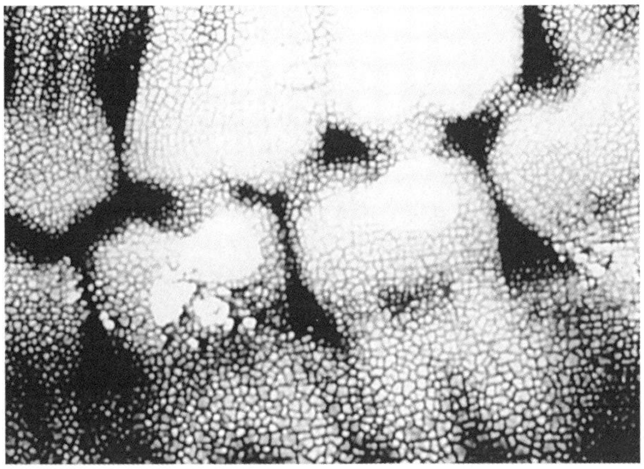

Fig 10-16 A film with a damaged emulsion appears cracked.

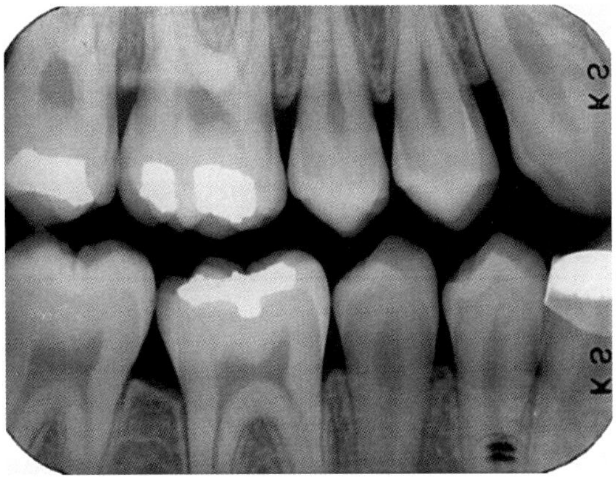

Fig 10-15 An overdeveloped film appears dark.

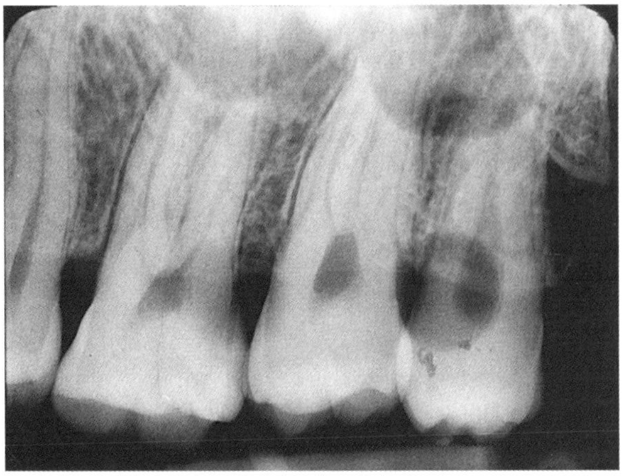

Fig 10-17 Developer spots appear dark or black.

Film Handling

Developer Cutoff

Appearance. A straight white border appears on the film (Figure 10-20).

Type of processing. Manual.

Problem. Developer cutoff results from a low level of developer solution and represents an undeveloped portion of the film. If the developer solution level is low, the films clipped at the very top of the film rack may not be completely immersed in the developer solution.

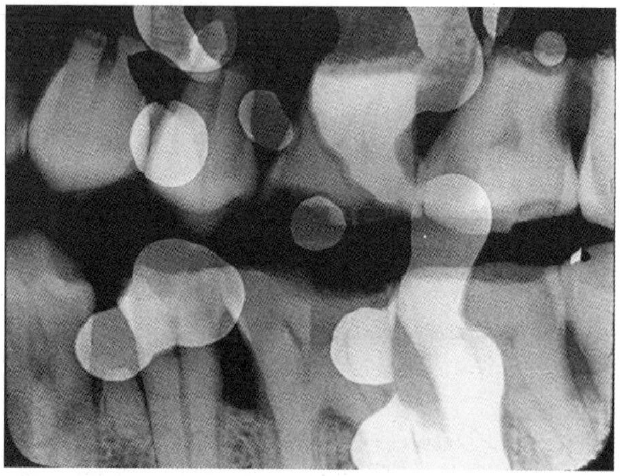

Fig 10-18 Fixer spots appear light or white.

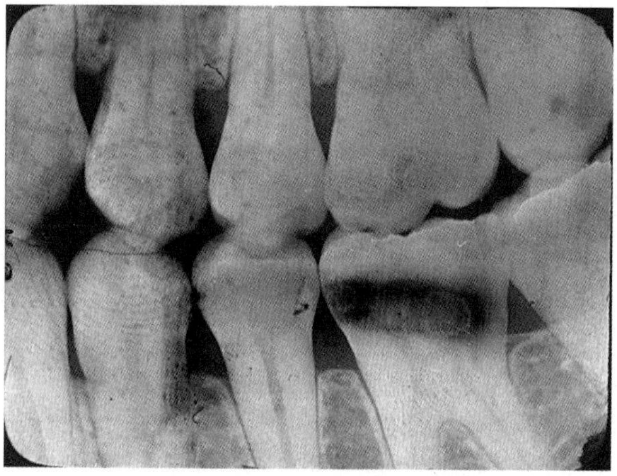

Fig 10-19 A number of processing errors may result in a yellow-brown film.

Solution. To avoid developer cutoff, do the following:

- Check the developer level before processing films.
- Add proper replenisher solution, if necessary.
- Make certain that all films on the film rack are completely immersed in the developer solution.

Fixer Cutoff

Appearance. A straight black border appears on the film (Figure 10-21).

Type of processing. Manual.

Problem. Fixer cutoff results from a low level of fixer solution and represents an unfixed portion of the film. If the fixer solution is low, the films clipped at the very top of the film rack may not be completely immersed in the fixer solution.

Solution. To avoid fixer cutoff, do the following:

- Check the fixer level before processing films.
- Add proper replenisher solution if necessary.
- Make certain that all films on the film rack are completely immersed in the fixer solution.

Overlapped Films

Appearance. White or dark areas appear on films where overlap has occurred (Figures 10-22 and 10-23).

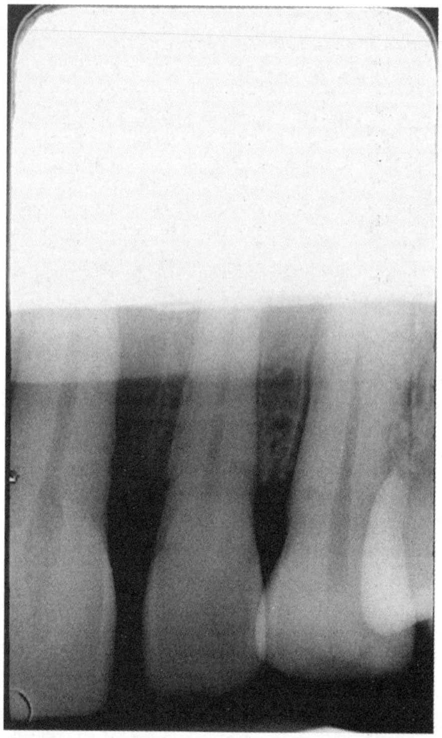

Fig 10-20 Developer cutoff appears as a straight white border on a film.

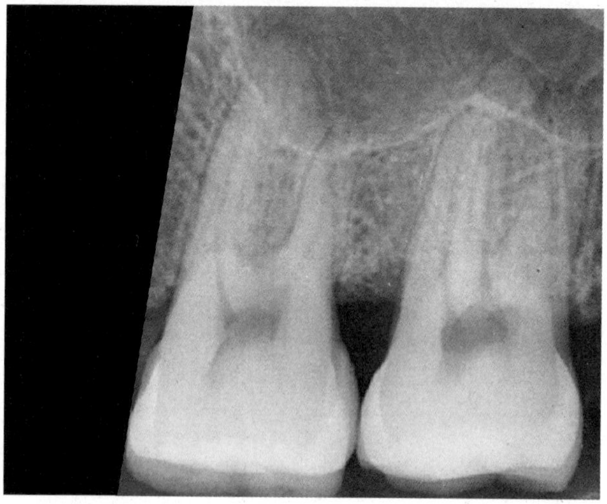

Fig 10-21 Fixer cutoff appears as a straight black border on a film.

Type of processing. Automatic or manual

Problem. Overlapped films occur when two films come into contact with each other during processing techniques. Films that overlap in the developer have white areas that represent an undeveloped portion of the film. Films that overlap in the fixer have black areas that represent an unfixed portion of the film.

Solution. To avoid overlapped films, care should be taken to ensure that no film is permitted to come into contact with another film during processing.

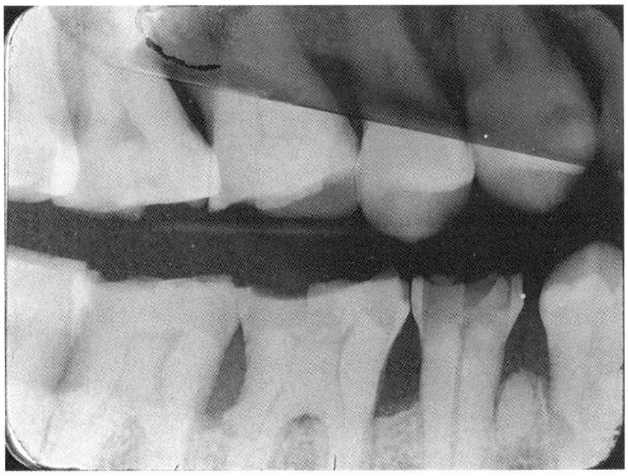

Fig 10-22 An overlapped film.

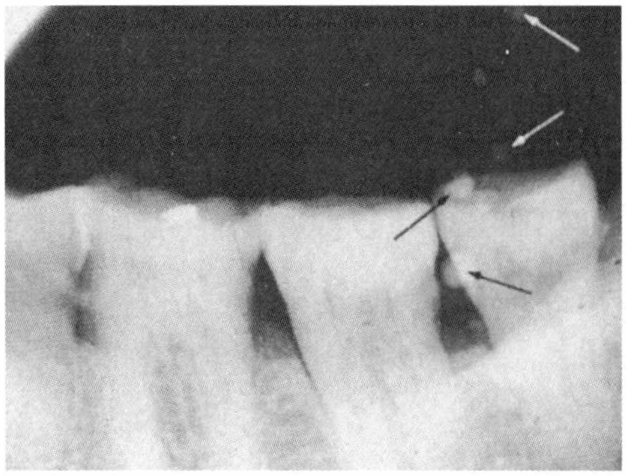

Fig 10-24 Air bubbles appear as tiny white spots *(arrows)*. (Courtesy Langlais RP: *Exercises in oral radiology and interpretation*, ed 4, St Louis, 2004, Saunders.)

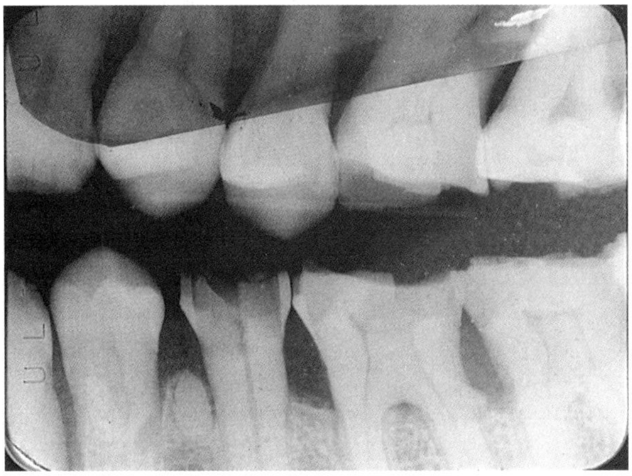

Fig 10-23 An overlapped film.

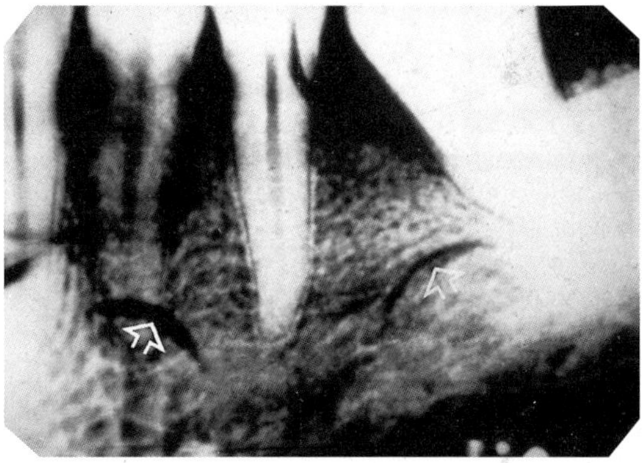

Fig 10-25 A fingernail artifact appears as a black, crescent-shaped mark *(arrowhead)*.

HELPFUL HINT

Film Handling

Avoid Overlapped Films

- Make certain the films are **straight** as they are inserted.
- Allow at least **10 seconds between insertions** of films.
- **Alternate sides** or slots whenever possible.

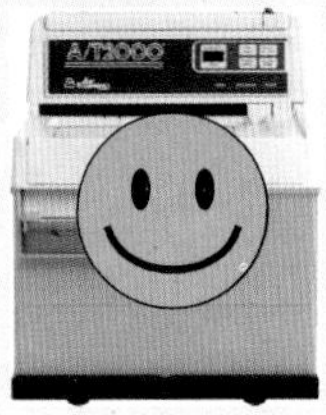

Air Bubbles

Appearance. White spots appear on the film (Figure 10-24).

Type of processing. Manual.

Problem. Air bubbles are seen when air is trapped on the film surface after the film is placed in the processing solution. Air bubbles prevent the chemicals from affecting the emulsion in that area.

Solution. To avoid air bubbles, gently agitate and stir film racks after placing them in the processing solution.

Fingernail Artifact

Appearance. Black, crescent-shaped marks appear on the film (Figure 10-25).

Type of processing. Automatic or manual.

Problem. A fingernail artifact is seen when the film emulsion is damaged by the operator's fingernail during rough handling of the film.

Solution. To prevent a fingernail artifact, handle the film gently, holding it on the edges only.

Fingerprint Artifact

Appearance. A black fingerprint appears on the film (Figure 10-26).

Type of processing. Manual.

Problem. A fingerprint artifact is seen when fingers contaminated with fluoride or processing solutions have touched the film. A fingerprint artifact may also be seen if a wet film is touched too soon or not handled carefully by the edges.

Solution. To prevent fingerprint artifacts, do the following:

- Wash and dry hands thoroughly before processing films.
- Work in a clean area to avoid contaminating the hands.
- Handle the films by holding on the edges only.
- Do not handle until the films are totally dry.

HELPFUL HINT
Film Handling

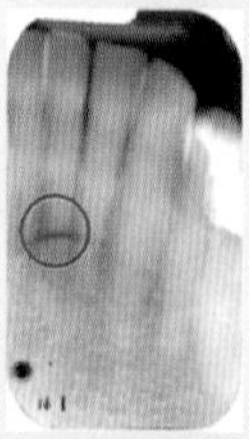
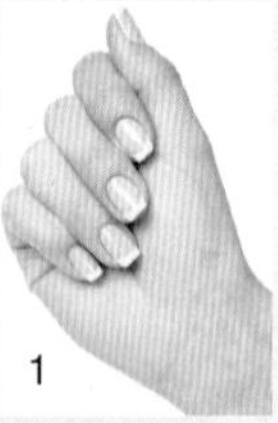

Fingernail
Black crescent shape

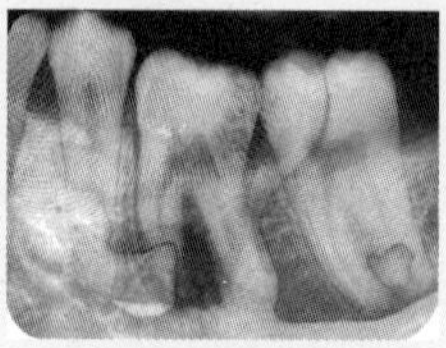

Fingerprint
Looks like a fingerprint

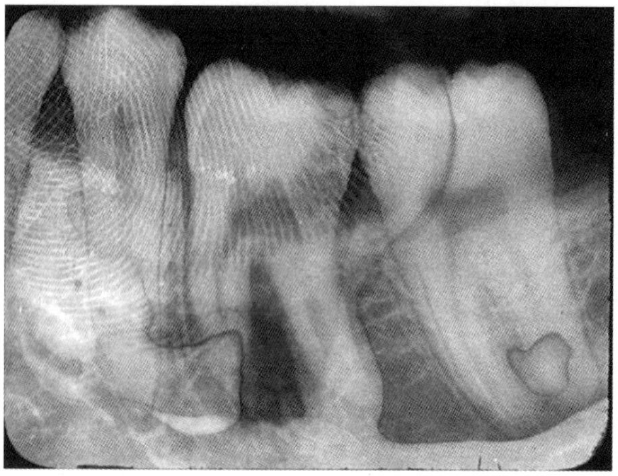

Fig 10-26 A black fingerprint artifact appears on the film.

Static Electricity

Appearance. Thin, black branching lines appear on the film (Figure 10-27).

Type of processing. Automatic or manual.

Problem. Static electricity may result from the following:

- Opening a film packet quickly
- Opening a film packet before touching another object such as the film processor or countertop in a carpeted office

Static electricity occurs most frequently during periods of low humidity.

Solution. To prevent static electricity, do the following:

- Always open film packets slowly.
- In a carpeted office, touch a conductive object before unwrapping films.

Scratched Film

Appearance. White lines appear on the film (Figure 10-28).

Type of processing. Manual.

Problem. A scratched film results when the soft film emulsion is removed from the film base by a sharp object, such as a film clip or film hanger.

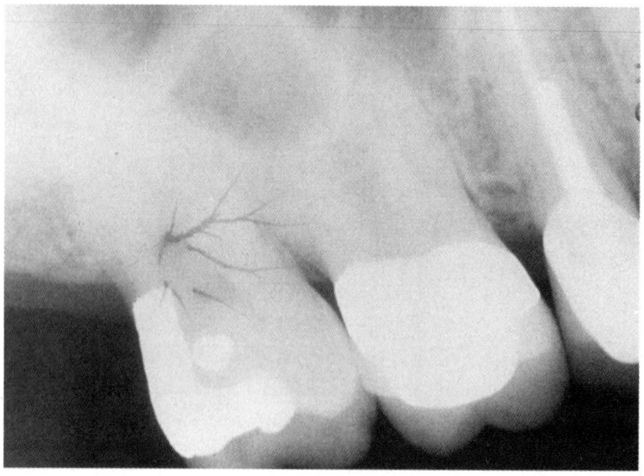

Fig 10-27 Static electricity appears as black branching lines.

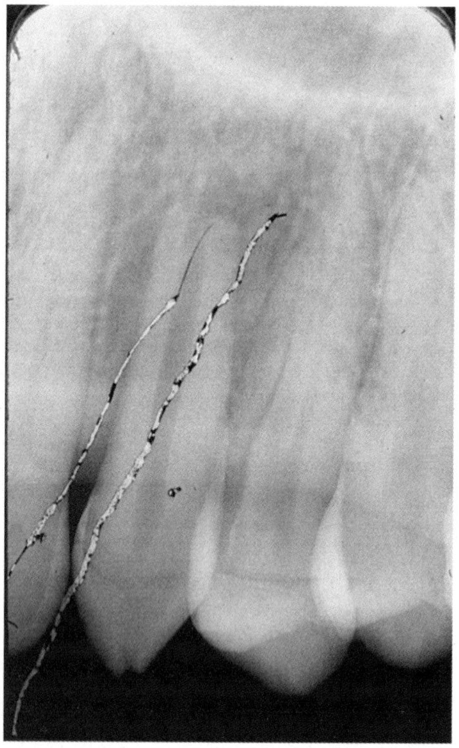

Fig 10-28 Scratches appear as thin white lines.

Solution. To prevent a scratched film, do the following:

- Use care when placing a film rack in the processing solutions.
- Avoid contact with other film hangers.

Lighting

Light Leak

Appearance. The exposed area appears black (Figure 10-29).

Type of processing. Automatic or manual.

Problems. A light leak results from the following:

- Accidental exposure of the film to white light
- Torn or defective film packets that expose a portion of the film to light

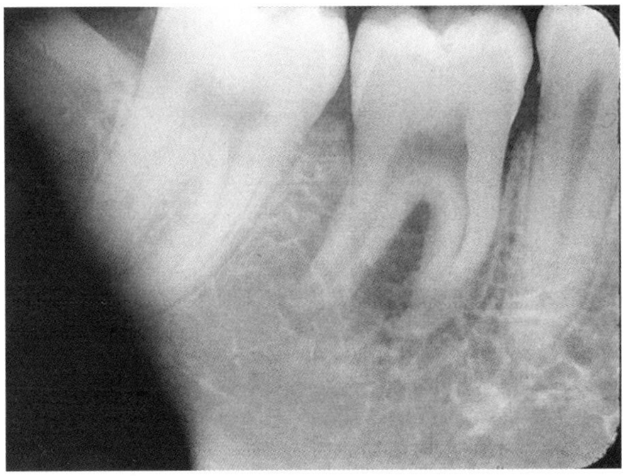

Fig 10-29 Portion of the film exposed to light appears black.

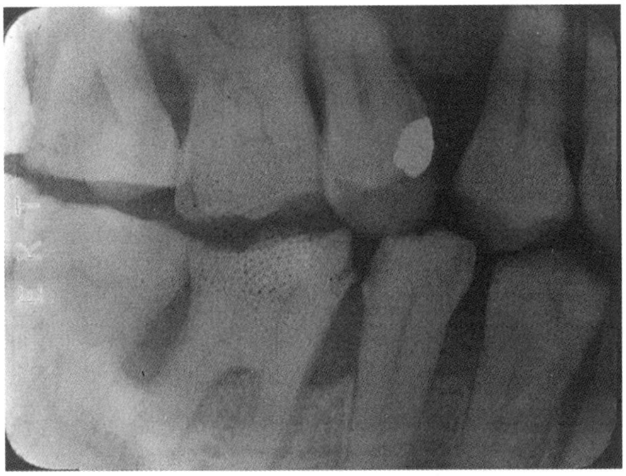

Fig 10-30 A fogged film appears gray and lacks detail and contrast.

Solution. To prevent light leaks, do the following:

- Examine film packets for minute tears or defects before use.
- Do not use film packets that are torn or defective.
- Never unwrap films in the presence of white light.

Fogged Film

Appearance. The film appears gray and lacks image detail and contrast (Figure 10-30).

Type of processing. Automatic or manual.

Problems. Fogged films result from the following:

- Improper safelighting and light leaks in the darkroom
- Improper film storage
- Outdated films
- Contaminated processing solutions
- High developer temperature

Solution. To prevent fogged films, do the following:

- Check the filter and bulb wattage of the safelight.
- Minimize film exposure to the safelight and check the darkroom for light leaks.
- Check the expiration date on film packages and store films in a cool, dry, protected area.
- Avoid contamination of processing solutions by replacing tank covers after each use.
- Always check the temperature of the developer before processing films.

SUMMARY

- *Film processing* refers to a series of steps that produce a visible permanent image on a dental radiograph.
- The pattern of stored energy on an exposed film is termed the *latent image;* this image remains invisible until it undergoes processing.
- The visible image that results on a dental radiograph is made up of black, white, and gray areas.
- Automatic processing is a simple way to process dental x-ray film. The essential equipment required is the automatic processor, which automates all film processing steps.
- Automatic processing includes four steps: (1) development, (2) fixing, (3) washing, and (4) drying.
- Advantages of automatic processing include the following: less processing time is required, time and temperatures are automatically controlled, less equipment is used, and less space is required.
- Manual film processing includes five steps: (1) development, (2) rinsing, (3) fixing, (4) washing, and (5) drying.
- Manual processing is a simple method used to develop, rinse, fix, and wash dental x-ray films. The essential piece of equipment needed is a processing tank, which is divided into compartments for the developer solution, water bath, and fixer solution.
- A darkroom is a completely darkened room where x-ray film can be handled and processed. The ideal darkroom should be conveniently located, of adequate size, equipped with correct lighting and ventilation, and arranged with ample work space and storage.
- The darkroom must be light-tight and must include proper safelighting.
- Safelighting provides illumination in the darkroom to perform processing activities safely without exposing or damaging the film.
- An identical copy of an intraoral or extraoral radiograph is made through the process of film duplication. Duplication of film requires the use of a film duplicator and special duplicating film.
- A number of processing problems may result in nondiagnostic films. Processing problems may result from time and temperature errors (see Table 10-4), chemical contamination errors (see Table 10-5), film handling errors (see Table 10-6), and lighting errors (see Table 10-7).
- The dental radiographer must be able to recognize the appearance of common processing errors, identify the potential causes of such errors, and know what steps are necessary to correct such errors.

BIBLIOGRAPHY

Frommer HH, Stabulas-Savage JJ: Film processing: the darkroom. In Radiology for the dental professional, ed 9, St Louis, 2011, Mosby.

Haring JI, Lind LJ: Film exposure, processing, and technique errors. In Radiographic interpretation for the dental hygienist, Philadelphia, 1993, Saunders.

Johnson ON: Dental x-ray film processing. In Essentials of dental radiography for dental assistants and hygienists, ed 9, Upper Saddle River, NJ, 2011, Prentice Hall.

Koneru J, Mahajan N, Mahalakshmi M: Management of dental radiographic waste, Dent J Adv Studies 2(II):55, 2014.

Miles DA, Van Dis ML, Jensen CW, et al: Film processing and quality assurance. In Radiographic imaging for the dental team, ed 4, St Louis, 2009, Saunders.

Mallya SM, Lam EWN: Film imaging. In White and Pharoah's oral radiology: principles and interpretation, ed 8, St. Louis, 2019, Elsevier.

Mallya SM, Lam EWN: Digital imaging. In White and Pharoah's oral radiology: principles and interpretation, ed 8, St. Louis, 2019, Elsevier.

QUIZ QUESTIONS

Multiple Choice

____ 1. The first step in manual film processing is:
- a. development
- b. rinsing
- c. fixing
- d. washing
- e. drying

____ 2. In manual film processing, the rinsing step is necessary because it:
- a. removes the silver halide crystals from the emulsion
- b. slows down the fixing process
- c. removes the developer from the film and stops the development process
- d. thoroughly removes all excess chemicals from the emulsion
- e. reduces the energized silver halide crystals to black metallic silver

____ 3. The film emulsion is hardened during:
- a. development
- b. rinsing
- c. fixing
- d. washing
- e. drying

____ 4. The hydroquinone in the developer brings out the _________ tones, whereas the Elon in the developer brings out the _________ tones on a dental radiograph.
- a. black; white
- b. white; black
- c. gray; gray
- d. white; gray
- e. black; gray

____ 5. In manual film processing, the optimal temperature for the developer solution is:
- a. 55° F
- b. 68° F
- c. 78° F
- d. 80° F
- e. 90° F

____ 6. The size of a darkroom is determined by all the following factors except:
- a. volume of radiographs processed
- b. type of processing equipment used
- c. humidity level of the room
- d. space required for duplication of films
- e. number of persons using the room

____ 7. Any leaks of white light into the darkroom will cause:
- a. film fogging
- b. film reticulation
- c. overdeveloped films
- d. underexposed films
- e. any of the above

____ 8. The safelight must be placed a minimum of how many feet from the film and the work area?
- a. 1
- b. 2
- c. 3
- d. 4
- e. 5

____ 9. A universal safelight filter such as the GBX-2 by Carestream Health is recommended for:
- a. intraoral films only
- b. extraoral screen films only
- c. extraoral nonscreen films only
- d. intraoral and extraoral films
- e. none of the above

____ 10. Unopened boxes of radiographic film should not be stored in the darkroom because:
- a. chemical fumes from processing solutions may fog the film
- b. continued exposure to the safelight is not recommended
- c. the box may have a tear that may expose the film
- d. processing solutions could splash onto the boxes of film
- e. all of the above

____ 11. The thermometer for manual processing should be placed in the:
- a. developer solution
- b. water bath
- c. fixer solution
- d. either a or c
- e. all of the above

____ 12. At 68° F, what is the optimal development time in minutes for manual film processing?
- a. 2
- b. 3
- c. 4
- d. 5
- e. 6

____ 13. All factors affect the life of the processing solutions except:
- a. number of films processed
- b. care in preparation of solutions
- c. type of safelight filter used
- d. age of solutions
- e. proper care and maintenance of the automatic processor

____ 14. A replenisher is added to the processing solution to:
- a. compensate for the loss of solution strength
- b. ensure uniform results between solution changes
- c. compensate for the loss of volume of solution
- d. compensate for oxidation
- e. all of the above

____ 15. How often should the processing tank be cleaned?
- a. once per week
- b. once per month
- c. once per day
- d. whenever solutions are changed
- e. none of the above

____ 16. Which can be used to clean the processing tank?
- a. commercial tank cleaner
- b. hydrochloric acid and water solution
- c. abrasive-type cleansers
- d. both a and b
- e. all of the above

____ 17. A breakdown of chemicals in the processing solution that results from exposure to air is termed:
- a. reduction
- b. selective reduction

c. oxidation
d. replenishment
e. none of the above

____ 18. The superconcentrated solution that is added to the processing solution to compensate for the effects of oxidation is termed the:
a. acidifier
b. hardener
c. oxidizer
d. replenisher
e. emulsifier

Matching

For questions 19 to 28, match each component part of the automatic processor with its function.

a. Opening used to insert films
b. Opening where processed films emerge
c. Holds fixer solution
d. Heated air is used to dry wet films
e. Holds developer solution
f. Solutions used to maintain proper concentration and levels of developer and fixer
g. Moves the film through the automatic processor
h. Encases component parts of automatic processor
i. Delivers developer and fixer solution to compartments
j. Holds circulating water

____ 19. processor housing
____ 20. film/feed slot
____ 21. roller film transporter
____ 22. film recovery slot
____ 23. drying chamber
____ 24. water compartment
____ 25. fixer compartment
____ 26. developer compartment
____ 27. replenisher solutions
____ 28. replenisher pump

Fill in the Blank

29. List the two equipment requirements for film duplication.

____
____
____
____

30. Discuss how exposure time affects the density of duplicating film.

____
____
____
____

Matching

For questions 31 to 36, describe the appearance of the processing error using one of the following words:

a. light
b. white
c. black
d. dark
e. gray

____ 31. fogged film
____ 32. overdeveloped film
____ 33. underdeveloped film
____ 34. light leak
____ 35. developer cutoff
____ 36. fixer cutoff

IDENTIFICATION

For questions 37 to 45, describe or identify the processing error that causes the following:

37. Black spots

____
____
____
____

38. White spots

____
____
____
____

39. Yellow-brown stains

____
____
____
____

40. Cracked appearance

____
____
____
____

41. Straight white border

____
____
____
____

42. Straight black border

____
____
____
____

43. Black, crescent-shaped marks

____
____
____
____

44. Thin, black branching lines

____
____
____
____

45. White lines

____
____
____
____

TRUE OR FALSE

For questions 46 to 50, identify each statement as true or false.

____ **46.** Film fogging results from improper safelighting.

____ **47.** Yellow-brown stains result from insufficient development time.

____ **48.** Developer cutoff appears as a straight black border across the film.

____ **49.** To avoid static electricity, touch a conductive object before unwrapping a film.

____ **50.** Torn or defective film packets may allow a portion of the film to be exposed to light.

11

Film Mounting and Viewing

LEARNING OBJECTIVES

After completion of this chapter, the student will be able to do the following:

1. Define the key terms associated with film mounting and viewing.
2. Do the following related to film mounting:
   - Define film mounting.
   - List the individuals who are qualified to mount and view dental radiographs.
   - Describe when and where films are mounted.
   - List several reasons to use a film mount.
   - Describe what information is placed on a film mount.
   - Describe how mounts are used with digital imaging.
3. Discuss the importance of normal anatomy in film mounting.
4. Describe how the identification dot is used to determine film orientation.
5. List and describe two methods of film mounting and identify the preferred method.
6. List and describe the step-by-step procedures for film mounting.
7. Do the following related to viewing film:
   - List the individuals who are qualified to view film.
   - List and describe the necessary equipment for film viewing.
   - Discuss the importance of masking extraneous viewbox light seen around a film mount.
   - Describe optimal viewing conditions, as well as when and where images should be viewed.
   - Explain the importance of examining images in an established viewing sequence.
8. List and describe the step-by-step procedures for film viewing and explain why multiple viewings of dental images are necessary, as well as list the areas, diseases, and abnormalities that must be included in the examinations.

Film mounting is an essential step in the interpretation of dental radiographs; the dental radiographer must be able to mount dental radiographs in correct anatomic order. To mount dental radiographs properly, the radiographer must have a thorough knowledge of the normal anatomy of the maxilla, the mandible, and related structures (see Chapter 28). Film viewing is also essential in the interpretation of dental radiographs; the dental radiographer must understand the importance of examining films under optimal viewing conditions.

The purpose of this chapter is to present the basic concepts of film mounting and film viewing and to describe the step-by-step procedures that must be followed to prepare for the interpretation of radiographs.

FILM MOUNTING

Mounted radiographs, or radiographs placed in a film holder in anatomic order, are essential to the dental professional. Compared with individual films, a series of mounted radiographs can be viewed more efficiently and are easier to interpret.

Basic Concepts

The term **mount** can be defined as "to place in an appropriate setting, as for display or study." In dental radiography, **film mounting** is the placement of radiographs in a supporting structure or holder.

What Is a Film Mount? A film mount is a cardboard, plastic, or vinyl holder that is used to support and arrange dental radiographs in anatomic order (Figure 11-1). **Anatomic order** refers to how teeth are arranged within the dental arches. Each film mount has a number of windows or frames in which the individual radiographs are placed, or "mounted." A film mount may be opaque or clear (Figure 11-2). An opaque film mount is preferred because it masks the light around each radiograph. Subtle changes in density and contrast are easier to detect when extraneous light is eliminated. To minimize extraneous viewbox light, each window of a film mount should contain a radiograph. When all the windows are not filled with radiographs, black opaque paper can be placed in the unused frames.

Film mounts are commercially available in many sizes and configurations and accommodate any number of films; mounts are available for single films, bite-wing films, a complete mouth series (CMS) of films, and countless other combinations of films (Figure 11-3). The overall size and shape of the film mounts are designed to fit a variety of viewboxes found in the dental office; the size of the film mount should correspond to the size of the viewbox.

Who Mounts Films? Any trained dental professional (dentist, dental hygienist, dental assistant) with knowledge of the normal anatomic landmarks of the maxilla, the mandible, and related structures is qualified to mount dental radiographs. In most dental offices, mounting films is the responsibility of the dental radiographer.

When and Where Are Films Mounted? The dental radiographer should always mount films immediately after processing. Films should be mounted in an area designated for film mounting. This area should consist of a clean, dry, light-colored work surface in front of an illuminator or viewbox.

Why Use a Film Mount? The use of a film mount is strongly recommended for the following reasons:

- Mounted radiographs are quicker and easier to view and interpret.
- Mounted radiographs are easily stored in the patient record and are readily accessible for interpretation.
- Film mounts decrease the chances of error in determining the patient's right and left sides because each film is mounted in anatomic order.
- Film mounts decrease the handling of individual films and prevent damage to the emulsion (e.g., fingerprint marks and scratches).

- Film mounts mask illumination immediately adjacent to individual radiographs and aid in interpretation.

What Information Is Placed on a Film Mount? The dental radiographer should label the film mount before the films are mounted. A special marking pencil designed to write on paper, plastic, or vinyl can be used to label film mounts. Radiographs are easily identified when the film mount has been clearly and legibly labeled with the following information:

- Patient's full name
- Date of exposure
- Dentist's name
- Radiographer's name

The patient's name and date of exposure are essential, the dentist's name is useful if the radiographs are sent to a third party (e.g., insurance company), and the radiographer's name is important if any questions should arise about the exposure of the images.

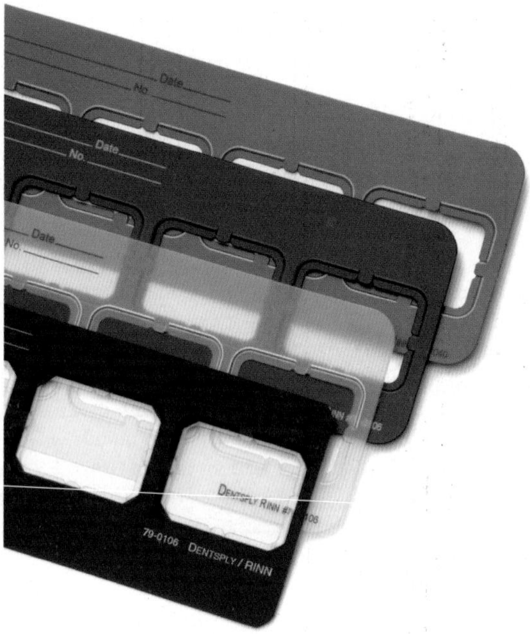

Fig 11-1 Examples of various film mounts. (Courtesy Dentsply Rinn, York, PA.)

Are Mounts Used with Digital Imaging? Similar to conventional radiography, digital images observed on the computer monitor must also be arranged correctly in anatomic order for proper viewing and interpretation. Most digital imaging software allows the dental radiographer to choose the appropriate-size mount, whether it be one periapical image, four bite-wing images, a full mouth series, or a panoramic image (Figures 11-4 and 11-5). For example, with a full mouth series of radiographs, the dental radiographer must "click and drag" each image to the correct corresponding window or frame on the mount on the computer monitor screen (Figure 11-6).

Some digital manufacturers include software that automatically saves each image exposed and places the image in the appropriate section of the mount. For example, before exposure of the right premolar bite-wing image, the dental radiographer highlights a section of the image mount in the appropriate anatomic location. Upon exposure, a digital image appears within moments and is logically placed in the mount in the area of the right premolar bite-wing image.

The images should be saved with the patient's full name and date of exposure. Digital systems vary from each manufacturer, but information regarding the name of the radiographer, amount of radiation the patient received during exposure, and the dentist's name may also be recorded. Once the mounting has been completed and verified, the images are saved in the patient's electronic file.

PRACTICE, PRACTICE, PRACTICE

Access the Evolve interactive exercises for this text to practice mounting digital images.

Evolve Interactive Exercises

- 10 practice mounts

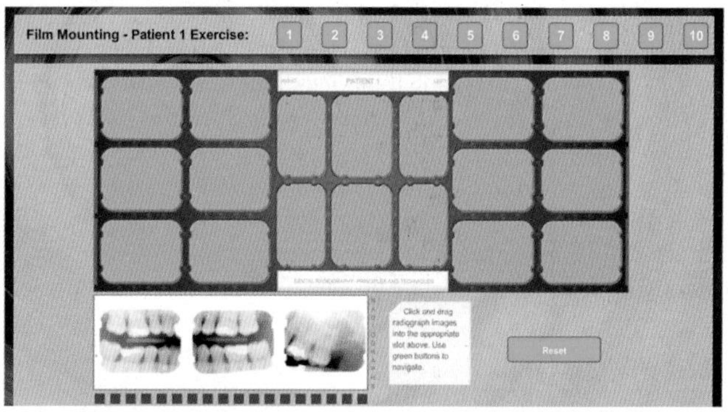

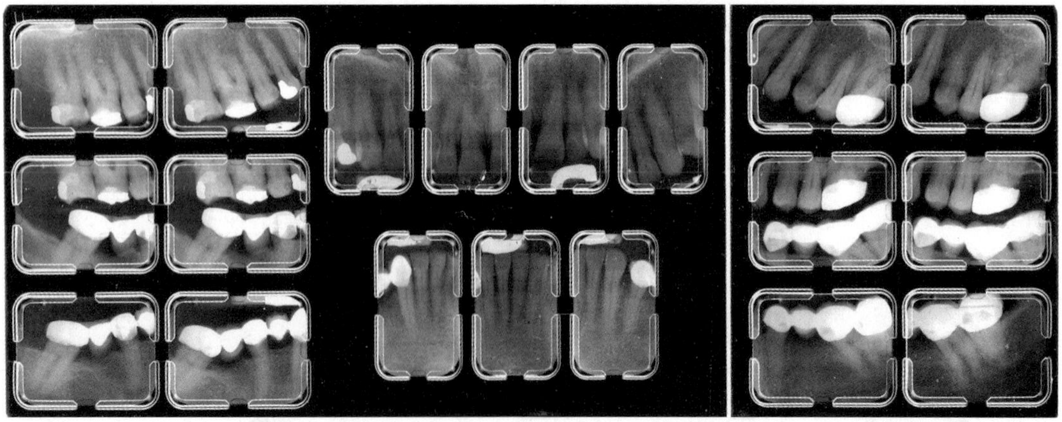

Fig 11-2 A complete series mounted using an opaque mount.

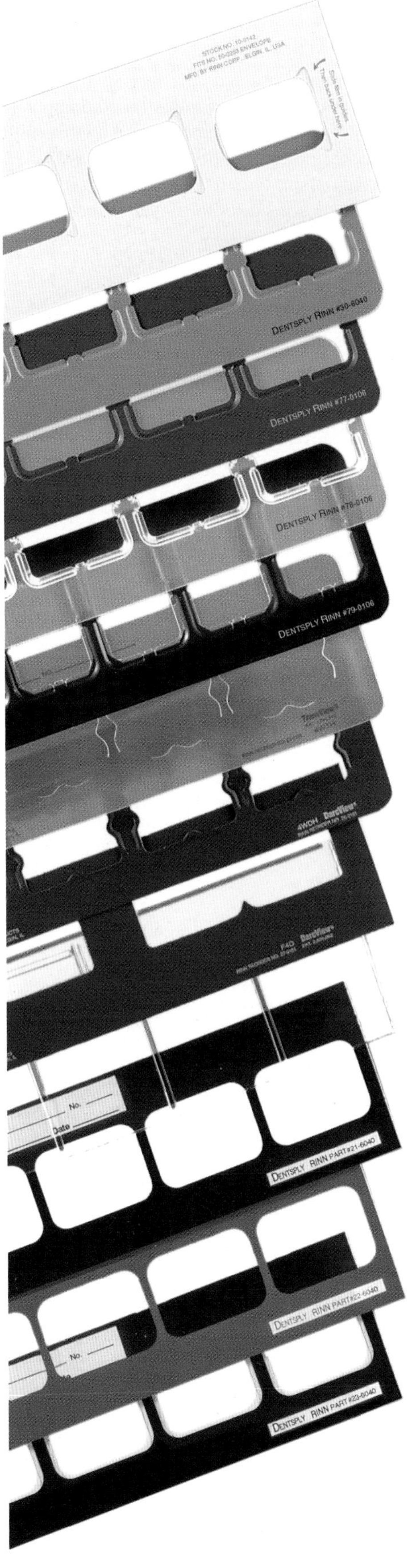

Fig 11-3 A variety of film mounts are available in many sizes and film combinations. (Courtesy Dentsply Rinn, York, PA.)

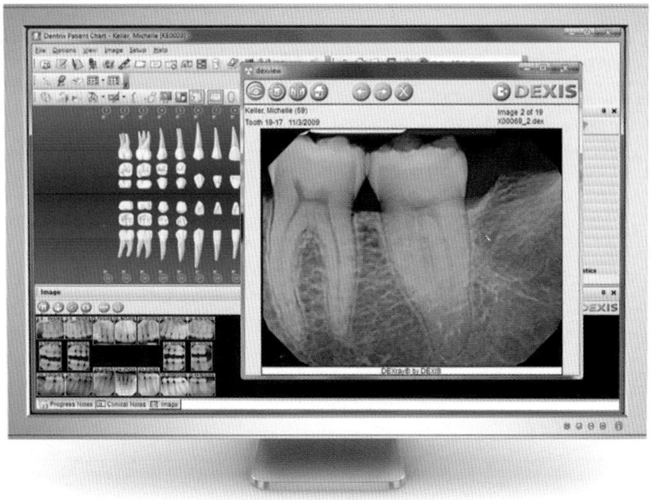

Fig 11-4 Digital images viewed on a computer monitor. (Courtesy KaVo Imaging, Brea, CA.)

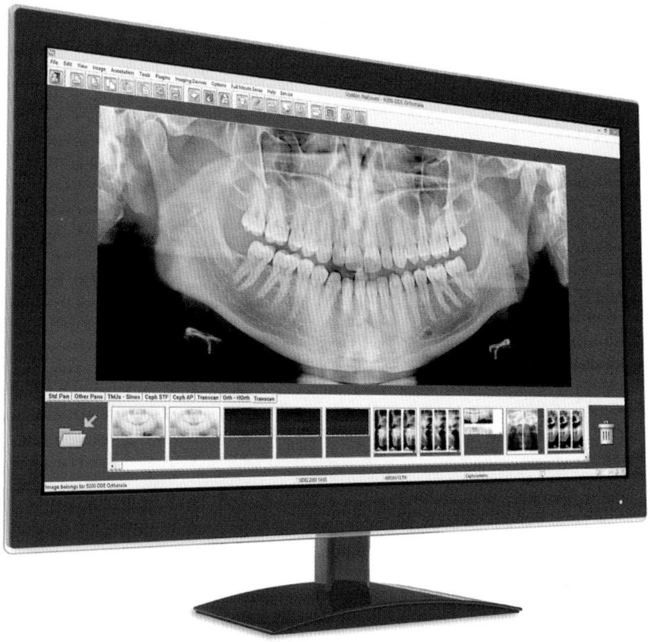

Fig 11-5 A panoramic image viewed on a computer monitor. (Courtesy KaVo Imaging, Brea, CA.)

Normal Anatomy and Film Mounting

Chapter 28 emphasizes that knowledge of normal anatomy is necessary to mount dental radiographs properly. The dental radiographer must be familiar with the characteristic anatomic landmarks seen in each region of the jaws. Identification of landmarks aids in distinguishing maxillary from mandibular periapical images, as shown in Figure 11-7.

It is important to note the curve of Spee when mounting bite-wing radiographs. The anterior-posterior anatomic curvature of the occlusal surfaces of the teeth, or curve of Spee, begins at the tip of the lower canine and follows the buccal cusps of the posterior teeth to the anterior border of the ramus. The curve of the maxillary arch is rounded or convex, while the curve of the mandibular arch is caved in or concave.

HELPFUL HINT

Normal Anatomy and Film Mounting

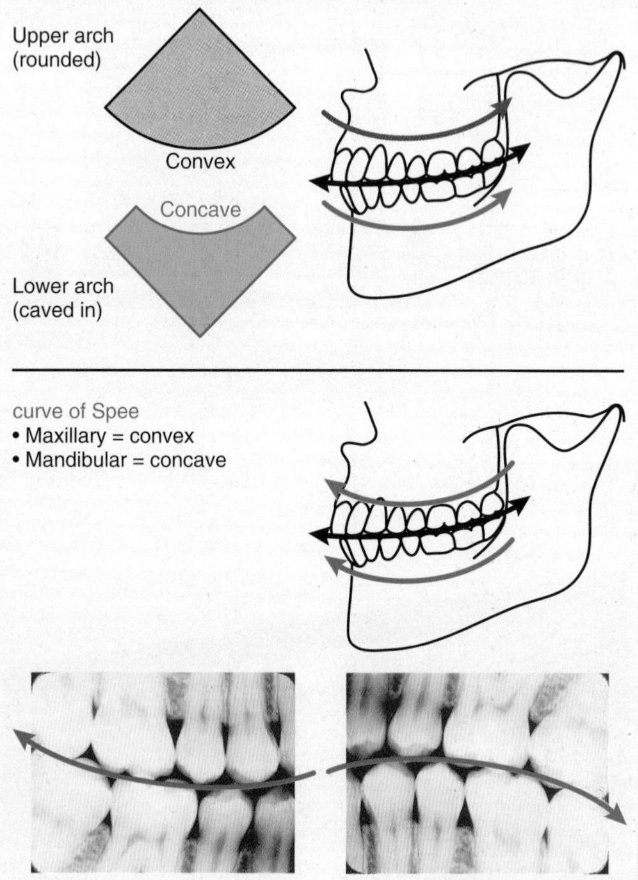

Film Mounting Methods

Two methods are used to mount films: (1) labial and (2) lingual. Both methods rely on identification of the embossed dot found on the film. As described in Chapter 9, a small, raised bump, known as the **identification dot**, is seen in one corner of each intraoral film packet; the dot on the packet indicates the location of the embossed identification dot on the radiograph (Figure 11-8). The film is positioned in the packet such that the raised side of the dot faces the x-ray beam during exposure.

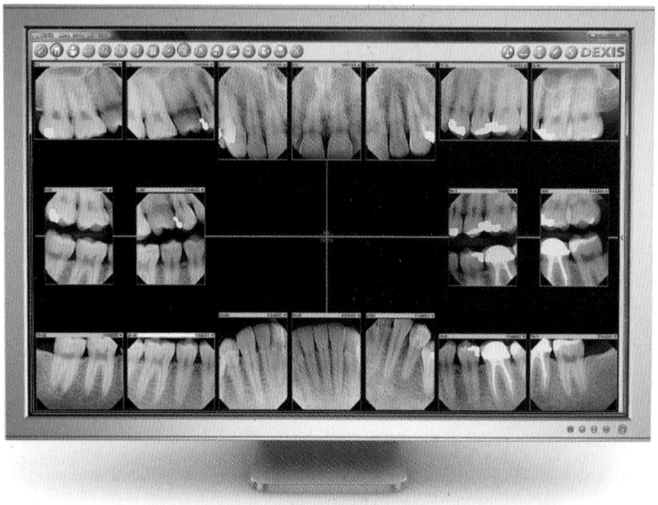

Fig 11-6 A full mouth series of radiographs exposed using digital imaging. Each image is placed in the appropriate window on the mount, arranged in anatomic order. (Courtesy KaVo Imaging, Brea, CA.)

Normal Anatomy on Intraoral Images

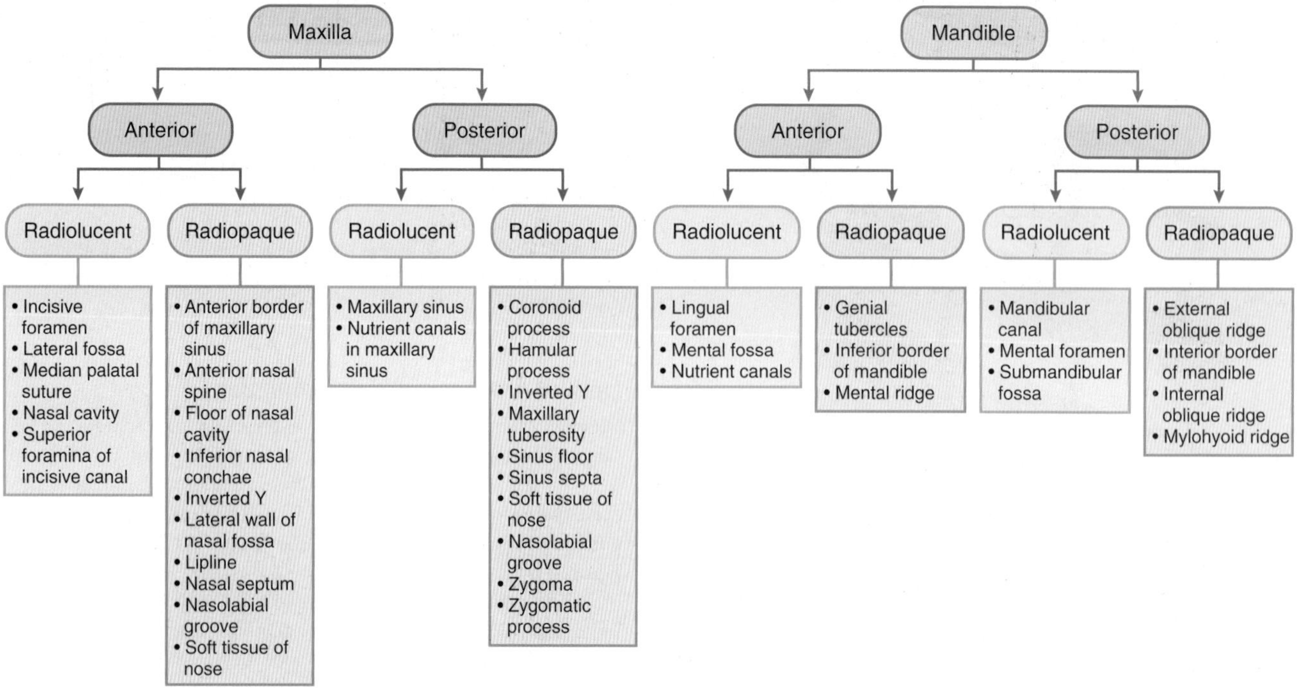

Fig 11-7 Landmarks distinguishing maxillary from mandibular periapical images.

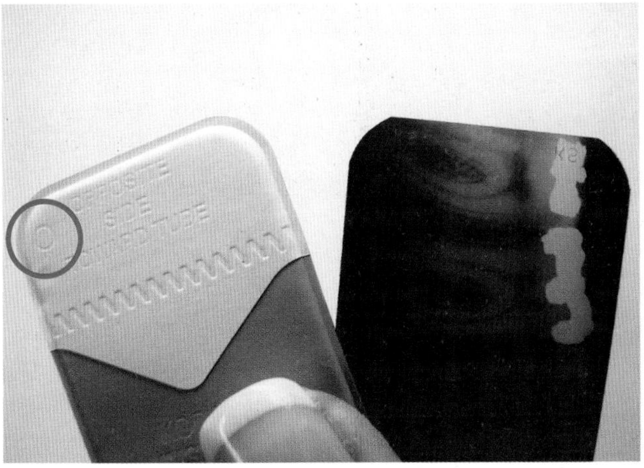

Fig 11-8 The dot on the packet indicates the relative location of the embossed identifying dot on the radiograph. (Courtesy Allyson Bowcutt.)

The identification dot is used to determine film orientation (i.e., determining the patient's right and left sides). After processing, the films should be placed in the film mount so that all the embossed dots are either raised (labial mounting) or depressed (lingual mounting); all the embossed dots must face in the same direction. The dental radiographer can then distinguish between the right and left sides of the patient. Either labial or lingual mounting can be used.

Labial Mounting. Labial mounting is the preferred method of mounting dental radiographs and is recommended by the American Dental Association. In the labial mounting method, radiographs are placed in the film mount with the *raised* (convex) side of the identification dot *facing the viewer* (dental radiographer). The radiographs are then viewed from the labial aspect (thus the term *labial mounting*). With this method, the radiographs are viewed as if the viewer is looking directly at the patient; the patient's left side is on the viewer's right, and the patient's right side is on the viewer's left (Figure 11-9). Images of teeth are mounted in anatomic order and have the same relationship to the viewer as they do when facing the patient.

Lingual Mounting. *Lingual mounting* can be used as an alternative method. Although some practitioners still use lingual mounting, this system of film mounting is not recommended. In the lingual mounting method, radiographs are placed in the film mount with the *depressed* (concave) side of the identification dot *facing the viewer*. The dental radiographer then views the radiographs from the lingual aspect (thus the term *lingual mounting*). With this method, the radiographs are viewed as if the dental radiographer is inside the patient's mouth and looking out; the patient's left side is on the viewer's left, and the patient's right side is on the viewer's right (Figure 11-10).

Step-by-Step Procedure

The dental radiographer in training can use the steps for film mounting listed in Procedure 11-1. As the mounting skills of the radiographer improve, simpler and faster techniques may be used.

HELPFUL HINTS

For mounting radiographs:

- **DO** master the normal anatomy of the maxilla, the mandible, and adjacent structures. A working knowledge of normal anatomy is necessary to correctly mount films.
- **DO** label and date the film mount before mounting the films; always include the patient's full name, the date of exposure, the dentist's name, and the radiographer's name.
- **DO** mount films immediately after processing.
- **DO** mount radiographs in a designated area; use a light-colored working surface in front of a viewbox.
- **DO** use an opaque film mount to block out extraneous light around each film.
- **DO** use clean dry hands to mount radiographs, and hold each radiograph by the edges only.
- **DO** identify the embossed dot on each film; always mount radiographs with the raised side of the dot facing the same direction. For labial mounting, all the raised dots must face the viewer.
- **DO** sort the radiographs before mounting them.
- **DO** use normal anatomic landmarks to distinguish maxillary images from mandibular images.
- **DO** use the order of teeth to distinguish the right side from the left side.
- **DO** use a definite order for mounting films. For example, begin with bite-wing images, then mount maxillary anterior periapical films, proceed to mandibular anterior periapical films, and then finish with maxillary posterior periapical films and mandibular posterior periapical films.
- **DO** mount bite-wing radiographs with the curve of Spee directed upward toward the distal.
- **DO** recognize the differences between maxillary and mandibular teeth (e.g., maxillary anterior teeth have larger crowns and longer roots than do mandibular anterior teeth).
- **DO** remember that most mandibular molars have two roots, whereas most maxillary molars have three.
- **DO** recognize that most roots curve toward the distal.
- **DO** verify the following points after mounting the radiographs: all the embossed dots are oriented correctly, the radiographs are arranged in anatomic order, the radiographs are mounted securely, and the film mount is labeled and dated.
- **DO** place the mounted radiographs in the patient's file as soon as possible to eliminate the possibility of loss or mix-up.

FILM VIEWING

Film viewing is essential in the interpretation of dental radiographs. The dental radiographer must be knowledgeable about optimal film viewing conditions and the recommended evaluation sequence for film viewing.

Basic Concepts

The term viewing means "examining or inspecting." In dental radiography, film viewing is the examination of dental radiographs.

Who Views Films? Any trained dental professional (dentist, dental hygienist, dental assistant) with knowledge of the normal anatomic landmarks of the maxilla, the mandible, and related structures is qualified to view dental radiographs. Although all members of the dental team may interpret dental radiographs, it is the responsibility of the dentist to establish a final or definitive interpretation and diagnosis. Interpretation, or the explanation of what is viewed on a dental radiograph, is discussed in Chapter 30.

What Equipment Is Required for Film Viewing? An adequate light source and magnification are required for optimal film viewing; both a viewbox and a magnifying glass are necessary.

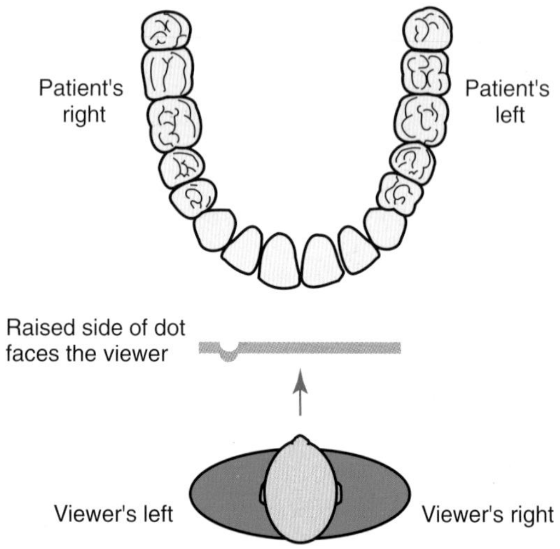

Fig 11-9 With the labial mounting method, the radiographs are viewed as if the dental radiographer were looking directly at the patient.

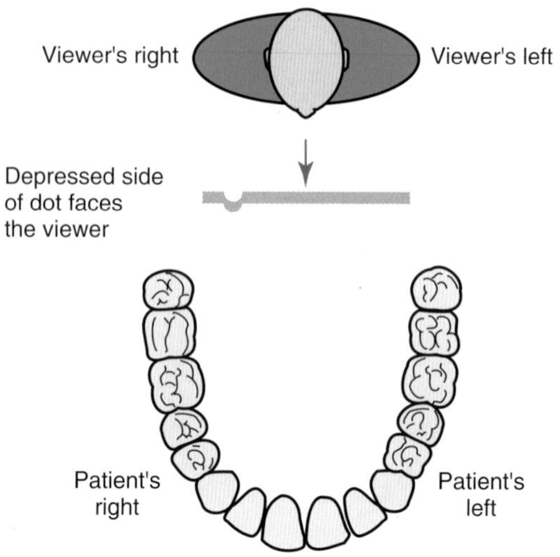

Fig 11-10 With the lingual mounting method, the radiographs are viewed as if the dental radiographer were inside the patient's mouth and looking out.

PROCEDURE 11-1 Mounting Dental Radiographs

1. Prepare for film mounting by placing a clean, light-colored paper towel over the work surface in front of the viewbox.
2. Turn on the viewbox.
3. Label and date the film mount (Figure 11-11).
4. Wash and dry your hands.
5. Examine each radiograph, identify the embossed dot, and then place each radiograph on the work surface with the raised side of the dot facing up (for labial mounting, as recommended by the American Dental Association). All radiographs must be mounted with the raised side of the dot facing in the same direction. Hold radiographs by the edges only (Figure 11-12).
6. Sort the radiographs into three groups: bite-wings, anterior periapicals, and posterior periapicals. Bite-wing images can be distinguished from periapical images because the crowns of both maxillary and mandibular teeth are seen on the image (Figure 11-13). Anterior periapical images can be distinguished from posterior periapical images because of the orientation of the film: in anterior periapical images, the long axis of the film is oriented vertically, and in posterior periapical images, the long axis is oriented horizontally (Figure 11-14).
7. Arrange the radiographs on the work surface in anatomic order. The normal anatomic landmarks can be used to distinguish maxillary images from mandibular images. In addition, all maxillary radiographs must be oriented with the roots of teeth pointing upward, and all mandibular radiographs must be oriented with the roots pointing downward (Figure 11-15). The order of teeth can be used to distinguish the right side from the left side (Figure 11-16).
8. Place each film in the corresponding frame of the film mount, and secure it (Figure 11-17). The following order for film mounting is suggested:
   a. Bite-wings
   b. Maxillary anterior periapicals

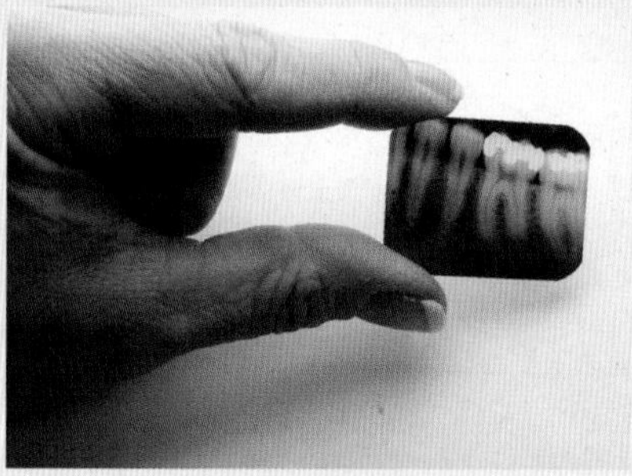

Fig 11-12 The dental radiographer should hold film by the edges only.

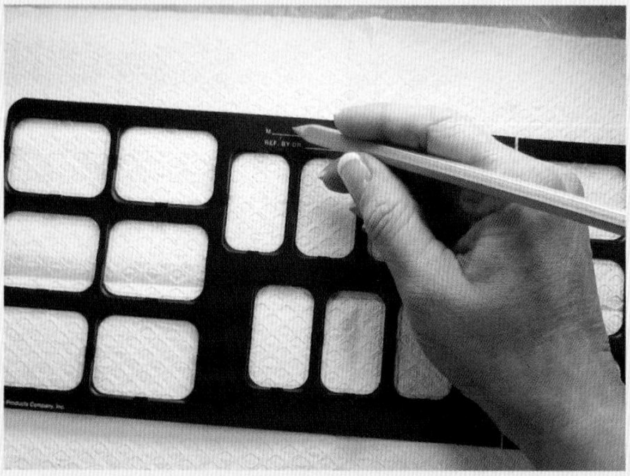

Fig 11-11 The dental radiographer must label and date the film mount before mounting the films.

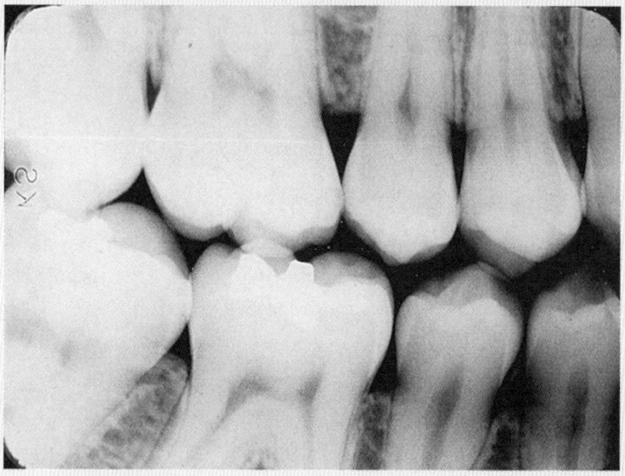

Fig 11-13 A bite-wing image shows the crowns of both maxillary and mandibular teeth on one film.

Continued

PROCEDURE 11-1 Mounting Dental Radiographs—cont'd

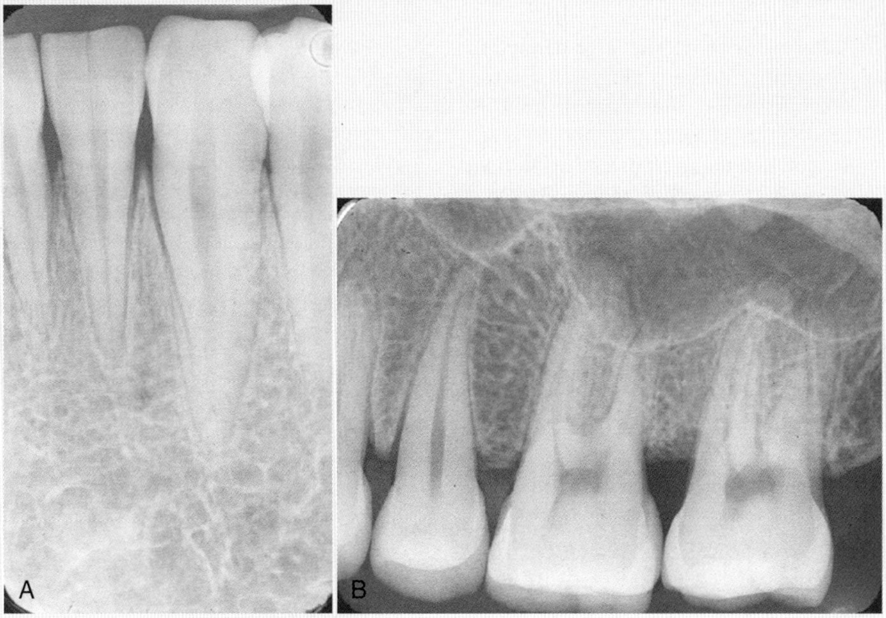

Fig 11-14 **A,** An anterior periapical film is oriented vertically. **B,** A posterior periapical film is oriented horizontally.

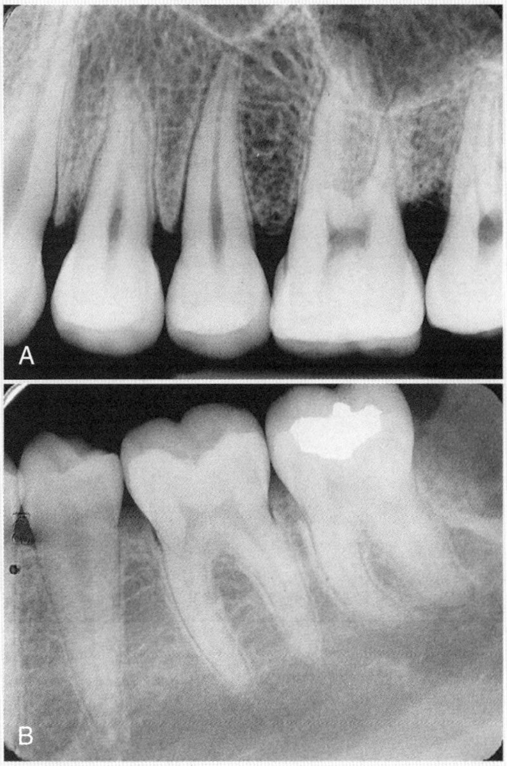

Fig 11-15 **A,** A maxillary periapical film is mounted with the roots pointing upward. **B,** A mandibular periapical film is mounted with the roots pointing downward.

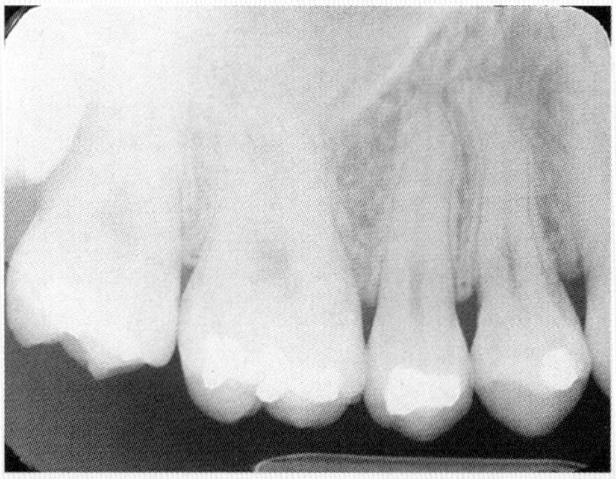

Fig 11-16 The order of teeth can be used to distinguish right from left; premolars are located in front of molars; therefore this is a maxillary right periapical image.

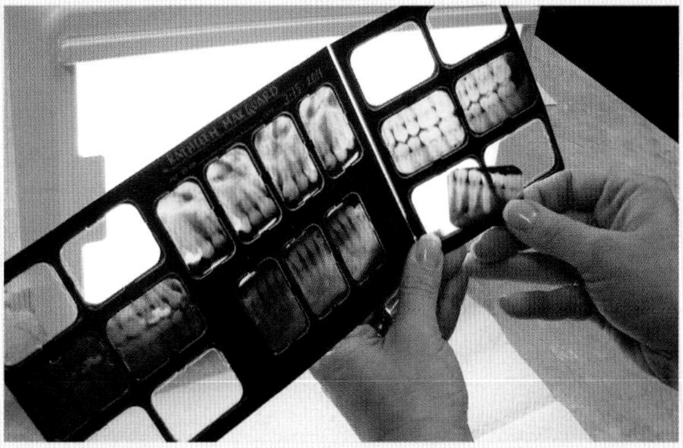

Fig 11-17 After the films have been arranged in proper order, the dental radiographer can place each film in the corresponding frame of the film mount.

c. Mandibular anterior periapicals
d. Maxillary posterior periapicals
e. Mandibular posterior periapicals

9. Check radiographs by verifying the following:
a. All embossed dots are oriented correctly.
b. All films are properly arranged in anatomic order.
c. All films are mounted securely.
d. The film mount is properly labeled and dated.

- *Light source:* A light source known as the viewbox, or *illuminator* (see Chapter 17), is required to view dental radiographs accurately and assist in the interpretation of images (Figure 11-18). The viewing area of the illuminator should be large enough to accommodate a variety of mounted films and unmounted extraoral films. The light from the viewbox should be of uniform intensity and evenly diffused. If the screen of the viewbox is not completely covered by the mounted radiographs, the harsh light around the mounted films must be masked to reduce glare and intensify the detail and contrast of the radiographic images (Figure 11-19).
- *Magnification:* The use of a pocket-sized magnifying glass is useful in interpretation. Magnification aids the viewer in evaluating slight changes in density and contrast in radiographic images (Figure 11-20).

When and Where Are Films Viewed? The dental radiographer should view radiographs immediately after mounting. Immediate film viewing is necessary to verify the correct arrangement of the images in the mount.

Films are best viewed by the dental radiographer on a viewbox in a room with dimmed lighting. When interpreting dental radiographs, an area free of distractions with subdued lighting provides optimal conditions for film viewing. Because such viewing conditions are typically present only in a medical facility, most films are examined on the viewbox at chairside in the dental setting.

Step-by-Step Procedure

Mounted radiographs must be viewed in sequential order. The dental radiographer must have an established viewing sequence to prevent errors in interpretation. The steps shown in Procedure 11-2 can be used to examine a CMS of dental radiographs (Figure 11-21).

The dental radiographer must use this recommended viewing sequence to examine films for each of the following:

- Unerupted, missing, and impacted teeth
- Dental caries and the size and shape of the pulp cavities
- Bony changes, the level of alveolar bone, and calculus
- Roots and periapical areas
- All areas not previously examined (e.g., remaining areas of the jaws, sinuses)

Many examinations of dental radiographs are necessary to check for all the problems listed. For example, the dental radiographer should first view the images quickly for evidence of unerupted, bony, or impacted teeth. Next, the examination sequence should be repeated for caries, pulp size, and pulp shape. The sequence must be repeated as many times as necessary to evaluate all surfaces of teeth and supporting structures for evidence of disease and abnormalities.

After film viewing, the dental professional must note any findings in the patient record. A standard diagram is included in the patient record and can be used to record significant findings (Figure 11-22). Although all dental professionals may note significant findings, it is important to remember that the final interpretation and diagnosis are the responsibility of the dentist.

HELPFUL HINTS

For viewing radiographs:

- **DO** use a viewbox to examine radiographs; avoid holding mounted films "up to the room light" to view.

PROCEDURE 11-2 Viewing Mounted Radiographs

1. Begin with maxillary teeth on the patient's right side (maxillary periapical films on the upper left side of the film mount).
2. Move horizontally across to maxillary teeth on the patient's left (maxillary periapical films on the upper right side of the mount).
3. Move down to mandibular teeth on the patient's left side (mandibular periapical films on the lower right side of the mount).
4. Move horizontally across to mandibular teeth on the patient's right (mandibular periapical films on the lower left side of the mount).
5. Move up to bite-wing films. View bite-wings on the left side of the mount, and then move to bite-wings on the right side of the mount.

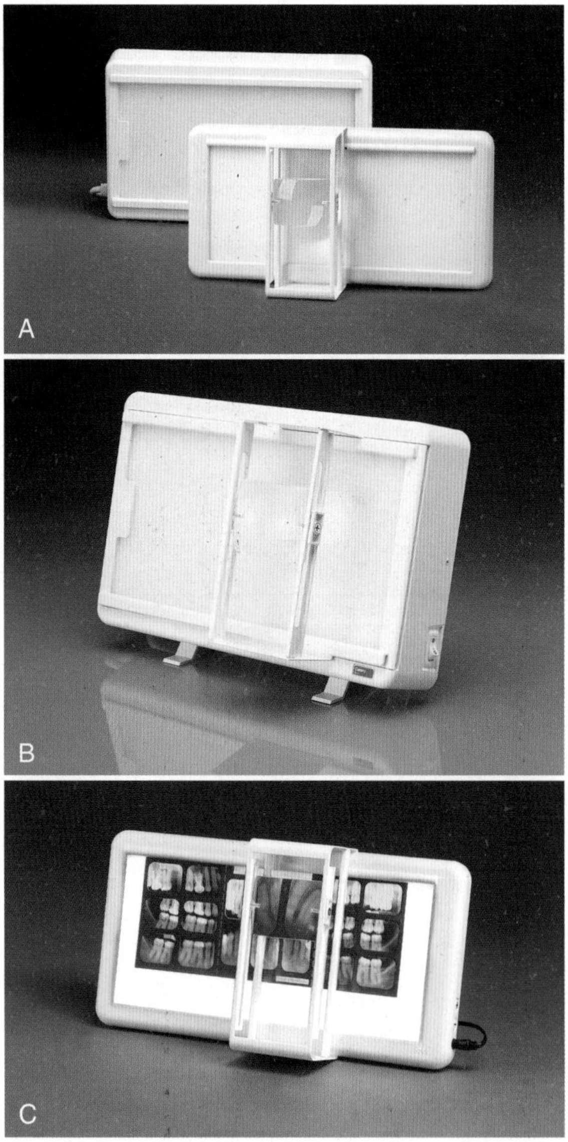

Fig 11-18 Examples of various viewboxes. (Courtesy Dentsply Rinn, York, PA.)

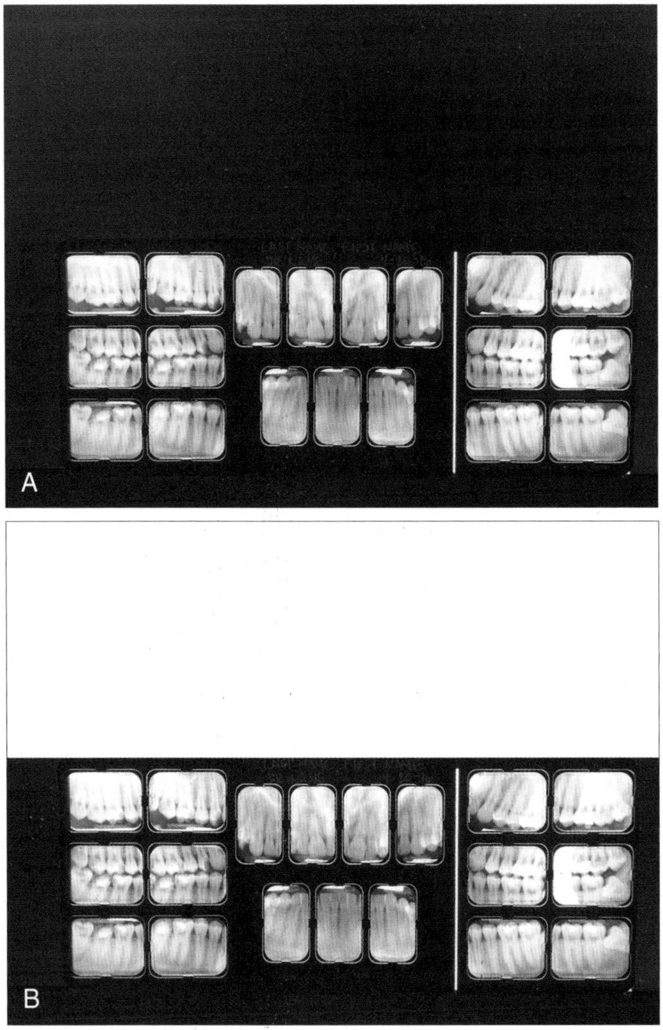

Fig 11-19 **A,** Extraneous light should be masked (black area above CMS) to reduce glare and intensify the contrast of images. **B,** When light is not masked (white area above CMS), it results in glare.

- **DO** block out the harsh light on a viewbox that occurs around the edges of the film mount; harsh light must be masked to reduce glare.
- **DO** use a magnifying glass to evaluate slight changes in density and contrast in radiographic images.
- **DO** view films immediately after mounting.
- **DO** view films under optimal viewing conditions whenever possible; use an area free of distractions with dimmed lighting.
- **DO** use a definite order for film viewing. To view a CMS, start with the films on the upper left side of the mount, move horizontally to the upper right, down to the lower right, across the lower left, up to the bite-wings, and then view the bite-wings from left to right.
- **DO** examine radiographs using the recommended viewing sequence as many times as necessary to evaluate them for (1) unerupted, impacted, and missing teeth; (2) dental caries, pulp size, and pulp shape; (3) bony changes, level of alveolar bone, and calculus; (4) roots and periapical areas; and (5) all areas not previously examined.
- **DO** record all radiographic findings in the patient record.

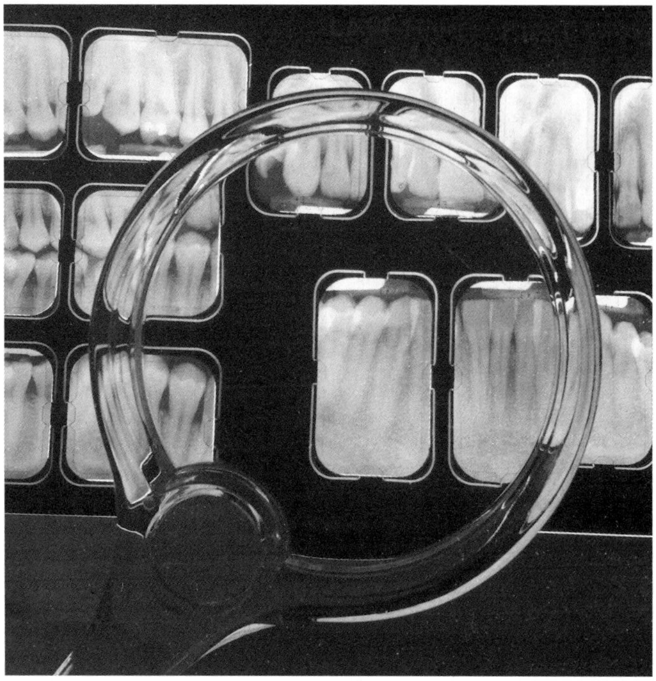

Fig 11-20 A magnifying glass aids the viewer in the evaluation of subtle changes in density and contrast.

SUMMARY

- Film mounting is the placement of radiographs in a supporting structure or holder.
- A film mount is a plastic or cardboard holder used to arrange radiographs in anatomic order (i.e., the order in which teeth are arranged in the dental arches).
- Any trained dental professional with knowledge of normal anatomy is qualified to mount dental radiographs. In most offices, the dental radiographer is responsible for the mounting of films.
- Dental radiographs should always be mounted immediately after processing in an area designated for film mounting.
- Mounted radiographs are quicker and easier to view and interpret and are more easily stored in the patient record. Mounted radiographs also decrease the chances of error in determining the patient's right and left sides, and they decrease the handling of films.
- A film mount should be labeled before mounting the films. The label includes patient's full name, date of exposure, dentist's name, and radiographer's name.
- Digital images should also be arranged correctly on the computer monitor and properly labeled with patient's name and date of exposure. The images must be saved in the electronic file of the patient.
- The two methods of mounting radiographs based on the orientation of the embossed dot are labial mounting and lingual mounting. The labial mounting method is recommended by the American Dental Association.

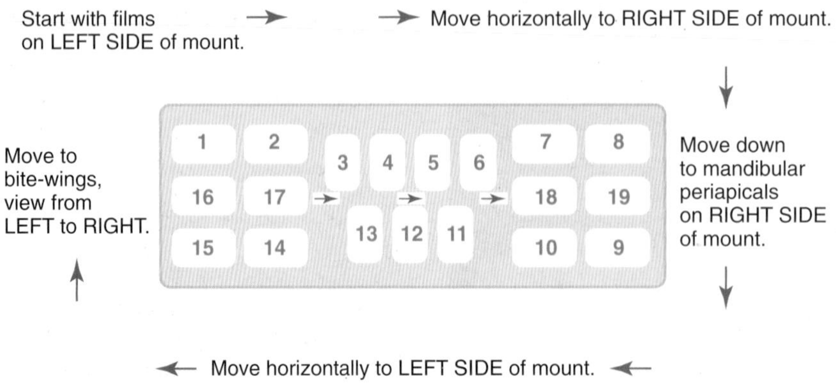

Fig 11-21 The dental radiographer must use a definite order for viewing radiographs. The sequence illustrated here is recommended. **Note that the numbers on the mount represent the viewing *order* and *not* tooth numbers**.

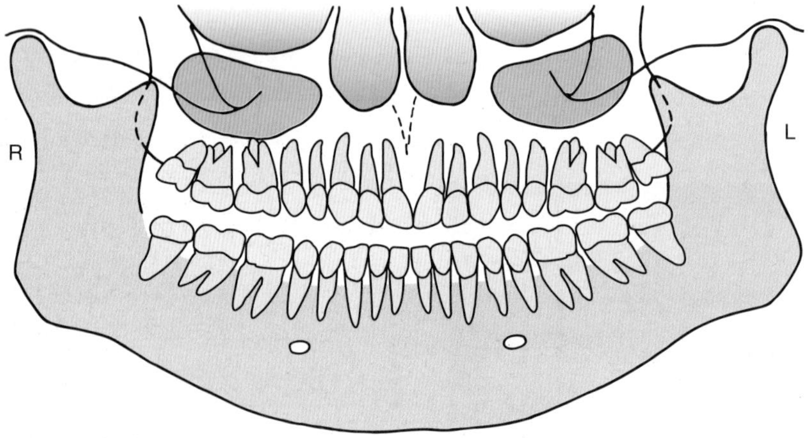

Fig 11-22 Standard diagram for recording radiologic findings. This diagram is used for panoramic and intraoral radiographs, but a similar arrangement can be used for other images.

- After films are mounted, the following must be verified: all embossed dots are oriented correctly, all films are arranged in anatomic order, all films are mounted securely, and the film mount is properly labeled and dated.
- Film viewing is the examination of radiographs. Films are best viewed on a viewbox (light source) in a room with dimmed lighting. Radiographs can be viewed by any trained dental professional and should be viewed immediately after mounting.
- Radiographs should be viewed in a sequential order as many times as necessary and should be examined for (1) unerupted, impacted, and missing teeth; (2) dental caries, pulp size, and pulp shape; (3) bony changes, level of alveolar bone, and calculus; (4) roots and periapical areas; and (5) all areas not previously examined.
- After film viewing, all significant findings must be noted in the patient record.

BIBLIOGRAPHY

Frommer HH, Stabulas-Savage JJ: Film mounting and radiographic anatomy. In Radiology for the dental professional, ed 9, St Louis, 2011, Mosby.

Haring JI, Lind LJ: The importance of dental radiographs and interpretation. In Radiographic interpretation for the dental hygienist, Philadelphia, 1993, Saunders.

Johnson ON: Identification of anatomical landmarks for mounting radiographs. In Essentials of dental radiography for dental assistants and hygienists, ed 9, Upper Saddle River, NJ, 2011, Prentice Hall.

Mallya SM, Lam EWN: Film imaging. In White and Pharoah's oral radiology: principles and interpretation, ed 8, St. Louis, 2019, Elsevier.

Miles DA, Van Dis ML, Razmus TF: Radiographic processing and processing quality assurance. In Basic principles of oral and maxillofacial radiology, Philadelphia, 1992, Saunders.

Miles DA, Van Dis ML, Williamson GF, et al: Film processing and quality assurance. In Radiographic imaging for the dental team, ed 4, St Louis, 2009, Saunders.

How to Mount a Complete Series

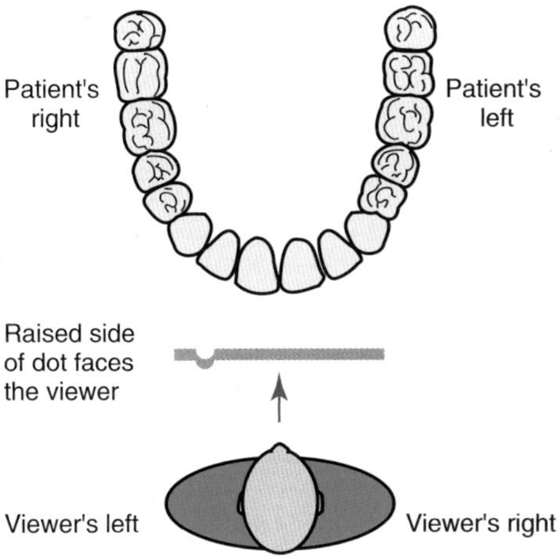

PREP
- Label mount.
- Work on a light-colored surface.
- Use a viewbox.

ARRANGE
- **Dot:** place all films with embossed **dot facing up.**
- **Sort: sort films** into BW's, anterior PA's, and posterior PA's.
- **Arrange:** arrange in **anatomic order.**

MOUNT
- Mount each film.
- Start on left of mount.
- Work from L to R.
- For each film:
  - Slide film under middle two tabs (1).
  - Then slide under left tab (2).
  - Then click film into right tab (3).

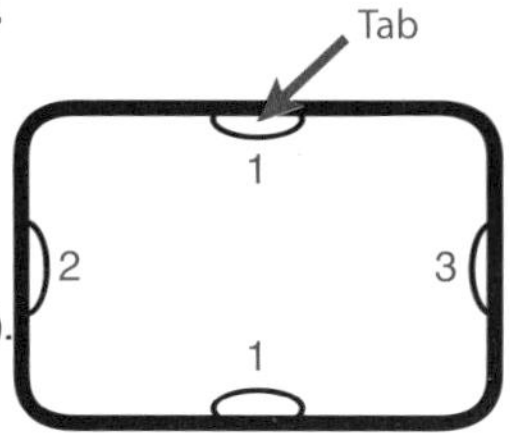

ORDER (see below/color coded)
- **First:** mount **Bite-wings** from L to R.
- **Second:** mount MAXILLARY **Anterior PA's** from L to R.
- **Next:** mount MANDIBULAR **Anterior PA's** from L to R.
- **Next:** mount MAXILLARY **Posterior PA's** from L to R.
- **Last:** mount MANDIBULAR **Posterior PA's** from L to R.

CHECK—CHECK—CHECK
- **Dots facing up?** All embossed dots are facing up.
- **Correct location?** Each film is placed in correct mount location.
- **Films secured?** Each film is secured with four plastic tabs.

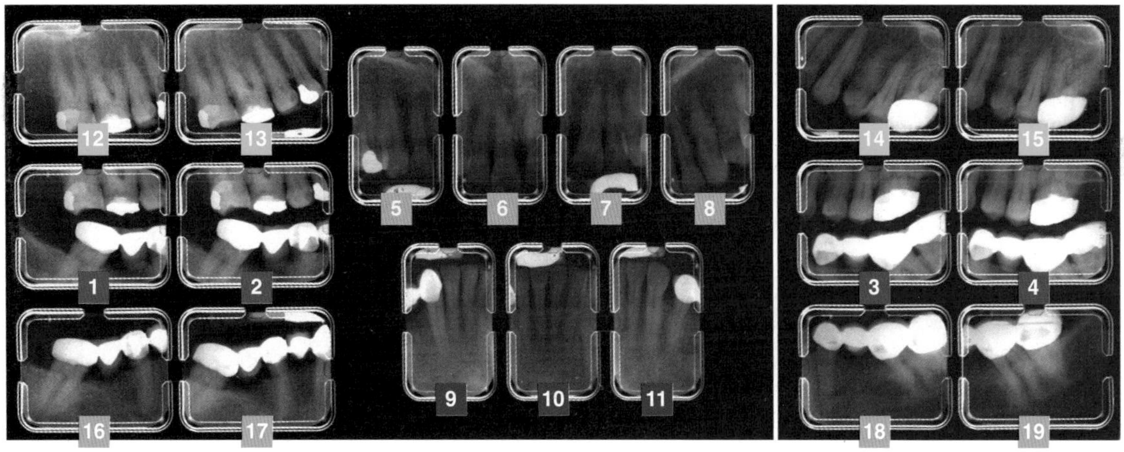

QUIZ QUESTIONS

True or False

_____ 1. *Anatomic order* refers to how teeth are arranged in the dental arches.

_____ 2. A clear film mount is preferred (instead of an opaque film mount) for better interpretation of radiographs.

_____ 3. Only the dentist is qualified to mount dental radiographs.

_____ 4. Films may be mounted at any time after processing.

_____ 5. Mounted films are quicker and easier to view and interpret.

_____ 6. Mounted films decrease the chances of error in distinguishing the patient's right and left sides.

_____ 7. Film mounts decrease the handling of individual films and prevent damage to the emulsion.

_____ 8. In the labial film mounting method, all the embossed identification dots are placed in the film mount with the raised (convex) side facing the viewer.

_____ 9. The lingual mounting method is widely used and is recommended by the American Dental Association.

_____ 10. Bite-wing radiographs must be mounted with the curve of Spee directed downward toward the distal.

_____ 11. *Film viewing* refers to the placing of films in a supporting structure.

_____ 12. Although all members of the dental team may view films, it is the responsibility of the dentist to establish a final, or definitive, interpretation and diagnosis.

_____ 13. Mounted radiographs may be viewed by holding the film mount up to the room light.

_____ 14. If the viewbox screen is not completely covered by the mounted radiographs, the harsh light around the mounted films must be masked to reduce glare and for better interpretation.

How to Mount Bite-Wings

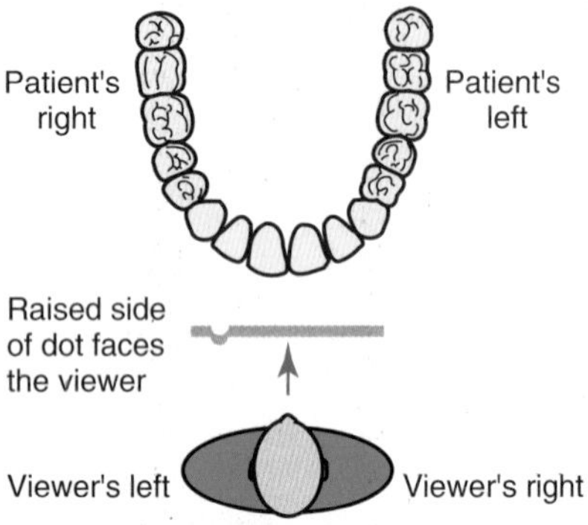

PREP
- Label mount.
- Work on a light-colored surface.
- Use a viewbox.

ARRANGE
- **Dot:** place films with embossed **dot facing up.**
- **Arrange:** arrange in **anatomic order.**
  Note **CURVE OF SPEE.**

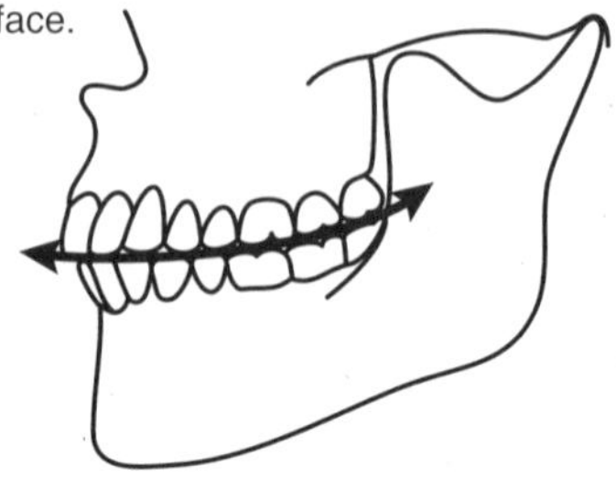

MOUNT
- Mount each BW film.
- Start on left of mount.
- Work from left to right.
- For each film:
  - Slide film under middle two tabs (1).
  - Then slide under left tab (2).
  - Then click film into right tab (3).

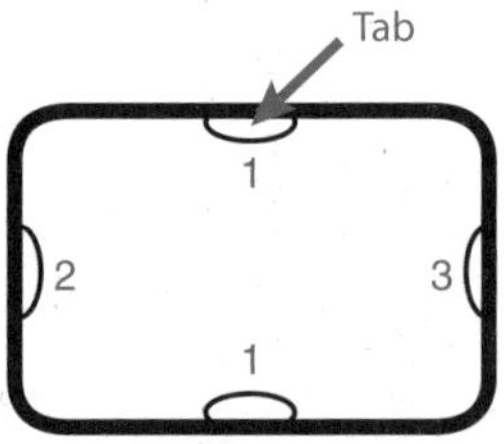

CHECK—CHECK—CHECK
- **Dots facing up?**
  All embossed dots are facing up.
- **Correct location?**
  Each film is placed in correct mount location.
- **Films secured?**
  Each film is secured with four plastic tabs.

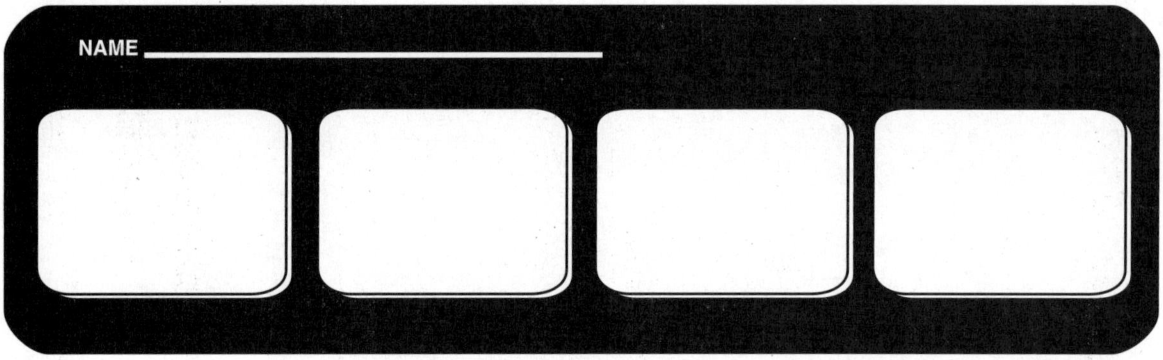

____ **15.** When interpreting dental radiographs, an area free of distractions and with dimmed room lighting provides optimal viewing conditions.

____ **16.** Optimal viewing conditions are typically present in the dental setting.

____ **17.** Mounted radiographs must be viewed in an established sequence to prevent errors in interpretation.

____ **18.** The dental radiographer must examine mounted radiographs many times to check for the presence of disease and abnormalities.

____ **19.** After film viewing, all positive findings must be noted in the patient record.

____ **20.** A viewbox is not necessary to examine dental radiographs.

Essay

21. List several reasons for using a film mount.

22. List and describe the two methods of film mounting.

23. Describe the step-by-step procedure for film mounting.

24. List and describe the necessary pieces of equipment for film viewing.

25. Describe the step-by-step procedure for film viewing.

12

Dental Images and the Dental Radiographer

LEARNING OBJECTIVES

After completion of this chapter, the student will be able to do the following:

1. Define the key terms associated with dental images.
2. Discuss the importance of dental images.
3. List the uses of dental images.
4. Discuss the benefits of dental images.
5. List examples of common dental conditions that may be evident on a dental image.
6. Discuss the knowledge and skill requirements of the dental radiographer.
7. List the duties and responsibilities that may be assigned to the dental radiographer.
8. Discuss the professional goals of the dental radiographer.

The dental radiographer must understand the importance of dental images and the reasons why imaging is a necessary component of comprehensive patient care. As discussed throughout this text, the dental radiographer must have both sufficient background knowledge and technical skills to perform dental imaging procedures. In addition, an understanding of the responsibilities and professional goals of the dental radiographer is necessary.

This chapter reviews the importance and benefits of dental images and the knowledge and skill requirements of the dental radiographer. The role of the dental radiographer is defined, and his or her duties and responsibilities are described. In addition, the professional goals of the dental radiographer are outlined.

DENTAL IMAGES

A dental image is a two-dimensional representation of a three-dimensional object produced by the passage of x-rays through teeth and supporting structures. The dental radiographer must have a thorough understanding of the value and importance of dental images. In addition, the dental radiographer must be familiar with the uses of dental images, the benefits of dental images, and the information that can be found on dental images.

Importance of Dental Images

Dental images are a necessary component of comprehensive patient care. In dentistry, dental images are essential for diagnostic purposes. Images enable the dental professional to identify many conditions that may otherwise go undetected and to see many conditions that are not apparent clinically (Figure 12-1). An oral examination without dental images limits the dental practitioner's knowledge to what is seen clinically: that is, teeth and soft tissues. With the use of dental images, the dental professional gains a great deal of information about teeth and supporting bone structures.

Uses of Dental Images

Dental images have many and varied uses. One of the most important uses of dental images is for detection of diseases, lesions, and conditions of the teeth and bones that cannot be identified by clinical examination alone. Many diseases and conditions produce no clinical signs or symptoms and are typically discovered only through the use of dental images (Figure 12-2).

Dental images are also used for confirming suspected diseases and for assisting in the localization of lesions and foreign objects. Images provide essential information during routine dental treatment; for example, the dentist relies on images during root canal procedures. Dental images can be used to examine the status of teeth and bone during growth and development. Dental images are indispensable for showing changes secondary to trauma, caries, and periodontal disease.

Dental images are an essential component of the patient record. An image contains a vast amount of information, much more than a written record does. Dental images provide the practitioner with baseline information about the patient. Each image serves to document the patient's condition at a specific time. Any subsequent images can be used for comparative purposes. Follow-up images can be compared with initial images and examined for changes resulting from treatment, trauma, or disease.

Benefits of Dental Images

The primary benefit of dental images to the patient is detection of disease, as mentioned earlier. When images are properly prescribed (see Chapter 4) and exposed, their benefit far outweighs the risk of small doses of x-radiation (Figure 12-3) (see Chapter 3). The use of dental images assists the dental professional in identifying and preventing problems, such as tooth-related pain or the need for surgical procedures.

Information Found on Dental Images

A number of conditions related to teeth and jaws produce no clinical signs or symptoms and can only be detected on dental images. Some of the more common diseases, lesions, and conditions found on dental images include the following:

- Missing teeth
- Extra teeth
- Impacted teeth
- Dental caries

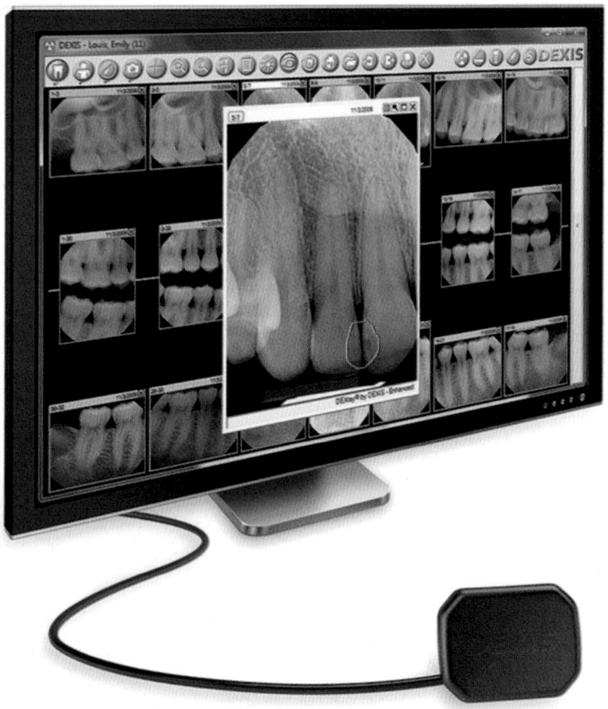

Fig 12-1 Dental images allow the practitioner to see conditions that clinically cannot be identified. (Courtesy KaVo Imaging, Brea, CA.)

- Periodontal disease
- Tooth abnormalities
- Retained roots
- Cysts and tumors

Images can be used to educate the dental patient about some of these common conditions that are only detected through the use of dental images.

THE DENTAL RADIOGRAPHER

The dental radiographer is any person who positions, exposes, and processes dental x-ray image receptors. In the typical dental practice, the dental radiographer is a dental auxiliary, either a dental hygienist or a dental assistant. The dental radiographer must have sufficient knowledge and technical skills to perform dental imaging procedures and must have a thorough understanding of his or her responsibilities and professional goals.

Knowledge and Skill Requirements

To be a competent dental radiographer, background knowledge of dental imaging is essential. The purpose of the first eleven chapters of this text has been to provide the dental radiographer with adequate background information to perform dental imaging procedures. The dental radiographer must have a basic understanding of radiation history (Chapter 1) and a working knowledge of radiation physics (Chapter 2), radiation biology (Chapter 3), radiation protection (Chapter 4), and radiation and image characteristics (Chapters 5 and 6). In addition, the dental radiographer must be familiar with dental x-ray equipment (Chapter 7), digital imaging sensors and dental x-ray film (Chapters 8 and 9), as well as dental x-ray film processing, mounting, and viewing (Chapters 10 and 11).

In addition to background information, the dental radiographer must master the knowledge of patient management basics (Chapters 12 to 16). A quality assurance plan ensures the production of diagnostic images (Chapter 17).

Most important, the dental radiographer must be proficient in technique concepts and the technical skills used in both film-based and digital imaging (Chapters 18 to 24).

Duties and Responsibilities

The dental auxiliary is a member of the dental team and has an important role in the practice. Each auxiliary employed in the dental office is assigned specific duties and responsibilities that vary depending on the size and nature of the dental practice and the individual qualifications of the auxiliary. Assigned responsibilities in regard to dental imaging may include the following (Figure 12-4):

- Positioning and exposure of dental x-ray imaging receptors
- Processing of dental x-ray films
- Data retrieval of digital images
- Mounting and identification of dental images
- Education of patients about dental imaging
- Maintenance of darkroom and processing equipment
- Implementation and monitoring of quality control tests
- Ordering of dental x-ray equipment and related supplies

Professional Goals

The dental radiographer must have pride in his or her work, always strive for professional improvement, have defined professional goals, and be committed to achieving those goals (Figure 12-5). Priority goals for the dental radiographer include patient and operator protection, patient education, operator competence and efficiency, and production of quality images.

Patient Protection. Patient protection must be a top priority and a primary concern of the dental radiographer. Whenever the dental radiographer performs imaging procedures on patients, the lowest possible level of x-radiation must be used. Retakes resulting in unnecessary patient exposure to x-radiation must be avoided at all times. Patient protection techniques used before exposure includes the proper prescribing of dental images and the use of proper equipment. During exposure, use of the thyroid collar and lead apron, a fast film or digital sensor, and beam alignment devices can limit patient exposure to radiation. In addition, proper selection of exposure factors and excellent technique also limit patient exposure. Specific to film-based imaging, meticulous handling and processing techniques are critical for the production of diagnostic images. Patient protection techniques are discussed in Chapter 4.

Operator Protection. Operator protection must also be a primary concern for the dental radiographer. To avoid occupational exposure to x-radiation, the dental radiographer must always avoid the primary beam and maintain an adequate distance, proper position, and proper shielding from x-rays during the procedure. A radiation-monitoring badge can be used to measure the amount of x-radiation received by the dental radiographer and to identify any excessive occupational exposure. Specific operator protection recommendations are discussed in Chapter 4.

Patient Education. Patient education is another priority for the dental radiographer. The dental radiographer must play an active role in the education of patients concerning radiation exposure, patient protection, and the value and uses of dental images (see Chapter 14).

Operator Competence. Operator competence must always be a concern of the dental radiographer, who must strive to maintain or

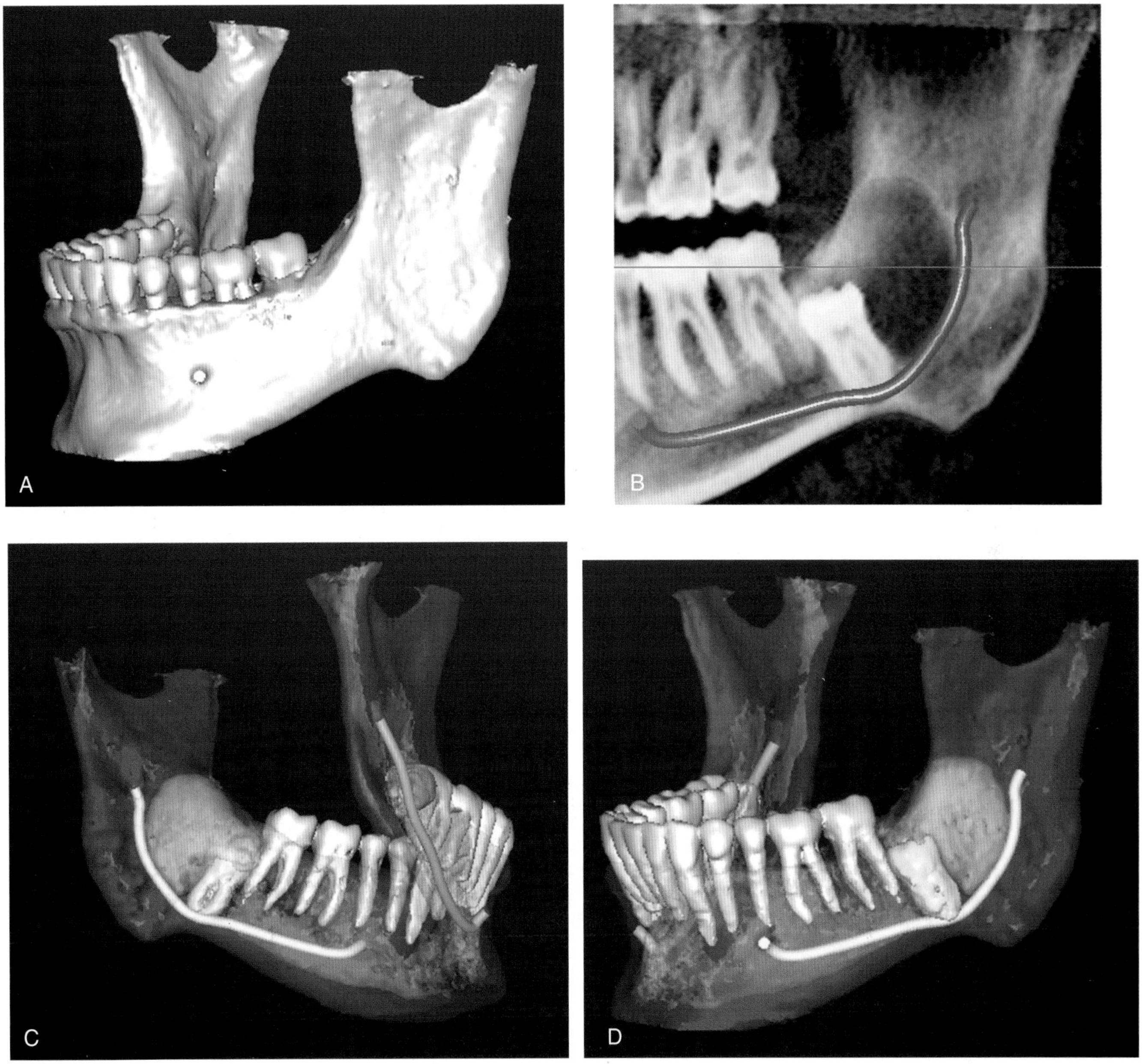

Fig 12-2 A young adult patient presented to the dental office for a routine preventive appointment. **A,** Clinical view of a three-dimensional image of patient. **B,** A panoramic image reveals an impacted tooth #17 associated with a corticated, unilocular radiolucent lesion. **C,** The transparent facial view reveals the exact location of the impacted tooth, mandibular canal, and dentigerous cyst. **D,** The lingual view reveals the extent of the dentigerous cyst and its proximity to tooth #18. (Courtesy Carolina OMF Imaging, W. Bruce Howerton Jr, DDS, MS, Franklinton, NC.)

improve professional competence by attending continuing education courses and lectures, studying professional books and journals, and reviewing and updating dental imaging techniques.

Operator Efficiency. The dental radiographer must be committed to performing his or her assigned duties in a time-efficient manner. He or she must always work carefully but quickly when positioning and exposing dental x-ray image receptors. Patients always appreciate the auxiliary who does not waste time and who works in a competent and efficient manner.

Production of Quality Images. The dental radiographer must be committed to producing high-quality, diagnostic dental images. To produce a diagnostic dental image, the radiographer must properly position and expose the receptor. The dental radiographer can take great professional pride in producing diagnostic dental images.

Quality Care. When the dental radiographer attains professional goals such as those detailed in this chapter, the patient receives the highest quality of care possible. Quality care benefits not only the patient but the profession of dentistry as well.

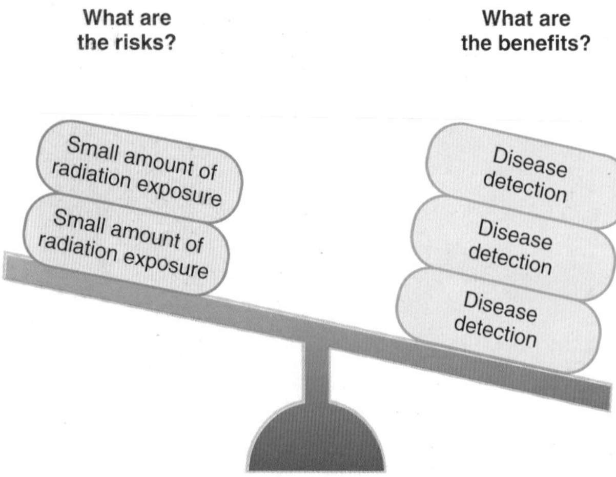

Fig 12-3 When dental images are properly prescribed, the benefits of disease detection outweigh the risk associated with dental x-ray exposure.

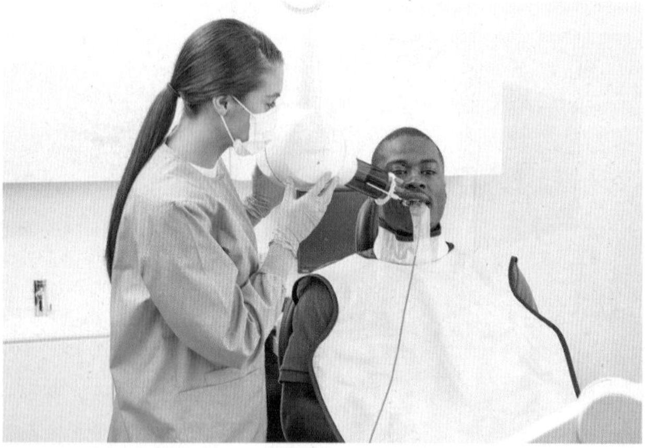

Fig 12-4 The dental radiographer is responsible for proper patient positioning and exposure of image receptors. (Courtesy Dentsply Sirona USA, Charlotte, NC.)

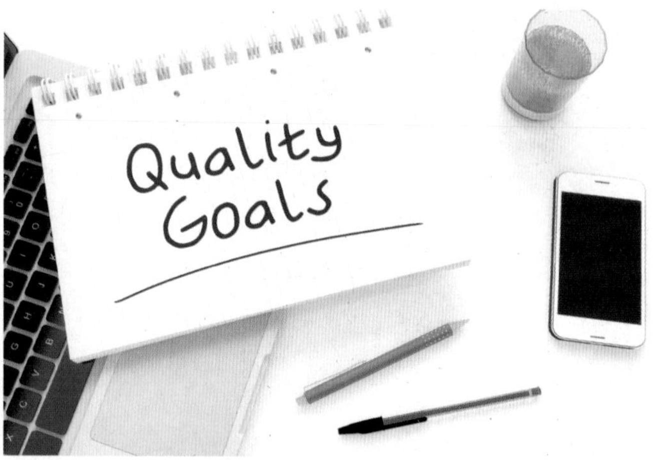

Fig 12-5 The dental radiographer, as a professional, must have defined professional goals and be committed to achieving them. Copyright Mathias Rosenthal/Shutterstock.com.

SUMMARY

- The dental radiographer must understand the importance of dental images and why dental images are a necessary component of comprehensive patient care.
- Dental images are essential for diagnostic purposes and enable the dental professional to identify many conditions that may otherwise go undetected.
- Although dental images have many uses, the primary use is detection of diseases, lesions, and conditions of the teeth and bones.
- Dental images are obtained to benefit the patient. The primary benefit is disease detection; the benefit of disease detection far outweighs the risk of small doses of radiation.
- Much information can be obtained from dental imaging. Numerous conditions related to teeth and jaws produce no clinical signs or symptoms and can only be detected on dental images.
- The dental radiographer is any person who positions, exposes, and processes dental x-ray image receptors. The dental radiographer must have both sufficient knowledge and technical skills to perform dental imaging procedures.
- Responsibilities of the dental radiographer include positioning, exposure, and retrieval of digital images or processing of films; mounting and identification of images; education of patients; maintenance of darkroom facilities and equipment; implementation and monitoring of quality control procedures; and ordering of equipment and supplies.
- Priority goals for the dental radiographer include patient protection, operator protection, patient education, operator competence, operator efficiency, and production of high-quality images.

BIBLIOGRAPHY

Frommer HH, Stabulas-Savage JJ: Patient management and special problems. In Radiology for the dental professional, ed 9, St Louis, 2011, Mosby.

Haring JI, Lind LJ: The importance of dental radiographs and interpretation. In Radiographic interpretation for the dental hygienist, Philadelphia, 1993, Saunders.

Johnson ON: Patient relations and education. In Essentials of dental radiography for dental assistants and hygienists, ed 9, Upper Saddle River, NJ, 2011, Prentice Hall.

QUIZ QUESTIONS

True or False

____ 1. Localization of foreign objects is the most important use of dental images.

____ 2. When images are properly prescribed, the benefit of disease detection does not outweigh the risk of small doses of x-radiation.

____ 3. Through the use of dental images, the dental professional can detect diseases, lesions, and conditions of the jaws that cannot be identified clinically.

____ 4. A dental image contains less information than a written record.

____ 5. Missing, extra, and impacted teeth can be identified on a dental image.

____ 6. The dental radiographer is any person who positions, exposes, and processes dental x-ray receptors.

____ 7. The dental radiographer is assigned only to position and expose dental x-ray imaging receptors.

____ 8. The dental radiographer may be assigned to monitor and implement quality control procedures.

____ 9. Patient and operator protection must be primary concerns of the dental radiographer.

____ 10. Operator competence is maintained by repeatedly performing dental imaging duties.

13

Patient Relations and the Dental Radiographer

LEARNING OBJECTIVES

After completion of this chapter, the student will be able to do the following:

1. Define the key terms associated with patient relations.
2. Discuss verbal, nonverbal, and listening skills, and explain how each can be used to enhance communication.
3. Discuss how facilitation skills can be used to enhance patient trust.
4. Define a relationship of trust between the dental professional and the patient.
5. Discuss the importance of first impressions, chairside manner, and attitude and explain how each can enhance patient relations.

Patient relations are important for all dental professionals. The dental radiographer needs good interpersonal skills to communicate with patients and establish trusting relationships (Figure 13-1). Communicating with dental patients may be the most demanding professional challenge that a dental radiographer encounters. The purpose of this chapter is to discuss specific interpersonal skills that enhance communication between the dental radiographer and the patient and to review the importance of patient relations.

INTERPERSONAL SKILLS

Skills that promote good relationships between individuals are termed **interpersonal skills**. (The term *interpersonal* is defined as "between persons.") The dental radiographer must have effective interpersonal skills not only to establish trusting relationships with dental patients but also to promote patient confidence. Technical skills alone are not sufficient for providing optimal patient care. Interpersonal skills must be used in conjunction with technical skills to enhance the quality of patient care.

HELPFUL HINT

Note

Technical skills alone are not sufficient for providing optimal patient care.

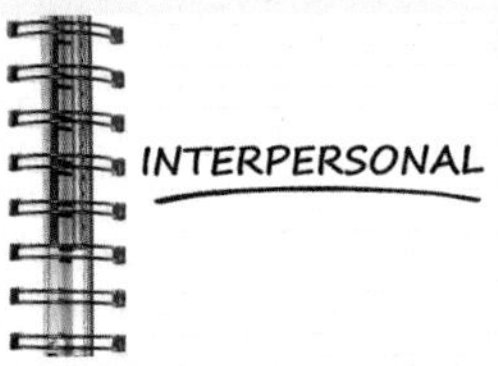

Copyright Underverse/Shutterstock.com

Communication Skills

Communication is a crucial interpersonal skill. **Communication** can be defined as the process by which information is exchanged between two or more persons. Effective communication is the basis for developing a successful radiographer-patient relationship.

Verbal Communication Skills. Verbal communication involves the use of language. The dental radiographer's choice of words is important when talking with the dental patient. Common phrases used informally in conversation can be off-putting in the professional setting and should be avoided (Box 13-1). Certain words detract from the professional image of the dental radiographer. For example, the term *pull* sounds less professional than *extract*, and the word *fix* sounds less professional than *repair* or *restore*. Some words used in the dental setting (e.g., *cut, drill, scrape, zap*) are associated with negative images and must be avoided. In addition, excessive use of technical words may cause confusion and result in miscommunication. The dental radiographer should always choose words that can be easily understood by the patient.

HELPFUL HINT

Verbal Skills

Skilled use of language involves:

- Word choice
- Delivery

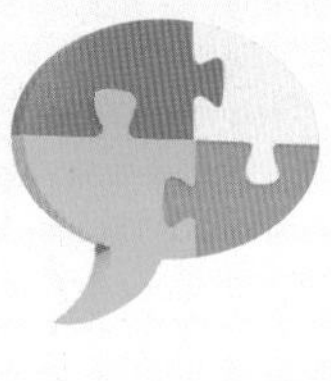

Copyright Klenger/Shutterstock.com

Careless use of language can contribute to miscommunication between the dental radiographer and the patient. The use of unnecessary words (e.g., "you know," "it's like," "I mean") may make it difficult for the patient to understand exactly what the radiographer is saying. Excessive use of slang can also increase the chance of misunderstanding.

The delivery of speech is important in verbal communication. The dental radiographer should always speak in a pleasant and relaxed manner. In the dental clinical setting, patients prefer the use of a soft tone of voice, as it is soothing and effective in conveying warmth and concern. A loud tone of voice is not appropriate and is often associated with fear, anger, or excitement. The dental radiographer should avoid speaking in a rushed or tense manner as well.

Nonverbal Communication Skills. *Nonverbal* communication involves the use of body language (Figure 13-2). Nonverbal messages that the dental radiographer conveys through posture, body movement, eye contact, and facial expression are important when working with patients in the dental clinical setting.

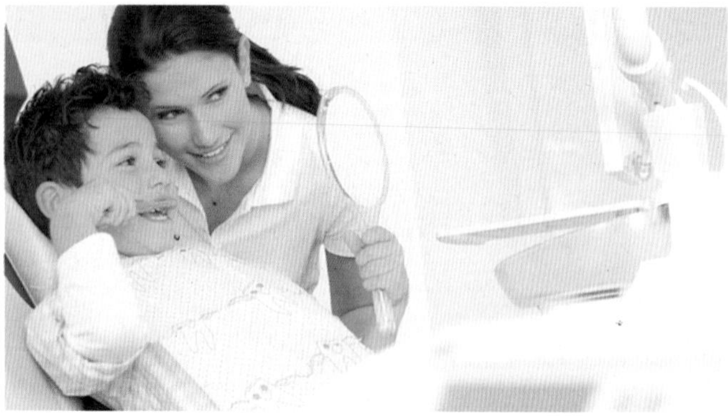

Fig 13-1 Interpersonal skills promote a good relationship between persons. (Courtesy Sirona Dental Systems, LLC, Charlotte, NC.)

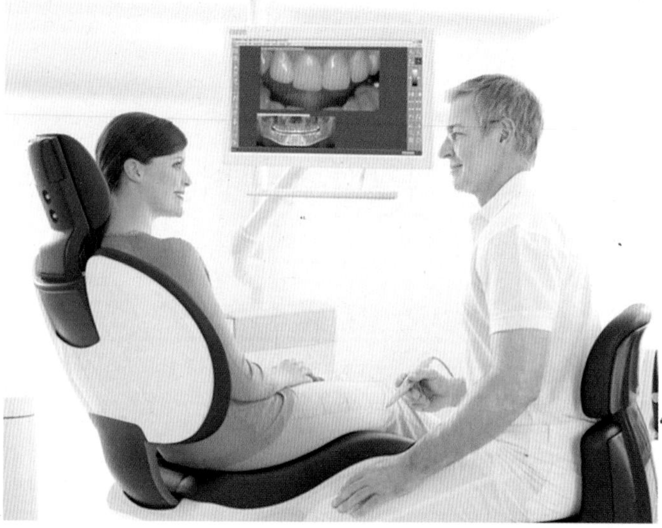

Fig 13-2 Body language, eye contact, and facial expression are all nonverbal skills used to communicate. (Courtesy Sirona Dental Systems, LLC, Charlotte, NC.)

BOX 13-1 Phrases to Avoid

"Sorry 'bout that."
If this phrase is said quickly and with no eye contact, it implies insincerity and that you do not really have time for a true apology.

"Just relax."
The underlying message of this phrase, often used with nervous patients, does not comfort the patient but adds to the anxiety that is already present.

"Calm down."
Using this phrase is similar to saying, "You are out of control and have lost all credibility" and serves to further agitate the patient.

"I don't know."
This phrase can be interpreted as, "It is up to you to figure it out." When you do not know something, the appropriate response is, "I don't know, but let me find out for you."

"Not a problem."
This phrase indicates there could have been a problem and negates the person's appreciation. When someone thanks you, it is best to respond with "You're welcome" or "My pleasure."

"It's crazy around here today."
This comment implies that chaos reigns in your office setting and is not comforting to the patient. It serves no purpose to convey this message to a patient.

Nonverbal messages can be substituted for verbal messages. For example, a nod of the head indicates agreement, whereas a shake of the head signals disagreement. Nonverbal behavior can also be used to enhance communication. For example, if the statement "It's nice to see you" is accompanied by a smile, consistency exists between the verbal and nonverbal messages; the verbal message is enhanced by the nonverbal message. When nonverbal messages are consistent with verbal messages, the patient is more likely to relax and trust the dental professional. When nonverbal messages are not consistent with verbal messages, however, the patient is more likely to respond with apprehension and mistrust.

Posture and *body movement* are important nonverbal cues that convey the attitude of the dental radiographer. An attentive posture and leaning slightly toward the patient, with relaxed, still hands, are nonverbal cues associated with interest and warmth. Conversely, a slumped posture and leaning away from the patient, with arms folded across the chest and fingers tapping, are nonverbal cues that signal indifference and coldness (Figure 13-3). Patients are more likely to understand and remember information presented by an interested health professional than by a professional whose nonverbal cues signal indifference.

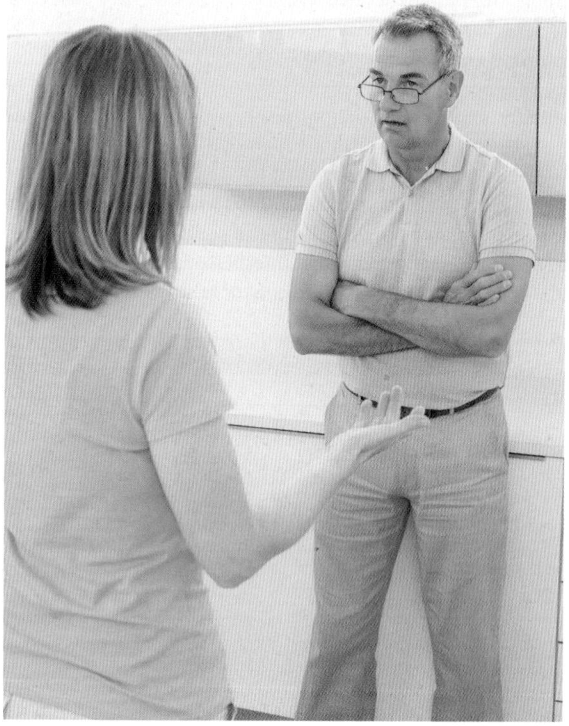

Fig 13-3 Standing with folded arms is a type of posture that signals indifference and coldness, the principal negative barrier to communication. © shutterstock / lightwavemedia

Eye contact is another nonverbal means of communication that is important in the dental setting. When listening to a patient, the dental radiographer should always maintain direct eye contact with the

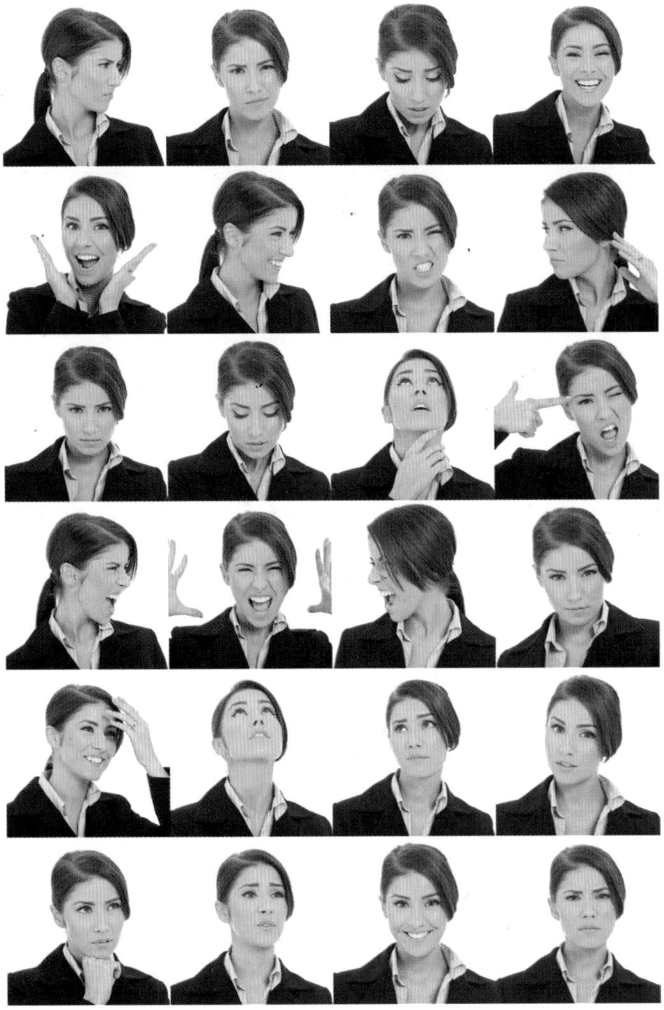

Fig 13-4 Facial expressions convey a variety of emotions. Copyright Viorel Sima/Shutterstock.com

patient; the eyes should not wander. Direct eye contact is associated with interest and attention and plays a powerful role in the initiation and development of interpersonal relationships. A lack of eye contact is often interpreted as indifference or lack of concern. It is important to note that different cultures have different rules for eye contact. For example, individuals in East Asia make less eye contact than do individuals from Western European or North American cultures.

Facial expressions are also a very important part of nonverbal communication and indicate much about a person's mood. Facial expressions convey a variety of emotions—some examples include confusion, surprise, focus, exhaustion, happiness, sadness, fear, anger, and disgust (Figure 13-4). The interpretations assigned to these facial expressions vary greatly based on an individual's culture and experience. When interacting with patients, the dental radiographer should use appropriate facial expressions to convey the apt emotional response.

Listening Skills. Listening involves more than just hearing; *listening* refers to the receiving and understanding of messages. When listening to a patient, the dental radiographer must receive and understand the information being presented. Careful listening results in better communication and less chance for misunderstandings. The radiographer with good listening skills understands what the patient has said and, in turn, is able to communicate that understanding to the patient.

HELPFUL HINT

Listening Tips

- Do not interrupt.
- Do not finish a patient's sentences.
- Give your undivided attention.

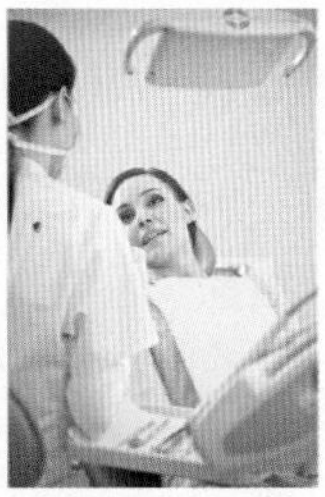

Copyright Izabela Habur/iStock.com

The good listener communicates attention and interest. When listening to a patient, the dental radiographer can use nonverbal cues such as a nod of the head or facial expressions to convey appropriate emotional responses. To communicate interest, the dental radiographer can paraphrase what the patient has just stated to confirm what has been heard.

To enhance communication, sometimes the dental radiographer may want to summarize the feelings of the patient rather than paraphrase the information that has been presented. When a patient is fearful and upset, the dental radiographer conveys interest and concern for the patient when he or she can summarize and emphasize the patient's feelings.

When listening to a patient, the dental radiographer should give undivided attention to that patient. The dental radiographer should never interrupt or correct the patient, finish the patient's sentences, look at a clock or watch, or distract the patient by fidgeting or playing with objects.

Facilitation Skills

Facilitation skills are interpersonal skills used to ease communication and develop a trusting relationship between the dental professional and the patient. (The term *facilitation* is defined as "the act of making something easier.") In a trusting relationship, the patient feels cared for and understood by the dental professional. In the dental clinical setting, trust means that the patient believes that the dental professional will interact in a beneficial way and not in a harmful way. A trusting relationship facilitates the delivery of patient care by reducing worry and psychological stress in the patient. When a patient trusts the dental professional, the patient is more likely to provide information, cooperate during procedures, comply with prescribed treatment, and return for further treatment.

HELPFUL HINT

Facilitation Skills

Facilitation skills are used to **ease communication** and to **develop a trusting relationship**.

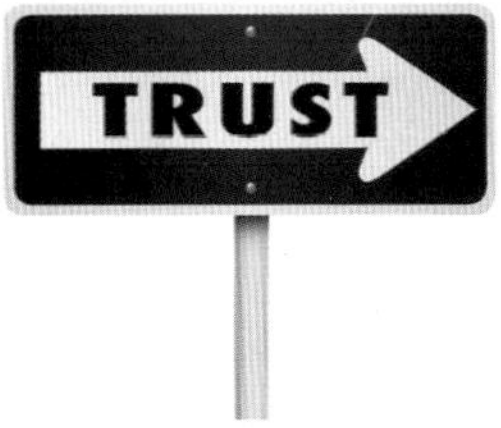

Copyright iQoncept/Shutterstock.com

Facilitation skills that enhance patient trust include encouraging questions, answering questions, responding with action, and expressing warmth. The dental radiographer must encourage each patient to ask questions. Many patients may be hesitant to ask questions because they may be feeling intimidated by the dental professional or apprehensive about the dental visit. Inviting a patient to ask questions enhances communication. In addition, the dental radiographer must be prepared to answer the patient's questions directly. Whenever a patient asks a question, the dental radiographer should respond with accurate information in a direct manner and use language that the patient can easily understand.

The dental radiographer must be prepared to respond with action or carry out patient requests. For example, if a patient requests a glass of water, the dental radiographer can respond by providing a glass of water to the patient. The patient feels cared for when the dental radiographer responds to requests with the desired action. In addition, the dental radiographer must respond to patients with *warmth*, which can be communicated through voice and facial expression. The dental radiographer who responds to patients with warmth is friendly and smiling and shows interest in the patient. Warmth communicates that the professional cares for the patient as a person.

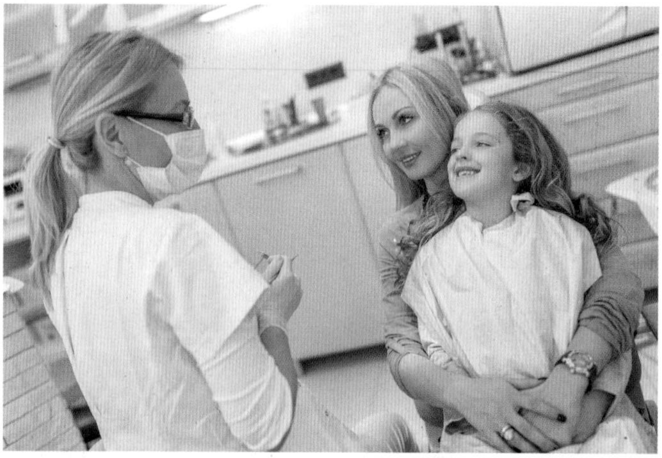

Fig 13-5 The dental auxiliary is often responsible for establishing a positive first impression with the patient. Copyright BraunS/iStock.com

PATIENT RELATIONS

In dentistry, the term patient relations refer to the relationship between the patient and the dental professional. Patient relations are important to all dental professionals: the dentist, the dental hygienist, and the dental assistant.

First Impressions and Patient Relations

The relationship between the patient and the dental professional begins with first impressions. The patient's first impression of the dental team most often involves the dental auxiliary, specifically the auxiliary's appearance and greeting (Figure 13-5).

The professional appearance of the dental auxiliary is important. The dental auxiliary should always wear clean clothing and be well groomed. Strict attention must be paid to personal hygiene, including handwashing and maintaining fresh breath. In addition, the dental auxiliary should never eat, drink, or chew gum while working with patients (Boxes 13-2 and 13-3).

BOX 13-2 Helpful Hints

Personal grooming	Hair and nails should be neat and clean. Use of a deodorant is a must. In addition, dental professionals must pay careful attention to maintaining fresh breath.
Clothing	All clothing should be clean—without stains—and pressed.
Shoes/socks	Pay attention to your shoes. Shoes should be polished and clean. Always wear socks with shoes. Open-toed shoes are inappropriate for health professional environments.
Eating and drinking	Never chew gum, eat mints, eat, or drink while working with patients.
Manners	To make sure your manners are appropriate, take a business etiquette class.

HELPFUL HINT

First Impressions

First impressions are formed by:
- Appearance
- Hygiene
- Greeting

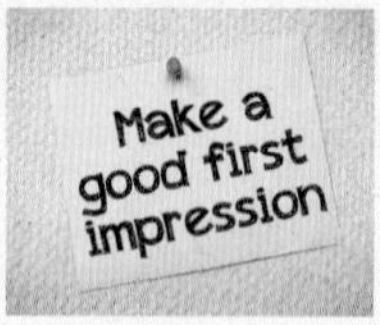

Copyright Constantin Stanciu/Shutterstock.com

In many offices, the dental auxiliary is the first dental professional to meet and greet the patient. The dental auxiliary should always greet patients in the reception room before escorting them to the treatment area. Patients should always be greeted by name. The dental auxiliary should address the patient using the patient's proper title (Miss, Ms., Mrs., Mr., Dr., Rev., etc.) and last name. If uncertain about the correct pronunciation of the name, the dental auxiliary should find out the correct pronunciation from the patient. The dental auxiliary should always introduce himself or herself to the patient, using both name and title. Here is a typical first greeting:

Hello, Mrs. Davis. My name is Kate Miller, and I'm the dental assistant who will be working with you today. It's a pleasure to meet you. If you'll follow me to the patient treatment area, we can get started with today's appointment.

HELPFUL HINT

Greeting

- Address the patient by title.
- Welcome the patient.
- Introduce yourself and describe your role.
- Say, "It's a pleasure to meet you."
- Tell the patient where you are going.
- Depending on policy, offering a handshake may not be an appropriate gesture considering social distancing. Check with office or school protocol for other greeting options that do not involve touching as personal contact.

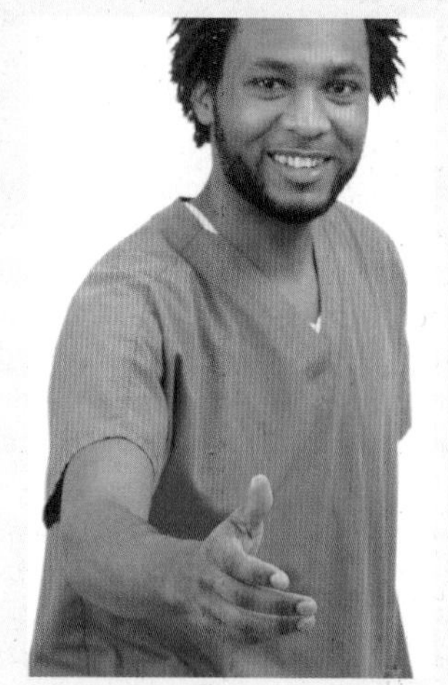

Copyright Val Lawless/Shutterstock.com

BOX 13-3 First Impressions Checklist

- Find out the patient's preferred name, and use it.
- When the patient arrives, offer a warm welcome—both verbally and through body language.
- Introduce yourself to each patient with a smile and a handshake, taking into consideration social distancing guidelines.
- Introduce other staff members to the new patient.
- Wear a name tag; knowing your name gives the patient a sense of belonging.
- Ask your patient questions, and then *listen.*

When seeing the same patient for the second or third visit, it is appropriate to recall certain facts about the patient to show that the dental auxiliary remembers not only the patient's name, but also some events that are important to the patient. For example, it would be considerate to ask patients about their grandchildren, a recent vacation, or a work promotion the patient had mentioned on a previous visit. This type of conversation enhances patient relations and conveys a sense of caring to the patient.

Chairside Manner and Patient Relations

The relationship between the patient and the dental professional develops as the professional works with the patient. Chairside manner refers to the way a dental professional conducts himself or herself at the patient's chairside. The dental auxiliary must develop a relaxing chairside manner that makes the patient feel comfortable and at ease.

The dental auxiliary must also convey a confident chairside manner. The patient must be confident about the auxiliary's ability to perform radiographic procedures. The dental radiographer must avoid comments such as "Oops!" or "Uh oh" and other statements that indicate a mistake or a lack of control. The patient must feel that the operator is in control of all procedures being performed. Instead of stating, "This won't hurt at all," it is better for the dental radiographer to say, "I will work as quickly as possible to minimize any discomfort that may occur." One way to convey operator confidence is to explain to the patient exactly which procedures are about to be performed and then answer any questions the patient may have about the procedures.

In most dental offices, the dental auxiliary is responsible for performing radiographic procedures. However, some patients may be apprehensive about allowing a dental auxiliary to perform such procedures because they are accustomed to the dentist performing all procedures. As a result, these patients may object to a dental auxiliary performing any services for them. In such cases, the dental auxiliary must try to establish a relationship with the patient by explaining the concept of the dental team. The dental auxiliary can educate and orient the patient to the dental team members and their respective roles and responsibilities. The dentist may then reinforce such information and reassure the patient before the dental auxiliary performs the radiographic procedures.

Patient relations and management skills with regard to persons with specific dental needs are discussed further in Chapter 24, specifically patients with physical or developmental disabilities, as well as pediatric, endodontic, and edentulous patients.

Attitude and Patient Relations

The attitude of the dental auxiliary will affect patient relations. Attitude can be defined as "a position of the body, or manner of carrying oneself, indicative of a mood." The attitude of all dental auxiliaries must be professional and should include such attributes as courtesy, patience, and honesty. The dental auxiliary must be courteous and polite toward all patients at all times. Patience, which includes both tolerance and understanding, is important, especially when dealing with an uncooperative or difficult patient. Honesty is also a vital part of a professional attitude. Some procedures are uncomfortable in dental imaging, and the dental auxiliary must be honest and inform the patient of the potential discomfort.

HELPFUL HINT

Attitude

- Professional
- Courteous
- Patient
- Honest

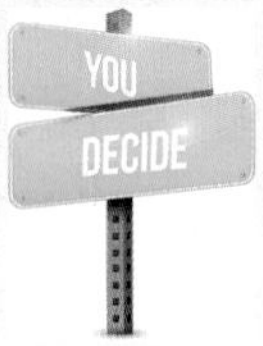

© shutterstock/alexmillos

SUMMARY

- Communication is an important interpersonal skill and the basis for developing a successful radiographer-patient relationship.
- Verbal communication involves the use of language. The dental radiographer's choice of words is very important; words that detract from the professional image of dentistry and words associated with negative images must be avoided.
- Nonverbal communication involves the use of body language and includes messages conveyed by posture, body movement, eye contact, and facial expression. A patient will respond positively to the dental professional whose nonverbal cues signal interest and warmth; a patient is less likely to respond to a dental professional whose nonverbal cues signal indifference and coldness.
- Communication also involves listening skills. The dental radiographer with good listening skills understands what the patient has said and is able to communicate that understanding to the patient. The good listener communicates both attention and interest.
- Facilitation skills make communication easier and develop a trusting relationship between the patient and the dental professional. Facilitation skills include encouraging patient questions, answering patient questions, responding to patient requests, and communicating with warmth.
- *Patient relations* refer to the relationship between the patient and the dental professional. The dental auxiliary must develop a relaxing and confident chairside manner that makes the patient feel comfortable.

BIBLIOGRAPHY

Boswell S: How to succeed in turning off patients without even trying: 8 taboo phrases to avoid!, Dent Pract Rep, 2004.

Frommer HH, Stabulas-Savage JJ: Patient management and special problems. In Radiology for the dental professional, ed 9, St Louis, 2011, Mosby.

Johnson ON: Patient relations and education. In Essentials of dental radiography for dental assistants and hygienists, ed 9, Upper Saddle River, NJ, 2011, Prentice Hall.

Levin R: Interpersonal communication, JADA 137:239, 2006.

Levin R: The interpersonal factor, JADA 139:986, 2008.

Levin R: Who has time for effective communication? JADA 139:195, 2008.

QUIZ QUESTIONS

True or False

____ 1. Skills that promote a good relationship between individuals are termed *facilitation skills*.

____ 2. Technical skills alone are sufficient for providing optimal patient care.

____ 3. The excessive use of technical words may confuse the patient and result in miscommunication.

____ 4. The delivery of speech is important in verbal communication; the dental radiographer should speak in a pleasant, relaxed manner.

____ 5. Nonverbal behavior cannot be used to enhance communication.

____ 6. If verbal messages are consistent with nonverbal messages, the patient is likely to respond with apprehension and mistrust.

____ 7. Patients are more likely to understand a dental professional whose nonverbal cues signal indifference.

____ 8. Eye contact plays a powerful role in the development of interpersonal relationships.

____ 9. Listening involves only hearing.

____ 10. When listening to a patient, the dental radiographer can use facial expressions to convey appropriate emotional responses.

____ 11. Interpersonal skills are skills that are used to make communication easier and develop a trusting relationship between the patient and the dental professional.

____ 12. When a patient trusts the dental professional, the patient is more likely to comply with the prescribed treatment and return for further treatment.

____ 13. The appearance of the dental auxiliary is important.

____ 14. In many offices, the dental auxiliary is the first person to meet and greet the patient.

____ 15. A patient should always be greeted by his or her first name.

____ 16. It is appropriate for the dental auxiliary to chew gum while working with patients.

____ 17. The dental auxiliary must develop a fast-paced, confident chairside manner.

____ 18. In most dental offices, the dental auxiliary is responsible for performing radiographic procedures.

____ 19. The attitude of the dental radiographer affects patient relations.

____ 20. The dental radiographer does not need to be courteous if a patient is uncooperative or difficult.

Role Playing

21. In the classroom or laboratory setting, ask students to work in pairs and to take turns role playing as a dental radiographer and a nervous patient.

14

Patient Education and the Dental Radiographer

LEARNING OBJECTIVES

After completion of this chapter, the student will be able to do the following:

1. Define the key terms associated with patient education.
2. Summarize the importance of educating patients about dental images.
3. List the three methods that can be used by the dental radiographer to educate patients about dental images.
4. Answer common patient questions about the need for dental images, x-ray exposure, the safety of dental x-rays, digital imaging, and other miscellaneous concerns.

The dental radiographer must be able to educate patients about the importance of dental images and also be prepared to answer common questions about the need for dental images, x-ray exposure, the safety of dental x-rays, and miscellaneous concerns. The purpose of this chapter is to discuss the importance of patient education, to describe different methods of patient education, and to review common patient questions and answers about dental imaging.

IMPORTANCE OF PATIENT EDUCATION

Educating dental patients about the importance of dental images is critical, yet patient education is often overlooked by dental professionals. Many patients do not understand the value of dental images. Often, the patient is simply told that "dental x-rays are needed by the dentist," and little additional information is provided. Some patients fear the use of x-radiation, while others believe that dental images are a way for the dentist to charge additional fees. To address such fears and misconceptions, the dental radiographer must be prepared to educate the patient about the value of dental images.

Many patients have heard or read about the damaging effects of x-radiation. Newspapers, magazines, and television shows often highlight the damaging effects of radiation and cast doubt on the necessity and benefit of dental imaging examinations. Such reports are often misleading and are not well researched. As a result, these reports cause patients to fear the use of x-radiation and to avoid all radiation exposure.

Because of such misinformation, the dental radiographer must take the time to educate the patient. In some instances, the patient may have to be completely re-educated. The dental radiographer must be prepared to explain exactly why dental images are important, how dental images are used, and how such images benefit the patient. In addition, the dental professional must be able to discuss common conditions and lesions that can be detected only through the use of dental images (see Chapter 12).

Comprehensive dental health education is one of the greatest services that a dental professional can provide to the patient. Education enhances understanding. A patient who is knowledgeable about the importance of dental images is more likely to realize the benefit of such images, accept the prescribed treatment, and follow prevention plans. Patient education is also likely to decrease fears of x-ray exposure, increase cooperation, and increase motivation for regular dental visits.

HELPFUL HINT

Importance of Patient Education

- Patient education concerning dental imaging is likely to result in decreased fears of x-ray exposure.
- A knowledgeable patient is more likely to accept prescribed treatment.

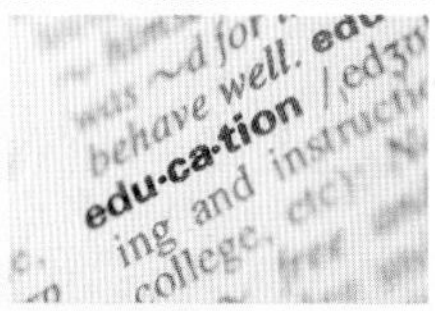

METHODS OF PATIENT EDUCATION

Patients can be educated about dental images in a number of ways. The dental radiographer can use an oral presentation, a video, printed literature, or a combination of these methods to educate the dental patient.

An oral presentation, in conjunction with sample dental images, can be used to communicate the importance of dental images. For example, the dental radiographer can show the patient a prepared series of images illustrating typical normal and abnormal conditions. This includes a visual component in the educational process; visual aids enhance patient comprehension. A prepared oral presentation with visual aids allows the patient to develop greater confidence in the expertise of the dental radiographer. A prepared presentation also communicates to the patient that the dental radiographer is organized and competent.

The use of digital imaging may further aid in patient education. This helps patients view their own periapical, bite-wing, or extraoral images on a computer monitor or television screen instead of looking at detailed information on mounted radiographs. The use of digital imaging helps explain concepts such as caries, periodontal changes, or oral diseases (Figure 14-1).

Videos and printed information about dental images are useful to educate the dental patient as well. Video messages can be played in the patient reception area, and brochures can be either placed in the reception area or provided to patients before the imaging examination. Two brochures, *Dental X-Ray Exams* and *Digital X-Rays*, are available for purchase online from the American Dental Association (ADA) at http://ebusiness.ada.org/default.aspx. These brochures discuss the value of the dental image as a diagnostic tool and spotlight the benefits of digital imaging. Customized brochures can be created to these brochures discuss the value of the dental image as a diagnostic

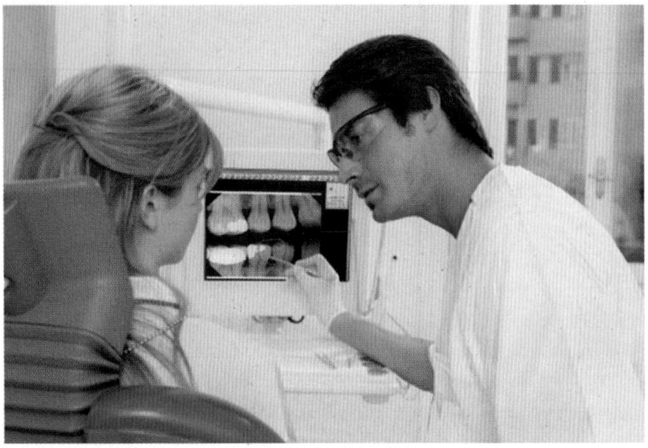

Fig 14-1 Dentist and patient reviewing digital images on a large computer monitor helps to facilitate patient education. (Courtesy Kavo Imaging, Brea, CA.)

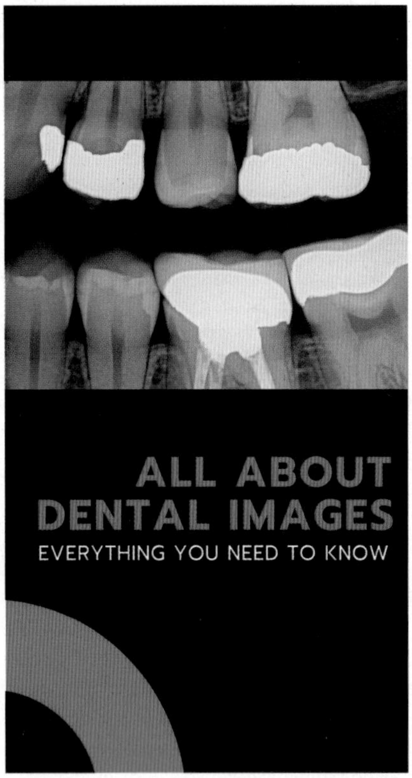

Fig 14-2 With a wide range of computer software platforms now available for designing visual content, customized patient education brochures can be created for use in dental practice settings.

tool and spotlight the benefits of digital imaging (Figure 14-2). Printed literature about dental images can also be custom designed by the dental professional and then printed for use in the dental office.

A combination of an oral presentation and printed literature is probably the most effective method of educating the dental patient about dental images. The use of both approaches can stimulate a question-and-answer type of discussion about dental images.

FREQUENTLY ASKED QUESTIONS

The dental radiographer must be prepared to answer frequently asked questions about the need for dental images, x-ray exposure, the safety of dental x-rays, digital imaging, and other concerns (Figure 14-3). Many patients ask the dental auxiliary, rather than the dentist, questions about x-radiation. The dental radiographer can answer many of the patient's questions. However, some questions must be answered only by the dentist; this restriction must be established by the dentist and understood by all members of the dental team. For example, only the dentist may answer questions about any diagnosis related to a dental image.

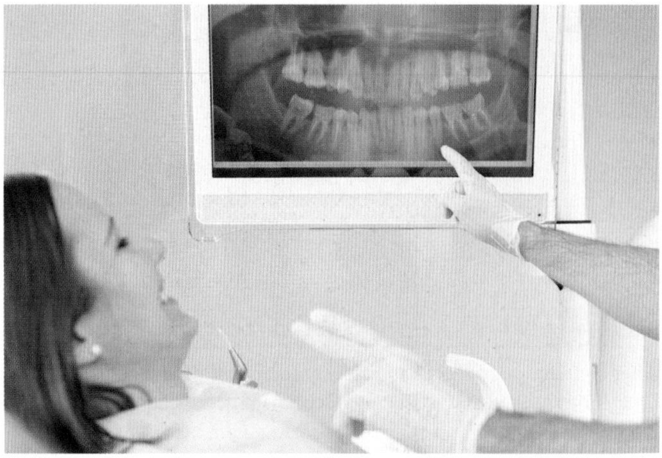

Fig 14-3 The dental radiographer must be familiar with frequently asked questions concerning dental imaging. (Copyright Microgen/iStock.com.)

Necessity Questions

Patients often ask questions about the need for dental x-ray images, the frequency of dental x-ray images for adults and children, the refusal of dental x-ray images, and the use of dental x-ray images from a previous dentist. Examples of questions and answers follow:

Question: **Are dental x-ray images really necessary?**

Answer: Yes. Many diseases and conditions such as tooth decay, gum disease, cysts, and tumors cannot be detected simply by looking into your mouth. Many diseases and conditions produce no signs or symptoms. Without dental x-ray images, these conditions may go unnoticed for a long time. As these conditions progress, extensive damage and pain may occur; these, in turn, may result in more extensive and costly treatment. Some oral diseases can even affect your general health or become life threatening.

Dental images are always prescribed to benefit the patient; the primary benefit is disease detection. Through the use of dental images, conditions and diseases that cannot be detected in any other way can be identified early. Early identification and treatment minimize and prevent problems, such as pain and the need for surgical procedures.

The treatment plan outlined by the dentist will be primarily based on the information we retrieve from your dental images. Dental images allow us to determine which teeth, if any, need restorative care. Therefore the images are necessary to correctly plan your treatment.

Question: **How often do I need dental x-ray images?**

Answer: The first step to limiting the amount of radiation that you receive is the proper prescribing, or ordering, of dental images. Decisions about the number, type, and frequency of dental x-ray images are determined by the dentist based on individual needs (Figure 14-4). Guidelines published by the American Dental Association are used by the dentist to aid in prescribing the number, type, and frequency of dental images for each patient.

Because every patient's dental condition is different, the frequency of dental imaging examinations is also different. The frequency of a dental imaging examination is based on the patient's individual needs. No set interval exists between x-ray examinations. For example, a patient with tooth decay or gum disease most likely will need more frequent dental imaging than a patient without such diseases.

Question: **How often do children need dental x-ray images?**

Answer: The interval between dental imaging examinations should be based on the individual needs of the child. Because every child's dental condition is different, the frequency of imaging examinations is different as well. There is no set interval between x-ray examinations. For example, a child with tooth decay most likely needs frequent dental imaging compared with a child without tooth decay. Guidelines published by the American Dental Association are used by the dentist to aid in prescribing the number, type, and frequency of dental images for your child.

Question: **Can I refuse x-ray images and be treated without them?**

Answer: No. When you refuse the prescribed dental x-ray images, the dentist cannot treat you. The standard of care requires that the dentist decline to treat a patient who refuses necessary x-ray images. Treatment without necessary images is considered negligent. No document can be signed to release the dentist from liability. For example, if you were to sign a paper stating refusal of dental x-ray images but releasing the dentist from any and all liability, you would be consenting to negligent care. Legally, patients cannot consent to negligent care.

Question: **Instead of exposing additional images, can you use the dental images from my previous dentist?**

Answer: Yes. Previous dental images can be used, provided the images are recent and of acceptable diagnostic quality. Additional dental images may be necessary, however, based on individual patient needs. If previous dental images, even if recent, are not of diagnostic quality, additional images will need to be exposed.

Exposure Questions

Patients often ask questions about how x-ray exposure is limited, the use of the lead apron during exposure, dental x-radiation during pregnancy, and the reason for the dental radiographer leaving the room during exposure. Examples of questions and answers follow:

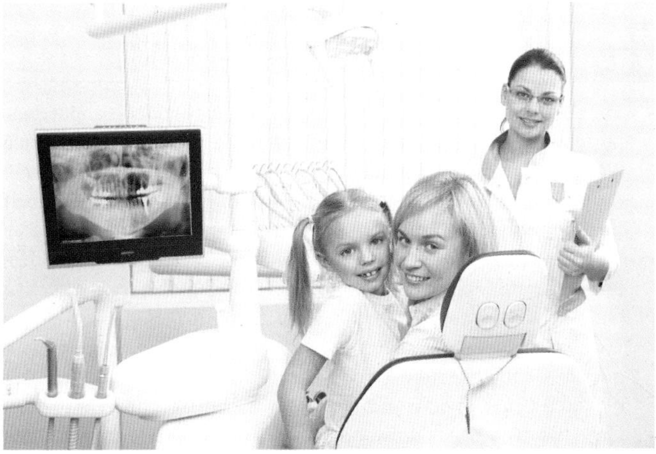

Fig 14-4 Dental images are ordered by the dentist based on the individual needs of the patient. (Copyright Deklofenak/iStock.com.)

Question: **How is patient exposure to x-rays limited?**

Answer: Because no amount of radiation is considered safe, strict guidelines are followed to limit the amount of x-radiation. For example, the dentist custom-orders patient x-ray images on the basis of individual needs. During exposure, a thyroid collar and lead apron, fast film or a digital sensor, and a beam alignment device will be used to protect the patient from excess radiation. Good exposure technique is also used to limit exposure to x-radiation.

The actual amount of x-radiation received will vary depending on the receptor used, the technique used, and exposure factors. Radiation exposure can be reduced by using digital sensors. The use of sensors instead of film can reduce the exposure time 50% to 90% compared with film-based imaging. When using film, radiation exposure can be limited by using F-speed, the fastest film currently available.

Question: **Why use a lead apron?**

Answer: A lead apron and a thyroid collar are used to protect reproductive, blood-forming, and thyroid tissues from scatter radiation. Lighter, lead-free aprons made of alloy sheeting are also an option (Figure 14-5). The use of an apron acts as a shield, prevents radiation from reaching radiosensitive organs, and protects from unnecessary radiation exposure.

Question: **Should dental x-ray exposure be avoided during pregnancy?**

Answer: When a lead apron is used during dental imaging procedures, the amount of radiation received in the gonadal region is nearly zero. No detectable exposure to the embryo or fetus occurs with the use of the lead apron. The American Dental Association, together with the Food and Drug Administration, has stated in the most recent Guidelines for Prescribing Dental Radiographs that the recommended guidelines "do not need to be altered because of pregnancy." Although scientific evidence indicates that dental x-ray procedures can be performed during pregnancy, some dentists elect to postpone such x-ray procedures because of patient concerns.

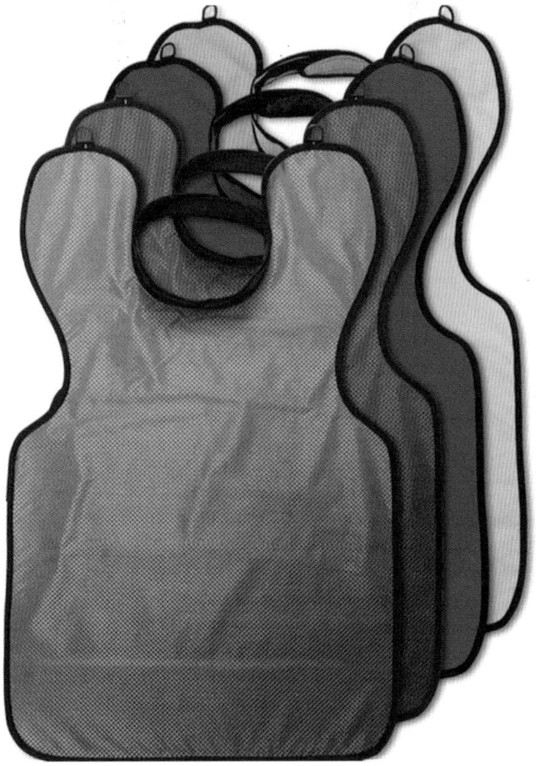

Fig 14-5 Lead-free x-ray aprons with thyroid collars provide protection for patients during x-ray exposure without the weight of lead. (Courtesy DUX Dental, Oxnard, CA.)

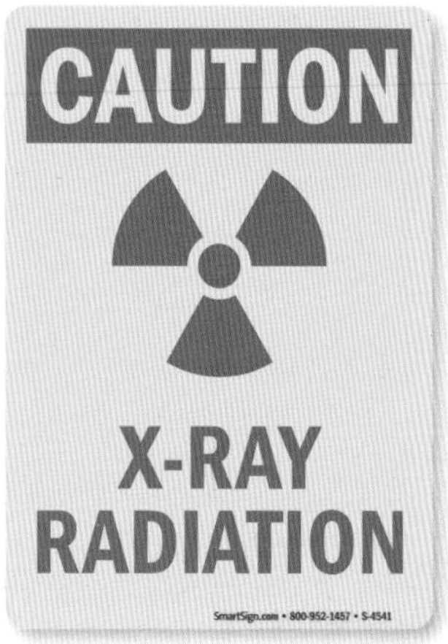

Fig 14-6 All radiation is harmful to living tissue. (Courtesy MySafetySign.com, Brooklyn, NY.)

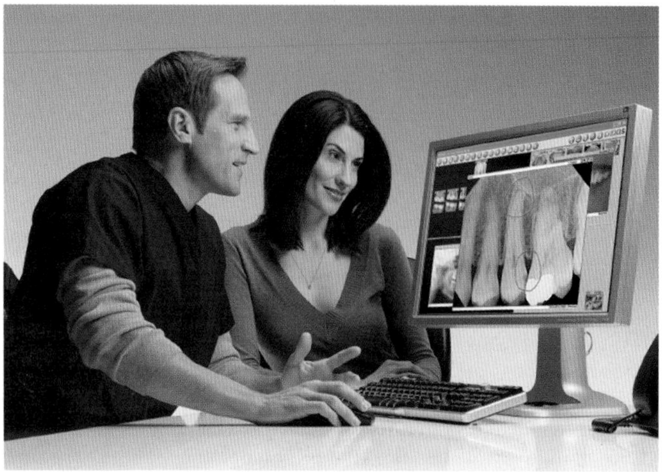

Fig 14-7 Digital images can be manipulated electronically. (Courtesy Kavo Imaging, Brea, CA.)

Question: **Why does the radiographer leave the room when x-rays are produced?**

Answer: When patients are exposed to x-rays, they receive the diagnostic benefit of the dental images; the radiographer does not receive any benefit. An individual should be exposed to x-radiation only when the benefit of disease detection outweighs the risk of exposure. Because the radiographer does not benefit from patient x-ray exposure, the radiographer must use proper protection measures. One of the most effective ways to limit x-ray exposure is to maintain adequate distance and shielding, which is why the radiographer steps out of the operatory during x-ray exposure.

Safety Questions

Patients often ask questions about the safety of dental x-rays and wonder whether dental x-rays cause cancer. Examples of questions and answers follow:

Question: **Are dental x-rays safe?**

Answer: All x-rays are harmful to living tissue (Figure 14-6). The term *safe* is defined as "no harm done." X-rays cannot be harmful and safe at the same time. The amount of x-radiation used in dental imaging is small, but biologic damage does occur. No amount of radiation is considered safe. As a result, dental x-rays must be prescribed only when the benefit of disease detection outweighs this risk of harm.

Question: **Will dental x-rays cause cancer?**

Answer: Not a single recorded case of a patient developing cancer from diagnostic dental x-ray exposure exists. The radiation exposure that occurs during a dental x-ray examination is very small, and the chance that it will contribute to or cause cancer is exceedingly small. For example, the potential risk of dental imaging inducing a fatal cancer has been estimated to be 3 in 1 million. The risk of a person developing cancer spontaneously is much higher, or 3300 in 1 million. When these two numbers are compared, it is evident that when cancer occurs, it is over 1000 times more likely to be unrelated to radiation exposure.

Digital Imaging Questions

Question: **What are the advantages of digital imaging?**

Answer: Digital imaging requires less exposure to radiation, which benefits the patient. Digital information can be stored, transmitted, and manipulated electronically (Figure 14-7). Digital imaging also allows for instant images that are environmentally friendly, as no film or processing chemicals are used.

Question: **Are there any risks associated with digital imaging?**

Answer: Because radiation is involved, a certain amount of risk does exist. With digital imaging, patient exposure is less than with film-based imaging. Radiation exposure time may be reduced by 50% to 90%.

Miscellaneous Questions

Question: **Can a panoramic image be exposed instead of a complete intraoral series?**

Answer: No. A panoramic image cannot be substituted for a complete series of dental images. A complete series of dental images is required when information about the details of the teeth and surrounding bone are needed. A panoramic image does not clearly reveal changes in teeth, as in tooth decay, or the details of the supporting bone. The panoramic image is useful for showing the general condition of a patient's teeth and bone.

Question: **Who owns a patient's dental images?**

Answer: All dental records, including the dental images, are the property of the dentist. However, patients have the privilege of reasonable access to their dental records. For example, patients can request a copy of their dental images or request that a copy is sent to a dentist of their choice. Digital images may also be electronically sent to a referring doctor. The dentist retains the original dental images as part of the patient record.

SUMMARY

- The dental radiographer must be able to educate patients about dental images. A patient who is knowledgeable about the importance of dental images is more likely to have reduced fears about x-ray exposure, realize the benefits of dental images, accept prescribed treatment, and follow prevention plans.
- The dental radiographer can use an oral presentation, a video, printed literature, or a combination (probably the most effective method) to educate the dental patient about images.
- The dental radiographer must be prepared to answer frequently asked questions about the need for dental images, x-ray exposure, the safety of dental x-rays, digital imaging, and miscellaneous concerns.
- Only the dentist may answer some patient questions, such as those about image-related diagnosis. These questions must be identified by the dentist and clearly communicated to all members of the dental team.

BIBLIOGRAPHY

Frommer HH, Stabulas-Savage JJ: Operator protection. In Radiology for the dental professional, ed 9, St. Louis, 2011, Mosby.

Frommer HH, Stabulas-Savage JJ: Patient protection. In Radiology for the dental professional, ed 9, St. Louis, 2011, Mosby.

Haring JI, Lind LJ: The importance of dental radiographs and interpretation. In Radiographic interpretation for the dental hygienist, Philadelphia, 1993, Saunders.

Johnson ON: Patient relations and education. In Essentials of dental radiography for dental assistants and hygienists, ed 9, Upper Saddle River, NJ, 2011, Prentice Hall.

Thunthy KH: X-rays: Detailed answers to frequently asked questions, Compend Contin Educ Dentistry 14(3):394, 1993.

QUIZ QUESTIONS

Essay

1. Summarize the importance of educating dental patients about dental images.
2. List the methods the dental radiographer can use to educate patients about dental images.

Short Answer

3. Are dental x-ray images really necessary?

4. How often should adults have dental x-ray images exposed?

5. How often should children have dental x-ray images exposed?

6. Can a patient refuse dental x-ray images and still be treated?

7. Can images from a previous dentist be used instead of exposing additional images?

8. How is x-ray exposure limited?

9. Why is a lead apron used during x-ray exposure?

10. Should x-ray exposure be avoided during pregnancy?

11. Why does the dental radiographer leave the room during x-ray exposure of the patient?

12. Are dental x-rays safe?

13. Do dental x-rays cause cancer?

14. Can a panoramic image be substituted for a complete intraoral series?

15. Who owns the dental images—the dentist or the patient?

15

Legal Issues and the Dental Radiographer

LEARNING OBJECTIVES

After completion of this chapter, the student will be able to do the following:

1. Define key terms associated with legal issues.
2. List federal and state regulations affecting the use of dental x-ray equipment and describe the general application of federal and state regulations relating to the dental auxiliary.
3. Describe licensure requirements for exposing dental images.
4. Discuss risk management and define the legal concept of informed consent.
5. Describe ways to obtain informed consent from a patient.
6. Discuss dental malpractice issues, including negligence and standard of care.
7. Discuss the concept of statute of limitations and the legal significance of the dental record.
8. Discuss how confidentiality laws affect the information in the dental record.
9. Describe the patient's rights with regard to the dental record.
10. Describe the legal implications of patient refusal to have dental x-ray images exposed.

The dental auxiliary must be aware of the legal implications of dental imaging. The dental auxiliary must be knowledgeable about, and comply with, laws that govern the use of ionizing radiation in dentistry. Furthermore, because dental imaging has implications for patient care, including the diagnosis of dental disease and treatment planning, the possibility of negligent care exists when dental images are not properly exposed or used.

The purpose of this chapter is to discuss general legal concepts, including various regulations as they apply to the dental radiographer who performs dental imaging procedures for patient care, as well as confidentiality and documentation.

HELPFUL HINT

Licensure Requirements

These may include:

- Obtaining additional certification or continuing education hours
- Exposing dental images only under direct supervision of a dentist
- Following restrictions concerning the types of dental images that may be legally exposed

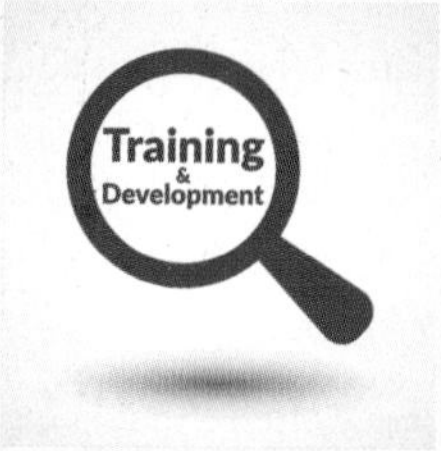

Copyright Nobelus/Shutterstock.com

LEGAL ISSUES AND DENTAL IMAGING

Federal and State Regulations

Both federal and state regulations control the use of dental x-ray equipment. The federal government has established requirements, including safety precautions, for the use of dental x-ray machines made and sold in the United States. For example, the Consumer-Patient Radiation Health and Safety Act outlines requirements for the safe use of dental x-ray equipment. This federal law also establishes guidelines for the proper maintenance of x-ray equipment and requires persons who perform dental imaging procedures to be properly trained and certified.

In addition to federal laws, state, county, and city laws may affect the use of dental x-ray equipment. Most states have laws that require regular inspection of dental x-ray equipment, for example, every 5 years. Some state laws also require that the dental radiographer be trained and certified or licensed to expose dental images.

Licensure Requirements

State laws regulate who is qualified to expose dental images. In most cases, the licensed dentist and the dental hygienist are not legally required to obtain additional certification to perform dental imaging procedures. The certification required for dental assistants to perform dental imaging varies from state to state. Consequently, it is the responsibility of the dental auxiliary to become informed about the specific requirements relating to dental imaging in his or her particular state. These requirements may include the following:

1. Obtaining additional certification in dental imaging
2. Performing dental imaging procedures only under the direct supervision of the dentist
3. Following restrictions concerning the types of dental images that may be legally used

LEGAL ISSUES AND THE DENTAL PATIENT

Risk Management

Risk management is extremely important in dental imaging. *Risk management* refers to the policies and procedures that should be followed by the dental radiographer to reduce the chances of a patient taking legal action against the dental radiographer or the supervising dentist.

HELPFUL HINT

Self-determination

Persons seeking dental care have the legal right to make choices about the care they receive, including the opportunity to consent to, or refuse, treatment.

Informed Consent. Persons seeking health care services, including dental care, have the right to self-determination; persons have the legal right to make choices about the care received, including the opportunity to consent to or to refuse treatment. Therefore before receiving treatment, the dental patient should be informed of the various aspects of the proposed treatment, including diagnostic procedures such as dental imaging.

It is the responsibility of the dentist to discuss both diagnostic and treatment procedures with the patient. All patients must be informed of the need for dental images. Information provided to the patient should include the following:

1. Purpose and potential benefits of the images
2. Person responsible for performing the imaging procedure
3. Number and type of images used
4. Possible harm that may result if dental images are not exposed
5. Risks associated with x-ray exposure
6. Alternative diagnostic aids that may serve the same purpose as dental images

HELPFUL HINT

Risk Management

Disclosure

The process of informing the patient about the particulars of exposing dental images

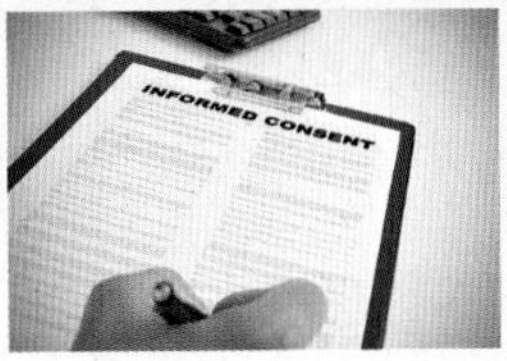

Informed Consent

Consent given by the patient following complete disclosure

Liability

Dentists are legally accountable or **liable to supervise** the performance of dental auxiliaries

This process of informing the patient about the particulars of dental imaging is termed disclosure. A competent dental professional must conduct the disclosure process. In many states, the prescription of dental images is the responsibility of the dentist, and the auxiliary is the person who performs the imaging procedures under the dentist's supervision. In such cases, the dentist should be involved in the disclosure process and should be available to answer any patient questions.

It is important to standardize the disclosure process so that patients receive enough information to make informed choices. Patients must also be given the opportunity to ask questions and have their questions answered before the procedure. Informed consent must be obtained from all patients. In the case of a patient who is a minor (generally, those under 18 years of age) or declared to be "legally incompetent," informed consent must be obtained from a legal guardian. It is important that the person who provides the disclosure not misrepresent any of the information disclosed or threaten the patient into giving consent. The person disclosing information should use language that the patient can understand easily.

After the disclosure process has been completed, the patient may give or withhold consent for the dental imaging procedure. Informed consent is defined as consent given by a patient after complete disclosure. Although the governing standards for informed consent may vary from state to state, certain recognized elements of informed consent can be summarized as follows:

1. Purpose of the procedure and who will perform it
2. Potential benefits of receiving the procedure
3. Possible risks involved in having the procedure performed, as well as the possible risks of not having it performed
4. Opportunity for the patient to ask questions and obtain complete information

A written consent form including these four elements may be used in obtaining informed consent.

If informed consent is not obtained from a patient before the dental imaging procedure, a patient may legally claim malpractice or negligence. A patient's consent to dental procedures is generally presumed valid if it is obtained in a manner consistent with state laws, if it follows disclosure rules, and if it is obtained freely from the appropriate individual. The following may show a lack of informed consent:

- Complete lack of consent from the patient
- Consent obtained from an individual who has no legal right to give it (e.g., minor, incompetent adult)
- Consent obtained from an individual who is under the influence of drugs or alcohol
- Consent obtained by misrepresentation or fraudulent means
- Consent given by an individual under duress
- Consent obtained after incomplete disclosure

Liability. When a dental auxiliary performs procedures, legal accountability (liability) is presumed to lie with both the supervising dentist and the dental auxiliary. According to state laws, dentists are legally accountable (liable) to supervise the performance of dental auxiliaries. Even though dental auxiliaries work under the supervision of a licensed dentist, auxiliaries are also legally liable for their own actions. The trend in dental negligence or malpractice actions has historically been to sue the supervising dentist alone; however, the dentist and the dental auxiliary may both be sued for the actions of the dental auxiliary.

Malpractice Issues

Dental malpractice results when the dental practitioner is negligent in the delivery of dental care. Negligence in dental treatment occurs when the diagnosis made or the dental treatment delivered falls below the standard of care. The standard of care can be defined as the quality of care that is provided by dental practitioners in a similar locality under the same or similar conditions.

Negligent care may result from the action or lack of action of either the dentist or the dental auxiliary. Because dental images are an essential part of diagnosis and treatment planning, negligence may result from the action or inaction of the dental radiographer. For example, if informed consent is not obtained from the patient before a dental imaging procedure begins, negligence may be claimed, except in the case of implied consent. Negligence may also be claimed if dental images are exposed improperly and the patient is injured in some way as a direct result. Examples of such negligence include the exposing of an incorrect number of images, lost or misplaced images, or nondiagnostic images requiring retakes.

HELPFUL HINT

Malpractice Issues

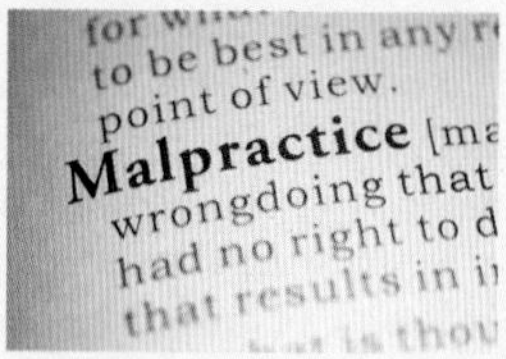

Malpractice

Results when the dental practitioner is negligent in the delivery of dental care

Negligence

When the diagnosis made or the dental treatment delivered falls below the standard of care

Standard of Care

Quality of care provided by dental practitioners in a *similar* locality under *similar* conditions

Statute of Limitations

Time period during which a patient may bring a malpractice action against the dentist or auxiliary

Copyright Feng Yu/Shutterstock.com

State laws govern the duration of time within which a patient may bring a malpractice action against the dentist or the auxiliary. This time period is known as the statute of limitations. In many states, this time period begins when the patient discovers (or should have discovered) that an injury has occurred as a result of dental negligence. In such cases, the statute of limitations may not begin until years after the dental negligence occurred. Frequently, it is not until a patient seeks care from another dental professional that he or she becomes aware that previous dental treatment may have been negligent. For example, if dental images are not exposed properly, or if all of the information presented on the images is not interpreted or recorded accurately, dental disease may go undiagnosed and untreated. Years later, the patient may be informed that he or she has an irreversible condition (e.g., advanced periodontal disease, root fracture, change in size of a tumor or other growth), which might have been prevented or more successfully treated with early detection. Even though such a dental disease is not life threatening, the lack of diagnosis and treatment may result in significant harm to the patient. Examples of harm may include loss of self-esteem, emotional distress, loss of income, and expenses incurred in seeking additional dental treatment.

It is the responsibility of the dentist to review and report *all* information presented on dental images and acquired data sets. For example, a bite-wing image demonstrating interproximal caries associated with tooth #4 must be reported even though the patient's symptoms were related to tooth #30. The same is true for extraoral images and data generated with cone-beam computer tomography (CBCT). If the dentist is uncertain or uncomfortable interpreting data within the field of view, a board-certified oral and maxillofacial radiologist should review and interpret the images.

Patient Records

A dental record must be established for every patient, and dental images are an integral part of such a record. The dental record must accurately reflect all aspects of patient care. Complete dental records are important to ensure continuity of patient care and to provide legal documentation of a patient's condition.

Documentation

It is essential that the dental record include the following:

1. Informed consent
2. Number and type of dental images exposed (including retakes)
3. Rationale for these dental images
4. An imaging report including diagnostic information obtained from the interpretation of the images

The prescription and the evaluation of images are typically the responsibility of the dentist; therefore entries in the dental record should be made by the dentist or under the dentist's supervision. Entries made in the dental record should never be erased or blacked out. If an error is made, a clean line should be drawn through the error and initialed by the radiographer, and the correct entry should be added to the record.

HELPFUL HINT

Patient Records

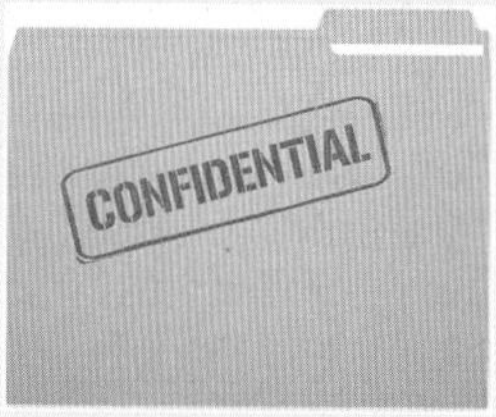

Documentation

- Informed consent
- Number and type of images exposed
- Rationale for exposing images
- Diagnostic information obtained from the interpretation of images

Confidentiality

- All the information in the patient record is confidential/private
- This includes dental images

Copyright Axstokes/Shutterstock.com

Confidentiality. All the information contained in the dental record, including information found on dental images, is *confidential*, or private, to the extent that state laws do not otherwise require disclosure. State confidentiality laws protect this information and generally prohibit the transfer of this information to nonprivileged persons. A *nonprivileged person* is an individual who is not directly involved in the treatment of the patient. It is not appropriate for any dental professional to discuss a patient's care with another patient or with office staff members who are not involved in the treatment of the patient. Likewise, sharing dental images with others not involved in the patient's care is considered a violation or breach of confidentiality laws.

Ownership and Retention of Dental Images. Legally, dental images are the property of the dentist, even though the patient or an insurance company may have paid for them. The basis for this ownership of dental images is that images are indispensable to the dentist as part of the patient's record.

HELPFUL HINT

Patient Records

Ownership and Retention

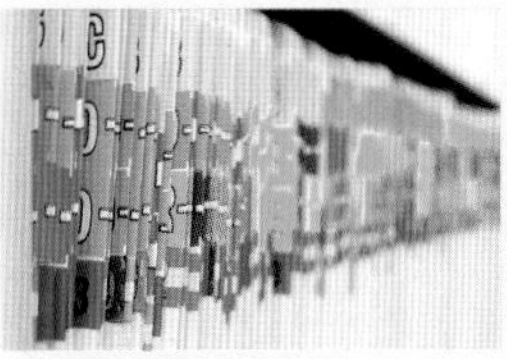

- The dental record is a **legal document**.
- Dental images are the **property of the dentist**.
- Patients do have the **right of reasonable access** to their records.
- Patients must request **in writing** to have copies of the record forwarded.
- Dental records and dental images should be **retained indefinitely**.

Patients do have a right to reasonable access to their records. This includes the right to have their complete dental records, including copies of the images, forwarded to another dentist. When transferring to another dentist, a patient can request in writing that his or her dental records be forwarded to that dentist. Duplicates of the images should be created and forwarded and the original dental images retained. Digital images may be copied and sent electronically, and the patient's written request should be placed in the dental record as evidence of the patient's directive. It is generally not advisable to release a copy of the dental record, including dental images, directly to the patient. Instead, this information should be forwarded directly to the dentist or specialist who is assuming responsibility for the patient's care.

Dental records and dental images should be retained indefinitely. Because of varying state laws on the statute of limitations, it is not often possible to know when to destroy or discard a patient record. Therefore patient records should be stored carefully to maintain the integrity of these materials. All dental professionals must be aware of the importance and significance of maintaining patient records in good condition.

Patients Who Refuse Exposure of Dental Images

Some patients may refuse dental imaging procedures. When this occurs, the dentist must carefully consider the situation. The dentist must then decide whether an accurate diagnosis can be made and treatment provided without a dental image. In most cases, patient refusal of dental images compromises the patient's diagnosis and treatment, and the dentist may not be able to provide treatment for the patient.

As discussed in Chapter 14, every effort should be made to educate the patient about the importance and usefulness of dental images. No document can be signed to release the dentist from liability. For example, if the patient signs a release or waiver that states that he or she is taking responsibility for any injury that may result, and then an injury does result from negligence (e.g., failure to expose dental images), the patient's consent may be invalidated. Legally, the patient cannot consent to negligent care; such consent is invalid.

Table 15-1 lists several websites that provide specific information on topics presented in this chapter.

HELPFUL HINT

If a Patient Refuses Dental Images...

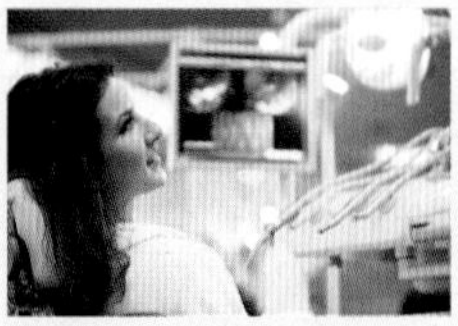

- The situation must be carefully considered by the dentist.
- The dentist must decide whether an accurate diagnosis can be made and whether treatment can be provided.

TABLE 15-1 Internet Resources

Organization	Website
American Academy of Oral and Maxillofacial Radiology	www.aaomr.org
American Dental Assistants Association	www.dentalassistant.org
American Dental Association	www.ada.org
American Dental Hygiene Association	www.adha.org
Dental Assisting National Board	www.danb.org
U.S. Department of Labor, Occupational Safety and Health Administration	www.osha.gov
U.S. Food and Drug Administration	www.fda.gov

SUMMARY

- Dental auxiliaries must understand their legal obligations with regard to dental imaging.
- The dentist is responsible for prescribing and interpreting dental images, whereas the dental auxiliary is most often responsible for the exposure and processing or retrieval of such images.
- The dental auxiliary may also be responsible for disclosing the requisite information and obtaining informed consent from the patient before performing the imaging procedure.
- In many states, dental auxiliaries are employees who work under the supervision of a licensed dentist, who is liable for the actions of these dental personnel. Dental auxiliaries are responsible for their own actions in providing patient care.
- The dental record must include documentation of informed consent and the imaging procedure (e.g., number and type of images exposed, rationale for exposure, interpretation report).
- Legally, dental images are the property of the dentist. The patient does have reasonable access to his or her dental images.
- In most cases, the dentist cannot treat a patient who refuses dental imaging; refusal compromises diagnosis and treatment. No document can be signed that releases the dentist from liability.

BIBLIOGRAPHY

American Dental Association: Survey of legal provisions for delegating expanded functions to dental assistants and dental hygienists, Chicago, 1995, American Dental Association.

Bundy AL: Radiology and the law, Rockville, MD, 1988, Aspen.

Frommer HH, Stabulas-Savage JJ: Legal considerations. In Radiology for the dental professional, ed 9, St. Louis, 2011, Mosby.

Miles DA, Van Dis ML, Jensen CW, et al: Radiation biology and protection. In Radiographic imaging for the dental team, ed 4, St. Louis, 2009, Saunders.

QUIZ QUESTIONS

Multiple Choice

_____ 1. Informed consent is based on the concept that a patient receives:
   a. some disclosure
   b. no disclosure
   c. complete disclosure
   d. enough disclosure

_____ 2. The process of informing the patient about the particulars of exposing dental images is termed:
   a. consent
   b. liability
   c. disclosure
   d. discussion

_____ 3. A dental assistant may have to take an additional certification or licensure examination to expose dental images.
   a. true
   b. false

_____ 4. The right to self-determination means that the patient has the right to consent to or refuse treatment.
   a. true
   b. false

_____ 5. Which person(s) may be liable for the actions of a dental auxiliary?
   a. dentist
   b. dental auxiliary
   c. both a and b
   d. neither a nor b

_____ 6. The improper exposure of dental images may result in:
   a. phobia
   b. malpractice
   c. standard of care
   d. malfeasance

_____ 7. It is best to retain dental records for 6 years.
   a. true
   b. false

_____ 8. The following must be disclosed to the patient before obtaining informed consent:
   a. the purpose of the procedure and who will perform it
   b. the potential benefits of receiving the procedure
   c. the possible risks in having the procedure performed, as well as the risk of not having the procedure performed
   d. all of the above

_____ 9. Incomplete disclosure to the patient before obtaining his or her informed consent may:
   a. validate the consent
   b. serve as partial consent
   c. invalidate the consent
   d. none of the above

_____ 10. The dental record is a legal document.
   a. true
   b. false

16

Infection Prevention and the Dental Radiographer

LEARNING OBJECTIVES

After completion of this chapter, the student will be able to do the following:

1. Define the key terms associated with infection prevention.
2. Describe the rationale for infection prevention.
3. Describe the three possible routes of disease transmission.
4. Describe the conditions that must be present for disease transmission to occur.
5. Discuss personal protective equipment (PPE), hand hygiene, sterilization and disinfection of instruments, and the cleaning and disinfection of the dental unit and environmental surfaces.
6. Describe the infection prevention procedures that are necessary before x-ray exposure.
7. Describe the infection prevention procedures that are necessary during x-ray exposure.
8. Describe the infection prevention procedures that are necessary after x-ray exposure.
9. Describe the infection prevention procedures that are necessary for digital imaging.
10. Describe the infection prevention procedures that are necessary for film processing.
11. Discuss film handling in the darkroom—with and without barrier envelopes.
12. Discuss film handling without barrier envelopes using the daylight loader of an automatic processor.

Infectious diseases present a significant hazard in the dental environment, and dental professionals are at an increased risk for acquiring such diseases. Therefore infection prevention is a major concern in dentistry. Infection prevention protocols are used in dentistry to minimize the potential for disease transmission. To protect themselves and their patients, dental professionals must understand and use infection prevention protocols.

The infection prevention practices used in dentistry apply to imaging procedures as well. The purpose of this chapter is to present the rationale for infection prevention and the associated terminology, to review the guidelines from the Centers for Disease Control and Prevention (CDC), and to describe in detail the step-by-step infection prevention procedures used in dental imaging.

INFECTION PREVENTION BASICS

To understand infection prevention practices, the dental professional must first understand the purpose of infection prevention and the terminology that is frequently used in infection prevention protocols.

Rationale for Infection Prevention

The primary purpose of infection prevention procedures is to prevent the transmission of infectious diseases. Infectious diseases may be transmitted from a patient to the dental professional, from the dental professional to a patient, and from one patient to another patient. The use of recommended infection prevention guidelines can greatly reduce the transmission of infectious diseases.

Before the dental professional can use infection prevention practices to prevent disease transmission, an understanding of how disease transmission occurs in the dental environment is necessary. Disease transmission involves pathogens; a **pathogen** is a microorganism capable of causing disease. Dental professionals and dental patients may be exposed to a variety of pathogens that are present in oral or respiratory secretions. These pathogens may include the following:

- Cold and flu viruses and bacteria
- Coronavirus (COVID-19)
- Cytomegalovirus (CMV)
- Hepatitis B virus (HBV)
- Hepatitis C virus (HCV)
- Herpes simplex virus (HSV-1, HSV-2)
- Human immunodeficiency virus (HIV)
- *Mycobacterium tuberculosis*

In the dental environment, the general routes of disease transmission can be described as follows:

- Direct contact with pathogens present in saliva, blood, respiratory secretions, or lesions
- Indirect contact with contaminated objects or instruments
- Direct contact with airborne contaminants present in spatter or aerosols of oral and respiratory fluids

For an infection to occur by one of these routes of transmission, the following three conditions must be present:

1. A susceptible host
2. A pathogen with sufficient infectivity and numbers to cause infection
3. A portal through which the pathogen may enter the host

Effective infection prevention practices are intended to alter one of these three conditions, thereby preventing disease transmission.

Infection Prevention Terminology

An understanding of the terminology related to infection prevention is important for the dental professional. The following terms are frequently used in discussions of infection prevention, in the infection prevention literature, and in infection prevention protocols:

Antiseptic: A substance that inhibits the growth of bacteria. This term is often used to describe handwashing or wound-cleansing procedures.

Asepsis: The absence of pathogens, or disease-causing microorganisms. This term is often used to describe procedures that prevent infection (e.g., aseptic technique).

Bloodborne pathogens: Pathogens present in blood that cause diseases in humans.

Disinfect: Use a chemical or physical procedure to inhibit or destroy pathogens. Highly resistant bacterial and mycotic (fungal) spores are not killed during disinfection procedures.
Disinfection: The act of disinfecting.
Exposure incident: A specific incident that involves contact with blood or other potentially infectious materials and that results from procedures performed by the dental professional.
Infectious waste: Waste that consists of blood, blood products, contaminated sharps, or other microbiologic products.
Occupational exposure: Contact with blood or other infectious materials that involves the skin, eye, or mucous membranes and that results from procedures performed by the dental professional.
Parenteral exposure: Exposure to blood or other infectious materials that results from piercing or puncturing the skin barrier (e.g., a needle-stick injury results in parenteral exposure).
Personal protective equipment (PPE): Includes protective attire, gloves, mask, and eyewear.
Sharps: Any objects that can penetrate the skin, including, but not limited to, needles and scalpels.
Standard precautions: Measures that include a standard of care designed to protect health care personnel and patients from pathogens that can be spread by blood or any other body fluid, excretion, or secretion.
Sterilize: The use of a physical or chemical procedure to destroy all pathogens, including highly resistant bacteria and mycotic spores.
Sterilization: The act of sterilizing.

GUIDELINES FOR INFECTION PREVENTION PRACTICES

The CDC released a publication entitled *Guidelines for Infection Control in Dental Health Care Settings* (2003), which provides infection prevention practices for dentistry. The CDC evidence-based recommendations are currently used to guide infection prevention practices in dental offices. In 2016 the CDC supplemented these guidelines with a *Summary of Infection Prevention Practices in Dental Practices – Basic Expectations for Safe Care*, and *Infection Prevention Checklist for Dental Settings*. For the most current CDC *Infection Prevention & Control in Dental Settings*, please visit the CDC website at https://www.cdc.gov/oralhealth/infectioncontrol/index.html

The recommended infection prevention practices are applicable to *all* settings in which dental treatment is provided (Box 16-1). These guidelines must be observed in conjunction with the practices and procedures for worker protection required by the Occupational Safety and Health Administration (OSHA) in its final rule on *Occupational Exposure to Bloodborne Pathogens*. The recommended infection prevention practices that directly relate to dental imaging procedures include the following:

- PPE
- Hand hygiene
- Respiratory hygiene / Cough etiquette
- Sterilization or disinfection of instruments
- Cleaning and disinfection of dental unit and environmental surfaces before and after the procedure

BOX 16-1 Infection Prevention Practices in Dental Health Care Settings

- Vaccination of dental professionals
- Use of protective attire and barrier techniques
- Hand hygiene
- Proper use and care of sharp instruments and needles
- Sterilization or disinfection of instruments
- Cleaning and disinfection of the dental unit and environmental surfaces
- Disinfection of the dental laboratory
- Use and care of handpieces, anti-retraction valves, and other intraoral dental devices attached to air and water lines of dental units
- Single use of disposable instruments
- Proper handling of biopsy specimens
- Proper use of extracted teeth in dental educational settings
- Proper disposal of waste materials
- Implementation of recommendations

Personal Protective Equipment

Protective Clothing. All dental professionals must wear protective clothing (e.g., reusable or disposable gown, laboratory coat, uniform) to prevent skin and mucous membrane exposure when contact with blood or other body fluids is anticipated. Protective clothing must be changed daily or changed more frequently if it is visibly soiled. Dental professionals must remove all protective garments before leaving the dental office, and the garments should be laundered according to the manufacturer's instructions.

Gloves. All dental professionals must wear medical gloves to prevent skin contact with blood, saliva, or mucous membranes. The dental professional must wear new gloves for each patient. Gloves must also be worn when touching contaminated items or surfaces. Nonsterile gloves are recommended for examinations and nonsurgical procedures; sterile gloves are recommended for all surgical procedures.

In preparation for treating each patient, hand hygiene must be completed before gloves are worn. After treating each patient or after exiting the patient treatment area, the dental professional must remove and discard the gloves and wash hands or use an antiseptic hand rub immediately. Hand hygiene must be completed, and new gloves must be used for each patient. During treatment, gloves must be removed and changed whenever tears, cuts, or punctures occur. Gloves should never be washed before use or disinfected for reuse. Washing or disinfection of gloves causes defects and diminishes the barrier protection provided by the gloves.

Masks and Protective Eyewear. Whenever spatter and aerosolized sprays of blood and saliva are likely, all dental professionals must use surgical masks and protective eyewear, or chin-length plastic face shields, to protect the eyes and face. The mask, when used, must be changed between patients or during treatment if it becomes wet or moist. After treatment, face shields and protective eyewear must be washed with appropriate cleaning agents. When visibly soiled, such equipment should be disinfected between patients.

The N95 filtering facepiece respirator (FFR) has become a popular choice for personal protective equipment since the onset of the COVID-19 pandemic. The number "95" indicates that this respirator filters at least 95% of airborne particles, including bacteria and viruses. This respirator (mask) may or may not include an exhalation valve. The N95 FFR protects against airborne particle transmission and liquids that could contaminate the face. At the time of publication, the Occupational Safety and Health Administration (OSHA) requires health care workers to use respiratory protection if treating patients with suspected or confirmed infection with COVID-19.

For the most current information on PPE in the dental setting, please visit the CDC at https://www.cdc.gov/oralhealth/infectioncontrol/faqs/personal-protective-equipment.html.

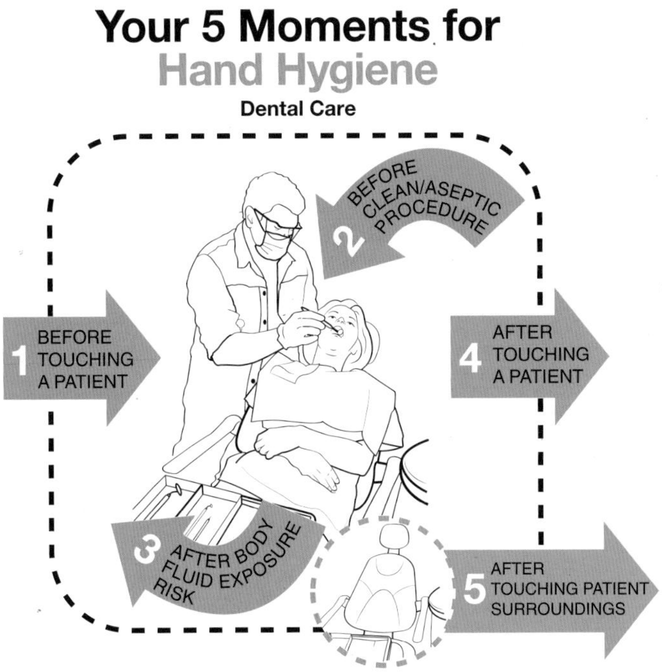

Fig 16-1 Based on "Your 5 Moments for Hand Hygiene," http://www.who.int/gpsc/5may/dental-care.pdf. World Health Organization 2012. All rights reserved.

Hand Hygiene

In dental imaging, *hand hygiene* is a general term that applies to routine hand-washing, antiseptic hand-wash, and antiseptic hand-rub techniques. Indications for hand hygiene include the following:

- Before and after treating each patient (e.g., before glove placement and after glove removal)
- After removing gloves that are torn, cut, or punctured and before putting on new gloves
- After contact of bare hands with inanimate objects likely to be contaminated by blood, saliva, or respiratory secretions
- Before leaving the dental operatory
- When hands are visibly soiled or contaminated

Figure 16-1 shows the World Health Organization's tips for hand hygiene in dental care; Figure 16-2 shows step-by-step instructions on how to hand wash; and Figure 16-3 shows step-by-step instructions on how to hand rub.

In dental imaging, three different types of hand hygiene may be practiced.

- *Routine hand wash:* Water and non-antimicrobial soap (i.e., plain soap) for 40 to 60 seconds
- *Antiseptic hand wash:* Water and antimicrobial soap (e.g., chlorhexidine, iodine and iodophors, chloroxylenol [PCMX], triclosan) for 15 seconds
- *Antiseptic hand rub:* Alcohol-based product until the hands are dry

For the most current information on hand hygiene, including hand lotions and how to store hand care products, please visit the CDC at https://www.cdc.gov/oralhealth/infectioncontrol/faqs/hand-hygiene.html.

Care of Hands

All dental professionals must take precautions to avoid hand injuries during dental procedures. Dental professionals with exudative or "weeping" lesions on their hands must refrain from all direct patient contact and from handling patient care equipment until the condition has resolved.

Respiratory Hygiene / Cough Etiquette

Respiratory hygiene and cough etiquette were added to the Standard Precautions of the Centers for Disease Control in 2007. The infection prevention measures are designed to limit the transmission of disease spread by respiratory pathogens via droplet or airborne route. Recommendations include signage to patients with respiratory conditions to cover their mouths and noses when sneezing, proper disposal of tissues, and hand-washing after contacting respiratory secretions (Figure 16-4). No-touch receptacles for the disposal of tissues should be available, as well as hand-washing stations for patients. Masks should be offered to coughing patients in the dental setting and ample space accessible to be seated away from other patients.

Sterilization and Disinfection of Instruments

All instruments in the dental practice can be classified into one of the following categories, depending on the risk of transmitting infection and the need to sterilize the instrument between uses:

Critical instruments: Instruments that are used to penetrate soft tissue or bone are considered *critical* and must be sterilized after each use. Examples include forceps, scalpels, bone chisels, scalers, and surgical burs. In dental imaging procedures, no critical instruments are used.

Semicritical instruments: Instruments that contact but do not penetrate soft tissue or bone are classified as *semicritical*. These devices must also be sterilized after each use. If the instrument can be damaged by heat and sterilization is not feasible, high-level disinfection is required. Beam alignment devices are examples of semicritical instruments used in dental imaging procedures.

Noncritical instruments: Instruments or devices that do not come in contact with mucous membranes are considered *noncritical*. Because little risk of transmitting infection from noncritical devices exists, intermediate-level or low-level infection techniques are required for their care between patients. Examples in dental imaging procedures include the position-indicating device (PID), the dental x-ray tubehead, the exposure button, the x-ray control panel, the lead apron, and, with digital imaging, the computer keyboard/mouse.

Acceptable methods of sterilization include steam under pressure (autoclave), dry heat, and chemical vapor. The instructions of the manufacturers of the instruments and sterilizer must be followed. Proper functioning of sterilization cycles must be verified by periodic use of a biologic indicator, such as the spore test.

The U.S. Environmental Protection Agency (EPA) has classified certain chemicals as "sterilants-disinfectants." These EPA-registered chemicals are classified as high-level disinfectants and can be used to disinfect heat-sensitive semicritical dental instruments.

Cleaning and Disinfection of Dental Unit and Environmental Surfaces

After each patient has been treated, dental unit surfaces and countertops that may have been contaminated with blood or saliva must be thoroughly cleaned with disposable toweling, using an appropriate cleaning agent and water as necessary. All surfaces must then be disinfected with a suitable chemical germicide, including door, faucet or cabinet handles, the patient chair, and dental equipment.

EPA-registered chemical germicides labeled as both hospital disinfectants and tuberculocidals are classified as intermediate-level disinfectants and are recommended for all surfaces that have been

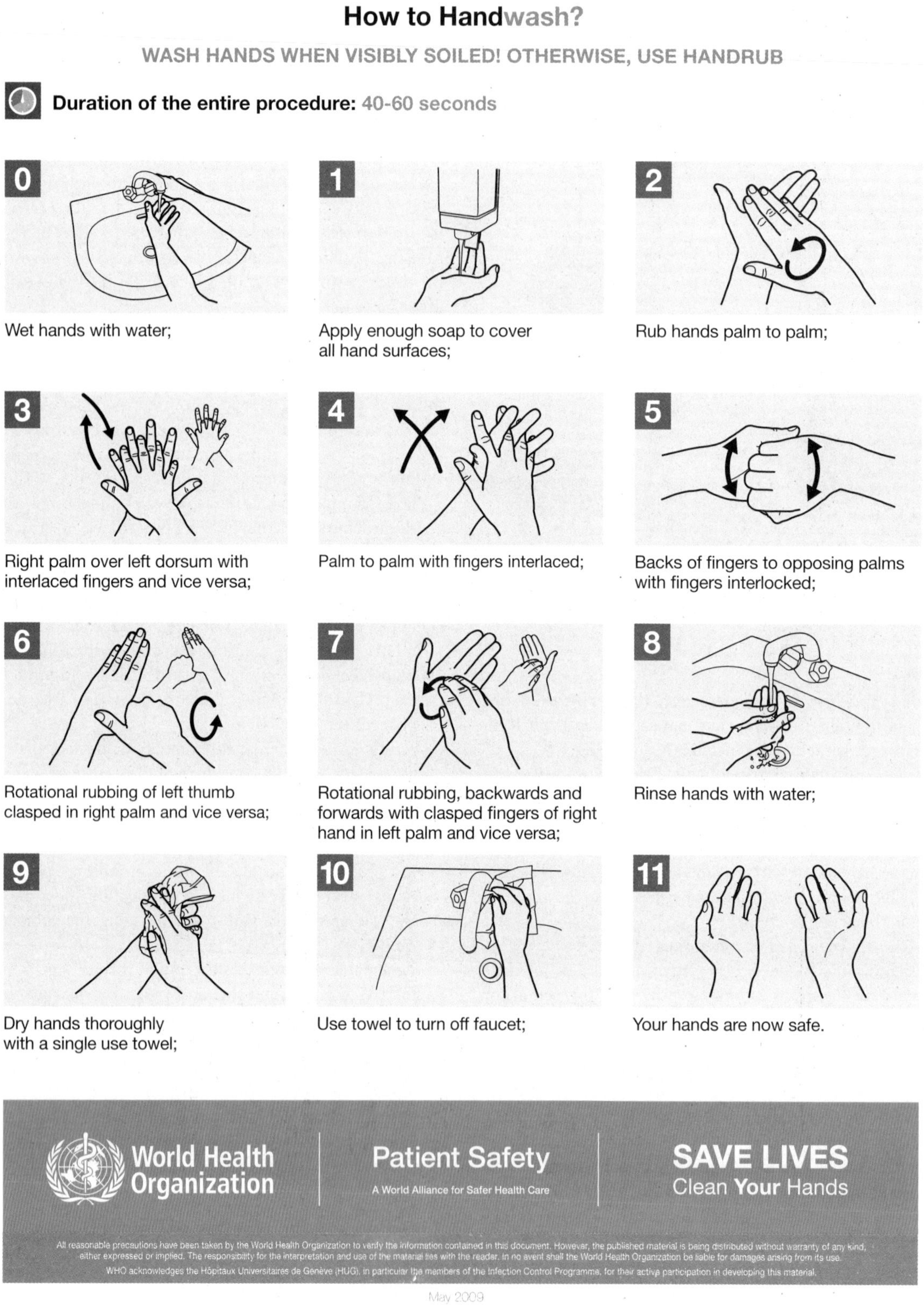

Fig 16-2 "How to Handwash". (Courtesy World Health Organization (WHO).)

contaminated. Intermediate-level disinfectants include phenolics, iodophors, and chlorine-containing compounds.

EPA-registered chemical germicides that are labeled only as hospital disinfectants are classified as **low-level disinfectants** and are recommended for general housekeeping purposes, such as cleaning floors and walls.

INFECTION PREVENTION IN DENTAL IMAGING

In dentistry, standard precautions are required when treating all patients. Standard precautions include a standard of care designed to protect health care personnel and patients from pathogens that can be spread by blood or any other body fluid, excretion, or secretion.

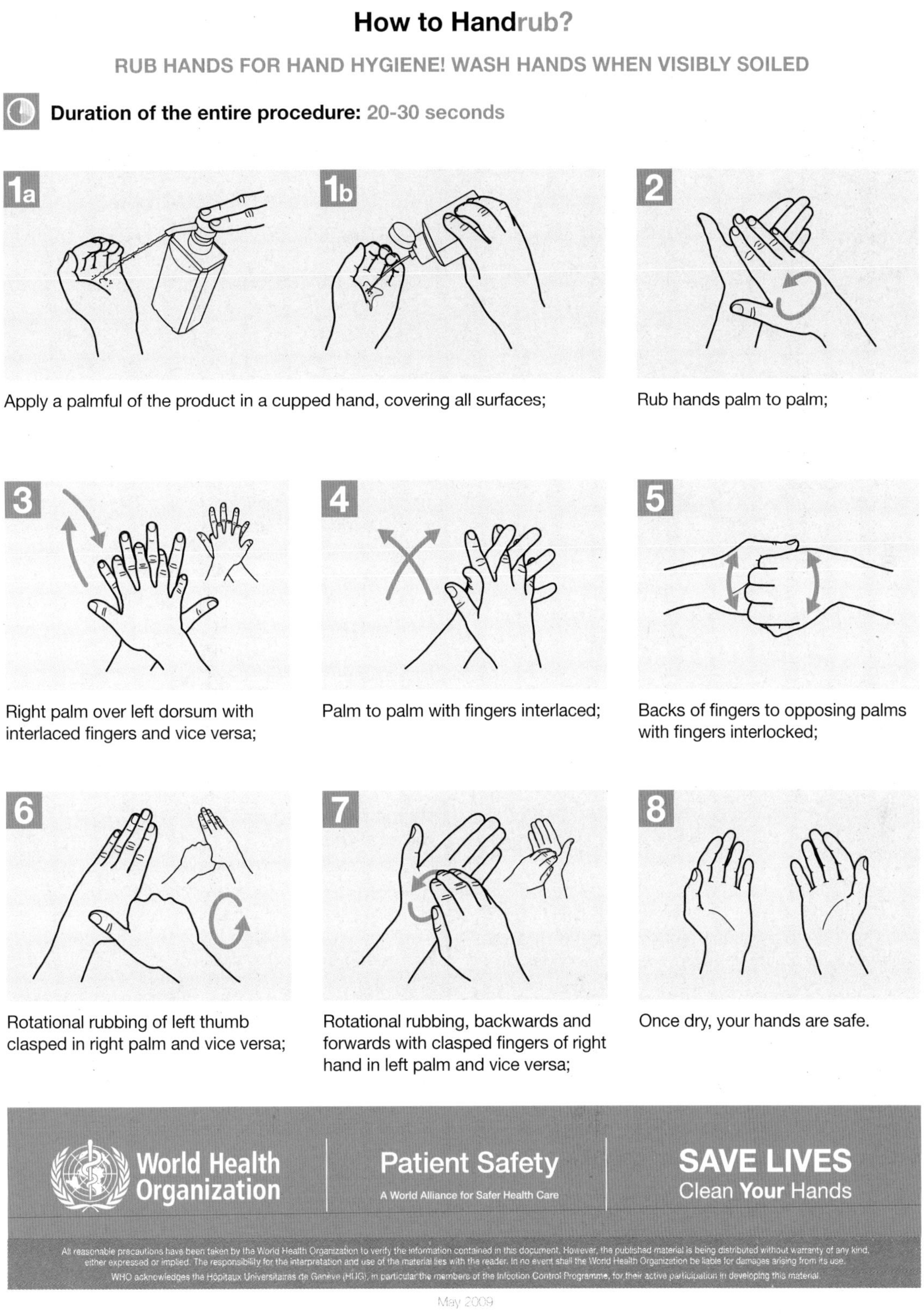

Fig 16-3 "How to Handrub". (Courtesy World Health Organization (WHO).)

The same infection prevention procedures must be used for each patient. No exceptions exist, and no "extra" precautions should be used on any patients. Specific infection prevention procedures pertain to dental imaging and must be used for each patient.

The areas designated for the exposure and processing of dental images are not routinely associated with the spatter of blood or saliva; however, transmission of infectious diseases is still possible if the equipment, supplies, film packets, digital sensors, or cassettes used for the imaging procedure are contaminated. Therefore specific infection prevention procedures that pertain to dental imaging must be used before, during, and after exposure (Box 16-2) and, when film is being used, during film processing (Procedure 16-1).

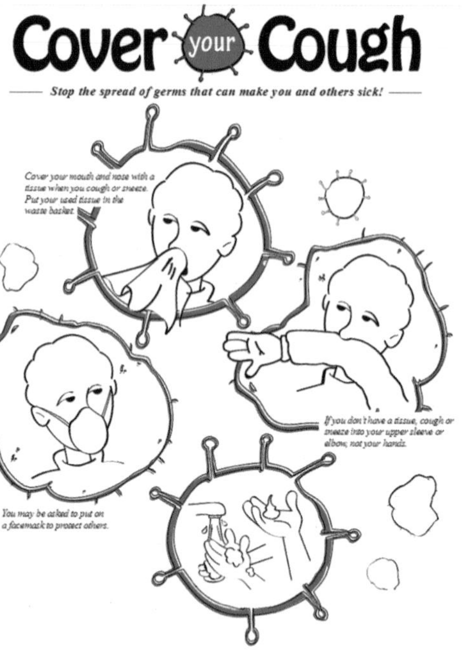

Fig 16-4 "Cover Your Cough". (Courtesy Centers for Disease Control (CDC).)

Infection Prevention Procedures Used Before Exposure

Before dental x-ray receptors are exposed, the treatment area must be prepared using aseptic techniques. Necessary supplies and equipment must also be prepared. After these preparations, the dental radiographer can seat the patient. At that time, the dental radiographer can also complete the final infection prevention procedures that are necessary before exposure.

Preparation of Treatment Area. The dental professional must prepare the surfaces that are likely to be touched during the imaging procedure. All these surfaces should be covered with impervious, disposable materials such as plastic wrap, plastic-backed paper, or aluminum foil. This provides adequate protection while eliminating the need for surface cleaning and disinfection between patients. If disposable materials are not used, after the imaging procedures have been completed, all contaminated areas must be disinfected with disinfecting products, following the manufacturer's instructions. Examples of surfaces that must be covered or disinfected include the following:

X-Ray Machine. The tubehead, PID, control panel, and exposure button must all be covered or disinfected.

Dental Chair. The headrest and the headrest adjustment and chair adjustment controls must be covered or disinfected.

Work Area. The area where x-ray supplies (e.g., film, sensors) are placed during exposure must be covered or disinfected.

Lead Apron. If contaminated, the lead apron must be wiped with a disinfectant between patients.

Preparation of Supplies and Equipment. The dental professional must also have ready all anticipated supplies and equipment, such as film, sensors, sterilized beam alignment devices, and other miscellaneous items, and must make these available in the work area.

Digital Sensors. The sensors (see Chapter 8) used in direct digital imaging (wired or wireless) cannot be heat sterilized. In order to avoid cross-contamination, both barrier techniques and disinfection are required. Dental offices using direct digital imaging require plastic disposable barrier sheaths to cover both the sensor and the wire connection (Figure 16-5). The supplemental use of a finger cot covering the sensor provides added protection and is often recommended. The CDC recommends cleaning and disinfecting the sensor with an EPA-registered intermediate-level disinfectant after removing the barrier and before using the sensor on another

BOX 16-2 Checklist for Infection Prevention in Dental Imaging

Before Exposure

Treatment Area

The following must be covered or disinfected:

- X-ray machine
- Dental chair
- Work area
- Lead apron

Supplies and Equipment

The following must be prepared before seating the patient:

- Image receptors
- Beam alignment devices
- Cotton rolls
- Paper towel
- Disposable container

Patient Preparation

The following must be performed before putting on gloves:

- Adjusting height of chair
- Adjusting position of headrest
- Placing lead apron on patient
- Removing metallic objects in the head and neck area of patient
- Pretreatment rinse

Radiographer Preparation

The following must be completed before exposure:

- Washing hands
- Putting on gloves
- Preparing beam alignment devices

During Exposure

Receptor Handling

Procedures must include the following:

- Drying receptor with paper towel after exposure
- Placing dried receptor in disposable container

Beam Alignment Devices

Handling of devices includes the following:

- Transferring beam alignment device from work area to mouth and back to work area; disassembling over a protected work area
- Never placing beam alignment devices on uncovered countertop

After Exposure

Before Glove Removal

- Disposing of all contaminated items
- Placing beam alignment devices in area designated for contaminated instruments

After Glove Removal

- Washing hands
- Removing lead apron

PROCEDURE 16-1 Steps for Film Handling During Processing

With Barrier Envelopes

- Place a disposable towel on the work surface in the darkroom.
- Place the container with contaminated films next to the towel.
- Put on gloves.
- Take one contaminated film out of the container.
- Tear open the barrier envelope.
- Allow the film to drop on the paper towel.
- Do not touch the film with gloved hands.
- Dispose of the barrier envelope.
- After all barrier envelopes have been opened, dispose of the container.
- Remove gloves, and wash hands.
- Turn out the darkroom lights, and secure the door.
- Unwrap and process films.
- Label the film mount, paper cup, or envelope with the patient's name, and use it to collect processed films.

Without Barrier Envelopes

- Place a disposable towel on the work surface in the darkroom.
- Place the container with contaminated films next to the towel.
- Put on gloves.
- Turn out the darkroom lights, and secure the door.
- Take one contaminated film out of the container.
- Open the film packet tab, and slide out the lead foil backing and black paper. Discard the film packet wrapping.
- Rotate the foil away from the black paper, and discard it.
- Without touching the film, open the black paper wrapping.
- Allow the film to drop on the paper towel.
- Do not touch the film with gloved hands.
- Discard the black paper wrapping.
- Remove gloves, and wash hands.
- Process the films.
- Label the film mount, paper cup, or envelope with the patient's name, and use it to collect processed films.

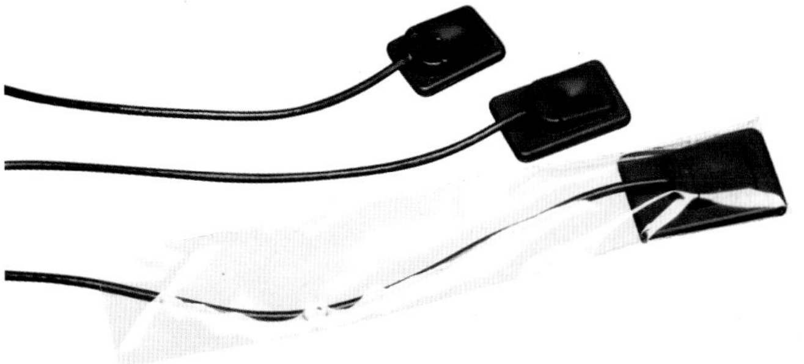

Fig 16-5 A plastic disposable sleeve covers both the wire and the sensor in direct digital imaging. (Courtesy KaVo Imaging, Brea, CA.)

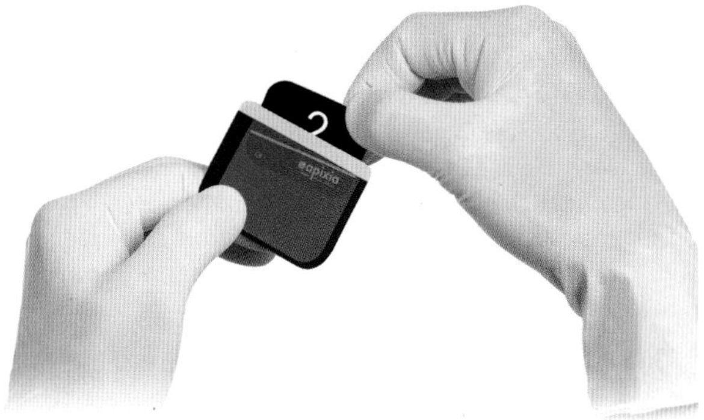

Fig 16-6 A plastic hygienic barrier envelope surrounds and protects this intraoral photostimulable phosphor (PSP) plate. (Courtesy Apixia Digital Imaging, Industry, CA.)

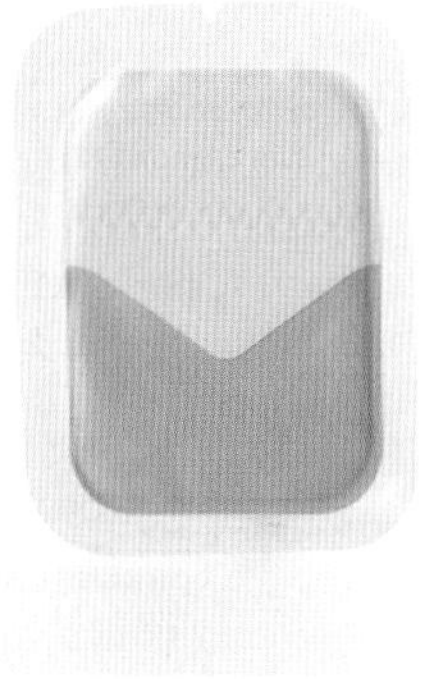

Fig 16-7 ClinAsept barrier films are easy to use. Exposure and processing procedures are completed in the same manner as with other intraoral films. Complete instructions are included with every carton. (Courtesy Carestream Dental, Rochester, NY.)

patient. Because sensors and digital imaging components vary by manufacturer and are expensive, manufacturers should be consulted regarding specific disinfection products and procedures.

PSP Sensors. As with dental x-ray film, photo-stimulable phosphor (PSP) imaging sensors used in indirect digital imaging should also be dispensed from a central supply area. Each sensor must be wrapped in plastic barrier envelopes to protect the sensor from saliva and contamination, much like the barriers used for intraoral films (Figure 16-6).

Film. Dental x-ray films should be dispensed from a central supply area in a disposable container (e.g., coin envelope, paper cup). Commercially available plastic barrier envelopes that fit over intraoral films can be used to protect the film packets from saliva and minimize contamination after exposure of the film. Intraoral films may be inserted and sealed in plastic barrier envelopes (e.g., ClinAsept Barrier Envelopes, manufactured by Carestream Dental) before dispensing films from a central supply area (Figure 16-7).

Beam Alignment Devices. Beam alignment devices should be packaged, sterilized in bags, and dispensed from a central supply area.

Miscellaneous Items. Disposable items include cotton rolls that can be used to stabilize receptor placement and paper towels that can be used to remove saliva from exposed receptors. A disposable container (e.g., paper cup or bag) labeled with the patient's name is necessary to collect the exposed receptors. All miscellaneous disposable items should be dispensed from a central supply area.

Preparation of the Patient. The dental professional can seat the patient after preparation of the treatment area, supplies, and equipment. After seating the patient, the dental radiographer must complete the procedures discussed next *before* completing hand hygiene and putting on gloves.

Chair Adjustment. The chair must be positioned so that the patient is seated upright. The height of the chair should be adjusted to a comfortable working height for the dental radiographer.

Headrest Adjustment. The headrest must be adjusted to support the patient's head. The patient's head should be positioned with the maxillary arch parallel to the floor.

Lead Apron. The lead apron with the thyroid collar must be placed on the patient and secured before any x-ray exposure.

Miscellaneous Objects. Miscellaneous objects may interfere with exposure (e.g., eyeglasses, chewing gum, dentures, earrings) and should be removed by the patient at this time.

Prerinse. Some dental offices may require patients to use a pretreatment rinse solution to disinfect and clean the mouth.

Preparation of the Dental Radiographer. After patient preparation and before x-ray exposure of the patient, the dental radiographer must complete some final infection prevention procedures.

Hand hygiene. Hands must be washed with soap or an antiseptic hand-rub product must be used in the presence of the patient.

Gloves. Immediately after hand hygiene, gloves must be worn.

Mask and Eyewear. Because no aerosolized contaminants are typically created during imaging exposures, the use of a surgical mask and protective eyewear is optional yet highly recommended.

Beam Alignment Devices. If beam alignment devices are to be used during exposure, remove the instruments from sterilized packages with gloved hands in the presence of the patient and assemble over a covered work area.

Infection Prevention Procedures Used During Exposure

Once gloves have been put on and exposure begins, the dental radiographer should take special care to touch only covered surfaces. The best way the dental radiographer can minimize contamination is to touch as few surfaces as possible, including the face. During and immediately after exposure, the dental radiographer must handle each receptor in a manner consistent with comprehensive infection control guidelines.

Drying of Exposed Receptors. After each receptor has been placed in the patient's mouth, exposed to radiation, and removed, it must be dried with a paper towel to reduce any excess saliva. If using a wired digital sensor, dry the plastic sheath to remove excess saliva as needed when exposing multiple images.

Collection of Exposed Receptors. Once dried, each receptor must be placed in a disposable container (paper bag or cup) labeled with the patient's name. This container is used to collect and transport the exposed films to the darkroom or PSP sensors to the scanning area and must *not* be touched by gloved hands. To prevent fogging caused by scatter radiation, the container should not be placed in a room where additional receptors are being exposed. In addition, exposed receptors should never be placed in the dental radiographer's uniform pocket.

Beam Alignment Devices. During exposure, beam alignment devices should be transferred from the covered work area to the patient's mouth and then back to the same area. Contaminated instruments should never be placed on an uncovered countertop.

Interruptions During Exposure. If the dental radiographer is interrupted and must leave the room during exposure of receptors, the radiographer must remove the gloves and wash hands before leaving the area. Before resuming the procedure, the hands must be rewashed and new gloves put on.

Infection Prevention Procedures Used After Exposure

Immediately after the completion of receptor exposures, all contaminated items must be discarded, and any uncovered areas must be disinfected. Contaminated items must be handled in a manner consistent with recommended infection control guidelines.

Disposal of Contaminated Items. All contaminated items (cotton rolls, bite-wing tabs, cups, bags, and protective coverings) must be disposed of following local and state environmental regulations. Contaminated items must be discarded while the dental radiographer is still wearing gloves; this includes disposable materials found on protected surfaces as well. The dental radiographer must carefully unwrap all covered surfaces; gloved hands should not touch the surfaces that are wrapped. Ideally, the disposal of all contaminated items should take place in the presence of the patient.

Beam Alignment Devices. While still wearing gloves, the dental radiographer must remove the contaminated beam alignment devices from the treatment area and place them in an area designated for contaminated instruments.

Hand Hygiene. After removal and disposal of all contaminated items, the radiographer must remove the gloves and discard them. Hands must be washed with soap, or an antiseptic hand-rub gel must be used.

Lead Apron Removal. After hand hygiene, the radiographer can remove the lead apron from the patient. It is suggested that the lead apron be handled by clean hands only; it is very difficult to disinfect the lead apron. After this, the patient can be dismissed from the area.

Surface Disinfection. Any uncovered areas that were contaminated during treatment must be cleaned and disinfected using an EPA-registered hospital-grade intermediate-level disinfectant and utility gloves.

Infection Prevention Procedures Used for Digital Imaging

After the exposure of digital sensors, specific infection control guidelines must be followed. Neither wired sensors nor PSP plates can be placed into an autoclave or submerged in a disinfecting solution. Therefore protective barriers and disinfecting wipes must be used to meet infection control standards.

Wired Sensors. Unlike film that is used one time only, the same wired sensor is used for each intraoral projection on every patient. It is therefore important to completely cover the sensor and the wired connection with a plastic sheath (Figure 16-8). Literature has reported that the plastic sheaths can tear or leak after several exposures. As a result, latex finger cots used in conjunction with the standard plastic sleeves more effectively prevent cross-contamination than does the plastic sheath alone. After exposures are complete, remove the finger cot and plastic sheath from the wired sensor. Wipe the sensor with a disinfectant approved by the imaging manufacturer. Inspect the connection between the wire and the sensor to ensure that it is not damaged. Wired sensors are delicate, expensive, and nonsterilizable and must be handled carefully.

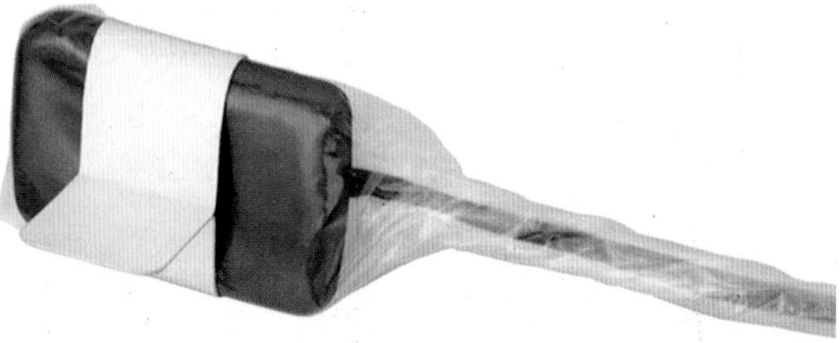

Fig 16-8 A wired digital sensor ready for a bite-wing exposure. (Courtesy Dentsply Rinn, York, PA.)

PSP Sensors. PSP plates can be a potential source of cross-contamination because this type of receptor is used on multiple patients. Similar to the ClinAsept barrier used with film, phosphor plates should always be covered with individual barrier sheaths (Figure 16-9). After exposure, wipe each plate with a paper towel to remove excess saliva. Transfer the plates in a labeled disposable container to the laser scanning area. Wearing a new pair of gloves, remove each plate and tear away the barrier, allowing the plate to drop onto the countertop. Do not touch the plate with gloved hands. Once all plates have been unwrapped and the plastic barriers removed, place all waste material into the disposable container and remove gloves. Continue with the scanning procedures, handling each plate by the edges only. Intermediate-level disinfectants may be used to clean the phosphor plate after scanning procedures are complete (Figure 16-10). Once dry, the plates are placed into new barrier covers.

Infection Prevention Procedures Used for Film Processing

After the exposure of x-ray films, specific infection prevention guidelines must be followed while transporting the films to the darkroom, handling them, and processing them.

Film Transport. As previously described, films contaminated with saliva must be placed in a labeled disposable container after exposure. The disposable container should never be touched by gloved hands. Only after removing gloves, washing hands, dismissing the patient, and cleaning the area should the dental radiographer carry the disposable container holding the contaminated films to the darkroom.

Darkroom Supplies. Paper towels and gloves, which are necessary for handling films before they are processed, must be available in the darkroom. Paper envelopes, paper cups, or film mounts labeled with the patient's name are used to hold films after processing, and these also should be available in the darkroom.

Film Handling with and without Barrier Envelopes. Commercially available barrier envelopes help minimize contamination in the darkroom. Procedure 16-1 lists the recommended film-handling steps when exposed films are protected by barrier envelopes (Figure 16-11) and when films are not protected by barrier envelopes (Figure 16-12). These same steps can be applied to the handling and scanning of PSP sensors used with indirect digital imaging.

Disinfection of Darkroom. Darkroom countertops and any areas touched by gloved hands must be disinfected with an EPA-registered hospital-grade intermediate-level disinfectant.

Daylight Loader Procedures. Infection prevention procedures for processing film without barrier envelopes in automatic film processors equipped with daylight loaders include the following:

1. Place the paper cup and the vinyl or nonpowdered gloves in the daylight loader compartment.
2. Place the container with contaminated films next to the cup.
3. Close the daylight loader lid, and push hands through openings.
4. Put on gloves.
5. Take one contaminated film out of the container.
6. Open film packets as described in Film Handling without Barrier Envelopes (see Procedure 16-1).
7. Allow the film to drop onto the processor film feed slot area. (Do not touch the film with gloved hands.)
8. Dispose of film packet wrappings in the paper cup.

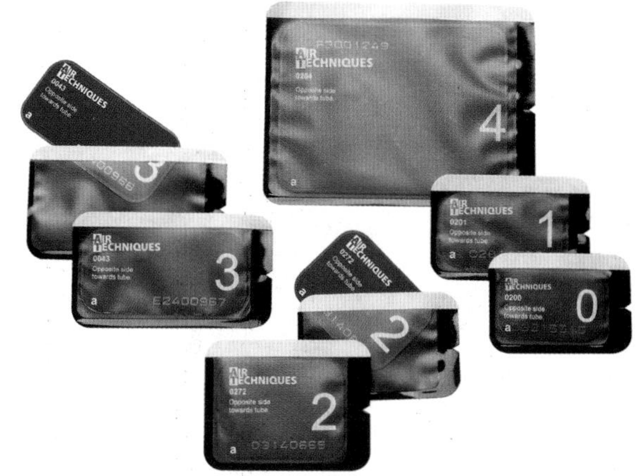

Fig 16-9 Various sizes of barrier envelopes for PSP sensors. (Courtesy Air Techniques, Melville, NY.)

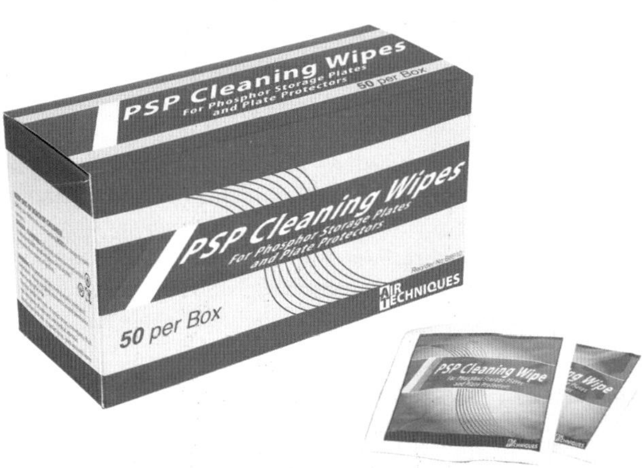

Fig 16-10 Cleaning wipes for PSP sensors. (Courtesy Air Techniques, Melville, NY.)

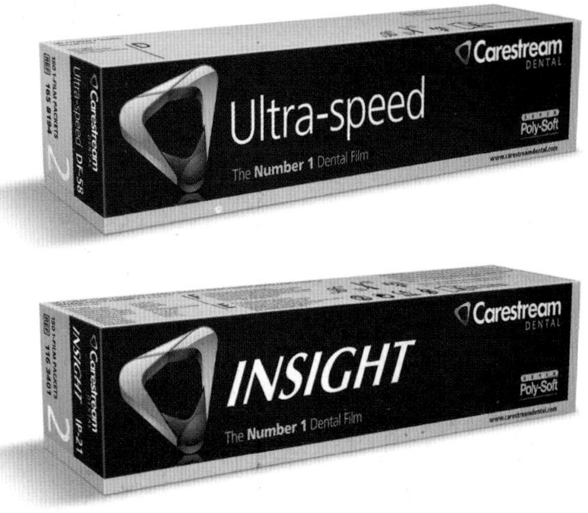

Fig 16-11 Packaging for barrier film. (Courtesy Carestream Dental, Rochester, NY.)

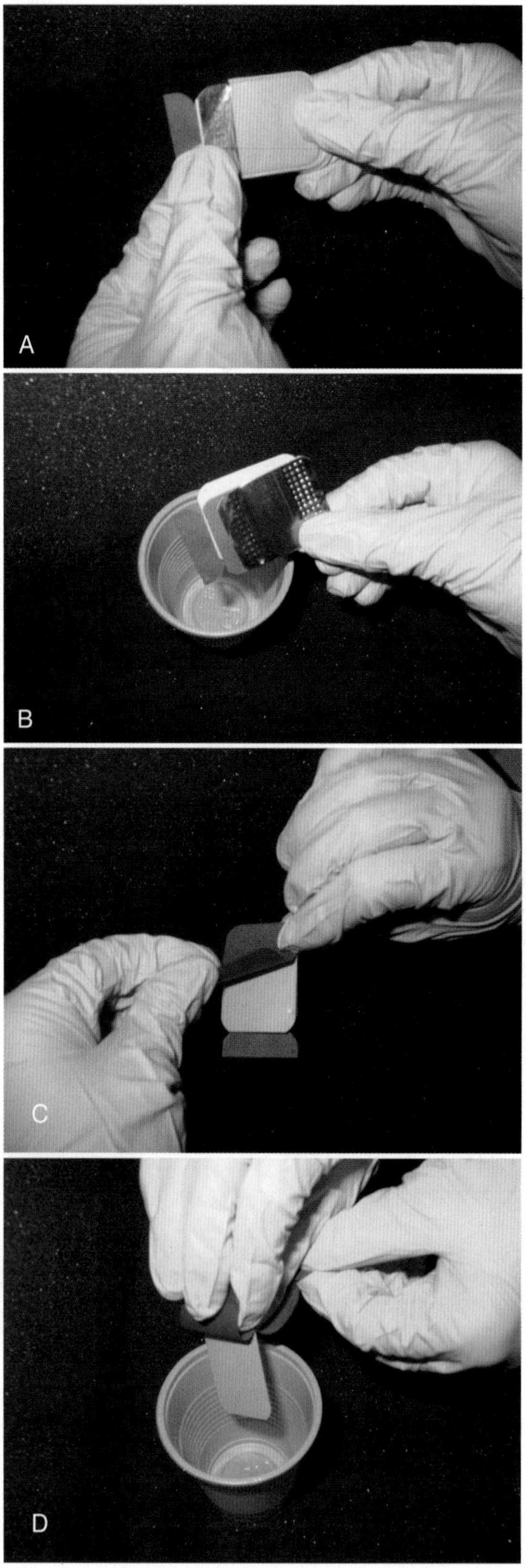

Fig 16-12 Steps used to open a size 2 film packet without contaminating film. **A**, Method for removing films from packet and not touching them with contaminated gloves. Open tab, and slide lead foil and black interleaf paper from wrapping. **B**, Rotate contaminated film packet away from black paper and foil and discard. **C**, Peel back paper wrapping away from film. **D**, Allow film to fall into a clean cup.

9. After all film packets have been opened, remove gloves and place them in the cup.
10. Feed all unwrapped films into the processor.
11. Remove hands from the daylight loader.
12. Wash hands.
13. Lift the daylight loader lid to remove and discard the cup with contaminated wrappings and the container that held contaminated films.
14. Label the film mount, paper cup, or envelope with the patient's name, and use it to collect processed films.

SUMMARY

- To protect themselves and their patients, dental professionals must understand and use infection prevention protocols. The primary purpose of infection prevention procedures is to prevent the transmission of infectious diseases.
- Disease transmission involves pathogens, or microorganisms, that are capable of causing disease. In dentistry, disease transmission may occur as a result of one of the following:
  - Direct contact with pathogens in saliva, blood, respiratory secretions, or lesions
  - Indirect contact with contaminated objects or instruments
  - Direct contact with airborne contaminants present in spatter or aerosols or oral and respiratory fluids
- For infection to occur, three conditions must be present: (1) susceptible host, (2) pathogen with sufficient infectivity and numbers to cause infection, and (3) portal of entry for pathogen to infect host.
- The CDC's *Guidelines for Infection Control in Dental Health Care Settings* (2003) outlines specific infection prevention measures that pertain to dentistry, including PPE, hand hygiene, respiratory hygiene and sterilization and disinfection of instruments. The CDC's *Summary of Infection Prevention Practices in Dental Settings: Basic Expectations for Safe Care*, and *Infection Prevention Checklist for Dental Settings* (2016) can both be used to supplement the 2003 CDC Guidelines.
- The recommended infection prevention practices are applicable to all settings in which dental treatment is provided. The same infection prevention procedures must be used for each patient, with no exceptions and no extra precautions for select patients.
- Infection prevention procedures before x-ray exposure include the preparation of (1) the treatment area (x-ray machine, dental chair, work area, lead apron), (2) the supplies and equipment (film, PSP sensors, direct digital sensors, beam alignment devices, other items), (3) the patient (chair and headrest adjustment, lead apron), and (4) the radiographer (hand hygiene, gloves).
- Infection prevention practices during exposure involve drying and collecting exposed receptors, reassembly of beam alignment devices, and dealing with interruptions properly.
- Infection prevention procedures after exposure include disposal of contaminated items, removal of beam alignment devices, hand hygiene, lead apron removal, and surface disinfection.
- Infection prevention practices during processing involve film transport, darkroom supplies, film handling with and without barrier envelopes, disinfection of the darkroom, and daylight loaders.

BIBLIOGRAPHY

American Academy of Oral and Maxillofacial Radiology: Infection control guidelines for dental radiographic procedures, Oral Surg Oral Med Oral Pathol 73:248, 1992.

Centers for Disease Control and Prevention: Guidelines for infection control in dental health care settings, MMWR 52(RR–17):1, 2003.

Centers for Disease Control and Prevention. Summary of Infection Prevention Practices in Dental Settings: *Basic Expectations for Safe Care*. Atlanta GA: Centers for Disease Control and Prevention, US Dept of Health and Human Services; October 2016.

Centers for Disease Control and Prevention. *Infection Prevention Checklist for Dental Settings: Basic Expectations for Safe Care*. Atlanta GA: Centers for Disease Control and Prevention, US Dept of Health and Human Services; October 2016.

Cottone JA, Terezhalmy GT, Molinari JA: Infection control in dental radiology. In Practical infection control in dentistry, Philadelphia, 1991, Lea & Febiger.

Cottone JA, Terezhalmy GT, Molinari JA: Rationale for practical infection control in dentistry. In Practical infection control in dentistry, Philadelphia, 1991, Lea & Febiger.

Cottone JA, Terezhalmy GT, Molinari JA: Appendix B. In Practical infection control in dentistry, Philadelphia, 1991, Lea & Febiger.

Frommer HH, Stabulas-Savage JJ: Infection control in dental practice. In Radiology for the dental professional, ed 9, St Louis, 2011, Mosby.

Hokett SD, et al: Assessing the effectiveness of direct digital radiography barrier sheaths and finger cots, J Am Dent Assoc 131:463, 2000.

Mallya SM, Lam EWN: Quality assurance and infection control. In White and Pharoah's oral radiology: principles and interpretation, ed 8, St. Louis, 2019, Elsevier.

WEBSITES

American Dental Association: ADA Statement on Infection Control in Dentistry. http://www.ada.org/en/member-center/oral-health-topics/infection-control-resources.

Centers for Disease Control: Infection Control in Dental Settings. http://www.cdc.gov/oralhealth/infectioncontrol/.

CDC https://www.cdc.gov/flu/pdf/protect/cdc_cough.pdf

CDC 2007 Guideline for Isolation Precautions.
http://www.cdc.gov/hicpac/pdf/isolation/isolation2007.pdf

CDC Infection Prevention and Control in the Dental Settings. https://www.cdc.gov/oralhealth/infectioncontrol/index.html

OSAP: Dentistry's Resource for Infection Control and Safety. http://www.osap.org.

OSAP: Infection Control Checklists. http://www.osap.org/?page=ChartsChecklists.

World Health Organization: Hand Hygiene.
https://www.osha.gov/video/respiratory_protection/medevaluations_transcript.html
http://www.who.int/gpsc/5may/How_To_HandWash_Poster.pdf?ua=1 http://www.who.int/gpsc/5may/How_To_HandRub_Poster.pdf?ua=1 http://www.who.int/gpsc/tools/Five_moments/en/.

QUIZ QUESTIONS

Matching

For questions 1 to 10, match each definition with one term.

a. Disinfect
b. Sterilize
c. Asepsis
d. Infectious waste
e. Pathogen
f. Noncritical instrument
g. Critical instrument
h. Semicritical instrument
i. Parenteral exposure
j. Occupational exposure
k. Antiseptic

____ **1.** Use of a chemical or physical procedure to destroy all pathogens, including spores
____ **2.** Microorganism capable of causing disease
____ **3.** Exposure to infectious materials resulting from procedures performed by the dental professional
____ **4.** Exposure to infectious materials that results from piercing or puncturing the skin
____ **5.** Use of a chemical or physical procedure to destroy all pathogens, except spores
____ **6.** Instrument used to penetrate soft tissue or bone
____ **7.** Instrument that contacts but does not penetrate soft tissue or bone
____ **8.** Instrument that does not contact mucous membranes
____ **9.** Waste that consists of blood, blood products, contaminated sharps, and other microbiologic products
____**10.** Absence of pathogens

Short Answer

11. What is the primary purpose of infection prevention?

____
____
____
____

12. List the three possible routes of disease transmission.

____
____
____
____

13. List the three conditions that must be present for disease transmission to occur.

____
____
____
____

Multiple Choice

____ **14.** Identify the false statement concerning protective clothing:
a. It must be worn by all dental professionals.
b. It must be worn to prevent contact with infectious materials.
c. It must be changed weekly.
d. It must be removed before leaving the dental office.

____ **15.** Identify the false statement concerning gloves:
a. Gloves must be worn by all dental professionals.
b. Gloves must be washed before use.
c. Gloves must be worn for each patient.
d. Gloves must be sterile for surgical procedures.

____ **16.** Identify the false statement concerning masks and protective eyewear:
a. Masks and protective eyewear are optional, but highly suggested, for dental radiographic procedures.
b. Masks must be changed between patients.
c. When visibly soiled, protective eyewear must be disinfected between patients.
d. Protective shield must be worn during radiographic procedures.

____ 17. Identify the true statements concerning hand hygiene. Hands must be washed:
a. before and after gloving
b. before and after each patient
c. after touching contaminated surfaces
d. with plain soap for routine dental procedures
1. a, b, c, and d
2. a, b, and c
3. a, b, and d
4. b, c, and d

____ 18. Examples of critical instruments include:
a. beam alignment device
b. scalpel
c. scaler
d. amalgam condenser
1. a, b, c, and d
2. a, b, and c
3. b, c, and d
4. b and c

____ 19. EPA-registered chemical germicides labeled as both hospital disinfectants and tuberculocidal agents are classified as:
a. high-level disinfectants
b. sterilant disinfectants
c. low-level disinfectants
d. intermediate-level disinfectants

____ 20. EPA-registered chemical germicides labeled only as hospital disinfectants are classified as:
a. high-level disinfectants
b. sterilant disinfectants
c. low-level disinfectants
d. intermediate-level disinfectants

Essay

21. Describe the infection prevention procedures that are necessary before x-ray exposure.
22. Describe the infection prevention procedures that are necessary during x-ray exposure.
23. Describe the infection prevention procedures that are necessary after x-ray exposure.
24. Describe the infection prevention procedures that are necessary with digital imaging equipment.
25. Describe the infection prevention procedures that are necessary for film processing.
26. Discuss film handling in the darkroom, with and without barrier envelopes.

17

Quality Assurance in the Dental Office

LEARNING OBJECTIVES

After completion of this chapter, the student will be able to do the following:

1. Define the key terms associated with quality assurance in the dental office.
2. List quality control tests and quality administration procedures that should be included in the quality assurance plan.
3. Discuss the purpose and frequency of testing dental x-ray machines.
4. Describe the tests used to check for fresh film and adequate screen-film contact; discuss the frequency of testing and the interpretation of test results.
5. Describe the test used to check for darkroom light leaks and proper safelighting; discuss the frequency of testing and the interpretation of test results.
6. Describe the test used to check the automatic processor; discuss the frequency of testing and the interpretation of test results.
7. List the three tests used to check the strength of the developer solution.
8. Describe the preparation of the reference radiograph and the standard stepwedge radiograph; discuss the use of these radiographs to compare densities and to monitor the strength of the developer solution.
9. Describe the test used to check the strength of the fixer; discuss the frequency of testing and the interpretation of test results.
10. Discuss quality control tests needed for digital imaging procedures.
11. Discuss the basic elements of a quality administration program.
12. Detail the importance of operator competence in dental radiographic procedures.

Quality assurance refers to special procedures that are used to ensure the production of high-quality diagnostic images. A quality assurance plan includes both quality control tests and quality administration procedures (Box 17-1). Although the dentist is ultimately responsible for the overall quality assurance plan, the dental radiographer can play an important role in the implementation and administration of such a plan. The dental radiographer must be knowledgeable about the quality assurance program used in the dental office.

The purpose of this chapter is to introduce the dental radiographer to quality control tests that are used to monitor dental x-ray units, supplies, film processing, and digital imaging equipment. Quality administration procedures and operator competence for the dental office are also discussed.

QUALITY CONTROL TESTS

Quality control tests are specific tests that are used to maintain and monitor dental x-ray units, supplies, film processing, and digital imaging equipment. To avoid excess exposure of patients and personnel to x-radiation, the dental radiographer must have a clear understanding of the quality control procedures used to test x-ray units, supplies, film processing, and digital imaging equipment in the dental office.

Equipment and Supplies

Quality control tests are necessary to monitor dental x-ray machines, dental x-ray film, screens and cassettes, and viewing equipment. To produce diagnostic-quality images consistently, dental x-ray equipment and supplies must always function properly and be kept in good repair.

Dental X-Ray Machines. All dental x-ray machines must be inspected and monitored periodically. Some state and local regulatory agencies provide dental x-ray equipment inspection services as part of their registration and licensing procedures. Dental x-ray machines must also be calibrated—or adjusted for accuracy—at regular intervals. A qualified technician must calibrate dental x-ray equipment to ensure consistent x-ray machine performance and the production of diagnostic radiographs.

The American Academy of Oral and Maxillofacial Radiology (AAOMR) recommends a number of annual tests for dental x-ray machines. These tests are designed to identify minor malfunctions, including machine output variations, inadequate collimation, tubehead drift, timing errors, and inaccurate kilovoltage and milliamperage readings (Box 17-2).

Annual tests for dental x-ray machines can be performed by the dentist, dental hygienist, dental assistant, or manufacturer's service representative. Most of the tests require some basic testing materials, film, and test logs to record the results.

Dental X-Ray Film. As discussed in Chapter 9, the dental x-ray film must be properly stored, protected, and used before the expiration date. For quality control purposes, when each box of film is opened, it should be tested for freshness.

> **APPLICATION TO PRACTICE**
>
> ***Fresh Film Test***
>
> **Steps**
>
> 1. *Prepare the film.* Unwrap one unexposed film from a newly opened box.
> 2. *Process the film.* Use fresh chemicals to process the unexposed film.
>
> **Results**
>
> - *Fresh film.* If the processed film appears clear with a slight blue tint, the film is fresh and has been properly stored and protected. Proceed with the use of this film.
> - *Fogged film.* Film that has expired, has been improperly stored, or has been exposed to radiation appears fogged. If the film is fogged, it should not be used.

BOX 17-1 Quality Assurance Plan

Quality Control Tests
- Dental x-ray machines
- Dental x-ray film
- Screens and cassettes
- Darkroom lighting
- Processing equipment
- Processing solutions
- Digital imaging equipment

Quality Administration Procedures
- Description of plan
- Assignment of duties
- Monitoring schedule
- Maintenance schedule
- Record-keeping logs
- Evaluation and revision plan
- In-service training

BOX 17-2 Checklist: Annual Quality Control Tests for Dental X-Ray Machines
- X-ray output
- Kilovoltage (kV) calibration
- Half-value layer (HVL)
- Timer
- Milliamperage (mA)
- Collimation
- Beam alignment
- Tubehead stability

Screens and Cassettes. Extraoral intensifying screens used within a cassette holder should be periodically examined for the presence of any dirt and scratches. Screens should be cleaned on a monthly basis with commercially available cleaners recommended by the screen manufacturer. After the screen is cleaned, an antistatic solution should be applied to it. Screens that have scratches or visible wear should be replaced.

Cassette holders must be examined every month for worn closures, light leaks, and warping, all of which may result in fogged and blurred images; these cassettes must be repaired or replaced. Cassettes must also be checked for adequate screen-film contact.

APPLICATION TO PRACTICE

Screen-film Contact Test

Steps
1. *Load the cassette.* Insert one film between the screens in the cassette holder and close.
2. *Place test object.* Place a wire mesh test object on top of the loaded cassette.
3. *Position the PID.* Position the position-indicating device (PID) using a 40-inch target-receptor distance while directing the central ray perpendicular to the cassette.
4. *Expose the cassette.* Expose the cassette using 10 mA, 70 kV, and 0.25 seconds.
5. *Process the film.* Process the exposed film
6. *View.* Check the film on a viewbox in a dimly lit room at a distance of 6 feet.

Results
- *Adequate contact.* If the "wire mesh" image seen on the film exhibits a uniform density, good screen-film contact has taken place. Proceed with cassette and screen use.
- *Inadequate contact.* If the wire mesh image seen on the film exhibits varying densities, poor screen-film contact has taken place. Areas of poor screen-film contact appear darker than good contact areas (Figure 17-1). Cassettes that provide inadequate screen-film contact must be repaired or replaced.

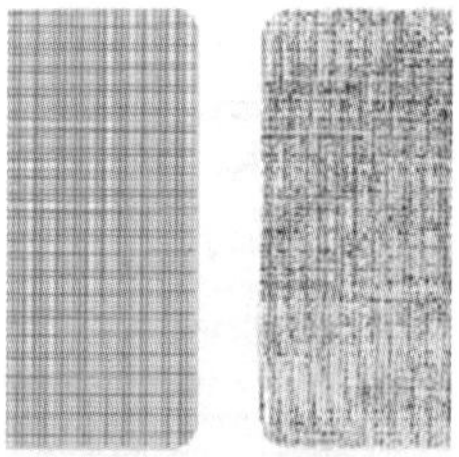

Fig 17-1 Illustrations of screen-film contact. *Left,* Cassette exhibiting good film-screen contact. *Right,* Cassette exhibiting poor film-screen contact. (Courtesy Carestream Health, Inc., Rochester, NY.)

Viewing Equipment. The viewbox, or illuminator, is a light source that is used to view processed films (Figure 17-2). A working viewbox is a necessary piece of equipment for the interpretation of dental images. Depending on the type of digital imaging equipment in the dental office, a viewbox may also be used to clear the images from exposed sensors. The viewbox contains fluorescent lightbulbs that emit light through an opaque plastic or Plexiglas front. The viewbox should emit a uniform and subdued light when it is functioning properly. A photographic light meter can be used to determine proper viewing brightness.

The viewbox should be periodically examined for the presence of dirt on the Plexiglas surface and any discoloration. The surface of the viewbox should be wiped clean every week. Permanently discolored Plexiglas surfaces must be replaced. Any blackened fluorescent lightbulbs must also be replaced.

Film Processing

Film processing is one of the most critical areas in quality control and requires daily monitoring. Processing problems have the potential to result in a large number of nondiagnostic images. Quality control tests must be performed routinely to determine whether the conditions for film processing are acceptable.

Darkroom Lighting. The darkroom must be checked for light-tightness every month, and for proper safelighting every 6 months. Only *after* the light-tightness of the darkroom has been established can the safelighting be checked.

APPLICATION TO PRACTICE

Light Leak Test

Steps
1. *Prepare the darkroom.* Close the darkroom door, and turn off all lights, including the safelight.
2. *Examine the darkroom.* Once your eyes become accustomed to the darkness, observe the areas around the door, the seams of the walls and ceiling, the vent areas, and the keyhole for light leaks.

Results
- *No light leaks.* If the darkroom is light-tight, no visible light is seen. Proceed with film processing.
- *Light leaks.* Light leaks, if present, are seen around the door, through the seams of the walls or ceiling, or through a vent or keyhole. Using weather stripping or black tape before proceeding with film processing must be completed to eliminate light leaks.

APPLICATION TO PRACTICE

Safelighting Test (Coin Test)

Steps

1. *Prepare the darkroom.* Turn off all the lights in the darkroom, including the safelight.
2. *Prepare the film.* Unwrap one unexposed film. Place it on a flat surface at least 4 feet from the safelight. Place a coin on top of the film.
3. *Turn on the safelight.* Allow the film and the coin to be exposed to the safelight for 3 to 4 minutes.
4. *Process the film.* Remove the coin, and process the film.

Results

- *Proper safelighting.* If no visible image is seen on the processed film, the safelight is correct. Proceed with film processing.
- *Improper safelighting.* If the image of the coin and a fogged background appear on the processed film, the safelight is not safe to use with that type of film (Figure 17-3). As discussed in Chapter 10, to avoid safelighting problems, the dental radiographer must use the film manufacturer's recommended safelight filters and bulb wattages. In addition, the film must be unwrapped at least 4 feet away from the safelight. Safelighting problems must be corrected before proceeding with film processing.

Processing Equipment. Processing equipment must be meticulously maintained and monitored daily. As discussed in Chapter 10, the thermometer and timer must be checked for accuracy with manual processing techniques. The temperature and level of the water bath, the developer, and the fixer solutions must also be monitored when manual processing techniques are used. The processing time and temperature recommendations of the film manufacturer must be strictly followed.

If automatic processing equipment is used, the water circulation system must be checked, and the solution level, the replenishment system, and the temperatures must be monitored. The manufacturer's procedure and maintenance directions must be followed carefully. Each day, two test films should be processed in the automatic processor.

APPLICATION TO PRACTICE

Automatic Processor Test

Steps

1. *Prepare the films.* Unwrap two unexposed films; expose one to light.
2. *Process both films* in the automatic processor.

Results

- *Functioning processor.* If the unexposed film appears clear and dry, and if the film exposed to light appears black and dry, the automatic processor is functioning properly. Proceed with processing.
- *Nonfunctioning processor.* If the unexposed film does not appear clear and dry, and if the exposed film does not appear completely black and dry, the processing solutions and dryer temperature must be checked. Corrections must be made before proceeding with processing.

Processing Solutions. The most critical component of film processing quality control is the monitoring of the processing solutions. As discussed in Chapter 10, the processing solutions must be replenished daily and changed every 3 to 4 weeks as recommended by the manufacturer. As an alternative to using the calendar to determine the freshness of solutions, quality control tests can be used to monitor the strength of the developer and fixer solutions. Processing solutions must be evaluated each day before any patient films are processed.

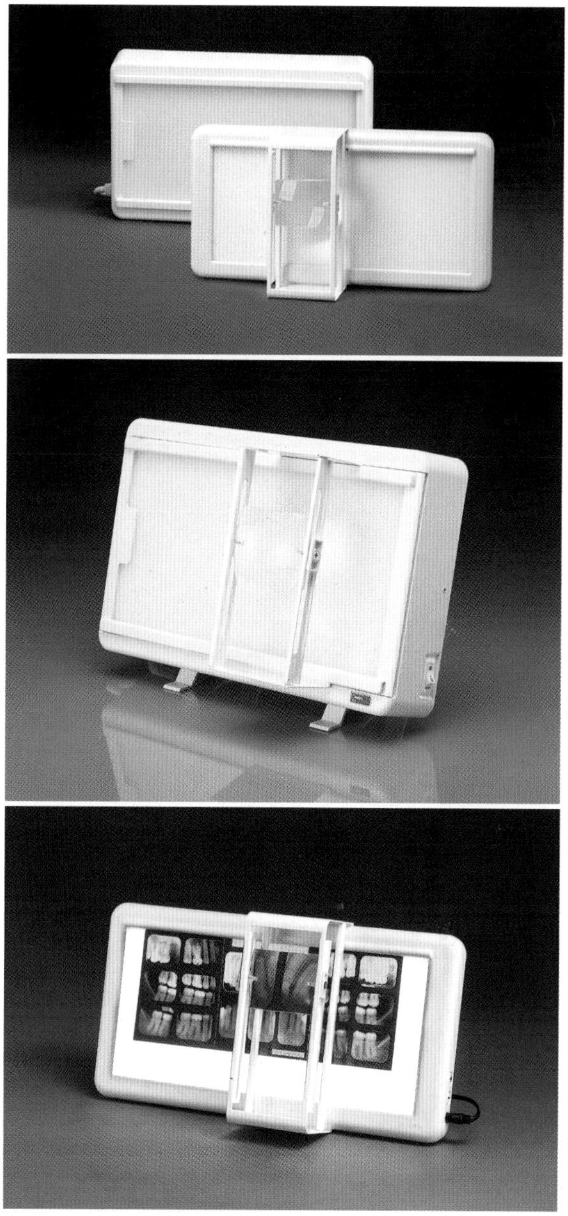

Fig 17-2 Examples of viewboxes in sizes to accommodate most dental viewing needs. (Courtesy Dentsply Rinn, York, PA.)

Developer strength. When the developer solution loses strength, the time-temperature recommendations of the manufacturer can no longer be used as the standard of measurement. An easy way to check the strength of the developer solution is to compare film densities to a standard. One of the following tests can be used (Table 17-1):

- Reference radiograph
- Stepwedge radiographs
- Normalizing device

Reference radiograph. A reference radiograph is one that is processed under ideal conditions and then used to compare the film densities of radiographs that are processed daily. An intraoral film prepared in this manner yields a high-quality image that can be used as a comparative radiograph. Each day, one processed film (daily radiograph) is selected to compare to the reference radiograph. The daily radiograph is compared side by side on a viewbox to the reference radiograph. Minor or major changes in densities indicate problems with exposure or processing, and corrective action must be taken.

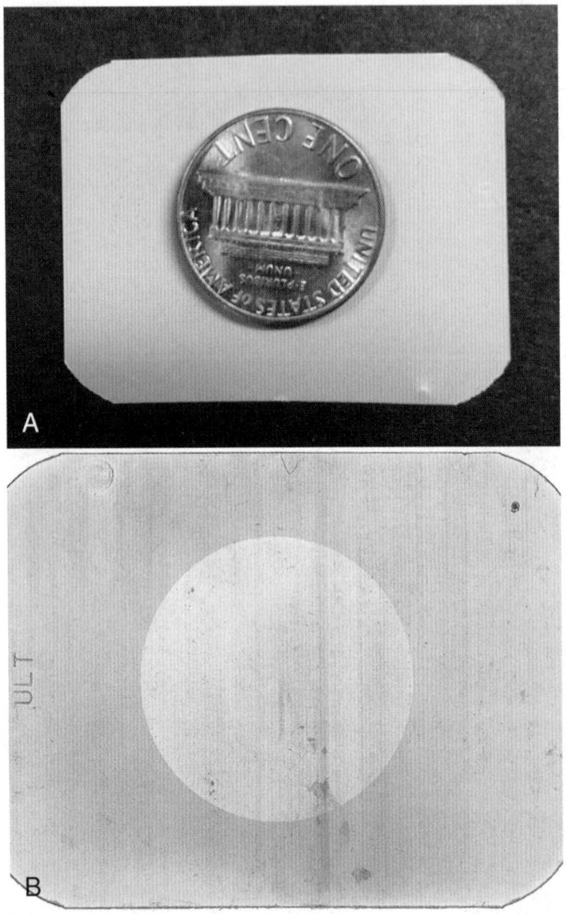

Fig 17-3 Coin test for safelighting. **A,** Coin placed on unexposed film under safelight. **B,** Developed film showing outline of coin indicating that safelight intensity is too great and is not safe. (From Bird DL, Robinson DS: *Modern dental assisting*, ed 10, St Louis, 2012, Saunders.)

APPLICATION TO PRACTICE

Reference Radiograph

Steps

1. *Prepare the film.* Use fresh film to make a reference radiograph. Place an aluminum stepwedge on top of the film.
2. *Expose the film,* using correct exposure factors. With INSIGHT film, use 65 kV, 7 mA, and an exposure time of 0.13 to 0.14 seconds.
3. *Process the film,* using fresh chemicals at the recommended time and temperature.

Results

- *Matched densities.* If the densities seen on the reference radiograph match the densities seen on the daily radiographs, the developer solution strength is adequate. Proceed with processing.
- *Unmatched densities.* If the densities seen on the daily radiographs appear *lighter* than those seen on the reference radiograph, the developer solution is either weak or cold. If the densities seen on the daily radiographs appear *darker* than those seen on the reference radiograph, the developer solution is either too concentrated or too warm. Weakened or concentrated developer solution must be replaced. If the developer solution is too cool or too warm, the temperature must be adjusted.

Stepwedge radiographs. As described in Chapter 6, a **stepwedge** is a device constructed of layered aluminum steps. Aluminum stepwedges are commercially available and may be purchased from a number of sources, including Margraf Dental Manufacturing Inc. (www.margrafcorp.com). When a stepwedge is placed on top of a film and then exposed to x-rays, the different steps absorb varying amounts of x-rays. When processed, different film densities are seen on the dental radiograph as a result of the stepwedge (see Figure 6-8).

APPLICATION TO PRACTICE

Stepwedge Radiographs

Steps

1. *Prepare the films.* Use a total of 20 fresh films to create a 1-month supply of films for daily testing. Place an aluminum stepwedge on top of one film.
2. *Expose the film.* Repeat with the remaining films using the same stepwedge, same target-receptor distance, and same exposure factors. With INSIGHT film, use 65 kV, 7 mA, and an exposure time of 0.13 to 0.14 seconds.
3. *Using fresh chemicals, process only one of the exposed films.* This processed radiograph is known as the **standard stepwedge radiograph**.
4. *Store the remaining 19 exposed films in a cool, dry area protected from x-radiation.*
5. *Each day, after the chemicals have been replenished, process one of the exposed stepwedge films.* This film is known as the *daily radiograph.*
6. *View the standard radiograph and the daily radiograph side by side on a viewbox.* Compare the densities seen on the daily radiograph with the densities seen on the standard radiograph.

Results

- *Matched densities.* Use the middle density seen on the standard stepwedge radiograph for comparison. If the density seen on the standard radiograph matches the density seen on the daily radiograph, the developer solution strength is adequate (Figure 17-4). Proceed with processing.
- *Unmatched densities.* If the density on the daily radiograph differs from that on the standard radiograph by more than two steps on the stepwedge, the developer solution is depleted (Figure 17-5). The developer solution must be changed before proceeding with processing.

Normalizing device. A dental radiographic normalizing and monitoring device can be used to monitor developer strength and film density. The **normalizing device** is commercially available. A current source for the dental radiographic normalizing and monitoring device is XQC/Xray Quality Control (www.xrayqc.com).

Fixer strength. As discussed in Chapter 10, the fixer solution removes the unexposed silver halide crystals on the film that result in "clear" areas on the processed dental image. When the fixer solution loses strength, the film takes a longer time to clear or becomes transparent in the unexposed areas. When the fixer is at full strength, a film should clear within 2 minutes, without agitation.

APPLICATION TO PRACTICE

Clearing Test

Steps

1. *Prepare the film.* Unwrap one film and immediately place it in the fixer solution.
2. *Check the film for clearing.* Measure the amount of time the film takes to clear.

Results

- *Fast clearing.* If the film clears in 2 minutes, the fixer is of adequate strength. Proceed with processing.
- *Slow clearing.* If the film is not completely clear after 2 minutes, reimmerse it in the fixer solution. If the film does not completely clear in 3 to 4 minutes, the fixer solution is depleted. The fixer solution must be replaced before proceeding with processing.

TABLE 17-1 Quality Control Tests for Film Processing

Day	Solution Strength	Quality Control Tests	Test Results
1	Use fresh, full-strength processing solutions.	*Reference radiograph:* Using a stepwedge and correct exposure factors, expose and process one film. This film becomes the **"reference radiograph."**	The **reference radiograph** demonstrates optimal film contrast and density.
	—OR—	*Stepwedge radiographs:* Expose 20 stepwedge films; process one film. This film becomes the **"standard stepwedge radiograph."**	The **standard stepwedge radiograph** demonstrates optimal film contrast and density.
2, 3, etc.	Fresh processing solutions weaken with time and use; exhausted solutions result.	*Reference radiograph:* Each day, choose one processed film (daily radiograph) to compare with the reference radiograph.	Compare the **daily radiograph** with the **reference radiograph:**
			If densities match, continue processing.
			If densities do not match, replace processing solutions.
	—OR—	*Stepwedge radiograph:* Each day, process one of the previously exposed stepwedge films (daily stepwedge radiograph).	Compare the **daily stepwedge radiograph** with the **standard stepwedge radiograph:**
			If densities match, continue processing.
			If the densities differ by more than two steps on the stepwedge, replace processing solutions.

Digital Imaging

Just as quality assurance procedures for conventional x-ray film and processing solutions are necessary, quality assurance protocols for offices that use digital imaging are also required. Quality assurance for digital imaging equipment, including the x-ray unit, sensors, and computer, is important to ensure that diagnostic images are consistently produced. The American Dental Association (ADA) Technical Report 1094 describes the essential quality assurance elements required for digital imaging in dentistry.

Dental X-ray Machines. As mentioned earlier, all dental x-ray machines must be inspected and monitored on a periodic basis. Images exposed annually with fixed settings (mA, kVp, exposure time, distance) on a phantom head may be reviewed in a side-by-side comparison. This test may reveal discrepancies with image sharpness, density, or contrast. Images may become "grainy" over time and require inspection by a technician recommended by the equipment manufacturer.

Sensor. Along with annual tests for the calibration of the imaging equipment, the receptors (whether for direct or indirect imaging) also require periodic examination for scratching, bending, and general wear and tear. Because the traditional x-ray film is used one time and the digital sensors and imaging plates are reused multiple times, greater care in handling and infection control of the sensors is necessary. Digital receptors must be handled carefully, avoiding shock to the sensors from being dropped or pulled excessively by the wired attachment. Imaging sensors and plates that are damaged by debris, bite marks, or bending show the same artifacts repeatedly because the sensors are reexposed to radiation on various patients. Dental professionals who use direct digital imaging must inspect the wired connection for any signs of separation from the sensor or deterioration, as well as overbending of the wire; patients should also be discouraged from biting on the cable itself.

Computer. It is recommended to perform a back-up of the digital data on the computer on a daily basis, especially in offices with high patient volume. Update and maintenance of computers and laser scanning devices should adhere to manufacturer's instructions, as discussed in Chapter 8. Imaging software systems used with digital imaging may recommend periodic updates that should be adhered to for maximum efficiency and performance.

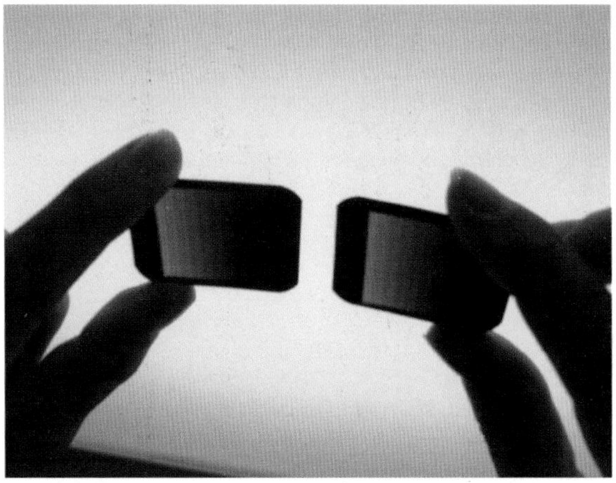

Fig 17-4 The daily stepwedge film should appear identical to the control (standard) film. (From Miles DA, Van Dis ML, Razmus TF: *Basic principles of oral and maxillofacial radiology*, Philadelphia, 1992, Saunders.)

Performance testing and monitoring of digital imaging equipment must be done in accordance with equipment manufacturer specifications. Commercial kits that are available include a set of test objects, which can be used quickly and easily on an ongoing basis to check imaging performance, particularly those aspects that are subject to deterioration. Such kits allow for the following checks: erasure cycle efficiency, image retention, sensitivity, uniformity, scaling errors, blurring artifacts, contrast, and resolution. Kits may be obtained from CSP Medical (www.cspmedical.com).

QUALITY ADMINISTRATION PROCEDURES

Quality administration refers to the management of the quality assurance plan in the dental office. Although many of the technical aspects of the quality assurance plan (e.g., quality control tests) may be delegated to the dental radiographer, the dentist is ultimately responsible for overall quality assurance. The basic elements of a quality administration program include the following:

- Description of the plan
- Assignment of duties
- Monitoring schedule

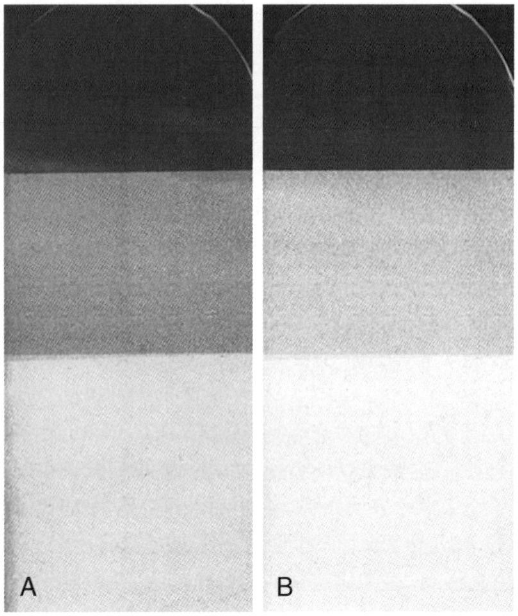

Fig 17-5 Two radiographs of stepwedges that were exposed at the same time and processed at different times. **A,** Radiograph processed when the processing chemicals were fresh and complete development of image was obtained. **B,** Radiograph processed later, when developer solution was weaker. (From Miles DA, Van Dis ML, Williamson GF, Jensen CW: *Radiographic imaging for the dental team,* 4e, St. Louis, 2009, Saunders.)

- Maintenance schedule
- Record-keeping log
- Plan for evaluation and revision
- In-service training

A detailed written description of the quality assurance plan used in the dental office should be on file and made available to all participating staff members. The dentist must outline the standards of quality. Each staff member involved in the quality assurance plan must understand the standards of quality, as well as the purpose and importance of maintaining quality control of radiographic procedures. A detailed written assignment of quality assurance duties should also be on file and made available to all participating staff members. Each staff member assigned to perform a duty must understand the purpose and importance of that specific duty. Although the dentist may serve as the administrator of the quality assurance program, an assigned staff member may oversee the daily quality control testing and results.

A written monitoring schedule detailing all quality control tests and the frequency of testing for all dental x-ray equipment, supplies, film processing, and digital imaging should be posted in the office. A written maintenance schedule for the routine service and inspection of dental x-ray machines and processing and computer equipment should also be posted in the office.

A record-keeping log of all quality control tests, including the specific test performed, the date performed, and the test results, should be carefully maintained and kept on file in the dental office. In addition, a log for processing solutions, which lists the dates of solution replacement, replenishment, and processor or tank cleaning, should be maintained. A written plan for the periodic evaluation and revision of the existing quality assurance program should also be part of the quality administration plan. Finally, periodic in-service training of staff members to upgrade and improve x-ray exposure techniques, film processing procedures, and digital imaging is recommended.

OPERATOR COMPETENCE

The dentist is ultimately responsible for the diagnostic quality of *all* dental images exposed in his or her office, regardless of who actually exposes the images. Therefore the dentist relies on the competence of the dental radiographers. Each dental radiographer must be competent in exposure, processing, and imaging retrieval techniques.

If the operator (dental radiographer) produces a nondiagnostic image, the image must be retaken. Because all retakes expose the patient to additional x-radiation, the number of retakes must be kept to an absolute minimum. Operator errors that require retakes should all be recorded. The use of a log to record retakes aids in identifying recurring problems that require attention. Continuing education courses or individualized instruction are useful to upgrade and improve the competence of the dental radiographer.

SUMMARY

- A quality assurance plan ensures the production of high-quality images and includes both quality control tests and quality administration procedures.
- Quality control tests are used to monitor dental x-ray equipment, supplies, film processing, and digital imaging. The following quality control tests are recommended:
  1. *X-ray machines.* Dental x-ray machines should be tested for minor malfunctions, output variations, collimation problems, tubehead drift, timing errors, and inaccurate kilovoltage and milliamperage readings (Box 17-2). These tests should be performed once a year.
  2. *X-ray film.* The fresh film test can be used to determine whether dental x-ray film is fresh and has been properly stored and protected. This test should be performed each time a new box of film is opened.
  3. *Screens and cassettes.* Cassettes should be examined for adequate closure, light leaks, and warping. The screen-film contact test can be used to determine the adequacy of contact. This test should be performed monthly. More frequent testing is required if the screens and cassettes are used often.
  4. *Darkroom lighting.* The light leak test can be used to evaluate the darkroom for light leaks and should be performed every month. The safelighting test can be used to check for proper safelighting conditions and should be performed every 6 months.
  5. *Processing equipment.* Processing equipment must be carefully maintained and monitored daily for potential problems. With manual processing techniques, the thermometer and timer must be accurate, and the temperature and level of the water bath, developer, and fixer solutions must be checked. The automatic processor test can be used to check the functioning of the automatic processor. These tests and checks must be performed daily.
  6. *Processing solutions.* The developer strength can be monitored by a reference radiograph, stepwedge radiographs, or a normalizing device. The fixer solution can be checked by performing a clearing test. These tests must be performed daily.
- Quality assurance plans also include equipment used in digital imaging, including the x-ray machine, sensors, and computer.
- Quality administration procedures include a description of the quality assurance plan, the assignment of duties, a monitoring schedule (Table 17-2), a maintenance schedule, record-keeping logs, a plan for evaluation and revision, and in-service training.
- The dentist is ultimately responsible for the overall quality assurance plan. In addition, the dentist is responsible for the diagnostic quality of all images.

TABLE 17-2 Monitoring Schedule

	Daily	Weekly	Monthly	Yearly	Other	Comments
Dental X-Ray Machines						
All quality-control tests (see Box 17-2)				X		Upon installation, inspection by a qualified expert
Dental X-Ray Film						
Rotate stock					X	As new film arrives
Fresh film test					X	As a new box of film is opened
Screens and Cassettes						
Clean			X			
Inspect			X			
Contact test			X			
Darkroom						
Light leak test			X			
Safelight test					X	Every 6 months
Processing Equipment and Solutions						
Temperature check–solutions	X					
Quality control tests	X					
Replenish solutions	X					
Drain and clean					X	At regular intervals, at least every 3 weeks
Change solutions					X	As indicated by quality control tests
Viewbox						
Plexiglas surface					X	Inspect periodically
Lightbulbs					X	Inspect periodically
Clean		X				
Digital Imaging Equipment						
Computer data backup	X					
Sensors					X	Frequent inspections needed
Imaging plates					X	Frequent inspections needed
Wired attachments					X	Frequent inspections needed

- To ensure the production of diagnostic images, the dentist depends on the skill of knowledgeable dental radiographers who are competent in exposure, processing, and image retrieval techniques.

BIBLIOGRAPHY

American Dental Association Council on Scientific Affairs: The use of dental radiographs: update and recommendations, JADA 137(9):1304, 2006.

American Dental Association Technical Report. No. 1094 - 2017. Quality assurance for digital intraoral radiographic systems.

Frommer HH, Stabulas-Savage JJ: Film processing: The darkroom. In Radiology for the dental professional, ed 9, St Louis, 2011, Mosby.

Frommer HH, Stabulas-Savage JJ: Patient protection. In Radiology for the dental professional, ed 9, St Louis, 2011, Mosby.

Johnson ON: Identifying and correcting faulty radiographs. In Essentials of dental radiography for dental assistants and hygienists, ed 9, Upper Saddle River, NJ, 2011, Prentice Hall.

Johnson ON: Quality assurance in dental radiography. In Essentials of dental radiography for dental assistants and hygienists, ed 9, Upper Saddle River, NJ, 2011, Prentice Hall.

Johnson ON: Radiation protection. In Essentials of dental radiography for dental assistants and hygienists, ed 9, Upper Saddle River, NJ, 2011, Prentice Hall.

Lusk LT: Peak performance, RDH Natl Mag Dent Hygiene Professionals 14(3):32, 1994.

Mallya SM, Lam EWN: Quality assurance and infection control. In White and Pharoah's oral radiology: principles and interpretation, ed 8, St. Louis, 2019, Elsevier.

Miles DA, Van Dis ML, Jensen CW, et al: Film processing and quality assurance. In Radiographic imaging for the dental team, ed 4, St Louis, 2009, Saunders.

QUIZ QUESTIONS

Multiple Choice

____ 1. Calibration of dental x-ray equipment can be performed by a dentist, dental hygienist, or dental assistant.
   a. True
   b. False

____ 2. Annual tests for dental x-ray machines can be performed by a dentist, dental hygienist, or dental assistant.
   a. True
   b. False

____ 3. For quality control purposes, each new box of unopened film should be tested for film freshness and fogging before it is used.
   a. True
   b. False

____ 4. After processing, fresh film that has been properly stored and protected will appear ________.
a. fogged
b. clear with a slight blue tint
c. clouded with a blue tint
d. dark blue
e. totally black

____ 5. After performing the screen-film contact test, a wire mesh image of uniform density appears. These results indicate ________.
a. adequate film-screen contact
b. inadequate film-screen contact

____ 6. When functioning properly, a viewbox should emit a uniform and intense light.
a. true
b. false

____ 7. One of the most critical areas of quality control that requires daily monitoring is ________.
a. examination of the fluorescent bulbs inside the viewbox
b. cleaning the extraoral intensifying screens
c. examination of the darkroom for light-tightness
d. processing of films
e. all of the above

____ 8. The coin test is used to check ________.
a. proper safelighting
b. strength of the processing solution
c. film density
d. screen-film contact
e. beam collimation

____ 9. The following must be closely monitored with manual processing techniques:
a. temperature of the water bath
b. levels of the processing solutions
c. accuracy of the timer
d. accuracy of the thermometer
e. all of the above

____10. On the average, processing solutions should be changed ________.
a. once daily
b. once weekly
c. every 3 to 4 weeks
d. every 8 to 10 weeks
e. every 3 to 4 months

____11. On the average, processing solutions should be replenished ________.
a. once daily
b. once weekly
c. every 3 to 4 weeks
d. every 8 to 10 weeks
e. every 3 to 4 months

____12. Fresh films and fresh chemicals must be used when preparing reference radiographs.
a. True
b. False

____13. A reference radiograph is used to check ________.
a. proper safelighting
b. light-tightness of the darkroom
c. strength of the fixer solution
d. strength of the developer solution
e. none of the above

____14. The densities seen on the daily image appear lighter than the densities seen on the reference radiograph; this result indicates that ________.
a. the developer solution is too weak
b. the developer solution is too concentrated
c. the developer solution is too cold
d. either a or c
e. either b or c

____15. The clearing test is used to monitor ________.
a. developer strength
b. fixer strength
c. accuracy of the timer
d. film density
e. none of the above

____16. Regardless of who actually exposes the patient to radiation, the dentist is ultimately responsible for the diagnostic quality of all dental images.
a. True
b. False

18

Introduction to Dental Imaging Examinations

LEARNING OBJECTIVES

After completion of this chapter, the student will be able to do the following:

1. Define the key terms associated with dental imaging examinations.
2. List the three types of intraoral imaging examinations.
3. Describe the purpose, the type of receptor, and the technique used for each of the three types of intraoral imaging examinations.
4. List the various projections that constitute a complete mouth series (CMS).
5. List the general diagnostic criteria for intraoral images.
6. List examples of extraoral imaging examinations.
7. Discuss the prescribing of dental images.
8. Describe when prescribing a CMS for a new patient is warranted.

The dental radiographer must have a working knowledge of dental imaging techniques. Before the discussion of the basics of the techniques, an understanding of the different types of dental imaging examinations is necessary. Dental imaging examinations may involve either intraoral projections (placed inside the mouth) or extraoral projections (placed outside the mouth).

The purpose of this chapter is to introduce the dental radiographer to the different intraoral imaging examinations used in dentistry, to define the complete mouth series, and to describe in detail the diagnostic criteria of intraoral images. In addition, the extraoral imaging examinations used in dentistry are introduced.

INTRAORAL IMAGING EXAMINATION

The intraoral imaging examination is an inspection used to examine the teeth and intraoral adjacent structures. Such intraoral examinations are the foundation of dental imaging. The intraoral imaging examination requires the use of intraoral receptors (see Chapters 8 and 9). Intraoral receptors are placed inside the mouth to examine the teeth and supporting structures.

Types of Intraoral Imaging Examinations

Three types of intraoral imaging examinations are used in dentistry:

- Periapical examination
- Interproximal examination
- Occlusal examination

Each of these examinations has a certain purpose and requires the use of a specific type of imaging receptor and technique.

Periapical Examination

Purpose. Periapical examination is used to examine the entire tooth (crown and root) and supporting bone.

Type of Imaging Receptor. The periapical receptor is used in periapical examination. The term *periapical* is derived from the Greek prefix *peri-* (meaning "around") and the Latin word *apex* (referring to the terminal end of a tooth root). Periapical images show the terminal end of the tooth root and surrounding bone, as well as the crown (Figure 18-1).

Technique. Two methods are used for obtaining periapical images: (1) the paralleling technique (see Chapter 19) and (2) the bisecting technique (see Chapter 20).

HELPFUL HINT

Intraoral Imaging Exam

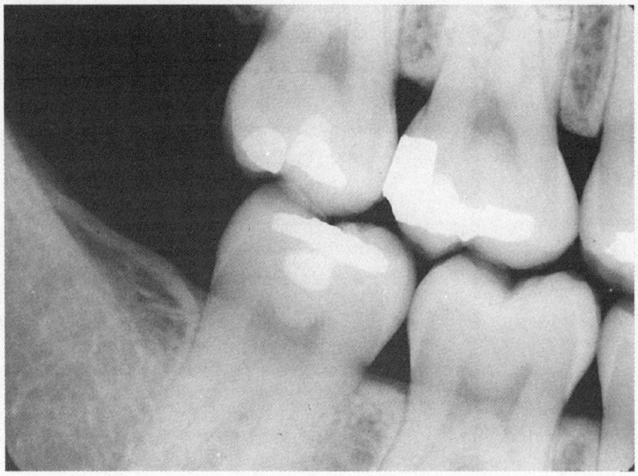

- An inspection used to examine **teeth and adjacent structures**
- Requires the use of an **intraoral image receptor** (film or sensor)
- Receptor is placed **inside the mouth**

Interproximal Examination

Purpose. Interproximal examination is used to examine the crowns of both maxillary and mandibular teeth on a single image. As the term *proximal* suggests, this examination is useful in examining adjacent tooth surfaces and crestal bone (Figure 18-2).

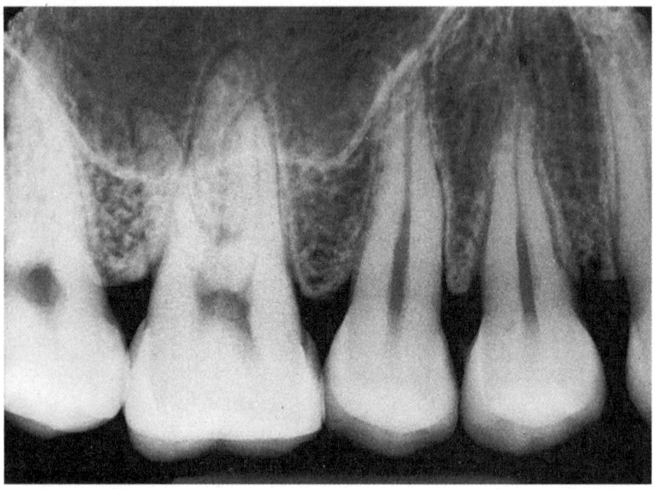

Fig 18-1 A periapical image.

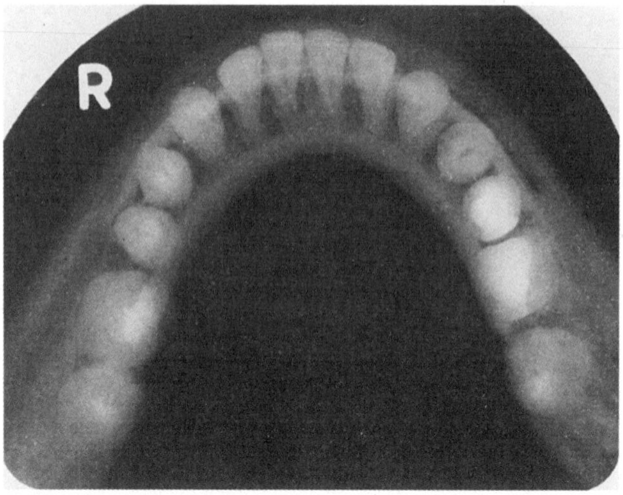

Fig 18-3 An occlusal image. (Courtesy Carestream Health, Rochester, NY.)

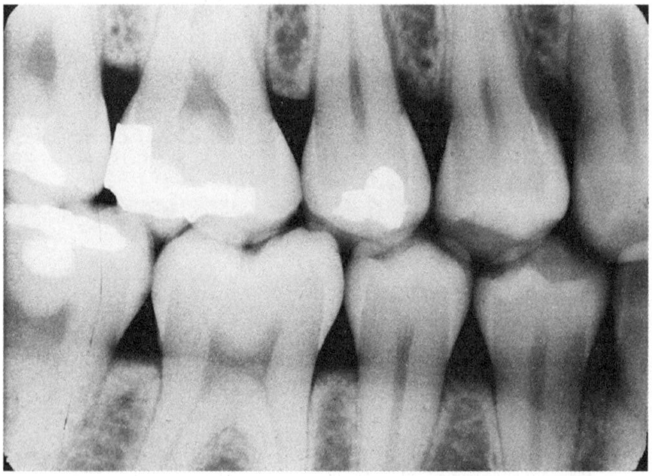

Fig 18-2 A bite-wing image.

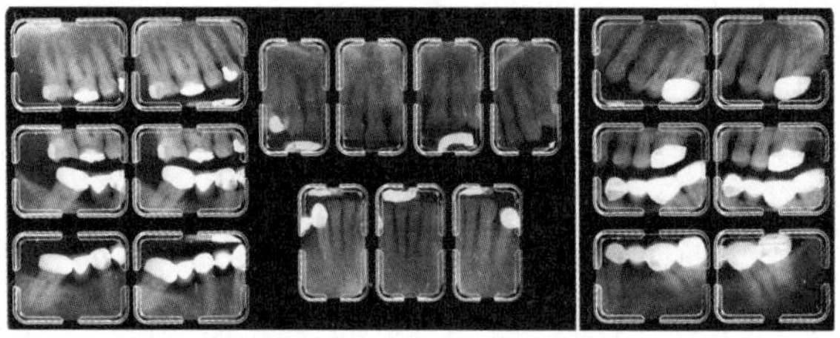

Fig 18-4 A complete mouth series.

Type of Imaging Receptor. The bite-wing receptor is used in interproximal examination. The bite-wing receptor has a "wing" or tab attached to it; the patient "bites" on the wing to stabilize the receptor.

Technique. The bite-wing technique (see Chapter 21) is used in interproximal examination.

Occlusal Examination

Purpose. Occlusal examination is used to examine large areas of the maxilla or the mandible on one image (Figure 18-3).

Type of Imaging Receptor. The occlusal receptor is used in occlusal examination. As the term *occlusal* suggests, the patient "occludes," or bites on, the entire receptor. Although the major portion of the receptor is inside of the mouth, a section of the receptor remains outside of the mouth.

Technique. The occlusal technique (see Chapter 23) is used in occlusal examination.

Complete Mouth Series/Full Mouth Series

The complete mouth series (CMS) is also known as the full mouth series (FMS or FMX) or the complete series (Figure 18-4). The CMS can be defined as a series of intraoral dental images that show all the tooth-bearing areas of both jaws. Tooth-bearing areas are the regions of the maxilla and the mandible where the 32 teeth of the human dentition are normally located. Tooth-bearing areas include dentulous areas, or areas that exhibit teeth, and edentulous areas, or areas where teeth are no longer present.

The CMS consists of periapical images alone or a combination of periapical (PA) and bite-wing (BW) images. Bite-wing images should be prescribed only in areas where teeth have interproximal contact with other teeth to examine the contact areas for caries (decay). To include every tooth and all tooth-bearing areas, a range of 14 to 20 images may be included in the CMS.

The number of images is dictated by the dental imaging technique used for exposure and the number of teeth present. For example, in the patient without teeth, 14 periapical images are usually sufficient to cover the edentulous arches. In the dentulous patient, the number of periapical images varies, depending on which technique—paralleling or bisecting—is used. Receptor size is also dictated by the technique used.

Diagnostic Criteria for Intraoral Images

A diagnostic image, as described in Chapter 6, provides a great deal of information. Specific diagnostic criteria for each intraoral image exposure are described in Chapters 19, 20, 21, and 23 (paralleling, bisecting, bite-wing, and occlusal, respectively). General diagnostic criteria for intraoral images are listed in Box 18-1.

EXTRAORAL IMAGING EXAMINATION

The extraoral imaging examination is an inspection used to examine large areas of the skull or jaws. The extraoral imaging examination

BOX 18-1 General Diagnostic Criteria for Intraoral Images

1. Dental images must display optimal density, contrast, definition, and detail.
2. Dental images must display the least amount of distortion possible; images must be of the same shape and size as the object being imaged.
3. The complete mouth series (CMS) must include images that show all tooth-bearing areas, including dentulous and edentulous regions.
4. Periapical images must show the entire crowns and roots of the teeth being examined, as well as 2 to 3 mm beyond the root apices.
5. Bite-wing images must show open contacts, or interproximal tooth surfaces that are not overlapped.

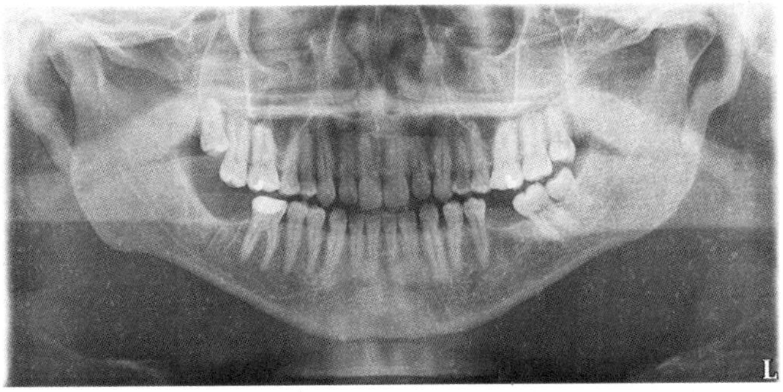

Fig 18-5 A panoramic image.

HELPFUL HINT

Complete Mouth Series

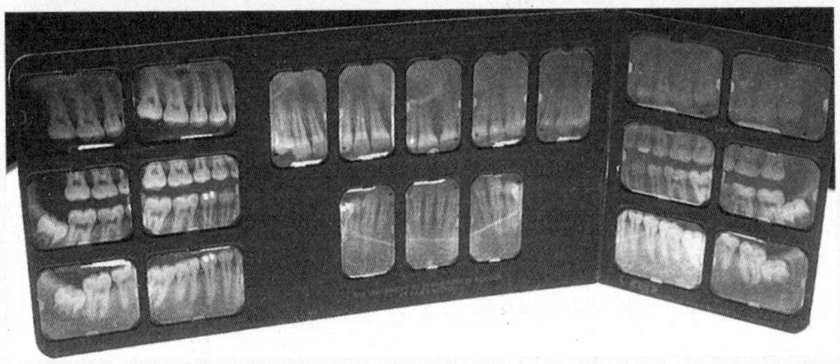

From Miles DA, Van Dis ML, Williamson GF, Jensen CW: Radiographic imaging for the dental team, 4e, St. Louis, 2009, Saunders.

- "Full mouth" series **CMS, FMS, FMX**
- Shows **all** tooth-bearing areas
- Includes **dentulous** and **edentulous** areas
- Includes combo of **PAs and BWs**, or **all PAs**
- A total of **14 to 20 images** may be included
- An **edentulous** patient requires **14 images**

requires the use of extraoral imaging receptors (see Chapter 9). Extraoral receptors are placed outside the mouth. Examples of common extraoral images include the panoramic image (Figure 18-5), as well as the lateral jaw, lateral cephalometric, posteroanterior, Waters, submentovertex, reverse Towne, transcranial, tomographic projections and cone-beam computer tomography (CBCT). Each of these extraoral examinations has a specific purpose and requires the use of certain receptors and techniques. The purposes, receptors, and techniques used in extraoral imaging are described in Chapters 25, 26, and 27.

HELPFUL HINT

Extraoral Imaging Exam

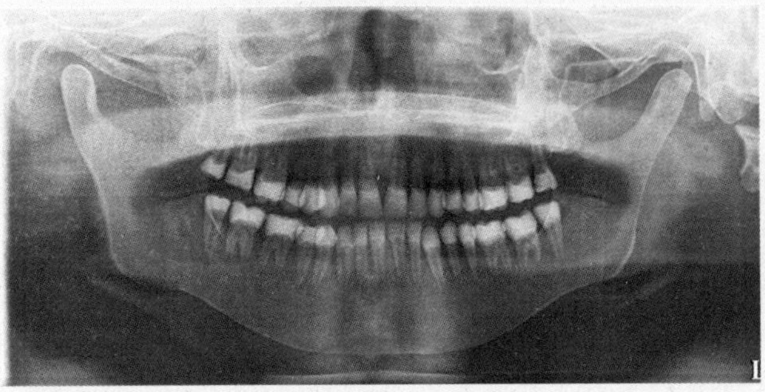

- An inspection used to examine large areas of the skull or jaws
- Requires the use of an extraoral image receptor
- Receptor is placed outside the mouth

PRESCRIBING DENTAL IMAGES

As discussed in Chapter 4, the prescribing or ordering of dental images is based on the individual needs of the patient. The dentist uses professional judgment to make decisions about the number, type, and frequency of dental images. Every patient's dental condition is different, and therefore every patient must be evaluated for dental images on an individual basis.

For example, not all patients need a CMS. As detailed in the Recommendations for Prescribing Dental Radiographs (see Table 4-1), a CMS is appropriate when a new adult patient presents with clinical evidence of generalized dental disease or a history of extensive dental treatment. Otherwise, a combination of bite-wings, selected periapicals, a panoramic image, or a CBCT scan should be prescribed on the basis of a patient's individual needs.

SUMMARY

- Dental imaging examinations may involve either intraoral projections (placed inside the mouth) or extraoral projections (placed outside the mouth).
- The intraoral imaging examination is an inspection of teeth and intraoral structures using x-rays. The three common types of intraoral examinations are periapical, interproximal, and occlusal examinations.
- Periapical examination is used to inspect the crowns and roots of teeth, as well as the supporting bone. Periapical receptors are used in periapical examination. Either the paralleling technique or the bisecting technique can be used to expose periapical receptors.
- Interproximal examination is used to examine the crowns of maxillary and mandibular teeth on a single image. The bite-wing receptor and the bite-wing technique are used in interproximal examination.
- Occlusal examination is used to examine large areas of the maxilla or mandible on one image. Occlusal receptors and the occlusal technique are used.
- The complete mouth series (CMS), or full-mouth series (FMS or FMX), is an intraoral series of dental images that shows all the tooth-bearing areas of the maxilla and the mandible and consists of 14 to 20 images (periapical images alone or combination of periapical and bite-wing images), depending on imaging technique and number of teeth present.

- An intraoral image is considered diagnostic if it exhibits optimal density, contrast, definition and detail, and minimal distortion. In addition, a diagnostic periapical image shows the entire crowns and roots of the teeth being examined, and a diagnostic bite-wing image should show open contacts.
- The extraoral imaging examination is an inspection of large areas of the skull or jaws using x-rays.

BIBLIOGRAPHY

Johnson ON: Intraoral radiographic procedures. In Essentials of dental radiography for dental assistants and hygienists, ed 9, Upper Saddle River, NJ, 2011, Prentice Hall.

Mallya SM, Lam EWN: Intraoral projections. In White and Pharoah's oral radiology: principles and interpretation, ed 8, St. Louis, 2019, Elsevier.

Miles DA, Van Dis ML, Jensen CW, et al: Intraoral radiographic technique. In Radiographic imaging for the dental team, ed 4, St. Louis, 2009, Saunders.

QUIZ QUESTIONS

Matching

For questions 1 to 10, match each definition with one term.

a. Dentulous
b. Edentulous
c. Periapical receptor
d. Bite-wing receptor
e. Occlusal receptor
f. Intraoral receptor
g. Extraoral receptor
h. Maxilla
i. Mandible
j. Occlude
k. Occlusion

_____ **1.** A receptor placed inside the mouth
_____ **2.** The lower jaw
_____ **3.** Without teeth
_____ **4.** To close or to bite
_____ **5.** A receptor used to examine a large area of the maxilla or mandible in one image
_____ **6.** A receptor used to examine the crowns of the maxillary and mandibular teeth on a single image
_____ **7.** A receptor placed outside the mouth
_____ **8.** With teeth
_____ **9.** The upper jaw
_____ **10.** A receptor used to examine the entire tooth and supporting bone

Essay

11. List the three types of intraoral imaging examinations.
12. Describe the purpose, type of receptor, and technique used for each of the three types of intraoral imaging examinations.
13. List the general diagnostic criteria for intraoral images.
14. List examples of extraoral imaging examinations.
15. Discuss the prescribing of dental images.

19

Paralleling Technique

LEARNING OBJECTIVES

After completion of this chapter, the student will be able to do the following:

1. Define the key terms associated with the paralleling technique.
2. State the basic principle of the paralleling technique and illustrate the placement of the receptor, beam alignment device, position-indicating device (PID), and central ray.
3. Discuss how object-receptor distance affects the image and how target-receptor distance is used to compensate for such changes.
4. Describe why a beam alignment device is necessary with the paralleling technique.
5. List the beam alignment devices that can be used with the paralleling technique.
6. Identify and label the parts of the Rinn XCP instruments.
7. Describe the different sizes of receptors used with the paralleling technique and how each receptor is placed in the bite-block.
8. State the five basic rules of the paralleling technique.
9. Describe the patient and equipment preparations that are necessary before using the paralleling technique.
10. Discuss the exposure sequence for 15 periapical receptor placements using the paralleling technique; describe each of the 15 periapical receptor placements recommended for use with the Rinn XCP instruments.
11. Summarize the guidelines for periapical receptor positioning.
12. Explain the modifications in the paralleling technique that are used for a patient with a shallow palate, bony growths, or a sensitive premolar region.
13. List the advantages and disadvantages of the paralleling technique.

In dentistry, the radiographer must master a variety of intraoral imaging techniques. The paralleling technique is important for obtaining dimensionally accurate periapical images. Before the dental radiographer can use the paralleling technique, an understanding of the basic concepts and required equipment is necessary. In addition, the dental radiographer must understand patient preparation, equipment preparation, exposure sequencing, and the receptor placement procedures used in the paralleling technique.

The purpose of this chapter is to present basic concepts and to describe patient preparation, equipment preparation, and receptor placement procedures used in the paralleling technique. This chapter also describes modifications of this technique that can be used in patients with certain anatomic conditions, outlines the advantages and disadvantages of the paralleling technique, and reviews helpful hints.

BASIC CONCEPTS

The paralleling technique (also known as the *extension cone paralleling [XCP] technique, right-angle technique,* and *long-cone technique*) is one method that can be used to expose periapical and bite-wing image receptors. Before the dental radiographer can competently use the paralleling technique, a thorough understanding of the terminology, principles, and basic rules is necessary. Knowledge of the beam alignment devices and receptors used with the paralleling technique is also required.

Terminology

An understanding of the following basic terms is necessary before describing the paralleling technique:

Parallel: Moving or lying in the same plane, always separated by the same distance and not intersecting (Figure 19-1, A).

Intersecting: To cut across or through (Figure 19-1, B).

Perpendicular: Intersecting at or forming a right angle (Figure 19-1, C).

Right angle: An angle of 90 degrees formed by two lines perpendicular to each other (Figure 19-1, D).

Long axis of the tooth: An imaginary line that divides the tooth longitudinally into two equal halves (Figure 19-2).

Central ray: The central portion of the primary beam of x-radiation.

Principles of Paralleling Technique

As the term *paralleling* indicates, this technique is based on the concept of *parallelism*. The basic principles of the paralleling technique can be described as follows (Figure 19-3):

1. The receptor is placed in the mouth *parallel* to the long axis of the tooth being radiographed.
2. The central ray of the x-ray beam is directed *perpendicular* (at a right angle) to the receptor and the long axis of the tooth.
3. A beam alignment device must be used to keep the receptor parallel with the long axis of the tooth. The patient *cannot* hold the receptor in this manner.

To achieve parallelism between the receptor and the tooth, the receptor must be placed *away* from the tooth and toward the middle of the oral cavity. Because of the anatomic configuration of the oral cavity (e.g., curvature of palate), the object-receptor distance (distance between tooth and receptor) must be increased to keep the receptor parallel with the long axis of the tooth (Figure 19-4). Because the receptor is placed away from the tooth, image magnification and loss of definition result. As discussed in Chapter 6, increased object-receptor distance results in increased image magnification.

To compensate for image magnification, the target-receptor distance (distance between source of x-rays and receptor) must also be increased to ensure that only the most parallel rays will be directed at the tooth and the receptor. As a result, a long (16-inch) target-receptor distance must be used with the paralleling technique. The paralleling technique is sometimes referred to as the "long-cone technique"; *long* refers to the length of the cone, or position-indicating device (PID), that is used. The use of a long target-receptor distance in the paralleling

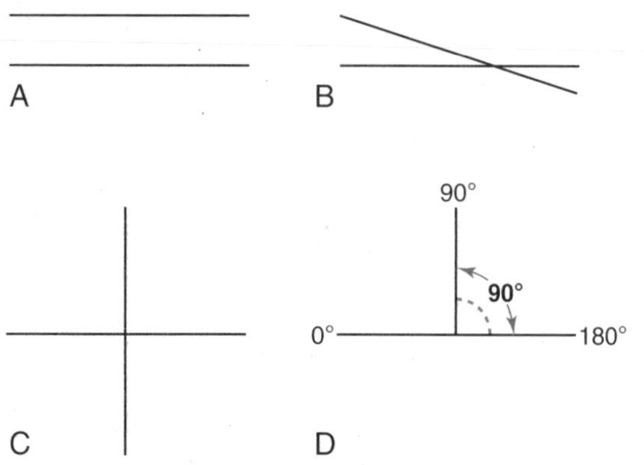

Fig 19-1 **A,** Parallel lines are always separated by the same distance and do not intersect. **B,** Intersecting lines cross one another. **C,** Perpendicular lines intersect one another to form right angles. **D,** A right angle measures 90 degrees and is formed by two perpendicular lines.

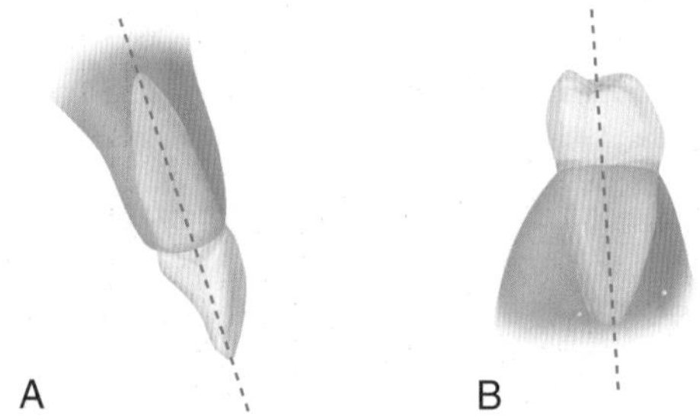

Fig 19-2 **A,** The long axis of the maxillary incisor divides the tooth into two equal halves. **B,** The long axis of a mandibular premolar divides the tooth into two equal halves.

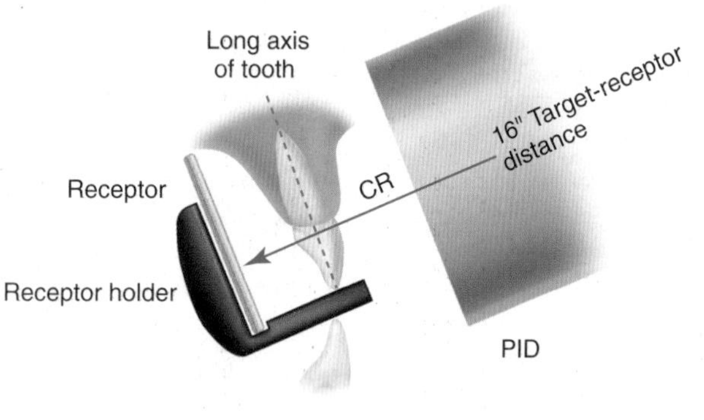

Fig 19-3 Positions of the receptor, teeth, and central ray (*CR*) of the x-ray beam in the paralleling technique. The receptor and the long axis of the tooth are parallel. The central ray is perpendicular to the tooth and the receptor. An increased target-receptor distance (16 inches) is required. *PID*, position-indicating device.

technique results in less image magnification and increased definition. As presented in Chapter 6, the longer PID is preferred but may be bulky or difficult to maneuver around the patient. Current x-ray machines are manufactured with a recessed focal spot, meaning the x-ray tube is recessed, or placed in the rear section of the tubehead. This allows for the use of a shorter PID while still maintaining the 16-inch extended target-receptor distance.

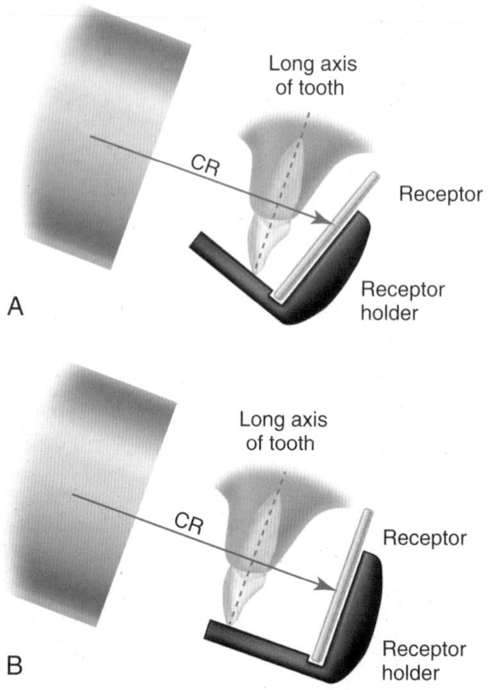

Fig 19-4 **A,** The receptor is placed close to the tooth and is not parallel to the long axis of the tooth. **B,** Increased object-receptor distance. The receptor is placed away from the tooth and is now parallel with the long axis of the tooth. *CR*, central ray.

The American Dental Association (ADA) and the American Academy of Oral and Maxillofacial Radiology both recommend the use of a rectangular collimator to reduce the amount of radiation the patient receives. Limiting the size of the x-ray beam not only reduces the amount of skin that is exposed but also results in a significant reduction of radiation to the patient, by as much as 70%. The receptor placement procedures illustrated in this chapter use a rectangular collimator attached to the end of the PID.

Beam Alignment Devices and Receptor Holding Devices

The paralleling technique requires the use of a beam alignment instrument or a receptor holding device to position the receptor parallel to the long axis of the tooth. Beam alignment devices are used to position an intraoral receptor in the mouth and maintain the receptor in position during exposure (see Chapter 7). Examples of commercially available intraoral beam alignment devices include the following Dentsply Rinn products (Dentsply Rinn Corporation, York, PA):

- The *Rinn XCP Extension Cone Paralleling System* includes three plastic bite-blocks, three plastic aiming rings, and three metal indicator arms. Different bite-blocks are available that accommodate film and PSP sensors, as well as digital sensors (Figure 19-5, A). The plastic bite-blocks and aiming rings are color-coded to aid in assembly: blue instruments are used in the anterior regions, yellow instruments are used in the posterior regions, red instruments are used for bite-wing projections, and green instruments are used in endodontic procedures.
- The *Rinn XCP-ORA One Ring & Arm Positioning System* includes a reduced number of component parts—one ring and one arm. Different bite-blocks are available that accommodate film and PSP sensors, as well as digital sensors (Figure 19-5, B).

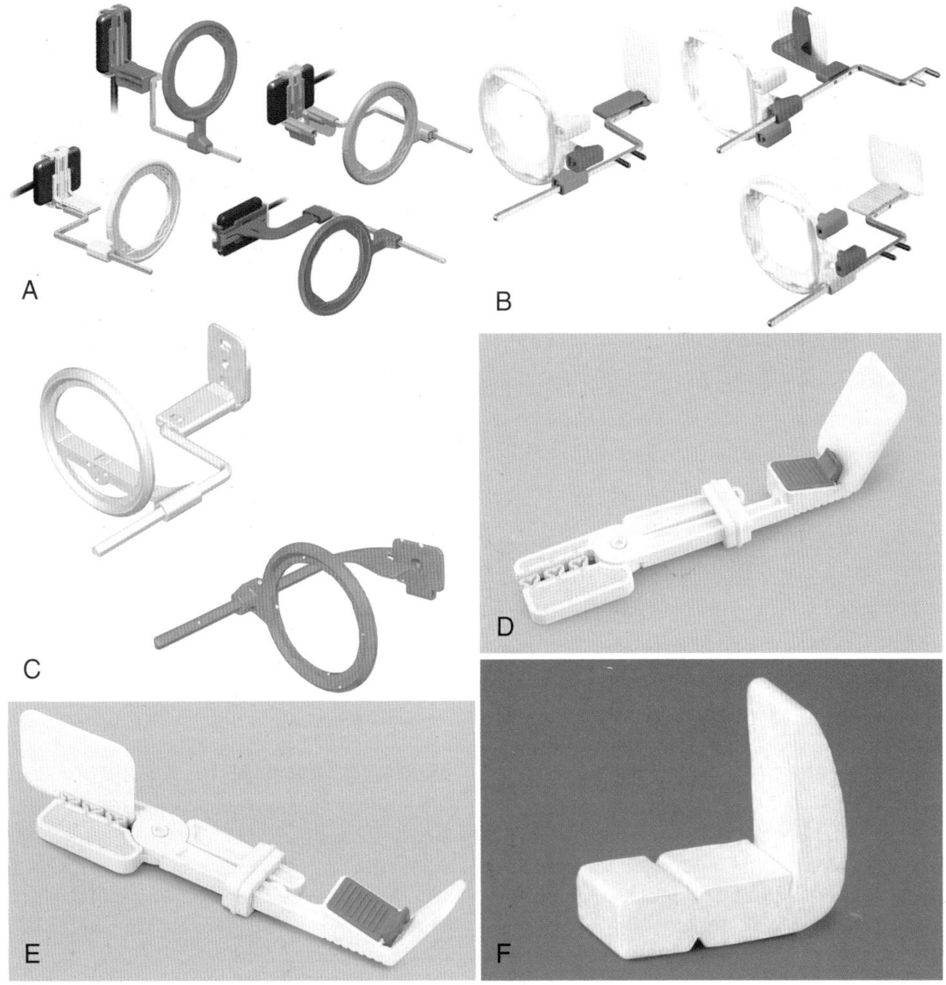

Fig 19-5 Beam alignment devices. **A,** Rinn XCP instruments: blue instruments are used in the anterior region, yellow instruments are used in the posterior region, red instruments are used in the bite-wing technique, and green instruments are used for endodontic procedures. **B,** Rinn XCP-ORA beam alignment devices provide accurate positioning in a system with one ring and one arm for anterior, posterior, and bite-wing projections. **C,** The Rinn Flip-Ray system uses a rotating bite-block and ring to eliminate multiple beam alignment devices. **D, E,** The Rinn Snap-A-Ray Xtra intraoral receptor holder is color coded for the anterior and posterior regions. **F,** An example of a disposable Stabe Bite-block. (**A, C, D, E,** Courtesy Dentsply Rinn Corporation, York, PA.)

- The *Rinn XCP-DS FIT Universal Sensor Holder* is a bite-block that includes a self-adjusting clip that stretches to accommodate the size of the digital sensor, regardless of brand or size. These bite-blocks may be used with the Rinn XCP or Rinn XCP-ORA systems.
- The *Rinn Flip-Ray System* uses a rotating bite-block and ring to eliminate multiple positioning parts. It may be used with film or PSP sensors (Figure 19-5, C).

Examples of receptor holding devices that are used with the paralleling technique to position an intraoral receptor include the following:

- The Rinn Snap-A-Ray Holder comes in two versions, one for film and one for digital sensors. This receptor holding device can be used in both anterior and posterior areas (Figure 19-5, D and E).
- The Stabe Bite-block is a disposable receptor holder made of Styrofoam and is designed for one-time use only (Figure 19-5, F).

Some receptor holders are disposable (e.g., Stabe Bite-block) and are designed for one-time use only. Other receptor holders are reusable (e.g., Snap-A-Ray Holder) and must be sterilized after each use.

Digital sensors come in a variety of sizes and thicknesses. Different digital sensor brands work with specific beam alignment devices. A 20-page publication entitled the *Rinn Digital Sensor Guide* is available on the Rinn website and details what holder works with what brand of sensor (www.rinncorp.com).

The Rinn XCP beam alignment instruments (XCP or XCP-ORA) are recommended for exposure of periapical receptors. These beam alignment devices are recommended because the aiming rings aid in the alignment of the PID with the receptor. These instruments are simple to position and easy to sterilize.

Receptors Used for Paralleling Technique

The size of the intraoral receptor used with the paralleling technique depends on the teeth being radiographed, as follows:

Anterior. In the anterior regions, a size 1 receptor is used; this narrow size is needed to permit placement high in the palate without bending or curving. Size 1 is always positioned with the long portion of the receptor in a *vertical* (upright) direction. Some practitioners prefer to use a size 2 receptor instead.

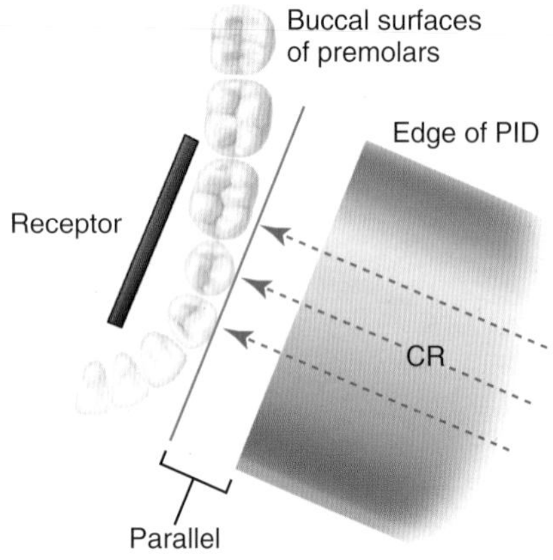

Fig 19-6 In this diagram, x-rays pass through the contact areas of the premolars because the central ray (*CR*) is directed through the contacts and perpendicular to the receptor. If the central ray is not directed through the contacts, overlap of the premolar contacts occurs.

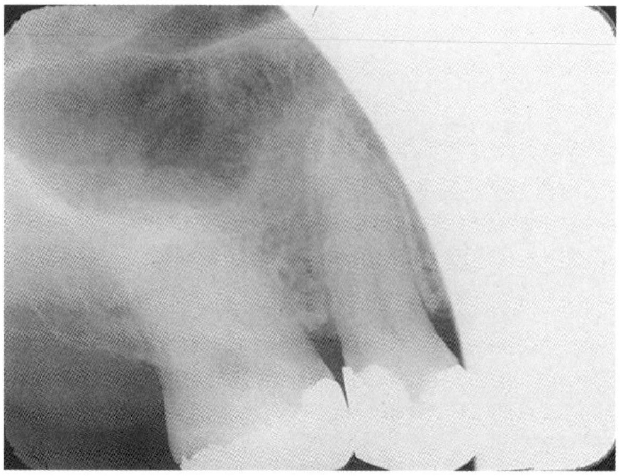

Fig 19-7 This image demonstrates a cone-cut, or clear, unexposed area on the image. The position-indicating device (PID) was positioned too far distally, and therefore the anterior portion of the receptor received no exposure.

Posterior. In the posterior regions, a size 2 receptor is used. Size 2 is always placed with the long portion of the receptor in a *horizontal* (sideways) direction.

Rules for Paralleling Technique

Five basic rules should be followed when using the paralleling technique.

1. *Receptor placement.* The receptor must be positioned to cover the prescribed area of teeth to be examined. Specific placements are detailed in the procedure sections of this chapter.
2. *Receptor position.* The receptor must be positioned parallel to the long axis of the tooth. The receptor and beam alignment device must be placed away from the teeth and toward the middle of the oral cavity (see Figure 19-3).
3. *Vertical angulation.* The central ray of the x-ray beam must be directed perpendicular (at a right angle) to the receptor and the long axis of the tooth (see Figure 19-3).
4. *Horizontal angulation.* The central ray of the x-ray beam must be directed through the contact areas between teeth (Figure 19-6).
5. *Receptor exposure.* The x-ray beam must be centered on the receptor to ensure that all areas are exposed. Failure to center the x-ray beam results in a partial image on the receptor or a "cone-cut." Cone-cuts can be produced with either a round PID or a rectangular PID (Figure 19-7). Cone-cuts are discussed in Chapter 22.

STEP-BY-STEP PROCEDURES

Step-by-step procedures for the exposure of periapical receptors using the paralleling technique include patient preparation, equipment preparation, and receptor placement methods. Exposure of bite-wing receptors using the paralleling technique is discussed in Chapter 21. Before exposing any receptors using the paralleling technique, infection prevention procedures (as detailed in Chapter 16) must be completed.

Patient Preparation

After completion of infection prevention procedures and preparation of the treatment area and supplies, the patient should be seated. After seating the patient, the dental radiographer must prepare the patient before the exposure of any receptors (Procedure 19-1).

Equipment Preparation

After patient preparation, equipment must also be prepared before the exposure of any receptors (Procedure 19-2).

Exposure Sequence for Receptor Placements

When using the paralleling technique, an exposure sequence, or definite order for periapical receptor placement and exposure, must be followed. The dental radiographer must have an established exposure routine to prevent errors and to use time efficiently. Working without an exposure sequence may result in omitting an area or in exposing an area to x-radiation twice.

Anterior Exposure Sequence. When exposing periapical receptors with the paralleling technique, *always* begin with the anterior teeth (canines and incisors), for the following reasons:

- The size 1 receptor used for anterior exposures is small, less uncomfortable, and easier for the patient to tolerate. Some practitioners prefer to use a size 2 receptor instead, which may be more difficult to place, depending on the size of the patient's mouth.
- The more tolerable anterior placements allow the patient to become accustomed to the beam alignment device used in the paralleling technique.
- Anterior placements are less likely to cause the patient to gag. Once the gag reflex is stimulated, the patient may gag on receptor placements that might normally be tolerated. Management of the patient with a hypersensitive gag reflex is discussed in Chapter 24.

PROCEDURE 19-1 Patient Preparation for Paralleling Technique

1. Briefly explain the imaging procedures to the patient.
2. Adjust the chair so that the patient is positioned upright and the level of the chair is at a comfortable working height.
3. Adjust the headrest to support and position the patient's head. Position the patient's head such that the maxillary arch is parallel to the floor and the midsagittal (midline) plane is perpendicular to the floor.
4. Place and secure the lead apron with thyroid collar on the patient.
5. Request that the patient remove eyeglasses and any objects in the mouth (e.g., dentures, retainers) that may interfere with the procedure.

PROCEDURE 19-2 Equipment Preparation for Paralleling Technique

1. Set the exposure control factors (kilovoltage, milliamperage, and time) on the x-ray unit according to the manufacturer recommendations.
2. Open the sterilized packaging containing the beam alignment devices, and assemble the devices over a covered work area. Anterior Rinn XCP instrument assembly is illustrated in Figure 19-8; posterior Rinn XCP instrument assembly is illustrated in Figure 19-9. For assembly instructions on other beam alignment devices, refer to manufacturer instructions.

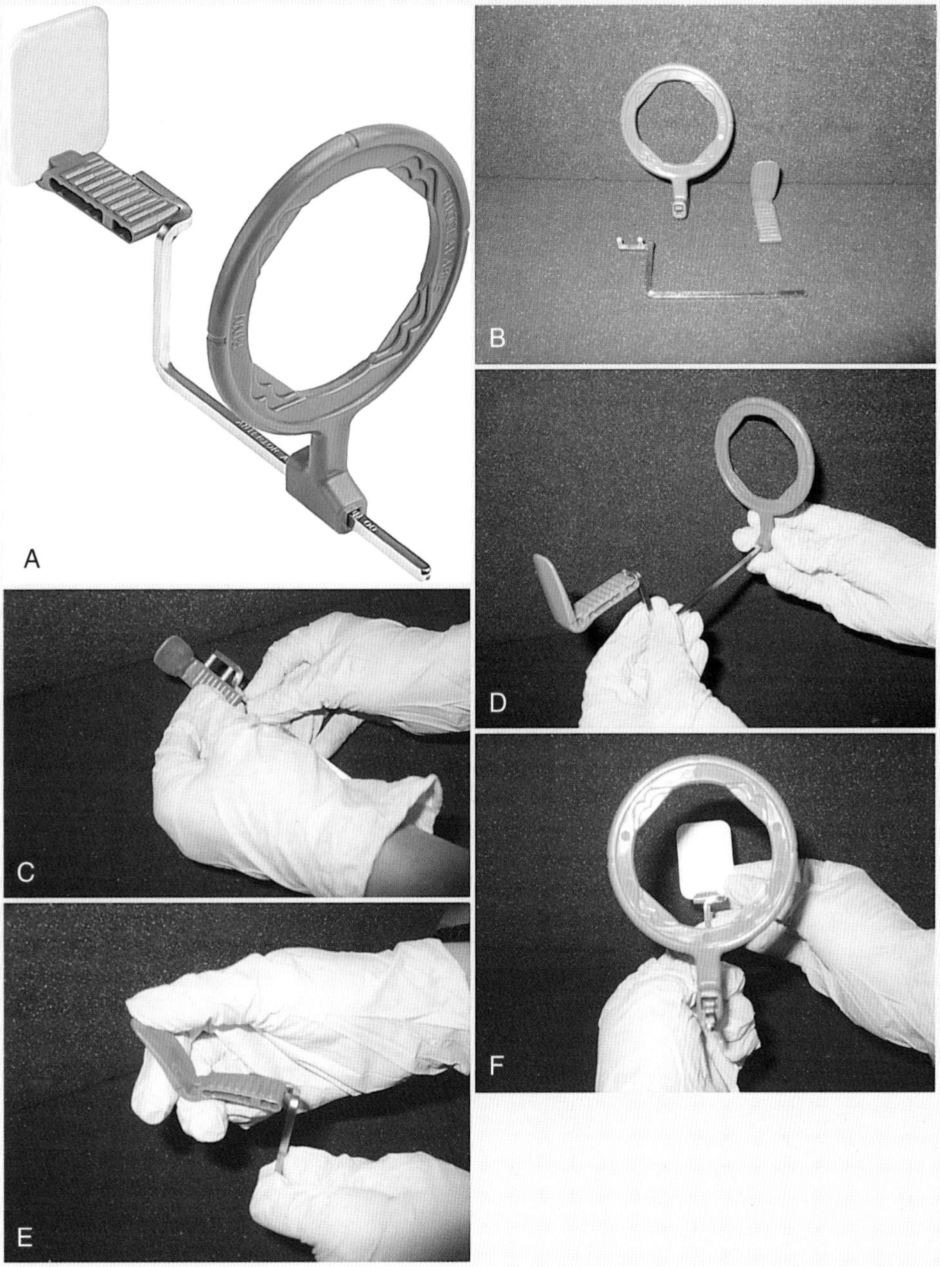

Fig 19-8 **A,** The correct assembly of the anterior Rinn XCP instrument holding an intraoral film. **B,** Parts of anterior Rinn XCP instrument. **C,** Assembly of anterior Rinn XCP instrument. The two prongs of the anterior indicator arm are inserted into the openings in the anterior bite-block, as shown. **D,** The anterior indicator arm is inserted into the opening on the anterior aiming ring, as shown. **E,** The plastic backing of bite-block is flexed to open the film slot for easy insertion of the anterior film packet. **F,** The anterior Rinn XCP instrument is correctly assembled when the film is seen centered in the middle of the aiming ring.

Continued

PROCEDURE 19-2 Equipment Preparation for Paralleling Technique—cont'd

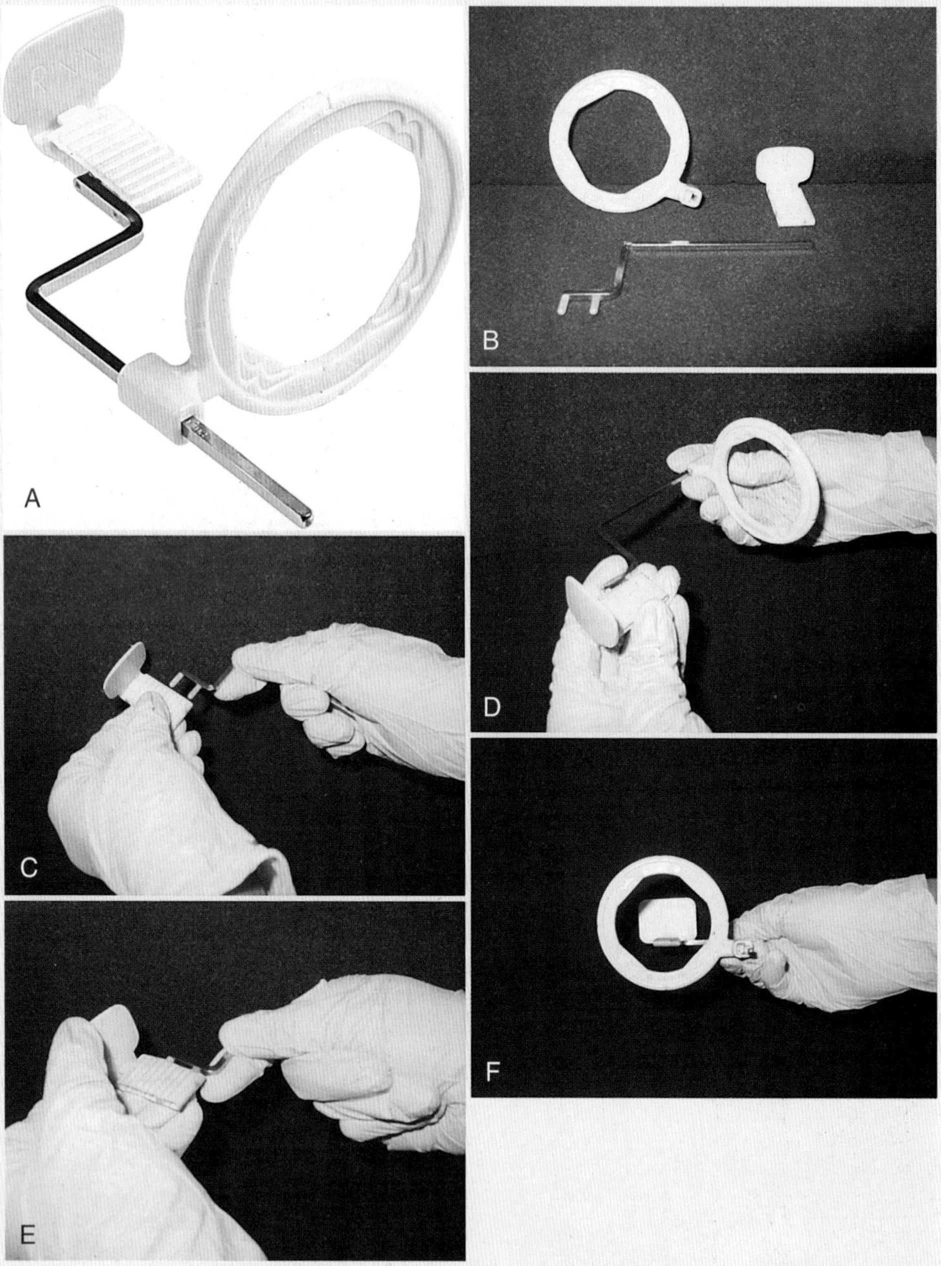

Fig 19-9 **A,** The correct assembly of the posterior XCP instrument for the maxillary left quadrant or the mandibular right quadrant. **B,** Parts of posterior XCP instrument. **C,** Assembly of posterior XCP instrument. The two prongs of the posterior indicator arm are inserted into the openings in the posterior bite-block, as shown. **D,** The posterior indicator arm is inserted into the opening on the posterior aiming ring, as shown. **E,** The plastic backing of the bite-block is flexed to open the slot for easy insertion of the posterior film packet. **F,** The posterior XCP instrument is correctly assembled when the film is seen centered in the middle of the aiming ring.

With the size 1 receptor, a total of 7 anterior placements may be used in the paralleling technique: 4 maxillary exposures and 3 mandibular exposures. If the size 2 receptor is used instead, 6 anterior placements are used: 3 maxillary exposures and 3 mandibular exposures. The authors recommend the use of size 1 receptors; the recommended anterior periapical exposure sequence for the Rinn XCP beam alignment instruments illustrated in this text is as follows (Table 19-1):

1. Assemble the anterior Rinn XCP instrument.
2. Begin with the maxillary right canine (tooth #6).
3. Expose the maxillary anterior teeth working from the patient's right to the patient's left.
4. End with the maxillary left canine (tooth #11).
5. Next, move to the mandibular arch.
6. Begin with the mandibular left canine (tooth #22).
7. Expose all the mandibular anterior teeth working from the patient's left to the patient's right.
8. Finish with the mandibular right canine (tooth #27).

TABLE 19-1 Exposure Sequence for Anterior Receptor Placements (with Rinn XCP Instruments): Paralleling Technique

Exposure Number	Arch	Side	Tooth	Tooth Number
1	Maxillary	Right	Canine	6
2	Maxillary	Right	Lateral incisor	7
	Maxillary	Right	Central incisor	8
3	Maxillary	Left	Central incisor	9
	Maxillary	Left	Lateral incisor	10
4	Maxillary	Left	Canine	11
5	Mandibular	Left	Canine	22
6	Mandibular	Left	Lateral incisor	23
	Mandibular	Left	Central incisor	24
	Mandibular	Right	Central incisor	25
	Mandibular	Right	Lateral incisor	26
7	Mandibular	Right	Canine	27

When the dental radiographer works from the patient's right to the patient's left in the maxillary arch and then from the patient's left to the patient's right in the mandibular arch, no wasted movement or shifting of the PID occurs (Figure 19-10).

In addition, when working from right to left and then from left to right, teeth are radiographed in ascending numerical order, as follows:

Teeth 6 → 7 → 8 → 9 → 10 → 11

and then ↘

Teeth 27 ← 26 ← 25 ← 24 ← 23 ← 22

This exposure sequence allows the dental radiographer to keep track of exposures easily, even when interruptions occur during the procedure.

Posterior Exposure Sequence. After the anterior exposures are completed, the posterior teeth (premolars and molars) are radiographed. In each quadrant, *always* expose the premolar receptor first followed by the molar receptor, for the following reasons:

- Premolar placements are easier for the patient to tolerate.
- Premolar placements are less likely to evoke the gag reflex.

Eight posterior placements may be used in the paralleling technique: 4 maxillary exposures and 4 mandibular exposures. The recommended exposure sequence for the posterior receptor placements varies, depending on the beam alignment device used. The recommended posterior periapical exposure sequence for the Rinn XCP beam alignment instruments illustrated in this text is as follows (Table 19-2):

1. Begin with the maxillary right quadrant.
2. Assemble the posterior Rinn XCP instrument for this area.
3. First, expose the premolar receptor (teeth #4 and 5), then expose the molar receptor (teeth #1, 2, and 3).
4. Without reassembling the posterior Rinn XCP instrument, move to the mandibular left quadrant.
5. Expose the premolar receptor (teeth #20 and 21), then expose the molar receptor (teeth #17, 18, and 19).
6. Reassemble the posterior Rinn XCP instrument over a covered work surface.
7. Next, move to the maxillary left quadrant.
8. Expose the premolar receptor (teeth #12 and 13), then expose the molar receptor (teeth #14, 15, and 16).
9. Finish with the mandibular right quadrant.
10. Expose the premolar receptor (teeth #28 and 29), and finish with the exposure of the molar receptor (teeth #30, 31, and 32).

Receptor Placement for Paralleling Technique

In a complete mouth series (CMS) using the paralleling technique, each periapical exposure has a prescribed placement. The specific teeth and their surrounding structures that must be included on the resultant image dictate receptor placement, or the specific area where the receptor must be positioned before exposure. Prescribed receptor placements for the anterior teeth are described in Box 19-1 and illustrated in Figure 19-11. Posterior placements are described in Box 19-2 and illustrated in Figure 19-12.

The specific placements described in this chapter are for a 15-receptor periapical series using size 1 receptors for anterior exposures and size 2 receptors for posterior exposures. Other reference sources or individual practitioners may recommend variations in receptor placement or the number and size of receptors used. Box 19-3 lists guidelines for periapical positioning used with the paralleling technique.

Anterior Receptor Placement. The anterior Rinn XCP instrument is used for all anterior receptor placements. After the anterior Rinn XCP instrument has been assembled, a size 1 receptor is inserted vertically into the bite-block and secured in the slot. A total of 7 anterior placements include the following:

- Two maxillary canine exposures (Procedure 19-3)
- Two maxillary incisor exposures (Procedure 19-4)
- Two mandibular canine exposures (Procedure 19-5)
- One mandibular incisor exposure (Procedure 19-6)

Posterior Receptor Placement. The posterior Rinn XCP instrument is used for all posterior receptor placements. After the posterior Rinn XCP instrument has been assembled, a size 2 receptor is inserted horizontally into the bite-block and secured in the slot. A total of 8 posterior placements include the following:

- Two maxillary premolar exposures (Procedure 19-7)
- Two maxillary molar exposures (Procedure 19-8)
- Two mandibular premolar exposures (Procedure 19-9)
- Two mandibular molar exposures (Procedure 19-10)

MODIFICATIONS IN PARALLELING TECHNIQUE

Modifications in the paralleling technique may be used to accommodate variations in anatomic conditions. Such modifications may be necessary when a patient has a shallow palate, bony growths, or a sensitive mandibular premolar region.

Shallow Palate

Parallelism between the receptor and the long axis of the tooth is difficult to accomplish in a patient with a shallow palate (roof of the mouth), also known as a *low palatal vault*. In a patient with a shallow palate, tilting of the bite-block occurs, which results in a lack of parallelism between the receptor and the long axis of the tooth. If the lack of parallelism between the receptor and the long

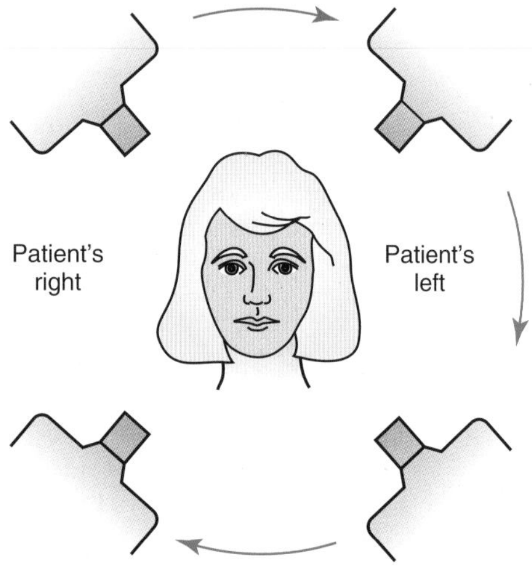

Fig 19-10 When exposing the maxillary anterior region, begin on the patient's right and work to the left. Then, expose the mandibular anterior receptors from the left to the right. No unnecessary movements of the PID result.

TABLE 19-2 Exposure Sequence for Posterior Receptor Placements (with Rinn XCP Instruments): Paralleling Technique

Exposure Number	Arch	Side	Teeth	Teeth Numbers
1	Maxillary	Right	Premolars	4, 5
2	Maxillary	Right	Molars	1, 2, 3
3	Mandibular	Left	Premolars	20, 21
4	Mandibular	Left	Molars	17, 18, 19
5	Maxillary	Left	Premolars	12, 13
6	Maxillary	Left	Molars	14, 15, 16
7	Mandibular	Right	Premolars	28, 29
8	Mandibular	Right	Molars	30, 31, 32

axis of the tooth does not exceed 20 degrees, the resultant image is generally acceptable (Figure 19-21). When the lack of parallelism is greater than 20 degrees, a modification in technique is necessary, as follows:

- *Cotton rolls.* To position the receptor parallel to the long axis of the tooth, two cotton rolls can be placed, one on each side of the bite-block (Figure 19-22). As a result, however, periapical coverage is reduced.
- *Vertical angulation.* To compensate for the lack of parallelism, the vertical angulation can be increased by 5 to 15 degrees more than the Rinn XCP instrument indicates. However, image distortion occurs as a result.

Bony Growths

A torus (plural, tori) is a bony growth seen in the oral cavity. A maxillary torus (torus palatinus) is a nodular mass of bone seen along the midline of the hard palate (Figure 19-23). Mandibular tori (singular, torus mandibularis) are bony growths along the lingual aspect (tongue side) of the mandible (Figure 19-24). When using the paralleling technique, maxillary and mandibular tori can cause problems with receptor placement, and modifications in technique are necessary, as follows:

- For a maxillary torus, the receptor must be placed on the far side of the torus (not *on* the torus) and then exposed (Figure 19-25, A).

BOX 19-1 Prescribed Placements for Anterior Periapical Exposures: Paralleling Technique

Maxillary Canine

- The entire crown and root of the canine, including the apex and the surrounding structures, must be visible.
- The interproximal alveolar bone and mesial contact of the canine must also be visible.
- The lingual cusp of the first premolar usually obscures the distal contact of the canine.

Maxillary Incisor

- The entire crowns and roots of one lateral and one central incisor, including the apices of the teeth and the surrounding structures, must be visible.
- The interproximal alveolar bone between the central and lateral and the mesial and distal contact areas, as well as the surrounding regions of bone, must also be visible.
- The mesial contact of the adjacent central incisor and the mesial contact of the adjacent canine should also be visible.

Mandibular Canine

- The entire crown and root of the canine, including the apex and the surrounding structures, must be visible.
- The interproximal alveolar bone and mesial and distal contacts must also be visible.

Mandibular Incisor

- The entire crowns and roots of the four mandibular incisors, including the apices of the teeth and the surrounding structures, must be visible.
- The contacts between the central incisors and those between the central and lateral incisors must also be visible.

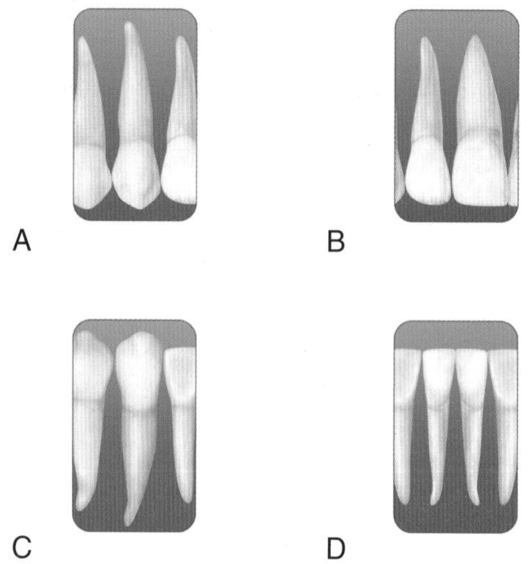

Fig 19-11 Prescribed placements for anterior periapical receptors. **A,** Exposure of the maxillary canine. **B,** Exposure of the maxillary lateral and central incisors. **C,** Exposure of the mandibular canine. **D,** Exposure of the mandibular lateral and central incisors.

BOX 19-2 Prescribed Placements for Posterior Periapical Exposures: Paralleling Technique

Maxillary Premolar

- All crowns and roots of the first and second premolars and of the first molar, including the apices, alveolar crests, contact areas, and surrounding bone, must be visible.
- The distal contact of the maxillary canine must also be visible.

Maxillary Molar

- All crowns and roots of the first, second, and third molars, including the apices, alveolar crests, contact areas, surrounding bone, and tuberosity region, must be visible.
- The distal contact of the maxillary second premolar must also be visible.

Mandibular Premolar

- All crowns and roots of the first and second premolars and of the first molar, including the apices, alveolar crests, contact areas, and surrounding bone, must be visible.
- The distal contact of the mandibular canine must also be visible.

Mandibular Molar

- All crowns and roots of the first, second, and third molars, including the apices, alveolar crests, contact areas, and surrounding bone, must be visible.
- The distal contact of the mandibular second premolar must also be visible.

BOX 19-3 Guidelines for Receptor Placement with Paralleling Technique

1. If using film, the white side of the film always faces the teeth ("white in sight"), and the identification dot is placed at the incisal or occlusal edge. When using a sensor, position the sensor toward the x-ray tube according to manufacturer directions.
2. The anterior receptors are always placed vertically.
3. The posterior receptors are always placed horizontally.
4. When placing the receptor in the mouth, always lead with the apical end of the receptor, and then rotate the beam alignment device.
5. When positioning the beam alignment device, always place the receptor away from the teeth and toward the middle of the oral cavity.
6. When positioning the beam alignment device, always center the receptor over the area to be examined (as defined in the prescribed placements).
7. When positioning the beam alignment device, ask the patient to "slowly close" on the bite-block. Always make certain that the teeth and not the lips stabilize the bite-block.

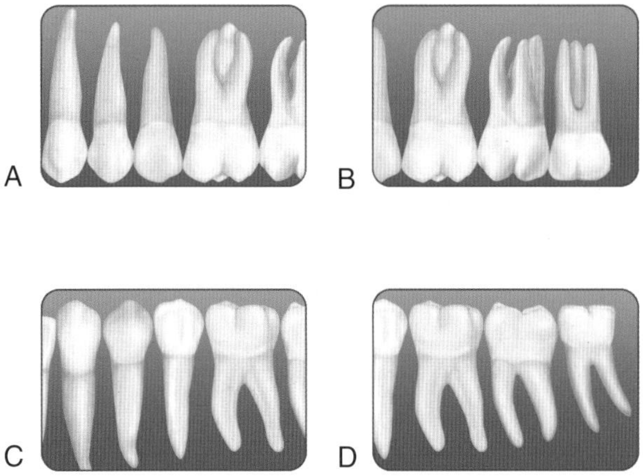

Fig 19-12 Prescribed placements for posterior periapical receptors. **A,** Exposure of the maxillary premolar. **B,** Exposure of the maxillary molar. **C,** Exposure of the mandibular premolar. **D,** Exposure of the mandibular molar.

A maxillary torus appears as a radiopacity on the dental image (Figure 19-25, B).

- For mandibular tori, the receptor must be placed between the tori and the tongue (not *on* the tori) and then exposed (Figure 19-26, A). Mandibular tori also appear radiopaque on the dental image (Figure 19-26, B).

Mandibular Premolar Region

The anterior floor of the mouth area can be a very sensitive region. When periapical placements cause discomfort in the mandibular premolar region, a modification in technique is necessary, as follows:

- *Receptor placement.* The receptor must be placed under the tongue to avoid impinging on muscle attachments and the sensitive soft tissues on the floor of the mouth. When inserting the beam alignment device into the mouth, the receptor is tipped away from the tongue and toward the teeth being examined while the bite-block is placed firmly on the mandibular premolars. As the patient slowly closes and gently bites on the bite-block, the receptor is gently moved into the proper position (Figure 19-27).
- *Film.* If using film, the lower edge of the film can be gently curved, or softened, to prevent discomfort. Bending or creasing the film, however, must be avoided.

ADVANTAGES AND DISADVANTAGES

As with all intraoral techniques, the paralleling technique has both advantages and disadvantages. The advantages of the paralleling technique, however, outweigh the disadvantages.

Advantages of Paralleling Technique

The primary advantage of the paralleling technique is that it produces an image without dimensional distortion. In addition, it is uncomplicated and can be easily repeated when serial images are indicated. The advantages of the paralleling technique can be summarized as follows:

- *Accuracy.* The paralleling technique produces an image that has dimensional accuracy; the image is highly representative of the actual tooth. The image is free of distortion and exhibits maximum detail and definition.
- *Simplicity.* The paralleling technique is simple and easy to learn and use. The use of a beam alignment device eliminates the need for the dental radiographer to determine horizontal and vertical angulations and also eliminates the chances of dimensional distortion.
- *Duplication.* The paralleling technique is easy to standardize and can be accurately duplicated, or repeated, when serial images are indicated. As a result, comparisons of serial images exposed using the paralleling technique have great validity.

Disadvantages of Paralleling Technique

The primary disadvantage of the paralleling technique is receptor placement. Patient discomfort may also be a problem. The disadvantages of the paralleling technique can be summarized as follows:

- *Receptor placement.* Because a beam alignment device must be used with the paralleling technique, receptor placement may be difficult for the dental radiographer. Difficulties may be encountered with the pediatric patient or with the adult patient who has a small

Text to continue on page 184

PROCEDURE 19-3 Maxillary Canine Exposure: Paralleling Technique (Figure 19-13)

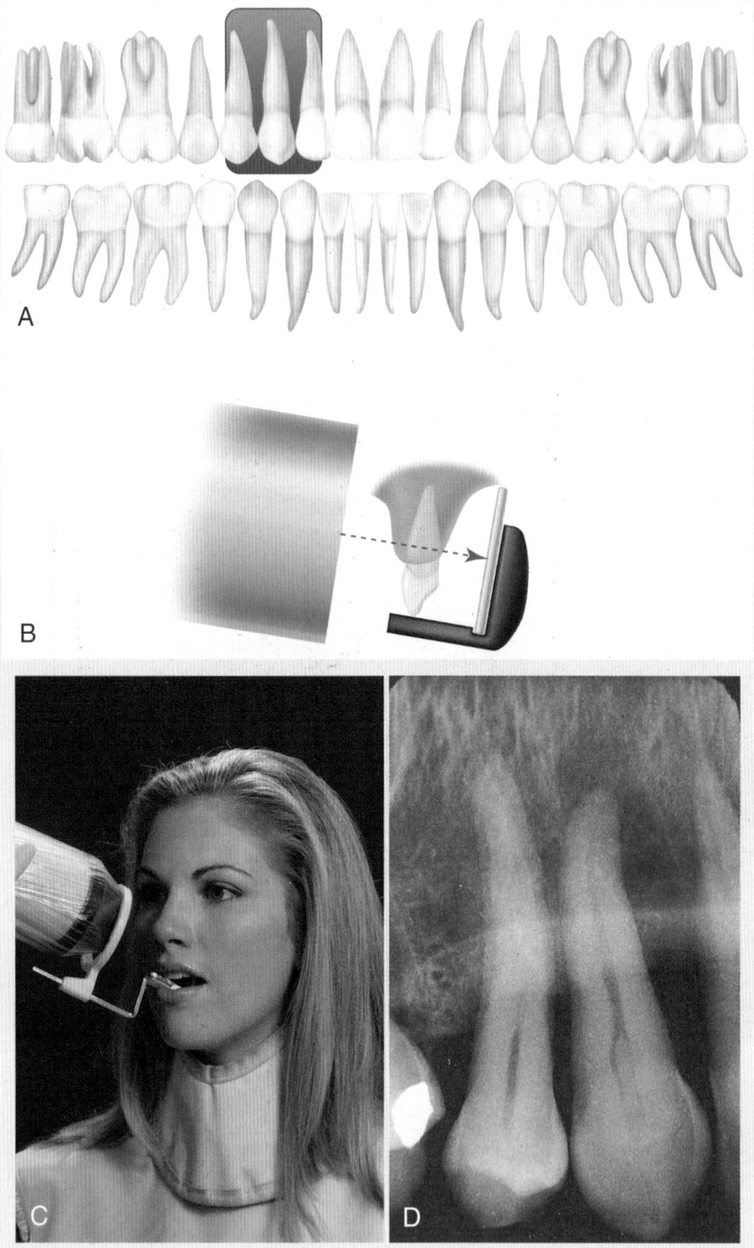

Fig 19-13 Exposure of the maxillary canine. **A,** Receptor placement. **B,** Positions of the receptor, tooth, and central ray. **C,** Exposure of the receptor with rectangular collimation. **D,** Resultant image.

1. Center the anterior Rinn XCP with receptor on the maxillary canine.
2. Position the receptor as far away from the teeth as possible.
3. Instruct the patient to "slowly close" and gently bite on the bite-block.
4. Slide the aiming ring down the indicator arm to the skin surface.
5. Align the PID with the aiming ring.
6. Expose the receptor.

PROCEDURE 19-4 Maxillary Incisor Exposure: Paralleling Technique (Figure 19-14)

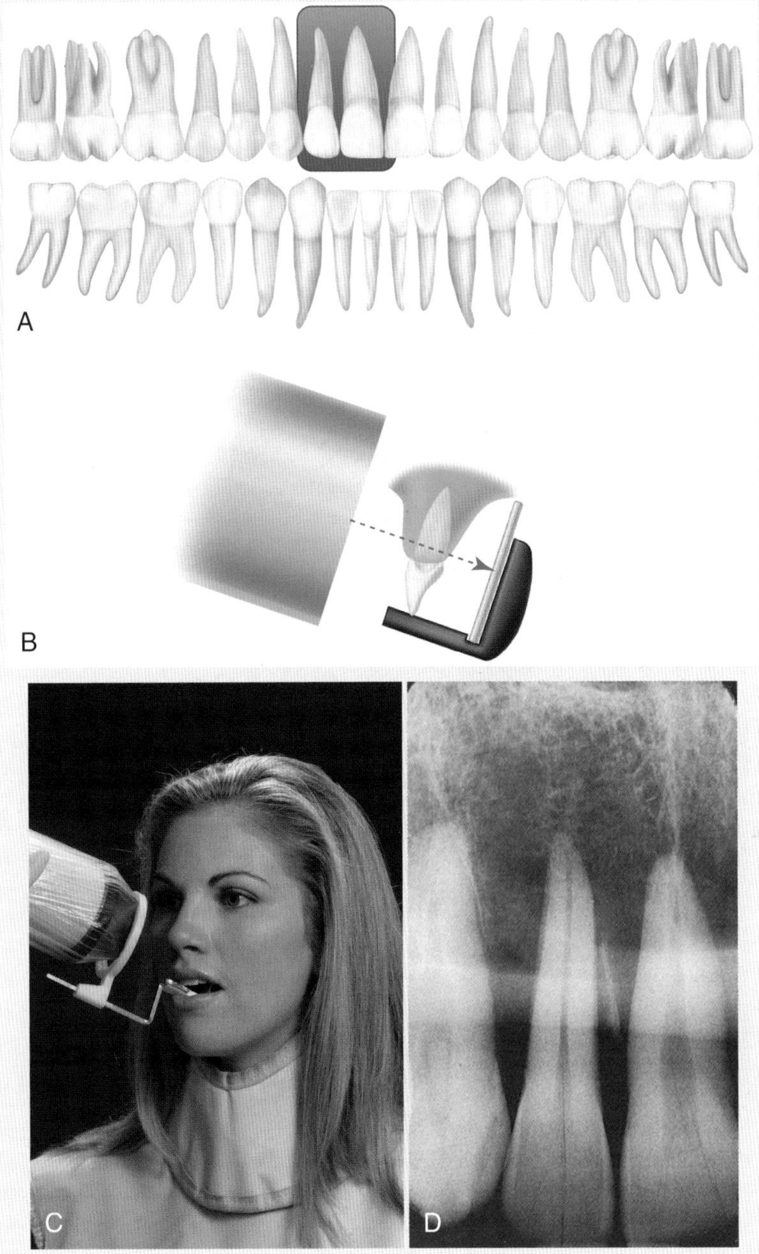

Fig 19-14 Exposure of the maxillary incisors. **A,** Receptor placement. **B,** Positions of the receptor, teeth, and central ray. **C,** Exposure of the receptor with rectangular collimation. **D,** Resultant image.

1. Center the anterior Rinn XCP with receptor on the contact between the maxillary central incisor and the lateral incisor.
2. Position the receptor as far away from the teeth as possible.
3. Instruct the patient to "slowly close" and gently bite on the bite-block.
4. Slide the aiming ring down the indicator arm to the skin surface.
5. Align the PID with the aiming ring.
6. Expose the receptor.

PROCEDURE 19-5 Mandibular Canine Exposure: Paralleling Technique (Figure 19-15)

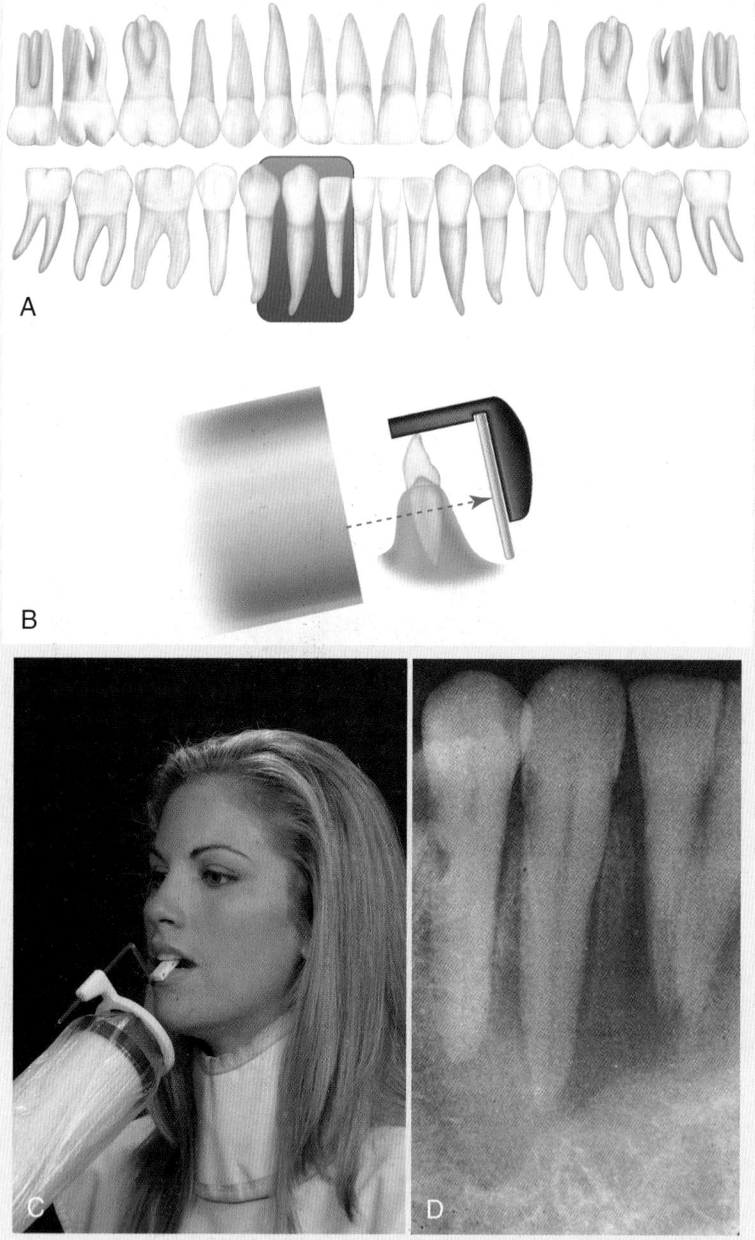

Fig 19-15 Exposure of the mandibular canine. **A,** Receptor placement. **B,** Positions of the receptor, tooth, and central ray. **C,** Exposure of receptor with rectangular collimation. **D,** Resultant image.

1. Center the anterior Rinn XCP with receptor on the mandibular canine.
2. Position the receptor as far away from the teeth as possible.
3. Instruct the patient to "slowly close" and gently bite on the bite-block.
4. Slide the aiming ring down the indicator arm to the skin surface.
5. Align the PID with the aiming ring.
6. Expose the receptor.

PROCEDURE 19-6 Mandibular Incisor Exposure: Paralleling Technique (Figure 19-16)

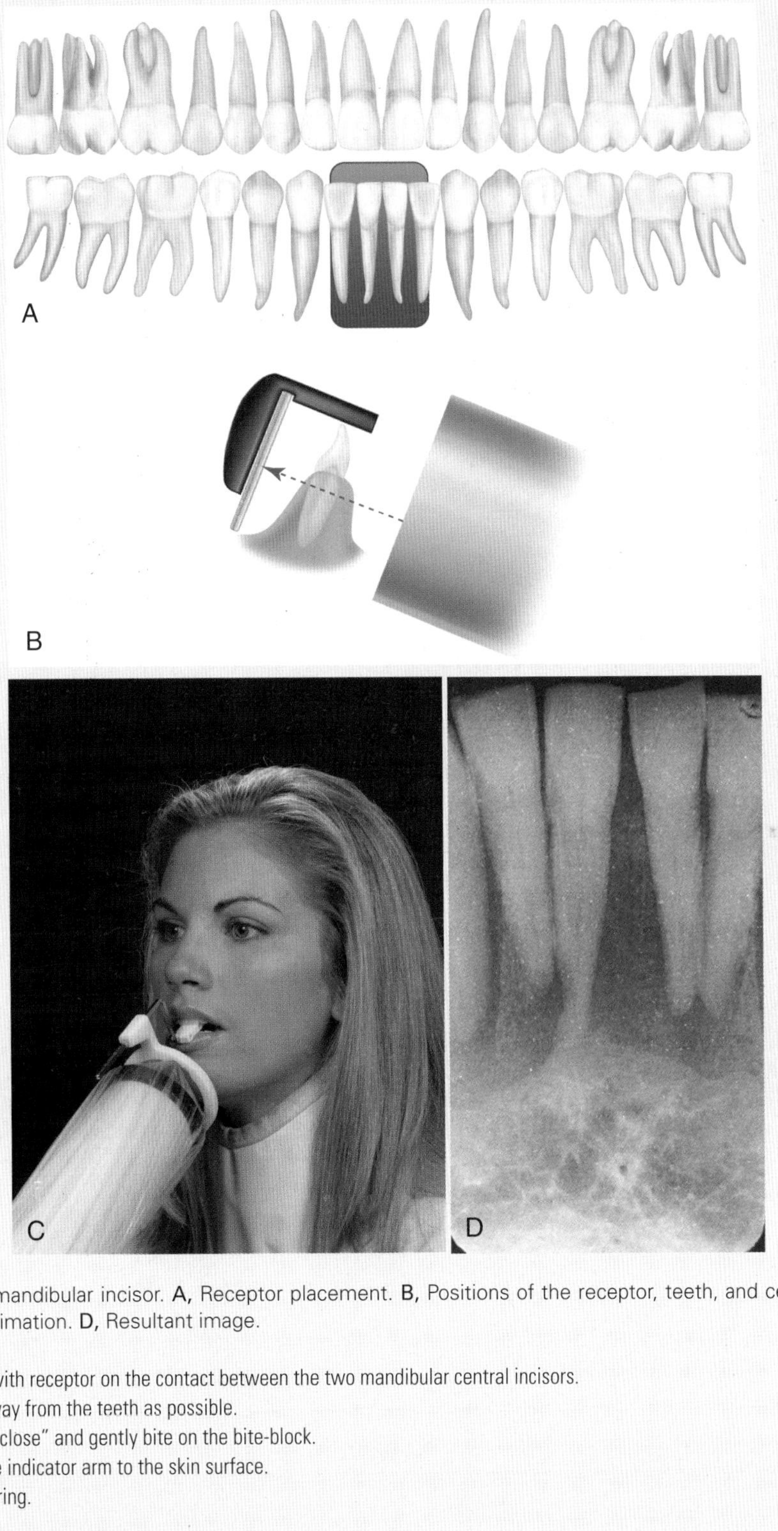

Fig 19-16 Exposure of the mandibular incisor. **A,** Receptor placement. **B,** Positions of the receptor, teeth, and central ray. **C,** Exposure of the receptor with rectangular collimation. **D,** Resultant image.

1. Center the anterior Rinn XCP with receptor on the contact between the two mandibular central incisors.
2. Position the receptor as far away from the teeth as possible.
3. Instruct the patient to "slowly close" and gently bite on the bite-block.
4. Slide the aiming ring down the indicator arm to the skin surface.
5. Align the PID with the aiming ring.
6. Expose the receptor.

PROCEDURE 19-7 Maxillary Premolar Exposure: Paralleling Technique (Figure 19-17)

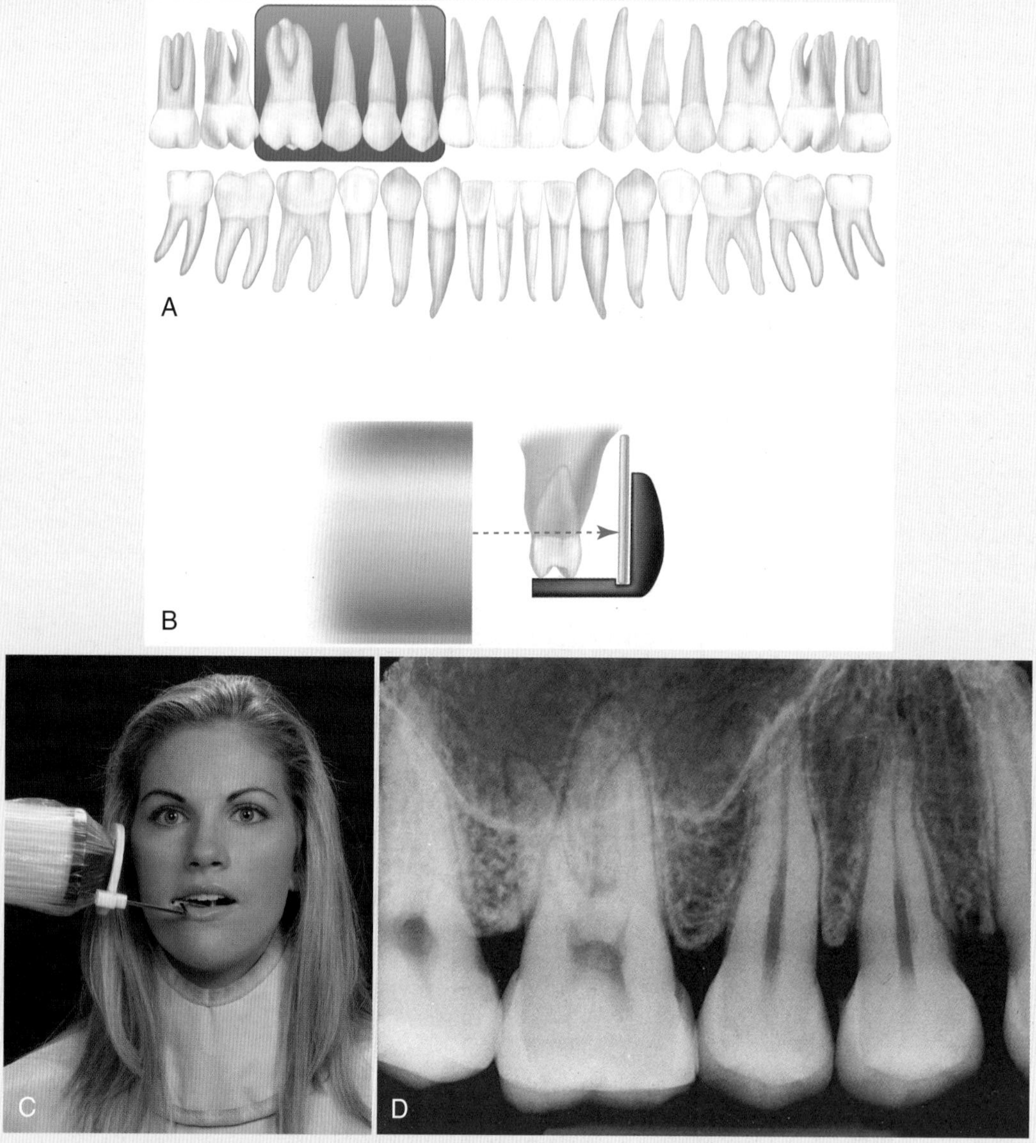

Fig 19-17 Exposure of the maxillary premolar. **A,** Receptor placement. **B,** Positions of the receptor, teeth, and central ray. **C,** Exposure of the receptor with rectangular collimation. **D,** Resultant image.

1. Center the posterior Rinn XCP with receptor on the maxillary second premolar; the front edge of the receptor should cover the distal half of the maxillary canine.
2. Position the receptor as far away from the teeth as possible.
3. Instruct the patient to "slowly close" and gently bite on the bite-block.
4. Slide the aiming ring down the indicator arm to the skin surface.
5. Align the PID with the aiming ring.
6. Expose the receptor.

PROCEDURE 19-8 Maxillary Molar Exposure: Paralleling Technique (Figure 19-18)

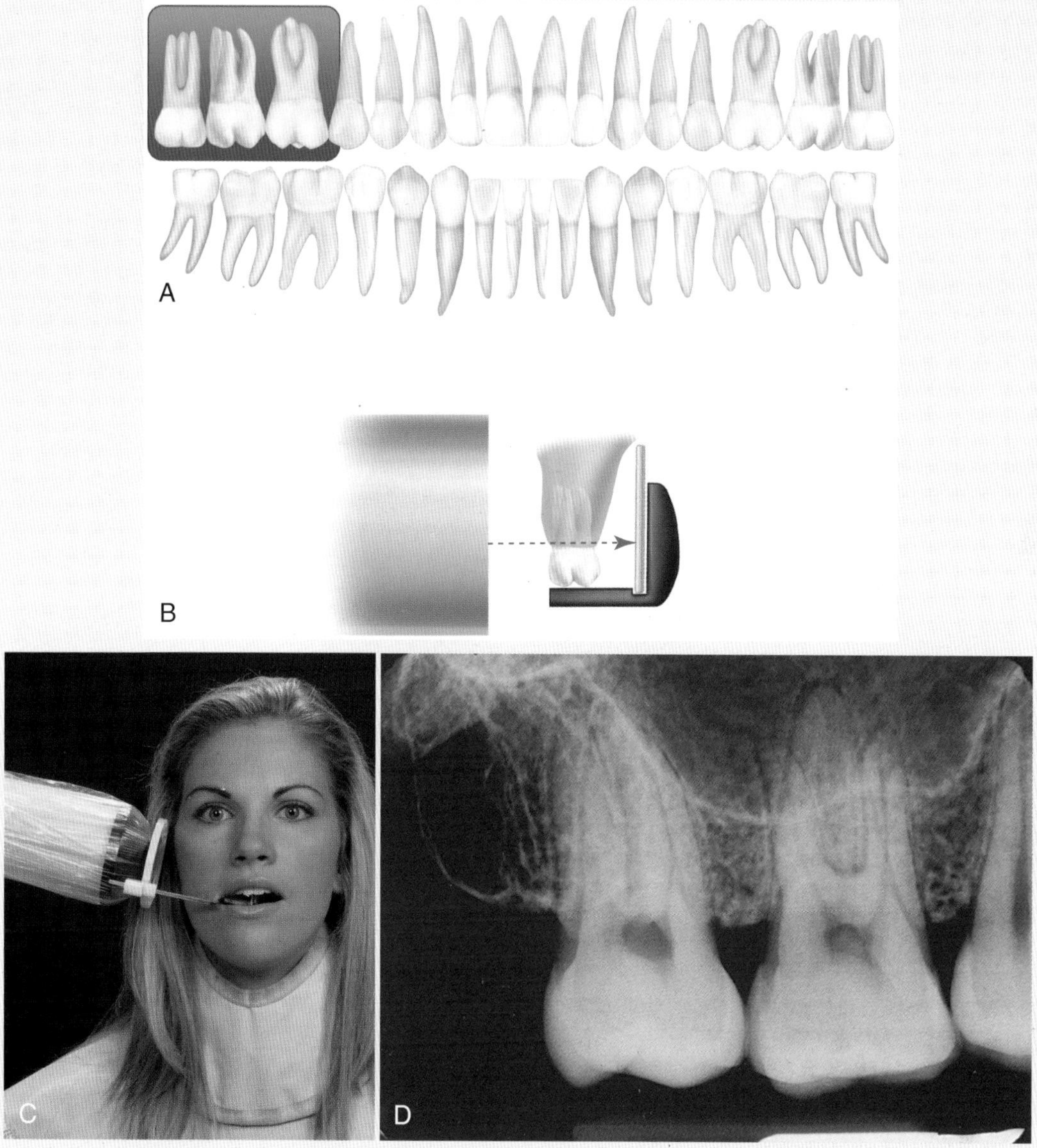

Fig 19-18 Exposure of the maxillary molar. **A,** Receptor placement. **B,** Positions of the receptor, teeth, and central ray. **C,** Exposure of the receptor with rectangular collimation. **D,** Resultant image.

1. Center the posterior Rinn XCP with receptor on the maxillary second molar; the front edge of the receptor should cover the distal half of the maxillary second premolar.
2. Position the receptor as far away from the teeth as possible.
3. Instruct the patient to "slowly close" and gently bite on the bite-block.
4. Slide the aiming ring down the indicator arm to the skin surface.
5. Align the PID with the aiming ring.
6. Expose the receptor.

PROCEDURE 19-9 Mandibular Premolar Exposure: Paralleling Technique (Figure 19-19)

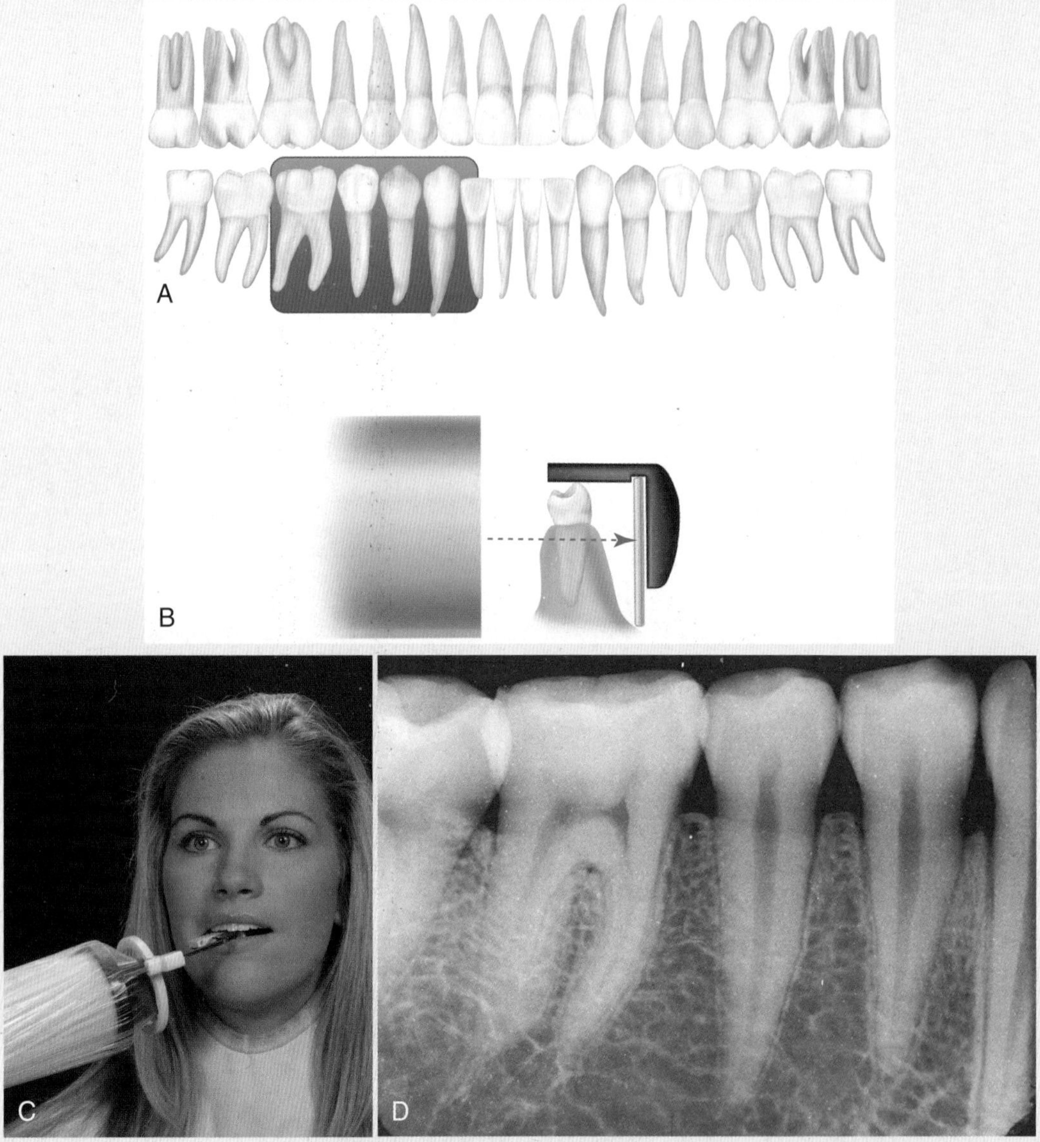

Fig 19-19 Exposure of the mandibular premolar. **A,** Receptor placement. **B,** Positions of the receptor, teeth, and central ray. **C,** Exposure of the receptor with rectangular collimation. **D,** Resultant image.

1. Center the posterior Rinn XCP with receptor on the mandibular second premolar; the front edge of the receptor should cover the distal half of the mandibular canine.
2. Position the receptor as far away from the teeth as possible.
3. Instruct the patient to "slowly close" and gently bite on the bite-block.
4. Slide the aiming ring down the indicator arm to the skin surface.
5. Align the PID with the aiming ring.
6. Expose the receptor.

PROCEDURE 19-10 Mandibular Molar Exposure: Paralleling Technique (Figure 19-20)

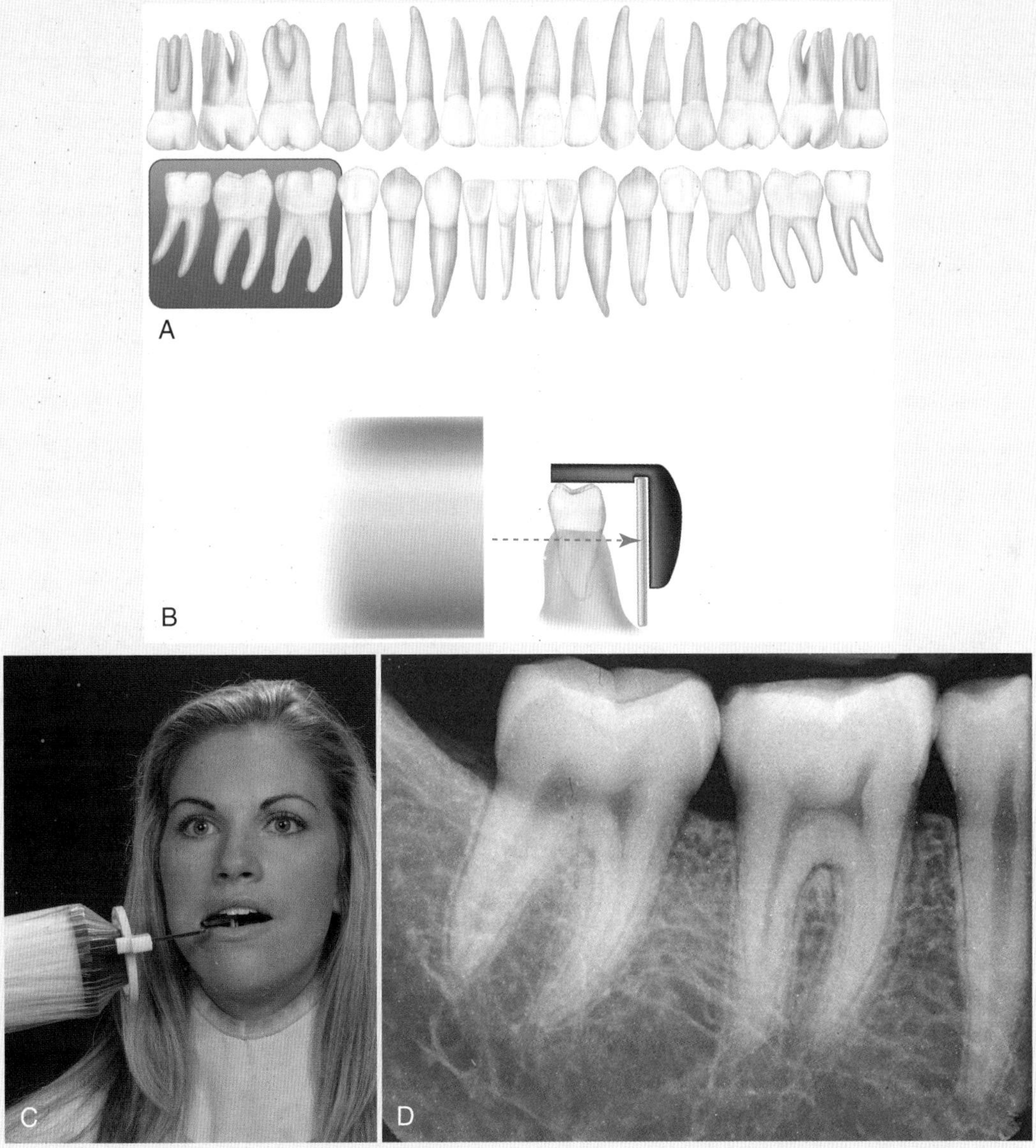

Fig 19-20 Exposure of the mandibular molar. **A,** Receptor placement. **B,** Positions of the receptor, teeth, and central ray. **C,** Exposure of the receptor with rectangular collimation. **D,** Resultant image.

1. Center the posterior Rinn XCP with receptor on the mandibular second molar; the front edge of the receptor should cover the distal half of the mandibular second premolar.
2. Position the receptor as far away from the teeth as possible.
3. Instruct the patient to "slowly close" and gently bite on the bite-block.
4. Slide the aiming ring down the indicator arm to the skin surface.
5. Align the PID with the aiming ring.
6. Expose the receptor.

Continued

PROCEDURE 19-10 Mandibular Molar Exposure: Paralleling Technique (Figure 19-20)—cont'd

An example of a charting note for a full-mouth series using the paralleling technique is provided below.

CHARTING A FULL-MOUTH SERIES

Date	ADA Procedure Code	Provider	Charting Notes	Comments
12/1/21	0210	LJH	Dr. Smith prescribed a complete mouth series of 19 images; paralleling technique used with Rinn XCP instruments; 15 periapicals and 4 bite-wings exposed; 1 right molar bite-wing retaken because of patient movement; Digital PSP plates used (20 total exposures)	Patient tolerated procedure fairly well; mandibular premolar region was difficult to place receptor because presence of bilateral tori; used the Stabe Bite-block for both mandibular premolar periapical projections; patient opened her mouth before the right molar bite-wing was exposed (retake required)

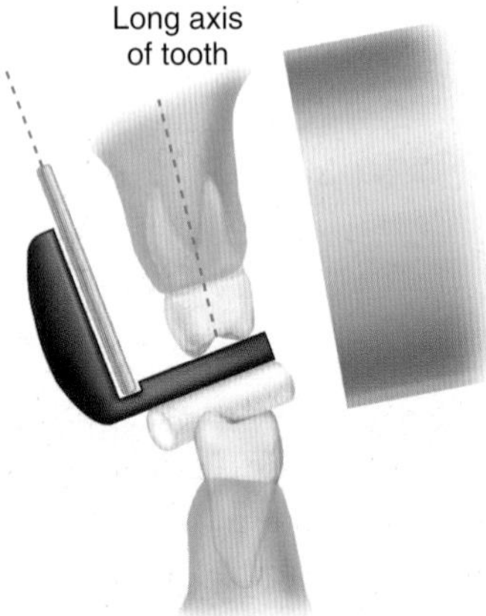

Fig 19-21 Tilting of the bite-block results in a lack of parallelism between the receptor and the long axis of the tooth. When the lack of parallelism is less than 20 degrees (*as shown in this diagram*), the image is generally acceptable.

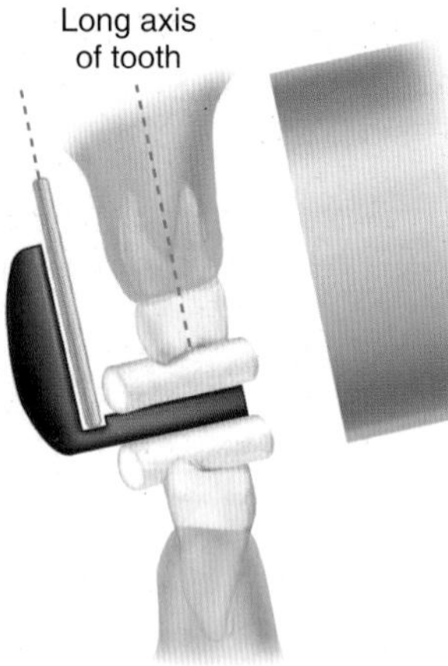

Fig 19-22 Two cotton rolls can be used to position the receptor parallel to the long axis of the tooth.

mouth or a shallow palate. Such placements become less problematic as the dental radiographer becomes more proficient at using the paralleling technique.

- *Discomfort.* The beam alignment device used to position the receptor in the paralleling technique may impinge on the oral tissues and cause discomfort for the patient.

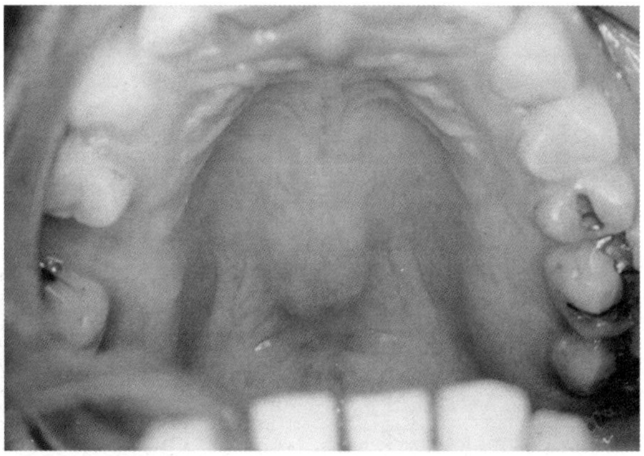

Fig 19-23 A maxillary torus.

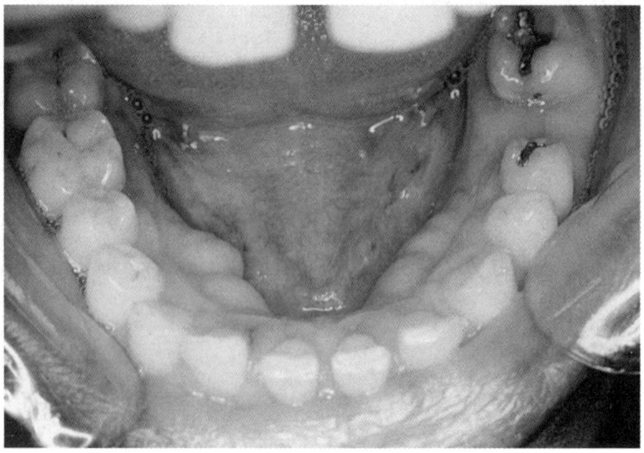

Fig 19-24 Mandibular tori.

HELPFUL HINTS

In using the paralleling technique:

- **DO** set all exposure control factors (kilovoltage, milliamperage, time) before placing any receptors in the mouth.
- **DO** ask patients to remove eyeglasses and all intraoral objects before placing any receptors in the mouth.
- **DO** use a definite order (exposure sequence) when exposing receptors to avoid errors and to make efficient use of time.
- **DO** place each film in the bite-block with the "dot in the slot." The identification dot must be located at the occlusal or incisal

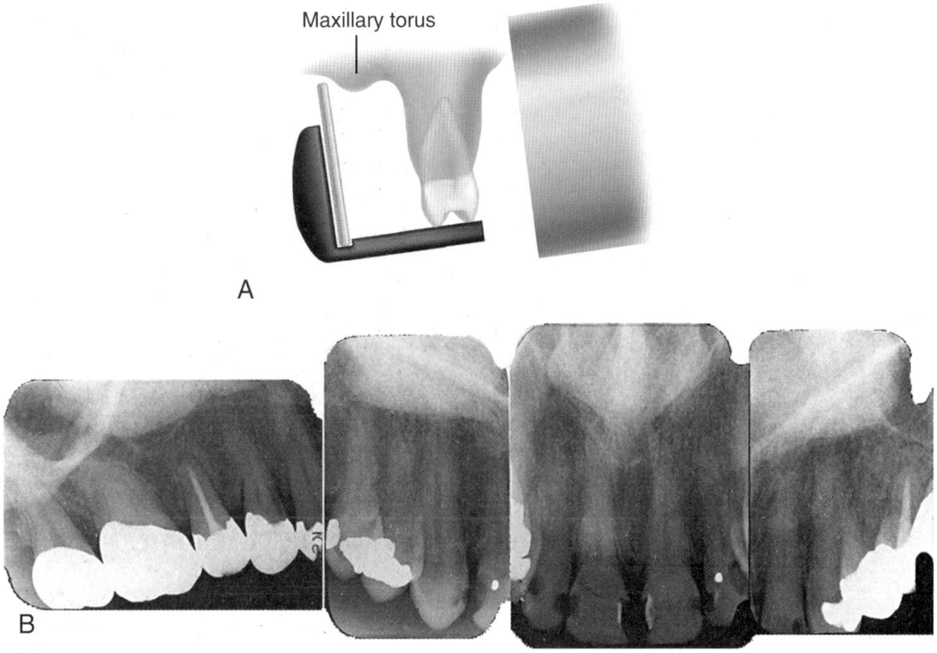

Fig 19-25 A, If a maxillary torus is present, the receptor must be placed on the far side of the torus and then exposed. B, Periapical radiographs reveal a maxillary torus as seen by the radiopaque areas superior to the apices of the teeth. (B, Courtesy Mallya SM, Lam EWN: *White and Pharoah's oral radiology: principles and interpretation, ed 8, St. Louis, 2019, Elsevier.*)

end of the film; this facilitates film mounting and ensures that the dot will not interfere with the diagnosis in the periapical area.

- **DO** explain the imaging procedures that will be performed; instruct patients on how to close and remain still during the exposure.
- **DO** communicate clearly with patients; patients are more likely to be tolerant of discomfort when they understand why a receptor must be placed in a specific area.
- **DO** use the word *please;* say, "Open, please."
- **DO** use praise; tell cooperative patients how much they are helping to simplify and speed the imaging procedure.
- **DO** instruct patients to "slowly close" and gently bite on the bite-block; when patients close slowly, the musculature relaxes and thus discomfort is reduced.
- **DO** align the PID such that the opening of the PID and the rectangular collimator are flush with the aiming ring of the Rinn XCP instrument.
- **DO NOT** bend or crimp a film packet or PSP digital sensors; excessive bending causes distortion of the image.
- **DO NOT** use words such as *hurt*. Instead, inform patients that the procedure will be "momentarily uncomfortable."
- **DO NOT** make comments such as "Oops" or other statements that indicate a lack of control in a situation. Patients will lose confidence in your abilities when hearing such comments.
- **DO NOT** pick up a receptor if you drop it. Leave it on the floor, as it has now become contaminated. Instead, remove it and dispose of it when you clean the treatment area.
- **DO NOT** allow patients to dictate how you should perform your imaging duties. Some patients need to be handled firmly. The dental radiographer must always remain in control of the procedures.
- **DO NOT** begin with posterior exposures; posterior placements may cause patients to gag. Instead, always begin with the easier anterior exposures.
- **DO NOT** position receptors on top of a torus (or tori); the apical regions of the teeth will not be seen on the resultant image. Instead, always position receptors behind the torus (or tori).

SUMMARY

- The paralleling technique is used to obtain periapical images. The receptor is placed in the mouth parallel to the long axis of the tooth, and the central ray is directed perpendicular to the receptor and the long axis of the tooth. To achieve parallelism between the receptor and the tooth, the receptor must be placed away from the tooth and toward the middle of the oral cavity.
- A beam alignment device must be used with the paralleling technique to position the receptor parallel to the long axis of the tooth. The sizes of intraoral receptors used in the paralleling technique depend on the teeth being imaged. With anterior teeth, size 1 receptors are used; with posterior teeth, size 2 receptors are used.
- The five basic rules with regard to the paralleling technique are as follows: (1) The receptor must cover the prescribed area of interest; (2) the receptor must be positioned parallel to the long axis of the tooth; (3) the central ray must be directed perpendicular to the receptor and the long axis of the tooth; (4) the central ray must be directed through the contact areas between teeth; and (5) the x-ray beam must be centered over the receptor to ensure that all areas of the receptor are exposed.
- Before imaging procedures using the paralleling technique begin, infection prevention measures must be completed, and the treatment area and the supplies must be prepared. After the patient is seated and the imaging procedures explained, adjustments to the chair and headrest are made, the lead apron is placed, and the patient is asked to remove eyeglasses and any intraoral objects. The exposure factors are then set and the beam alignment devices are assembled.

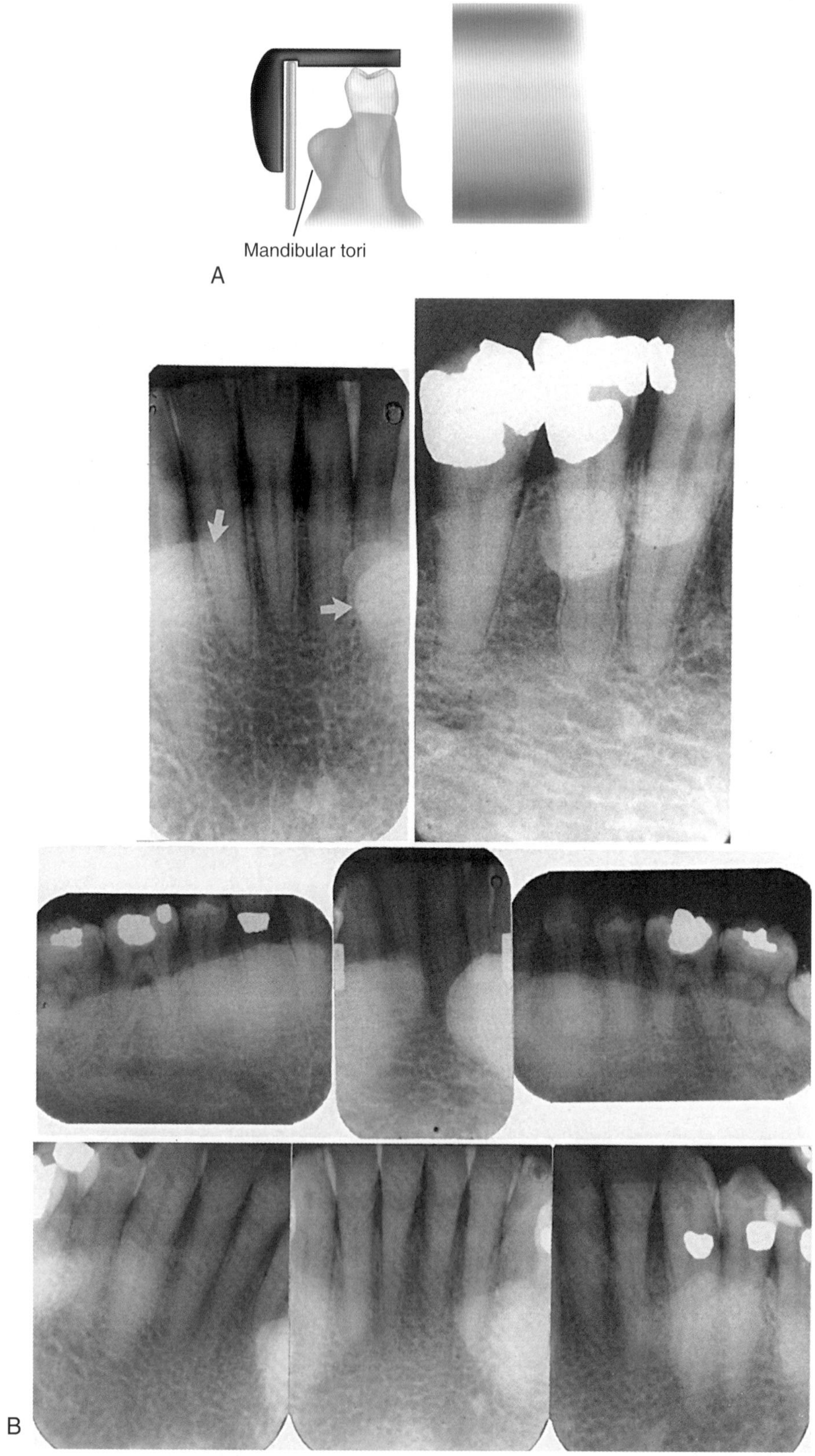

Fig 19-26 **A,** If mandibular tori are present, the receptor must be placed on the far side of the tori and then exposed. **B,** Bilateral mandibular tori are seen as dense radiopacities in the region of the canine and the first premolar. (**B,** Courtesy Mallya SM, Lam EWN: *White and Pharoah's oral radiology: principles and interpretation, ed 8, St. Louis, 2019, Elsevier.*)

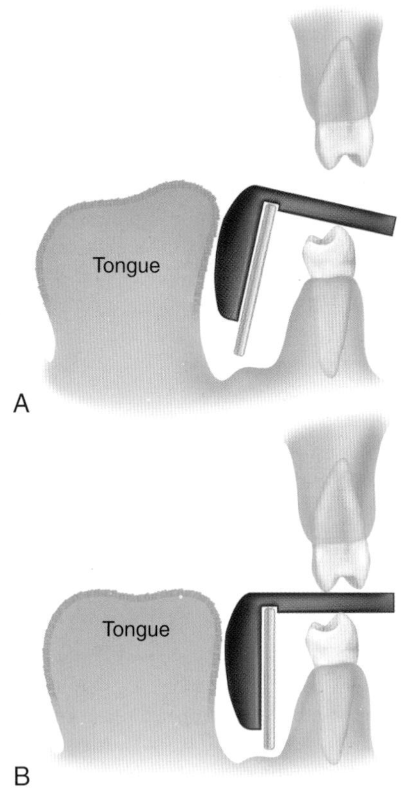

Fig 19-27 Positioning of the Rinn XCP instrument in the sensitive mandibular premolar area. **A,** The receptor is tipped away from the tongue while the bite-block is placed firmly on the mandibular premolars. **B,** When the patient closes on the bite-block, the receptor is moved into proper position.

- When using the paralleling technique, always begin with anterior exposures (easier for patient to tolerate, more comfortable, less likely to cause gagging), and then move on to the posterior regions. In each posterior quadrant, always expose the premolar receptor first and then the molar receptor.
- In a complete mouth series (CMS) using paralleling technique, each periapical exposure has a prescribed receptor placement (see Boxes 19-1 and 19-2 and Figs. 19-11 and 19-12).
- Modifications in paralleling technique may be necessary when a patient has a low or shallow palate, bony growths, or a sensitive mandibular premolar region.
- The advantages of the paralleling technique include the following: (1) it produces images with dimensional accuracy, (2) it is simple and easy to learn and use, (3) it is easy to standardize, and (4) it can be accurately repeated.
- The disadvantages of the paralleling technique are as follows: (1) placements of receptors may be difficult for the dental radiographer and (2) placement of the receptor in the patient's mouth may cause discomfort.

TECHNIQUE VIDEOS

View the Technique Videos and complete the accompanying Interactive Exercises that are available as part of the Student Resources on the companion Evolve website for this textbook.

BIBLIOGRAPHY

ADA Council on Scientific Affairs: Dental radiographic examinations: recommendations for patient selection and limiting radiation exposure, 2012.

Frommer HH, Stabulas-Savage JJ: Intraoral technique: the paralleling method. In Radiology for the dental professional, ed 9, St. Louis, 2011, Mosby.

Johnson ON: Intraoral radiographic procedures. In Essentials of dental radiography for dental assistants and hygienists, ed 9, Upper Saddle River, NJ, 2011, Prentice Hall.

Johnson ON: The periapical examination. In Essentials of dental radiography for dental assistants and hygienists, ed 9, Upper Saddle River, NJ, 2011, Prentice Hall.

Mallya SM, Lam EWN: Benign tumors and neoplasms. In White and Pharoah's oral radiology: principles and interpretation, ed 8, St. Louis, 2019, Elsevier.

Mallya SM, Lam EWN: Intraoral projections. In White and Pharoah's oral radiology: principles and interpretation, ed 8, St. Louis, 2019, Elsevier.

Miles DA, Van Dis ML, Jensen CW, et al: Intraoral radiographic technique. In Radiographic imaging for dental auxiliaries, ed 4, Philadelphia, 2009, Saunders.

Miles DA, Van Dis ML, Razmus TF: Intraoral radiographic techniques. In Basic principles of oral and maxillofacial radiology, Philadelphia, 1992, Saunders.

QUIZ QUESTIONS

Matching

For questions 1 to 8, refer to Figure 19-28. Match the letters (A to H) of the appropriate items with the descriptions below:

____ 1. size 1 receptor
____ 2. size 2 receptor
____ 3. Rinn XCP aiming ring, posterior
____ 4. Rinn XCP aiming ring, anterior
____ 5. Rinn XCP indicator arm, posterior
____ 6. Rinn XCP indicator arm, anterior
____ 7. Rinn XCP bite-block, posterior
____ 8. Rinn XCP bite-block, anterior

Short Answer

9. What happens to the image when the object-receptor distance is increased?

____
____
____
____

10. What piece of equipment is required to hold the receptor parallel to the long axis of the tooth in the paralleling technique?

____
____
____

11. What do the letters X, C, and P refer to?

____
____
____
____

12. What size receptor is typically used with the anterior Rinn XCP instrument?

____
____
____
____
____

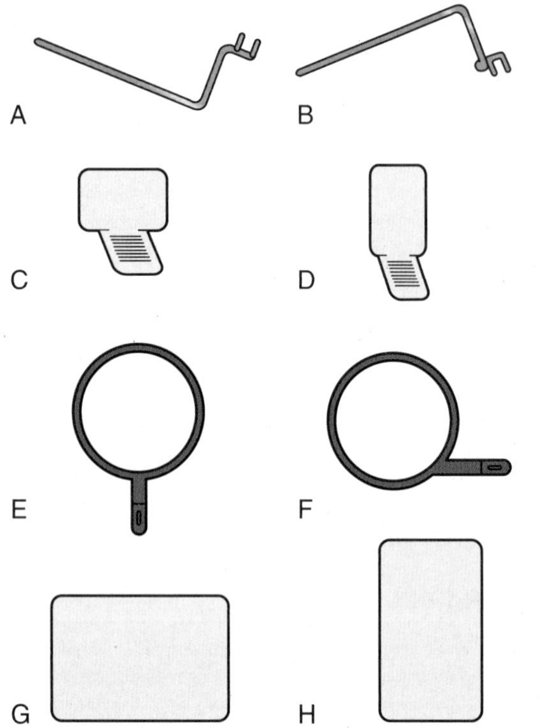

Fig 19-28

13. What size receptor is used with the posterior Rinn XCP instrument?

____
____
____
____

14. Which beam alignment devices are recommended for use with the paralleling technique to reduce radiation exposure of the patient?

____
____
____
____

15. How is the patient's head positioned before exposing receptors?

____
____
____
____
____

Multiple Choice

_____ **16.** Why is an increased target-receptor distance required in the paralleling technique?
- **a.** to avoid image magnification
- **b.** to avoid distortion
- **c.** to reduce scatter radiation
- **d.** to improve receptor placement

_____ **17.** Which describes the relationship of the central ray to the receptor in the paralleling technique?
- **a.** 20 degrees to the long axis of the tooth
- **b.** 90 degrees to the receptor and long axis of the tooth
- **c.** 75 degrees to the long axis of the tooth
- **d.** 15 degrees to the receptor and the long axis of the tooth

_____ **18.** Which definition is incorrect?
- **a.** *parallel:* always separated by the same distance
- **b.** *intersecting:* to cut through
- **c.** *right angle:* formed by two parallel lines
- **d.** *central ray:* central portion of the x-ray beam

_____ **19.** Which describes the relationship between the receptor and the long axis of the tooth in the paralleling technique?
- **a.** The receptor and the tooth are parallel to each other.
- **b.** The receptor and the tooth are at right angles to each other.
- **c.** The receptor and the tooth are perpendicular to each other.
- **d.** The receptor and the tooth are intersecting each other.

_____ **20.** Which describes the distance between the receptor and the tooth in the paralleling technique?
- **a.** The receptor is placed as close as possible to the tooth.
- **b.** The receptor is placed away from the tooth and toward the middle of the oral cavity.
- **c.** Either a or b.
- **d.** None of the above.

_____ **21.** Which are correct?
1. Anterior receptors are placed horizontally.
2. Anterior receptors are placed vertically.
3. Posterior receptors are placed horizontally.
4. Posterior receptors are placed vertically.
   - **a.** 1, 2, and 3
   - **b.** 2, 3, and 4
   - **c.** 2 and 3
   - **d.** 1 and 4

_____ **22.** Which is incorrect?
- **a.** Anterior receptors are always exposed before posterior receptors.
- **b.** Either anterior or posterior receptors may be exposed first.
- **c.** In posterior quadrants, the premolar receptor is always exposed before the molar receptor.
- **d.** When exposing anterior receptors, work from the patient's right to left in the maxillary arch, and then work from left to right in the mandibular arch.

_____ **23.** Which is correct?
- **a.** If the lack of parallelism is greater than 30 degrees, the image is generally acceptable.
- **b.** If the lack of parallelism is less than 20 degrees, the image is generally acceptable.
- **c.** If the lack of parallelism is less than 50 degrees, the image is generally acceptable.
- **d.** If the lack of parallelism is greater than 50 degrees, the image is generally acceptable.

_____ **24.** Which are advantages of the paralleling technique?
1. increased accuracy
2. simplicity of use
3. ease of duplication
4. ease of receptor placement
   - **a.** 1, 2, 3, and 4
   - **b.** 1, 2, and 3
   - **c.** 2, 3, and 4
   - **d.** 1, 3, and 4

_____ **25.** The advantages of the paralleling technique outweigh the disadvantages.
- **a.** true
- **b.** false

Essay

26. State the basic principle of the paralleling technique.
27. Describe why a beam alignment device must be used in the paralleling technique.
28. State the five rules of the paralleling technique.
29. Discuss the patient and equipment preparations that must be completed before using the paralleling technique.
30. Discuss the exposure sequence for 15 periapical receptor placements using the paralleling technique.
31. Describe each of the 15 periapical receptor placements that are recommended for use with the Rinn XCP instruments.
32. Summarize the guidelines for periapical receptor positioning with the paralleling technique.
33. Explain the modifications in the paralleling technique that are used for a shallow palate, bony growths, or a sensitive premolar region.

20

Bisecting Technique

LEARNING OBJECTIVES

After completion of this chapter, the student will be able to do the following:

1. Define the key terms associated with the bisecting technique.
2. State the rule of isometry.
3. State the basic principles of the bisecting technique and illustrate the locations of the receptor, tooth, imaginary bisector, central ray, and position-indicating device (PID).
4. List the beam alignment devices and receptor holders that can be used with the bisecting technique.
5. Describe the receptor size used with the bisecting technique.
6. Describe correct and incorrect horizontal angulation.
7. Describe correct and incorrect vertical angulation.
8. State each of the recommended vertical angulation ranges used for periapical exposures in the bisecting technique.
9. State the basic rules of the bisecting technique.
10. Describe patient and equipment preparations necessary before using the bisecting technique.
11. Discuss the exposure sequence used for the 14 periapical receptor placements used in the bisecting technique.
12. Describe each of the 14 periapical receptor placements recommended for use in the bisecting technique.
13. List the advantages and disadvantages of the bisecting technique.

The dental radiographer must master a variety of intraoral imaging techniques. As discussed in Chapter 19, the paralleling technique is the preferred method for exposing periapical images. Another intraoral method for exposing periapical images is the bisecting technique. Before the dental radiographer can use this technique, an understanding of the basic concepts, including terminology and principles, is necessary. In addition, the dental radiographer must understand patient preparation, equipment preparation, exposure sequencing, and receptor placement procedures used in the bisecting technique.

The bisecting technique was introduced as the original method for exposing periapical images. Years later, the long-cone paralleling technique was introduced as an additional method for exposing periapical images. Over time, the paralleling technique has become accepted as the preferred method, because this technique produces images that can be easily replicated. As the popularity of the paralleling technique has increased, the use of the bisecting technique has decreased.

The American Academy of Oral and Maxillofacial Radiology recommends the use of the paralleling technique for intraoral exposures because it provides the most accurate image with the least amount of radiation exposure to the patient. The bisecting technique is an alternative technique for exposing periapical images that is not recommended for routine use but, rather, only in limited circumstances. Such instances include the patient with specific oral anatomic configurations (e.g., extremely shallow palate) or when a patient finds it painful to close on a bite-block. It may also be used when a rubber dam is in place or when paralleling instruments are not available.

The rationale for devoting a chapter to the bisecting technique is to provide the dental radiographer with a step-by-step guide should this technique need to be used. Instructors using this text may choose to spend limited time on the topic of the bisecting technique.

The purpose of this chapter is to present basic concepts and to describe patient preparation, equipment preparation, and receptor placement procedures used in the bisecting technique. This chapter also describes the advantages and disadvantages of the bisecting technique and reviews helpful hints.

BASIC CONCEPTS

The **bisecting technique** (also known as the *bisecting-angle technique* or *bisection-of-the-angle technique*) is another method that can be used to expose periapical images.

Terminology

An understanding of the following basic terms is necessary before describing the bisecting technique:

Angle: In geometry, a figure formed by two lines diverging from a common point (Figure 20-1, A).

Bisect: To divide into two equal parts (noun, bisector) (Figure 20-1, B).

Triangle: In geometry, a figure formed by connecting three points not in a straight line by three straight-line segments (Figure 20-1, C). A triangle has three angles.

Triangle, equilateral: In geometry, a triangle with three equal sides (Figure 20-1, D).

Triangle, right: In geometry, a triangle with one 90-degree angle (right angle) (Figure 20-1, E).

Triangles, congruent: Triangles that are identical and correspond exactly when superimposed (Figure 20-1, F).

Hypotenuse: In geometry, the side of a right triangle opposite the right angle (Figure 20-1, G).

Isometry: Equality of measurement.

Long axis of the tooth: An imaginary line that divides the tooth longitudinally into two equal halves (Figure 20-2).

Central ray: The central portion of the primary beam of x-radiation.

Principles of Bisecting Technique

The bisecting technique is based on a simple geometric principle known as the **rule of isometry**. The rule of isometry states that two triangles are equal if the triangles have two equal angles and share a common side (Figure 20-3). In dental imaging, this geometric principle is applied to the bisecting technique to form two imaginary equal triangles (Figure 20-4). The bisecting technique can be described as follows:

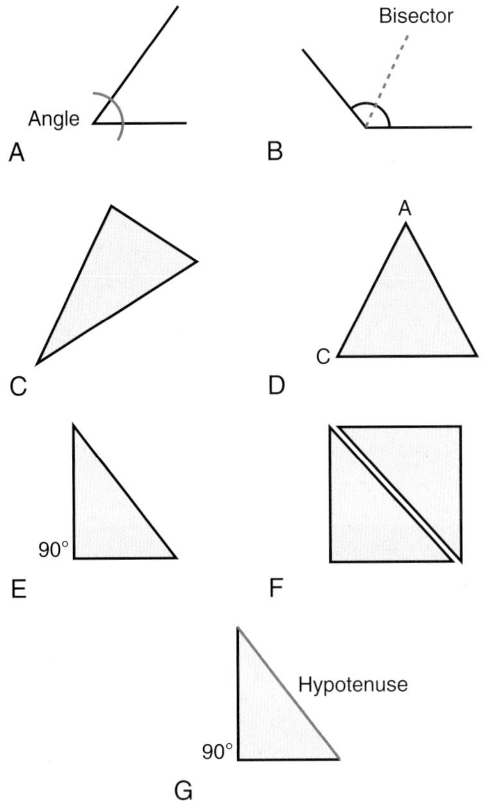

Fig 20-1 **A,** An angle is formed by two lines that diverge from a common point. **B,** A bisector divides an angle into equal angles. **C,** A triangle. **D,** An equilateral triangle has three equal sides (AB=BC=CA). **E,** A right triangle has one 90-degree angle. **F,** Congruent triangles are identical. **G,** The hypotenuse is the side of a right triangle opposite the right angle.

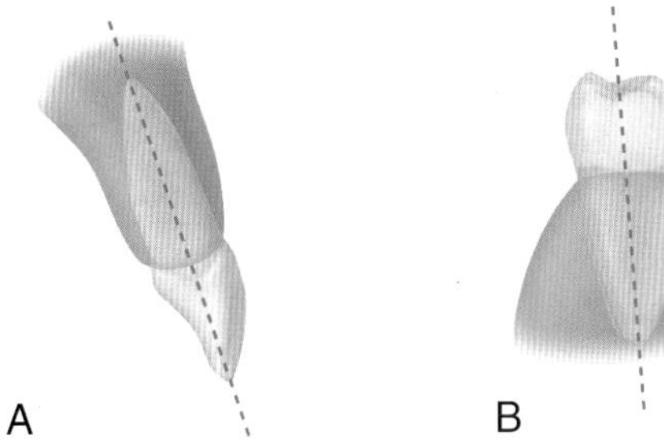

Fig 20-2 **A,** The long axis of the maxillary incisor divides the tooth into two equal halves. **B,** The long axis of a mandibular premolar divides the tooth into two equal halves.

1. The receptor must be placed along the lingual surface of the tooth.
2. At the point where the receptor contacts the tooth, the plane of the receptor and the long axis of the tooth form an angle.
3. The dental radiographer must visualize a plane that divides in half, or bisects, the angle formed by the receptor and the long axis of the tooth. This plane is termed the imaginary bisector. The imaginary bisector creates two equal angles and provides a common side for the two imaginary equal triangles.
4. The dental radiographer must then direct the central ray of the x-ray beam perpendicular to the imaginary bisector. When the central ray is directed at an angle of 90 degrees to the imaginary bisector, two imaginary equal triangles are formed.

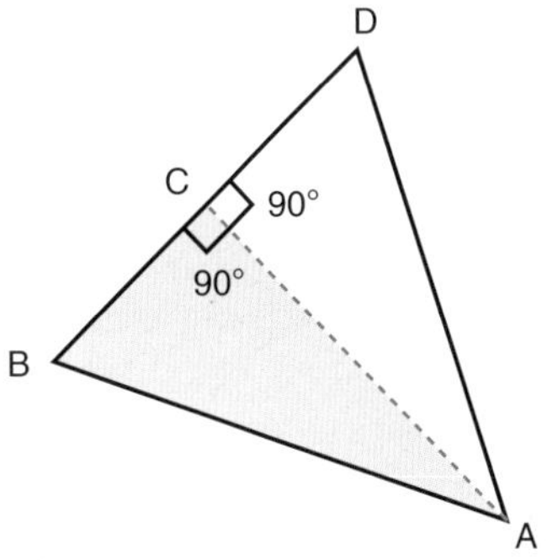

Fig 20-3 Angle A is bisected by line AC. Line AC is perpendicular to line BD. Angle BAC is equal to angle DAC. Angle ACB is equal to angle ACD. According to the rule of isometry, triangle BAC *(shaded)* is equal to triangle DAC.

5. The two imaginary triangles that result are right triangles and are congruent. The hypotenuse of one imaginary triangle is represented by the long axis of the tooth; the plane of the receptor represents the other hypotenuse.

When the rule of isometry is followed strictly, the image of the tooth will be accurate. When the angle formed by the plane of the receptor and the long axis of the tooth is bisected, and the x-ray beam is directed at a right angle to the imaginary bisector, the actual tooth and the image of the tooth are the same length (Figure 20-5).

As an analogy, think of the sun shining on a tree. As the sun rises, the angle of its rays changes throughout the morning. When the sun first rises, the rays come from low on the horizon (flat) and the shadow of the tree appears longer than the tree. At some point in the morning, as the sun continues to rise, it creates a shadow that is the same length as the tree. This occurs when the rays are perpendicular to an imaginary plane that bisects the angle formed by the tree and the ground. Then as the sun continues to rise to its highest point, the rays come from higher above the horizon (steep) and the shadow of the tree is very short.

In dental imaging, longer images occur when the beam angulation is too flat (e.g., the sun in early morning). Shorter images occur when the beam angulation is too steep (e.g., the sun at noon). When the dental x-ray beam is positioned perpendicular to the imaginary plane that bisects the angle formed by the tooth and the receptor, the tooth image on the receptor is the same length as the tooth.

Receptor Stabilization

In the bisecting technique, beam alignment devices or receptor holding devices may be used to position and stabilize the receptor.

Beam Alignment Devices. Beam alignment devices are used to position an intraoral receptor in the mouth and maintain it in position during exposure (see Chapter 7). The aiming rings allow for easy alignment of the position-indicating device (PID). An example of commercially available intraoral beam alignment devices that can be used with the bisecting technique is the following:

- *Rinn BAI System* (Dentsply Rinn Corporation, York, PA). The BAI (bisecting angle instrument) system includes plastic bite-blocks, plastic aiming rings, and metal indicator arms. To reduce the amount of radiation received by the patient, snap-on ring collimators can be added to the plastic aiming rings. The Rinn BAI has been designed to aid in the determination of horizontal and vertical angulations, prevent cone-cuts, and minimize distortion from receptor bending (Figure 20-6, A).

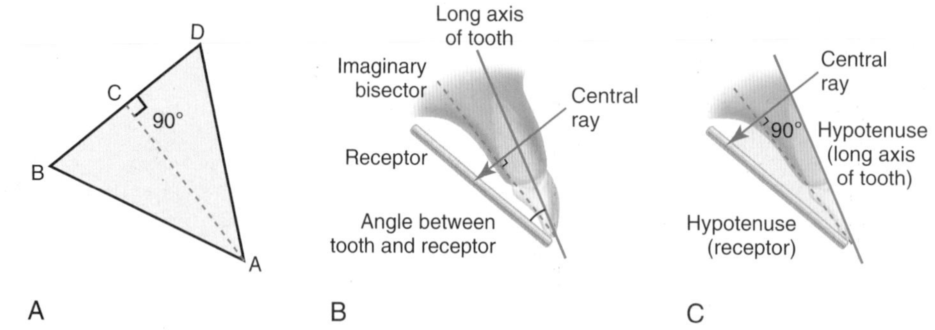

Fig 20-4 A, The receptor (line BA) is placed along the lingual surface of the tooth. At the point where the receptor contacts the tooth, the plane of the receptor and the long axis of the tooth (DA) form an angle (BAD). The imaginary bisector divides this angle into two equal angles (BAC and DAC). The central ray (BD) is directed perpendicular to the imaginary bisector and completes the third sides (BC and CD) of the two triangles. **B,** The central ray is directed at a right angle to the imaginary bisector. **C,** The two imaginary triangles that result are right triangles and congruent. The hypotenuse of each triangle is represented by the long axis of the tooth and the plane of the receptor.

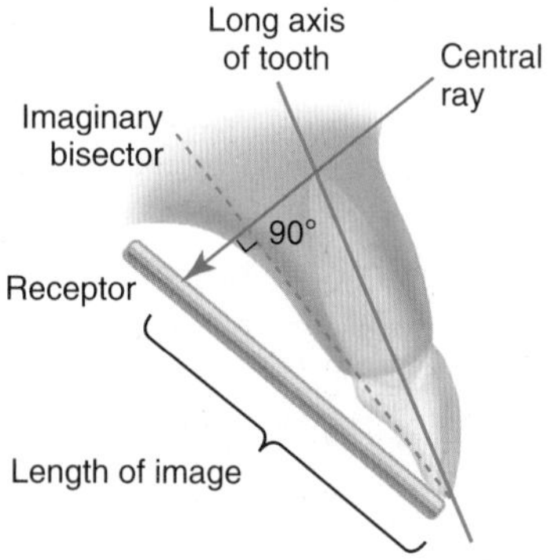

Fig 20-5 The image on the receptor is equal to the length of the tooth when the central ray is directed at 90 degrees to the imaginary bisector. A tooth and its image will be equal in length when two equal triangles are formed that share a common side (imaginary bisector).

Receptor Holding Devices. Receptor holding devices are used to position the receptor in the mouth and maintain it in position during exposure. No aiming rings are used with these receptor holders; the operator must determine the horizontal and vertical angulations. Examples of receptor holders include the following:

- *Stabe Bite-block (Rinn).* This styrofoam device can be used to hold a receptor with the paralleling technique or the bisecting technique. For use with the bisecting technique, the scored front section is removed, and the receptor is placed as close to the teeth as possible (Figure 20-6, B).
- *Rinn Snap-A-Ray Holder.* This device is used to stabilize a receptor when using either the paralleling technique or the bisecting technique (Figure 20-6, C). Along with being autoclavable, the Snap-A-Ray offers a universal design for digital sensors and film. Operators may prefer the length of the Snap-A-Ray handle compared with placing the bite-block alone, especially for molar projections.

The Rinn BAI and the Rinn Snap-A-Ray Holder are reusable instruments and must be sterilized after each use. The Stabe Bite-block is disposable and is designed for one-time use only.

When the Rinn BAI instruments are used with the bisecting technique, the addition of a rectangular collimator is recommended. The aiming ring aids in the alignment of the position-indicating device (PID), and the collimator significantly reduces the amount of patient exposure to x-radiation. The Rinn BAI instruments are simple to assemble and position. For information about the use of these instruments or

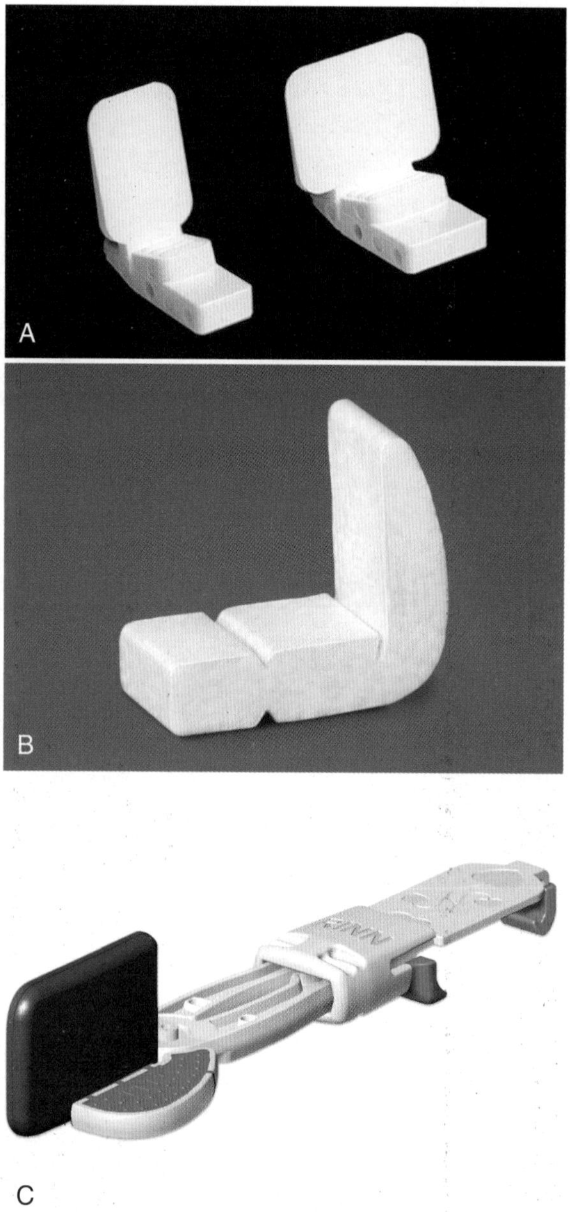

Fig 20-6 **A,** Rinn BAI bite-blocks used with the bisecting technique. **B,** Stabe disposable receptor holder. **C,** Dentsply Rinn Snap-A-Ray Holder. (Courtesy Dentsply Rinn Corporation, York, PA.)

other devices available for the bisecting technique, the dental radiographer should refer to manufacturer instructions.

Receptors Used for Bisecting Technique

Traditionally, a size 2 intraoral receptor is used for all periapical projections with the bisecting technique. In the anterior region, a size 2 receptor is always placed with the long portion of the receptor in a vertical (upright) direction. In the posterior region, a size 2 receptor is always placed with the long portion of the receptor in a horizontal (sideways) direction.

Position-Indicating Device Angulation

In the bisecting technique, the angulation of the PID is critical. **Angulation** is a term used to describe the alignment of the central ray of the x-ray beam in horizontal and vertical planes. Moving the PID in either a horizontal direction or a vertical direction can vary angulation. The use of the Rinn BAI system with aiming rings dictates the proper PID angulation. However, when a receptor holder without an aiming ring is employed, the dental radiographer must determine both horizontal and vertical angulations for each exposure.

Horizontal Angulation. **Horizontal angulation** refers to the positioning of the PID and the direction of the central ray in a horizontal, or side-to-side, plane (Figure 20-7). The horizontal angulation does not differ according to the technique used; paralleling, bisecting, and bitewing techniques all use the same principles of horizontal angulation.

Correct horizontal angulation. With correct horizontal angulation, the central ray is directed perpendicular to the curvature of the arch and through the contact areas of the teeth (Figure 20-8). As a result, the contact areas on the dental image appear "opened."

Incorrect horizontal angulation. Incorrect horizontal angulation results in overlapped ("unopened") contact areas (Figure 20-9). An image with overlapped interproximal contact areas cannot be used to examine the interproximal areas of the teeth and is thus nondiagnostic (Figure 20-10).

Vertical Angulation. **Vertical angulation** refers to the positioning of the PID in a vertical, or up-and-down, plane (Figure 20-11). Vertical angulation is measured in degrees and is registered on the outside of the tubehead. The vertical angulation differs according to the imaging technique used, as follows:

- With the paralleling technique, the vertical angulation of the central ray is directed perpendicular to the receptor and the long axis of the tooth (see Chapter 19).

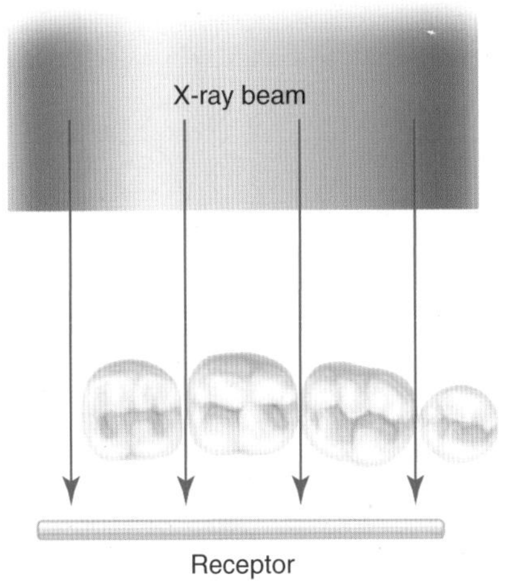

Fig 20-8 Correct horizontal angulation.

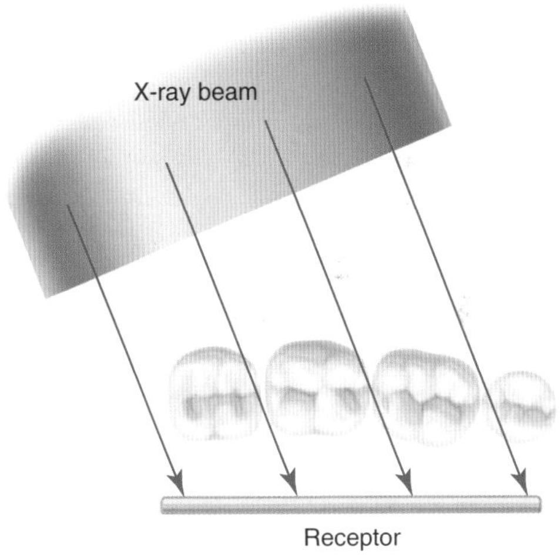

Fig 20-9 Incorrect horizontal angulation.

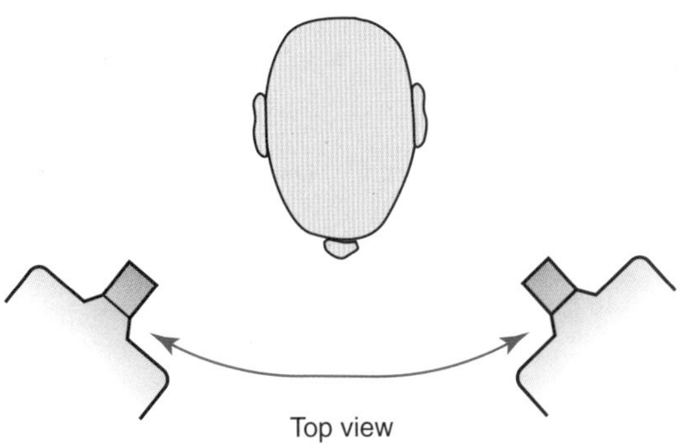

Fig 20-7 *Horizontal angulation* of the position-indicating device (PID) refers to PID placement in a side-to-side (ear-to-ear) direction. (From Haring JI, Lind LJ: *Radiographic interpretation for the dental hygienist*, Philadelphia, 1993, Saunders.)

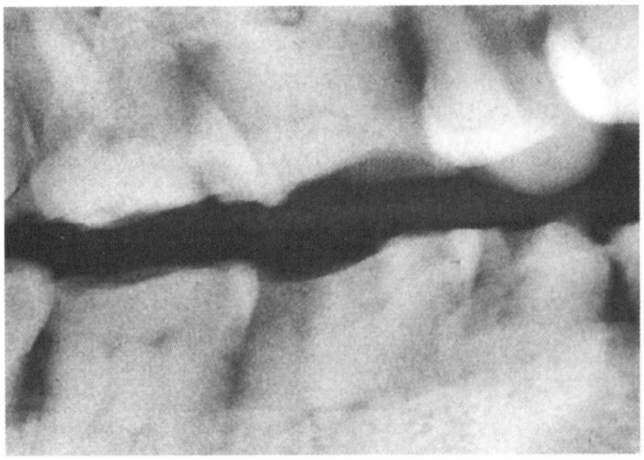

Fig 20-10 Overlapped contacts. (From Haring JI, Lind LJ: *Radiographic interpretation for the dental hygienist*, Philadelphia, 1993, Saunders.)

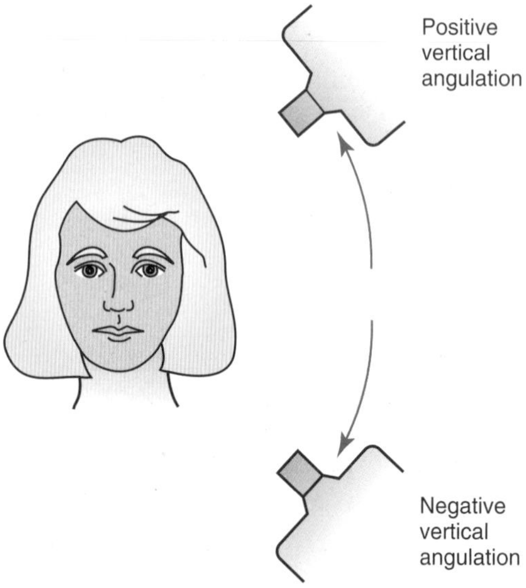

Fig 20-11 *Vertical angulation* of the position-indicating device (PID) refers to PID placement in an up-and-down (head-to-toe) direction. (From Haring JI, Lind LJ: *Radiographic interpretation for the dental hygienist*, Philadelphia, 1993, Saunders.)

TABLE 20-1 Recommended Vertical Angulation Ranges: Bisecting Technique

	Maxillary Teeth: Vertical Angulation (degrees)	Mandibular Teeth: Vertical Angulation (degrees)
Canines	+45 to +55	−20 to −30
Incisors	+40 to +50	−15 to −25
Premolars	+30 to +40	−10 to −15
Molars	+20 to +30	−5 to 0

- With the bisecting technique, the vertical angulation is determined by the imaginary bisector; the central ray is directed perpendicular to the imaginary bisector.
- With the bite-wing technique using tabs, the vertical angulation is predetermined; the central ray is directed at +10 degrees to the occlusal plane (see Chapter 21).

Correct vertical angulation. Correct vertical angulation results in a dental image that is the same length as the tooth. Table 20-1 lists recommended vertical angulation ranges for the bisecting technique.

Incorrect vertical angulation. Incorrect vertical angulation results in an image that is not of the same length as that of the tooth; instead, the image exhibits distortion and appears longer or shorter. Elongated or foreshortened images are not diagnostic.

Foreshortened images. *Foreshortened images* refer to images that appear shortened. Foreshortening of images results from excessive vertical angulation. When the vertical angulation is too steep, the image of the tooth appears shorter than the actual tooth (Figure 20-12). Foreshortening also occurs if the central ray is directed perpendicular to the plane of the receptor rather than to the imaginary bisector.

Elongated images. *Elongated images* refer to images of the teeth that appear too long. Elongation of images results from insufficient vertical angulation. When the vertical angulation is too flat, the image of the tooth appears longer than the actual tooth (Figure 20-13). Elongation also occurs if the central ray is directed perpendicular to the long axis of the tooth rather than to the imaginary bisector.

Rules for Bisecting Technique

Five basic rules should be followed when using the bisecting technique.

1. *Receptor placement.* The receptor must be positioned to cover the prescribed area of the tooth to be examined. Specific placements are described in the procedures.
2. *Receptor position.* The receptor must be placed against the lingual surface of the tooth. The occlusal end of the receptor must extend approximately one eighth of an inch beyond the incisal or occlusal surfaces (Figure 20-14). The apical end of the receptor must rest against the palatal or alveolar tissues.
3. *Vertical angulation.* The central ray of the x-ray beam must be directed perpendicular (at a right angle) to the imaginary bisector that divides the angle formed by the receptor and the long axis of the tooth.
4. *Horizontal angulation.* The central ray of the x-ray beam must be directed through the contact areas between teeth.
5. *Receptor exposure.* The x-ray beam must be centered on the receptor to ensure that all areas of the receptor are exposed. Failure to center the x-ray beam results in a partial image or a cone-cut.

STEP-BY-STEP PROCEDURES

Step-by-step procedures for the exposure of periapical images using the bisecting technique include patient preparation, equipment preparation, and receptor placement methods. Before exposing any receptors using the bisecting technique, infection prevention procedures (as detailed in Chapter 16) must be completed.

Patient Preparation

After completion of infection prevention procedures and preparation of the treatment area and supplies, the patient should be seated. After seating the patient, the dental radiographer must prepare the patient before the exposure of any receptors (Procedure 20-1).

Equipment Preparation

After patient preparation, equipment must also be prepared before the exposure of any receptors (Procedure 20-2).

Exposure Sequence for Receptor Placements

When using the bisecting technique, an exposure sequence, or definite order for periapical receptor placements and exposures, must be followed. The dental radiographer must have an established exposure routine to prevent errors and use time efficiently. Working without an exposure sequence may result in confusion, omitting an area, or exposing an area to x-radiation twice.

Anterior Exposure Sequence. When exposing periapical receptors with the bisecting technique, always begin with the anterior teeth (canines and incisors) for the following reasons:

- The more tolerable anterior placements allow the patient to become accustomed to the beam alignment device used in the bisecting technique.
- The anterior placements are less likely to cause the patient to gag. Once the gag reflex has been stimulated, the patient may gag on projections that could normally be tolerated. Management of the patient with a hypersensitive gag reflex is discussed in Chapter 24.

HELPFUL HINT

Incorrect Vertical Angulation

In FORE***SHORT***ENING:

- The PID is too ***STEEP***.
- ***SHORT*** image
- To correct this, you must **decrease** the PID angle.
- Compare the length of the **image** to the length of the **tooth**. (See red lines—the image is *shorter* than the tooth.)
- The image appears ***SHORT***.

  Too STEEP

  Too SHORT

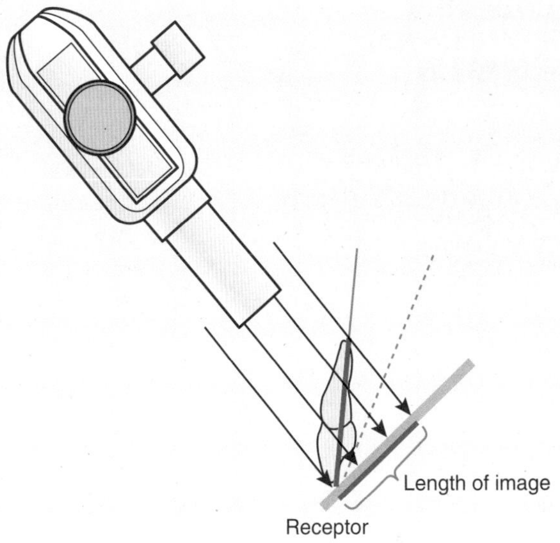

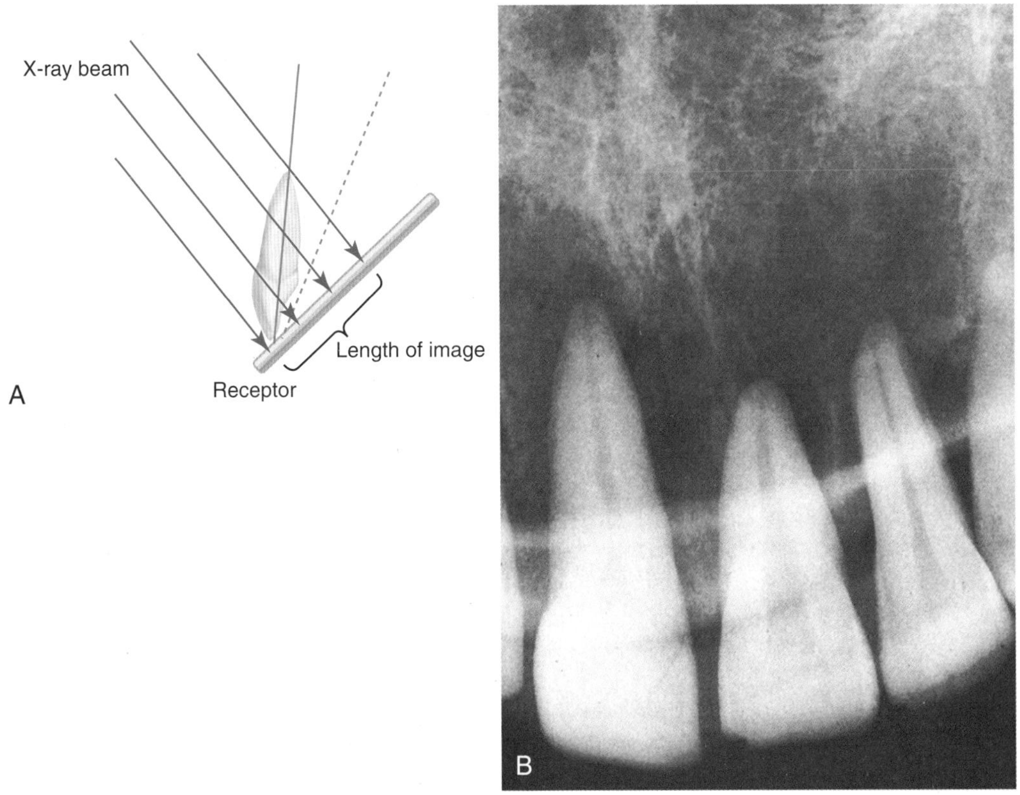

Fig 20-12 **A,** If the vertical angulation is too steep, the image is shorter than the actual tooth. **B,** A foreshortened image. (From Haring JI, Lind LJ: *Radiographic interpretation for the dental hygienist*, Philadelphia, 1993, Saunders.)

HELPFUL HINT

Incorrect Vertical Angulation

In E***LONG***ATION:

- The PID is too ***FLAT***.
- ***LONG*** image
- To correct this, you must **increase** the PID angle.
- Compare the length of the **image** to the length of the **tooth**. (See red lines—the image is *longer* than the tooth.)
- The image appears ***LONG*** (stretched).
  Too ***FLAT***
  Too ***LONG***

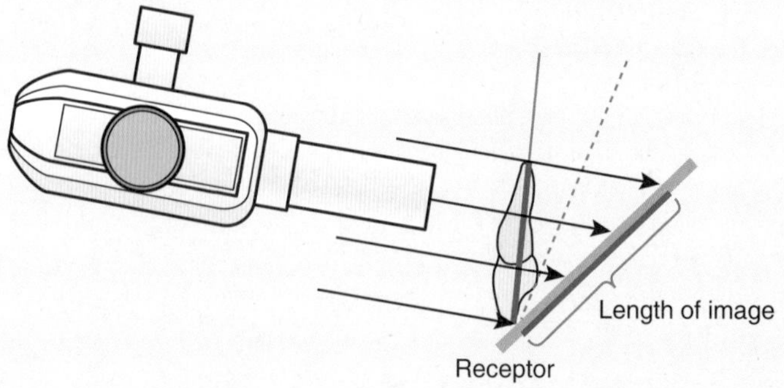

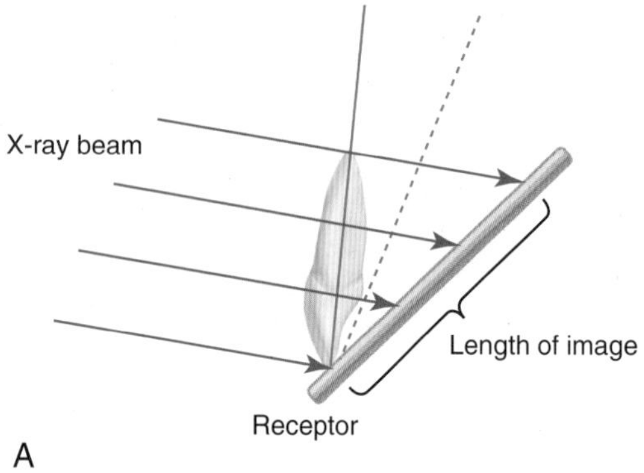

A

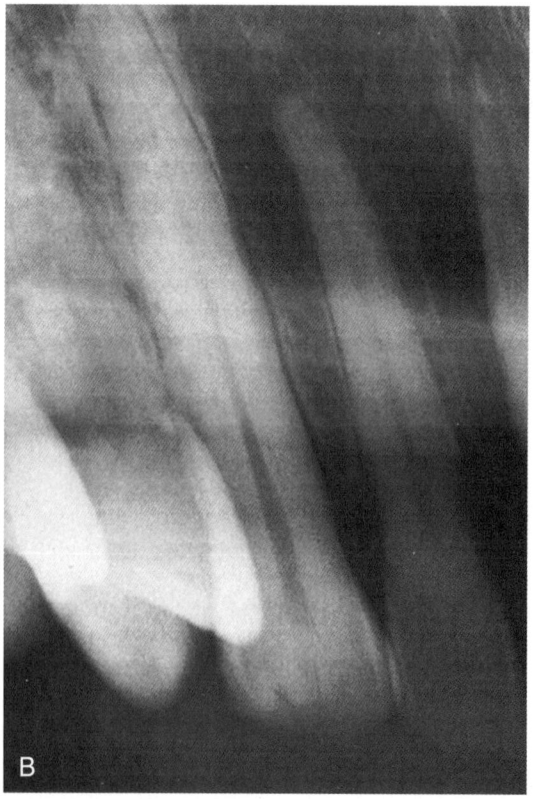

B

Fig 20-13 A, If the vertical angulation is too flat, the image is longer than the actual tooth. **B,** An elongated image. (From Haring JI, Lind LJ: *Radiographic interpretation for the dental hygienist*, Philadelphia, 1993, Saunders.)

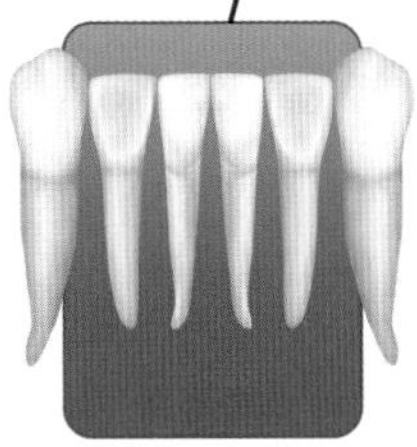

Fig 20-14 Approximately one eighth of an inch of the receptor must appear beyond the incisal edges of the teeth.

PROCEDURE 20-1 Patient Preparation for Bisecting Technique

1. Briefly explain the imaging procedures to the patient.
2. Adjust the chair so that the patient is positioned upright and the level of the chair is at a comfortable working height.
3. Adjust the headrest to support the patient's head. Position the patient's head such that the arch that is being imaged is parallel to the floor and the midsagittal plane is perpendicular to the floor.
4. Place and secure the lead apron with thyroid collar over the patient.
5. Request that the patient remove eyeglasses and any objects in the mouth (e.g., dentures, retainers, chewing gum) that may interfere with the procedure.

PROCEDURE 20-2 Equipment Preparation for Bisecting Technique

1. Set the exposure control factors (kilovoltage, milliamperage, and time) on the x-ray unit according to the recommendations of the receptor manufacturer. Either a short (8-inch) or long (16-inch) position-indicating device (PID) may be used with the bisecting technique; typically, the short PID is preferred.
2. If using a beam alignment device with the bisecting technique, open the sterilized package containing the device, and assemble the device over a covered work area.

With the size 2 receptor, a total of 6 anterior placements are used in the bisecting technique: 3 maxillary exposures and 3 mandibular exposures. The recommended anterior periapical exposure sequence for the bisecting technique is as follows (Table 20-2):

1. Begin with the maxillary right canine (tooth #6).
2. Expose the maxillary anterior teeth from the patient's right to the patient's left.
3. End with the maxillary left canine (tooth #11).
4. Next, move to the mandibular arch.
5. Begin with the mandibular left canine (tooth #22).
6. Expose all the mandibular anterior teeth from the patient's left to the patient's right.
7. Finish with the mandibular right canine (tooth #27).

As previously discussed in Chapter 19, when the dental radiographer works from the patient's right to the patient's left in the maxillary arch and then from the patient's left to the patient's right in the mandibular arch, no wasted movement or shifting of the PID occurs (see Figure 19-10). In addition, when working from right to left and then from left to right, the teeth are exposed in ascending numerical order.

TABLE 20-2 Exposure Sequence for Anterior Receptor Placement: Bisecting Technique

Exposure Number	Arch	Side	Tooth	Tooth Number
1	Maxillary	Right	Canine	6
2	Maxillary	Right	Lateral incisor	7
	Maxillary	Right	Central incisor	8
	Maxillary	Left	Central incisor	9
	Maxillary	Left	Lateral incisor	10
3	Maxillary	Left	Canine	11
4	Mandibular	Left	Canine	22
5	Mandibular	Left	Lateral incisor	23
	Mandibular	Left	Central incisor	24
	Mandibular	Right	Central incisor	25
	Mandibular	Right	Lateral incisor	26
6	Mandibular	Right	Canine	27

TABLE 20-3 Exposure Sequence for Posterior Receptor Placement: Bisecting Technique

Exposure Number	Arch	Side	Teeth	Teeth Numbers
1	Maxillary	Right	Premolars	4, 5
2	Maxillary	Right	Molars	1, 2, 3
3	Mandibular	Right	Premolars	28, 29
4	Mandibular	Right	Molars	30, 31, 32
5	Maxillary	Left	Premolars	12, 13
6	Maxillary	Left	Molars	14, 15, 16
7	Mandibular	Left	Premolars	20, 21
8	Mandibular	Left	Molars	17, 18, 19

This exposure sequence makes it easier for the dental radiographer to keep track of the last exposure if the imaging procedure is interrupted.

Posterior Exposure Sequence. After anterior exposures, the posterior teeth (premolars and molars) are exposed. In each quadrant, always expose the premolar receptor first and then the molar receptor. The rationale for exposing the premolar placement first is as follows:

- Premolar placements are easier for the patient to tolerate.
- Premolar exposures are less likely to evoke the gag reflex.

Eight posterior receptor placements are used in the bisecting technique: 4 maxillary exposures and 4 mandibular exposures. The recommended posterior periapical exposure sequence for the bisecting technique is as follows (Table 20-3):

BOX 20-1 Prescribed Placements for Anterior Periapical Receptors: Bisecting Technique

Maxillary Canine
- The entire crown and root of the canine, including the apex and the surrounding structures, must be seen on this image.
- The interproximal alveolar bone and mesial contact of the canine must also be visible.
- The lingual cusp of the first premolar usually obscures the distal contact of the canine.

Maxillary Incisor
- The entire crowns and roots of all four maxillary incisors, including the apices of the teeth and the surrounding structures, must be seen on this image.
- The interproximal alveolar bone between the central incisors and the central and lateral incisors must also be visible.

Mandibular Canine
- The entire crown and root of the canine, including the apex and the surrounding structures, must be seen on this image.
- The interproximal alveolar bone and mesial and distal contacts must also be visible.

Mandibular Incisor
- The entire crowns and roots of the four mandibular incisors, including the apices of the teeth and the surrounding structures, must be seen on this image.
- The contacts between the central incisors and between the central and lateral incisors must also be visible.

1. Begin with the maxillary right quadrant.
2. Expose the premolar receptor (teeth #4 and 5), then expose the molar receptor (teeth #1, 2, and 3).
3. Move to the mandibular right quadrant.
4. Expose the premolar receptor (teeth #28 and 29), then expose the molar receptor (teeth #30, 31, and 32).
5. Move to the maxillary left quadrant.
6. Expose the premolar receptor (teeth #12 and 13), then expose the molar receptor (teeth #14, 15, and 16).
7. Finish with the mandibular left quadrant.
8. Expose the premolar receptor (teeth #20 and 21) and finish the posterior periapical placements with the exposure of the molar receptor (teeth #17, 18, and 19).

Receptor Placement for Bisecting Technique

In a complete mouth series (CMS) using the bisecting technique, each periapical exposure has a prescribed placement. Receptor placement, or the specific area where the receptor must be positioned before exposure, is dictated by the teeth and surrounding structures that must be included on the resultant dental image. Prescribed placements for the anterior teeth are detailed in Box 20-1 and illustrated in Figure 20-15. Posterior placements are detailed in Box 20-2 and illustrated in Figure 20-16.

The specific placements described in this chapter are for a 14-receptor periapical series using size 2 receptors for all anterior and posterior exposures. Other reference sources or individual practitioners may recommend variations in receptor placement or the number and size of receptors used (Box 20-3).

BOX 20-2 Prescribed Placements for Posterior Periapical Receptors: Bisecting Technique

Maxillary Premolar
- All crowns and roots of the first and second premolars and first molar, including the apices, alveolar crests, contact areas, and surrounding bone, must be seen on this image.
- The distal contact of the maxillary canine must be visible in this projection.

Maxillary Molar
- All crowns and roots of the first, second, and third molars, including the apices, alveolar crests, contact areas, surrounding bone, and tuberosity region, must be seen on this image.
- The distal contact of the maxillary second premolar must be visible in this projection.

Mandibular Premolar
- All crowns and roots of the first and second premolars and first molar, including the apices, alveolar crests, contact areas, and surrounding bone, must be seen on this image.
- The distal contact of the mandibular canine should be visible in this projection.

Mandibular Molar
- All crowns and roots of the first, second, and third molars, including the apices, alveolar crests, contact areas, and surrounding bone, must be seen on this image.
- The distal contact of the mandibular second premolar must be visible in this projection.

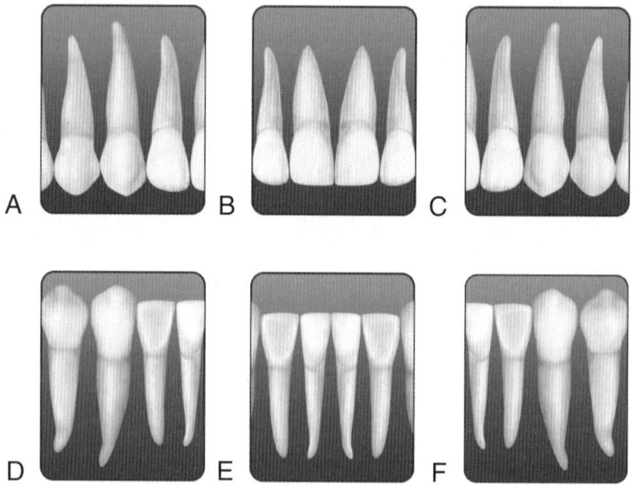

Fig 20-15 Prescribed placements for anterior periapicals. **A,** Exposure of the maxillary right canine. **B,** Exposure of the maxillary incisor. **C,** Exposure of the maxillary left canine. **D,** Exposure of the mandibular right canine. **E,** Exposure of the mandibular incisor. **F,** Exposure of the mandibular left canine.

Anterior Placement. A size 2 receptor is used for all anterior placements and is positioned vertically in the mouth. The size 2 receptor is inserted vertically into the Rinn BAI device and secured. A total of 6 anterior placements include the following:
- Two maxillary canine exposures (Procedure 20-3)
- One maxillary incisor exposure (Procedure 20-4)

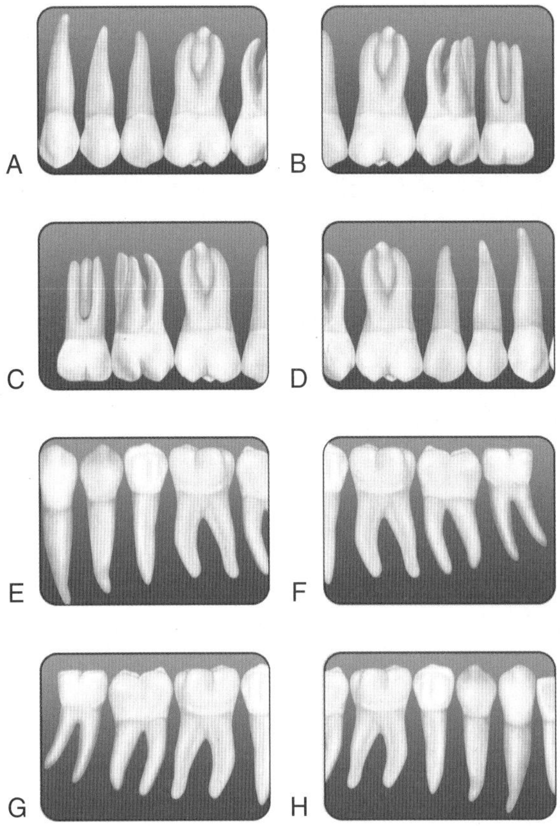

Fig 20-16 Prescribed placements for posterior periapicals. **A,** Exposure of the left maxillary premolar. **B,** Exposure of the left maxillary molar. **C,** Exposure of the right maxillary molar. **D,** Exposure of the right maxillary premolar. **E,** Exposure of the left mandibular premolar. **F,** Exposure of the left mandibular molar. **G,** Exposure of the right mandibular molar. **H,** Exposure of the right mandibular premolar.

BOX 20-3 Guidelines for Receptor Placement with Bisecting Technique

1. If using film, the white side of the film always faces the teeth ("white in sight"), and the identification dot is placed at the incisal or occlusal edge. When using a sensor, position the sensor toward the x-ray tube according to manufacturer directions.
2. The anterior receptors are always placed vertically.
3. The posterior receptors are always placed horizontally.
4. The incisal or occlusal edge of the receptor must extend approximately one eighth of an inch beyond the teeth.
5. When positioning the receptor, always center the receptor over the area to be examined (as defined in the prescribed placements).

- Two mandibular canine exposures (Procedure 20-5)
- One mandibular incisor exposure (Procedure 20-6)

Posterior Placement. A size 2 receptor is used for all posterior placements and is positioned horizontally in the mouth. The size 2 receptor is inserted horizontally into the Rinn BAI device and secured. A total of 8 posterior placements include the following:

- Two maxillary premolar exposures (Procedure 20-7)
- Two maxillary molar exposures (Procedure 20-8)
- Two mandibular premolar exposures (Procedure 20-9)
- Two mandibular molar exposures (Procedure 20-10)

ADVANTAGES AND DISADVANTAGES

As with all intraoral techniques, the bisecting technique has both advantages and disadvantages. The disadvantages of the bisecting technique outweigh the advantages. Therefore the paralleling technique is preferred over the bisecting technique for the exposure of periapical images and should be used whenever possible.

Advantages of Bisecting Technique

The primary advantage of the bisecting technique is that it eliminates the use of a beam alignment device. When the anatomy of the patient (shallow palate, bony growths, sensitive mandibular premolar areas) precludes the use of such a device, the bisecting technique is a good alternative approach. Another advantage is decreased exposure time. When a short (8-inch) PID is used with the bisecting technique, a shorter exposure time is recommended.

Disadvantages of Bisecting Technique

The primary disadvantage of the bisecting technique is dimensional distortion. The disadvantages of the bisecting technique can be summarized as follows:

- *Image distortion.* Distortion occurs when a short PID is used; a short PID causes an increased divergence of x-rays, resulting in image magnification. Distortion also occurs when a tooth (three-dimensional structure) is projected onto a receptor (two-dimensional structure); structures that are farther away from the receptor appear more elongated than those closer to the receptor.
- *Angulation problems.* Without the use of a beam alignment device and aiming ring, it is difficult for the dental radiographer to visualize the imaginary bisector and then determine the vertical angulation. Any error in vertical angulation will result in image distortion (elongation or foreshortening).

HELPFUL HINTS

In using the bisecting technique:

- **DO** set all exposure control factors (kilovoltage, milliamperage, time) before placing any receptors in the mouth.
- **DO** ask patients to remove eyeglasses and all intraoral objects before placing any receptors in the mouth.
- **DO** use a definite order (exposure sequence) when exposing receptors to avoid errors and to make efficient use of time.
- **DO** explain the imaging procedures that will be performed.
- **DO** instruct patients on exactly how to stabilize the bite-block and remain still during the exposure.
- **DO** memorize the recommended vertical angulation ranges for each periapical exposure, and use these ranges as a guide when determining PID placement.
- **DO** direct the central ray perpendicular to the imaginary bisector.
- **DO** align the opening of the PID parallel to the imaginary bisector.
- **DO** use the word *please;* say, "Open, please."
- **DO** use praise; tell cooperative patients how much they are helping to simplify and speed the imaging procedure.
- **DO** instruct patients to "slowly close" their teeth together on the bite-block; when patients close slowly, the musculature relaxes and thus discomfort is reduced.
- **DO NOT** bend or crimp a film packet or PSP digital sensors; excessive bending causes image distortion.

PROCEDURE 20-3 Maxillary Canine Exposure: Bisecting Technique (Figure 20-17)

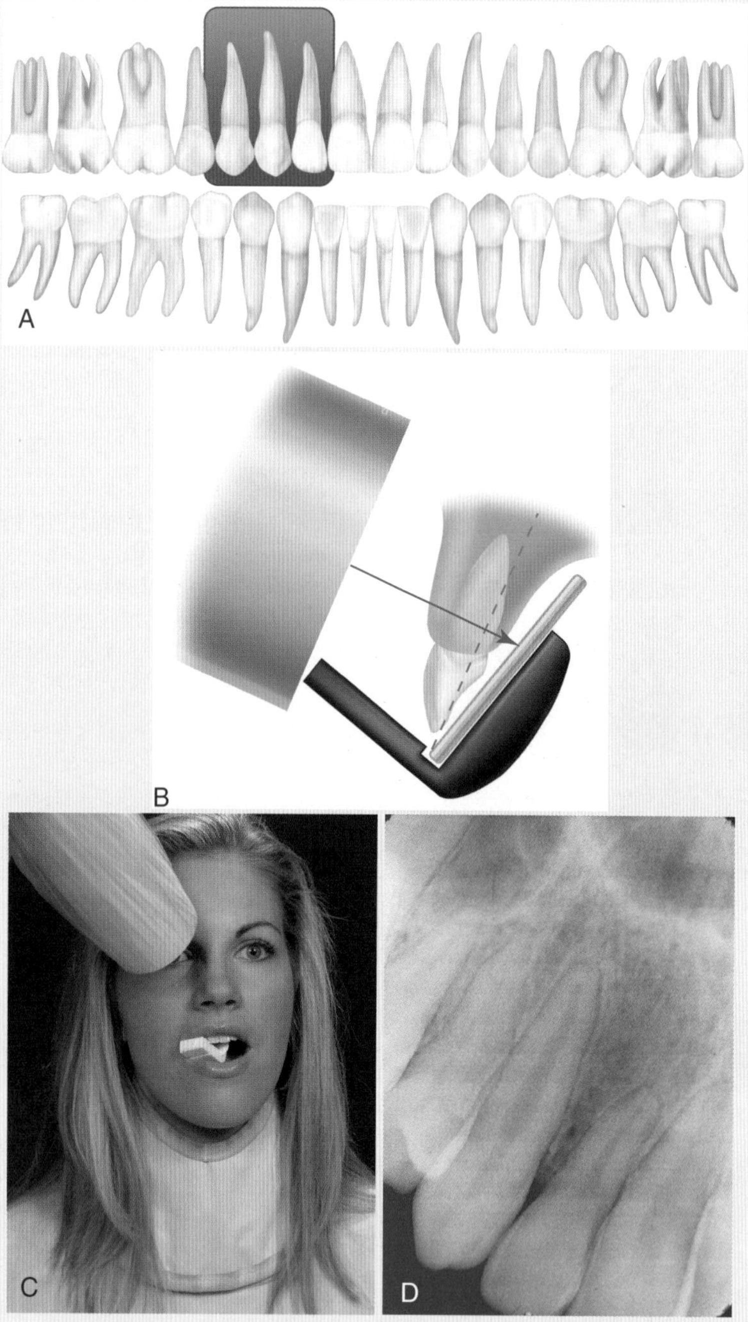

Fig 20-17 Exposure of the maxillary canine. **A,** Receptor placement. **B,** Imaginary bisector and central ray. **C,** Exposure of the receptor. **D,** Resultant image.

1. Center the receptor on the maxillary canine.
2. Position the lower edge of the receptor parallel to the occlusal plane so that one-eighth of an inch extends below the incisal edge of the canine.
3. Instruct the patient to "slowly close" and gently bite on the receptor holder or beam alignment device.
4. If not using a beam alignment device, establish the correct vertical angulation by bisecting the angle and directing the central ray perpendicular to the imaginary bisector.
5. If not using a beam alignment device, establish the correct horizontal angulation by directing the central ray between the contacts of the canine and the first premolar.
6. Position the position-indicating device (PID) using the correct vertical and horizontal angulations. Center the PID over the receptor to avoid cone-cutting.
7. Expose the receptor.

PROCEDURE 20-4 Maxillary Incisor Exposure: Bisecting Technique (Figure 20-18)

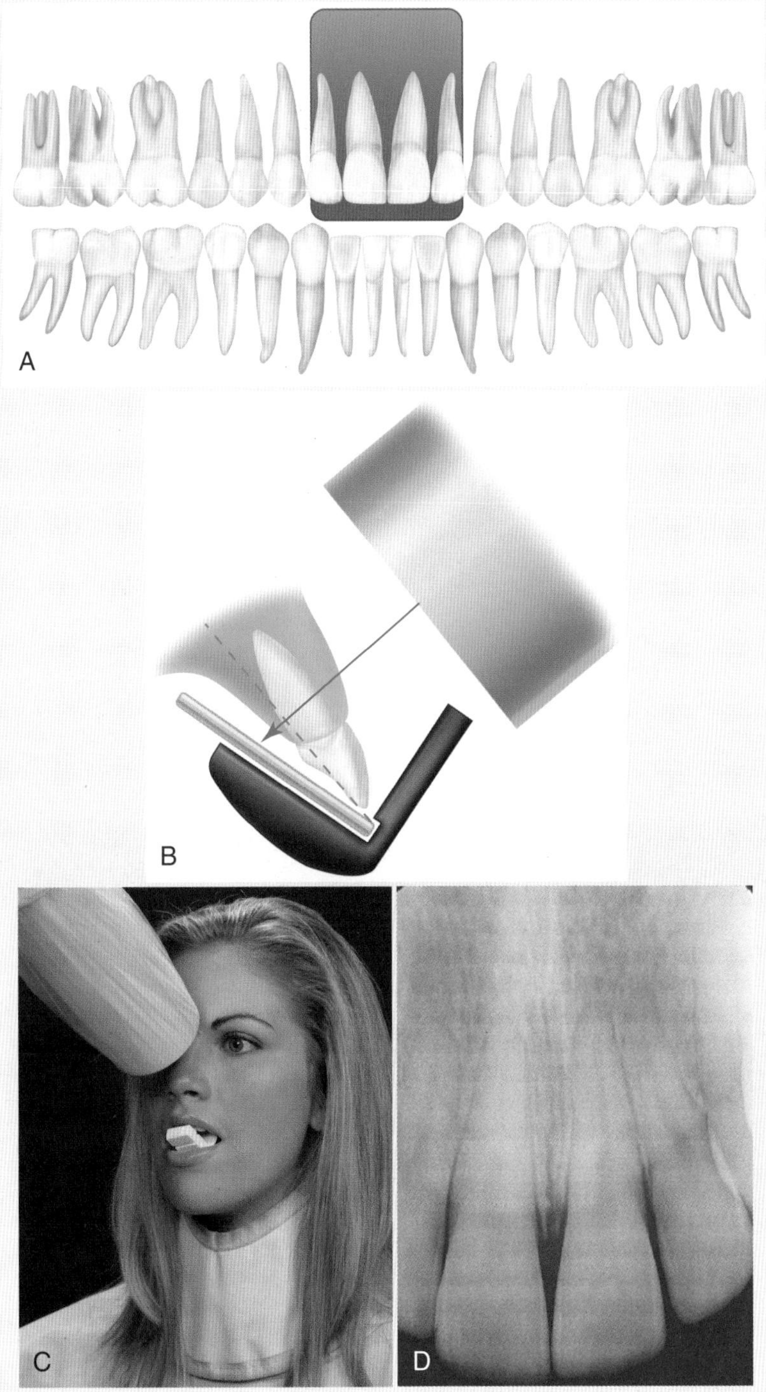

Fig 20-18 Exposure of the maxillary incisors. **A,** Receptor placement. **B,** Imaginary bisector and central ray. **C,** Exposure of the receptor. **D,** Resultant image.

1. Center the receptor on the contact between the two maxillary central incisors.
2. Position the lower edge of the receptor parallel to the occlusal plane so that one-eighth of an inch extends below the incisal edges of the teeth.
3. Instruct the patient to "slowly close" and gently bite on the receptor holder or beam alignment device.
4. If not using a beam alignment device, establish the correct vertical angulation by bisecting the angle and directing the central ray perpendicular to the imaginary bisector.
5. If not using a beam alignment device, establish the correct horizontal angulation by directing the central ray between the contacts of the central incisors.
6. Position the position-indicating device (PID) using the correct vertical and horizontal angulations. Center the PID over the receptor to avoid cone-cutting.
7. Expose the receptor.

PROCEDURE 20-5 Mandibular Canine Exposure: Bisecting Technique (Figure 20-19)

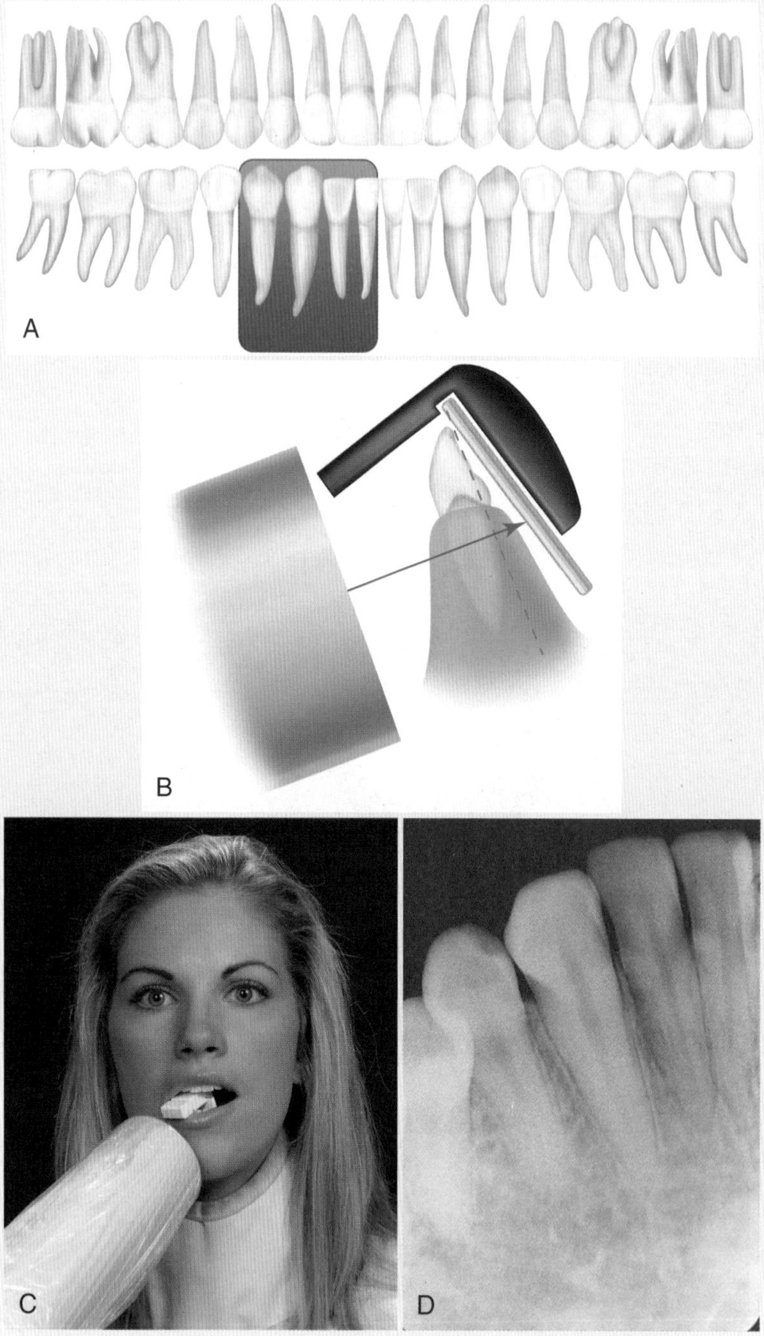

Fig 20-19 Exposure of the mandibular canine. **A,** Receptor placement. **B,** Imaginary bisector and central ray. **C,** Exposure of the receptor. **D,** Resultant image.

1. Center the receptor on the mandibular canine.
2. Position the upper edge of the receptor parallel to the occlusal plane so that one-eighth of an inch extends above the incisal edge of the canine.
3. Instruct the patient to "slowly close" and gently bite on the receptor holder or beam alignment device.
4. If not using a beam alignment device, establish the correct vertical angulation by bisecting the angle and directing the central ray perpendicular to the imaginary bisector.
5. If not using a beam alignment device, establish the correct horizontal angulation by directing the central ray between the contacts of the canine and first premolar.
6. Position the position-indicating device (PID) using the correct vertical and horizontal angulations. Center the PID over the receptor to avoid cone-cutting.
7. Expose the receptor.

PROCEDURE 20-6 Mandibular Incisor Exposure: Bisecting Technique (Figure 20-20)

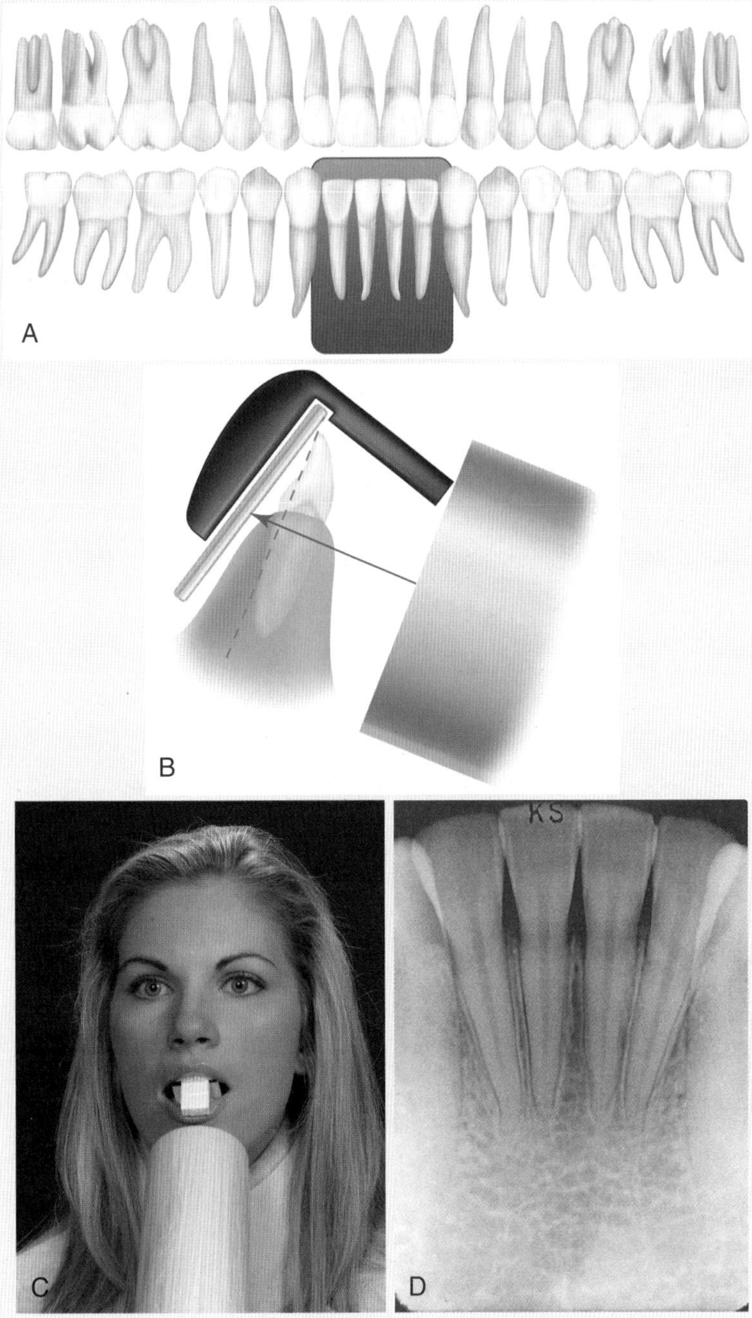

Fig 20-20 Exposure of the mandibular incisors. **A,** Receptor placement. **B,** Imaginary bisector and central ray. **C,** Exposure of the receptor. **D,** Resultant image.

1. Center the receptor on the contact between the two mandibular central incisors.
2. Position the upper edge of the receptor parallel to the occlusal plane so that one-eighth of an inch extends above the incisal edges of the teeth.
3. Instruct the patient to "slowly close" and gently bite on the receptor holder or beam alignment device.
4. If not using a beam alignment device, establish the correct vertical angulation by bisecting the angle and directing the central ray perpendicular to the imaginary bisector.
5. If not using a beam alignment device, establish the correct horizontal angulation by directing the central ray between the contacts of the central incisors.
6. Position the position-indicating device (PID) using the correct vertical and horizontal angulations. Center the PID over the receptor to avoid cone-cutting.
7. Expose the receptor.

PROCEDURE 20-7 Maxillary Premolar Exposure: Bisecting Technique (Figure 20-21)

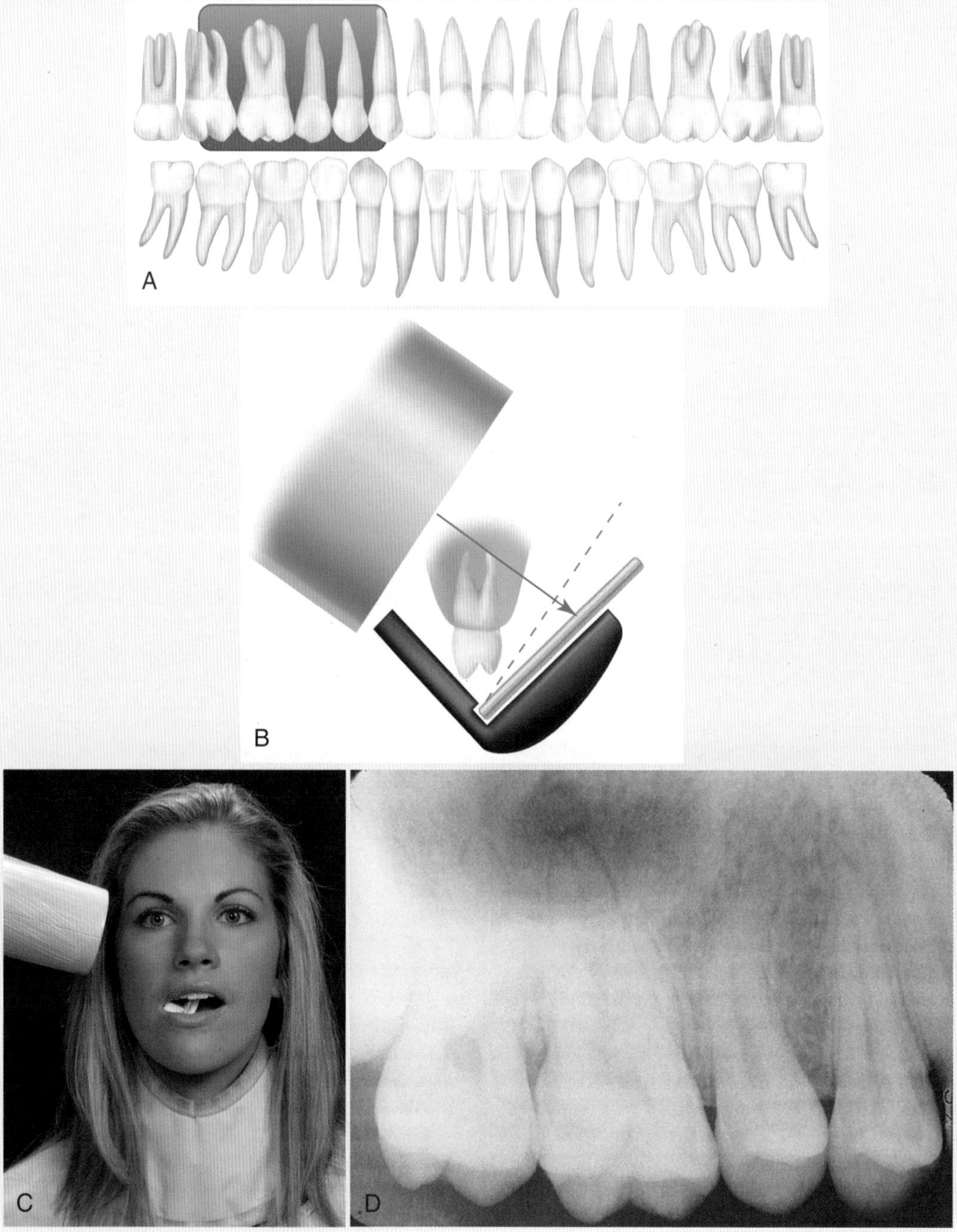

Fig 20-21 Exposure of the maxillary premolars. **A,** Receptor placement. **B,** Imaginary bisector and central ray. **C,** Exposure of the receptor. **D,** Resultant image.

1. Center the receptor on the maxillary second premolar; the front edge of the receptor should be aligned with the midline of the maxillary canine.
2. Position the lower edge of the receptor parallel to the occlusal plane so that one-eighth of an inch extends below the occlusal edges of the teeth.
3. Instruct the patient to "slowly close" and gently bite on the receptor holder or beam alignment device.
4. If not using a beam alignment device, establish the correct vertical angulation by bisecting the angle and directing the central ray perpendicular to the imaginary bisector.
5. If not using a beam alignment device, establish the correct horizontal angulation by directing the central ray between the contacts of the premolars.
6. Position the position-indicating device (PID) using the correct vertical and horizontal angulations. Center the PID over the receptor to avoid cone-cutting.
7. Expose the receptor.

PROCEDURE 20-8 Maximillary Molar Exposure: Bisecting Technique (Figure 20-22)

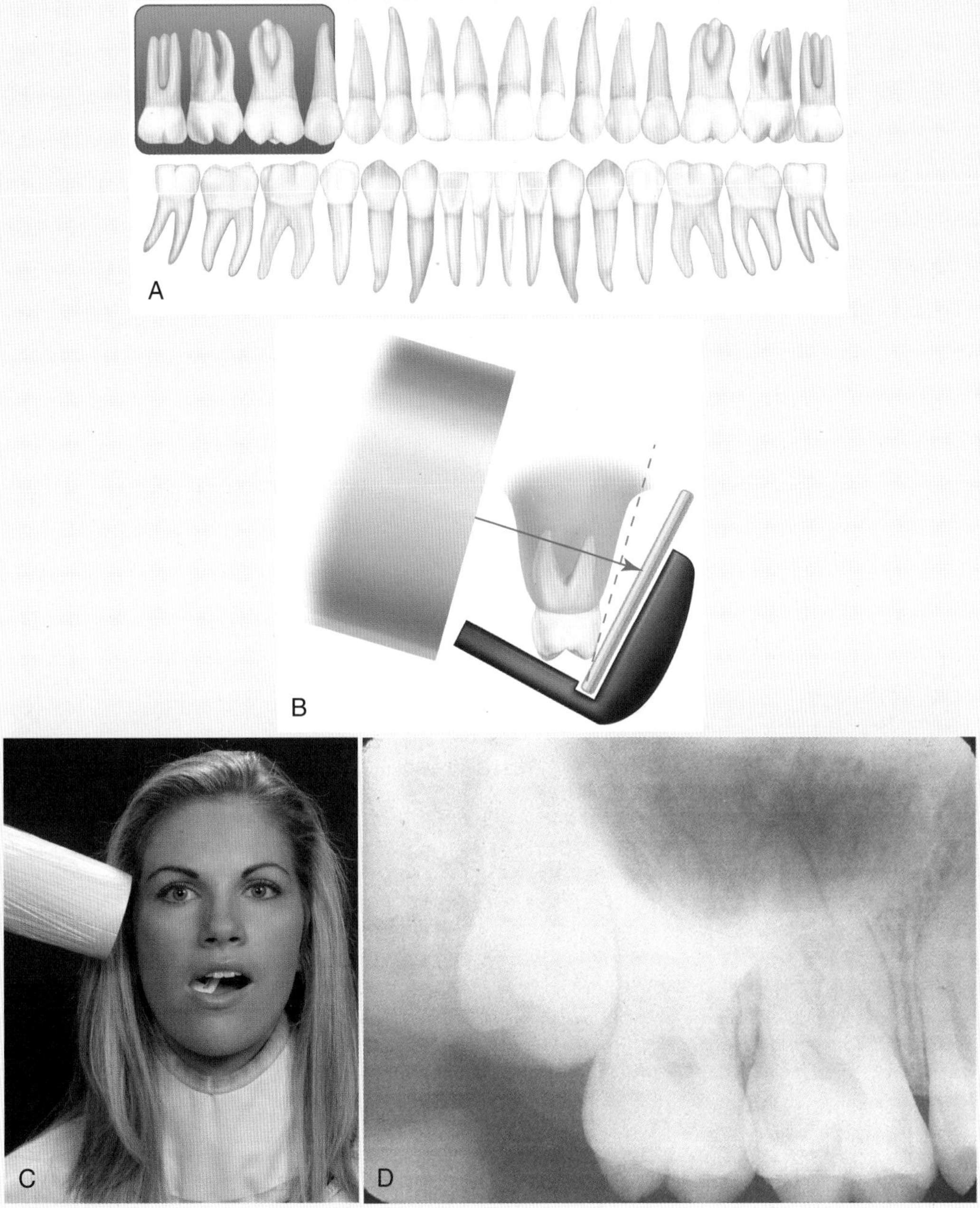

Fig 20-22 Exposure of the maxillary molars. **A,** Receptor placement. **B,** Imaginary bisector and central ray. **C,** Exposure of the receptor. **D,** Resultant image.

1. Center the receptor on the maxillary second molar; the front edge of the receptor should be aligned with the midline of the maxillary second premolar.
2. Position the lower edge of the receptor parallel to the occlusal plane so that one-eighth of an inch extends below the occlusal edges of the teeth.
3. Instruct the patient to "slowly close" and gently bite on the receptor holder or beam alignment device.
4. If not using a beam alignment device, establish the correct vertical angulation by bisecting the angle and directing the central ray perpendicular to the imaginary bisector.
5. If not using a beam alignment device, establish the correct horizontal angulation by directing the central ray between the contacts of the molars.
6. Position the position-indicating device (PID) using the correct vertical and horizontal angulations. Center the PID over the receptor to avoid cone-cutting.
7. Expose the receptor.

PROCEDURE 20-9 Mandibular Premolar Exposure: Bisecting Technique (Figure 20-23)

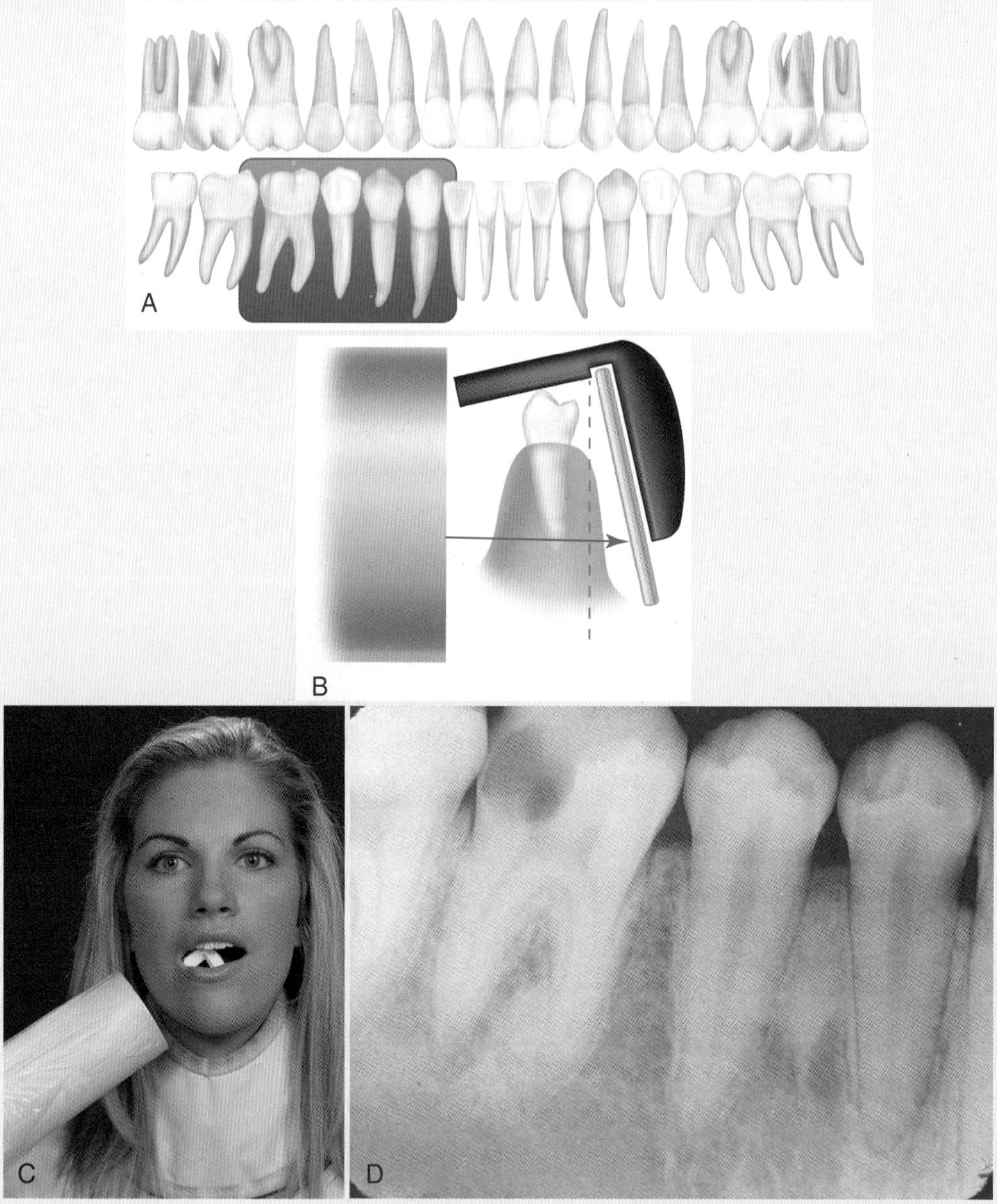

Fig 20-23 Exposure of the mandibular premolars. **A,** Receptor placement. **B,** Imaginary bisector and central ray. **C,** Exposure of the receptor. **D,** Resultant image.

1. Center the receptor on the mandibular second premolar; the front edge of the receptor should be aligned with the midline of the mandibular canine.
2. Position the upper edge of the receptor parallel to the occlusal plane so that one-eighth of an inch extends above the occlusal edges of the teeth.
3. Instruct the patient to "slowly close" and gently bite on the receptor holder or beam alignment device.
4. If not using a beam alignment device, establish the correct vertical angulation by bisecting the angle and directing the central ray perpendicular to the imaginary bisector.
5. If not using a beam alignment device, establish the correct horizontal angulation by directing the central ray between the contacts of the premolars.
6. Position the position-indicating device (PID) using the correct vertical and horizontal angulations. Center the PID over the receptor to avoid cone-cutting.
7. Expose the receptor.

PROCEDURE 20-10 Mandibular Molar Exposure: Bisecting Technique (Figure 20-24)

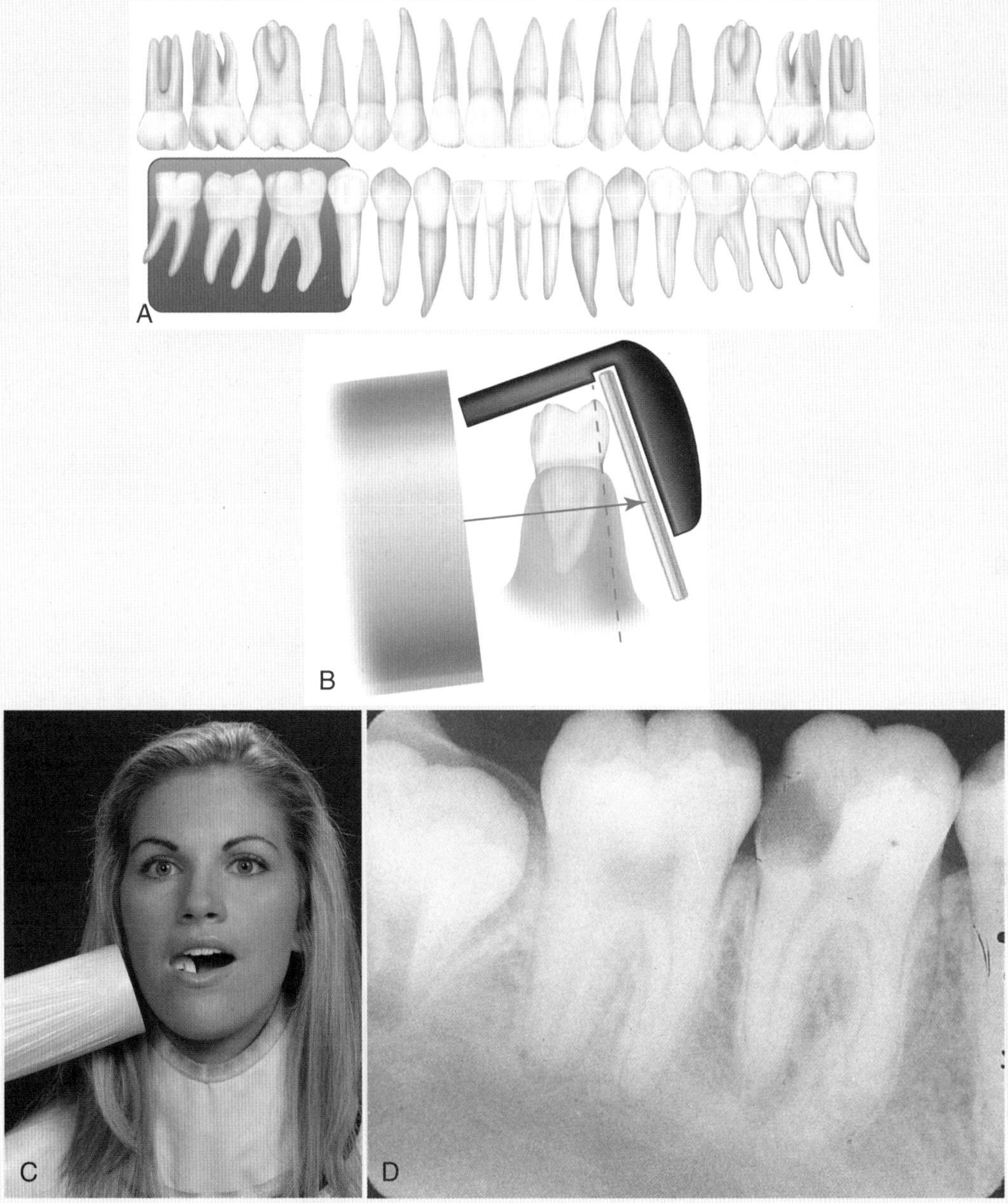

Fig 20-24 Exposure of the mandibular molars. **A,** Receptor placement. **B,** Imaginary bisector and central ray. **C,** Exposure of the receptor. **D,** Resultant image.

1. Center the receptor on the mandibular second molar; the front edge of the receptor should be aligned with the midline of the mandibular second premolar.
2. Position the upper edge of the receptor parallel to the occlusal plane so that one-eighth of an inch extends above the occlusal edges of the teeth.
3. Instruct the patient to "slowly close" and gently bite on the receptor holder or beam alignment device.
4. If not using a beam alignment device, establish the correct vertical angulation by bisecting the angle and directing the central ray perpendicular to the imaginary bisector.
5. If not using a beam alignment device, establish the correct horizontal angulation by directing the central ray between the contacts of the molars.
6. Position the position-indicating device (PID) using the correct vertical and horizontal angulations. Center the PID over the receptor to avoid cone-cutting.
7. Expose the receptor.

PROCEDURE 20-10 Mandibular Molar Exposure: Bisecting Technique (Figure 20-24)—cont'd

An example of a charting note for a full-mouth series using the bisecting technique is given below:

CHARTING A FULL-MOUTH SERIES

Date	ADA Procedure Code	Provider	Charting Notes	Comments
12/1/21	0210	LJH	Dr. Stewart prescribed a modified complete mouth series of images; bisecting technique used with Stabe Bite-block; 10 periapicals and 2 bite-wing images exposed; digital PSP plates used (12 total exposures)	Patient has had all molar teeth extracted; only anterior teeth and premolars are present; patient tolerated procedure well; prefers the styrofoam bite-block over the plastic beam alignment device; slight gag reflex noted on maxillary periapical placements; instructed patient to breathe through nose

- **DO NOT** use words such as *hurt*. Instead, inform patients that the procedure will be "momentarily uncomfortable."
- **DO NOT** make comments such as "Oops." Patients will lose confidence in your abilities when hearing such comments.
- **DO NOT** pick up a receptor if you drop it. Leave it on the floor; it has now become contaminated. Instead, remove it and dispose of it when you clean the treatment area.
- **DO NOT** allow patients to dictate how you should perform your imaging duties. The dental radiographer must always remain in control of the procedures.
- **DO NOT** begin with posterior exposures; posterior placements may cause patients to gag. Instead, always begin with the easier anterior exposures.

SUMMARY

- The bisecting technique is an intraoral technique used to expose periapical images. This technique is based on the concept of bisecting the angle formed by the receptor and the long axis of the tooth.
- The bisecting technique is an alternative method for exposing periapical images when the paralleling technique cannot be used.
- In the bisecting technique, (1) the receptor is placed along the lingual surface of the tooth; (2) at the point where the receptor contacts the tooth, the plane of the receptor and the long axis of the tooth form an angle; (3) an imaginary bisector divides the angle in half, or bisects it; and (4) the central ray of the x-ray beam is directed perpendicular to the imaginary bisector.
- In the bisecting technique, beam alignment devices are recommended to stabilize the receptor. A variety of beam alignment devices and receptor holders are commercially available.
- Before imaging procedures using the bisecting technique begin, infection prevention measures must be completed, and the treatment area and the supplies must be prepared. After the patient is seated and the imaging procedures explained, adjustments to the chair and headrest are made, the lead apron is placed, and the patient is asked to remove eyeglasses and any intraoral objects. The exposure factors are then set.
- A size 2 intraoral receptor is used with the bisecting technique. For anterior exposures, the receptor is always positioned vertically; for posterior exposures, the receptor is always positioned horizontally.
- *Horizontal angulation* refers to the positioning of the PID in a side-to-side plane. With correct horizontal angulation, the central ray is directed through the contact areas of the teeth, and thus the contact areas on the image appear "opened." Incorrect horizontal angulation results in overlapped ("unopened") contacts.
- *Vertical angulation* refers to the positioning of the PID in an up-and-down plane. With the bisecting technique, the vertical angulation is determined by the imaginary bisector; the central ray is directed perpendicular to the imaginary bisector. Correct vertical angulation results in a dental image that is of the same length as that of the tooth.
- Incorrect vertical angulation results in a dental image that is not of the same length as that of the tooth. Foreshortening of images occurs with excessive vertical angulation (too steep), whereas elongation of images results from insufficient vertical angulation (too flat).
- Five basic rules exist for the bisecting technique: (1) The receptor must cover the prescribed area of interest; (2) the receptor must be positioned with one eighth of an inch extending beyond the incisal or occlusal surfaces; (3) the central ray must be directed perpendicular to the imaginary bisector that divides the angle formed by the tooth and the receptor; (4) the central ray must be directed through the contact areas between teeth; and (5) the x-ray beam must be centered over the receptor to ensure that all areas of the receptor are exposed.
- When using the bisecting technique, the dental radiographer always begins with anterior exposures; anterior exposures are less likely to cause gagging. After anterior exposures, the posterior teeth are imaged. In each quadrant, the premolar region is always exposed first and then the molar region.
- When exposing a complete mouth series (CMS) using the bisecting technique, each of 14 periapical exposures has a prescribed placement (see Boxes 20-1 and 20-2 and Figures 20-15 and 20-16).
- The advantages of the bisecting technique are that it eliminates the need for beam alignment devices and that it requires a shorter exposure time.
- The disadvantages of the bisecting technique are image distortion and angulation problems.
- The paralleling technique is preferred over the bisecting technique and should be used whenever possible.

TECHNIQUE VIDEOS

View the Technique Videos and complete the accompanying Interactive Exercises that are available as part of the Student Resources on the companion Evolve website for this textbook.

BIBLIOGRAPHY

Frommer HH, Stabulas-Savage JJ: Accessory radiographic techniques: bisecting technique and occlusal technique. In Radiology for the dental professional, ed 9, St. Louis, 2011, Mosby.

Johnson ON: Intraoral radiographic procedures. In Essentials of dental radiography for dental assistants and hygienists, ed 9, Upper Saddle River, NJ, 2011, Prentice Hall.

Johnson ON: The periapical examination. In Essentials of dental radiography for dental assistants and hygienists, ed 9, Upper Saddle River, NJ, 2011, Prentice Hall.

Mallya SM, Lam EWN: Projection geometry. In White and Pharoah's oral radiology: principles and interpretation, ed 8, St. Louis, 2019, Elsevier.

Miles DA, Van Dis ML, Razmus TF: Intraoral radiographic techniques. In Basic principles of oral and maxillofacial radiology, Philadelphia, 1992, Saunders.

QUIZ QUESTIONS

Matching

For questions 1 to 4, refer to Figure 20-25. Match the letter (A to D) of the item shown with the description below.

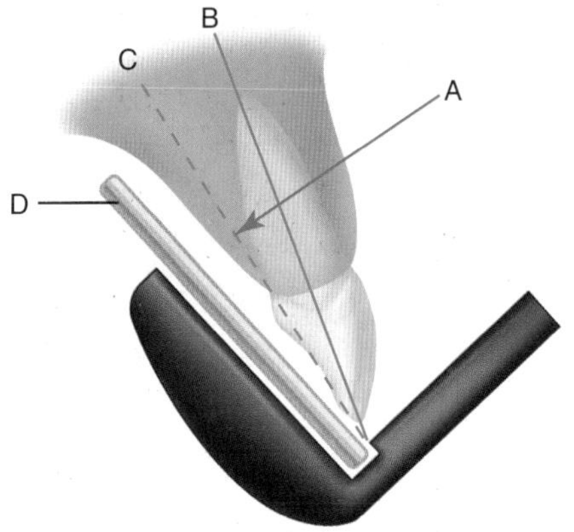

Fig 20-25

_____ 1. Plane of the receptor
_____ 2. Long axis of the tooth
_____ 3. Imaginary bisector
_____ 4. Central ray

Identification

For questions 5 to 10, refer to Figures 20-26, 20-27, and 20-28. Write in the letter of the item defined in each question.

_____ 5. In Figure 20-26, identify the angle that is bisected correctly.
_____ 6. In Figure 20-27, identify the central ray that is correctly positioned perpendicular to the imaginary bisector.
_____ 7. In Figure 20-28, identify the position-indicating device (PID) that is aligned correctly.
_____ 8. In Figure 20-28, identify the vertical angulation that results in foreshortening.
_____ 9. In Figure 20-28, identify the vertical angulation that results in elongation.
_____ 10. In Figure 20-28, identify the correct vertical angulation.

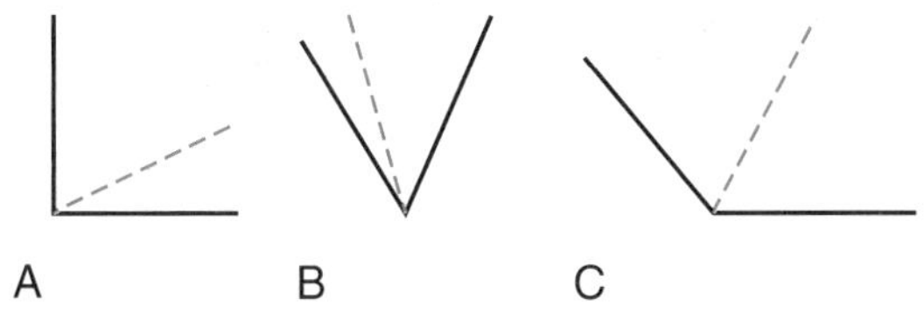

Fig 20-26

Short Answer

11. What happens to the dental image when a short (8-inch) PID is used?

____
____
____
____

12. Which size receptor is used with the bisecting technique?

____
____
____
____

13. Which beam alignment device is recommended for use with the bisecting technique because it aids in the alignment of the PID and reduces patient exposure?

____
____
____
____

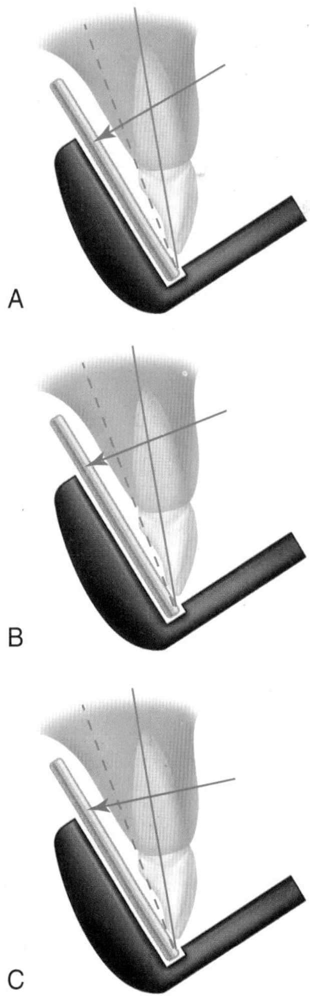

Fig 20-27

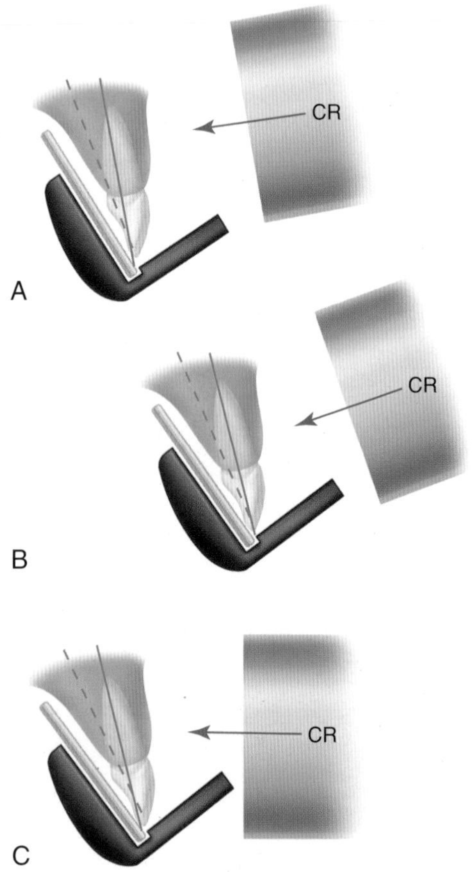

Fig 20-28

14. How is the patient's head positioned before exposing maxillary periapical images with the bisecting technique?

____

____

____

____

15 How is the patient's head positioned before exposing mandibular periapical images with the bisecting technique?

____

____

____

____

Multiple Choice

____ 16. Which describes the proper direction of the central ray in the bisecting technique?
- **a.** 90 degrees to the long axis of the tooth
- **b.** 90 degrees to the receptor and long axis of the tooth
- **c.** 90 degrees to the receptor
- **d.** 90 degrees to the imaginary bisector

____ 17. Which describes the distance between the receptor and the tooth in the bisecting technique?
- **a.** The receptor is placed as close as possible to the tooth.
- **b.** The receptor is placed away from the tooth and toward the middle of the oral cavity.
- **c.** The receptor is placed parallel to the tooth.
- **d.** None of the above.

____ 18. Which is/are advantages of the bisecting technique?
1. increased accuracy
2. simplicity of use
3. shorter exposure time
   - **a.** 1, 2, and 3
   - **b.** 1 and 2
   - **c.** 2 and 3
   - **d.** 3 only

____ 19. The disadvantages of the bisecting technique outweigh the advantages.
- **a.** true
- **b.** false

Essay

20. State the rule of isometry.
21. Discuss the significance of the shaded areas in Figure 20-29.

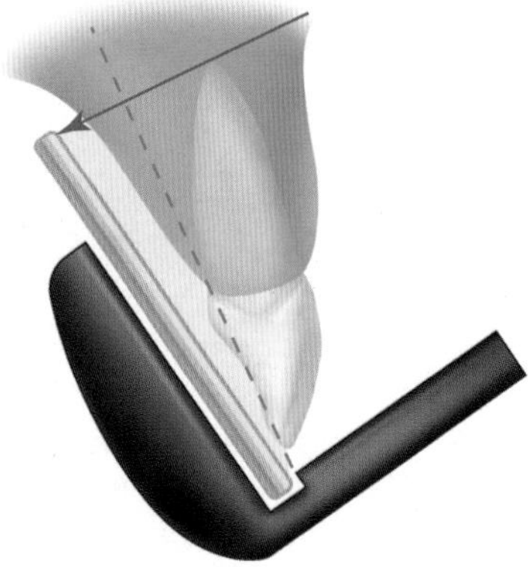
Fig 20-29

22. State the five rules for the bisecting technique.
23. Discuss the patient and equipment preparations that must be completed before using the bisecting technique.
24. Discuss the exposure sequence for the 14 periapical placements using the bisecting technique.
25. Describe each of the 14 periapical placements recommended for use with the bisecting technique.
26. Describe correct and incorrect horizontal angulation.
27. State the recommended vertical angulations for each maxillary periapical exposure using the bisecting technique.
28. State the recommended vertical angulations for each mandibular periapical exposure using the bisecting technique.

21

Bite-Wing Technique

LEARNING OBJECTIVES

After completion of this chapter, the student will be able to do the following:

1. Define the key terms associated with the bite-wing technique.
2. Describe the purpose and use of the bite-wing image.
3. Describe the appearance of opened and overlapped contact areas on a bite-wing image.
4. State the basic principles of the bite-wing technique.
5. List the two ways a receptor can be stabilized in the bite-wing technique and identify which one is recommended for bite-wing exposures.
6. List the three receptor sizes that can be used in the bite-wing technique and identify which size is recommended for exposures in the adult patient.
7. Describe correct and incorrect horizontal angulation.
8. Describe the difference between positive and negative vertical angulation.
9. State the recommended vertical angulation for all bite-wing exposures using a bite-wing tab.
10. State the basic rules for the bite-wing technique.
11. Describe patient and equipment preparations that are necessary before using the bite-wing technique.
12. Discuss the exposure sequence for a complete mouth series (CMS) that includes both periapical and bite-wing exposures.
13. Describe the correct premolar and molar bite-wing receptor placements.
14. Describe the purpose and use of vertical bite-wing images.
15. List the number of exposures and the size of receptor used in the vertical bite-wing technique.
16. Discuss modifications in the bite-wing technique for patients who have had teeth extracted for orthodontic purposes, or in patients with edentulous spaces or bony growths.

The dental radiographer must master a variety of intraoral imaging techniques. The bite-wing technique is used to examine the interproximal surfaces of teeth. A **bite-wing image** includes the crowns of maxillary and mandibular teeth, interproximal areas, and areas of crestal bone on the same image. Bite-wing images are primarily used to detect interproximal **caries** (tooth decay) and are particularly useful in detecting early carious lesions that are not clinically evident. Bite-wing images are also useful to monitor the progression of dental caries, assess existing restorations, and examine the crestal bone levels between teeth.

The bite-wing image derived its name from the original technique that required the patient to "bite" on a small "wing" of paper attached to a film packet. Currently, the need for a wing (now termed a "tab") is eliminated when a beam alignment device is used to hold the film or sensor. The choice to use a bite-wing beam alignment device is a matter of practitioner preference. Many dental practices still use bite-wing tabs. Regardless of whether a tab is used, this intraoral image is still referred to as a *bite-wing*.

Before the dental radiographer can use this important technique, an understanding of the basic concepts, including the terminology and principles relating to the bite-wing technique, is necessary. In addition, the dental radiographer must understand patient preparation, equipment preparation, exposure sequencing, and the receptor placement procedures used in the bite-wing technique.

The purpose of this chapter is to present basic concepts and to describe patient preparation, equipment preparation, and receptor placement procedures for the bite-wing technique. This chapter also outlines bite-wing technique modifications and reviews helpful hints.

BASIC CONCEPTS

The **bite-wing technique** (also known as the *interproximal technique*) is a method used to examine the interproximal surfaces of teeth. Before the dental radiographer can competently use this technique, a thorough understanding of the terminology, principles, and basic rules of the bite-wing technique is necessary. In addition, knowledge of the beam alignment devices, receptor sizes, and angulations of the position-indicating device (PID) used with the bite-wing technique is also required.

Terminology

An understanding of the following basic terms is necessary before describing the bite-wing technique:

- **Interproximal:** Between two adjacent surfaces.
- **Interproximal examination:** Intraoral examination used to inspect the crowns of both maxillary and mandibular teeth on a single image.
- **Bite-wing receptor:** Type of receptor used in interproximal examination. The bite-wing receptor has a "wing," or tab, and the patient "bites" on the wing to stabilize the receptor.
- **Alveolar bone:** Bone that supports and encases the roots of teeth (Figure 21-1).
- **Crestal bone:** Coronal portion of alveolar bone found between teeth; also known as the *alveolar crest* (Figure 21-2).
- **Contact areas:** The area of a tooth that touches an adjacent tooth; the area where adjacent tooth surfaces contact each other (Figure 21-3).
- **Horizontal bite-wing:** The bite-wing receptor is placed in the mouth with the long portion of the receptor in a horizontal direction.
- **Opened contacts:** On a dental image, opened contacts appear as thin radiolucent lines between adjacent tooth surfaces (Figure 21-4).
- **Overlapped contacts:** On a dental image, the area where the contact area of one tooth is superimposed over the contact area of an adjacent tooth is referred to as *overlapped contacts* (Figure 21-5).
- **Vertical bite-wing:** The bite-wing receptor is placed in the mouth with the long portion of the receptor in a vertical direction (Figure 21-6).

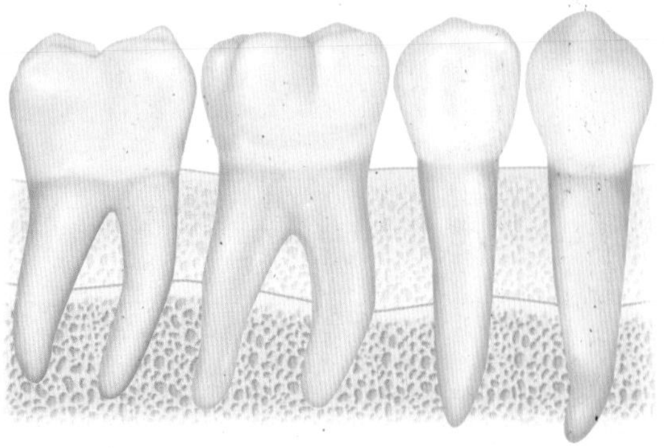

Fig 21-1 Alveolar bone.

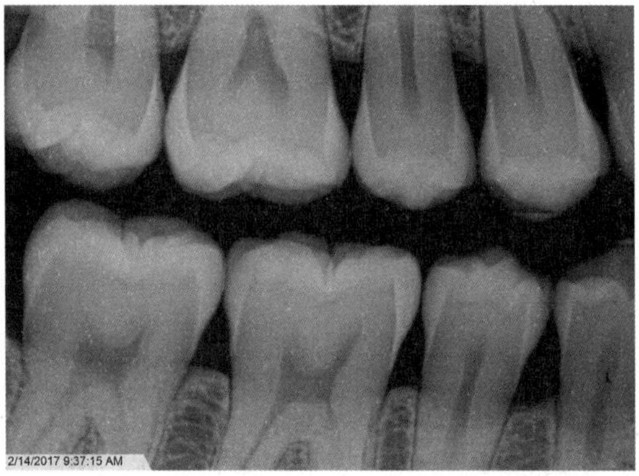

Fig 21-2 Crestal bone is the most coronal portion of alveolar bone found between teeth.

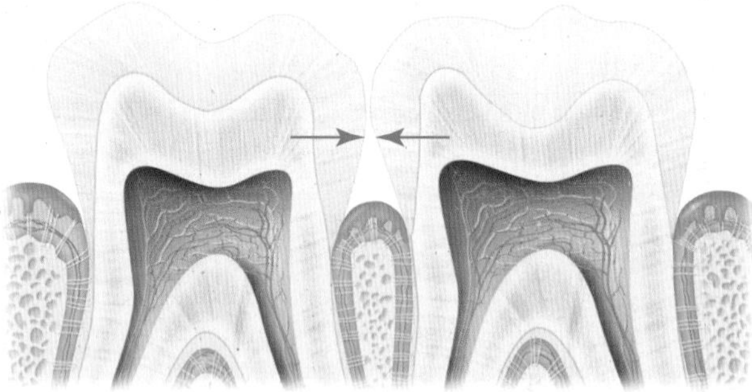

Fig 21-3 Contact areas are areas where adjacent tooth surfaces contact each other.

Principles of Bite-Wing Technique

The basic principles of the bite-wing technique can be described as follows (Figure 21-7):

The receptor is placed in the mouth *parallel* to the crowns of both maxillary and mandibular teeth.

The receptor is stabilized when the patient bites on the bite-wing tab or the bite-block of the beam alignment device.

When using a bite-wing tab on film or PSP sensors, the central ray of the x-ray beam is directed through the contacts of teeth, using a vertical angulation of +10 degrees.

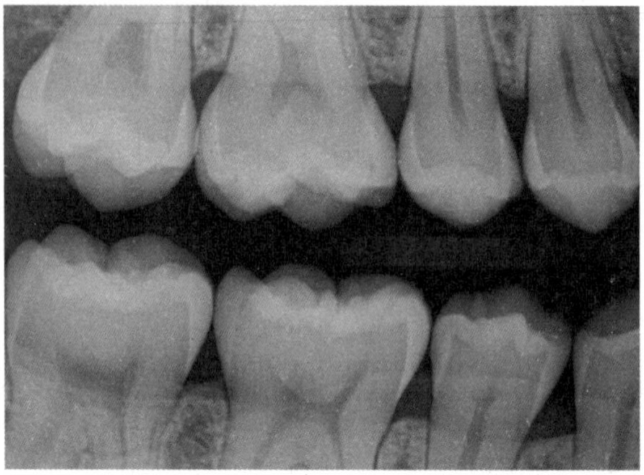

Fig 21-4 The opened contacts in the premolar region appear as thin radiolucent lines. Note that the occlusal plane is positioned horizontally along the midline of the long axis of the image.

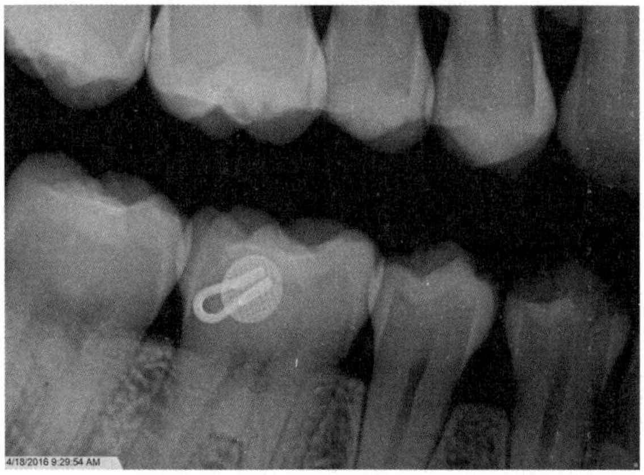

Fig 21-5 A nondiagnostic bite-wing image with overlapped interproximal contacts.

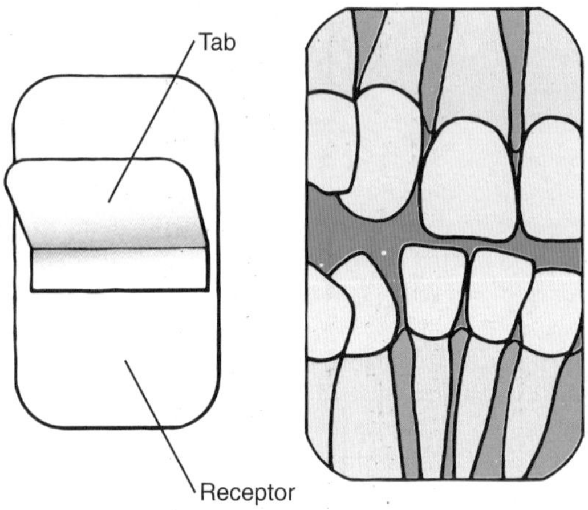

Fig 21-6 A vertical bite-wing image.

Beam Alignment Device and Bite-Wing Tab

In the bite-wing technique, either a beam alignment device or a bite-wing tab is used to stabilize the receptor.

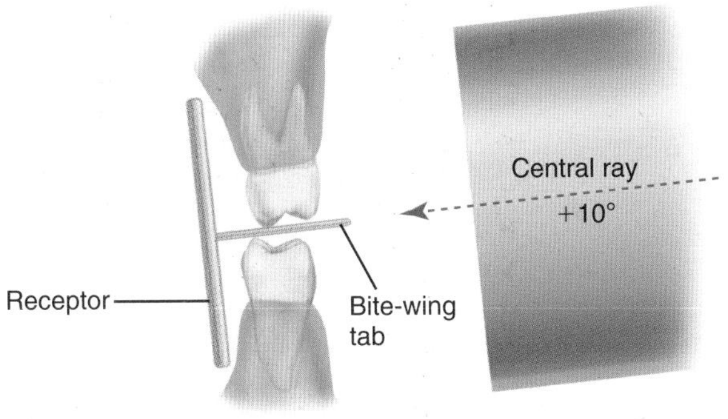

Fig 21-7 Positions of the receptor, bite-wing tab, and central ray in the bite-wing technique. The receptor is parallel to the crowns in the maxillary and mandibular teeth. The central ray is directed slightly downward (+10 degrees of vertical angulation).

HELPFUL HINT

Tabs or Beam Alignment Devices

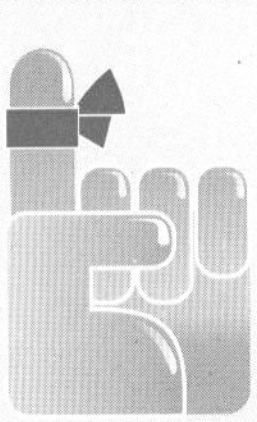

- If you can produce a diagnostic bite-wing using a tab, then you can easily produce a diagnostic one using a Rinn bite-wing instrument.
- Many dental practices use bite-wing tabs on digital sensors and films.
- Using tabs, you must be able to produce bite-wings with **open contacts** and **no cone-cuts**.

Bite-Wing Beam Alignment Device. A beam alignment device is a device used to position an intraoral receptor in the mouth and maintain the receptor in position during the imaging procedure (see Chapter 7). Beam alignment devices eliminate the need for the patient to stabilize the receptor with a bite-wing tab. As presented in Chapter 19, an example of a commercially available intraoral bite-wing beam alignment device is included with the *Rinn XCP Extension Cone Paralleling System* (Dentsply Rinn Corporation, York, PA). The Rinn XCP system is recommended for bite-wing projections. The Rinn XCP bite-wing instrument is color-coded and includes a red aiming ring, metal arm, and red plastic bite-blocks (Figure 21-8, A, B). The bite-blocks are available in sizes that accommodate film, PSP plates, or digital sensors and can be positioned in a horizontal or vertical orientation. This beam alignment device is simple to assemble and position. The Rinn XCP bite-wing instrument is reusable and must be sterilized after each use. For information about the use of the Rinn XCP bite-wing instruments, the dental radiographer should refer to manufacturer instructions.

To reduce the amount of radiation exposure to the patient, both the American Dental Association and the American Academy of Oral and Maxillofacial Radiology recommend the use of a rectangular collimator for all intraoral exposures (see Chapter 19). Consistent with the recommendations of these groups, when a rectangular collimator is used with the Rinn XCP bite-wing instrument, a significant reduction of radiation exposure occurs (Figure 21-8, C).

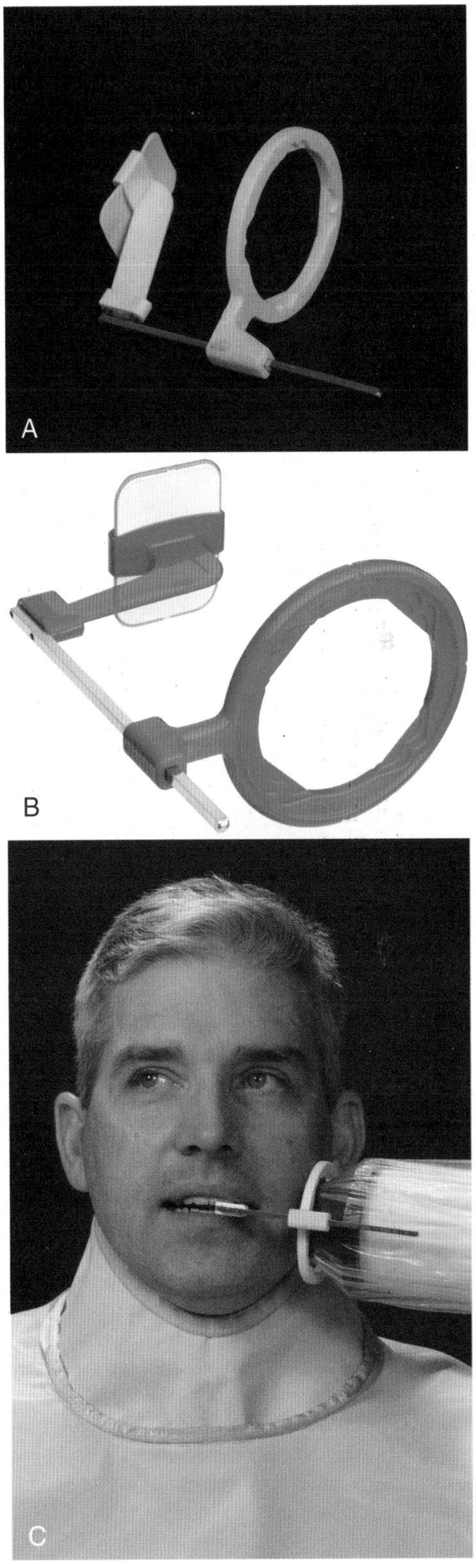

Fig 21-8 **A,** Beam alignment device for horizontal bite-wing images. Note aiming ring used for the positioning of the PID to ensure that the entire receptor is covered by the x-ray beam. **B,** Beam alignment device for vertical bite-wings. **C,** Rectangular collimation used with a bite-wing exposure.

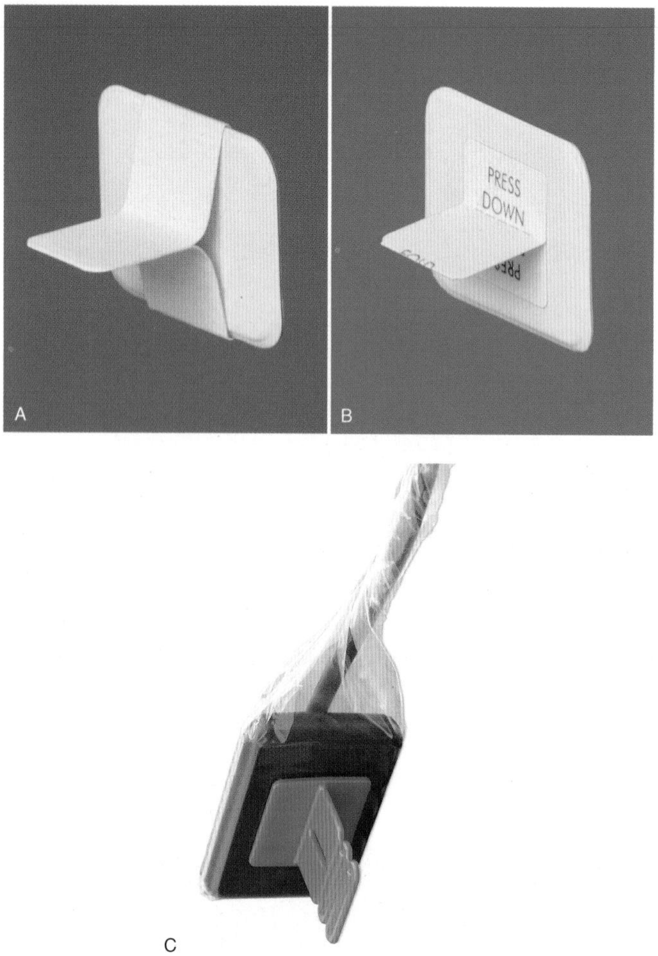

Fig 21-9 A, Paper bite-wing tabs. B, Adhesive paper bite-wing tabs. C. Adhesive plastic bite-wing tab used with a sensor. (Courtesy Dentsply Rinn, York, PA)

Bite-Wing Tab. It is not always possible to use a beam alignment device to expose a bite-wing image, especially in children or an individual with a small mouth or limited opening. Therefore the dental radiographer must be familiar with the original bite-wing technique of using a tab attached to the receptor for use with such patients.

As an alternative to a beam alignment device, a bite-wing tab may be used to stabilize the receptor during exposure. To prepare a bite-wing receptor, either a *bite tab* or *bite loop* is attached to a periapical film or sensor. If a bite tab is used, an adhesive tab made out of plastic or heavy paperboard is attached to the receptor. If a bite loop is used, a paper loop with a tab extension is slipped over the receptor. In both cases, the tab must be attached to, or extend from, the tube side of the film (white side) or sensor (Figure 21-9, A, B, C). Bite tabs and bite loops are available in various sizes. Bite-wing tabs may be used on horizontal or vertical bite-wing projections.

Bite-Wing Receptors

As described in Chapter 9, three sizes of bite-wing receptors (0, 2, and 3) are available.

HELPFUL HINT

Receptor Sizes

Size 0 Receptor
- Used with primary dentition
- Always placed horizontally

Size 2 Receptor
- Used in **adults**
- Placed horizontally or vertically

Size 3 Receptor
- Used in **adults**
- Always placed horizontally
- *Not* recommended

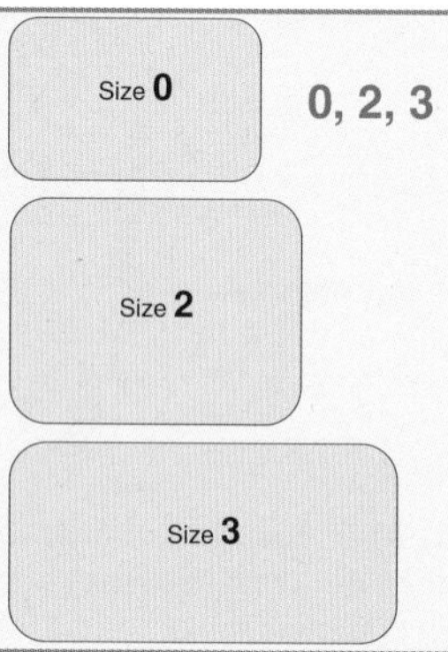

- *Size 0* is used to examine the posterior teeth of children with primary dentitions. This receptor is always placed with the long portion of the receptor in a *horizontal* (sideways) direction.
- *Size 2* is used to examine the posterior teeth in older children and adults and may be placed horizontally or vertically. For most bite-wing exposures, a size 2 receptor is placed with the long portion of the receptor in a *horizontal* direction. When a vertical posterior bite-wing exposure is indicated, a size 2 receptor is placed with the long portion of the receptor in a vertical direction.
- *Size 3* is longer and narrower than the standard size 2 receptor and is used *only* for bite-wing exposures. One receptor is exposed on each side of the arch to examine all the premolar and molar contact areas. A size 3 receptor is placed with the long portion of the receptor in a *horizontal* direction.

In the adult patient, a size 2 receptor is recommended for bite-wing exposures. The size 3 receptor is *not* recommended. With a size 3 receptor, overlapped contacts often result because of the difference in the curvature of the arch between the premolar and molar areas. In an adult patient, it is very difficult to open all posterior contacts with one exposure. In addition, the crestal bone areas may not be adequately seen on the dental images of patients with bone loss because of the narrow dimension of the receptor.

Position-Indicating Device Angulation

In the bite-wing technique, the angulation of the PID is critical. As defined in Chapter 20, angulation is a term used to describe the alignment of the central ray of the x-ray beam in both horizontal and vertical planes. Angulation can be varied by moving the PID in a horizontal or vertical direction. The position of the aiming ring of the Rinn XCP bite-wing instrument dictates the proper PID angulation. However, when a bite-wing tab is used without an aiming ring, the dental radiographer must determine both horizontal and vertical angulations for each exposure.

Horizontal Angulation. As described in Chapter 20, horizontal angulation refers to the positioning of the central ray in a horizontal, or side-to-side, plane (see Figure 20-7). The bite-wing, paralleling, and bisecting techniques all use the same principles of horizontal angulation.

Correct horizontal angulation. With correct horizontal angulation, the central ray is directed perpendicular to the curvature of the arch

HELPFUL HINT

PID Angulation

Horizontal Angulation

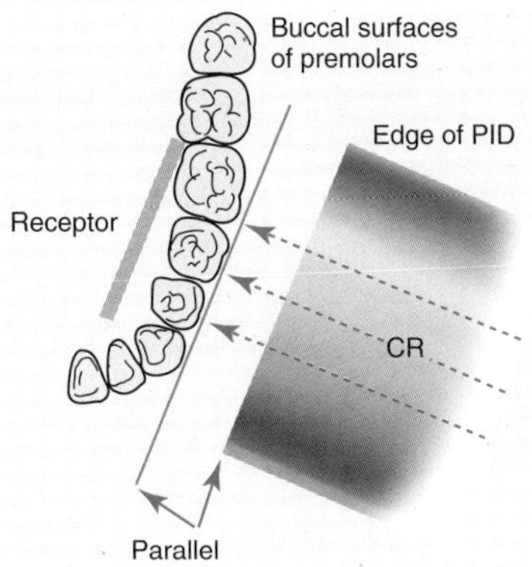

Vertical Angulation

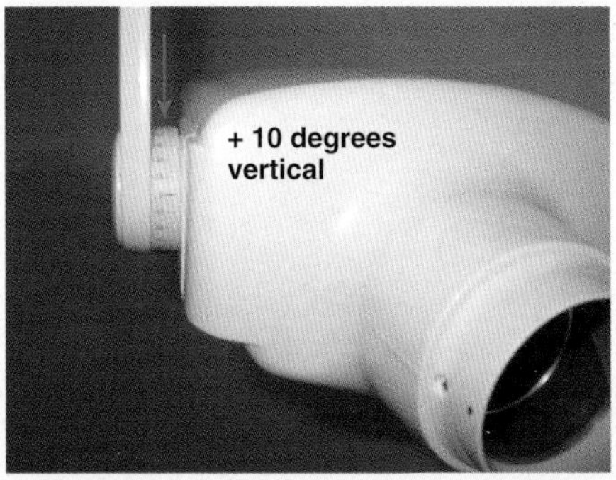

Open Contacts

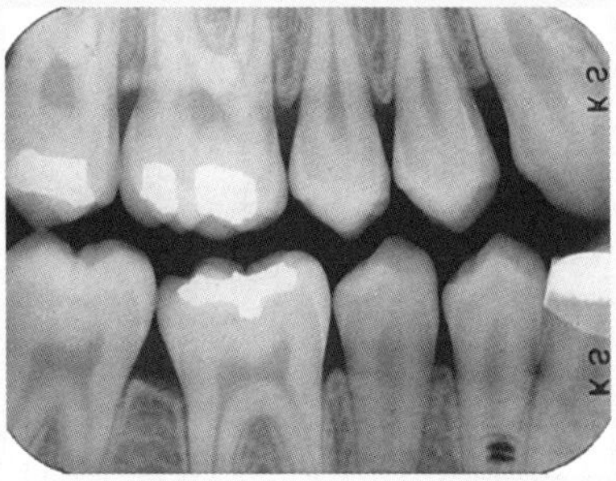

- **With tabs**, you must determine horizontal and vertical angulation.
- The goal is ***open* contacts**.

and through the contact areas of teeth (see Figure 20-8). As a result, the contact areas on the exposed image appear "opened" and can be examined for evidence of caries (see Figure 21-4).

Incorrect horizontal angulation. Incorrect horizontal angulation results in overlapped ("unopened") contact areas (see Figure 20-9). An image with overlapped interproximal contact areas cannot be used to examine the interproximal areas of teeth for evidence of caries and may require a retake (see Figure 21-5).

Vertical Angulation. As described in Chapter 20, vertical angulation refers to the positioning of the PID in a vertical, or up-and-down, plane (Figure 21-10). Vertical angulation may be positive or negative and is measured in degrees as labeled on the outside of the tubehead (Figure 21-11). If the PID is positioned above the occlusal plane and the central ray is directed downward, the vertical angulation is termed positive (+). If the PID is positioned below the occlusal plane and the central ray is directed upward, the vertical angulation is termed negative (−).

Correct vertical angulation. A vertical angulation of +10 degrees is recommended when a bite-wing tab is used with film or PSP sensors and without a beam alignment device. The +10 degree vertical angulation is used to compensate for the slight bend of the upper portion of the receptor and the slight tilt of maxillary teeth (Figure 21-12). Prior to positioning the PID with the correct vertical angulation, it is important to adjust the headrest to support the patient's head so that the occlusal plane is parallel with the floor.

Incorrect vertical angulation. Incorrect vertical angulation used in the exposure of a bite-wing results in a distorted image. For example, if a negative vertical angulation is used, the occlusal surfaces of maxillary teeth are evident, and the apical regions of mandibular teeth are seen (Figure 21-13). A bite-wing image exposed with an excessive negative vertical angulation is nondiagnostic.

Rules for Bite-Wing Technique

Five basic rules must be followed when using the bite-wing technique.

1. *Receptor placement.* The bite-wing receptor must be positioned to cover the prescribed area of teeth to be examined. Specific placements are detailed in the procedures section of this chapter.
2. *Receptor position.* The bite-wing receptor must be positioned parallel to the crowns of both maxillary and mandibular teeth. The receptor must be stabilized when the patient bites on the bite-wing tab or on the bite-block of the beam alignment device.
3. *Vertical angulation.* When a bite-wing tab is used with film or PSP sensors, the central ray of the x-ray beam must be directed at +10 degrees (see Figure 21-12).
4. *Horizontal angulation.* When a bite-wing tab is used, the central ray of the x-ray beam must be directed through the contact areas between teeth.
5. *Receptor exposure.* The x-ray beam must be centered on the receptor to ensure that all areas of the receptor are exposed. Failure to center the x-ray beam results in a partial image on the bite-wing receptor or a cone-cut. Cone-cuts are discussed in Chapter 22.

HELPFUL HINT

Rules for Bite-Wing Technique

Receptor Placement
- Cover prescribed teeth

Receptor Position
- Placed **parallel** to teeth
- Stabilized by patient **biting on tab** or Rinn XCP bite-block

Vertical Angulation
- +10 degrees (tabs) if using film or PSP sensors

Horizontal Angulation
- CR directed through contacts

Receptor Exposure
- CR centered on receptor

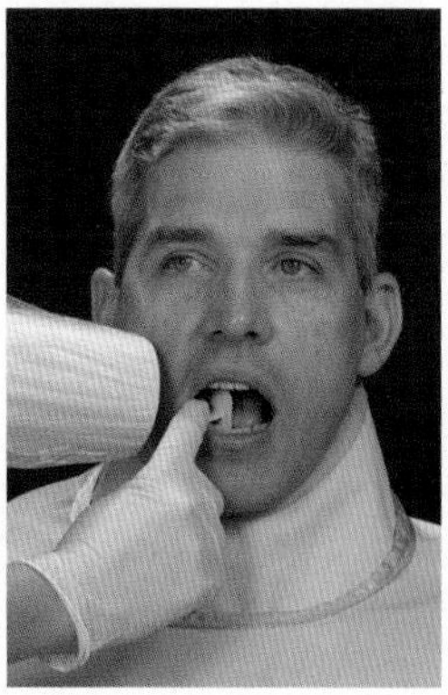

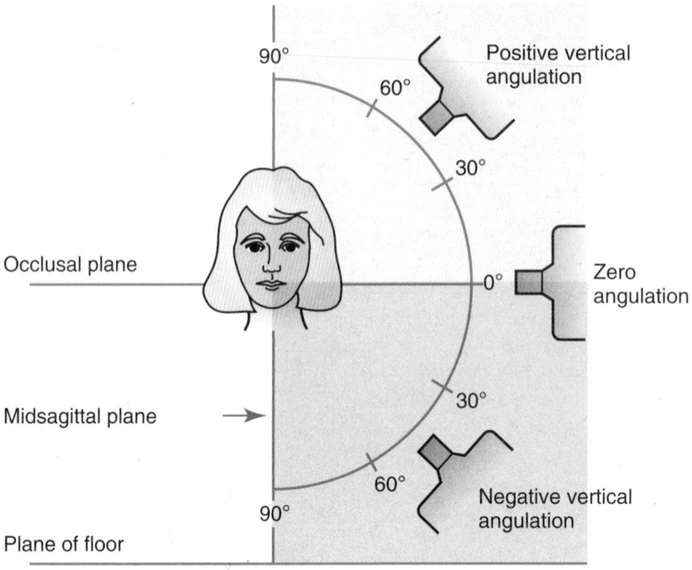

Fig 21-10 All vertical angulations above the occlusal plane are termed *positive*. Vertical angulations below the occlusal plane are termed *negative*. Zero angulation is achieved when the position-indicating device (PID) and the central ray are parallel to the floor.

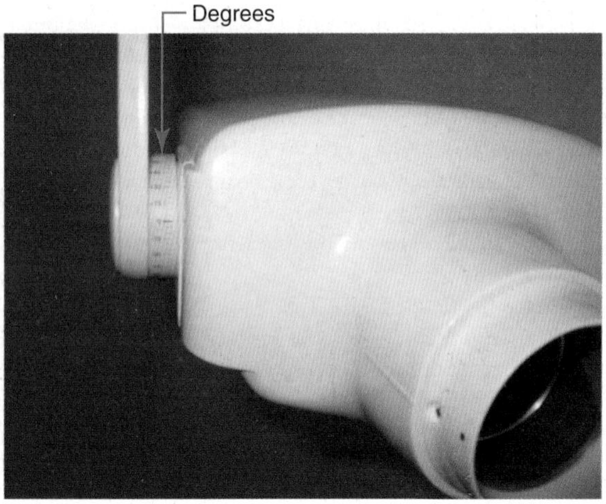

Fig 21-11 Vertical angulation is measured in degrees on the outside of the tubehead.

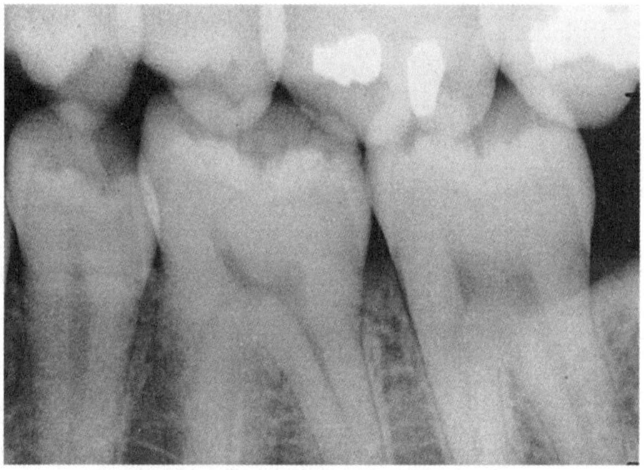

Fig 21-13 Negative vertical angulation.

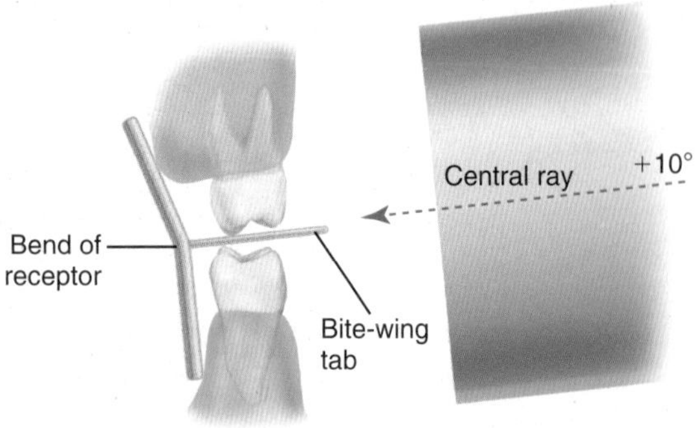

Fig 21-12 A vertical angulation of+10 degrees is used to compensate for the slight bend of the upper portion of the receptor (film or PSP plate) and the tilt of maxillary teeth.

Step-By-Step Procedures

Step-by-step procedures for the exposure of bite-wing receptors include patient preparation, equipment preparation, and receptor placement methods. Before exposing any bite-wing images, infection prevention procedures (as described in Chapter 16) must be completed.

Patient Preparation. After completion of infection prevention procedures and preparation of the treatment area and supplies, the patient should be seated. The dental radiographer must then prepare the patient before the exposure of any receptors (Procedure 21-1).

Equipment Preparation. After patient preparation, equipment must also be prepared before the exposure of any receptors begins (Procedure 21-2).

Exposure Sequence for Receptor Placements. When using the bite-wing technique, an exposure sequence, or definite order for receptor placements and exposure, must be followed. The dental radiographer must have an established exposure routine to prevent errors and

PROCEDURE 21-1 Patient Preparation for Bite-Wing Images

1. Briefly explain the imaging procedures to the patient.
2. Adjust the chair so the patient is positioned upright and the level of the chair is at a comfortable working height.
3. Adjust the headrest to support and position the patient's head. Position the patient's head such that the maxillary arch is parallel to the floor and the midsagittal (midline) plane is perpendicular to the floor.
4. Place and secure the lead apron with a thyroid collar on the patient.
5. Request that the patient remove eyeglasses and all objects from the mouth (e.g., dentures, retainers, chewing gum) that may interfere with the procedure.

PROCEDURE 21-2 Equipment Preparation for Bite-Wing Images

1. Set the exposure control factors (kilovoltage, milliamperage, and time) on the x-ray unit according to the manufacturer recommendations.
2. If a beam alignment device is used with the bite-wing technique, open the sterilized package containing the device, and assemble the device on a covered work area.
3. If a bite-wing tab is used, attach the tab to the white side of the film, or the correct side of the receptor.

make efficient use of time. Working without an exposure sequence may result in confusion, omitting an area, or exposing the same area to x-radiation twice.

As discussed in Chapter 18, a complete mouth series (CMS) is an intraoral series of dental images that shows all the tooth-bearing areas of the maxilla and the mandible. The CMS may consist of periapical images alone, anterior and posterior vertical bite-wings, or a combination of periapical and bite-wing images. Bite-wing exposures should be prescribed only for areas where teeth have interproximal contact with adjacent teeth.

The number of bite-wing images necessary for a patient is based on the curvature of the arch and the number of teeth present in the posterior region. The curvature of the arch often differs between the premolar and molar areas (Figure 21-14). If the curvature of the arch differs, it is impossible to open all the posterior contact areas on one bite-wing image. Consequently, two bite-wing receptors are typically exposed on each side of the arch. Because the curvature of the arch differs in most adult patients, a total of four bite-wing images are exposed in the following areas: right premolar, right molar, left premolar, and left molar.

When posterior teeth are missing (e.g., in patients in whom the premolars and third molars have been extracted as part of orthodontic treatment), one bite-wing exposure on each side of the arch (instead of two) may be sufficient to cover the number of teeth present. (See Modifications in Bite-wing Technique.)

Exposure Sequence for Bite-Wings and Periapicals. In the patient who requires both periapical and bite-wing exposures, the following exposure sequence is recommended:

1. First, expose all anterior periapical receptors (see Chapters 19 and 20).
2. Follow with exposure of posterior periapical receptors (see Chapters 19 and 20).
3. Finish with bite-wing exposures.

The sequence ends with bite-wing exposures because these receptors are relatively easy for the patient to tolerate. It is unwise to end the examination with difficult exposures (e.g., painful placements or maxillary posterior placements that elicit the gag reflex). Completing a CMS with bite-wing exposures may leave the patient with a more positive feeling regarding the series.

Exposure Sequence for Bite-Wings Only. In the patient who requires bite-wing images only, the following exposure sequence is recommended for each side of the mouth:

1. Expose the premolar bite-wing first. This receptor is easier for the patient to tolerate and is less likely to evoke the gag reflex.
2. Next, expose the molar bite-wing receptor.
3. Repeat on opposite side of mouth.

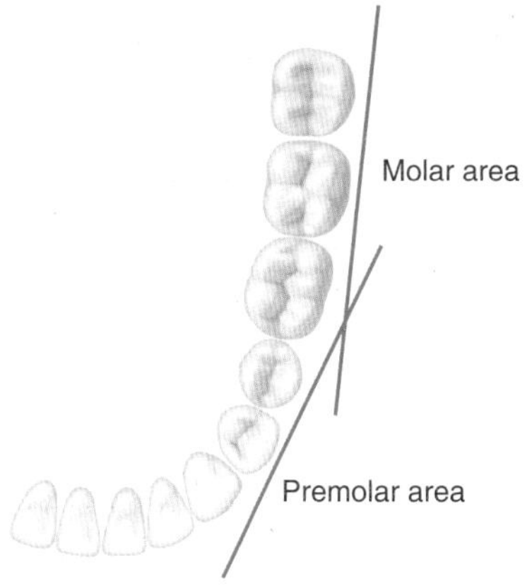

Fig 21-14 Note the difference in the curvature of the arch in premolar and molar areas.

Receptor Placement for Bite-Wing Images. When exposing bite-wing receptors, each exposure has a prescribed placement. **Receptor placement**, or the specific area where the receptor must be positioned before exposure, is dictated by the teeth and surrounding structures that must be included on the resulting bite-wing image. The specific placements described in this chapter are for a four-receptor posterior bite-wing series using size 2 receptors and bite-wing tabs. Variations in placement, receptor size, or total number of exposures may be recommended by other reference sources or individual practitioners (Box 21-1).

Posterior Receptor Placement. Placements for a four-receptor posterior bite-wing series include the following:

- Right and left premolar exposures (Procedure 21-3)
- Right and left molar exposures (Procedure 21-4)

It is important to note that in the procedures for premolar and molar bite-wing exposures, it is recommended that the receptor be placed into the patient's mouth after the exposure control factors on the x-ray unit have been chosen, as well as after both vertical and horizontal angulations have been set.

Vertical Bite-Wings

A vertical bite-wing image can be used to examine the level of alveolar bone in addition to caries detection. The vertical bite-wing is placed with the long portion of the receptor in an up-and-down, or vertical, direction (Figure 21-26). Vertical bite-wing images are often used as post-treatment or follow-up images for patients with bone loss caused by periodontal disease. Because of the extent of the periodontal condition, a horizontal bite-wing may not adequately show the amount of bone loss. Therefore either a vertical bite-wing or periapical image may be needed for thorough diagnostic purposes (Figures 21-27 and 21-28).

A modified CMS may be prescribed using vertical bite-wing images alone. A total of 7 projections (3 anterior and 4 posterior) are used to cover the anterior and posterior areas. Size 2 receptors may be used for all exposures, or a combination of size 1 (anterior teeth) and size 2 (posterior teeth) may be used. When tabs are used for projections in the anterior regions, a longer bite-wing tab is often necessary for the patient to be able to close completely on the tab. The patient should be instructed to bite on the tab in an end-to-end occlusal relationship (Figure 21-29).

Modifications in Bite-Wing Technique

Modifications in the bite-wing technique may be used to accommodate variations in anatomic conditions. Such modifications may be necessary in patients who have had teeth extracted prior to orthodontic treatment, or in patients with edentulous spaces or bony growths.

Extracted Teeth. Instead of the typical 32 teeth, patients may present with a total of 24 teeth as a result of the extraction of one set of premolars and all third molars; this is commonly seen in patients with previous orthodontic treatment. In this case four bite-wing exposures may not be necessary. Instead of a premolar and molar projection on each side, the dentist may decide that only one projection is necessary per side to adequately image all interproximal spaces. The bite-wing receptor is placed to capture the distal of the mandibular canine, and the premolar and molars are visible (Figure 21-30).

BOX 21-1 Guidelines for Bite-Wing Receptor Placement

1. If using film, the white side of the film always faces the teeth ("white in sight"). When using a sensor, position the sensor toward the x-ray tube according to the manufacturer instructions.
2. If using film, the identification dot has no significance in the bite-wing placement.
3. In posterior bite-wing series, receptors are placed horizontally or vertically.
4. When positioning the receptor, always center the receptor over the area to be examined (as defined in the prescribed placements).
5. When positioning the receptor, ask the patient to "slowly bite" on the bite-wing tab or on the bite-block of the beam alignment device. Always make certain that the teeth and not the lips alone stabilize the bite-block or tab.

PROCEDURE 21-3 Premolar Bite-Wing Exposure With Bite Tab (Figures 21-15 to 21-21)

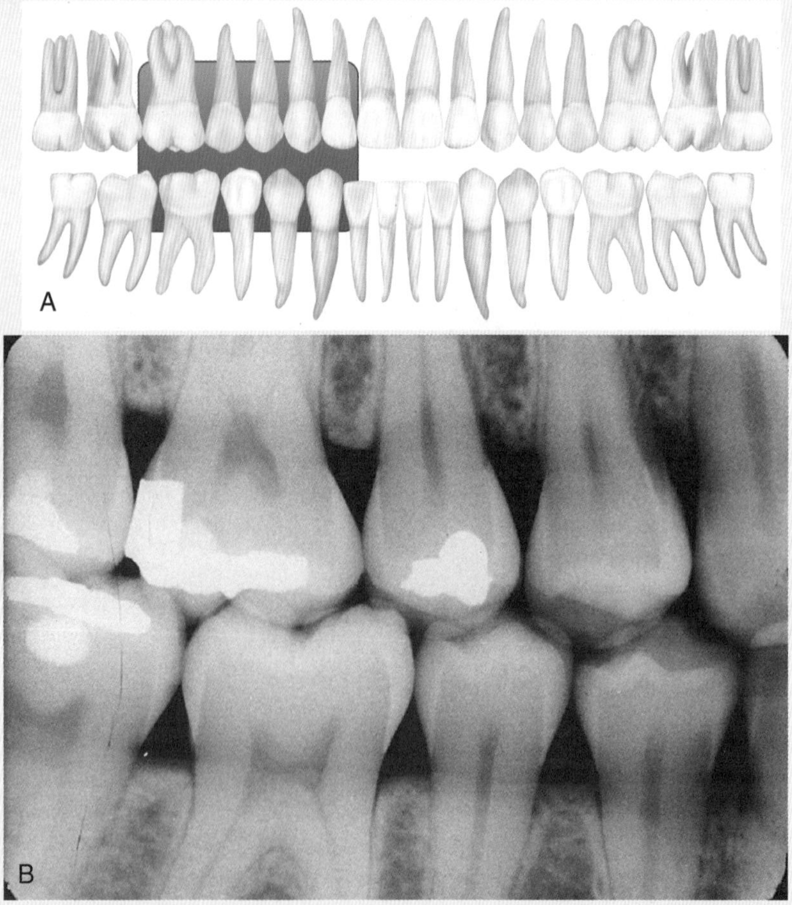

Fig 21-15 The premolar bite-wing. **A,** Receptor placement. **B,** Resultant image.

PROCEDURE 21-3 Premolar Bite-Wing Exposure With Bite Tab (Figures 21-15 to 21-21)—cont'd

1. Set vertical angulation at +10 degrees if using film or PSP sensors (Figure 21-16).
2. To set the horizontal angulation, stand in front of the patient. Examine the posterior curvature of the arch. To better visualize the curvature of the arch, place your index finger along the premolar area. Align the open end of the position-indicating device (PID) parallel to your index finger and the curvature of the arch in the premolar area, and direct the central ray through the contact areas (Figure 21-17).
3. Make certain that the PID is positioned far enough forward to cover both maxillary and mandibular canines and is positioned evenly over the mandibular and maxillary arches to avoid a cone-cut. The middle of the PID should be directed at the level of the occlusal plane (Figure 21-18). After the vertical angulation, horizontal angulation, and PID position have been established, the PID should not be adjusted, and the receptor should be placed without moving the PID.
4. Fold down one-third of the bite-wing tab, and crease it. Insert the receptor into the patient's mouth, and place the lower half of the receptor between the patient's tongue and teeth. Place the biting surface of the tab on the occlusal surfaces of mandibular teeth. Center the receptor on the mandibular second premolar; the front edge of the receptor should be aligned with the midline of the mandibular canine. Using your index finger, hold the folded portion of the bite-wing tab against the buccal surfaces of the premolars (Figure 21-19). Hold the tab in place during steps 5 and 6.
5. Make certain that the patient's occlusal plane is parallel to the floor. If necessary, ask the patient to lower the chin (Figure 21-20).
6. To check for a cone-cut, stand directly behind the tubehead and look along the side of the PID. No portion of the receptor should be visible; the receptor should be covered by the opening of the PID (Figure 21-21). If the receptor is not visible, ask the patient to "slowly close" and gently bite while still holding the bite-wing tab. If any portion of the receptor is visible, a cone-cut will result. In such cases, the PID must be adjusted to cover the receptor. After the PID has been positioned properly, ask the patient to "slowly close" and gently bite while still holding the bite-wing tab.
7. Expose the receptor.

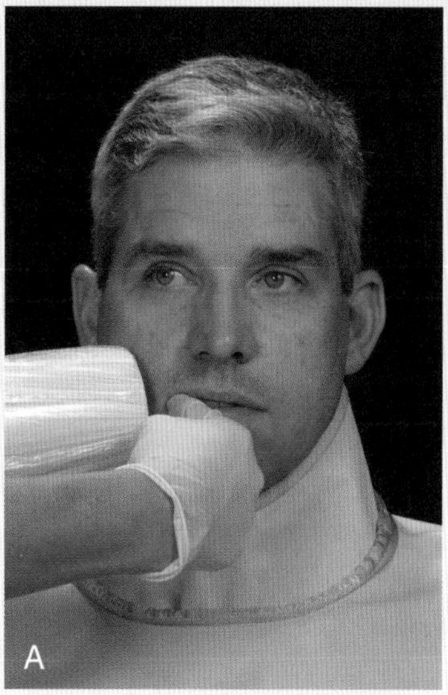

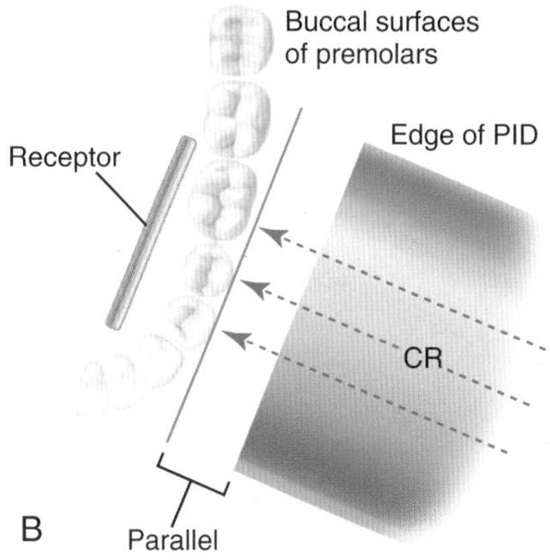

Fig 21-17 **A,** To better visualize the curvature of the arch, place the index finger along the premolar area. **B,** Correct horizontal angulation of the premolar area.

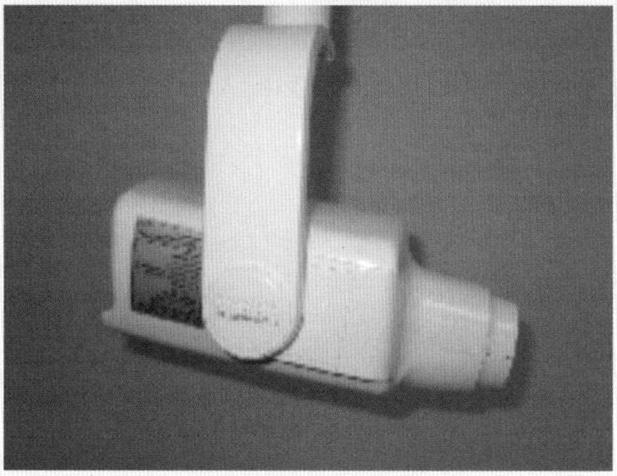

Fig 21-16 Vertical angulation is set at +10 degrees.

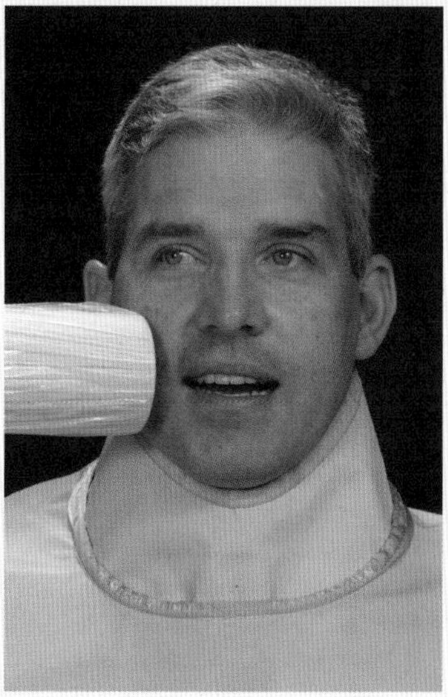

Fig 21-18 The middle of the position-indicating device (PID) should be directed at the level of the occlusal plane.

PROCEDURE 21-3 Premolar Bite-Wing Exposure With Bite Tab (Figures 21-15 to 21-21)—cont'd

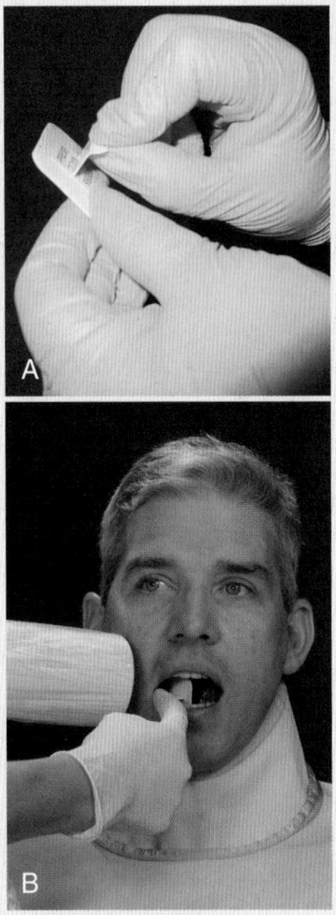

Fig 21-19 **A,** Fold down one-third of the bite-wing tab and crease it before placing the receptor in the patient's mouth. **B,** Place the biting area of the tab on the occlusal surfaces of teeth while holding the tab against the buccal surfaces of premolars. The front edge of the receptor should be aligned with the middle of the mandibular canine.

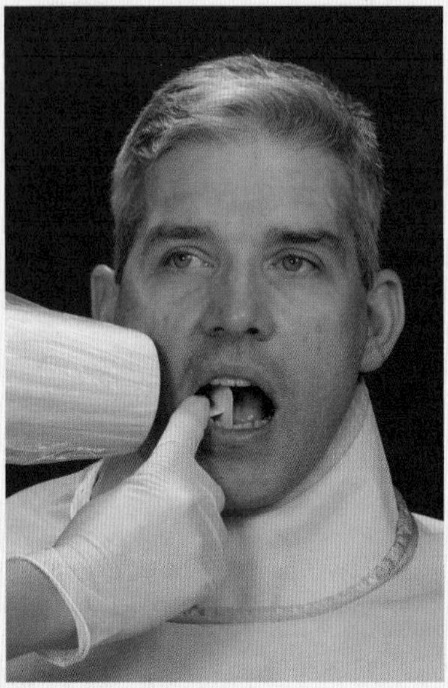

Fig 21-20 The patient's occlusal plane must be parallel to the floor for bite-wing exposures.

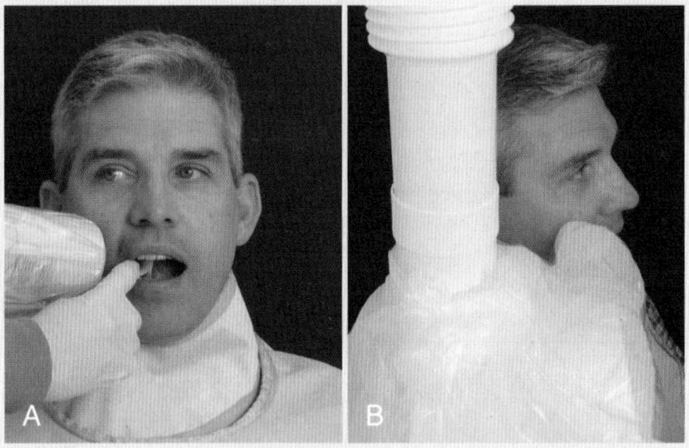

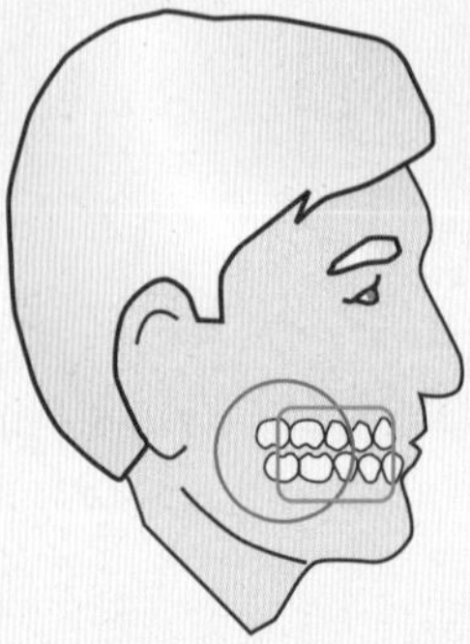

C

Fig 21-21 **A,** To check for cone-cuts, stand behind the tubehead and look along the side of the position-indicating device (PID). **B,** No portion of the receptor should be visible. **C,** A cone-cut results when any portion of the receptor is visible.

HELPFUL HINT

Molar Bite-Wing Placement Is Easy as 1, 2, 3

Step 1: Position PID
- Place **finger** parallel to lower molars
- Place opening of **PID** parallel to finger

Step 2: Place Receptor
- Place receptor
- Hold tab against teeth while patient bites

Step 3: Check for Cone-Cuts
- Stand behind the PID; **look down the PID**
- If you see the receptor, a cone-cut will result

HELPFUL HINT

Premolar Bite-Wing Checklist

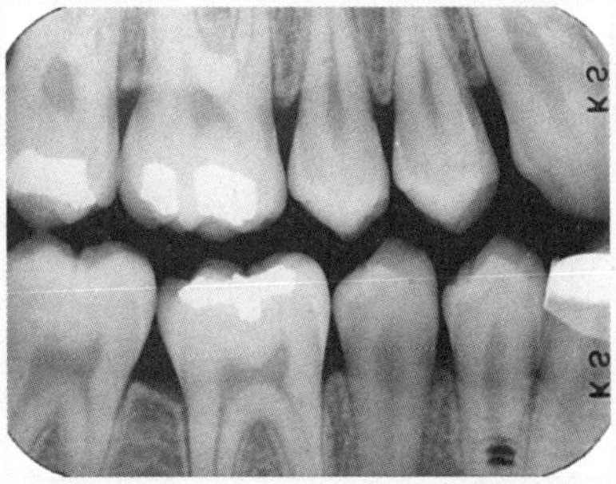

- ☐ Front edge in middle of lower mandibular canine
- ☐ Premolars visible
- ☐ Occlusal plane in middle of receptor
- ☐ Occlusal plane parallel with bottom receptor edge
- ☐ Correct horizontal = open premolar contacts
- ☐ Correct vertical angulation of +10 degrees
- ☐ No cone-cuts

Image from Miles DA, et al: *Radiographic imaging for the dental team,* ed 4, St. Louis, 2009, Saunders.

HELPFUL HINT

Premolar Bite-Wing Placement Is Easy as 1, 2, 3

Step 1: Position PID
- Place **finger** parallel to lower premolars
- Place opening of **PID** parallel to finger

Step 2: Place Receptor
- Place receptor
- Hold tab against teeth while patient bites

Step 3: Check for Cone-Cuts
- Stand behind the PID; **look down the PID**
- If you see the receptor, a cone-cut will result

PROCEDURE 21-4 Molar Bite-Wing Exposure With Bite Tab (Figures 21-16 to 21-25)

1. Set the vertical angulation at +10 degrees (see Figure 21-16) if using film or PSP sensors.
2. To set the horizontal angulation, stand in front of the patient. Examine the posterior curvature of the arch. To better visualize the curvature of the arch, place your index finger along the molar area. Align the open end of the position-indicating device (PID) parallel to your index finger and the curvature of the arch in the molar area, and direct the central ray through the contact areas (Figure 21-23).
3. Make certain that the PID is positioned far enough forward to cover both maxillary and mandibular second premolars and is positioned evenly over the mandibular and maxillary arches to avoid a cone-cut. The middle of the PID should be directed at the level of the occlusal plane (see Figure 21-18). After the vertical angulation, horizontal angulation, and PID position have been established, the PID should not be adjusted, and the receptor should be placed without moving the PID.
4. Fold down one-third of the bite-wing tab, and crease it. Insert the receptor into the patient's mouth, and place the lower half of the receptor between the patient's tongue and teeth. Place the biting surface of the tab on the occlusal surfaces of mandibular teeth. Center the receptor on the mandibular second molar; the front edge of the receptor should be aligned with the midline of the mandibular second premolar. Using your index finger, hold the folded portion of the bite-wing tab against the buccal surfaces of the molars (Figure 21-24). Hold the tab in place during steps 5 and 6.
5. Make certain that the patient's occlusal plane is parallel to the floor. If necessary, ask the patient to lower the chin (see Figure 21-20).
6. To check for a cone-cut, stand directly behind the tubehead and look along the side of the PID. No portion of the receptor should be visible; the receptor should be covered by the opening of the PID (Figure 21-25). If the receptor is not visible, instruct the patient to "slowly close" and gently bite while still holding the bite-wing tab. If any portion of the receptor is visible, a cone-cut will result. In such cases, the PID must be adjusted to cover the receptor. After the PID has been positioned properly, instruct the patient to "slowly close" and gently bite while still holding the bite-wing tab.
7. Expose the receptor.

PROCEDURE 21-4 Molar Bite-Wing Exposure With Bite Tab (Figures 21-16 to 21-25) —cont'd

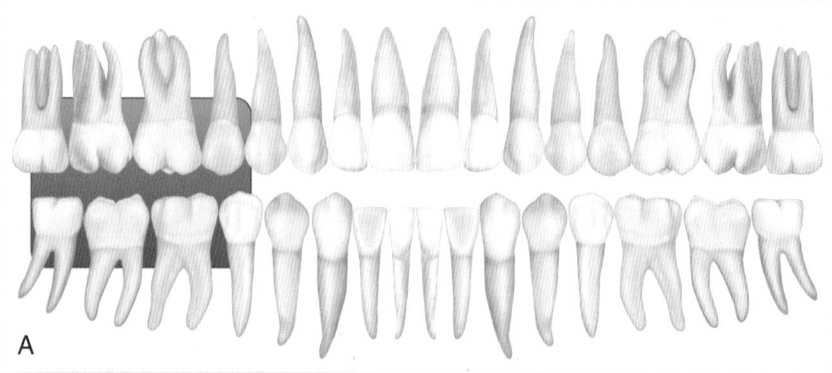

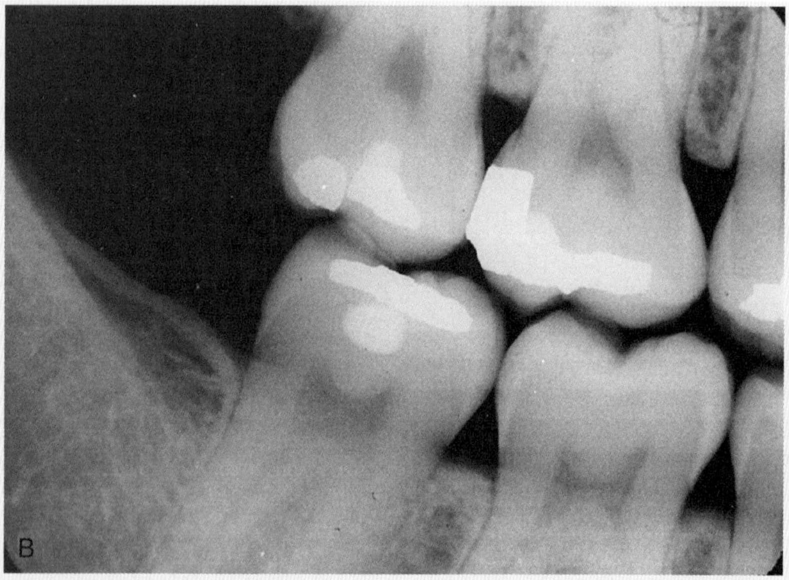

Fig 21-22 The molar bite-wing. **A**, Receptor placement. **B**, Resultant image.

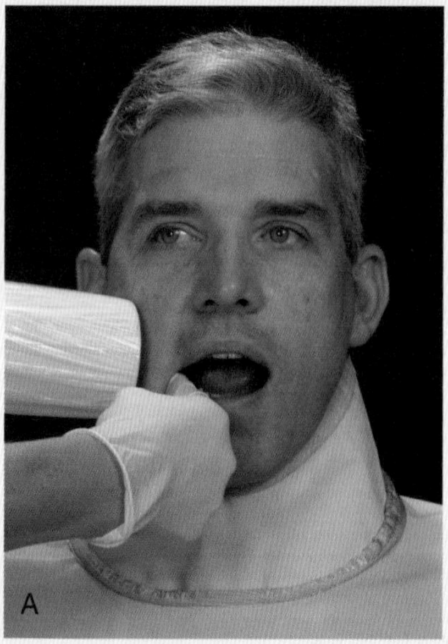

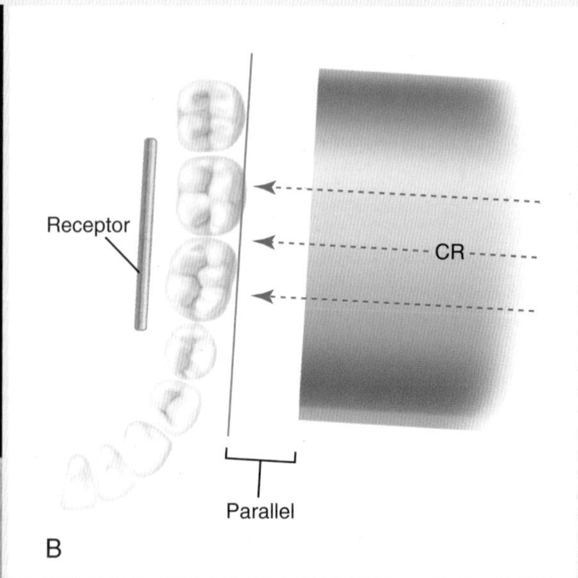

Fig 21-23 **A**, To better visualize the curvature of the arch, place the index finger along the molar area. **B**, Correct horizontal angulation of the molar area.

PROCEDURE 21-4 Molar Bite-Wing Exposure with Bite Tab (Figures 21-16 to 21-25) —cont'd

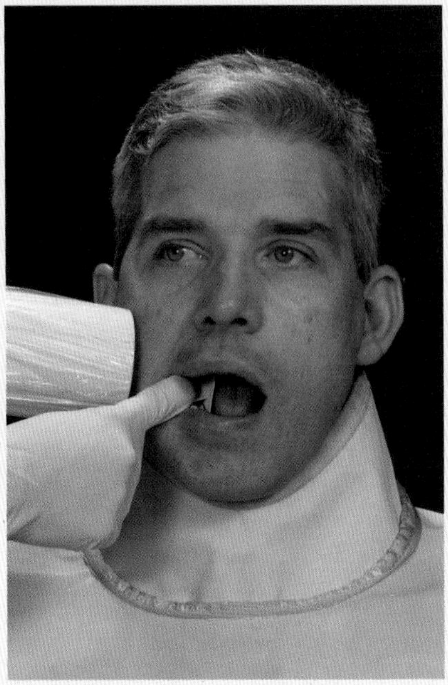

Fig 21-24 Place the biting area of the tab on the occlusal surfaces of teeth while holding the tab against the buccal surfaces of premolars. The front edge of the receptor should be aligned with the middle of the mandibular second premolar.

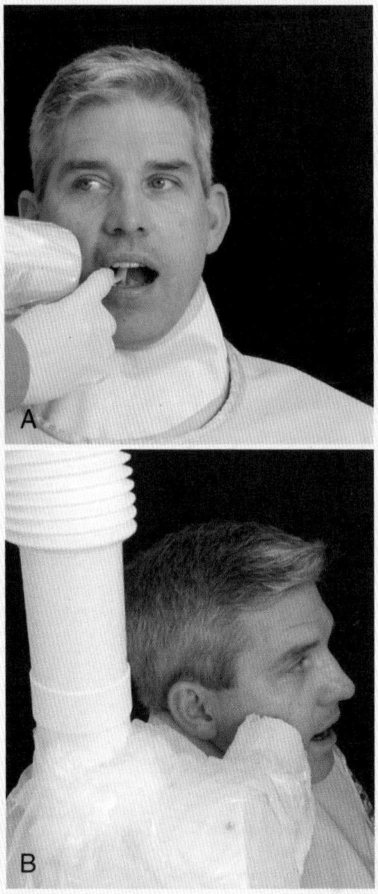

Fig 21-25 **A,** To check for cone-cuts, stand behind the tubehead and look along the side of the position-indicating device (PID). **B,** No portion of the receptor should be visible.

HELPFUL HINT

Molar Bite-Wing Checklist

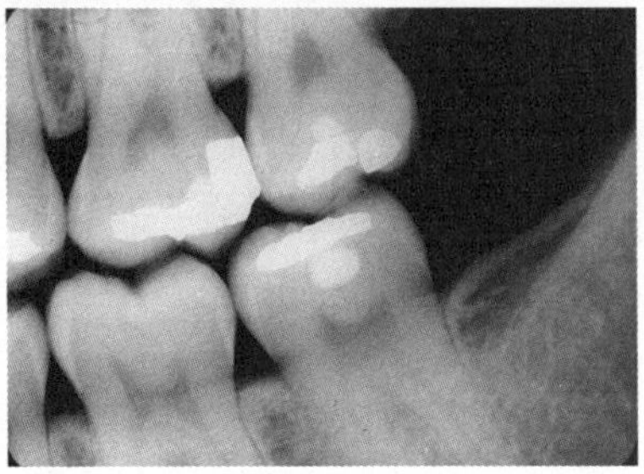

- ☐ Front edge in middle of lower mandibular 2nd premolar
- ☐ Molars visible
- ☐ Occlusal plane in middle of receptor
- ☐ Occlusal plane parallel with bottom receptor edge
- ☐ Correct horizontal = open molar contacts
- ☐ Correct vertical angulation of +10 degrees
- ☐ No cone-cuts

An example of a charting note to document a four-receptor posterior bite-wing series appears below:

CHARTING BITE-WING EXPOSURES

Date	ADA Procedure Code	Provider	Charting Notes	Comments
12/13/21	0274	LJH	Dr. Campbell prescribed four horizontal bite-wing exposures; digital sensors used (4 total exposures)	Patient recently had orthodontic appliances removed; slight cone-cut on the left premolar bite-wing but information is present on the left molar projection

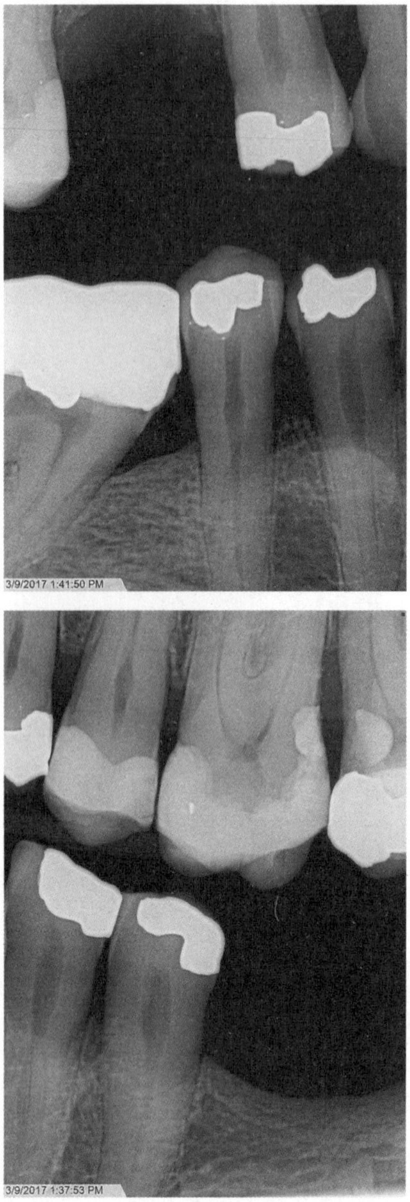

Fig 21-26 Right and left vertical bite-wing images of the same patient.

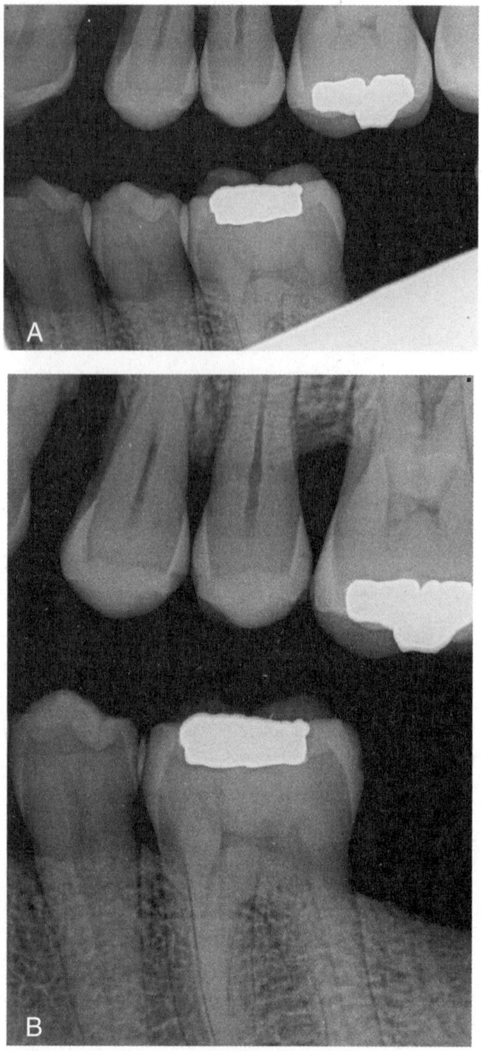

Fig 21-27 **A,** A horizontal bite-wing image does not adequately reveal the level of bone in the maxillary arch as a result of the periodontal condition. **B,** More information regarding the bone loss can be seen on a vertical bite-wing image of the same region.

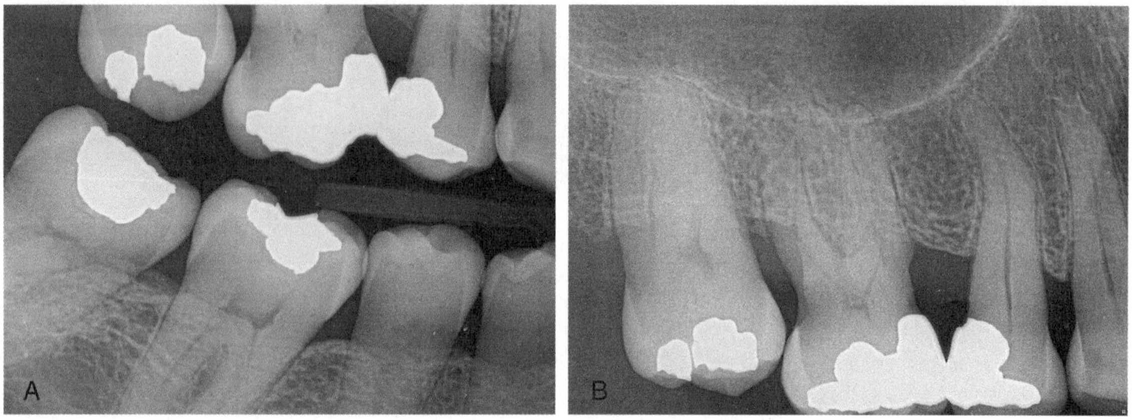

Fig 21-28 **A,** The horizontal bite-wing image does not allow the practitioner enough diagnostic information about the existing bone level. **B,** A periapical image of the same region is exposed.

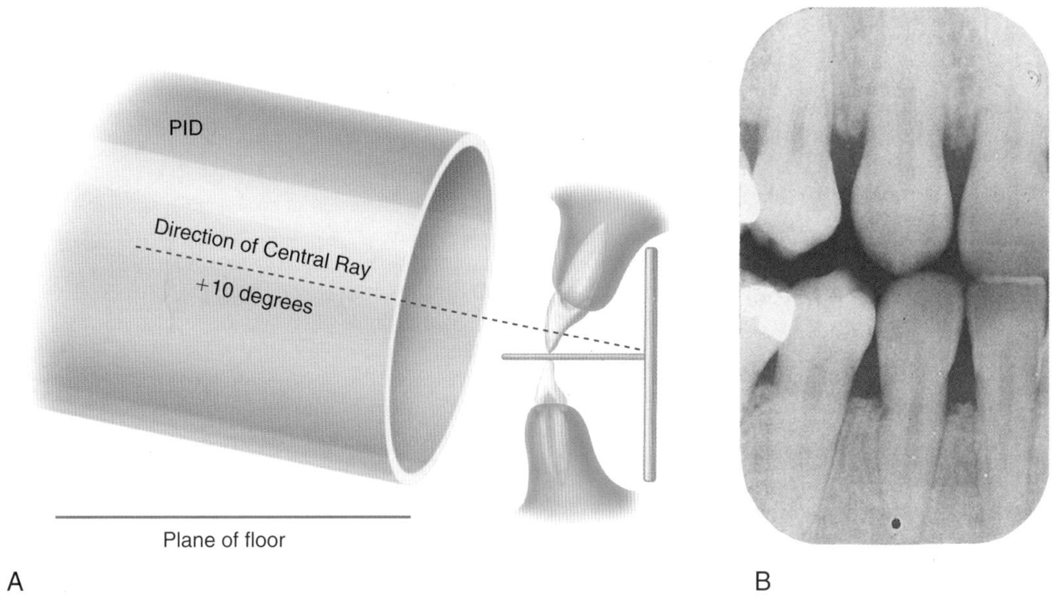

FIG 21-29 Anterior interproximal area. **A,** Center the receptor vertically at midline, and stabilize the patient by having him or her gently close on the tab at the incisal edges of teeth. Teeth meet the tab in the end-to-end position. When using film or PSP sensors, the suggested vertical angulation is + 10 degrees toward the center of the receptor; horizontally, the x-ray beam is directed through the interproximal spaces. **B,** Vertical bite-wing image of the right canine area.

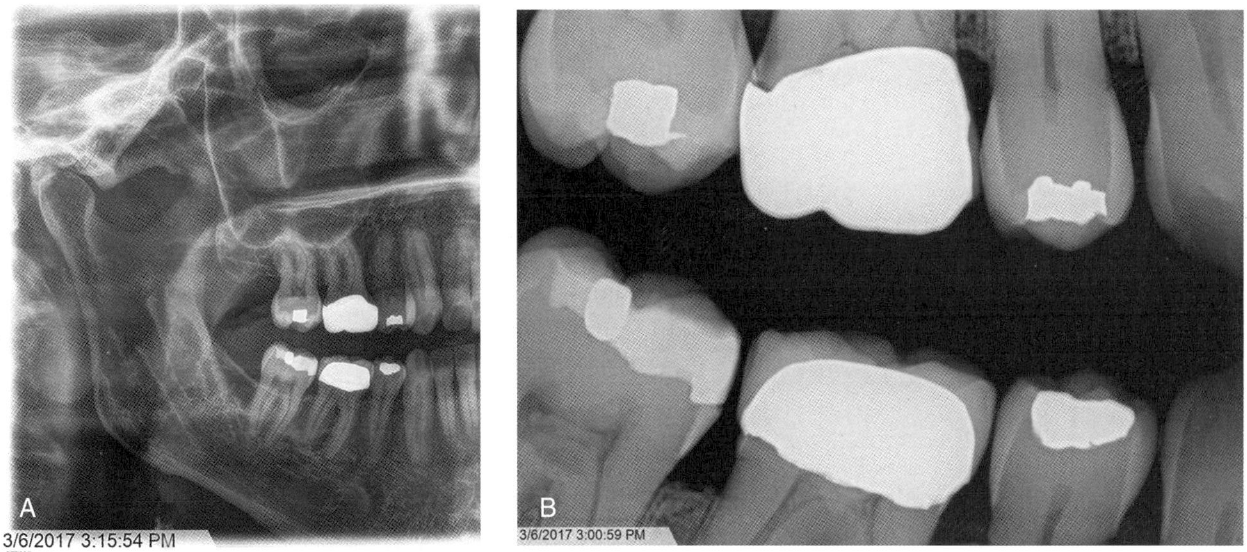

Fig 21-30 **A,** A sectioned panoramic image of a patient with missing premolars and third molars. **B,** Only one bite-wing image is needed per side to see all interproximal contact areas.

Edentulous Spaces. As described in Chapter 18, an edentulous space is an area where teeth are no longer present. An edentulous space may cause problems in bite-wing receptor placement, and a modification in technique is necessary. A cotton roll must be placed in the area of the missing tooth (or teeth) to support the bite-wing tab or the beam alignment device. When the patient closes, opposing teeth occlude on the cotton roll and support the bite-wing tab or the beam alignment device. Failure to support the bite-wing tab or the beam alignment device results in a tipped occlusal plane on the resulting image.

Bony Growths. As described in Chapter 19, a torus (plural, tori) is a bony growth in the oral cavity. Mandibular tori are bony growths along the lingual aspect (tongue side) of the mandible (Figure 21-31). When using the bite-wing technique, mandibular tori may cause problems in receptor placement, and a modification in technique is therefore necessary.

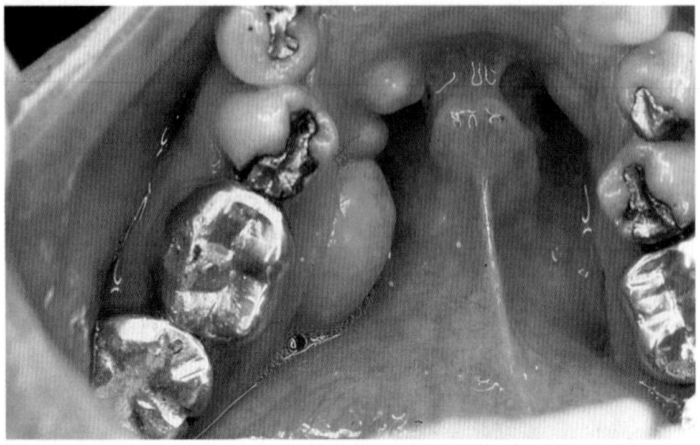

Fig 21-31 Mandibular tori.

HELPFUL HINT

Bite-Wing Technique Modifications

Edentulous Area

- Use cotton rolls where teeth are missing.
- Cotton rolls **prevent tipping** of the receptor.

Mandibular Tori

- Bite-wing must be placed between tori and tongue.
- Rinn **beam alignment device** is recommended.

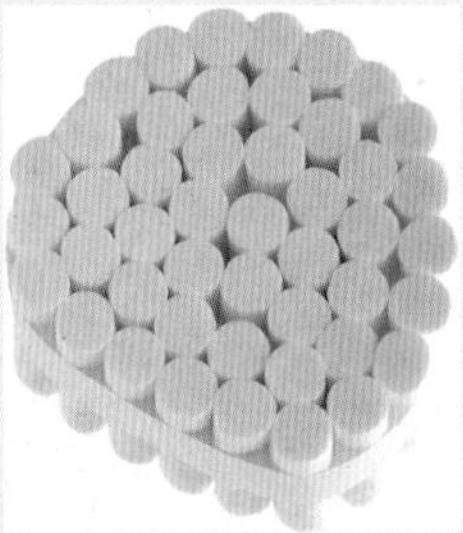

The receptor must be placed *between* the tori and the tongue (not *on* the tori) and then exposed. With large tori, the receptor is pushed away from teeth. As a result, the patient bites on the very end of the bite-wing tab to stabilize the receptor, thus making it difficult for the dental radiographer to achieve correct placement. In such cases, a bite-wing beam alignment device is recommended. PSP receptors should not be creased to accommodate bony growths. Once bent, these receptors exhibit the crease for the remainder of their use and need to be replaced. With film, bent corners cause distortion and may render the image nondiagnostic.

Helpful Hints

In using the bite-wing technique:

- **DO** set all exposure control factors (kilovoltage, milliamperage, time) before placing any receptors in the mouth.
- **DO** ask patients to remove eyeglasses and all intraoral objects before placing any receptors in the mouth.
- **DO** use a definite order (exposure sequence) when exposing receptors to avoid errors and to make efficient use of time.
- **DO** explain the imaging procedures that will be performed.
- **DO** set vertical and horizontal angulations before placing the receptor into the patient's mouth.
- **DO** set the vertical angulation at +10 degrees when using film or PSP sensors.
- **DO** direct the central ray through the contact areas of the teeth, and align the opening of the PID parallel with the curvature of the arch.
- **DO** check for cone-cuts before exposing the receptor.
- **DO** use the word *please;* say, "Open, please."
- **DO** use praise; tell cooperative patients how much they are helping to simplify and speed the imaging procedure.
- **DO** instruct patients to "slowly close" and gently bite on the bite-block or bite-wing tab and remain still during the exposure; make certain that the patient remains closed on the bite-wing tab during the exposure.
- **DO** make certain that the teeth and not the lips alone stabilize the bite-block or tab.
- **DO NOT** bend or crimp a film packet or PSP receptor; excessive bending causes distortion of the image.
- **DO NOT** use words such as *hurt*. Instead, inform patients that the procedure will be "momentarily uncomfortable."
- **DO NOT** make comments such as "Oops." Patients will lose confidence in your abilities when hearing such comments.
- **DO NOT** pick up a receptor if you drop it. Leave it on the floor; it has now become contaminated. Remove it and dispose of it when you clean the treatment area.
- **DO NOT** allow patients to dictate how you should perform your imaging duties. The dental radiographer must always remain in control of the procedures.
- **DO NOT** begin with the molar bite-wing exposure; molar placements may cause patients to gag. Instead, always begin with the easier premolar bite-wing exposure.
- **DO NOT** position a receptor on top of a torus (tori). Instead, always position the receptor between the torus and the tongue.

SUMMARY

- A bite-wing image includes crowns of maxillary and mandibular teeth, interproximal areas, and areas of crestal bone on the same image.
- Bite-wing images are useful for examining the interproximal surfaces of teeth, detecting caries, and examining crestal bone levels between teeth.
- The patient "bites" on the "wing" to stabilize the bite-wing receptor.
- The bite-wing receptor is placed parallel to the crowns of both maxillary and mandibular teeth; the receptor is stabilized when the patient bites on the tab or the beam alignment device; and the central ray of the x-ray beam is directed through contacts.
- A beam alignment device (Rinn XCP) is recommended, or a bite-wing tab may be used to stabilize the receptor.
- Three sizes of receptors (0, 2, and 3) can be used in the bite-wing technique; in the adult patient, a size 2 receptor is recommended.
- With correct horizontal angulation (side-to-side positioning of the PID), the central ray is directed through the contact areas of teeth; contact areas on the image appear "opened." Incorrect horizontal angulation results in overlapped ("unopened") contacts.
- A vertical angulation (up-and-down positioning of the PID) of +10 degrees is recommended for bite-wing receptors (film or PSP sensors) exposed with a tab to compensate for the slight bend of the upper portion of the receptor and the slight tilt of maxillary teeth.
- Five basic rules are followed in the bite-wing technique: (1) The receptor must cover the prescribed area of interest, (2) the receptor must be positioned parallel to the crowns of maxillary and mandibular teeth and stabilized by the tab or the beam alignment device, (3) the vertical angulation must be directed at +10 degrees for film or PSP sensors using bite tabs, (4) the central ray must be directed through the contact areas between teeth, and (5) the x-ray beam must be centered over the receptor to ensure that all areas are exposed.
- Before performing imaging procedures using the bite-wing technique, infection prevention procedures must be completed and the treatment area and supplies must be prepared. After the patient is seated and the imaging procedures explained, adjustments to the chair and headrest are made, the lead apron is placed, and the patient

is asked to remove eyeglasses and any intraoral objects. The exposure factors are then set and the beam alignment devices are assembled.

- When exposing bite-wing images only (instead of a CMS), the radiographer should always begin with premolar bite-wing exposures (easier for patients to tolerate and making gagging less likely). Premolar exposures are followed by molar exposures.
- Premolar and molar bite-wing exposures have prescribed receptor placements (see Procedures 21-3 and 21-4).
- Vertical bite-wing images can be used to examine the level of alveolar bone in addition to caries detection and are placed with the long portion of the receptor in a vertical direction. Vertical bite-wing images are often used as post-treatment exposures in the case of patients with bone loss caused by periodontal disease. Vertical bite-wing images may be exposed in both anterior and posterior regions.
- Modifications in the bite-wing technique may be necessary when a patient has extracted teeth, edentulous spaces, or bony growths.

TECHNIQUE VIDEOS

View the Technique Videos and complete the accompanying Interactive Exercises that are available as part of the Student Resources on the companion Evolve website for this textbook.

BIBLIOGRAPHY

ADA Council on Scientific Affairs: Dental radiographic examinations: recommendations for patient selection and limiting radiation exposure, 2012.

Frommer HH, Stabulas-Savage JJ: Intraoral technique: The paralleling method. In Radiology for the dental professional, ed 9, St Louis, 2011, Mosby.

Johnson ON: The bite-wing examination. In Essentials of dental radiography for dental assistants and hygienists, ed 9, Upper Saddle River, NJ, 2011, Prentice Hall.

Mallya SM, Lam EWN: Intraoral projections. In White and Pharoah's oral radiology: principles and interpretation, ed 8, St. Louis, 2019, Elsevier.

Miles DA, Van Dis ML, Jensen CW, et al: Intraoral radiographic technique. In Radiographic imaging for dental team, ed 4, Philadelphia, 2009, Saunders.

Miles DA, Van Dis ML, Razmus TF: Intraoral radiographic techniques. In Basic principles of oral and maxillofacial radiology, Philadelphia, 1992, Saunders.

QUIZ QUESTIONS

Short Answer

1. What does the term *bite-wing* refer to?

2. What size receptor is recommended for use with the bite-wing technique in the adult patient?

3. What size receptor is recommended for use with the bite-wing technique in the pediatric patient with primary dentition?

4. How is the patient's head positioned before exposing a bite-wing receptor?

5. What is the primary use of bite-wing images?

6. What size receptor is used to include all of the posterior teeth in one bite-wing exposure?

7. What type of angulation is determined by the up-and-down movement of the position-indicating device (PID)?

8. What type of angulation is determined by the side-to-side movement of the PID?

9. When the central ray of the x-ray is not directed through the contact areas of teeth, what error is seen on the resulting image?

10. When does a cone-cut result?

Multiple Choice

____ 11. Which examination area describes the primary use of the bite-wing image?
a. apical areas of teeth
b. apical and interproximal areas of teeth
c. interproximal areas of teeth
d. pulp chambers of teeth

____ 12. Which is the correct vertical angulation used with the bite-wing technique and the bite tab on film or PSP sensors?
a. −10 degrees
b. −20 degrees
c. +10 degrees
d. +15 degrees

____ 13. Which statement describes the relationship of the receptor to maxillary and mandibular teeth in the bite-wing technique?
a. The receptor and teeth are parallel to each other.
b. The receptor and teeth are at right angles to each other.
c. The receptor and teeth are perpendicular to each other.
d. The receptor and teeth intersect each other.

____ 14. Which statements about receptor placement are correct?
1. Anterior bite-wings may be placed horizontally.
2. Anterior bite-wings may be placed vertically.
3. Posterior bite-wings may be placed horizontally.
4. Posterior bite-wings may be placed vertically.
a. 1, 2, and 3
b. 2, 3, and 4
c. 2 and 3
d. 1 and 4

____ 15. Which statement about the exposure sequence for a CMS that includes periapical and bite-wing exposures is incorrect?
a. Anterior periapical receptors are always exposed first.
b. Posterior periapical receptors are exposed after anterior periapicals.
c. Bite-wing receptors are exposed last in the CMS.
d. None of the above.

Essay

16. State the basic principles of the bite-wing technique.
17. Describe the two ways to stabilize the receptor in the bite-wing technique.
18. State the basic rules for the bite-wing technique.
19. Discuss patient and equipment preparations necessary before using the bite-wing technique.
20. Discuss the exposure sequence for a CMS that includes both periapical and bite-wing exposures.
21. Describe premolar and molar bite-wing placements.
22. Explain the modifications in the bite-wing technique that are used for patients with edentulous spaces or bony growths.
23. Describe why a +10 degree vertical angulation is used with the bite-wing technique and a bite tab on film or PSP sensors.

Ordering

Arrange the following in the recommended order of exposure:

____ 24. periapicals, posterior
____ 25. bite-wing, molar
____ 26. bite-wing, premolar
____ 27. periapicals, maxillary anterior
____ 28. periapicals, mandibular anterior

22

Exposure and Technique Errors

LEARNING OBJECTIVES

After completion of this chapter, the student will be able to do the following:

1. Define the key terms associated with exposure and technique errors.
2. Identify and describe the appearance of the following exposure errors: unexposed receptor, film exposed to light, overexposed receptor, and underexposed receptor.
3. Identify and describe the appearances of the following periapical technique errors caused by receptor placement: absence of apical structures and dropped receptor corner.
4. Describe horizontal and vertical angulation.
5. Identify and describe the appearances of the following periapical technique errors caused by angulation problems: incorrect horizontal angulation (overlapped contacts), incorrect vertical angulation (foreshortened images and elongated images), and incorrect beam alignment (cone-cut images).
6. Describe and identify proper receptor placement for bite-wing images.
7. Identify and describe the appearances of the following bite-wing technique errors caused by receptor placement: incorrect placement of premolar bite-wing and incorrect placement of molar bite-wing.
8. Identify and describe the appearances of the following bite-wing technique errors caused by angulation problems: incorrect horizontal angulation (overlapped contacts), incorrect vertical angulation (distorted image), and incorrect position-indicating device (PID) alignment (cone-cut images).
9. Identify and describe the appearances of the following miscellaneous technique errors: bending, creasing, debris accumulation, phalangioma, double image, movement, reversed/backward placement, and wired cable issues.

The dental radiographer must remember that only *diagnostic* images are useful. A diagnostic dental image is one that has been properly placed, exposed, processed, or retrieved; errors in any one of these areas may result in nondiagnostic images. In many instances, nondiagnostic images must be retaken. Retakes result in additional exposure of the patient to x-radiation, which is harmful to the patient. Regardless of the receptor used, a digital sensor or film, a nondiagnostic image does not allow for a diagnosis to be established or for proper treatment to be provided.

Whichever type of imaging receptor is used, many exposure and technique errors are possible. Errors may occur with both sensors and film, whereas some errors are unique to film and other errors are unique to sensors. This chapter reviews common errors that occur with the use of digital sensors and/or film, and strategies for avoiding such errors.

The dental radiographer must have a working knowledge of receptor exposure, technique, and processing errors (processing errors are discussed in Chapter 10). The purpose of this chapter is to describe exposure problems and technique errors that involve periapical and bite-wing images.

RECEPTOR EXPOSURE ERRORS

Receptor exposure errors that result in nondiagnostic images include unexposed, overexposed, and underexposed receptors, as well as film that is accidentally exposed to light. All of these errors produce images that are too light or too dark. The dental radiographer must be able to recognize exposure errors, identify their causes, and know the necessary steps to correct such problems.

Exposure Problems

Unexposed Receptor

Receptor. This error may occur with digital sensors (direct or indirect) or film.

Appearance. When using film, the image appears clear (Figure 22-1). When using a digital sensor, the image appears blank or white with no anatomic structures recorded.

Cause. The receptor was not exposed to x-radiation. With film or sensors, causes include failure to turn on the x-ray machine, electrical failure, x-ray unit malfunction, or failure to align the PID over the receptor. With some digital imaging systems, a fixed time interval exists during which the receptor must be exposed, or the system "times out." If the exposure does not take place within that fixed time interval, no exposure of the receptor occurs and no image is produced.

Correction. To ensure proper exposure of the receptor, make certain that the x-ray machine is turned on, and listen for the audible exposure signal. Make certain the PID is centered over the receptor. With digital imaging systems, be aware of the time interval during which exposures must occur prior to the system "timing out."

Film Exposed to Light

Receptor. This error occurs only with film.

Appearance. The image appears black (Figure 22-2). This error is exclusive to film.

Cause. The film was accidentally exposed to white light.

Correction. To protect the film, do not unwrap the film packet in a room with white light. Check the darkroom for possible light leaks. Turn off all the lights in the darkroom (except for safelights) before unwrapping the film.

Time and Exposure Factor Problems

Overexposed Receptor

Receptor. This error may occur with digital sensors (direct or indirect) or film.

Appearance. The image appears dark or high in density (Figure 22-3).

Fig 22-1 An unexposed receptor appears clear.

Fig 22-2 A film exposed to light appears black. (From Haring JI, Lind LJ: *Radiographic interpretation for the dental hygienist*, Philadelphia, 1993, Saunders.)

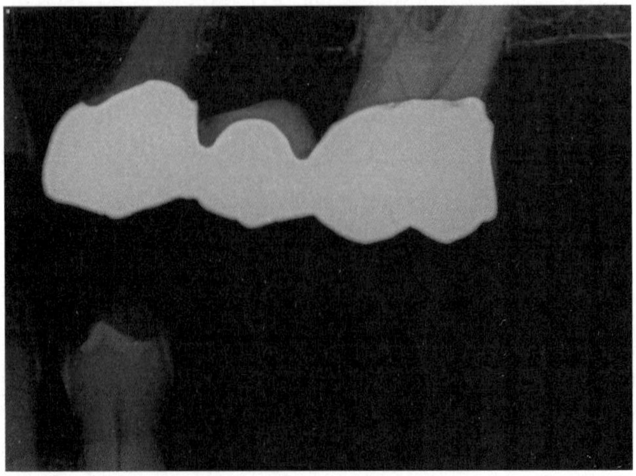

Fig 22-3 An overexposed receptor appears dark.

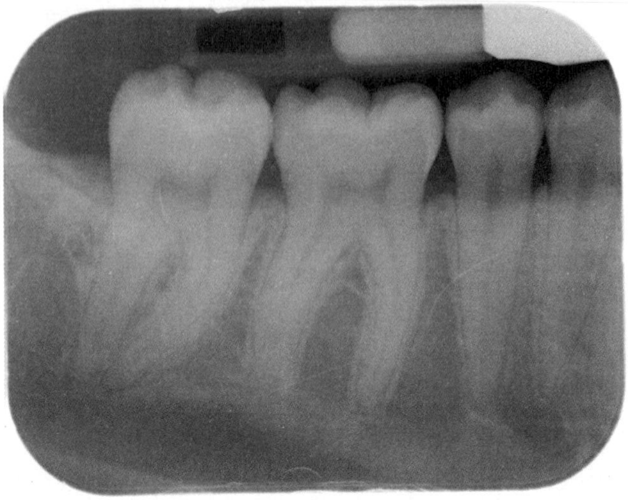

Fig 22-4 An underexposed receptor appears light.

Cause. The receptor was exposed to too much radiation. An overexposed image results from excessive exposure time, kilovoltage, or milliamperage, or a combination of these factors. Too much exposure time is the most common cause of overexposure.

Correction. To prevent overexposure, check the exposure time, kilovoltage, and milliamperage settings on the x-ray machine before exposing the receptor. If the patient is small, reduce exposure time, kilovoltage, or milliamperage as needed. With digital imaging, an overexposed image may not need to be retaken if it can be improved by using the image enhancement software to adjust the brightness and contrast.

Underexposed Receptor

Receptor. This error may occur with digital sensors (direct or indirect) or film.

Appearance. The image appears light or low in density (Figure 22-4).

Cause. The receptor was exposed to too little radiation. An underexposed image results from inadequate exposure time, kilovoltage, or milliamperage, or a combination of these factors. Too little exposure time is the most common cause of underexposure.

Correction. To prevent underexposure, check the exposure time, kilovoltage, and milliamperage settings on the x-ray machine before exposing the receptor. If the patient is large, increase the exposure time, kilovoltage, or milliamperage as needed. With digital imaging, an underexposed image may not need to be retaken if it can be improved by using the image enhancement software to adjust the brightness and contrast.

PERIAPICAL TECHNIQUE ERRORS

Just as exposure errors may result in nondiagnostic images, errors in technique may also result in nondiagnostic images. Periapical technique errors include problems with receptor placement, angulation, and beam alignment. The dental radiographer must be able to recognize periapical technique errors, identify their causes, and know the necessary steps to correct such problems.

Receptor Placement Problems

As described in Chapter 18, the periapical image shows the entire tooth, including the apex and surrounding structures (Figure 22-5). For a periapical image to be considered diagnostic, receptor placement

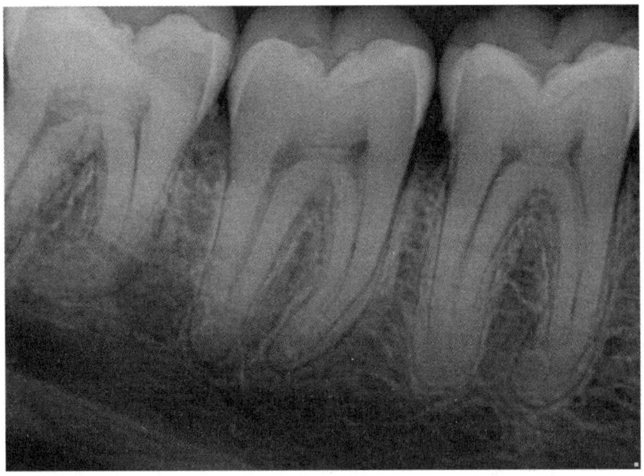

Fig 22-5 Correct periapical placement demonstrates the entire tooth, including the apex and surrounding structures.

must be correct. Specific periapical placements for incisors, canines, premolars, and molars are described in Chapters 19 and 20. Each periapical receptor must be positioned in a certain way to show specific teeth and related anatomic structures. In addition, the edge of the periapical receptor must be placed parallel to the incisal or occlusal surfaces of the teeth and extend one-eighth of an inch beyond the incisal or occlusal surfaces.

A nondiagnostic periapical image may result from improper placement of a receptor over the area of interest, inadequate coverage of the apical regions, or a dropped receptor corner.

Absence of Apical Structures

Receptor. This error may occur with digital sensors (direct or indirect) or film.

Technique. This error may occur with the paralleling or bisecting technique.

Appearance. No apices are seen on the image, and an excessive margin of receptor edge appears as a radiolucent band (Figure 22-6, A, B).

Cause. The receptor was not positioned in the patient's mouth to cover the apical regions of teeth.

Correction. To ensure that apical structures appear on the receptor, the teeth being imaged must be firmly in contact with the bite-block. Instruct the patient to stabilize the bite-block with the teeth and *not* the lips. Ask the patient to smile with the lips open in order to view the teeth in contact with the bite-block. In addition, make certain that no more than one-eighth of an inch of the receptor edge extends beyond the incisal-occlusal surfaces of teeth. It is important to note that some digital sensors have a smaller recording dimension than film, which may result in the absence of the tooth apices. To compensate for this issue when using a digital sensor, increase the vertical angulation slightly to capture the apices.

Dropped Receptor Corner

Receptor. This error may occur with digital sensors (direct or indirect) or film.

Technique. This error may occur with the paralleling or bisecting technique.

Appearance. The occlusal plane appears tipped or tilted (Figure 22-7).

Cause. The edge of the receptor was not placed parallel to the incisal-occlusal surfaces of teeth. A corner of the receptor may slip or drop if the patient is not firmly closed on the bite-block.

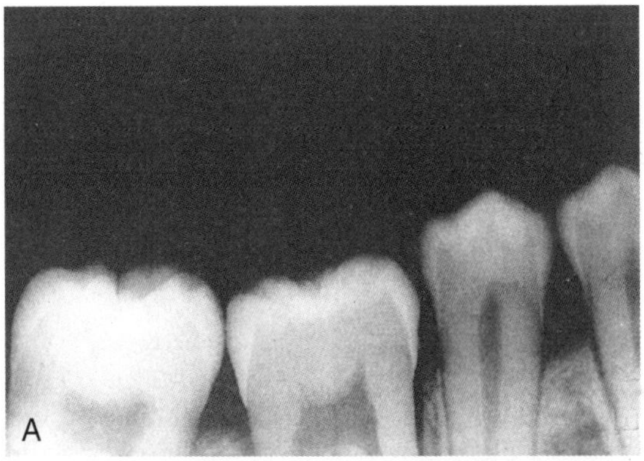

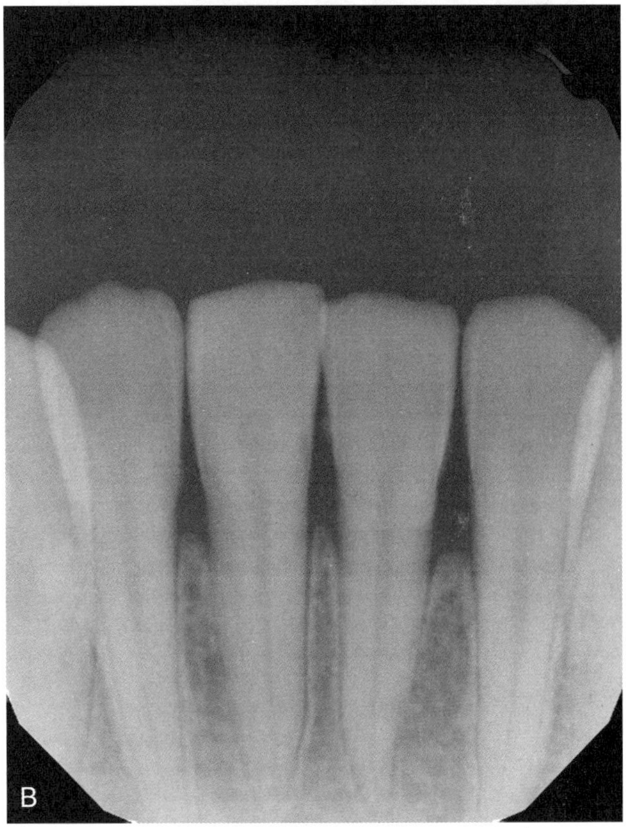

Fig 22-6 **A,** Improper placement; no apices are seen on this image. (From Haring JI, Lind LJ: *Radiographic interpretation for the dental hygienist*, Philadelphia, 1993, Saunders.) **B,** Improper placement; an image of the mandibular anterior region.

Correction. To prevent a dropped receptor corner, make certain that the edge of the receptor is placed parallel to the incisal-occlusal surfaces of teeth. Instruct the patient to bite firmly on the bite-block to stabilize the receptor.

Angulation Problems

Angulation is a term used to describe the alignment of the central ray of the x-ray beam in the horizontal and vertical planes. Angulation is varied by moving the position-indicating device (PID) in either a horizontal or a vertical direction. **Horizontal angulation** refers to the positioning of the PID in a horizontal, or side-to-side, plane. **Vertical angulation** refers to the positioning of the PID in a vertical, or up-and-down, plane. Correct horizontal and vertical angulations of periapical images are described in Chapter 20.

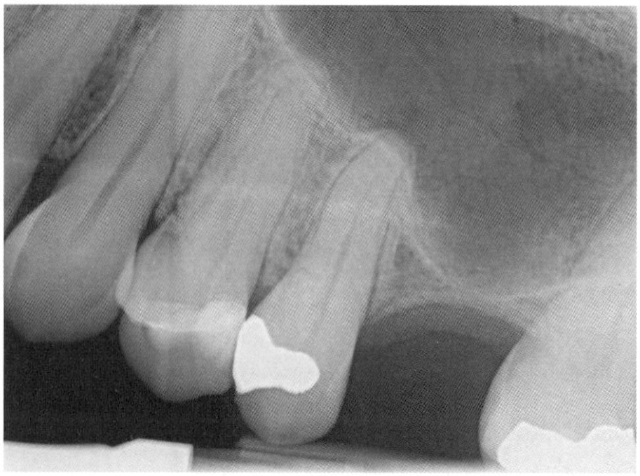

Fig 22-7 Improper placement; a dropped corner is seen when the edge of the receptor is not placed parallel to the incisal or occlusal surfaces of teeth.

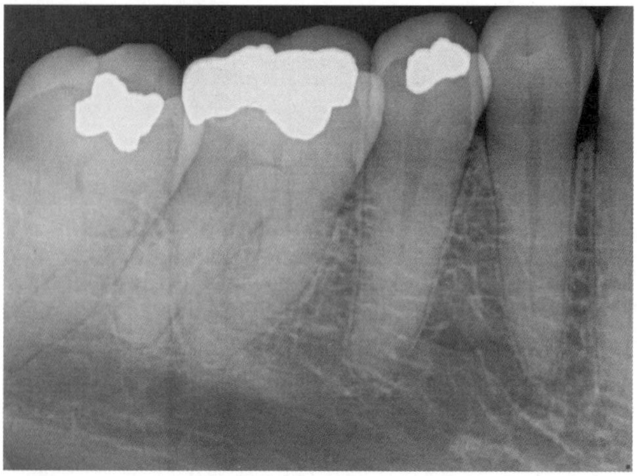

Fig 22-8 Incorrect horizontal angulation results in overlapped contact areas.

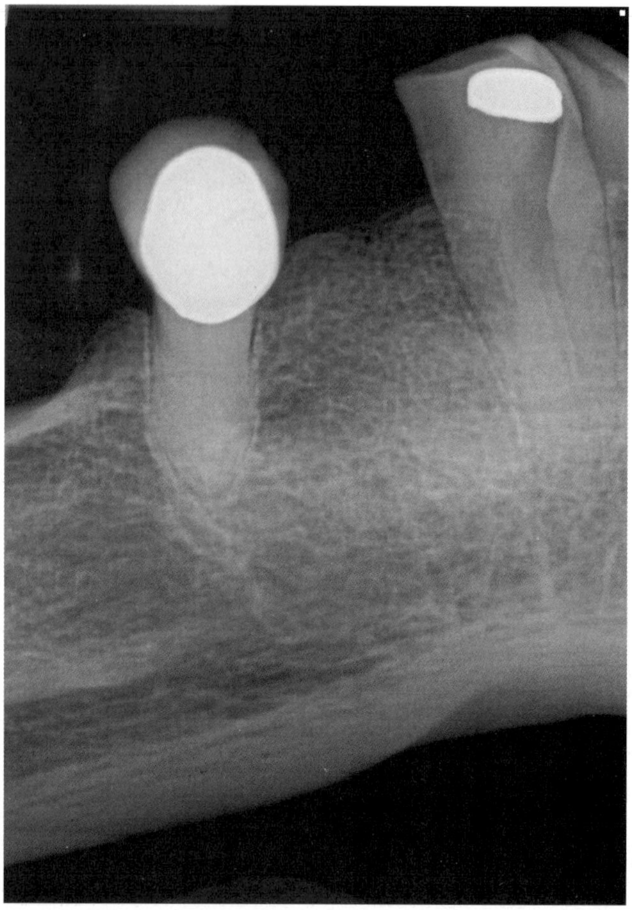

Fig 22-9 If the vertical angulation is too steep, the image of the tooth on the receptor is shorter than the actual tooth; the images are foreshortened.

Incorrect vertical angulation results in an image that is not the same length as that of the tooth; instead, the image appears either shorter or longer. Foreshortened or elongated images are nondiagnostic. Incorrect horizontal angulation results in an image with overlapped contacts. On a dental image, overlapped contacts can be defined as the area where the contact area of one tooth is superimposed over the contact area of an adjacent tooth.

Overlapped Contacts—Incorrect Horizontal Angulation

Receptor. This error may occur with digital sensors (direct or indirect) or film.

Technique. This error may occur with the paralleling or bisecting technique.

Appearance. The contact area of one tooth is superimposed over the contact area of an adjacent tooth (Figure 22-8).

Cause. The central ray was not directed through the interproximal spaces.

Correction. To avoid overlapped contacts on a periapical image, direct the central ray *through* the proximal contacts of the teeth. The use of Rinn XCP and BAI beam alignment devices minimizes errors in horizontal angulation.

Foreshortened Images—Incorrect Vertical Angulation

Receptor. This error may occur with digital sensors (direct or indirect) or film.

Technique. This error may occur with the bisecting technique when a beam alignment device is *not* used.

Appearance. Teeth appear short with blunted roots on the image (Figure 22-9).

Cause. The vertical angulation was excessive (too steep). A foreshortened image, one that is shorter than the actual tooth, results.

Correction. To avoid foreshortened images, do not use a steep vertical angulation with the bisecting technique. The use of a Rinn BAI beam alignment device minimizes errors in vertical angulation.

Elongated Images—Incorrect Vertical Angulation

Receptor. This error may occur with digital sensors (direct or indirect) or film.

Technique. This error may occur with the bisecting technique when a beam alignment device is not used.

Appearance. Teeth appear long and distorted on the image (Figure 22-10).

Cause. The vertical angulation was insufficient (too flat). An elongated image, one that is longer than the actual tooth, results.

Correction. To avoid elongated images, do not use a flat vertical angulation with the bisecting technique. The use of a Rinn BAI beam alignment device minimizes errors in vertical angulation.

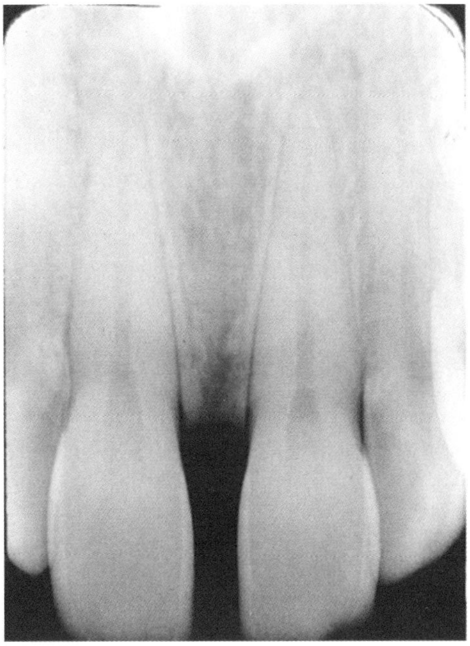

Fig 22-10 If the vertical angulation is too flat, the image of the tooth on the receptor is longer than the actual tooth; the images are elongated.

Position-Indicating Device Alignment Problems

If the PID is misaligned and the x-ray beam is not centered over the receptor, a partial image results. The PID, or "cone," is said to "cut" the image; the portion outside of the PID is not exposed and appears missing or cut. A cone-cut appears as a clear or white unexposed area on a dental image and may occur with a rectangular or round PID. If a rectangular PID is used, the cone-cut appears with a linear border. If a round PID is used, the cone-cut appears with a curved border.

Cone-Cut *With* Beam Alignment Device

Receptor. This error may occur with digital sensors (direct or indirect) or film.

Technique. This error may occur with either the paralleling or bisecting technique when a beam alignment device is used.

Appearance. A clear (unexposed) area is seen on the image (Figure 22-11).

Cause. The PID was not properly aligned with the beam alignment device, and the x-ray beam did not expose the entire receptor.

Correction. To avoid a cone-cut on a periapical receptor when using a beam alignment device, position the PID carefully. Make certain that the PID and the aiming ring are flush and aligned.

Cone-Cut *Without* Beam Alignment Device

Receptor. This error may occur with digital sensors (direct or indirect) or film.

Technique. This error may occur with the bisecting technique when a beam alignment device is *not* used.

Appearance. A clear (unexposed) area is seen on the image (Figure 22-12).

Cause. The PID was not directed at the center of the receptor, and the x-ray beam did not expose the entire receptor.

Correction. To avoid a cone-cut on a periapical receptor when *not* using a beam alignment device, position the PID carefully. Make certain that the x-ray beam is centered over the receptor and that the entire receptor is covered by the diameter of the PID.

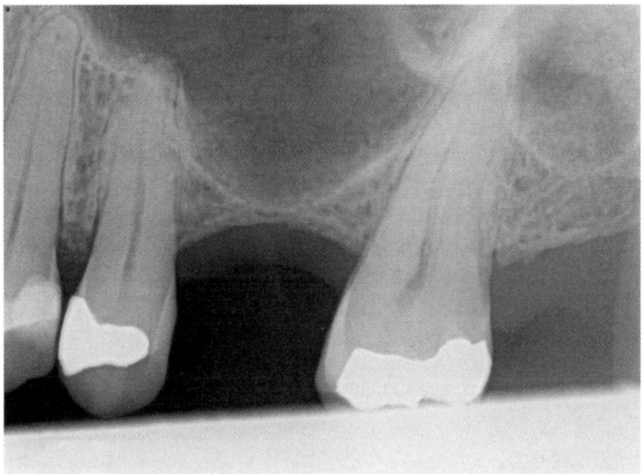

Fig 22-11 A cone-cut is seen when the position-indicating device (PID) is not properly aligned with the periapical beam alignment device.

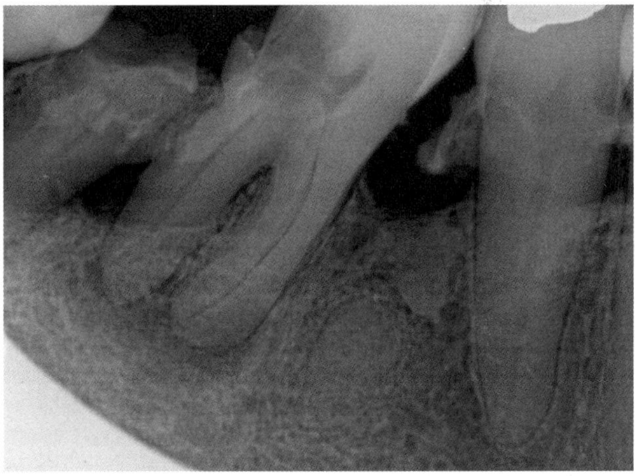

Fig 22-12 A cone-cut is seen as a curved unexposed (clear) area on the image.

BITE-WING TECHNIQUE ERRORS

Just as errors in the periapical technique may result in nondiagnostic images, errors in the bite-wing technique may also result in images that are nondiagnostic. Bite-wing technique errors include problems with receptor placement, angulation, and beam alignment. Such errors may occur when using a beam alignment device or bite-tab. The dental radiographer must be able to recognize bite-wing technique errors, identify their causes, and know the necessary steps to correct such problems.

Receptor Placement Problems

As described in Chapter 21, the bite-wing image includes the crowns of both maxillary and mandibular teeth, the interproximal contact areas, and crestal bone. For a bite-wing image to be considered diagnostic, receptor placement must be correct. Specific bite-wing placements for premolars and molars are described in Chapter 21. In addition to placement over the prescribed areas, the image must show an occlusal plane that is positioned horizontally and parallel to the long axis of the receptor. The premolar bite-wing must be positioned such that the resulting image shows both maxillary and mandibular premolars and the distal contact areas of both canines

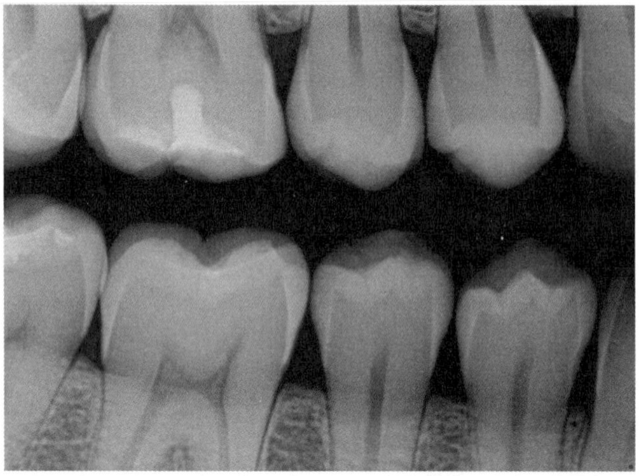

Fig 22-13 Correct receptor placement for the premolar bite-wing image.

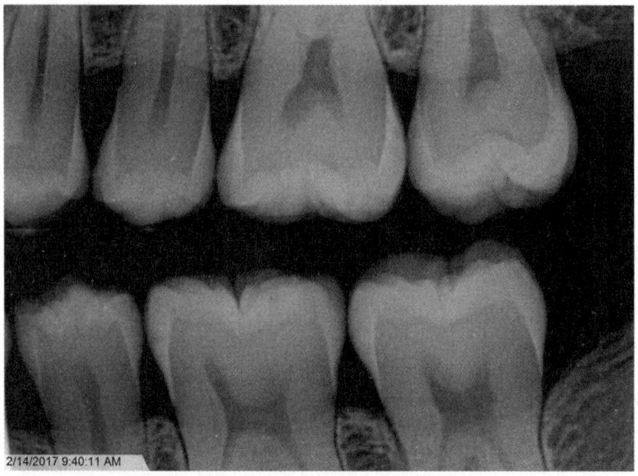

Fig 22-14 Correct receptor placement for the molar bite-wing image.

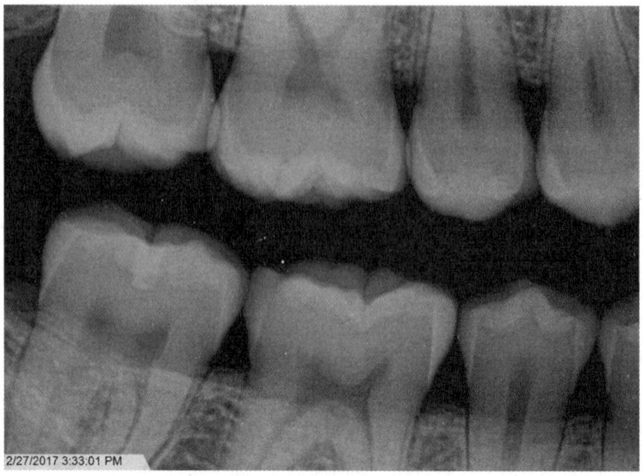

Fig 22-15 Incorrect receptor placement for the premolar bite-wing image.

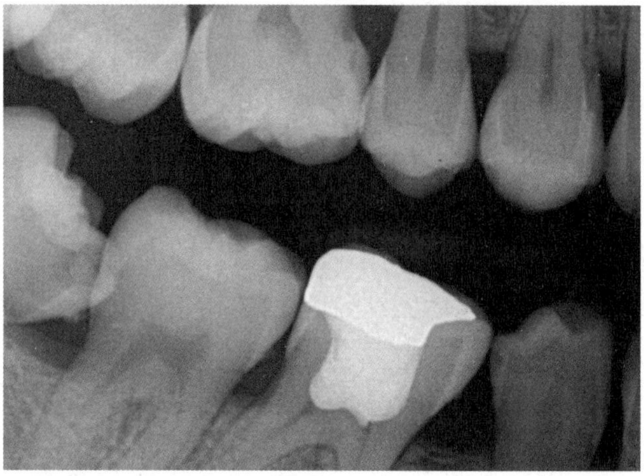

Fig 22-16 Incorrect receptor placement for the molar bite-wing image.

(Figure 22-13). The molar bite-wing must be positioned such that the resulting image shows both maxillary and mandibular molars. The molar bite-wing must be centered over the mandibular second molar (Figure 22-14).

Incorrect bite-wing receptor placement may result in absence of specific teeth or tooth surfaces on an image, a tipped occlusal plane, overlapped interproximal contacts, or a distorted image. Such errors may render a bite-wing image nondiagnostic.

Incorrect Placement of Premolar Bite-Wing

Receptor. This error may occur with digital sensors (direct or indirect) or film.

Technique. This error may occur with the bite-wing technique when a beam alignment device or bite-tab is used.

Appearance. The distal surfaces of canines are not visible on the image (Figure 22-15).

Cause. The bite-wing receptor was positioned too far back in the mouth; the anterior edge of the receptor was not placed to include the mandibular canine.

Correction. To prevent this error, make certain that the anterior edge of the bite-wing receptor is positioned at the midline of the mandibular canine, or positioned to cover the entire mandibular canine. When using a digital sensor, capturing the distal surfaces of the canines during a bite-wing exposure can be challenging. In such cases, position the anterior edge of the sensor away from the teeth and toward the canine on the opposite side of the arch.

Incorrect Placement of Molar Bite-Wing

Receptor. This error may occur with digital sensors (direct or indirect) or film.

Technique. This error may occur with the bite-wing technique when a beam alignment device or bite-tab is used.

Appearance. The third molar regions are not visible on the image (Figure 22-16).

Cause. The bite-wing receptor was positioned too far forward in the mouth; the anterior edge of the receptor was not placed at the midline of the mandibular second premolar.

Correction. To prevent this error, make certain that the anterior edge of the bite-wing receptor is positioned at the midline of the mandibular second premolar. *Always* center the molar bite-wing on the mandibular second molar, even when third molars are not present.

Angulation Problems

To produce diagnostic bite-wing images, the dental radiographer must be prepared to choose the correct horizontal and vertical angulations.

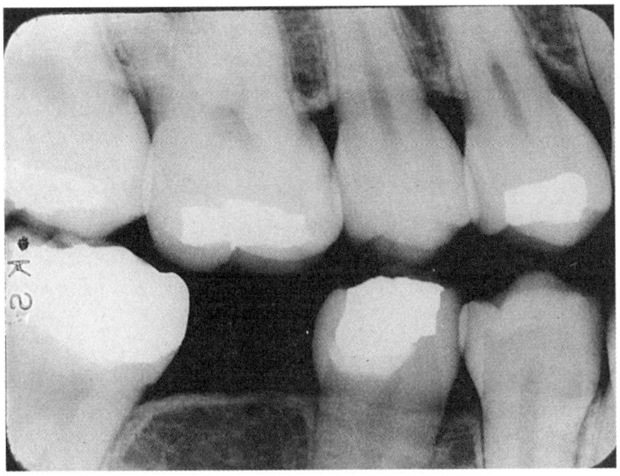

Fig 22-17 Overlapped interproximal contacts result from incorrect horizontal angulation.

Correct horizontal and vertical angulations of bite-wing images are described in Chapter 21. Incorrect horizontal angulation results in overlapped interproximal contacts, and incorrect vertical angulation results in distorted images.

Overlapped Contacts—Incorrect Horizontal Angulation

Receptor. This error may occur with digital sensors (direct or indirect) or film.

Technique. This error may occur with the bite-wing technique when a beam alignment device or bite-tab is used.

Appearance. Overlapped contacts are seen on the image (Figure 22-17).

Cause. The central ray was not directed through the interproximal spaces. When using a beam alignment device, overlapped contacts may occur if the receptor is not placed parallel to the teeth, or if the PID is not flush with the aiming ring. If the overlapping is more pronounced in the posterior half of the image, the PID was pointed too much from the mesial toward the distal. If the overlapping is more pronounced in the anterior half of the image, the PID was pointed too much from the distal toward the mesial.

Correction. To avoid overlapped contacts on a bite-wing image, direct the x-ray beam *through* the interproximal regions. When the contacts are opened, a thin radiolucent line is seen between the proximal surfaces of teeth. Proper use of a Rinn XCP bite-wing instrument minimizes errors in horizontal angulation.

Distorted Image—Incorrect Vertical Angulation

Receptor. This error may occur with digital sensors (direct or indirect) or film.

Technique. This error may occur with the bite-wing technique when a bite-tab is used.

Appearance. A distorted image is seen (Figure 22-18). In this case a negative vertical angulation was used. Note the occlusal surfaces of maxillary teeth and the apical regions of mandibular teeth.

Cause. The vertical angulation was negative instead of +10 degrees.

Correction. When using a bite-tab, always use a +10 degree vertical angulation. This positive vertical angulation compensates for the slight lingual tilt of both the maxillary teeth.

Position-Indicating Device Alignment Problems

As previously described in this chapter, if the PID is misaligned and the x-ray beam is not centered over the receptor, a partial image, known as a *cone-cut*, results.

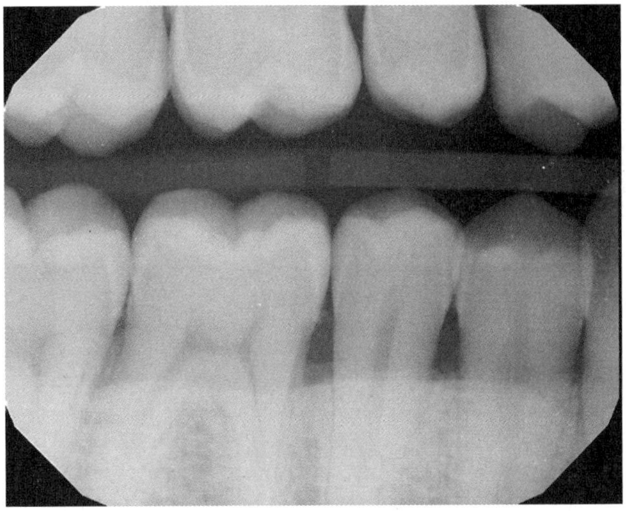

Fig 22-18 Incorrect vertical angulation causes the images to appear distorted.

Cone-Cut *With* Beam Alignment Device

Receptor. This error may occur with digital sensors (direct or indirect) or film.

Technique. This error may occur with the bite-wing technique when a beam alignment device is used.

Appearance. With a round PID, a curved, clear (unexposed) area is seen on the image (Figure 22-19, A). A cone-cut can occur with a rectangular PID and is seen as a linear clear area on the image (Figure 22-19, B).

Cause. The PID was not properly aligned with the bite-wing beam alignment device, and the x-ray beam did not expose the entire receptor.

Correction. To avoid a cone-cut on a bite-wing receptor when using a bite-wing beam alignment device, position the PID carefully. Make certain that the PID and the aiming ring are flush and aligned.

Cone-Cut *Without* Beam Alignment Device

Receptor. This error may occur with digital sensors (direct or indirect) or film.

Technique. This error may occur with the bite-wing technique when a bite-tab is used.

Appearance. A clear (unexposed) area is seen on the image (Figure 22-20).

Cause. The PID was not directed at the center of the receptor, and the x-ray beam did not expose the entire receptor.

Correction. To avoid a cone-cut on a bite-wing receptor when using a bite-tab, position the PID carefully. Make certain that the x-ray beam is centered over the receptor and that the entire receptor is covered by the diameter of the PID. A cone-cut is more likely to occur when a bite-tab is used because there is no aiming ring to guide PID placement. To avoid a cone-cut, ask the patient to smile with the lips open while biting on the tab in order to view the location of the tab and to aid in PID alignment.

MISCELLANEOUS TECHNIQUE ERRORS

Miscellaneous technique errors, which may be seen on both periapical and bite-wing images, include bending, creasing, debris accumulation, a phalangioma, a double image, patient movement, backward receptor placement, and issues with the wired cable. The dental radiographer must be able to recognize these miscellaneous errors, identify their causes, and know the necessary steps to correct such problems.

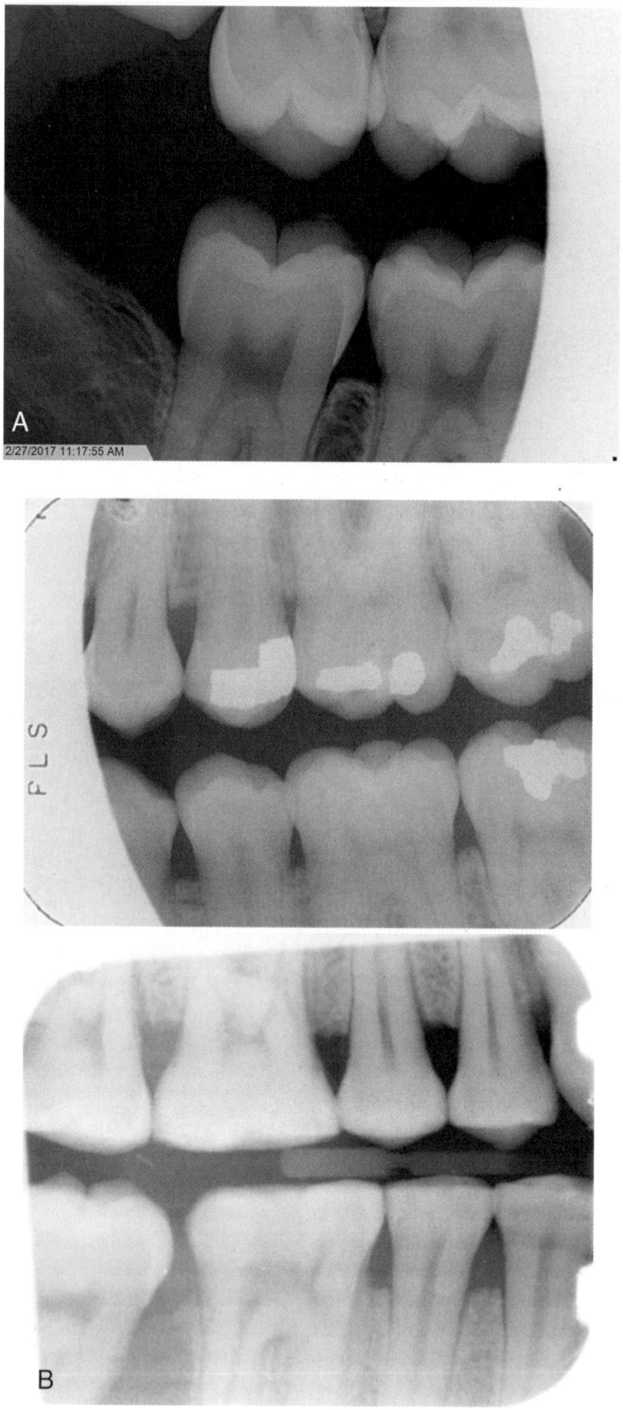

Fig 22-19 **A,** A cone-cut is seen when the position-indicating device (PID) is not properly aligned with the bite-wing beam alignment device. **B,** A cone-cut can also be produced with rectangular collimation; the PID is not properly aligned with the bite-wing beam alignment device.

Bending

Receptor. This error may occur with indirect digital sensors (PSP receptors) or film. Bending cannot occur with direct digital sensors.

Technique. This error may occur with the paralleling, bisection, or bite-wing techniques.

Appearance. The image appears stretched and distorted on a film (Figure 22-21) and on PSP receptors (Figure 22-22).

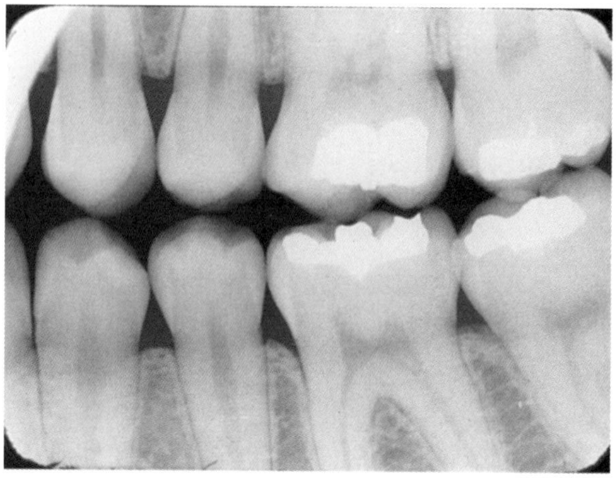

Fig 22-20 A cone-cut is seen as a curved unexposed *(clear)* area on the image.

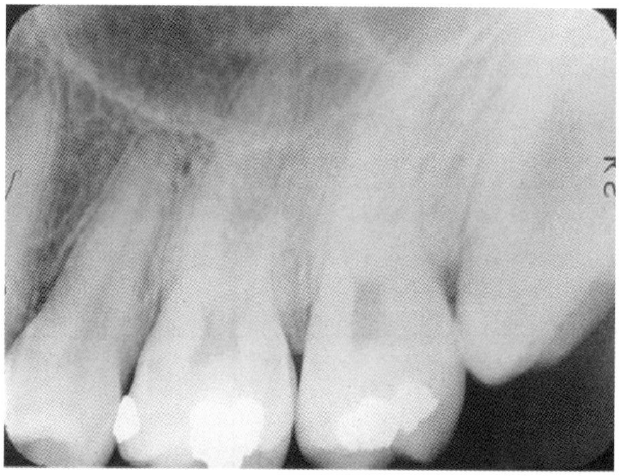

Fig 22-21 A bent film results in a distorted image.

Cause. During improper handling, the receptor was damaged. A receptor may be bent because of the curvature of the patient's hard palate, or as the result of rough and excessive handling.

Correction. To avoid bending, always check receptor placement before exposure. If the receptor is bent because of the curvature of the hard palate, cotton rolls can be used with the paralleling technique, or the bisecting technique can be used. Avoid handling and manipulating the receptor more than necessary. Use of a beam alignment device is helpful in preventing bending.

Creasing

Receptor. This error may occur with indirect digital sensors (PSP receptors) or film. Creasing cannot occur with direct digital sensors.

Technique. This error may occur with the paralleling, bisecting, or bite-wing techniques.

Appearance. When using film, a thin radiolucent line is seen on the image (Figure 22-23). When using a PSP receptor, a crease appears as a white line (Figure 22-24).

Cause. During improper handling, the receptor was creased.

Correction. To avoid creasing, do not overmanipulate the receptor in an attempt to increase patient comfort. Instead, gently soften the corners of the receptor before placement. Once a plate receptor is creased, a permanent artifact occurs and appears on each resultant image. Damaged plate receptors must be replaced.

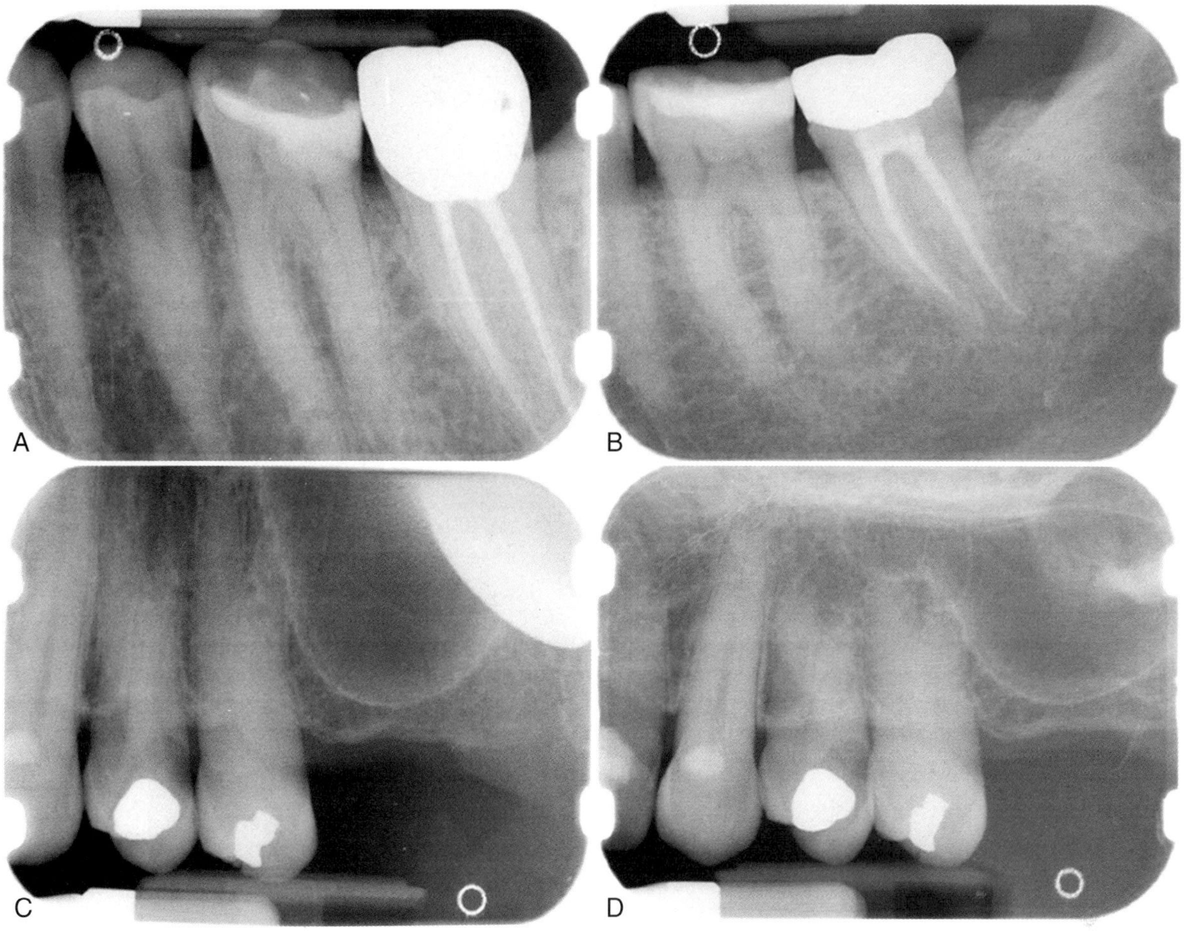

Fig 22-22 Bending of PSP plates during intraoral placement: **A,** Moderate bending. **B,** Retake of image. **C,** Severe bending. **D,** Retake of image. (From White SC, Pharoah MJ: *Oral radiology principles and interpretation*, St. Louis, 2014, Mosby.)

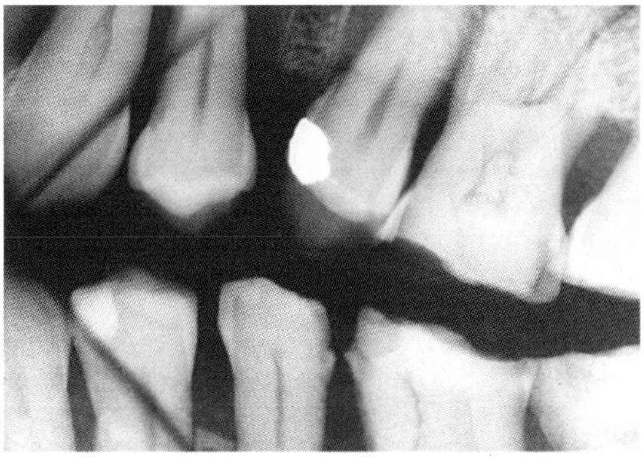

Fig 22-23 A film crease is seen as a thin radiolucent line on the image. (From Haring JI, Lind LJ: *Radiographic interpretation for the dental hygienist*, Philadelphia, 1993, Saunders.)

Debris Accumulation

Receptor. This error may occur with digital sensors.

Technique. This error may occur with the paralleling, bisecting, or bite-wing techniques.

Appearance. Debris on the surface of the sensor may cause permanent radiopaque artifacts or radiolucent scratch marks on the sensor (Figure 22-25).

Cause. If sensors are not handled carefully or wiped off between uses, debris such as dirt or dust particles may accumulate on the surface of the sensor.

Correction. Extreme care must be used when handling digital sensors. Sensors are expensive and not disposable (as film is), and therefore they must be handled carefully between patients. Correct infection prevention procedures and cleaning of sensors are important to prevent debris from accumulating or scratching the sensor.

Phalangioma

Receptor. This error may occur with digital sensors or film.

Technique. This error may occur with the bisecting technique when the finger-holding method is used. This method results in needless exposure of the patient's finger, and, based on the ALARA principle, is contraindicated. The authors of this text never recommend this technique to stabilize a receptor.

Appearance. An image of the patient's finger is seen on the image (Figure 22-26).

Cause. With the finger-holding technique, the patient's finger was incorrectly positioned in front of the receptor instead of behind it. As a result, a bone of the patient's finger is seen on the image. The term phalangioma refers to the distal phalanx of the finger seen in the image. (A *phalanx* [plural, *phalanges*] is any bone of a finger or toe.)

Correction. To avoid a phalangioma, never allow a patient to hold a receptor during exposure.

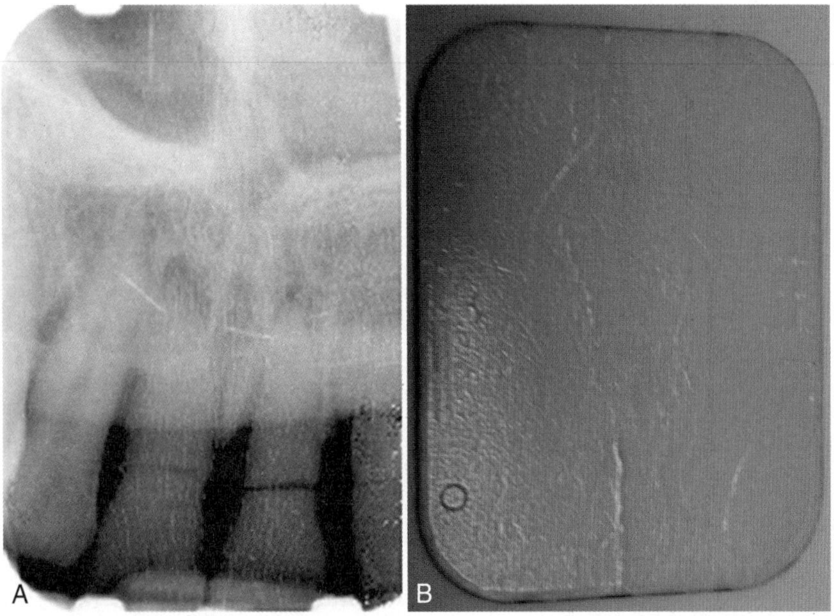

Fig 22-24 **A,** Image artifacts resulting from excessive creasing of PSP plate. **B,** Permanent damage seen on phosphor plate. (From White SC, Pharoah MJ: *Oral radiology principles and interpretation*, St. Louis, 2014, Mosby.)

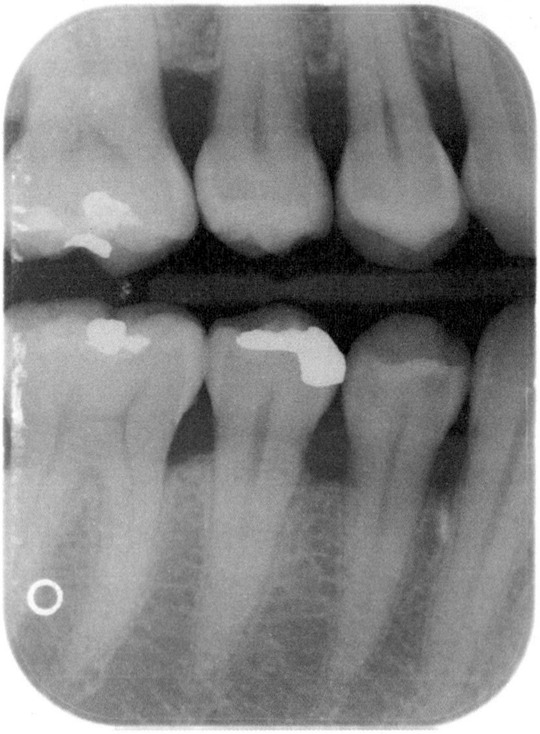

Fig 22-25 Radiopaque artifacts caused by debris seen on this vertical bite-wing image.

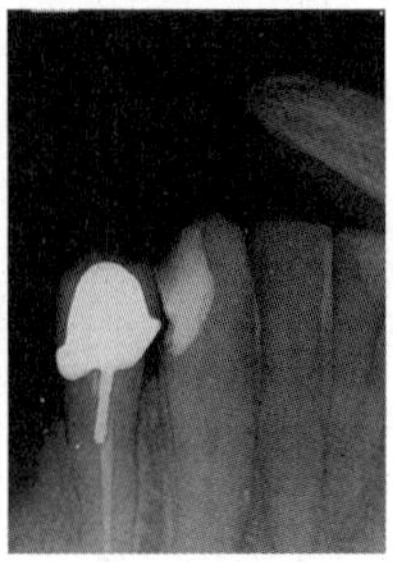

Fig 22-26 This example demonstrates a phalangioma; the image of the bones of a patient's finger is seen on the image.

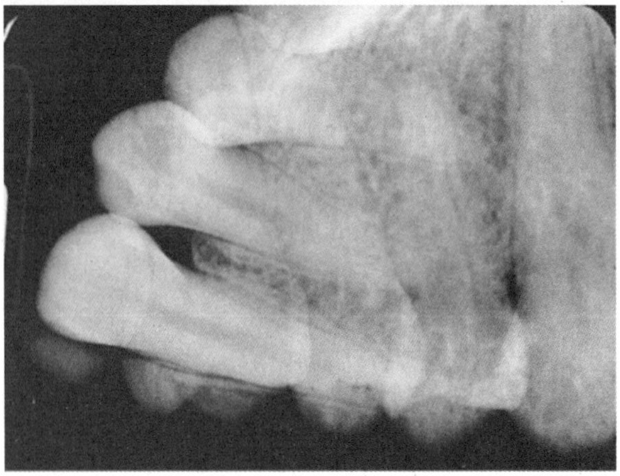

Fig 22-27 This image demonstrates double exposure of a receptor.

Double Image

Receptor. This error may occur with indirect digital sensors (PSP receptors) or film. A double image cannot be produced with a direct digital sensor.

Technique. This error may occur with the paralleling, bisecting, or bite-wing techniques.

Appearance. A double image results and appears dark with superimposed structures (Figures 22-27 and 22-28).

Cause. The same receptor was exposed twice in the patient's mouth. A double image is a serious error and necessitates two retakes, one for each of the two areas previously exposed.

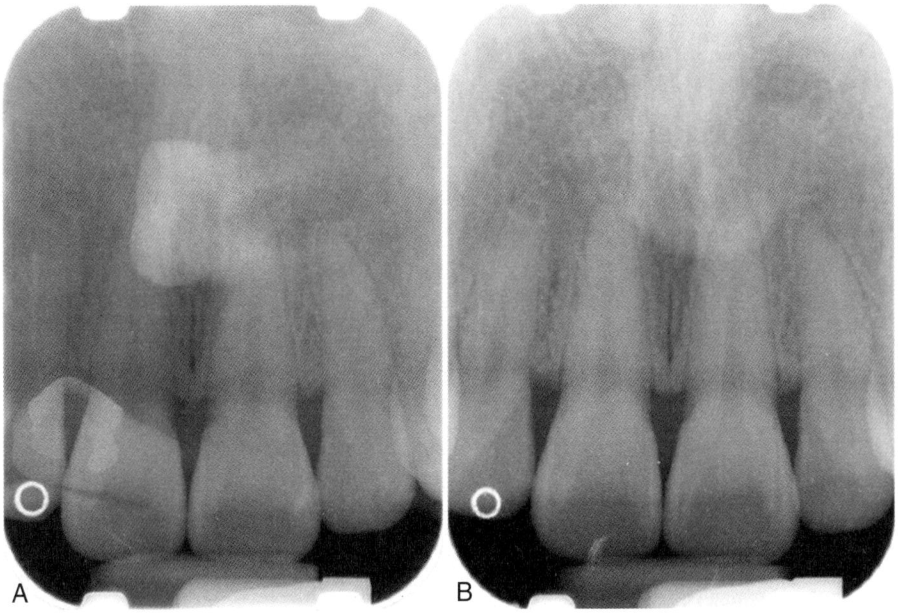

Fig 22-28 **A,** PSP double image resulting from incomplete erasure of previous image. **B,** Retake of image. (From White SC, Pharoah MJ: *Oral radiology principles and interpretation*, St. Louis, 2014, Mosby.)

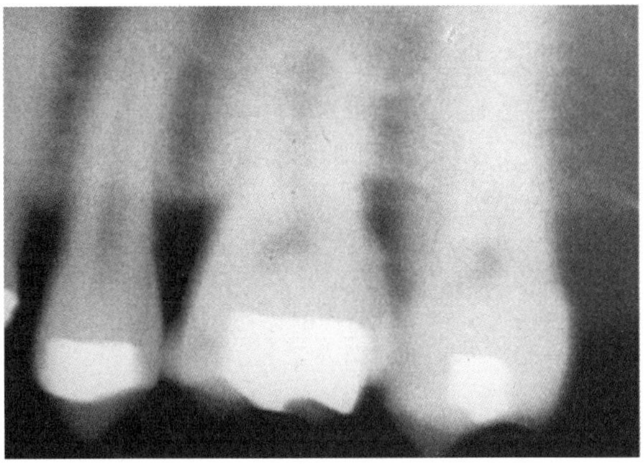

Fig 22-29 Movement results in a blurred image. (From Haring JI, Lind LJ: *Radiographic interpretation for the dental hygienist*, Philadelphia, 1993, Saunders.)

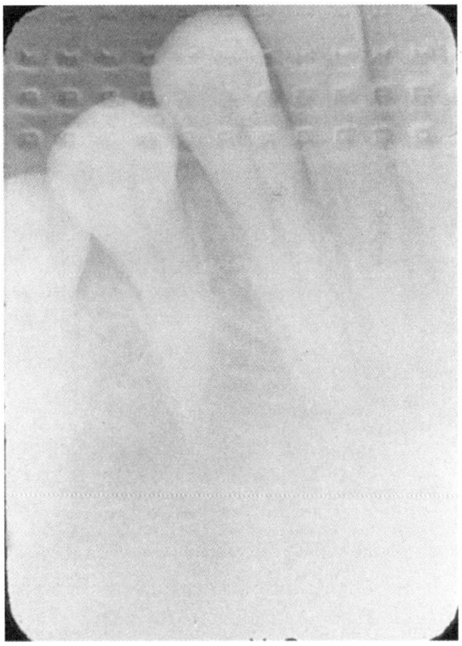

Fig 22-30 A reversed film (placed backward in the mouth) causes an image that appears light with a herringbone (or tire-track) pattern. The tire-track pattern is seen on the lead-foil backing within the film packet.

Correction. To avoid a double image, always separate exposed and unexposed receptors. Once a receptor has been exposed, place it in a designated area (e.g., a disposable cup or bag) away from unexposed receptors. If care is always taken to separate exposed receptors from unexposed receptors, this error will not occur. PSP receptors must be totally erased before reuse to avoid a remnant image left on the plate.

Movement/Motion Unsharpness

Receptor. This error may occur with digital sensors or film.

Technique. This error may occur with the paralleling, bisecting, or bite-wing techniques.

Appearance. A blurred image results (Figure 22-29).

Cause. The tubehead, receptor, or patient moved during the exposure. Patient movement is the most common cause of a blurred image.

Correction. To prevent movement errors, stabilize the tubehead and the patient's head before exposing the receptor, and instruct the patient to remain still. Never expose a receptor when a tubehead is drifting or a patient is moving. Reposition the tubehead, the patient, the receptor, or the PID as necessary, and then expose the receptor.

Reversed/Backward Placement

Receptor. This error may occur with digital sensors or film.

Technique. This error may occur with the paralleling, bisecting, or bite-wing techniques.

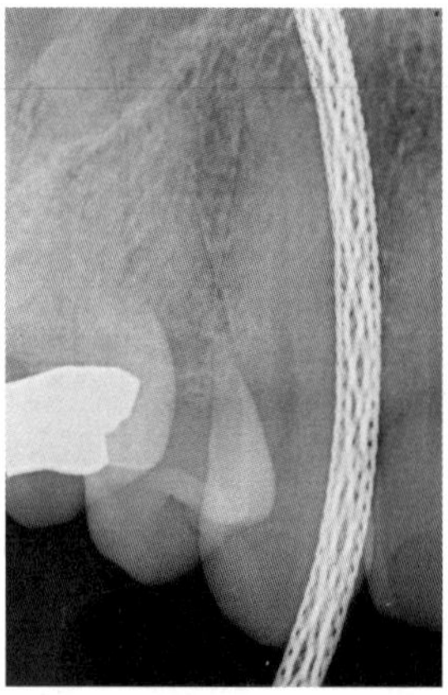

Fig 22-31 A wired sensor cable appears radiopaque.

Appearance. With film, a light image with a herringbone pattern is seen (Figure 22-30). With a digital sensor, a blank or white image is seen with no anatomic structures recorded.

Cause. With film, the receptor was placed in the mouth backward (reversed) and then exposed. The x-ray beam was attenuated by the lead foil backing in the film packet; consequently, a decreased amount of the x-ray beam exposed the film. As a result, a light image with a herringbone pattern (also known as the *tire-track pattern*) is seen. The herringbone pattern is representative of the actual pattern embossed on the lead foil (see Chapter 9). With a digital sensor, the receptor was placed in the mouth backward (reversed) and then exposed. As the result of exposing the wrong side of the sensor, no x-ray interaction occurred, and no image was produced.

Correction. To avoid a reversed film, always place the white side of the packet adjacent to the teeth ("white in sight"). Always note the front and back sides of the film before placing it in the patient's mouth. For plate receptors, the emulsion side must be directed toward the x-ray beam. For direct digital sensors, the plain, flat non-wired side or the non-battery side of the receptor must be directed toward the x-ray beam.

Wired Cable Issues

Receptor. This error occurs exclusively with direct digital sensors.

Technique. This error may occur with the paralleling, bisecting, or bite-wing techniques.

Appearance. The wired cable appears as a radiopaque outline (Figure 22-31).

Cause. The intraoral sensor is linked to the computer via a fiber-optic cable. If the sensor is placed with the cable between the sensor and the source of radiation, an outline of the cable will be seen.

Correction. Most manufacturers of direct digital imaging systems provide a clamp on the metal indicator arm of the beam alignment device to securely hold the cable in place. It is important to check that the cable is secure, the patient is not biting on the cable, and that the cable is out of the beam of x-radiation before *each* exposure.

SUMMARY

- The dental radiographer must have a working knowledge of exposure technique errors that result in nondiagnostic images. Processing errors are discussed in Chapter 10.
- Receptor exposure errors that result in nondiagnostic images include unexposed, overexposed, and underexposed receptors and film that is accidentally exposed to white light.
- Periapical and bite-wing technique errors include receptor placement, angulation, and PID alignment problems.
- Miscellaneous technique errors include bending, creasing, debris accumulation, phalangioma, double exposure, patient movement, the reversed/backward placement of the receptor, and wired cable issues.
- The dental radiographer must be able to recognize and identify the causes of exposure and technique errors. In addition, the dental radiographer must know the necessary steps to correct such errors.

BIBLIOGRAPHY

Haring JI, Lind LJ: Film exposure, processing and technique errors. In Radiographic interpretation for the dental hygienist, Philadelphia, 1993, Saunders.

Johnson ON: Identifying and correcting faulty radiographs. In Essentials of dental radiography for dental assistants and hygienists, ed 9, Upper Saddle River, NJ, 2011, Prentice Hall.

Mallya SM, Lam EWN: Film Imaging. In White and Pharoah's Oral radiology: principles and interpretation, ed 8, St. Louis, 2019, Elsevier.

Miles DA, Van Dis ML, Razmus TF: Intraoral radiographic techniques. In Basic principles of oral and maxillofacial radiology, Philadelphia, 1992, Saunders.

Miles DA, Van Dis ML, Williamson GF, et al: Technique/processing errors and troubleshooting. In Radiographic imaging for the dental team, ed 4, St. Louis, 2009, Saunders.

Williamson GF: Digital imaging techniques and error correction. Continuing education course. 2014. www.dentalcare.com.

QUIZ QUESTIONS

Identification

For questions 1 to 10, refer to Figures 22-32 through 22-41. Identify the exposure technique error seen in each image.

1. ______________________
2. ______________________
3. ______________________
4. ______________________
5. ______________________
6. ______________________
7. ______________________
8. ______________________
9. ______________________
10. ______________________

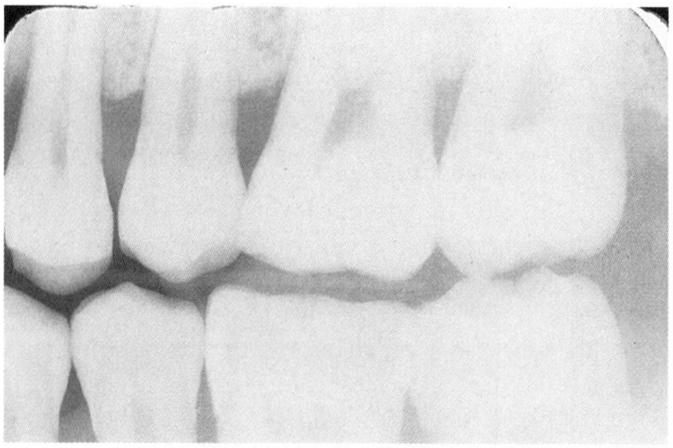

Fig 22-32

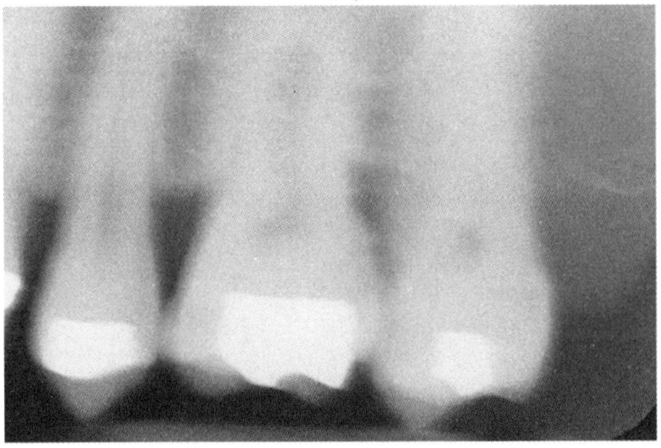

Fig 22-33

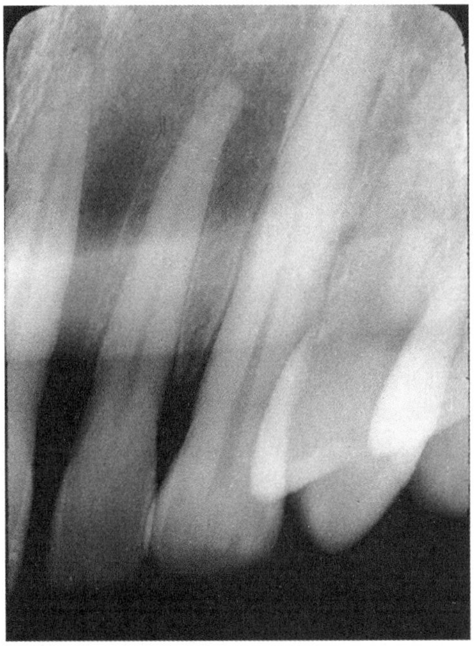

Fig 22-34

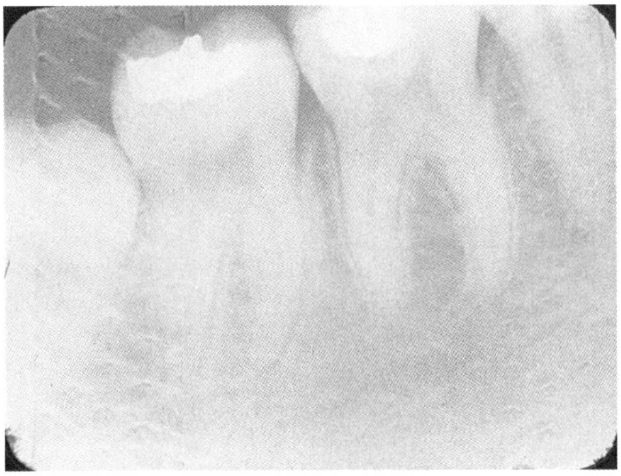

Fig 22-35

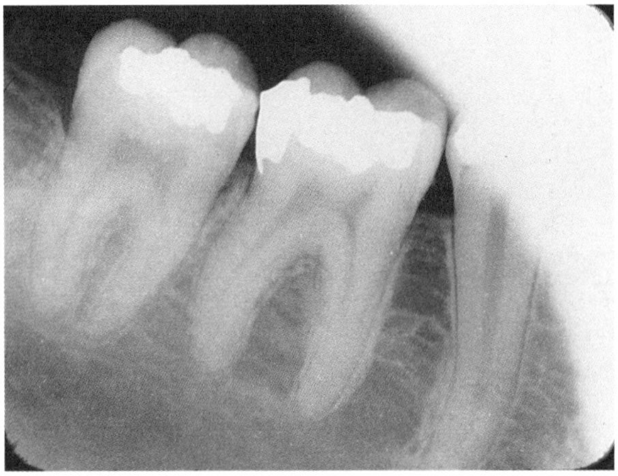

Fig 22-36

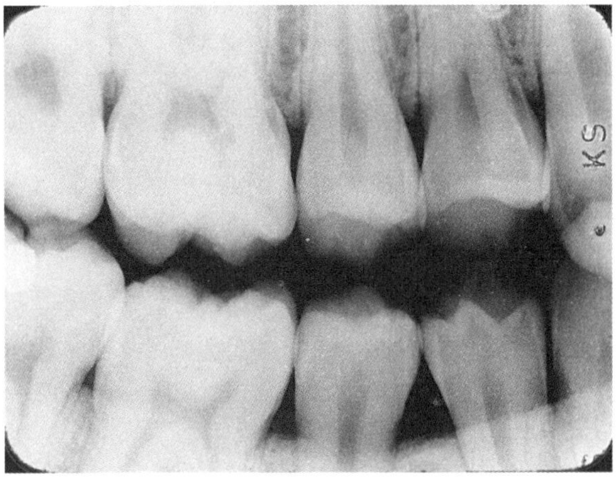

Fig 22-37

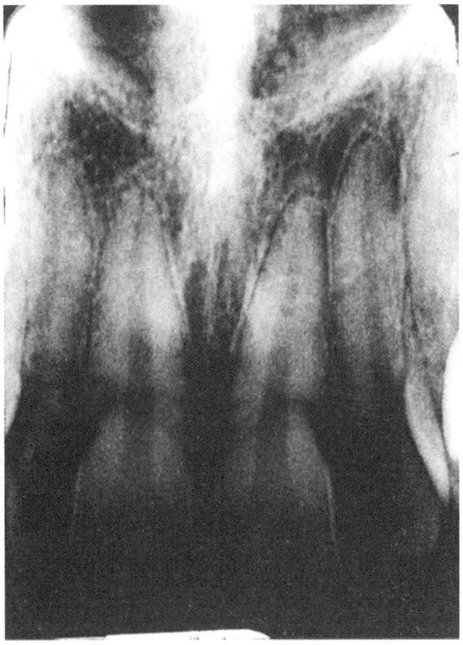

Fig 22-38

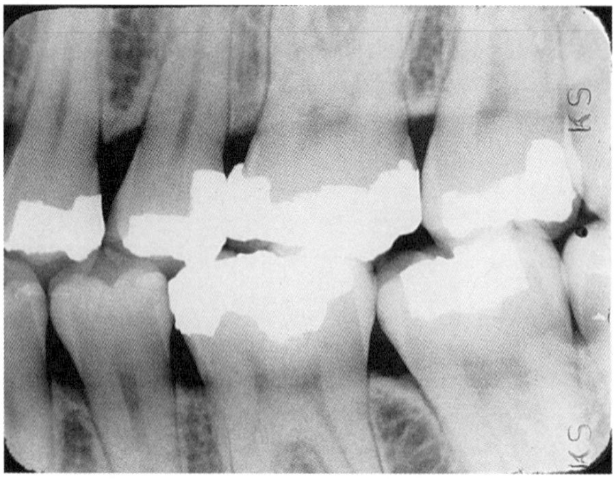

Fig 22-39

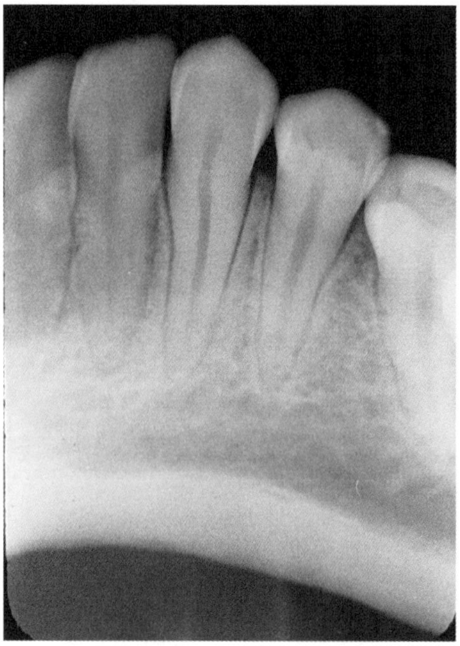

Fig 22-40

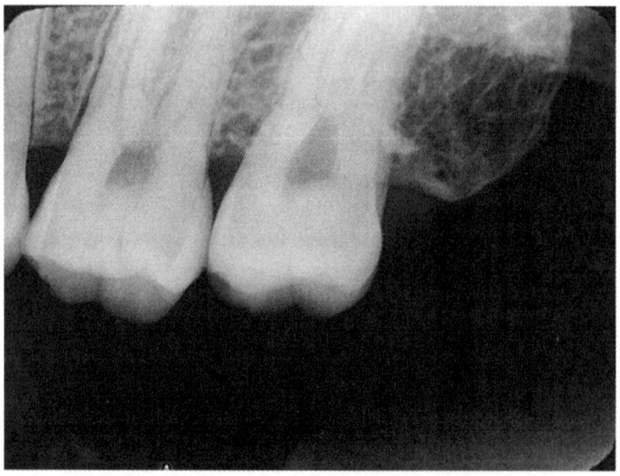

Fig 22-41

MATCHING

For questions 11 to 15, describe the appearance of each error using one of these terms:

Clear
Black
Light
Dark

____ **11.** Overexposed image
____ **12.** Underexposed image
____ **13.** Film exposed to light
____ **14.** Unexposed receptor
____ **15.** Reversed receptor

Multiple Choice

____ **16.** Too much vertical angulation results in images that are:
- **a.** elongated
- **b.** foreshortened
- **c.** overlapped
- **d.** none of the above

____ **17.** Too little vertical angulation results in images that are:
- **a.** elongated
- **b.** foreshortened
- **c.** overlapped
- **d.** none of the above

____ **18.** Incorrect horizontal angulation results in images that are:
- **a.** elongated
- **b.** foreshortened
- **c.** overlapped
- **d.** none of the above

____ **19.** Which error(s) can occur with the bite-wing technique?
1. elongation
2. overlapped contacts
3. cone-cut
4. phalangioma
- **a.** 1, 2, 3, and 4
- **b.** 1, 2, and 3
- **c.** 2 and 4
- **d.** 2 and 3

____ **20.** Which error(s) can occur with the bisecting technique?
1. elongation
2. overlapped contacts
3. cone-cut
4. phalangioma
- **a.** 1, 2, 3, and 4
- **b.** 1, 2, and 3
- **c.** 2 and 4
- **d.** 2 and 3

23

Occlusal and Localization Techniques

LEARNING OBJECTIVES

After completion of this chapter, the student will be able to do the following:

1. Define the key terms associated with occlusal and localization techniques.
2. Describe the purpose of occlusal examination.
3. List the uses of occlusal examination and discuss the basic principles involved.
4. Describe the patient and equipment preparations that are necessary before using the occlusal technique.
5. State the recommended vertical angulations for the following maxillary occlusal projections: topographic, lateral (right or left), and pediatric.
6. State the recommended vertical angulations for the following mandibular occlusal projections: topographic, cross-sectional, and pediatric.
7. State the purpose of localization techniques and list their uses.
8. Describe the buccal object rule.
9. Describe the right-angle technique.
10. List the patient and equipment preparations that are necessary before using the buccal object rule or the right-angle technique.
11. Describe receptor placements for the buccal object rule and compare the resulting images.
12. Describe receptor placements for the right-angle technique and compare the resulting images.

In addition to mastering periapical and interproximal examination techniques, the dental radiographer must also master occlusal and localization techniques. Before the dental radiographer can use these important techniques, an understanding of the basic concepts, patient preparation, equipment preparation, and receptor placement procedures is necessary.

The purpose of this chapter is to present basic concepts and to describe patient preparation, equipment preparation, and receptor placement procedures for both occlusal and localization techniques.

OCCLUSAL TECHNIQUE

The occlusal technique is used to examine large areas of the maxilla or the mandible. Before the dental radiographer can use the occlusal technique, a thorough understanding of basic concepts is necessary. In addition, knowledge of step-by-step procedures is required.

Basic Concepts

Terminology. Before describing the principles of the occlusal technique, a number of basic terms must be defined, as follows:

Occlusal surfaces: Chewing surfaces of posterior teeth.

Occlusal examination: A type of intraoral radiographic examination to inspect large areas of the maxilla or the mandible on one image.

Occlusal technique: Method used to expose a receptor in occlusal examination.

Occlusal receptor: In the occlusal technique, a size 4 intraoral receptor is used. The receptor is so named because the patient "occludes," or bites, on the entire receptor. Size 4 receptors are the largest size of intraoral receptors, measuring 3×2.25 inches. In the adult, a size 4 receptor is used in occlusal examination. In the child with a primary dentition, a size 2 receptor is typically used.

Purpose and Use. The occlusal technique is a supplementary imaging technique that is usually used in conjunction with periapical or bitewing images. The occlusal technique is used when large areas of the maxilla or the mandible must be visualized. The occlusal image is preferred when the area of interest is larger than a periapical receptor may cover or when the placement of intraoral receptors is too difficult for the patient. Occlusal imaging can be used for the following purposes:

- To locate retained roots of extracted teeth
- To locate supernumerary (extra), unerupted, or impacted teeth
- To locate foreign bodies in the maxilla or the mandible
- To locate salivary stones in the duct of the submandibular gland
- To locate and evaluate the extent of lesions (e.g., cysts, tumors, malignancies) in the maxilla or the mandible
- To evaluate the boundaries of the maxillary sinus
- To evaluate fractures of the maxilla or the mandible
- To aid in the examination of patients who cannot open their mouths more than a few millimeters
- To examine the area of a cleft palate
- To measure changes in the size and shape of the maxilla or the mandible

Principles. The basic principles of the occlusal technique can be described as follows:

1. The receptor is placed with the tube side facing the arch that is being exposed. When using film, it is positioned with the white side facing the arch that is being exposed. When using a digital sensor, the flat non-wired or non-battery side of the sensor must face the arch that is being exposed.
2. The receptor is placed in the mouth between the occlusal surfaces of maxillary and mandibular teeth.
3. The receptor is stabilized when the patient gently bites on the surface of the receptor. It is important to stress to the patient to *gently* bite on the receptor to avoid seeing permanent bite marks on the surface of the sensor.

Step-by-Step Procedures

Step-by-step procedures for the exposure of occlusal images include patient preparation, equipment preparation, and receptor placement methods. Before exposing any occlusal receptors, infection prevention procedures (as described in Chapter 16) must be completed.

Patient Preparation. After completion of infection prevention procedures and preparation of the treatment area and supplies, the patient should be seated. After seating the patient, the dental radiographer must prepare the patient before the exposure of any receptors (Procedure 23-1).

Equipment Preparation. After patient preparation, equipment must also be prepared before the exposure of any receptors begins (Procedure 23-2).

Maxillary Occlusal Projections. Three maxillary occlusal projections are commonly used: (1) topographic, (2) lateral (right or left), and (3) pediatric.

1. *Topographic projection.* The maxillary topographic occlusal projection is used to examine the palate and the anterior teeth of the maxilla (Procedure 23-3).
2. *Lateral (right or left) projection.* The maxillary lateral occlusal projection is used to examine the palatal roots of molar teeth. It may also be used to locate foreign bodies or lesions in the posterior maxilla (Procedure 23-4).
3. *Pediatric projection.* The maxillary pediatric occlusal projection is used to examine the anterior teeth of the maxilla and is recommended for use in children 5 years or younger (Procedure 23-5).

PROCEDURE 23-1 Patient Preparation for Occlusal Technique

1. Briefly explain the imaging procedure to the patient.
2. Adjust the chair so that the patient is positioned upright and the level of the chair is at a comfortable working height.
3. Adjust the headrest to support the patient's head.
   - For maxillary occlusal exposures, the patient's head must be positioned with the maxillary arch parallel to the floor and the midsagittal (midline) plane perpendicular to the floor.
   - For some mandibular occlusal exposures, the patient's head must be reclined and positioned with the occlusal plane perpendicular to the floor. For others, the patient is positioned with the occlusal plane parallel to the floor.
4. Place and secure the lead apron with thyroid collar on the patient.
5. Request that the patient remove eyeglasses and any objects in the mouth (e.g., dentures, retainers, chewing gum) that may interfere with the procedure.

PROCEDURE 23-2 Equipment Preparation for Occlusal Technique

1. Set the exposure control factors (kilovoltage, milliamperage, and time) on the x-ray unit according to the recommendations of the receptor manufacturer.
2. Either a short (8-inch) or a long (16-inch) PID may be used with the occlusal technique.

Mandibular Occlusal Projections. Three mandibular occlusal projections are commonly used: (1) topographic, (2) cross-sectional, and (3) pediatric.

1. *Topographic projection.* The mandibular topographic occlusal projection is used to examine the anterior teeth of the mandible (Procedure 23-6).
2. *Cross-sectional projection.* The mandibular cross-sectional occlusal projection is used to examine the buccal and lingual aspects of the mandible. It is also used to locate foreign bodies or salivary stones in the region of the floor of the mouth (Procedure 23-7).
3. *Pediatric projection.* The mandibular pediatric occlusal projection is used to examine the anterior teeth of the mandible and is recommended for use in children 5 years or younger (Procedure 23-8).

Vertical Angulations. The recommended vertical angulations for all maxillary and mandibular occlusal exposures are summarized in Table 23-1.

LOCALIZATION TECHNIQUES

A localization technique is a method used to locate the position of a tooth or an object in the jaws. Before the dental radiographer can use localization techniques, a thorough understanding of basic concepts is necessary. In addition, knowledge of step-by-step procedures is required.

Basic Concepts

Purpose and Use. The dental image is a two-dimensional picture of a three-dimensional object. A dental image depicts an object in superior-inferior and anterior-posterior relationships. The dental image, however, does not depict the buccal-lingual relationship, or the depth, of an object. In dentistry, it may be necessary to establish the buccal-lingual position of a structure such as a foreign object or an impacted tooth within the jaws. Localization techniques can be used to obtain this three-dimensional information. Localization techniques may be used to locate the following:

- Foreign bodies
- Impacted teeth
- Unerupted teeth
- Retained roots
- Root positions
- Salivary stones
- Jaw fractures
- Broken needles and instruments
- Dental restorative materials

TABLE 23-1 Occlusal Projections and Corresponding Vertical Angulations

Occlusal Projection	Vertical Angulation (degrees)
Maxillary topographic	+65
Maxillary lateral (right or left)	+60
Maxillary pediatric	+60
Mandibular topographic	−55
Mandibular cross-sectional	90
Mandibular pediatric	−55

PROCEDURE 23-3 Maxillary Topographic Occlusal Projection (Figure 23-1)

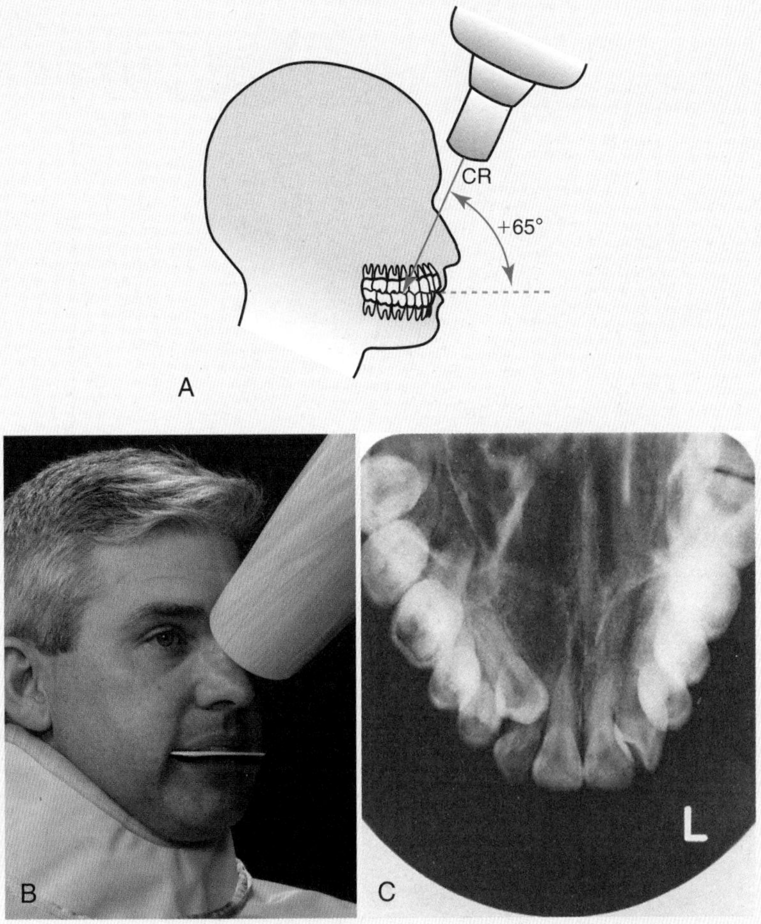

Fig 23-1 **A,** The central ray (CR) is directed at +65 degrees vertical angulation to the plane of the receptor. **B,** Relationship of the receptor and PID. **C,** Maxillary topographic occlusal projection. (**A** and **C,** Courtesy Carestream Health, Inc., Rochester, NY.)

1. Position the patient with the maxillary arch parallel to the floor.
2. Place a size 4 receptor with the tube side facing the maxilla and the long edge in a side-to-side direction. Insert the receptor into the patient's mouth, placing it as far posteriorly as the oral anatomy permits.
3. Instruct the patient to bite gently on the receptor, and hold the receptor in an end-to-end bite.
4. Position the PID with the central ray directed through the midline of the arch toward the center of the receptor.
5. Position the PID at +65 degrees vertical angulation toward the center of the receptor. Place the top edge of the PID between the patient's eyebrows on the bridge of the nose.

PROCEDURE 23-4 Maxillary Lateral Occlusal Projection (Figure 23-2)

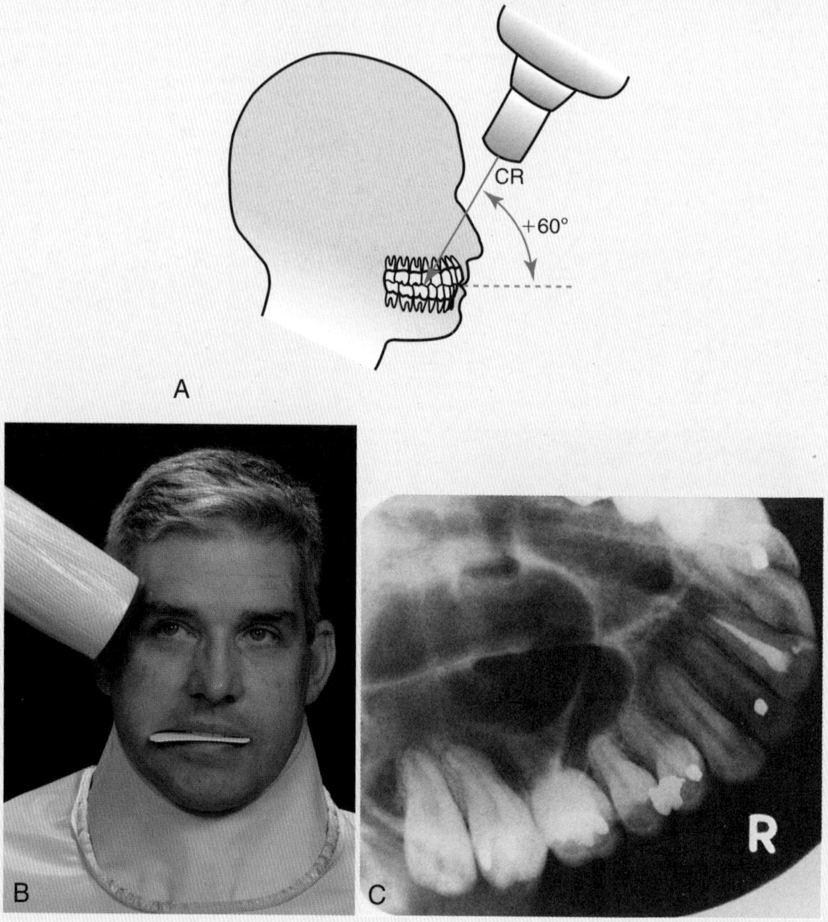

Fig 23-2 **A,** The central ray (CR) is directed at +60 degrees vertical angulation to the plane of the receptor. **B,** Relationship of the receptor and the PID. **C,** Maxillary lateral occlusal projection. (**A** and **C**, Courtesy Carestream Health, Inc., Rochester, NY.)

1. Position the patient with the maxillary arch parallel to the floor.
2. Place a size 4 receptor with the tube side facing the maxilla and the long edge in a front-to-back direction. Insert the receptor into the patient's mouth, and place it as far posteriorly as the oral anatomy permits. Shift the receptor to the side (right or left) of the area of interest. The long edge of the receptor should extend approximately ½ inch beyond the buccal surfaces of posterior teeth.
3. Instruct the patient to bite gently on the receptor, and hold the receptor in an end-to-end bite.
4. Position the PID with the central ray directed through the contact areas of interest.
5. Position the PID at +60 degrees vertical angulation toward the center of the receptor. Place the top edge of the PID above the corner of the patient's eyebrow.

PROCEDURE 23-5 Maxillary Pediatric Occlusal Projection (Figure 23-3)

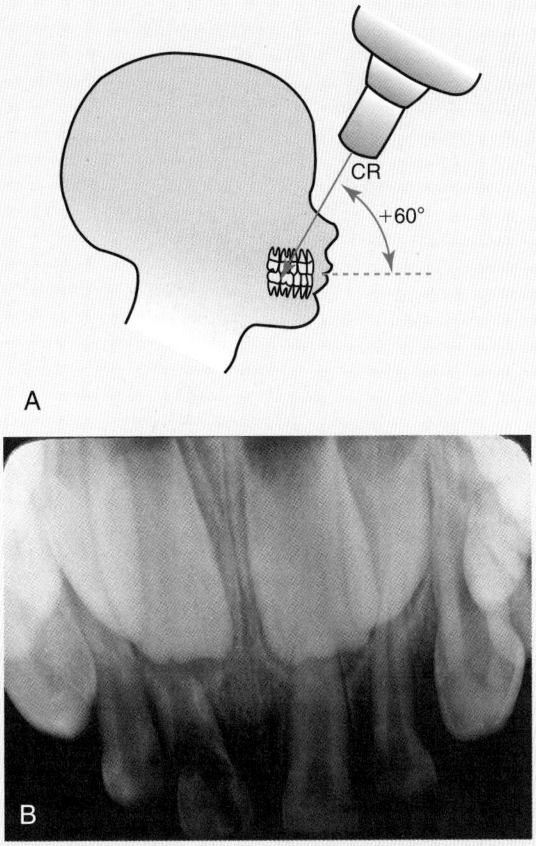

Fig 23-3 **A,** The central ray (CR) is directed at +60 degrees vertical angulation to the plane of the receptor. **B,** Maxillary pediatric occlusal projection.

1. Position the child such with maxillary arch parallel to the floor.
2. Place a size 2 receptor with the tube side facing the maxilla and the long edge in a side-to-side direction. Insert the receptor into the child's mouth.
3. Instruct the child to bite gently on the receptor, and hold the receptor in an end-to-end bite.
4. Position the PID with the central ray directed through the midline of the arch toward the center of the receptor.
5. Position the PID at +60 degrees vertical angulation toward the center of the receptor. Place the top edge of the PID between the child's eyebrows on the bridge of the nose.

PROCEDURE 23-6 Mandibular Topographic Occlusal Projection (Figure 23-4)

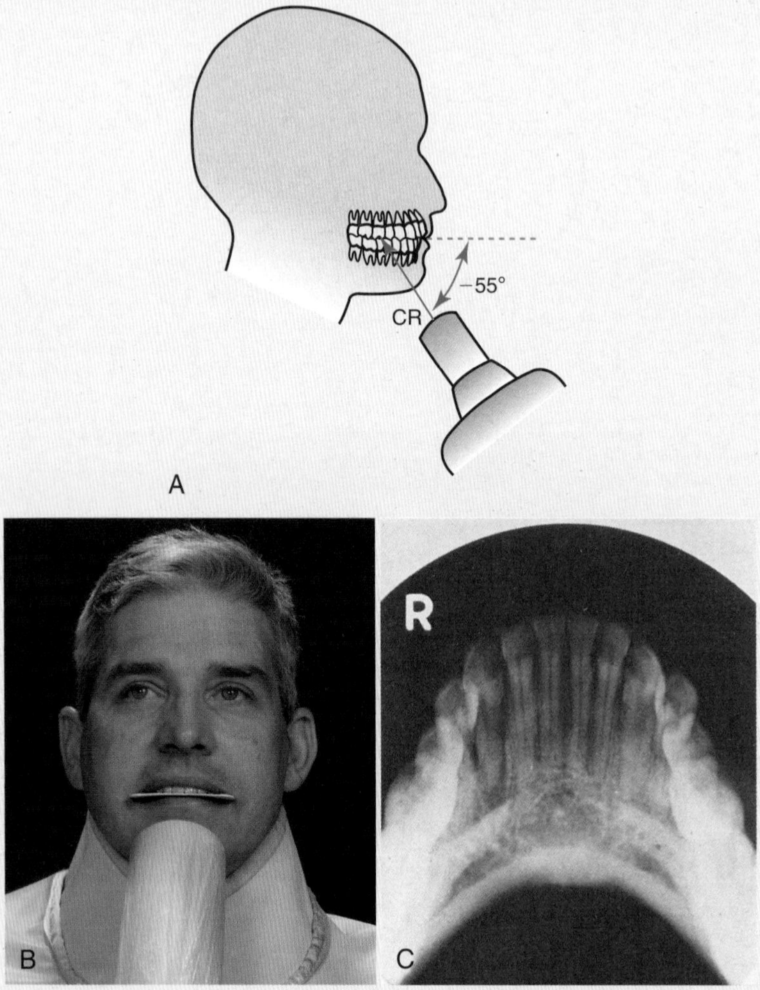

Fig 23-4 **A,** The central ray (CR) is directed at −55 degrees vertical angulation to the plane of the receptor. **B,** Relationship of the receptor and the PID. **C,** Mandibular topographic occlusal projection. (**A** and **C,** Courtesy Carestream Health, Inc., Rochester, NY.)

1. Position the patient with the mandibular arch parallel to the floor.
2. Place a size 4 receptor film with the tube side facing the mandible and the long edge in a side-to-side direction. Insert the receptor into the patient's mouth, placing it as far posteriorly as the oral anatomy permits.
3. Instruct the patient to bite gently on the receptor, and hold the receptor in an end-to-end bite.
4. Position the PID with the central ray directed through the midline of the arch toward the center of the receptor.
5. Position the PID at −55 degrees vertical angulation toward the center of the receptor. Center the PID over the patient's chin.

PROCEDURE 23-7 Mandibular Cross-Sectional Occlusal Projection (Figure 23-5)

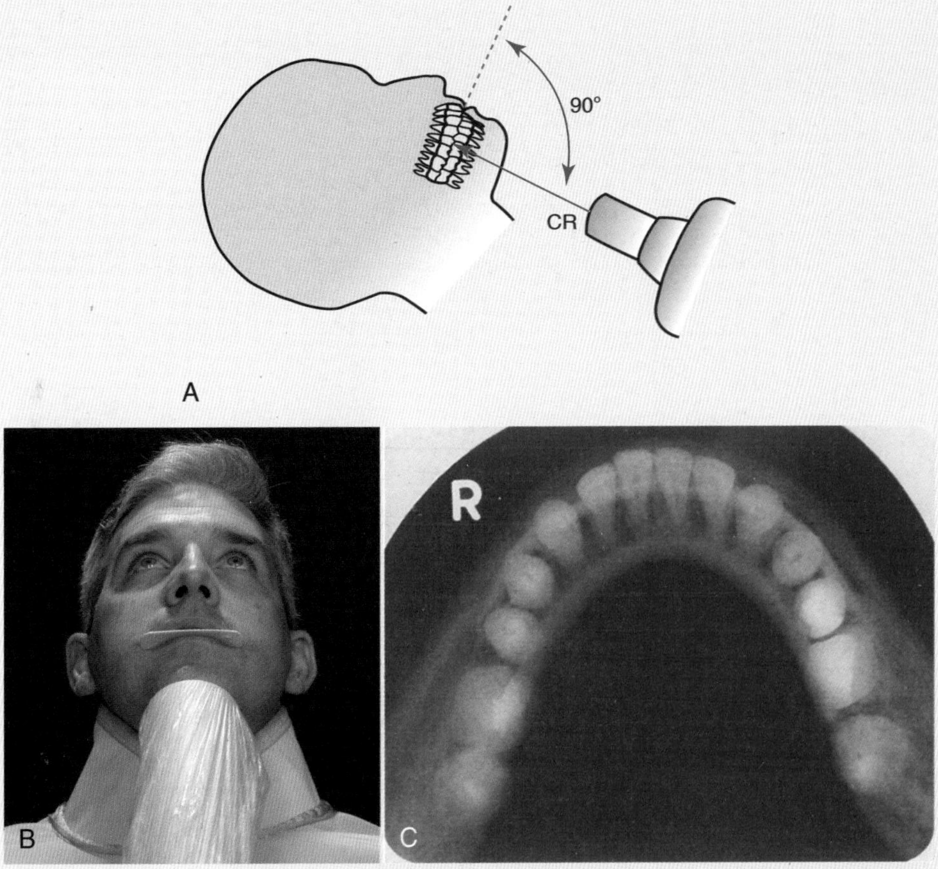

Fig 23-5 **A,** The central ray (CR) is perpendicular (90 degrees vertical angulation) to the plane of the receptor. **B,** Relationship of receptor and PID. **C,** Mandibular cross-sectional occlusal projection. (**A** and **C,** Courtesy Carestream Health, Inc., Rochester, NY.)

1. Recline the patient, and position the mandibular arch perpendicular to the floor.
2. Place a size 4 receptor with the tube side facing the mandible and the long edge in a side-to-side direction. Insert the receptor into the patient's mouth as far posteriorly as the oral anatomy permits.
3. Instruct the patient to bite gently on the receptor, and hold the receptor in an end-to-end bite.
4. Position the PID with the central ray directed through the midline of the arch toward the center of the receptor.
5. Position the PID at 90 degrees toward the center of the receptor. Place the PID approximately 1 inch below the patient's chin.

PROCEDURE 23-8 Mandibular Pediatric Occlusal Projection (Figure 23-6)

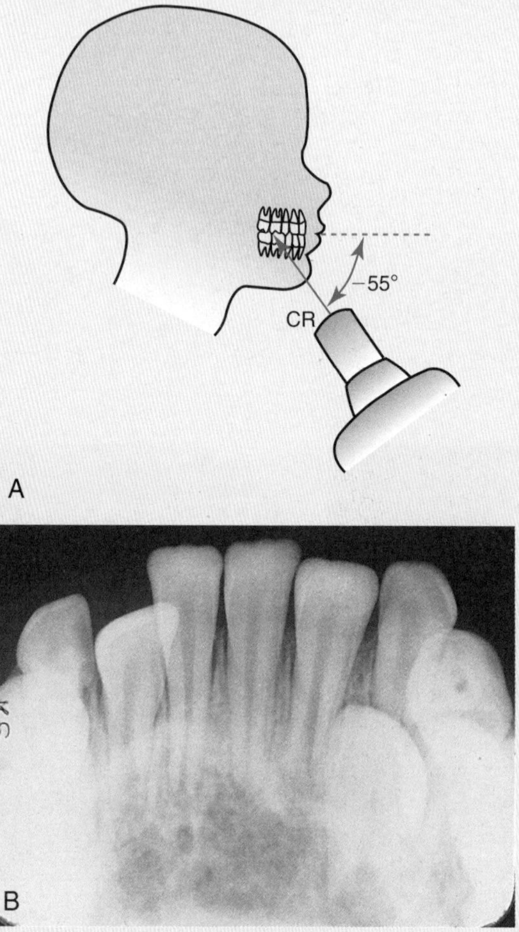

Fig 23-6 **A,** The central ray (CR) is directed at −55 degrees vertical angulation to the plane of the receptor. **B,** Mandibular pediatric occlusal projection.

1. Position the child with the mandibular arch parallel to the floor.
2. Place a size 2 receptor with the tube side facing the mandible and the long edge in a side-to-side direction. Insert the receptor into the child's mouth.
3. Instruct the child to bite gently on the receptor, and hold the receptor in an end-to-end bite.
4. Position the PID with the central ray directed through the midline of the arch toward the center of the receptor.
5. Position the PID at −55 degrees vertical angulation. Center the PID over the child's chin.

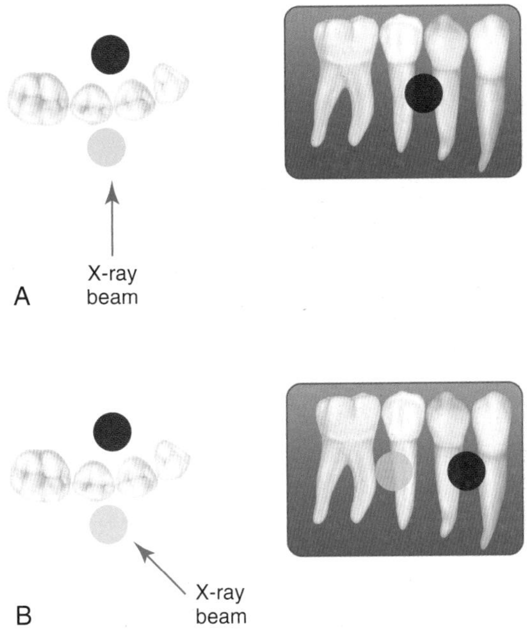

Fig 23-7 Buccal and lingual objects shift positions when the direction of the x-ray beam is changed. **A,** Buccal (*blue circle*) and lingual (*black circle*) objects are superimposed in the original image. **B,** If the tubehead is shifted in a mesial direction, the buccal object moves distally, and the lingual object moves mesially (same direction = lingual; opposite direction = buccal). (Redrawn from Haring JI, Lind LJ: *Radiographic interpretation for the dental hygienist,* Philadelphia, 1993, Saunders.)

Since the introduction of cone-beam computer tomography to dentistry, viewing anatomic structures in three dimensions may cause some of the localization techniques to be outdated (see Chapter 27). If three-dimensional digital imaging is not available in the dental practice, knowledge of these localization techniques is necessary.

Types of Localization Techniques. Two basic techniques are used to localize objects: (1) the buccal object rule and (2) the right-angle technique.

Buccal Object Rule. The buccal object rule governs the orientation of structures portrayed in two images exposed at different angulations. Using proper technique and angulation, a periapical or bite-wing receptor is exposed; then, after changing the direction of the x-ray beam, a second periapical or bite-wing receptor is exposed using a different horizontal or vertical angulation. For example, a different *horizontal angulation* is used when trying to locate *vertically aligned* images (e.g., teeth treated with root canal therapy), whereas a different *vertical angulation* is used when trying to locate a *horizontally aligned* image (e.g., the mandibular canal). After the two exposures are completed, the images are compared with each other.

When the dental structure or object seen in the second image appears to have moved in the *same direction as the shift of the PID,* the structure or object in question is positioned to the lingual (Figure 23-7). For example, if the horizontal angulation is changed by shifting the PID mesially, and the object in question moves mesially on the image, then the object lies to the lingual (lingual = same).

Conversely, when the dental structure or object seen in the second image appears to have moved in the *opposite direction opposite as the shift of the PID,* the structure or object in question is positioned to the *buccal* (Figure 23-8). For example, if the horizontal angulation is changed by shifting the PID distally, and the object in question moves mesially on the image, then the object lies to the buccal (buccal = opposite).

The mnemonic "SLOB" can be used to remember the buccal object rule, as follows:

Same = **L**ingual; **O**pposite = **B**uccal

In other words, when the two images are compared, the object that lies to the *lingual* appears to have moved in the *same* direction as the PID, and the object that lies to the *buccal* appears to have moved in the opposite direction as the PID. The buccal object rule is also referred to as the *SLOB rule.*

Right-Angle Technique. The right-angle technique is another rule for the orientation of structures seen in two images. One periapical receptor is exposed using the proper technique and angulation to show the position of the object in superior-inferior and anterior-posterior relationships. Next, an occlusal receptor is exposed directing the central ray at a right angle, or perpendicular (90 degrees), to the receptor. The occlusal image shows the object in buccal-lingual and anterior-posterior relationships. After the two receptors have been exposed and processed, the images are compared with each other to locate the object in three dimensions (Figure 23-9). This technique is primarily used for locating objects in the mandible.

HELPFUL HINT

Buccal Object Rule

If the object seen in the second image moves in the **same** direction as the shift of the PID, the structure or object in question is positioned to the **lingual**.

If the object seen in the second image moves in the **opposite** direction as the shift of the PID, the structure of object in question is positioned to the **buccal**.

S-L-O-B Rule

Same = **L**ingual
Opposite = **B**uccal

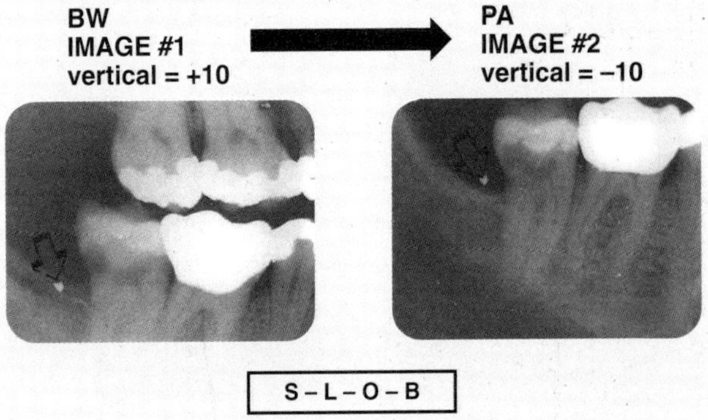

Step-by-Step Procedures

Step-by-step procedures for localization techniques include patient and equipment preparations and receptor placements and comparisons.

Patient and Equipment Preparations. Before exposing receptors using localization techniques, infection prevention procedures (as described in Chapter 16) and patient and equipment preparations (described earlier in this chapter) must be completed.

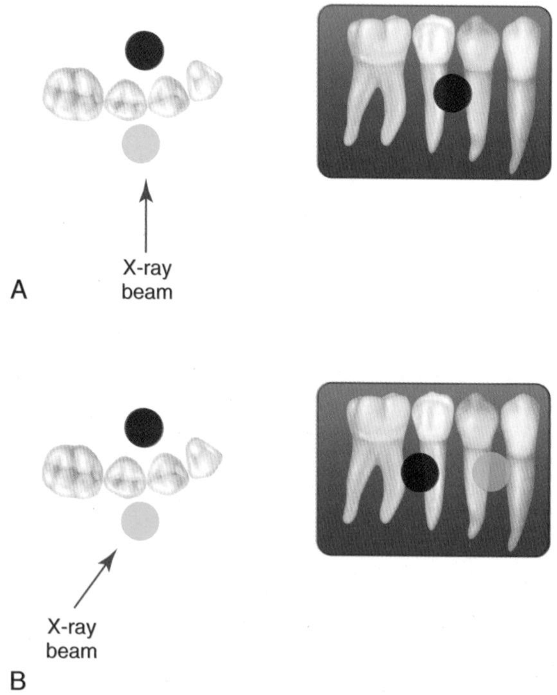

Fig 23-8 Buccal and lingual objects shift positions when the direction of the x-ray beam is changed. **A,** Buccal (*blue circle*) and lingual (*black circle*) objects are superimposed in the original image. **B,** If the tubehead is shifted in a distal direction, the buccal object moves mesially, and the lingual object moves distally (same direction = lingual; opposite direction = buccal). (Redrawn from Haring JI, Lind LJ: *Radiographic interpretation for the dental hygienist*, Philadelphia, 1993, Saunders.)

Receptor Placements and Image Comparisons.

Buccal Object Rule. The buccal object rule can be used to determine the position of a tooth treated endodontically with gutta percha (an endodontic filling material) in a maxillary second premolar (Figure 23-10).

1. Position the patient with the maxillary arch parallel to the floor.
2. Expose one molar periapical receptor using proper technique and angulation.
3. Shift the PID in a mesial direction, and then expose a premolar periapical receptor.
4. In the second image, when the PID was moved in a mesial direction, the gutta percha moved in the opposite direction. Therefore the location of the gutta percha is in the root that lies to the buccal (buccal = opposite).

The buccal object rule can be used to determine the location of an impacted supernumerary (extra) tooth (Figure 23-11).

1. Position the patient with the maxillary arch parallel to the floor.
2. Expose one central-lateral incisor periapical receptor using proper technique and angulation.
3. Shift the PID in a distal direction, and then expose the canine periapical receptor.
4. In the second image, when the PID was moved in a distal direction, the impacted tooth moved in the same direction. Therefore the tooth lies to the lingual (lingual = same).

Right-Angle Technique. The right-angle technique can be used to determine the position of a radiopaque foreign object (Figure 23-12).

1. Position the patient with the maxillary arch parallel to the floor.
2. Expose one periapical receptor using proper technique and angulation.
3. Expose an occlusal receptor, and direct the central ray perpendicular to the receptor.
4. In the occlusal image, the radiopaque foreign object is seen on the buccal side of the mandible.

Buccal Object Rule and Right-Angle Technique. The patient presents to the endodontist for root canal therapy on tooth #30. A small piece of clipped orthodontic wire is revealed by dental imaging. The wire was accidentally left behind during previous treatment and eventually was covered by the buccal mucosa. The buccal object rule is used to localize the orthodontic wire; the right-angle technique is also used to confirm the location, as follows:

1. Position the patient with the maxillary arch parallel to the floor.
2. Expose one periapical image of tooth #30. A radiopaque artifact is seen near the furcation area (Figure 23-13, A).

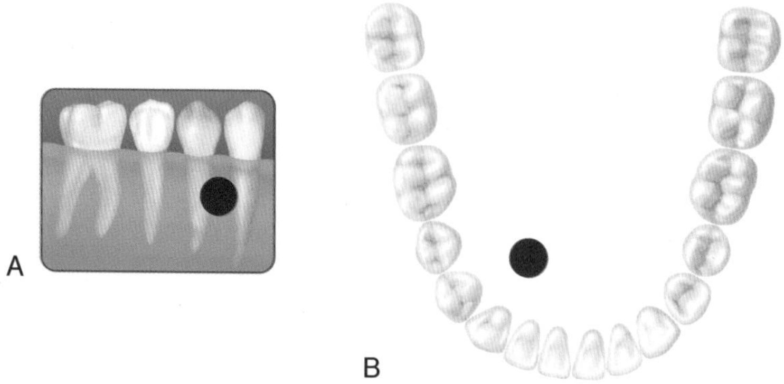

Fig 23-9 Right-angle technique. **A,** The object appears to be located in bone on the periapical image. **B,** The occlusal image reveals that the object is actually located in soft tissue lingual to the mandible.

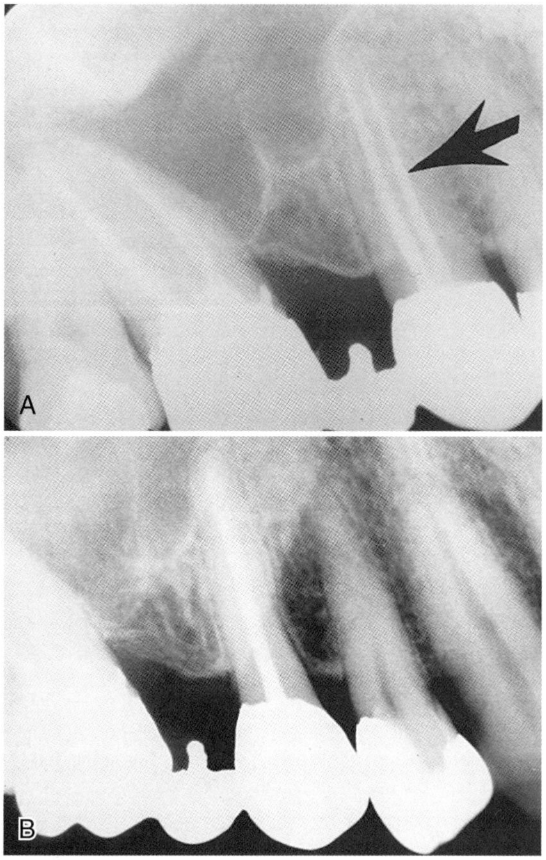

Fig 23-10 A, Note the two root canals filled with gutta percha in the maxillary second premolar (*arrow*). **B,** The PID was shifted in a mesial direction, so the gutta percha moved in a distal direction. The gutta percha in the original root labeled by the arrow is located on the buccal. (Images Courtesy Dr. Robert Jaynes, Columbus, OH. From Haring JI, Lind LJ: *Radiographic interpretation for the dental hygienist*, Philadelphia, 1993, Saunders.)

3. Shift the PID in a mesial direction, and then expose a second periapical image. The artifact appears to have moved in a distal direction in the second image (see Figure 23-13, B).
4. To confirm the location of the radiopaque artifact, expose a mandibular cross-sectional occlusal projection (see Figure 23-13, C).
5. By using both the buccal object rule and the right-angle technique, the orthodontic wire can be localized on the buccal side of the tooth and surgically removed (see Figure 23-13, D).

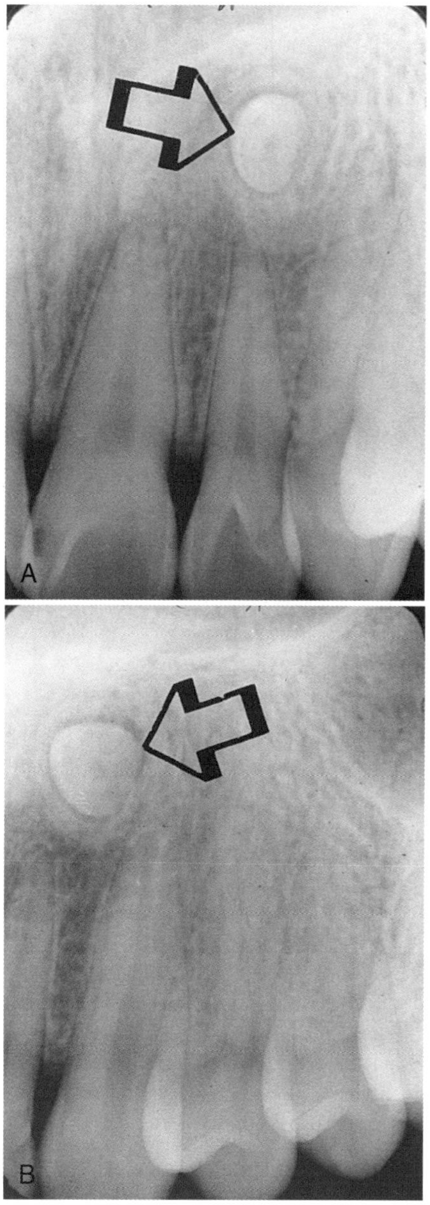

Fig 23-11 A, Note the impacted tooth (*arrow*). **B,** The position-indicating device (PID) was shifted in a distal direction, so the tooth moved in a distal direction. The tooth is located lingual to the adjacent teeth. (Images Courtesy Dr. Robert Jaynes, Columbus, OH.)

HELPFUL HINTS

For exposing occlusal projections:

- **DO** use the exposure factors recommended by the receptor manufacturer.
- **DO** set all exposure control factors (kilovoltage, milliamperage, time) before placing an occlusal receptor in the patient's mouth.
- **DO** ask the patient to remove eyeglasses and all intraoral objects before placing an occlusal receptor in the mouth.
- **DO** explain the imaging procedure that will be performed.
- **DO** instruct the patient on how to close gently on the occlusal receptor and remain still during the exposure.
- **DO** position the patient's head before placing the occlusal receptor into the mouth.
- **DO** position the occlusal receptor such that the tube side faces the arch being exposed.
- **DO** position the receptor such that a minimal receptor edge extends beyond the teeth being exposed.
- **DO** center the occlusal receptor directly over the area of interest so that all necessary information can be recorded.
- **DO** set the vertical angulation for each occlusal projection as recommended in this chapter.

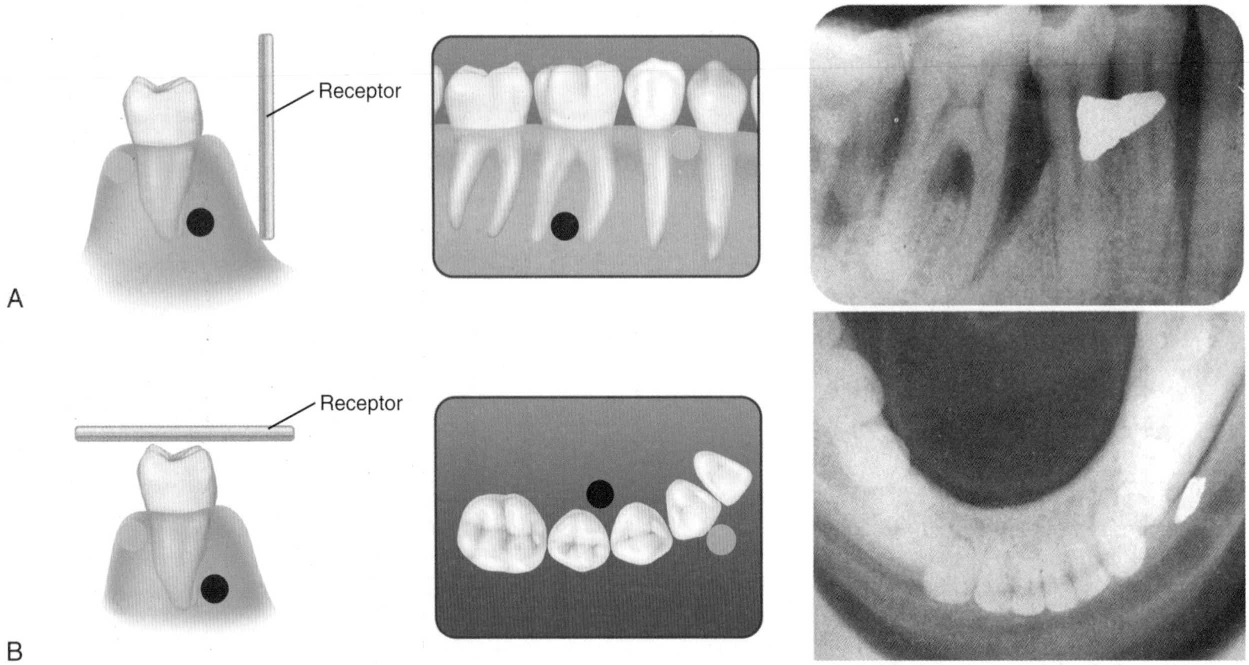

Fig 23-12 Right-angle localization technique. Two receptors are exposed at right angles to each other to identify the location of a foreign object. The periapical image **(A)** will demonstrate the superior-inferior and anterior-posterior positions of objects. A cross-sectional mandibular occlusal image **(B)** will demonstrate the anterior-posterior and buccal-lingual positions. These two views will demonstrate all three dimensions of an area, and the location of objects can thus be identified. (Redrawn from Olson SS: *Dental radiography laboratory manual*, Philadelphia, 1995, Saunders.)

SUMMARY

- The occlusal technique is a method used to examine large areas of the maxilla or the mandible. The technique is so named because the patient "occludes" or bites on the receptor.
- A size 4 intraoral receptor is used in the occlusal technique for the adult patient; a size 2 intraoral receptor is used for the child with a primary dentition.
- The occlusal image is preferred when the area of interest is larger than a periapical receptor may cover or when the placement of periapical receptors is too difficult for the patient.
- Uses for occlusal images include (1) localization of roots, impacted teeth, unerupted teeth, foreign bodies, and salivary stones; (2) evaluation of the sizes of lesions, boundaries of maxillary sinus, and jaw fractures; (3) examination of patients who cannot open their mouths; and (4) measurement of changes in the size and shape of the jaws.
- Occlusal receptor positioning includes the following: (1) the receptor is positioned with the tube side facing the arch being exposed, (2) the receptor is placed in the mouth between the occlusal surfaces of teeth, and (3) the receptor is stabilized when the patient gently bites on the surface of the receptor.
- Before imaging procedures using the occlusal technique begin, infection prevention procedures must be completed and the treatment area and supplies must be prepared. After the patient is seated and the imaging procedures explained, adjustments to the chair and headrest are made, the lead apron is placed, and the patient is asked to remove eyeglasses and any intraoral objects. The exposure factors are then set, and the beam alignment devices are assembled.
- A localization technique is used to locate the position of a tooth or an object in the jaws. It can be used to determine the buccal-lingual relationship of an object or to locate foreign bodies, impacted and unerupted teeth, retained roots, root positions, salivary stones, jaw fractures, broken needles and instruments, and filling materials.
- The buccal object rule—a rule for the orientation of structures seen in two images exposed at different angles—can be used as a localization technique.
- The right-angle technique—another rule for the orientation of structures seen in two images (one periapical, one occlusal)—can also be used as a localization technique.

BIBLIOGRAPHY

Frommer HH, Stabulas-Savage JJ: Accessory radiographic techniques: bisecting technique and occlusal technique. In Radiology for the dental professional, ed 9, St Louis, 2011, Mosby.

Frommer HH, Stabulas-Savage JJ: Patient management and special problems. In Radiology for the dental professional, ed 9, St Louis, 2011, Mosby.

Johnson ON: Mounting and introduction to interpretation. In Essentials of dental radiography for dental assistants and hygienists, ed 9, Upper Saddle River, NJ, 2011, Prentice Hall.

Johnson ON: The occlusal examination. In Essentials of dental radiography for dental assistants and hygienists, ed 9, Upper Saddle River, NJ, 2011, Prentice Hall.

Mallya SM, Lam EWN: Projection Geometry. In White and Pharoah's Oral radiology: principles and interpretation, ed 8, St. Louis, 2019, Elsevier.

Miles DA, Van Dis ML, Jensen CW, et al: Accessory radiographic techniques and patient management. In Radiographic imaging for the dental team, ed 4, Philadelphia, 2009, Saunders.

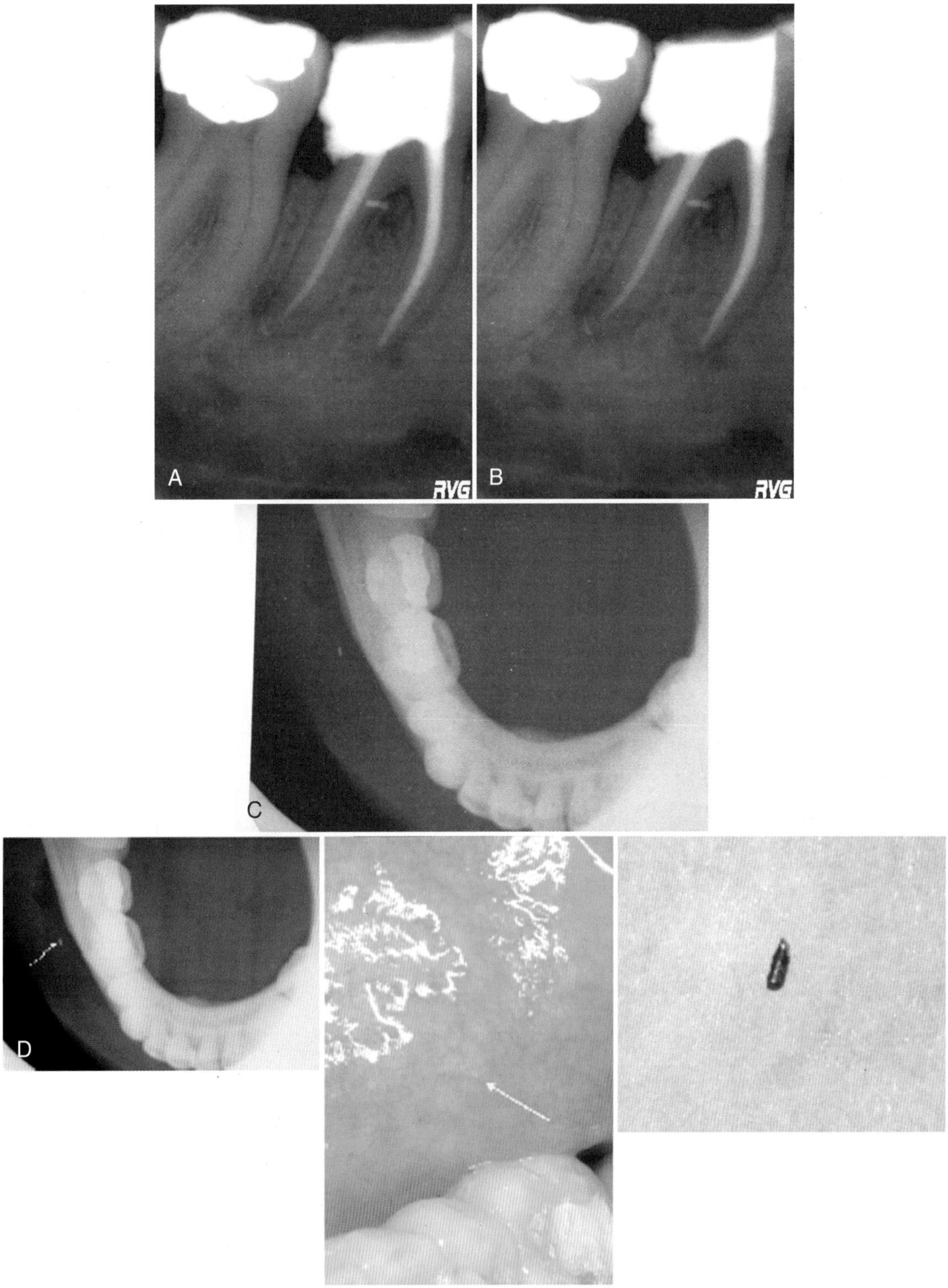

Fig 23-13 **A,** A radiopaque artifact seen on the image of tooth #30. **B,** The PID is shifted in a mesial direction, and a second image is exposed. **C,** A mandibular cross-sectional image of the same area. **D,** An arrow points to the location of the broken orthodontic wire, which is also seen in the mucosa and after surgical removal. (Courtesy S. Craig Rhodes, DMD, Orlando, FL.)

QUIZ QUESTIONS

Fill in the Blank

1. What does the term *occlusal* refer to?

2. What size receptor is recommended for use with the occlusal technique in the adult patient?

3. What size receptor is recommended for use with the occlusal technique in the pediatric patient with primary dentition?

4. How is the patient's head positioned before exposing a maxillary occlusal receptor?

5. What are the uses of the occlusal image?

6. State the vertical angulation used for the maxillary topographic occlusal projection.

7. State the vertical angulation used for the maxillary lateral occlusal projection.

8. State the vertical angulation used for the mandibular topographic occlusal projection.

9. State the vertical angulation used for the mandibular cross-sectional occlusal projection.

10. State the vertical angulations used for the maxillary and mandibular pediatric occlusal projections.

Short Answer

For questions 11 to 15, use the buccal object rule, and refer to the appropriate figures.

11. In Figure 23-14, is the labeled amalgam pit buccal or lingual? Why?

12. In Figure 23-15, is the amalgam fragment between the maxillary second and third molars buccal or lingual? Why?

13. In Figure 23-16, is the impacted canine located buccal or lingual to adjacent teeth? Why?

14. In Figure 23-17, is the gutta percha in the labeled canal located on the buccal or lingual side of the tooth? Why?

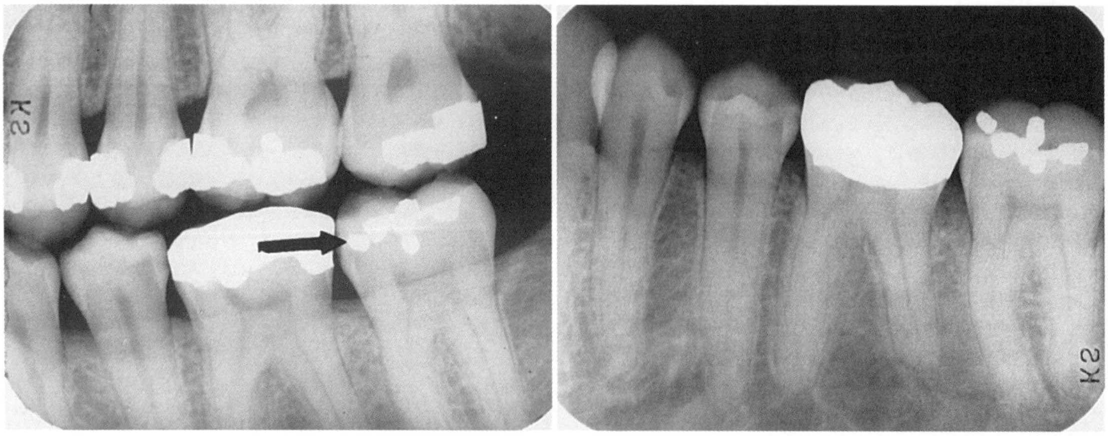

Fig 23-14 (Images courtesy Dr. Robert Jaynes, Columbus, OH. From Haring JI, Lind LJ: *Radiographic interpretation for the dental hygienist*, Philadelphia, 1993, Saunders.)

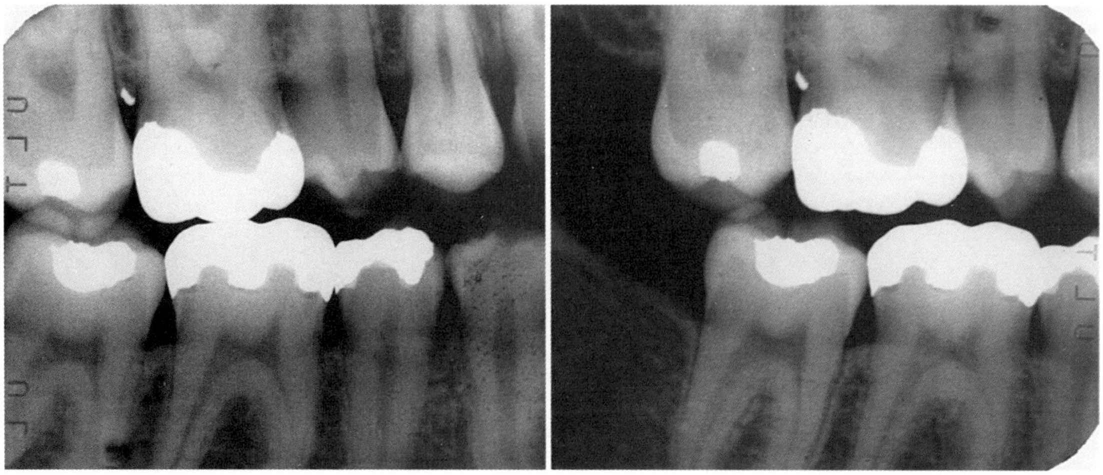

Fig 23-15 (Images courtesy Dr. Robert Jaynes, Columbus, OH. From Haring JI, Lind LJ: *Radiographic interpretation for the dental hygienist*, Philadelphia, 1993, Saunders.)

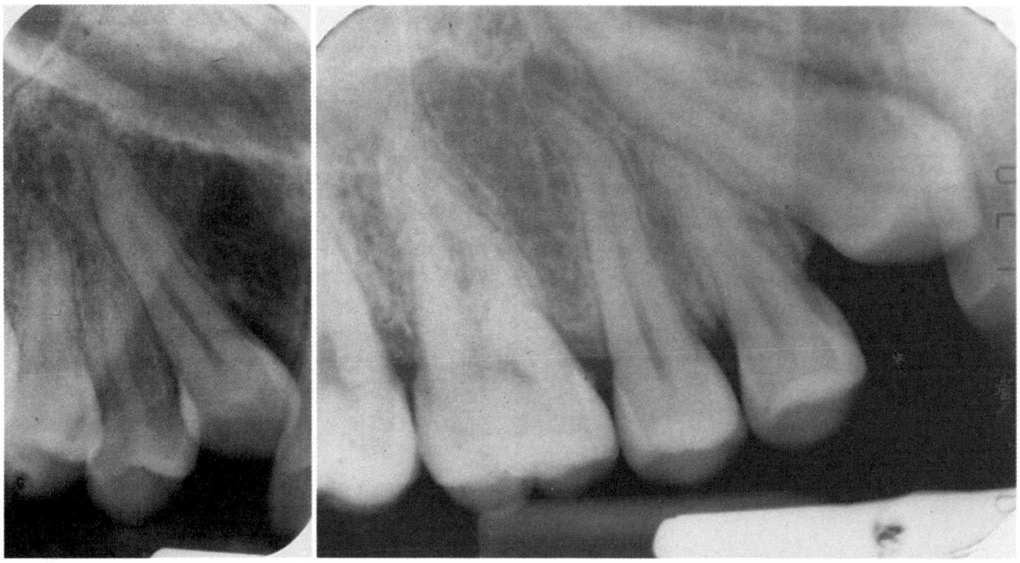

Fig 23-16 (Images courtesy Dr. Robert Jaynes, Columbus, OH. From Haring JI, Lind LJ: *Radiographic interpretation for the dental hygienist*, Philadelphia, 1993, Saunders.)

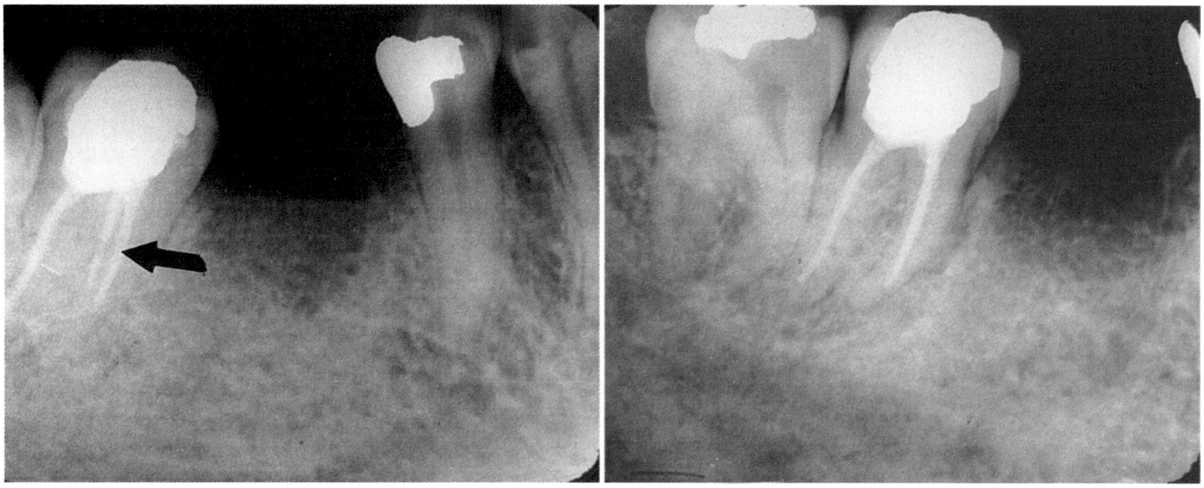

Fig 23-17 (Images courtesy Dr. Robert Jaynes, Columbus, OH.)

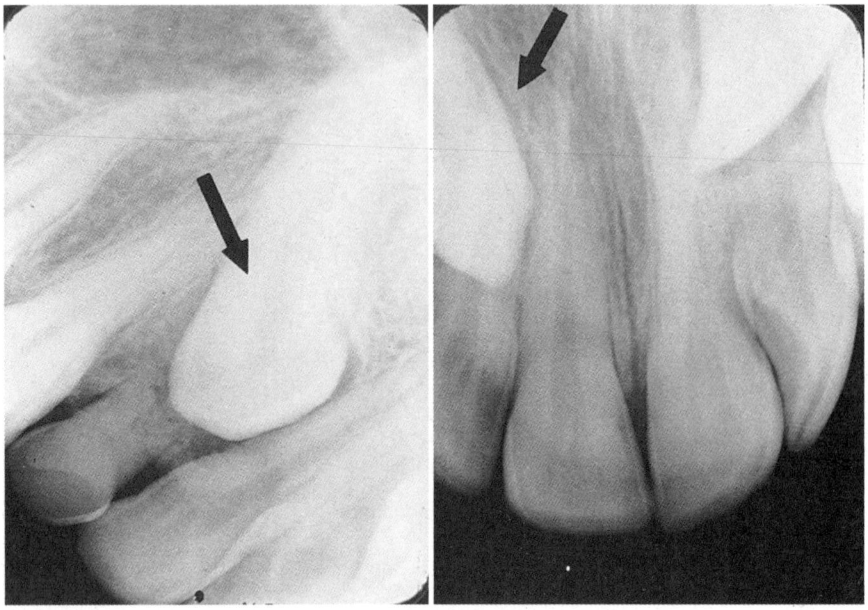

Fig 23-18 (Images courtesy Dr. Robert Jaynes, Columbus, OH.)

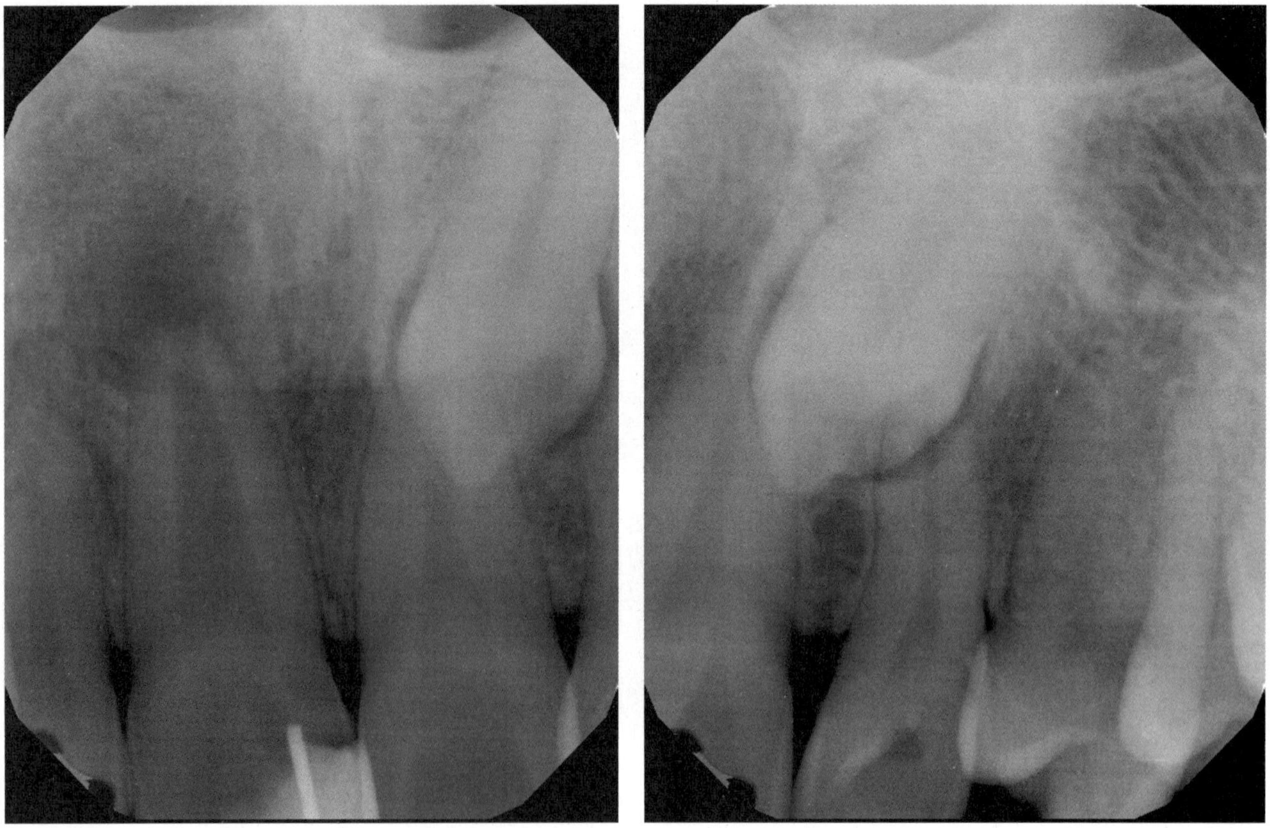

Fig 23-19

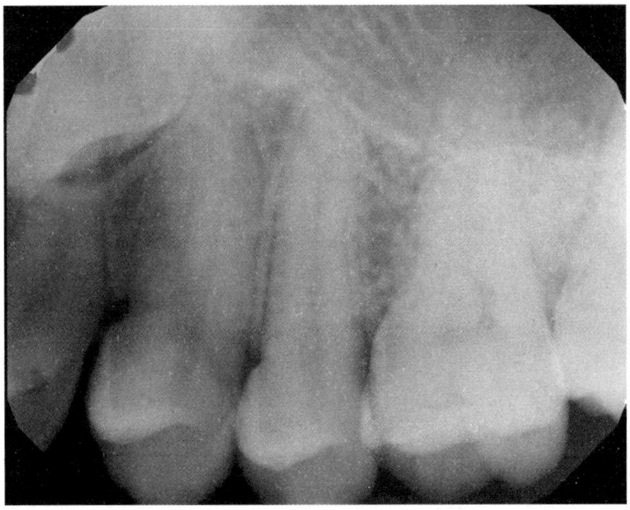

Fig 23-19 *Continued*

15. In Figure 23-18, is the impacted canine located buccal or lingual to adjacent teeth? Why?

____

____

____

____

____

____

16. In Figure 23-19, is the impacted canine located buccal or lingual to adjacent teeth? Why?

____

____

____

____

24

Imaging of Patients With Special Needs

LEARNING OBJECTIVES

After completion of this chapter, the student will be able to do the following:

1. Define the key terms associated with patients who have special needs.
2. List the areas of the oral cavity that are most likely to elicit the gag reflex when stimulated.
3. List two precipitating factors responsible for initiating the gag reflex.
4. Describe how to control the gag reflex using operator attitude, patient and equipment preparations, exposure sequencing, and receptor placement and technique.
5. Describe common physical disabilities and what modifications in technique may be necessary during the imaging examination.
6. Describe common developmental disabilities and what modifications in technique may be necessary during the imaging examination.
7. List helpful hints that can be used when treating a person with a disability.
8. Describe the tooth eruption sequences, prescribing of dental images, recommended techniques, types of examinations, digital sensor issues, patient and equipment preparation, and patient management pertaining to the pediatric dental patient.
9. Describe the use of receptor placement modifications and recommended periapical technique during endodontic (root canal) procedures.
10. Describe the purposes of the imaging examination in the edentulous patient.
11. List and describe the three types of imaging examination that may be used for the edentulous patient.

Not all dental imaging techniques can be successfully performed on all patients. Imaging examination techniques must often be modified to accommodate patients with special needs. The dental radiographer must be competent in altering the techniques to meet the specific diagnostic needs of individual patients.

The purpose of this chapter is to introduce the dental radiographer to the issues in treating patients with special needs. In addition, this chapter provides specific information on how to manage patients with a hypersensitive gag reflex, patients with physical or developmental disabilities, pediatric patients, endodontic patients, and edentulous patients.

PATIENTS WITH GAG REFLEX

The term **gagging** (also called *retching*) refers to the strong, involuntary effort to vomit. The **gag reflex** (also called the *pharyngeal reflex*) can be defined as retching that is elicited by stimulation of the sensitive tissues of the soft palate region. The gag reflex is a protective mechanism of the body that serves to clear the airway of obstruction. All patients have gag reflexes, although some are more sensitive than others. In dental imaging, a hypersensitive gag reflex is a problem that is commonly encountered.

The areas that are most likely to elicit the gag reflex when stimulated include the soft palate and the posterior lateral third of the tongue. Before the gag reflex is initiated, the following two reactions occur:

- Cessation of respiration
- Contraction of the muscles in the throat and abdomen

Precipitating factors for the initiation of the gag reflex include **psychogenic stimuli** (stimuli originating in the mind) and **tactile stimuli** (stimuli originating from touch). To suppress the gag reflex, the dental radiographer must eliminate or lessen these precipitating factors.

Patient Management

To effectively manage the patient with a hypersensitive gag reflex, the dental radiographer must be aware of the following:

- Operator attitude
- Patient and equipment preparations
- Exposure sequencing
- Receptor placement and technique

Operator Attitude. To prevent the gag reflex, the dental radiographer must convey a confident attitude. The patient must be confident of the radiographer's ability to perform imaging procedures and must be sure that the receptor will not slip and lodge in the throat. If the dental radiographer does not appear to be in complete control of the procedures, the patient interprets this as a lack of confidence. This lack of confidence may act as a psychogenic stimulus and elicit the gag reflex.

In addition, the dental radiographer must also convey patience, tolerance, and understanding. Every effort should be made to relax and reassure the patient with a hypersensitive gag reflex. It may be embarrassing for the patient with a gag reflex to proceed with imaging procedures, making the patient more uncomfortable in the dental setting. The dental radiographer should explain the imaging procedures about to be performed and then compliment the patient as each exposure is completed. As the patient becomes comfortable with the imaging procedures, he or she becomes more confident and, as a result, is less likely to gag.

Patient and Equipment Preparations. Patient and equipment preparations can help prevent the gag reflex (see Chapters 19, 20, and 21). In the patient with a hypersensitive gag reflex, every effort should be made to limit the amount of time that a receptor remains in the mouth. The longer a receptor stays in the mouth, the more likely the patient is to gag. When patient and equipment preparations are completed *before* receptor placement, valuable time is saved, and the likelihood of stimulating the gag reflex is reduced.

HELPFUL HINT

Gagging—Basic Concepts

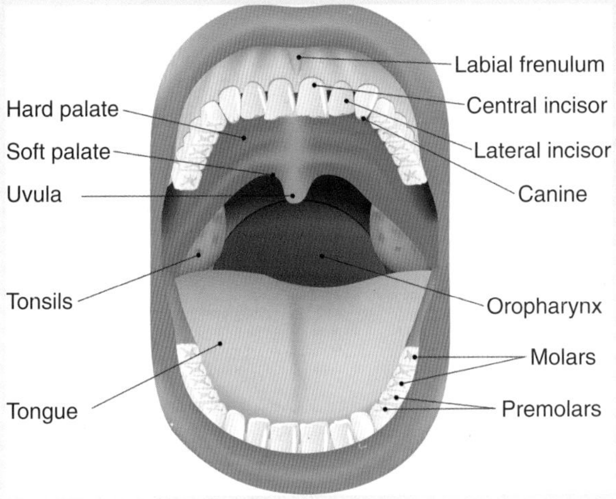

Gagging requires the following

- Cessation of respiration
- Contraction of muscles in throat and abdomen
- A person cannot gag and breathe at the same time.

Precipitating factors

- Psychogenic stimuli
- Tactile stimuli

Exposure Sequencing. Exposure sequencing plays an important role in preventing the gag reflex. As discussed in Chapters 19 to 21, the dental radiographer should always begin with anterior exposures. Anterior receptors are easier for the patient to tolerate and are less likely to elicit the gag reflex. With posterior receptor placements, the dental radiographer should always expose the premolar receptor before the molar receptor. Of all receptor placements, *the maxillary molar receptor is the most likely to elicit the gag reflex.* In the patient with a hypersensitive gag reflex, the exposure sequence should be altered so that the maxillary molar receptors are exposed at the end of the procedure.

Receptor Placement and Technique. Receptor placement and technique also play an important role in preventing the gag reflex. To avoid stimulating the gag reflex, *each receptor must be placed and exposed as quickly as possible.* Placement and technique modifications include the following:

- *Avoid the palate.* When placing receptors in the maxillary posterior areas, do not slide the receptor along the palate. Sliding the receptor along the palate stimulates this sensitive area and causes the gag reflex. Instead, position the receptor lingual to the teeth, and then firmly bring the receptor into contact with the palatal tissues using one decisive motion.
- *Demonstrate receptor placement.* In the areas that are most likely to elicit the gag reflex, rub a finger along the tissues near the intended area of receptor placement while telling the patient, "This is where the receptor will be positioned." Then place the receptor quickly. This technique demonstrates where the receptor will be placed and desensitizes the tissues in the area.

Extreme Cases of Gag Reflex

Occasionally the dental radiographer encounters a patient with a gag reflex that is uncontrollable. In such a patient, intraoral images are impossible to obtain. Instead, the dental radiographer must expose an extraoral image such as extraoral bite-wings or panoramic projection to obtain diagnostic information.

HELPFUL HINT

Gagging—Patient Management

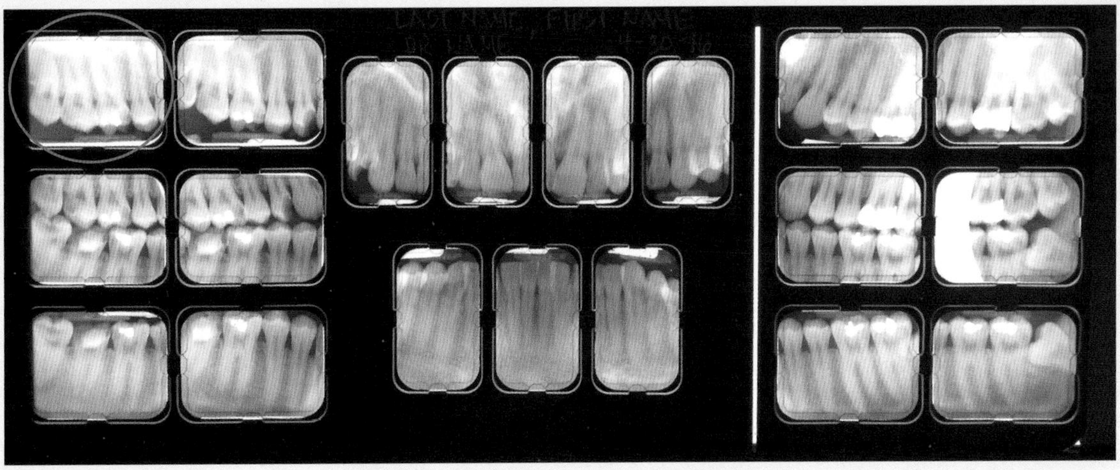

Exposure Sequence

- Start with **anterior exposures**.
- With posterior receptor placements, expose the premolar **before** the molar.
- The **maxillary molar receptor** is the *most likely to elicit the gag reflex.*

HELPFUL HINT

Gagging—Extreme Cases

If the gag reflex is uncontrollable, the dental radiographer must use **extraoral images** to obtain diagnostic information.

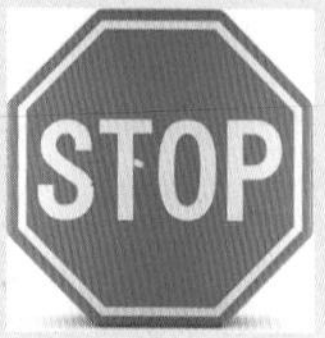

Helpful Hints

To reduce the gag reflex:

- **NEVER** suggest gagging. The dental radiographer must never bring up the subject of gagging or ask the patient such questions as "Are you a gagger?" or "Do you gag?" The power of suggestion can act as a strong psychogenic stimulus and can, in turn, elicit the gag reflex. When the patient brings up the subject of gagging, the dental radiographer must refrain from using the terms *gag, gagging,* and *gagger;* instead, the radiographer should refer to the gag reflex as "a tickle in the back of the throat" when discussing the topic with the patient.
- **DO** reassure the patient. If the patient gags, the dental radiographer must remove the receptor as quickly as possible and then reassure the patient. The patient with a hypersensitive gag reflex must be reassured that such a response is not unusual. Some patients are very embarrassed, and others may even cry. The dental radiographer must always maintain control of the situation while remaining calm and understanding.
- **DO** suggest deep breathing. The dental radiographer should instruct the patient to "breathe deeply" through the nose during receptor placement and exposure. The breathing should be audible, and the dental radiographer should demonstrate it to the patient. As previously stated, respiration must cease for the gag reflex to occur; therefore if the patient is breathing, the gag reflex cannot occur.
- **DO** try to distract the patient. Distraction often helps suppress the gag reflex. The dental radiographer can instruct the patient to do one of the following during receptor placement and exposure: (1) position a leg or arm in the air and hold it stationary; (2) close the thumb in the hand, make a fist, and squeeze tightly; or (3) hum a song (it is difficult to hum and gag at the same time). These acts help divert the patient's attention and lessen the likelihood of the gag reflex being elicited.
- **DO** try to reduce tactile stimuli. Reducing tactile stimuli helps prevent the gag reflex. The dental radiographer can try one of the following techniques before placing and exposing the receptor: (1) giving the patient a cup of ice water to drink or (2) placing a small amount of ordinary table salt on the tip of the tongue. These techniques help confuse the sensory nerve endings and lessen the likelihood of the gag reflex being stimulated.
- **DO** use a topical anesthetic. In the patient with a severe hypersensitive gag reflex, a topical anesthetic spray may be used. The spray is used to numb the areas that elicit the gag reflex. The dental radiographer should instruct the patient to exhale while the anesthetic is sprayed on the soft palate and posterior tongue. Caution must be used to ensure that the patient does not inhale the spray, which may cause inflammation of the lungs. The topical anesthetic spray takes effect after 1 minute and lasts for approximately 20 minutes. Topical anesthetic sprays should not be used in patients who are allergic to benzocaine.

HELPFUL HINT

Gagging – Patient Management

Exposure Sequence

- Try to distract the patient.
- Try to reduce tactile stimuli.
- Use a topical anesthetic.

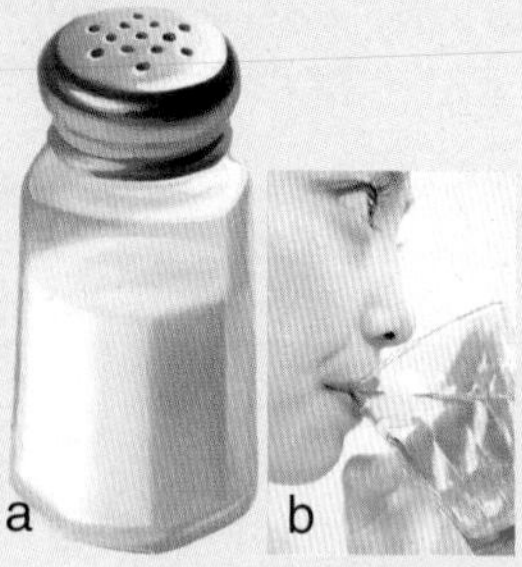

PATIENTS WITH DISABILITIES

A **disability** can be defined as a "physical or mental impairment that substantially limits one or more of an individual's major life activities." In the dental office, persons with both physical and developmental disabilities are encountered. It is important to remember that a person with a disability is still a person—and that the disability is simply a characteristic. Like all patients, a person with a disability should be treated with dignity and respect. The dental radiographer must be prepared to modify imaging techniques to accommodate persons with disabilities.

Physical Disabilities

A person with a **physical disability** may have problems with vision, hearing, or mobility. The dental radiographer must make every effort to meet the individual needs of such patients. A family member or other caregiver often accompanies the person with a physical disability to the dental office. Caregivers can be asked to assist the dental radiographer with communication or with the patient's physical needs. The dental radiographer must be aware of the common physical disabilities involving vision, hearing, and mobility and the necessary modifications to the procedure for patients who have such problems.

Vision Impairment. If a person is blind or visually impaired, the dental radiographer must communicate using clear verbal explanations. The dental radiographer must keep the patient informed of what is being done and explain each step of the procedure before performing it. In addition, the radiographer must inform the person when leaving the area. The dental radiographer must never gesture to another person in the presence of a person who is blind. A person who is blind is sensitive to this type of communication and may perceive this as the dental radiographer "talking behind his or her back."

Hearing Impairment. With a person who is deaf or hearing impaired, the dental radiographer has several options. The dental radiographer should ask the patient how they prefer to communicate and may ask the caregiver to act as an interpreter, use gestures or sign language, use assistive technology, or use written instructions. When the patient can read lips, the dental radiographer must face the patient and speak clearly and slowly. A face mask should not be used during treatment of a patient with a hearing impairment but may be replaced with a clear face shield.

Mobility Impairment. If a person is in a wheelchair and does not have use of the lower limbs, the dental radiographer should initially ask the patient how he or she would prefer to transfer to the dental chair. The dental radiographer may offer to help the person who needs mobility assistance in transferring to the dental chair or ask the caregiver to assist in the transfer. If a transfer is not possible, the dental radiographer may attempt to perform the necessary imaging procedures with the patient seated in the wheelchair. Extraoral imaging equipment has been manufactured to be wheelchair-friendly (Figure 24-1).

If a person does not have use of the upper limbs and a beam alignment device cannot be used to stabilize receptor placement, the dental radiographer may ask the caregiver to assist with the holding of the receptor. In such cases, the caregiver must wear a lead apron with thyroid collar and a lead glove (if available) during exposure of the receptors. In addition, the caregiver must be given specific instructions on how to hold the receptor for the patient. As stated in previous chapters, the dental radiographer must *never* hold a receptor for a patient during an x-ray exposure.

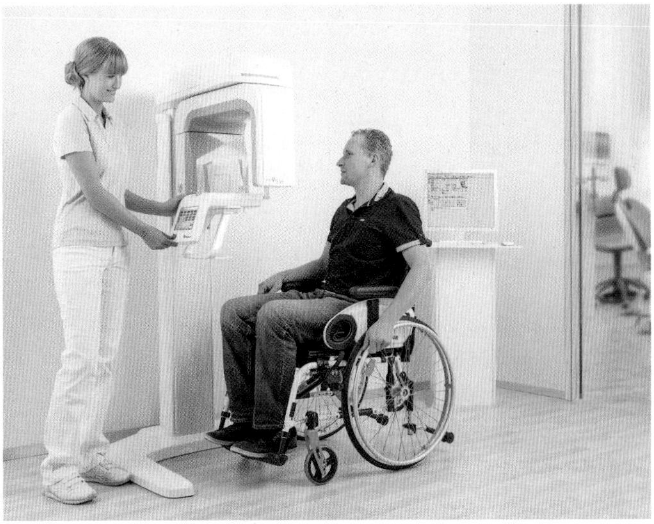

Fig 24-1 Patient in wheelchair with extraoral machine. (Courtesy Air Techniques, Melville, NY.)

Developmental Disabilities

A developmental disability is "a substantial impairment of mental or physical functioning that occurs before the age of 22 and is of indefinite duration." Examples include autism, cerebral palsy, epilepsy and other neuropathies, and mental retardation. The dental radiographer must make every effort to meet the individual needs of the patient with a developmental disability.

A person with a developmental disability may have problems with coordination or with comprehension of instructions. As a result, the dental radiographer may experience difficulties in obtaining intraoral images. If coordination is a problem, mild sedation may be useful. If comprehension is a problem, the radiographer should use clear, simple sentences. In some instances, the caregiver may be asked to assist with the holding of the receptor. When interacting with a patient who has a cognitive disability, allow extra time for communication and avoid finishing the patient's sentences.

It is important that the dental radiographer recognize situations in which the patient cannot tolerate intraoral exposures. In such cases, *no intraoral exposures should be exposed;* such exposures result only in nondiagnostic images and needless radiation exposure of the patient. In these cases, extraoral exposures (e.g., panoramic or three-dimensional imaging) may be used instead.

Patient Management Helpful Hints

The dental radiographer can use the helpful hints listed below in managing the patient with a disability:

- **DO** practice the *Golden Rule*. Treat the patient as you would like to be treated.
- **DO NOT** ask personal questions about a disability. Personal questions about a patient's disability are inappropriate in the dental setting.
- **DO** think before you speak. Always use *people first* language when speaking to a person with a disability. This empowers rather than marginalizes a person with a disability. For example, do not refer to a "blind person," but rather a person who is blind. Do not refer to a person as "wheelchair bound or confined to a wheelchair," but rather a person who uses a wheelchair or a person who needs mobility assistance.
- **DO** ask before assisting a person with a disability. The fact that a patient has a disability does not mean help or assistance is always welcomed or needed. Always ask before assisting a patient. For example, offer to push a wheelchair or to guide a person who is blind. The person with a disability will indicate whether help is needed or not and is often specific about how the assistance should be provided. For example, a person who is blind may prefer to hold the arm of a person offering guidance rather than having an arm held.
- **DO** talk directly to the person with a disability. When interacting with persons with disabilities, talk directly to them. It is inappropriate to talk to the caregiver instead of talking to the patient; for example, instead of asking the caregiver, "Can he [or she] transfer out of the wheelchair?" the radiographer should speak directly to the patient in the wheelchair. In addition, it is inappropriate to talk to the caregiver about a person with a disability as if that person were not present; the same is also true when an interpreter accompanies a deaf person.

PEDIATRIC PATIENTS

A pediatric patient is a child patient; the term pediatric is derived from the Greek word *pedia* meaning "child." Pediatric dentistry involves the diagnosis and treatment of dental diseases in children. In children, dental images are useful for detecting lesions as well as conditions of teeth and bones, for showing changes secondary to caries (tooth decay) and trauma, and for evaluating growth and development. When treating pediatric patients, the dental radiographer must be aware of the following:

- Tooth eruption sequences
- Prescribing of dental images
- Recommended techniques
- Types of examinations
- Digital sensor issues
- Patient and equipment preparations
- Patient management

Tooth Eruption Sequences

Twenty teeth make up the primary dentition—10 in the maxillary arch, and 10 mandibular in the mandibular arch (Figure 24-2). These 20 primary teeth are usually erupted by the age of 3 years. The typical ages for eruption of the 32 permanent teeth are detailed in Table 24-1. As permanent teeth erupt, a mixed dentition results. A mixed dentition, or combination of primary and permanent teeth, is present between

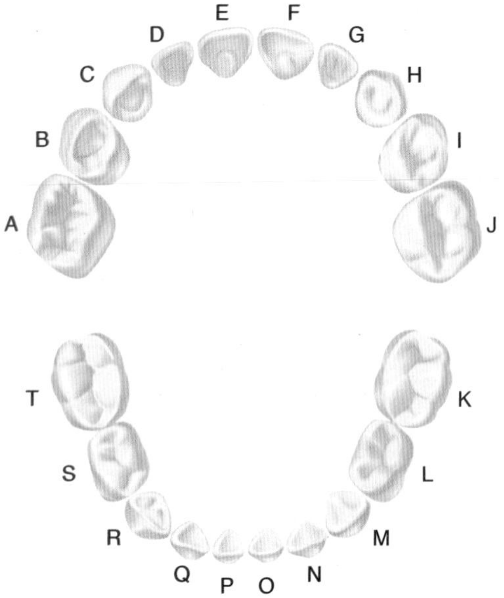

Fig 24-2 Primary teeth.

TABLE 24-1 Typical Age (in Years) at Eruption for Permanent Teeth

	AGE AT ERUPTION	
Tooth	**Maxillary**	**Mandibular**
Central incisor	7–8	6–7
Lateral incisor	8–9	7–8
Canine	11–12	9–10
1st premolar	10–11	10–12
2nd premolar	10–12	11–12
1st molar	6–7	6–7
2nd molar	12–13	11–13
3rd molar	17–21	17–21

the ages of 6 and 12 years. To better visualize what teeth erupt at what age, the erupting permanent teeth appear in white in Figure 24-3. By the age of 13, most adolescents have 28 permanent teeth in place. Four third molars are usually erupted by age 21. Knowledge of these normal eruption sequences is useful in determining what dental images are needed.

Prescribing of Dental Images

As described in Chapter 4, the prescribing of dental images is based on individual needs of the patient. The American Dental Association Recommendations for Prescribing Dental Radiographs (2012) include recommendations for both children and adults (see Table 4-1). For the pediatric patient, the prescribed number and type of dental images depends on the individual needs of the child including the number of teeth present, the age of the child, and the child's ability to cooperate during the procedures.

An imaging examination that includes all of the tooth-bearing areas is recommended at the early mixed dentition stage, after the first permanent tooth has erupted. This exam is used to assess the dental age of the patient and to aid in the early diagnosis of abnormalities. Another imaging exam that includes all tooth-bearing areas is indicated 2 years after the eruption of the permanent second molars.

In the pediatric patient, bite-wing images are needed whenever evidence of caries is suspected. In determining the time interval between bite-wing images, the more rapid progression of decay in primary teeth must be considered. In the absence of caries, bite-wing images are usually prescribed every 12 to 18 months *with primary interproximal tooth contact*, or every 24 months *with permanent interproximal tooth contact.*

Recommended Techniques

The imaging techniques used to expose intraoral projections in pediatric patients are similar to those used in adults. With periapical projections, either the bisecting technique or the paralleling technique can be used (see Chapters 19 and 20). In children with primary or transitional dentition, the bisecting technique is preferred because the small size of the mouth precludes the placement of a receptor beyond the apical regions of teeth. The bite-wing and occlusal techniques are also used in pediatric patients (see Chapters 21 and 23). Typical examinations of primary and transitional dentitions using these techniques are described in Table 24-2. Figures 24-4 through 24-8 provide examples of pediatric occlusal, bite-wing, and panoramic dental images.

Types of Examinations

When a pediatric patient is initially treated in the dental practice and does not have previous dental images, it is necessary to obtain a baseline series of images that show all tooth-bearing areas. These images are prescribed based on the individual needs of the child. These examinations may include the following:

- Four-image series:
  - 1 anterior occlusal/maxillary
  - 1 anterior occlusal/mandibular
  - 2 posterior bite-wings (right and left)
- Eight-image series:
  - 1 anterior periapical/maxillary
  - 1 anterior periapical/mandibular
  - 2 posterior periapicals/maxillary (right and left)
  - 2 posterior periapicals/mandibular (right and left)
  - 2 posterior bite-wings (right and left)
- Twelve-image series:
  - 1 incisor periapical/maxillary
  - 1 incisor periapical/mandibular
  - 2 canine periapicals/maxillary (right and left)
  - 2 canine periapicals/mandibular (right and left)
  - 2 posterior periapicals/maxillary (right and left)
  - 2 posterior periapicals/mandibular (right and left)
  - 2 posterior bite-wings (right and left)
- Sixteen-image series:
  - 1 incisor periapical/maxillary
  - 1 incisor periapical/mandibular
  - 2 canine periapicals/maxillary (right and left)
  - 2 canine periapicals/mandibular (right and left)
  - 2 premolar periapicals/maxillary (right and left)
  - 2 premolar periapicals/mandibular (right and left)
  - 2 molar periapicals/maxillary (right and left)
  - 2 molar periapicals/mandibular (right and left)
  - 2 posterior bite-wings (right and left)

Digital Sensor Issues

Based on the cooperation level, size of the mouth, and strength of the gag reflex, a pediatric patient may or may not be able to tolerate the use of a wired digital sensor. The size and thickness of a digital sensor

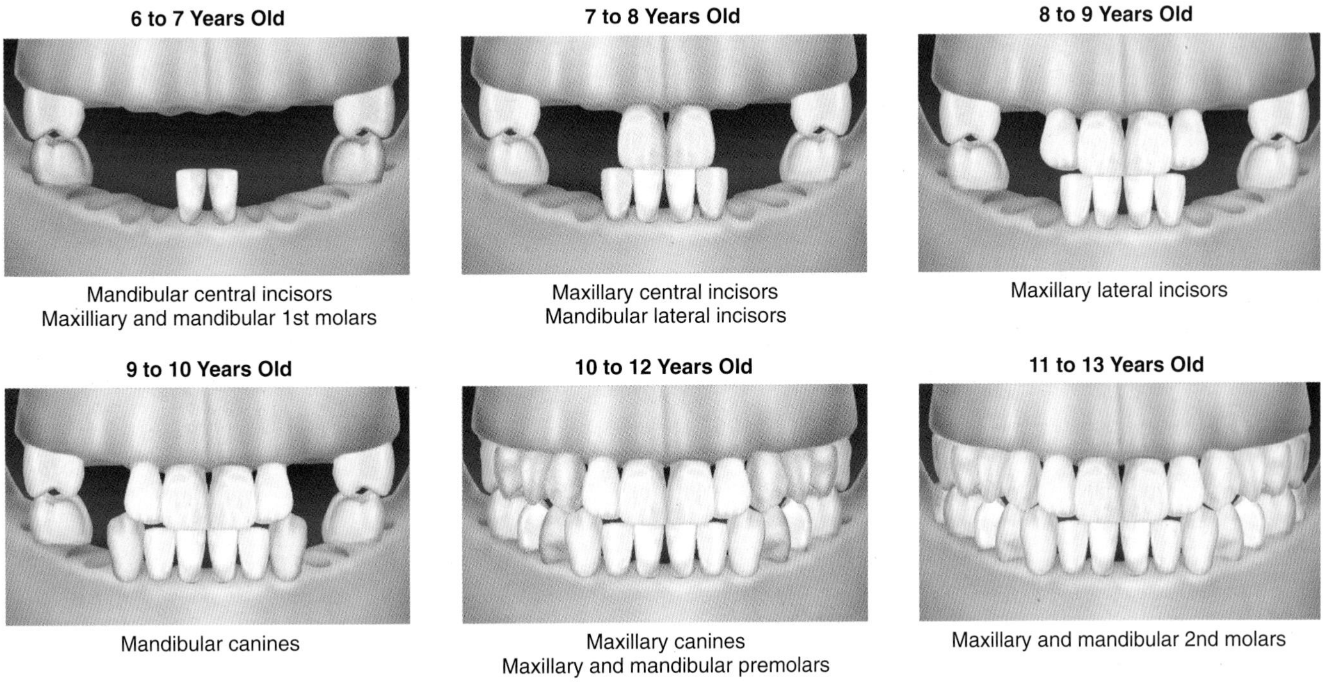

Fig 24-3 Use these diagrams to help remember what permanent teeth are present at what age. The erupting teeth are indicated in *blue*.

TABLE 24-2 Dental Imaging Examination of the Pediatric Patient

Dentition	Number of Projections	Type of Projection	Receptor Size
Primary (3–6 years)	1	Occlusal: maxillary	2
	1	Occlusal: mandibular	2
	2	Bite-wing	0
	2	Periapical: maxillary molar	0
	2	Periapical: mandibular molar	0
Mixed (6–12 years)	1	Periapical: maxillary incisor	1 or 2
	2	Periapical: maxillary canine	1 or 2
	1	Periapical: mandibular anterior	1 or 2
	2	Periapical: mandibular canine	1 or 2
	2	Bite-wing	2
	2	Periapical: maxillary molar	2
	2	Periapical: mandibular molar	2

may make intraoral placement difficult in young children. Using the correct-size sensor is critical; the smallest intraoral sensor (size 0 or size 1) should be used in young children.

Wireless sensors are preferred over wired sensors in pediatric dentistry. Most direct digital x-ray sensors have cables attached to the

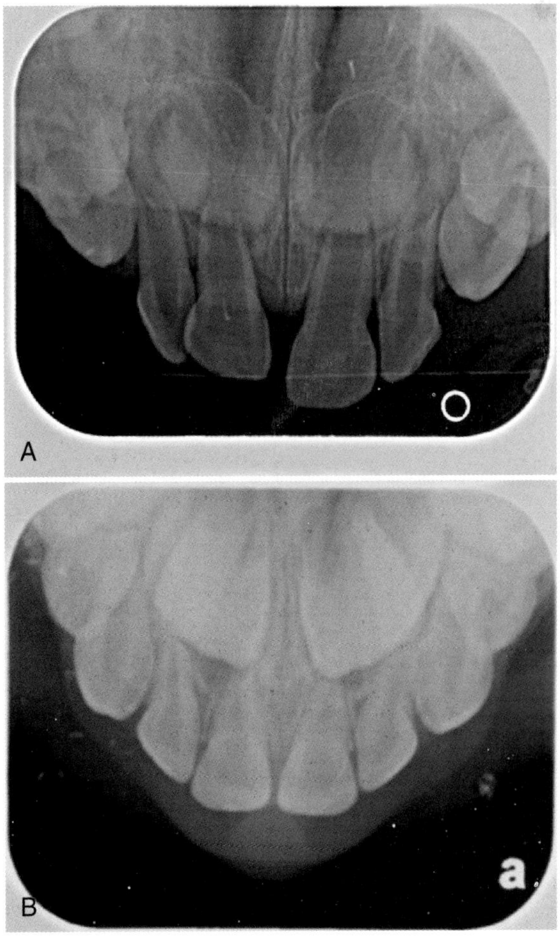

Fig 24-4 A, B, Examples of maxillary pediatric occlusal projections, each patient exposed with size 2 intraoral receptors. (Courtesy Cary Pediatric Dentistry, Cary, NC.)

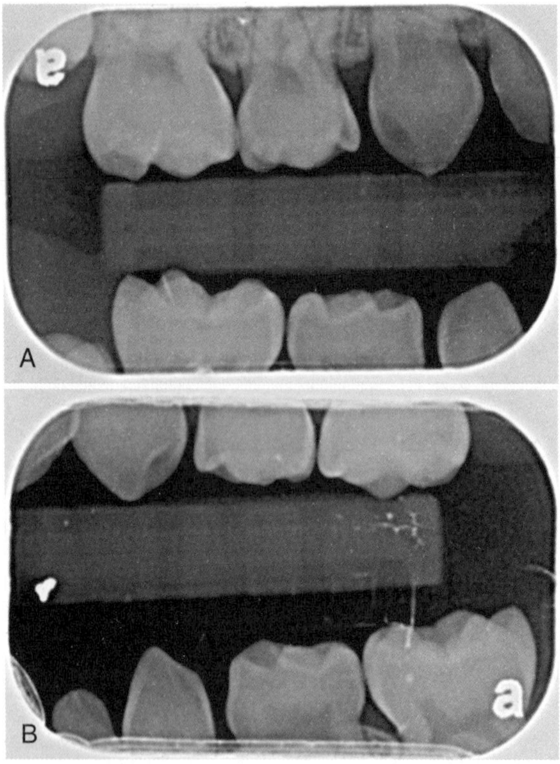

Fig 24-5 A, B, Right and left bite-wing images from a 5-year-old patient. (Courtesy Cary Pediatric Dentistry, Cary, NC.)

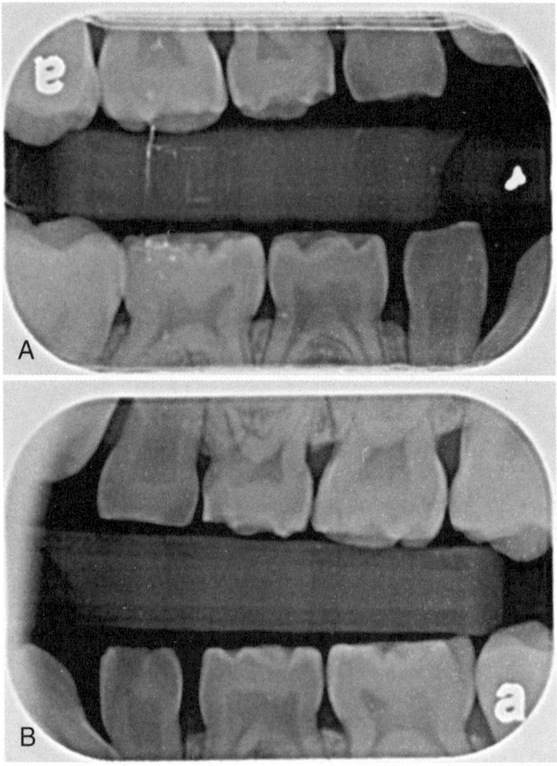

Fig 24-6 A, B, Right and left bite-wing images from a 6½-year-old patient. (Courtesy Cary Pediatric Dentistry, Cary, NC.)

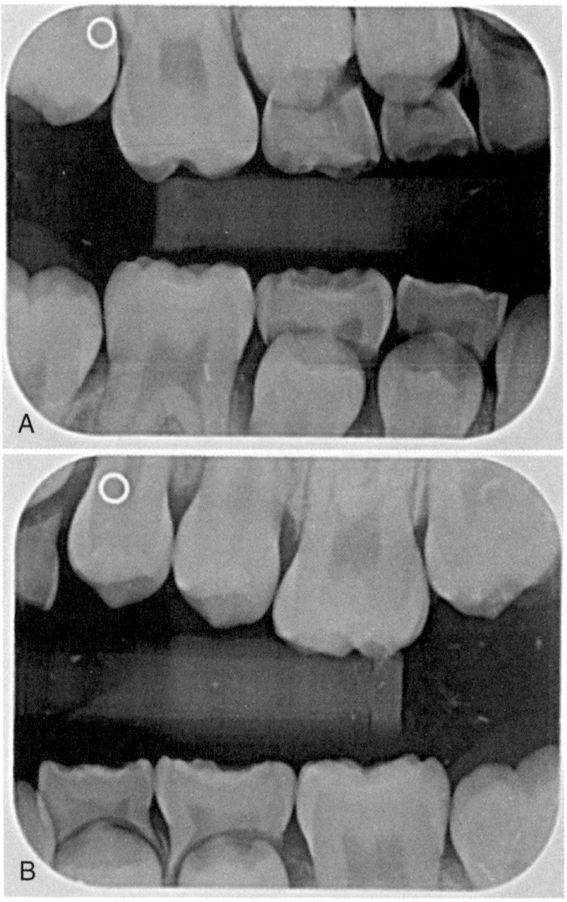

Fig 24-7 A, B, Right and left bite-wing images from a young teenage patient demonstrating mixed dentition. (Courtesy Cary Pediatric Dentistry, Cary, NC.)

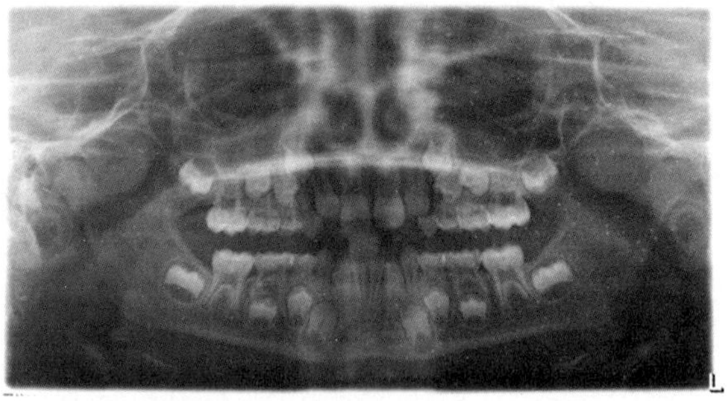

Fig 24-8 A panoramic dental image from a 7-year-old patient. (Courtesy Cary Pediatric Dentistry, Cary, NC.)

sensor. These wired sensors may be difficult to use in children who are younger than 4 years of age; such young children may not follow or understand instructions and may damage the sensor cable by chewing on it. As an alternative to digital sensors, less bulky PSP sensors may be used in young children. Remember that these sensors, are easily damaged by biting or bending.

Patient and Equipment Preparations

Patient and equipment preparations for the pediatric patient are identical to those described for the adult patient (see Chapters 19 to 21).

With the pediatric patient, however, special attention must be devoted to the following preparations:

- *Explanation of procedure.* The imaging procedures that are to be performed must be explained in terms that are easily understood by the child. For example, the dental radiographer can refer to the tubehead as a "camera," the lead apron as a "coat," and the image as a "picture."
- *Lead apron.* The growing tissues of a child are particularly vulnerable to the effects of ionizing radiation and must be protected. As a result, a lead apron and thyroid collar must be placed on a child before exposure to x-radiation.
- *Exposure factors.* Exposure factors (milliamperage, kilovoltage, time) must be reduced because of the size of the pediatric patient. A reduced exposure time is preferred; the shorter exposure time will reduce the chance of a blurred image should the child move. All exposure factors should be set according to the recommendations of the receptor manufacturer.
- *Receptor size.* Size 0 receptor is recommended for use in the pediatric patient with a primary dentition because of the small mouth size. In the child with a transitional dentition, a size 1 or size 2 receptor is recommended. As described in Chapter 23, a size 2 receptor is recommended for maxillary and mandibular occlusal exposures in children. In general, the largest size intraoral receptor that the child can tolerate should be used to obtain imaging information.

Patient Management Helpful Hints

Management of children requires that the dental radiographer be confident, patient, and understanding. The dental radiographer can use the helpful hints listed below in managing the pediatric patient.

- *Be confident.* Most children react favorably to the authority of a confident and capable operator. The dental radiographer must secure the child's confidence, trust, and cooperation. In addition, the dental radiographer must be patient and must not rush the imaging procedures.
- *Show and tell.* The typical child is curious. The dental radiographer can use a "show and tell" approach to prepare the patient for imaging procedures. Before beginning any exposures, the dental radiographer can show the child the equipment and materials that will be used and then describe to the child what will happen. The child should be encouraged to touch the tubehead, receptor, beam alignment device, and lead apron.
- *Reassure the patient.* The typical child has a fear of the unknown. Because a frightened child is not cooperative, the dental radiographer must reassure the child and allay any fears about the procedures.
- *Demonstrate behavior.* With the pediatric patient, the dental radiographer can demonstrate the desired behavior to show the child exactly what to do. For example, the radiographer can demonstrate "how to hold still" and then ask the child to do the same thing.
- *Request assistance.* If a child cannot hold still or stabilize the receptor, the dental radiographer can ask the parent or accompanying adult to provide assistance. The adult should wear a lead apron with thyroid collar and hold the receptor with a lead glove, or hold the child during the x-ray exposure.
- *Postpone the examination.* Only in emergencies should a child be forced to undergo dental imaging. It is much better to postpone the examination until the second or third visit rather than instill in the child a fear of visiting the dental office.

PATIENTS WITH SPECIFIC DENTAL NEEDS

Different patients have different diagnostic dental requirements based on specific needs. Dental imaging examination techniques must often be modified to accommodate patients with specific dental needs, including endodontic and edentulous patients.

Endodontic Patients

The term endodontic is derived from two Greek words, *endon*, meaning "within," and *odontos*, meaning "tooth." Endodontics is the branch of dentistry concerned with the diagnosis and treatment of diseases of the dental pulp within the tooth. Endodontic treatment usually involves removal of the dental pulp (nerve tissue) from the pulp chamber and canals within the tooth, then filling the empty pulp chamber and canals with a material such as gutta percha or silver points. This treatment is often referred to as a *root canal procedure* or *root canal therapy (RCT)*. The endodontic patient is one who has undergone root canal therapy.

The dental image is indispensable during root canal procedures and essential for diagnosing and managing pulpal problems. During a root canal procedure, a series of exposures is typically obtained of the same tooth; these exposures are used to evaluate the tooth before, during, and after treatment.

Receptor Placement. The dental radiographer must modify the receptor placement method for the endodontic patient. During a root canal procedure, receptor placement is difficult because of poor visualization of the tooth. The equipment used during a root canal procedure makes it difficult for the dental radiographer to visualize the area well in order to position and stabilize the receptor. Equipment used during a root canal procedure includes a rubber dam, rubber dam clamp, root canal instruments (files, reamers, broaches), and filling materials (gutta percha and silver points).

The EndoRay beam alignment device (see Chapter 7) can be used as an aid in positioning the receptor during a root canal procedure; this holder fits around a rubber dam clamp and allows space for root canal instruments and filling materials to protrude from the tooth. A hemostat may also be used to hold the receptor.

Recommended Technique. During a root canal procedure, the length of the pulp canals must be accurately measured without distortion (elongation or foreshortening). To avoid distortion, the paralleling technique (see Chapter 19) should be used whenever possible; the use of the bisecting technique (see Chapter 20) may result in elongated or foreshortened images. With the paralleling technique, the use of a beam alignment device (e.g., EndoRay) is strongly recommended.

Edentulous Patients

Edentulous means "without teeth." The edentulous patient, or patient without teeth, requires a dental imaging examination for the following reasons:

- To detect the presence of root tips, impacted teeth, and lesions (cysts, tumors)
- To identify objects embedded in bone
- To establish the position of normal anatomic landmarks (e.g., mental foramen) relative to the crest of the alveolar ridge
- To observe the quantity and quality of bone that is present

The dental imaging examination of the edentulous patient may include the following projections: panoramic, periapical, or a combination of occlusal and periapical images. Three-dimensional digital imaging may also be helpful in examining the edentulous jaw (see Chapter 27).

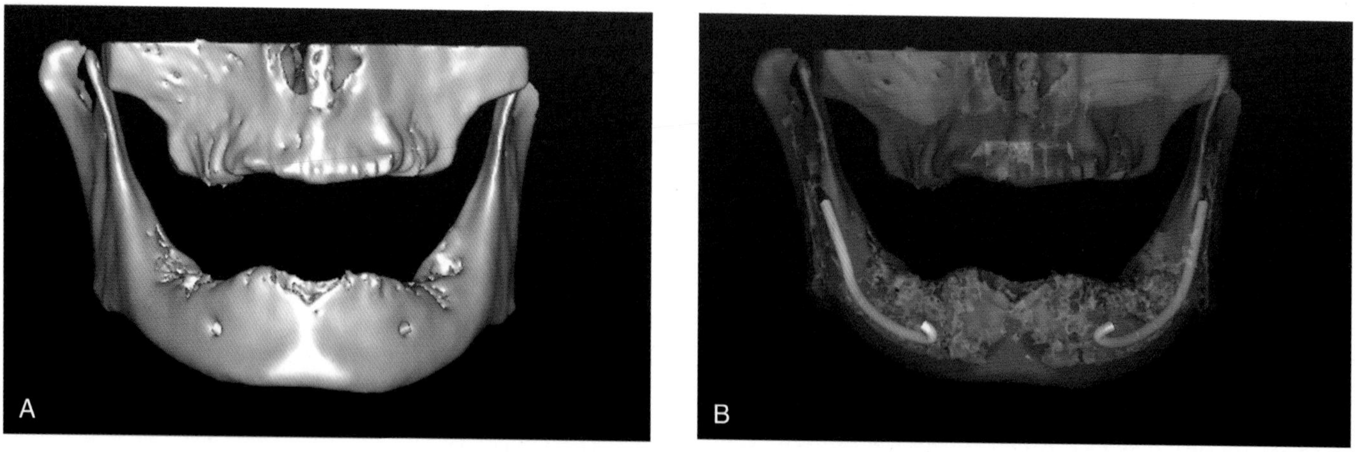

Fig 24-9 **A,** A three-dimensional volume rendering created with cone-beam computer tomography illustrates the edentulous maxilla and mandible. **B,** The transparent view of the same patient demonstrates the exact location of the mandibular nerve. (Courtesy Carolina OMF Imaging, W. Bruce Howerton Jr., DDS, MS, Franklinton, NC.)

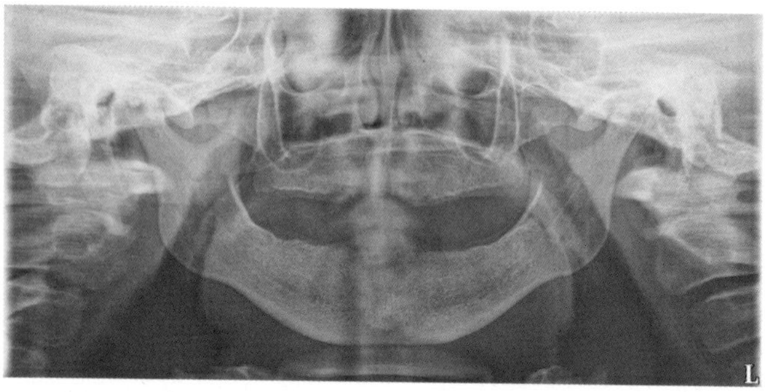

Fig 24-10 A panoramic image of an edentulous patient.

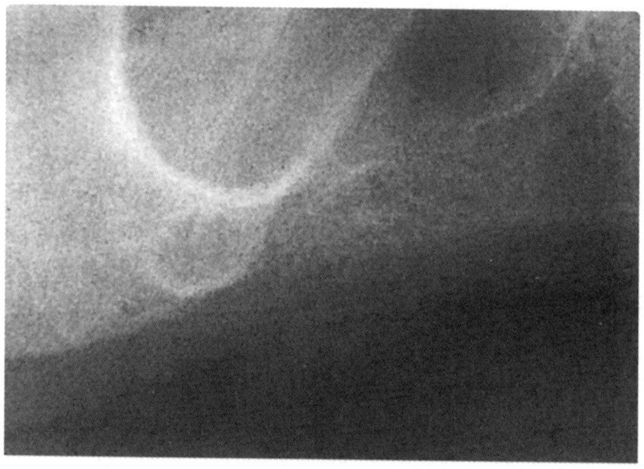

Fig 24-11 Projections must be exposed in all teeth-bearing areas of the mouth whether or not teeth are present. (From Olson SS: *Dental radiography laboratory manual*, Philadelphia, 1995, Saunders.)

An example of images created with cone-beam computer tomography techniques for the edentulous patient is seen in Figure 24-9.

Panoramic Examination. A panoramic image (see Chapter 25) is a common way of examining the edentulous jaw (Figure 24-10). The panoramic examination is quick and easy for the patient and requires only one exposure. If a panoramic image reveals any root tips, impacted teeth, foreign bodies, or lesions in the jaws, an intraoral periapical projection of that specific area should be exposed. The periapical image has more definition and permits the area in question to be examined in greater detail.

Periapical Examination. If a panoramic x-ray machine is not available, 14 periapical projections (6 anterior and 8 posterior) can be used to examine the edentulous arches (Figure 24-11). A size 2 receptor is typically used for the edentulous examination. Either the paralleling technique (see Chapter 19) or the bisecting technique (see Chapter 20) can be used for this periapical examination. If the paralleling technique is used, cotton rolls must be placed on both sides of the bite-block in place of the missing teeth. If the bisecting technique is used, the edentulous ridge and the receptor form the angle to be bisected (Figure 24-12). The receptor should be positioned such that approximately one-third of it extends beyond the edentulous ridge. If the alveolar ridges of the patient are severely resorbed, the bisecting technique is recommended.

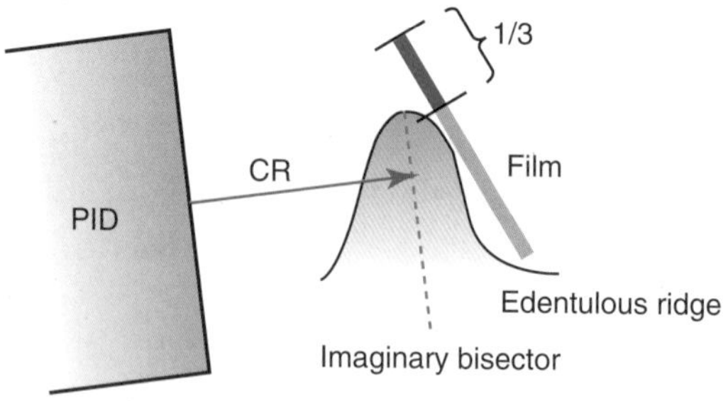

Fig 24-12 In the edentulous patient, the bisecting angle is formed by the ridge of bone and the receptor. The central ray (CR) is directed perpendicular to the imaginary bisector. Approximately one third of the receptor should extend beyond the edentulous ridge. *PID,* Position-indicating device.

Occlusal-Periapical Examination. Some practitioners prefer to use both occlusal and periapical projections to examine the edentulous patient. The combined occlusal and periapical examination consists of a total of six exposures (Figure 24-13): one maxillary topographic

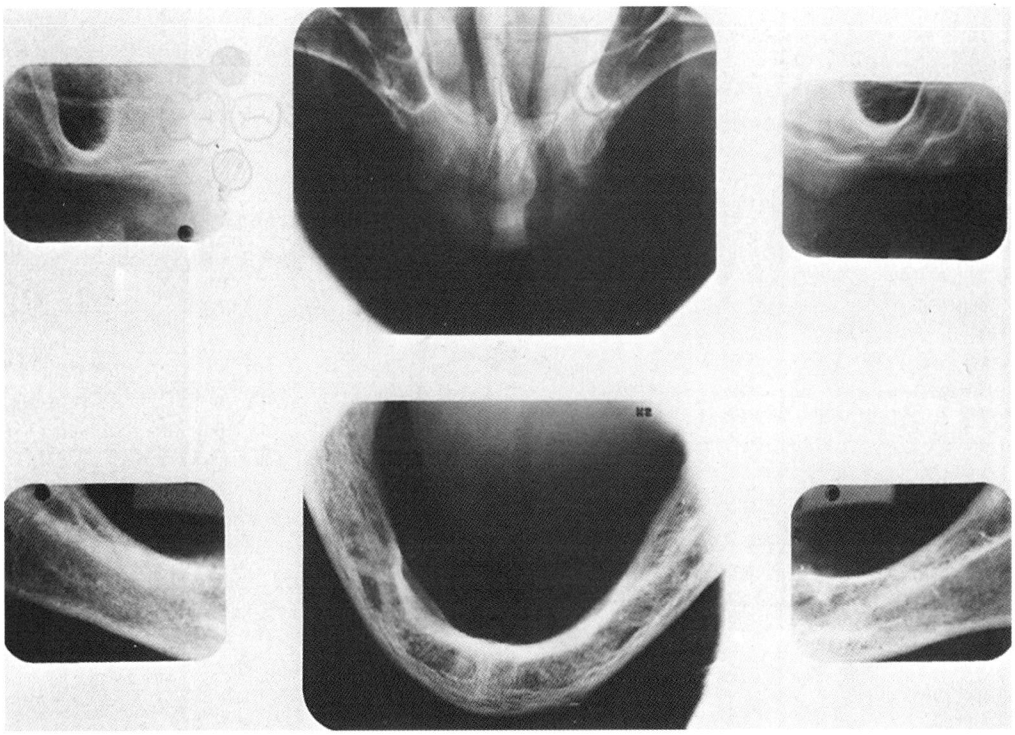

Fig 24-13 Mixed occlusal-periapical edentulous survey. (From Langland OE, Sippy FH, Langlais RP: *Textbook of dental radiology*, ed 2, Springfield, IL, 1984, Charles C Thomas. Courtesy Dr. Robert Langlais.)

occlusal projection (size 4 receptor), one mandibular cross-sectional occlusal projection (size 4 receptor), and four standard molar periapical exposures (size 2 receptor). As with the panoramic image, if an object is identified on an occlusal projection, a periapical projection of that specific area should be exposed.

SUMMARY

- Imaging techniques must often be modified to accommodate patients with special needs, including patients with a hypersensitive gag reflex, patients with physical or developmental disabilities, pediatric patients, endodontic patients, and edentulous patients.
- In dental imaging, the hypersensitive gag reflex is a commonly encountered problem. The areas most likely to elicit the gag reflex when stimulated include the soft palate and the posterior lateral third of the tongue.
- The dental radiographer can effectively manage the patient with a hypersensitive gag reflex by conveying a confident attitude, completing all patient and equipment preparations before receptor placement, using proper exposure sequencing, placing and exposing receptors as quickly as possible, and using modifications in technique as necessary.
- Helpful strategies to prevent gagging include avoiding the discussion or suggestion of gagging, reassuring the patient, suggesting breathing, distracting the patient, reducing tactile stimuli, and using a topical anesthetic.
- If the patient has an uncontrollable gag reflex, an extraoral projection (e.g., extraoral bite-wings or panoramic) can be used to obtain diagnostic information.
- The dental radiographer must be aware of the common physical disabilities (e.g., problems with vision, hearing, or mobility) and know the necessary modifications in technique to accommodate a person with a disability.
- The dental radiographer must also be aware of patients with specific dental needs, including pediatric patients, endodontic patients, and edentulous patients, and know the necessary modifications in technique to accommodate such patients.
- With the pediatric patient, special attention must be paid to the prescription of dental images, patient and equipment preparations, recommended techniques, and patient management.
- With the endodontic patient, the dental radiographer must be able to modify receptor placement and, at the same time, provide accurate images that measure the length of the pulp canals without distortion.
- With the edentulous patient also, the dental radiographer must be able to modify intraoral placements. Imaging is used in the edentulous patient to detect lesions, root tips, impacted teeth, and objects embedded in bone and to observe the quantity of bone present.

TECHNIQUE VIDEOS

View the Technique Videos and complete the accompanying Interactive Exercises that are available as part of the Student Resources on the companion Evolve website for this textbook.

BIBLIOGRAPHY

Dean JA, Avery DR, McDonald RE: McDonald and Avery's dentistry for the child and adolescent, ed 9, Maryland Heights, MD, 2011, Mosby.

Frommer HH, Stabulas-Savage JJ: Patient management and special problems. In Radiology for the dental professional, ed 9, St Louis, 2011, Mosby.

Johnson ON: Managing patients with special needs. In Essentials of dental radiography for dental assistants and hygienists, ed 9, Upper Saddle River, NJ, 2011, Prentice Hall.

Johnson ON: Radiography for children. In Essentials of dental radiography for dental assistants and hygienists, ed 9, Upper Saddle River, NJ, 2011, Prentice Hall.

Mallya SM, Lam EWN: Intraoral Projections. In White and Pharoah's Oral radiology: principles and interpretation, ed 8, St. Louis, 2019, Elsevier.

Miles DA, Van Dis ML, Jensen CW, et al: Accessory radiographic techniques and patient management. In Radiographic imaging for dental auxiliaries, ed 4, St Louis, 2009, Saunders.
Miles DA, Van Dis ML, Razmus TF: Intraoral radiographic techniques. In Basic principles of oral and maxillofacial radiology, Philadelphia, 1992, Saunders.
Ohio Governor's Council on People with Disabilities: Ten do's and don'ts when you meet a person with a disability, Catalog No G-16, Columbus, OH, 1990.
State of Illinois Department of Human Services: People first: a guide to interacting with people with disabilities, 2015 (online), http://www.dhs.gov/sites/default/files/publications/guide-interacting-with-people-who-have-disabilties_09-26-13.pdf.

QUIZ QUESTIONS

True or False

____ **1.** The area of the oral cavity that is most likely to elicit the gag reflex when stimulated is the anterior third of the tongue.
____ **2.** Breathing takes place simultaneously with the gag reflex.
____ **3.** Psychogenic and tactile stimuli are precipitating factors for the gag reflex.
____ **4.** Lack of operator confidence may act as a psychogenic stimulus and contribute to the gag reflex.
____ **5.** The longer a receptor stays in the mouth, the more likely the patient is to gag.
____ **6.** Exposure sequence does not play a role in preventing the gag reflex.
____ **7.** Posterior periapical projections are always exposed before anterior periapical projections.
____ **8.** The mandibular molar periapical projection is most likely to elicit the gag reflex.
____ **9.** A receptor that is dragged along the palatal tissues may stimulate the gag reflex.
____ **10.** The dental radiographer should ask the patient, "Are you a gagger?"
____ **11.** If a patient gags, the dental radiographer should remove the receptor as quickly as possible and reassure the patient.
____ **12.** If a patient is breathing during receptor placement and exposure, the gag reflex will not occur.
____ **13.** Distracting the patient often helps suppress the gag reflex.
____ **14.** Increasing tactile stimuli helps prevent the gag reflex.
____ **15.** The patient with a hypersensitive gag reflex should be instructed to inhale during the application of topical anesthetic spray.
____ **16.** It is appropriate for the dental radiographer to gesture to another person in the presence of a person who is blind.
____ **17.** In the case of a person with a disability, it is appropriate for the dental radiographer to hold a receptor during x-ray exposure.
____ **18.** If the dental radiographer determines that a person cannot tolerate intraoral projections, no intraoral receptors should be exposed.
____ **19.** It is appropriate for the dental radiographer to ask personal questions about a patient's disability.
____ **20.** The dental radiographer should talk to the caregiver of a patient with a disability instead of talking directly to the patient.
____ **21.** With the pediatric patient, the dental radiographer does not need to alter patient management techniques.
____ **22.** The radiographic examination should be performed on the pediatric patient regardless of the cooperation of the patient.
____ **23.** During an endodontic procedure, receptor placement is difficult because of poor visualization of the tooth.
____ **24.** The bisecting technique is recommended for the endodontic patient.
____ **25.** The panoramic examination is the imaging examination most often used in edentulous patients.

IDENTIFICATION

An example of a pediatric panoramic image is seen in Figure 24-14.
26. Identify the approximate age of the patient in Figure 24-15.
27. Identify the approximate age of the patient in Figure 24-16.
28. Identify the approximate age of the patient in Figure 24-17.
29. Identify the approximate age of the patient in Figure 24-18.
30. Identify the approximate age of the patient in Figure 24-19.
31. Identify the approximate age of the patient in Figure 24-20.
32. Identify the approximate age of the patient in Figure 24-21.
33. Identify the approximate age of the patient in Figure 24-22.
34. Identify the approximate age of the patient in Figure 24-23.

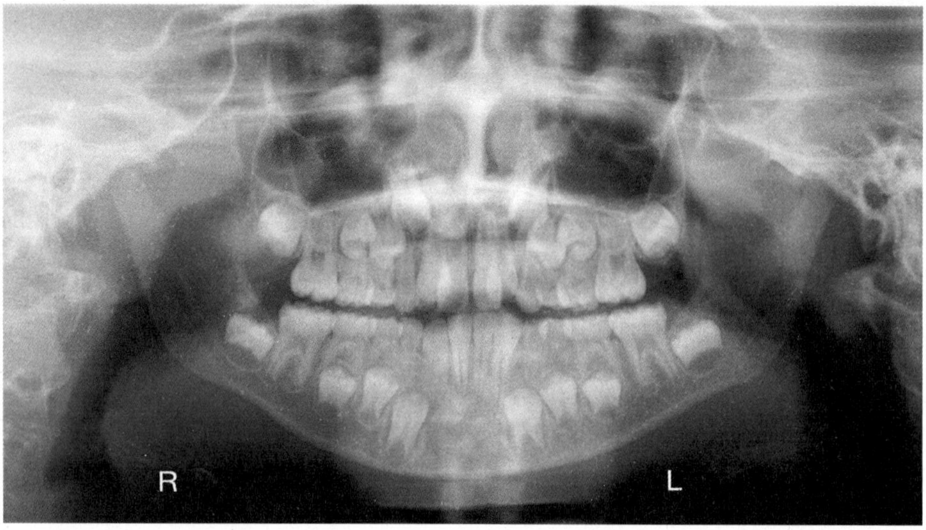

Fig 24-14 Panoramic image of a pediatric patient.

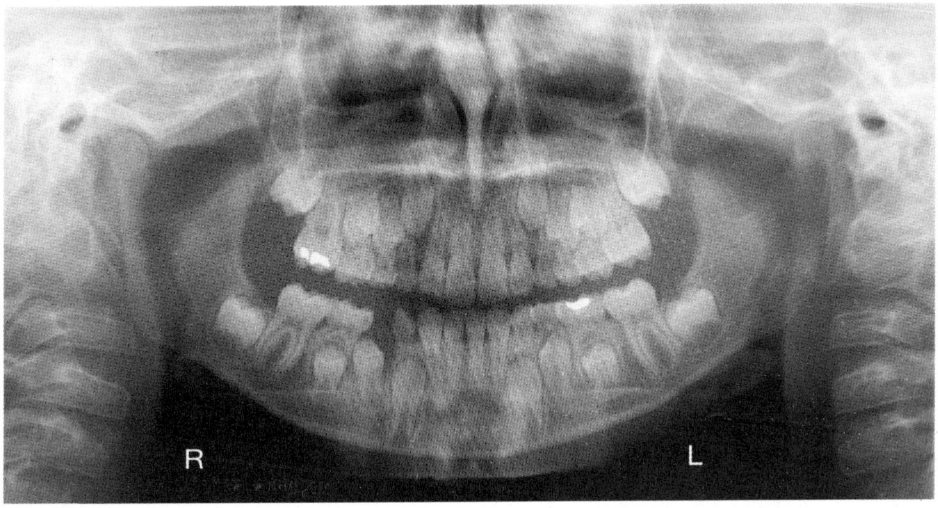

Fig 24-15 (Courtesy Cary Pediatric Dentistry, Cary, NC.)

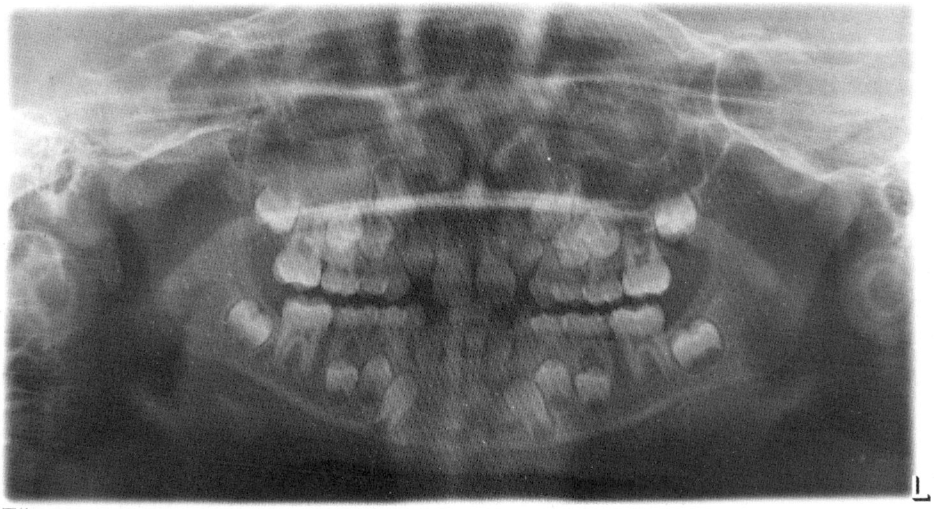

Fig 24-16 (Courtesy Cary Pediatric Dentistry, Cary, NC.)

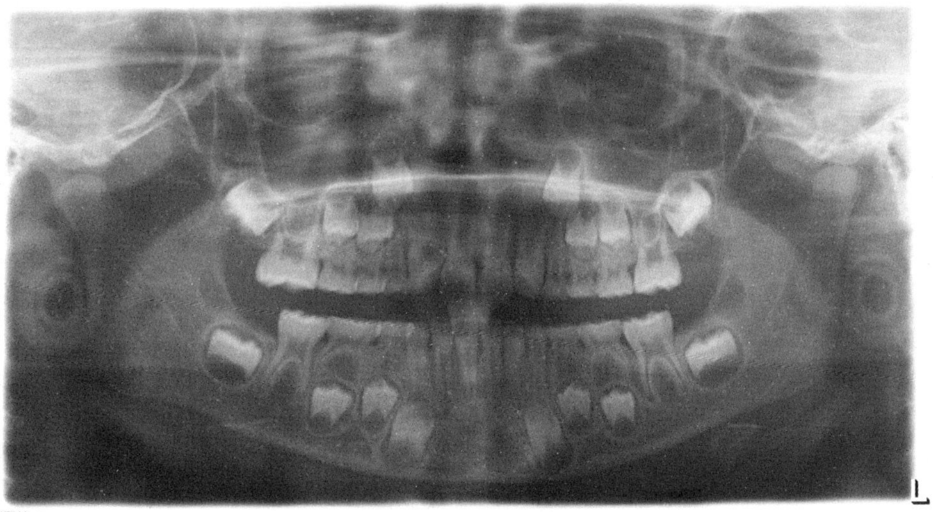

Fig 24-17 (Courtesy Cary Pediatric Dentistry, Cary, NC.)

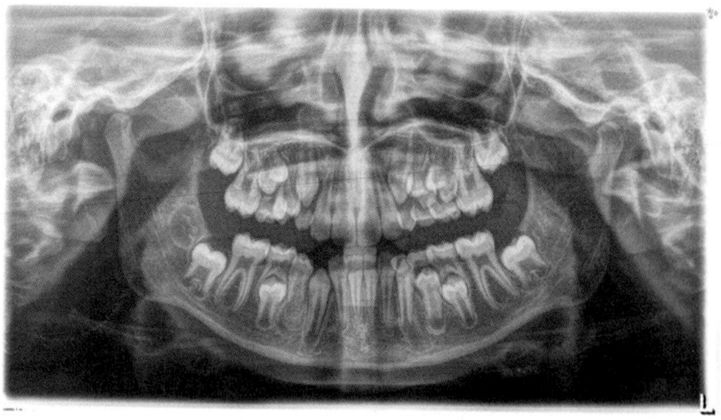

Fig 24-18

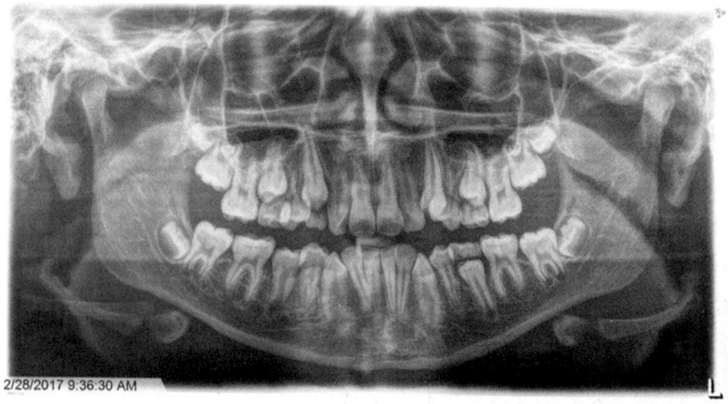

Fig 24-19

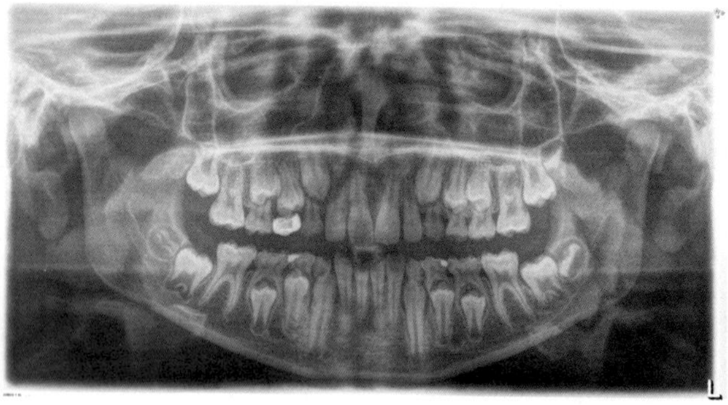

Fig 24-20

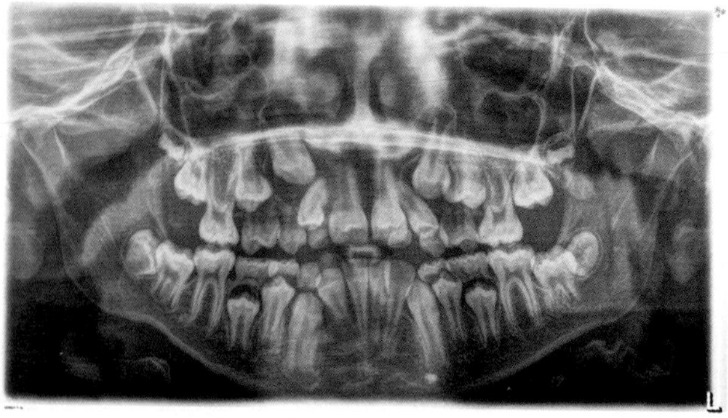

Fig 24-21

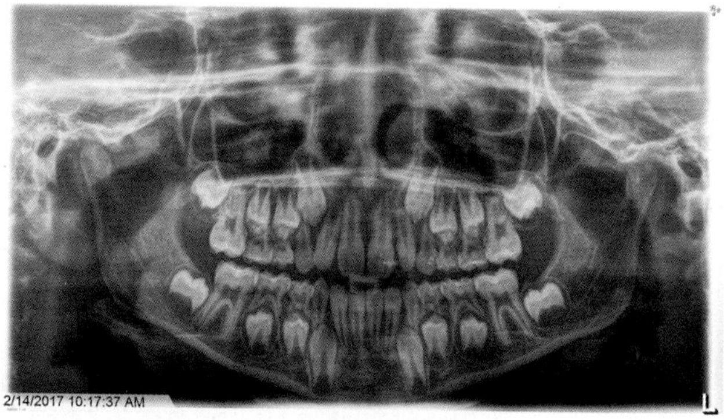

Fig 24-22

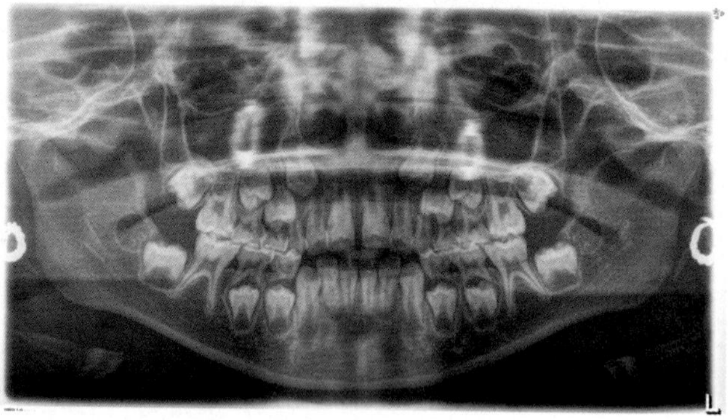

Fig 24-23

25

Panoramic Imaging

LEARNING OBJECTIVES

After completion of this chapter, the student will be able to do the following:

1. Define the key terms associated with panoramic imaging.
2. Describe the purpose and uses of panoramic imaging.
3. Describe the fundamentals of panoramic imaging.
4. Describe the equipment used in panoramic imaging.
5. Describe patient preparation, equipment preparation, and patient positioning procedures needed before exposing a panoramic projection.
6. Describe a diagnostic panoramic image.
7. Identify the patient preparation and patient positioning errors seen on panoramic images, discuss the causes of these errors, and describe the necessary measures needed to correct such errors.
8. Discuss the advantages and disadvantages of panoramic imaging.

It is often difficult, if not impossible, to obtain adequate diagnostic information from a series of intraoral images alone. Impacted third molar teeth, jaw fractures, and large lesions in the posterior mandible cannot be adequately examined on intraoral projections; in such cases, the panoramic image is preferred. The panoramic image allows the dental professional to view a large area of the maxilla and the mandible on a single projection.

Panoramic imaging has undergone major changes upon the introduction of digital imaging in dentistry. Panoramic x-ray machines are capable of acquiring not only the traditional panoramic image but also cone-beam computer generated images and cephalometric, temporomandibular joint, and extraoral bite-wing images. Although an increased number of dental practices have transitioned from film to digital, film-based panoramic imaging continues to be used in dental practices. Consequently, the dental radiographer must be familiar with both digital and film-based panoramic imaging in order to be prepared to work in a variety of offices.

The purpose of this chapter is to present basic concepts of panoramic imaging and to describe the patient preparation, equipment preparation, and patient positioning procedures needed to perform this procedure. In addition, this chapter describes the advantages and disadvantages of panoramic imaging and reviews helpful hints.

BASIC CONCEPTS

As the term panoramic suggests, a panoramic image shows a wide view of the maxilla and the mandible and surrounding structures (Figure 25-1). It allows for the visualization of the patient's oral and facial structures spread out across a flat surface.

Panoramic imaging is an extraoral technique that is used to examine the maxilla and the mandible on a single projection (Figure 25-2). As described in Chapter 7, an extraoral receptor is positioned *outside* the mouth during x-ray exposure. In panoramic imaging (also known as *rotational panoramic imaging*), both the receptor and the tubehead rotate around the patient, producing a series of individual images. When such images are combined, an overall view of the maxilla and the mandible is created.

Purpose and Use

The panoramic image provides the dental radiographer with an overall view of the maxilla and the mandible and is often used to supplement bite-wing and periapical images. The panoramic image is typically used for the following purposes:

- To evaluate the dentition and supporting structures
- To evaluate impacted teeth
- To evaluate eruption patterns, growth, and development
- To detect diseases, lesions, and conditions of the jaws
- To examine the extent of large lesions
- To evaluate trauma

The images on a panoramic projection are not as defined or sharp as the images produced with intraoral projections. Consequently, a panoramic image should not be used to diagnose caries (Chapter 33), periodontal disease (Chapter 34), or periapical lesions (Chapter 35). The panoramic image should not be used as a substitute for intraoral projections.

Fundamentals

When intraoral images (e.g., periapical and bite-wing images) are exposed, the receptor and the x-ray tubehead remain stationary. In panoramic imaging, the receptor and the x-ray tubehead move around the patient. The x-ray tube rotates around the patient's head in one direction, while the receptor rotates in the opposite direction (Figure 25-3). The patient may stand or sit in a stationary position, depending on the type of panoramic x-ray machine that is used. The movement of the receptor and the tubehead produces an image through the process known as *tomography. Tomo-* refers to section; tomography is an imaging technique that allows the imaging of one layer, or section, of the body while blurring the images of structures in other planes. In panoramic imaging, this image conforms to the shape of the dental arches.

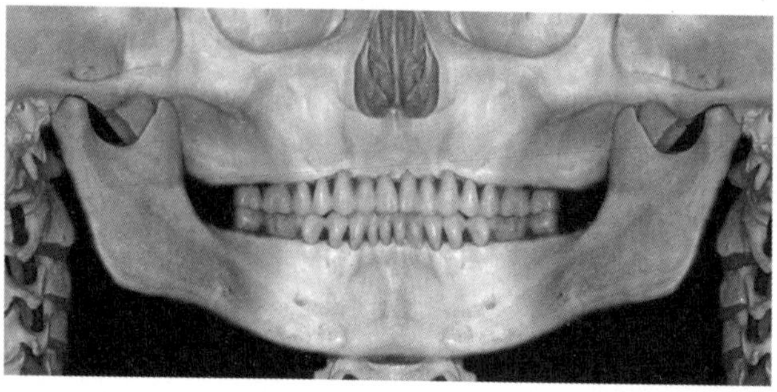

Fig 25-1 The bones of the skull on a panoramic image. From Mallya SM, Lam EWN: Panoramic Imaging. In White and Pharoah's Oral radiology: principles and interpretation, ed 8, St. Louis, 2019, Mosby.

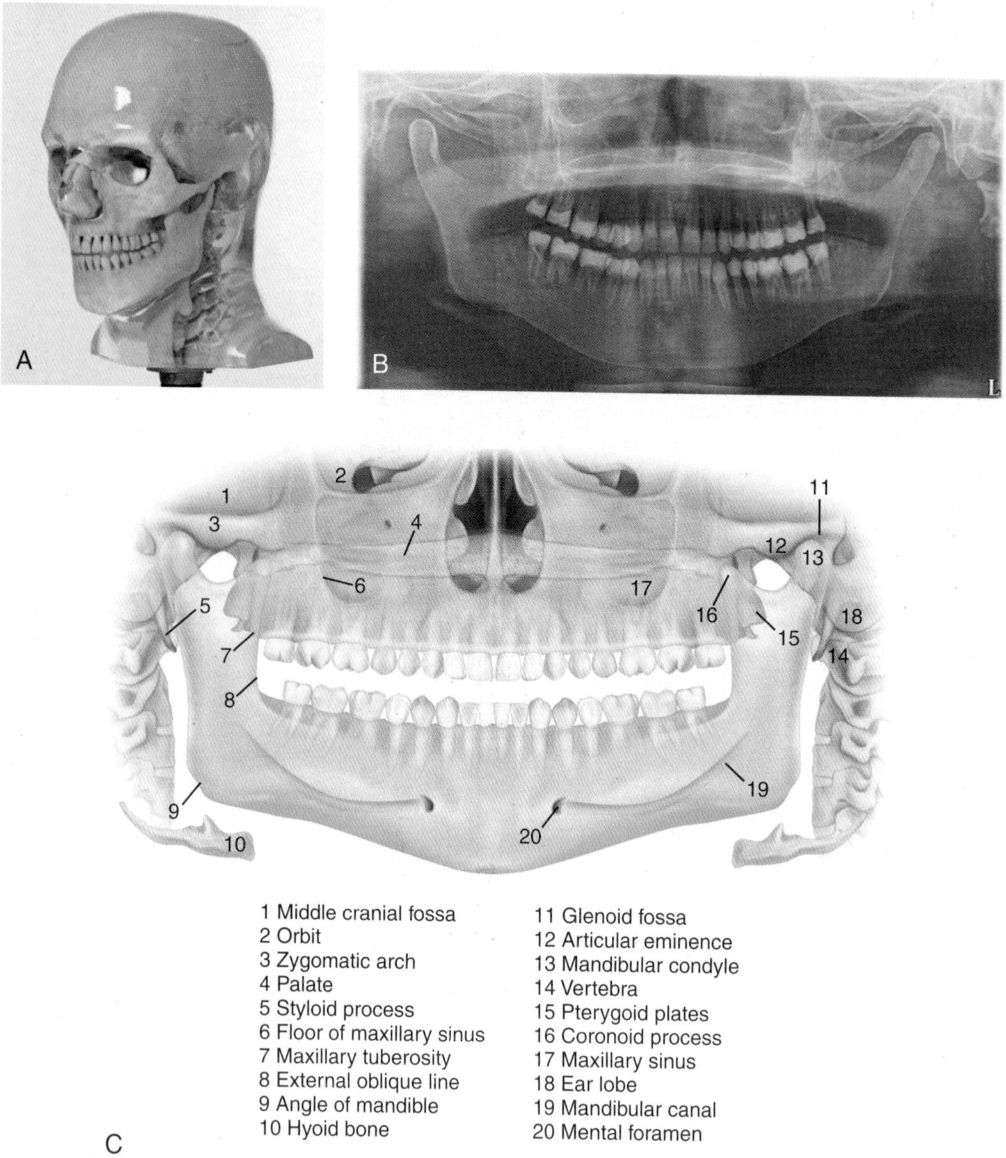

Fig 25-2 A, The CIRS ATOM Max Dental and Diagnostic Head Phantom is a standard of reference for diagnostic radiology of the head. **B,** Panoramic image of Diagnostic Head Phantom. **C,** Panoramic anatomy. (**A** and **B**, courtesy Fluke Biomedical, Cleveland, OH.)

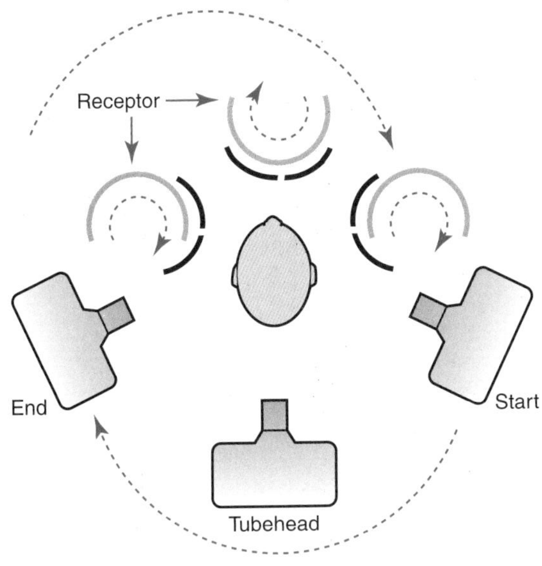

Fig 25-3 In panoramic imaging, the receptor and the x-ray tubehead move around the patient in opposite directions. (Courtesy Dr. Robert M. Jaynes, Columbus, OH.)

Rotation Center. In panoramic imaging, the receptor and the x-ray tubehead are connected and rotate simultaneously around a patient during exposure. The pivotal point, or axis, around which the receptor and the x-ray tubehead rotate is termed the rotation center. Modern panoramic x-ray units use a continuously moving center of rotation rather than multiple fixed center locations (Figure 25-4).

In all cases, the center of rotation changes as the receptor and the tubehead rotate around the patient. This rotational change allows the image layer to conform to the elliptical shape of the average dental arches. The moving x-ray source and receptor generate a zone known as the *focal trough.*

Focal Trough. In panoramic imaging, the focal trough is a theoretical concept used to determine where the dental arches must be positioned to obtain the sharpest image (Figure 25-5). The focal trough (also known as the *image layer*) can be defined as a three-dimensional curved zone in which structures are clearly demonstrated on a panoramic image. The structures located within the focal trough appear reasonably well defined on the resulting panoramic image. The structures positioned outside of the focal trough appear blurred or indistinct and are not readily visible on the panoramic image.

The size and shape of the focal trough vary, depending on the manufacturer of the panoramic x-ray unit. The closer the rotation center is to the teeth, the narrower the focal trough. In most panoramic x-ray machines, the focal trough is narrow in the anterior region and wide in the posterior region, conforming to the average patient size.

Each panoramic x-ray unit has a focal trough that is designed to accommodate the average jaw. Each manufacturer provides specific instructions about patient positioning to ensure that the teeth are positioned within the focal trough. The quality of the resulting panoramic image depends on the positioning of the patient's teeth within the focal trough and how closely the patient's maxilla and mandible conform to the focal trough designed for the average jaw.

Resultant Images. During the panoramic exposure cycle, some anatomic structures are penetrated twice by the x-ray beam because of the rotational imaging process. The location of these structures determines what type of image results: real, double, or ghost.

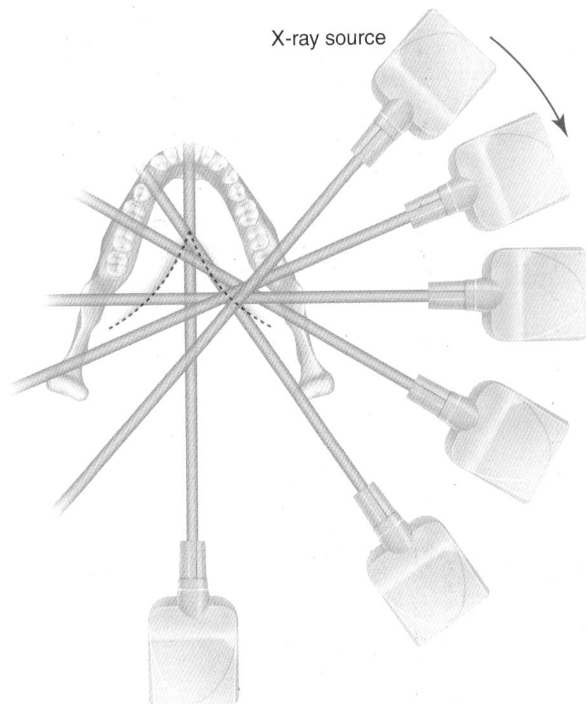

Fig 25-4 The center of rotation of the x-ray source moves continuously as the tubehead and receptor rotate around the patient. Initially, the x-ray beam rotates on the end of the dotted arc on the tube side of the patient. As the x-ray source moves behind the patient, the center of rotation moves forward along the arc (dotted line). The drawing shows the directions of the x-ray beam at various intervals for the first half of the exposure cycle. The x-ray source then continues to move around the patient to image the opposite side.

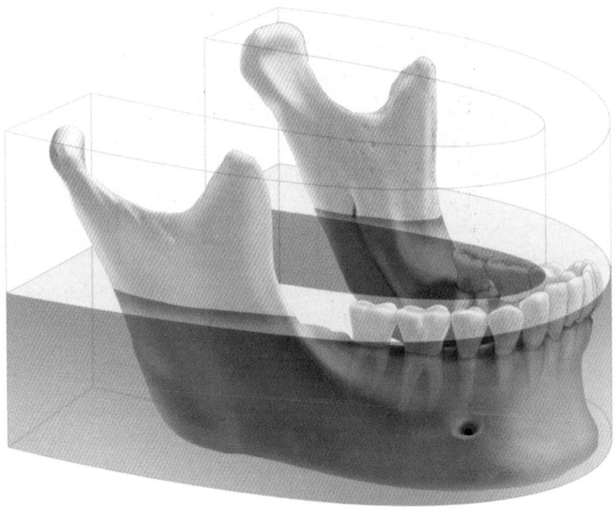

Fig 25-5 Example of a focal trough. (Courtesy Soredex, Finland, www.soredex.com.)

A real image results when a structure lies between the receptor and moving rotation center. A real image is a "true" image; it appears in the correct anatomic location with varying degrees of sharpness and distortion. Structures found within the focal trough appear sharp on the resultant image while structures outside of the focal trough appear blurred.

A double image results when an anatomic structure that is located *behind* the moving rotation center is penetrated twice by the x-ray beam. A double image has the same proportions as the real image and is located in the same location on the opposite side of the receptor. A double image appears as a mirror image, or the reverse of the real image. Examples include structures located at the midline such as the epiglottis, hyoid bone, and cervical spine. These structures appear as two images, or a double image, one on each side of the panoramic receptor.

A ghost image results when an anatomic structure or object is located outside of the focal plane and close to the x-ray source. A ghost image resembles its true image and is found on the opposite side of the receptor; it appears blurred, magnified, and higher than the actual counterpart. A ghost image appears in a different location than the true image; it appears on the opposite side because the receptor was on the opposite side when the x-rays passed through the structure. A ghost image appears blurred and distorted because the structure is far from the focal trough. A ghost image appears higher than the true image as the result of the negative vertical angulation of the x-ray beam. Anatomic structures that are located laterally, such as the ramus of the mandible, or located centrally, such as the hard palate, can produce ghost images. Objects located laterally such as metallic earrings can also produce ghost images. Ghost images created by earrings and other objects are discussed later in this chapter.

Equipment

The use of special equipment, including the panoramic x-ray unit, the receptor, and—when using film—intensifying screens and a cassette, is necessary in panoramic imaging.

Panoramic X-Ray Units. The panoramic x-ray units used in dental practices may be digital or film-based. Although dental practices continue to use film-based panoramic imaging, virtually all of the new panoramic units manufactured today are digital acquisition models.

A variety of panoramic x-ray units are available on the market today. One example is the digital Orthophos XG 3 (Sirona USA). Panoramic units may differ with regard to the size and shape of the focal trough and the type of receptor transport mechanism used. Although each manufacturer's panoramic unit is slightly different, all panoramic machines have similar components. The main components of the panoramic unit, whether digital or film-based, include the following (Figure 25-6):

- X-ray tubehead
- Head positioner
- Exposure controls

The panoramic x-ray tubehead is similar to an intraoral x-ray tubehead; each has a filament used to generate electrons and a target used to produce x-rays. The collimator used in the panoramic x-ray tubehead, however, differs from the collimator used in the intraoral x-ray tubehead. As described in Chapter 4, the collimator used in the intraoral x-ray machine is a lead plate with a small round or rectangular opening in the middle. The function of the collimator is to restrict the size and shape of the x-ray beam. The collimator used in the panoramic x-ray machine is a lead plate with an opening in the shape of a narrow vertical slit (Figure 25-7).

The x-ray beam emerges from the panoramic tubehead through the collimator as a narrow band. The beam passes through the patient and then exposes the receptor through another vertical slit in the receptor holder. The narrow x-ray beam that emerges from the collimator minimizes patient exposure to x-radiation.

The vertical angulation of the panoramic tubehead does not vary as in the case of the intraoral tubehead. The tubehead of the panoramic unit is fixed in position so that the x-ray beam is directed slightly upward (approximately −10 degrees). In addition, the tubehead of the panoramic unit always rotates *behind* the patient's head, while the receptor rotates in front of the patient.

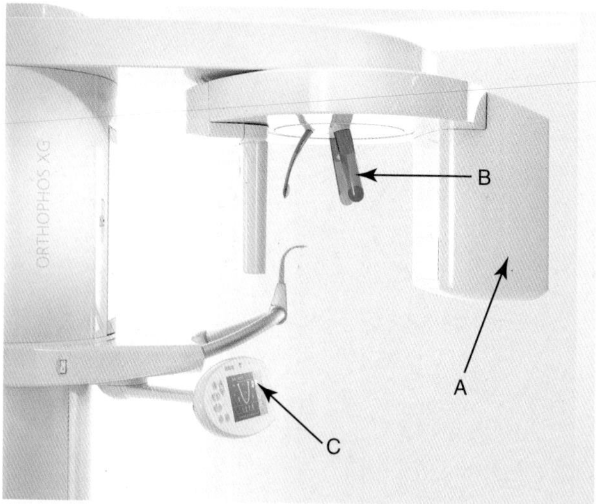

Fig 25-6 Main components of the panoramic x-ray unit Orthophos XG 3: A, x-ray tubehead; B, head positioner; C, exposure controls. (Courtesy Sirona USA, Charlotte, NC.)

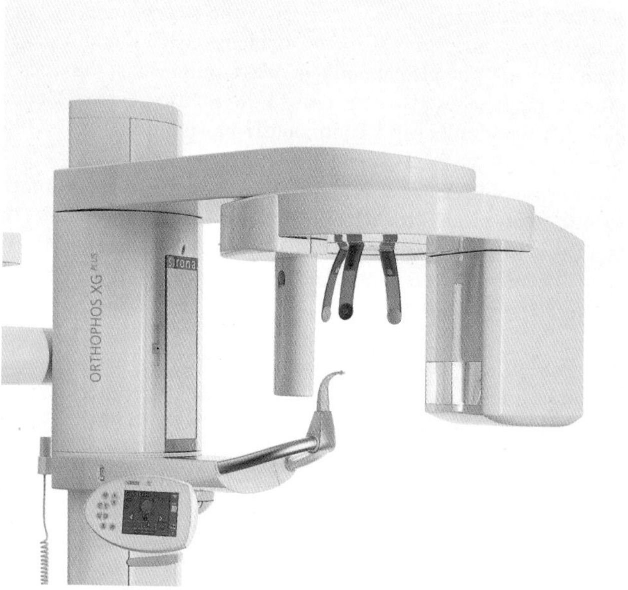

Fig 25-7 The collimator on the Orthophos XG Plus has a narrow slit opening. (Courtesy Sirona USA, Charlotte, NC.)

Each panoramic unit has a head positioner, which is used to align the patient's teeth as accurately as possible in the focal trough. The typical head positioner consists of a chin rest, notched bite-block, forehead rest, and lateral head supports or guides (Figure 25-8). The chin rest and bite-block are used to stabilize the patient's dentition in the anterior-posterior direction. The lateral head supports are used to stabilize the patient's head in both the vertical and horizontal planes. Each panoramic unit is different, and the operator must follow the manufacturer's instructions on how to position the patient's head in the focal trough. Many manufacturers incorporate the head positioner and the

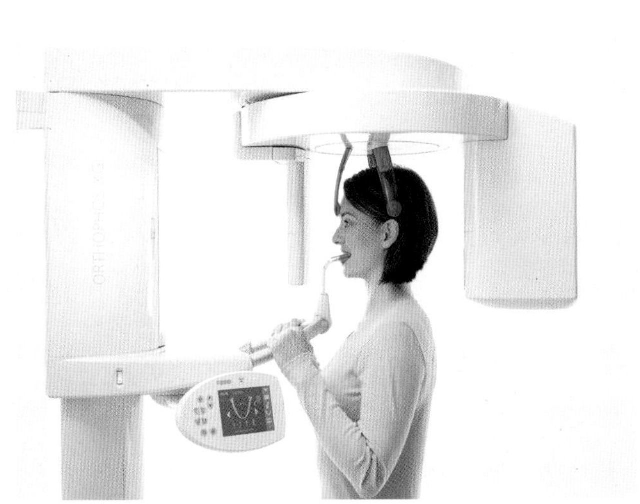

Fig 25-8 The head positioner (notched bite-block, forehead rest, and lateral head supports) is used to align the patient's teeth to the focal trough. (Courtesy Sirona USA, Charlotte, NC.)

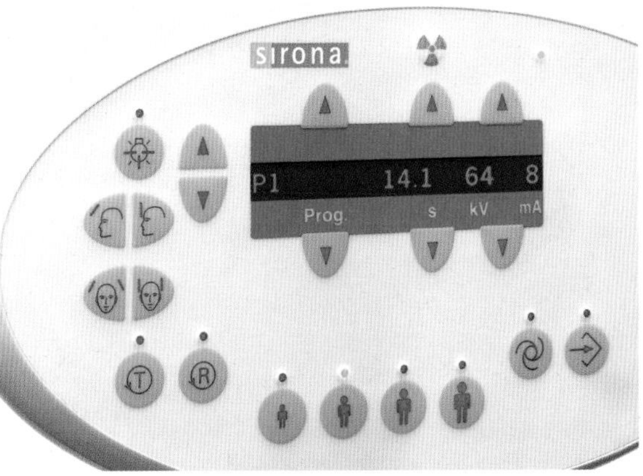

Fig 25-9 Exposure controls can be used to adjust exposure factors. (Courtesy Sirona USA, Charlotte, NC.)

focal trough together, allowing for simplicity in aligning the patient correctly into the machine.

Each panoramic unit has exposure factors (milliamperage, kilovoltage, and time) that are determined by the manufacturer and suggested in the instruction manual for the x-ray machine. Although predetermined exposure settings for panoramic imaging are available, the milliamperage and kilovoltage settings are adjustable and can be varied to accommodate patients of different sizes (Figure 25-9). The exposure time may be adjusted based on the type of image obtained (panoramic, extraoral bite-wing). The panoramic imaging exposure time varies depending on the receptor and the x-ray unit but typically ranges from 10 to 30 seconds.

Image Receptors. In panoramic x-ray units, the image receptor may be a direct digital sensor (CCD or CMOS), a PSP plate, or film. With digital imaging, imaging software downloads the patient information within seconds and can transmit the image to various computer workstations within the dental office. Innovative features of dental imaging software provide high-quality images with adjustable contrast and sharpness. More information on digital imaging is

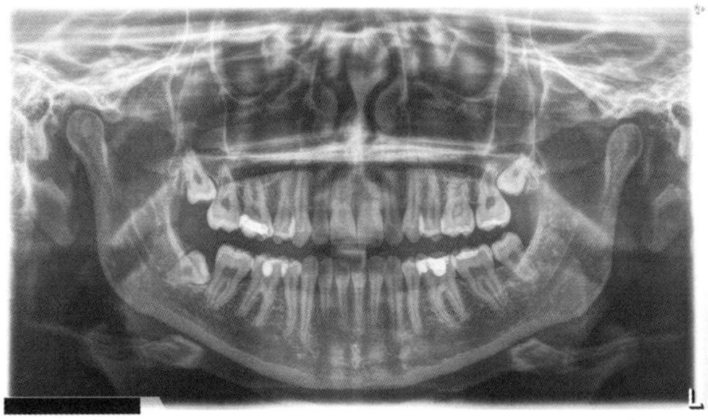

Fig 25-10 This digital panoramic image is labeled with the letter L to indicate the patient's left (L) side.

found in Chapter 8. Whether a digital sensor or film receptor is used, the image must clearly indicate the patient's right and/or left sides (Figure 25-10).

Extraoral screen film is used in film-based panoramic imaging; this film is sensitive to the light emitted from intensifying screens (see Chapter 9). A screen film is placed between two intensifying screens in a cassette holder. When the cassette holder is exposed to x-rays, the screens convert the x-ray energy into light, which, in turn, exposes the screen film. Some screen films are sensitive to green light (T-Mat film), whereas others are sensitive to blue light (X-Omat DBF films). Blue-sensitive film must be paired with screens that produce blue light, and green-sensitive film must be paired with screens that produce green light. The film used in panoramic imaging is available in two sizes: 5 × 12 inch and 6 × 12 inch.

Additional Equipment. In film-based panoramic imaging, intensifying screens and a cassette holder are required; these items are *not* used in digital panoramic imaging.

Two basic types of intensifying screens are used: calcium tungstate and rare earth (see Chapter 9). Calcium tungstate screens emit blue light, and the rare earth screens emit green light. Rare earth screens require less x-ray exposure than do calcium tungstate screens and are considered "faster." Consequently, rare earth screens are recommended in panoramic imaging because of less radiation exposure to the patient.

The cassette is a device that is used to hold the extraoral film and intensifying screens (see Chapter 9). The cassette may be rigid or flexible, curved or straight, depending on the panoramic x-ray unit. All cassettes must be "light-tight" to protect the film from exposure. One intensifying screen is placed on each side of the film and held in place when the cassette is closed.

The cassette must be marked to orient the finished image. Before exposure, a metal letter "R" can be attached to the front of the cassette to indicate the patient's right side; the letter "L" is used to identify the patient's left side. Special labeling may also be attached to indicate the patient's name and the exposure date. If the cassette is not labeled before exposure, the film must be labeled immediately after processing, using a marking pen or adhesive label.

STEP-BY-STEP PROCEDURES

Step-by-step procedures for the exposure of a panoramic receptor include equipment preparation, patient preparation, and patient positioning. Before exposing a panoramic receptor, infection prevention procedures (as described in Chapter 16) must be completed.

Equipment Preparation

The dental radiographer must complete the panoramic imaging equipment preparations *before* preparing the patient for exposure (Procedure 25-1). The equipment preparation varies depending on the receptor used (digital sensor or film), and the specific panoramic x-ray unit. The dental radiographer must be familiar with the manufacturer's specific directions for equipment preparation found in the instruction manual.

Patient Preparation

After preparing the panoramic x-ray unit, the dental radiographer must prepare the patient for the procedure (Procedure 25-2). Patient preparation is the same for digital and film-based panoramic imaging.

Patient Positioning

Patient positioning is extremely important in panoramic procedures because of the length of time needed to acquire the panoramic image. Therefore it is important that the patient be as comfortable as possible during the procedure. Contemporary panoramic machines are sleek and less bulky than older machines. Ergonomic handles and head positioning devices allow for patient comfort while maintaining the correct position for exposure. Most machines allow for patients to stand, sit, or use a wheelchair during exposure.

The dental radiographer must be familiar with the manufacturer's specific directions for patient positioning that are included in the instruction manual. Many panoramic manufacturers include laser alignment lights to offer guidance with patient positioning. These lighted lines allow the radiographer to easily visualize the midsagittal and Frankfort planes; some lights also indicate the correct position of the focal trough. Although each manufacturer's positioning and exposure instructions are slightly different, the patient positioning steps listed in this text are common to all panoramic imaging procedures, whether digital or film-based (Procedure 25-3).

DIAGNOSTIC PANORAMIC IMAGE

A diagnostic panoramic image results when the equipment preparation, patient preparation, and patient positioning are completed correctly. The ideal panoramic image should be free from all errors in exposure, technique, and positioning. Such an image is not always possible. Minor errors may be present that do not affect the diagnostic quality of the image. In such cases, a retake of the panoramic image is unnecessary.

A diagnostic panoramic image must demonstrate accurate anatomic features and proper exposure resulting in correct density and contrast.

Anatomic Features

A panoramic image must allow for the visualization of the maxillofacial anatomic features that it represents (Figure 25-15). The panoramic image may be divided into six areas for review: the dentition, ramus

PROCEDURE 25-1 **Equipment Preparation for Panoramic Imaging**

1. Prepare receptor
   - If using film, load the panoramic cassette in the darkroom under safelight conditions.
   - Place one extraoral film and two intensifying screens in the cassette and securely close.
   - Load the cassette into the cassette carrier of the panoramic unit.
2. Prepare bite-block
   - Cover the bite-block with a disposable plastic cover slip.
   - If not covered with an impervious material, the bite-block must be sterilized between patients.
3. Choose exposure settings
   - Set the exposure factors (kilovoltage, milliamperage, time) according to the manufacturer's recommendations.
   - Use size of the patient to determine exposure factors.
4. Adjust machine height
   - Adjust the machine to accommodate the height of the patient, and align all movable parts.

PROCEDURE 25-2 **Patient Preparation for Panoramic Imaging**

1. Explain the imaging procedure
   - Briefly explain the imaging procedure to the patient.
2. Place lead apron
   - Place and secure a lead apron without a thyroid collar on the patient.
   - Place the lead apron low around the neck so that it does not block the x-ray beam.
   - Use a double-sided lead apron to protect the patient (Figure 25-11).
3. Remove all objects
   - Request that the patient remove all objects from the head-and-neck area that may interfere with the procedure.
   - Items to remove include eyeglasses, earrings, intraoral and extraoral piercings, necklaces, napkin chains, hearing aids, hairpins, barrettes, and any intraoral prostheses (complete or partial dentures).

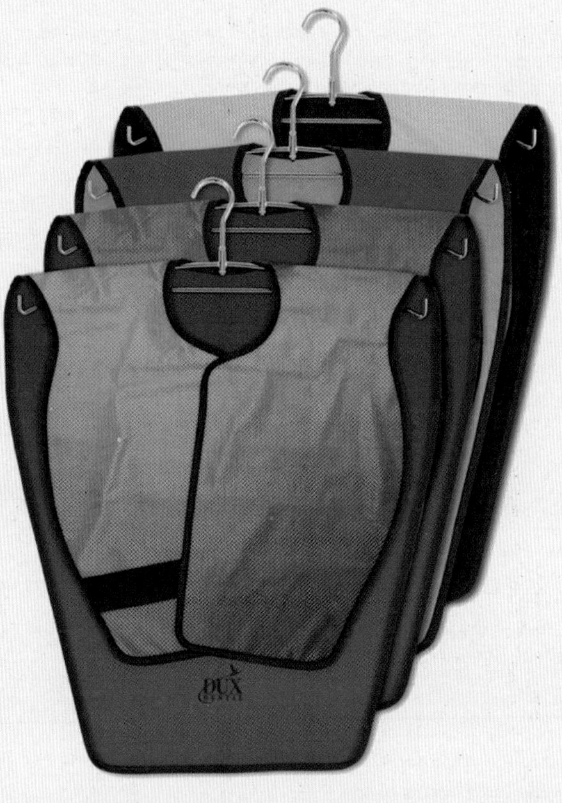

Fig 25-11 A double-sided lead apron is recommended for use during exposure of a panoramic receptor. (Courtesy DUX Dental, Oxnard, CA.)

PROCEDURE 25-3 Patient Positioning for Panoramic Imaging

1. Position spine
   - Instruct the patient to sit or stand "as tall as possible" with the shoulders back.
   - The spine must be perfectly straight.
2. Position teeth
   - Instruct the patient to bite in the groove located on the plastic bite-block; this aligns the teeth in the focal trough.
   - Position maxillary and mandibular anterior in an end-to-end position in the groove on the bite-block (Figure 25-12).
3. Position head
   - Position the midsagittal plane (an imaginary plane that divides the patient's face into right and left sides) perpendicular to the floor (Figure 25-13).
   - Position the Frankfort plane (an imaginary plane that passes through the top of the ear canal and the bottom of the eye socket) parallel to the floor (Figure 25-14).
   - The patient's head must not be tipped up or down.
4. Position lips and tongue
   - Instruct the patient to place the tongue on the roof of the mouth.
   - Suggest that the patient "swallow and feel the tongue rise up to the roof of the mouth" and keep the tongue in that position during the procedure.
   - Instruct the patient to close the lips around the bite-block.
5. Final instructions and exposure
   - Instruct the patient to remain still while the machine is rotating during exposure.
   - Expose the receptor.

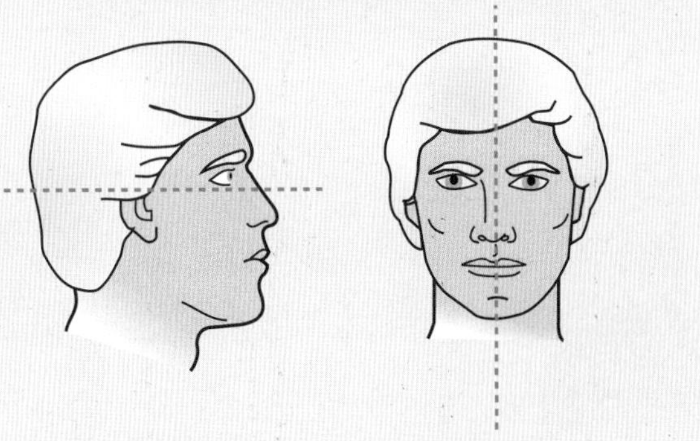

Fig 25-13 Frankfort and midsagittal planes. The Frankfort plane passes through the floor of the orbit and the external auditory meatus. The midsagittal plane divides the face in half into right and left sides. (From Olson SS: Dental radiography laboratory manual, Philadelphia, 1995, Saunders.)

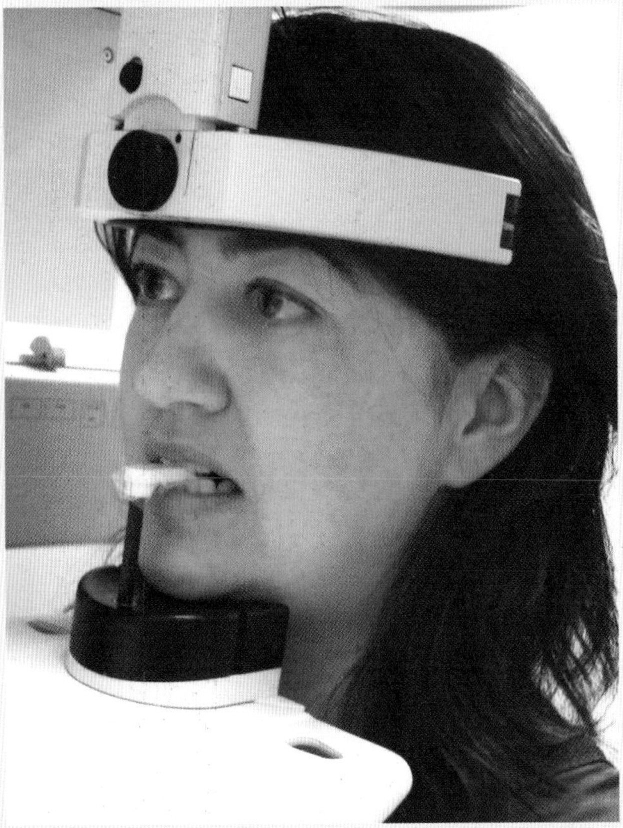

Fig 25-12 The patient must place his or her teeth in the grooves on the bite-block.

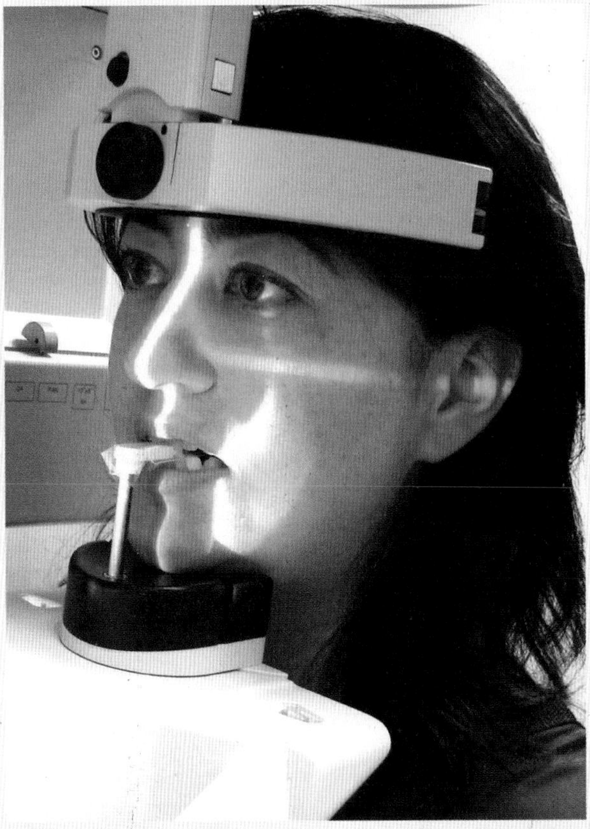

Fig 25-14 The patient's head must be positioned such that the Frankfort plane is parallel to the floor.

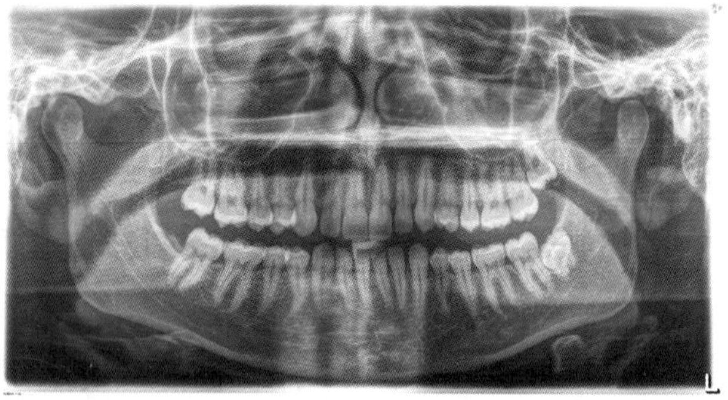

Fig 25-15 A diagnostic panoramic image. (Courtesy Sirona USA, Charlotte, NC.)

and cervical spine, nasal cavity and maxillary sinus, body of the mandible, condyle, and hyoid bone (Box 25-1). If any areas are obstructed, absent, or distorted, the image should be retaken.

Each panoramic image should be assessed to determine whether the dentition and bones of the maxillofacial region are representative. Assessment of acceptable dentition features includes the following: Anterior teeth are in focus with pulp chambers visible, anterior teeth are not excessively narrow or wide, and posterior teeth on right side appear similar in size to the posterior teeth on the left side. Assessment of bony anatomic accuracy includes the following: Both condyles appear on the image, the palate appears above the apices of the maxillary teeth and superimposed over the maxillary sinus, and the width of the right ramus is similar to the width of the left ramus.

Density and Contrast

The diagnostic panoramic image results from adequate exposure and exhibits proper density and contrast. Adequate exposure results from choosing the correct kilovoltage and milliamperage settings for the size of the patient. Smaller patients require less exposure, whereas larger patients require more. With an ideal panoramic image, the density, or overall darkness, is not excessive. An overexposed image appears excessively dark with areas of "burnout" (Figure 25-16). An underexposed image appears excessively light with areas of "whiteout" (Figure 25-17). An overexposed or underexposed panoramic image may cause problems with detection of unerupted teeth or bony lesions. It is important to note that with digital imaging, an overexposed image can be corrected with the use of software, but an underexposed image cannot. Proper contrast on a panoramic image is also critical, especially when multiple anatomic structures appear overlapped. Ideal contrast on a panoramic image should allow for the identification of the junction between enamel and dentin in the molar region (Figure 25-18). Inadequate contrast may lead to problems with the detection of unerupted or impacted teeth.

COMMON ERRORS

To produce a diagnostic panoramic image and minimize patient exposure, mistakes must be avoided. In addition to being familiar with how to create a diagnostic panoramic image, the dental radiographer must be able to recognize common patient preparation and patient positioning errors and understand the necessary steps to correct these errors.

Patient Preparation Errors

Proper patient preparation is critical in obtaining a diagnostic panoramic image. The two most common patient preparation errors are the ghost image and the lead apron artifact.

BOX 25-1 Diagnostic Panoramic Image Features

Each of these six areas can be reviewed to determine the diagnostic quality of the panoramic image.

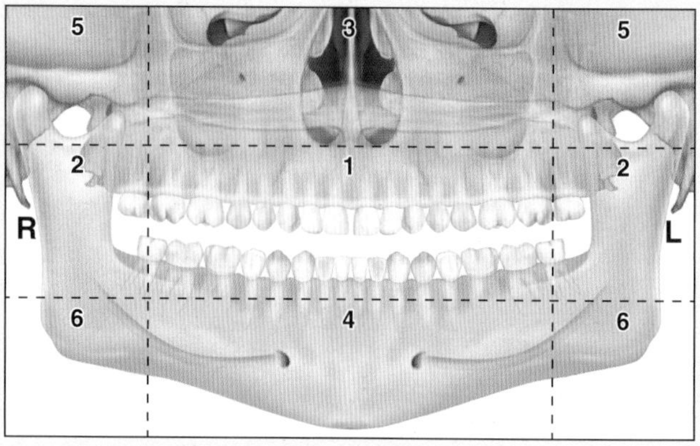

Area 1 Dentition
Teeth are arranged in a smile-like curve. Crowns and apices of all teeth visible.

Area 2 Ramus and Cervical Spine
Ramus should be the same width on each side. Cervical spine may be present along edges, but should not overlap the ramus.

Area 3 Nasal Cavity and Maxillary Sinus
Hard palate double image appears above the apices of the maxillary teeth.

Area 4 Body of Mandible
Inferior border of mandible appears smooth and continuous.

Area 5 Condyle
Condyle is centered, is of equal size on each side, and is on the same horizontal plane.

Area 6 Hyoid Bone
Hyoid bone double image appears. Hyoid bone may slightly overlap mandible.

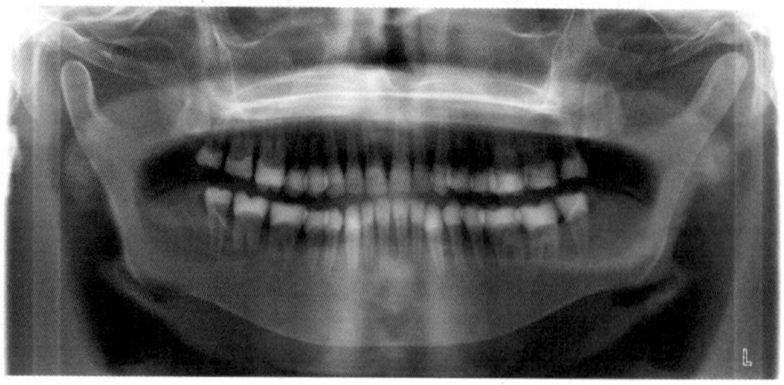

Fig 25-16 An overexposed panoramic image.

Ghost Images.

Problem. If all metallic or dense objects (e.g., eyeglasses, earrings, necklaces, intraoral and extraoral piercings, hairpins, removable partial dentures, complete dentures, orthodontic retainers, hearing aids, napkin chains) are not removed before the exposure of a panoramic receptor, a ghost image results that may obscure diagnostic information.

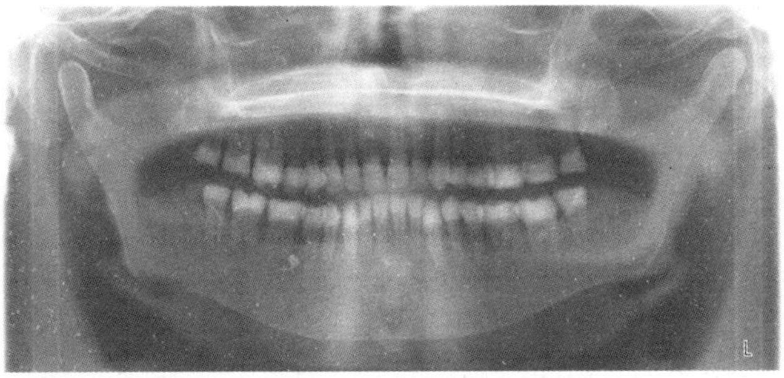

Fig 25-17 An underexposed panoramic image.

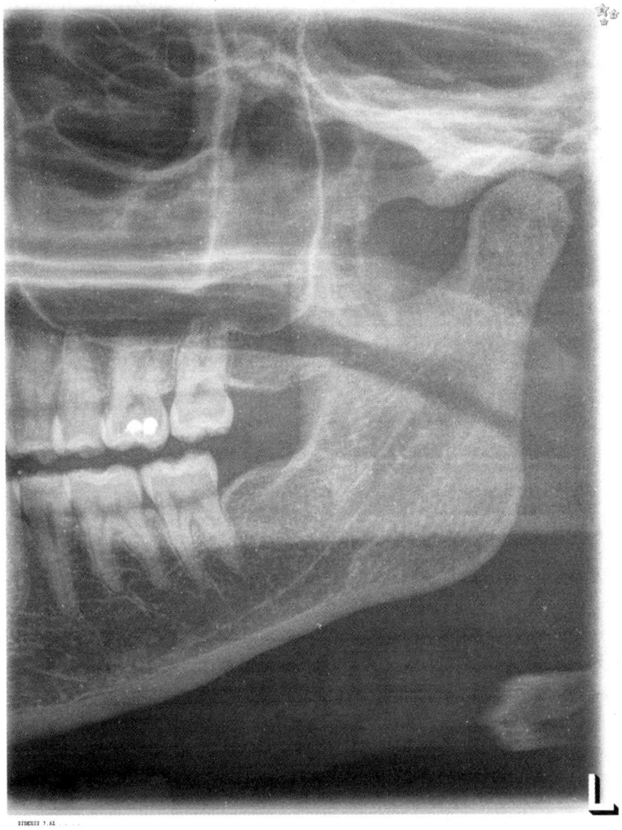

Fig 25-18 Ideal contrast allows for the identification of the junction between the enamel and dentin in the molar region. (Courtesy Sirona USA, Charlotte, NC.)

A ghost image, which is a radiopaque artifact seen on a panoramic image, is produced when a thick, dense object is located outside of the focal plane and close to the x-ray source. A ghost image resembles its real counterpart and is found on the opposite side of the image; it appears indistinct, larger, and higher than its actual counterpart. For example, a ghost image of a hoop earring appears on the opposite side of the image as a radiopacity that is larger and higher than the real image of the hoop earring. In addition, the ghost image of the hoop earring appears blurred in both horizontal and vertical directions (Figure 25-19). As previously detailed in this chapter, a ghost image may also be caused by normal anatomic structures. For example, the dense cortical bone of the ramus of the mandible or hard palate may produce ghost images; such ghost images cannot be avoided and seldom render the image nondiagnostic.

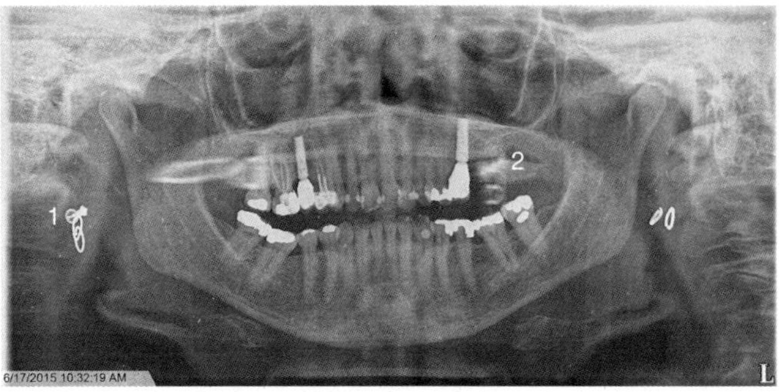

Fig 25-19 Hoop earrings (1) and ghost images (2). The ghost image of the earring appears on the opposite side of the image and is enlarged and laterally distorted.

Solution. To avoid a ghost image artifact, the dental radiographer must instruct the patient to remove all dense objects in the head-and-neck region before positioning the patient for panoramic radiography.

Lead Apron Artifact.

Problem. If the lead apron is incorrectly placed on the patient, a radiopaque cone-shaped artifact results that obscures diagnostic information. If a lead apron with a thyroid collar is used during the exposure of a panoramic projection, a bilateral radiopaque artifact results that obstructs the mandible (Figure 25-20).

Solution. To prevent such artifacts, the dental radiographer must always use a lead apron *without* a thyroid collar when exposing a panoramic projection. The lead apron without a thyroid collar must be placed low around the neck of the patient so that it does not block the x-ray beam. In addition, the primary beam in panoramic imaging is directed slightly upward, and the area of the thyroid gland receives little or no radiation dose.

Patient Positioning Errors

Patient positioning is of critical importance during exposure of a panoramic projection. Because the panoramic image does not show the fine anatomic details seen on intraoral radiographs, even the smallest patient positioning error can create a distorted image.

Positioning of Lips and Tongue.

Problem. If the patient's lips are not closed on the bite-block during the exposure of a panoramic projection, a dark radiolucent shadow results that obscures anterior teeth. This area of increased darkness occurs over the maxillary anterior region and may be mistaken for bone loss. If the tongue is not in contact with the palate during the exposure of a panoramic projection, a dark radiolucent shadow results that obscures the apices of the maxillary teeth (Figure 25-21). Although failure to position the tongue on the roof of the mouth is one of the most common patient positioning errors, it rarely requires a retake.

Solution. To prevent such errors, the dental radiographer must instruct the patient to close the lips around the bite-block. The patient must then be instructed to swallow once and to hold the tongue against the hard palate during the exposure of the projection.

Chin Tipped Up.

Problem. If the patient is positioned such that the chin is too high or is tipped up (Figure 25-22), the Frankfort plane is angled upward, and the following errors result:

- The condyles may not be visible or may appear near the lateral edge of the image.

HELPFUL HINT

Causes of Ghost Images

- Glasses
- Earrings, nose jewelry
- Necklaces
- Hair clips (in front of ears)
- Hearing aids
- Napkin chains
- Anything removable in mouth (dentures, retainers, etc.)

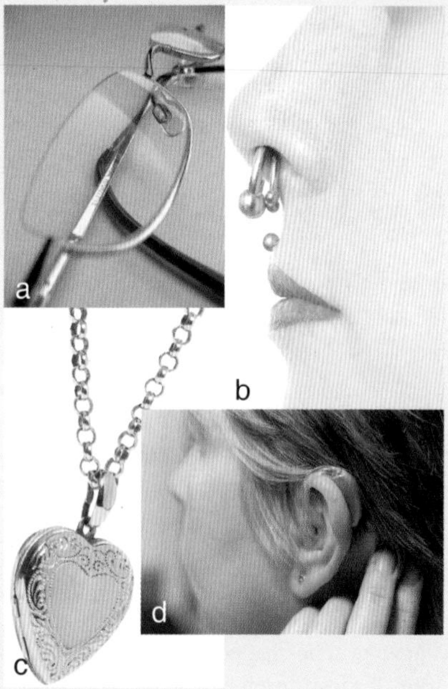

[a]Copyright Andreas Herpens/iStock.com
[b]Copyright Alexander Raths/Shutterstock.com
[c]Copyright PaulaConnelly/iStock.com
[d]Copyright Alexander Raths/Shutterstock.com

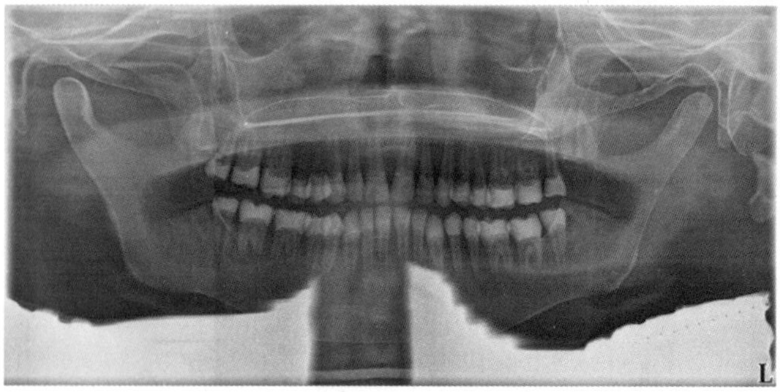

Fig 25-20 On a panoramic image, a thyroid collar artifact appears as a bilateral radiopaque artifact obscuring the mandible.

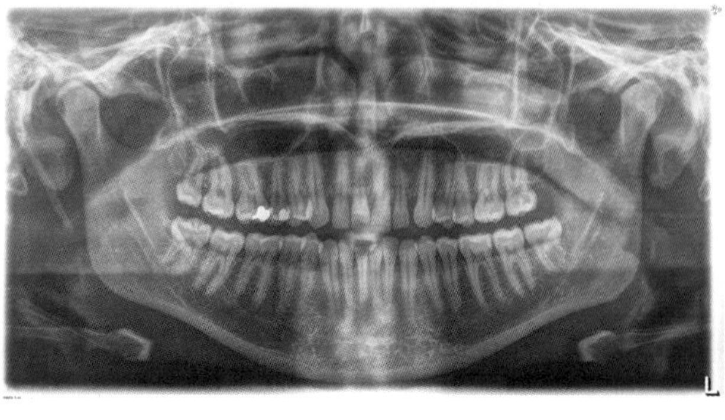

Fig 25-21 A radiolucent shadow will be superimposed over the apices of the maxillary teeth if the patient does not keep the tongue against the palate throughout the entire exposure.

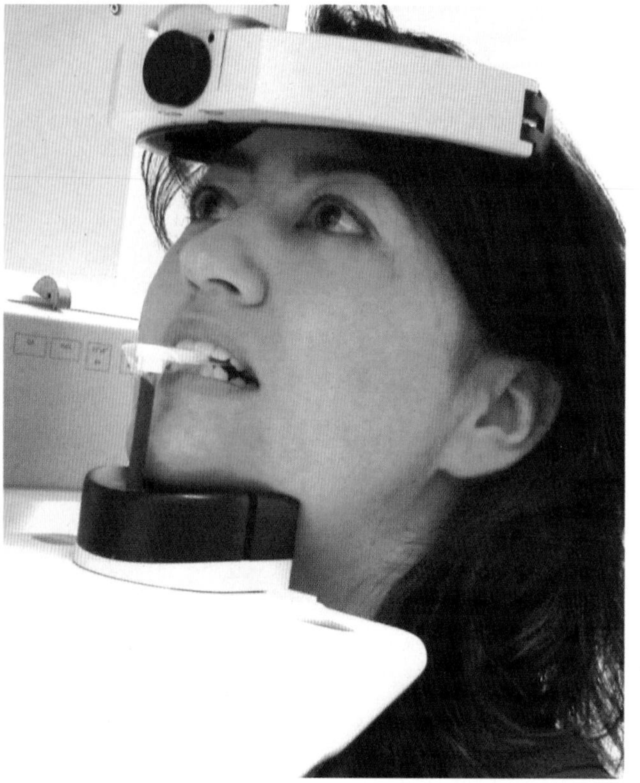

Fig 25-22 The patient's head is incorrectly positioned; the chin is tipped up.

- The hard palate and floor of the nasal cavity appear superimposed over the roots of the maxillary teeth.
- The maxillary incisors appear blurred and magnified.
- A loss of detail occurs in the maxillary incisor region.
- A "reverse smile line" (curved downward) is seen on the image (Figure 25-23).

Solution. To prevent such an error, the dental radiographer must carefully position the patient such that the Frankfort plane (imaginary plane that passes from the bottom of the eye socket through the top of the ear canal) is parallel to the floor.

Chin Tipped Down.

Problem. If the patient is positioned such that the chin is too low or is tipped down (Figure 25-24), the Frankfort plane is angled downward, and the following errors result:

- The condyles are positioned higher on the image.
- The hyoid bone forms a single widened line.
- The mandibular incisors appear blurred; roots may appear short.
- A loss of detail occurs in the anterior apical region.
- An "exaggerated smile line" or "jack-o'-lantern" appearance (curved upward) is seen on the image (Figure 25-25).

When the chin is tipped down too far, these anatomic features described may be severe, requiring a retake of the image.

Solution. To prevent such an error, the dental radiographer must carefully position the patient such that the Frankfort plane is parallel to the floor.

Teeth Anterior to the Focal Trough.

Problem. If the patient is positioned such that the anterior teeth are not positioned in the focal trough, as indicated by the groove in the bite-block, teeth appear blurred. If the patient's teeth are too far forward

HELPFUL HINT

The Frankfort Plane—Tipped Up

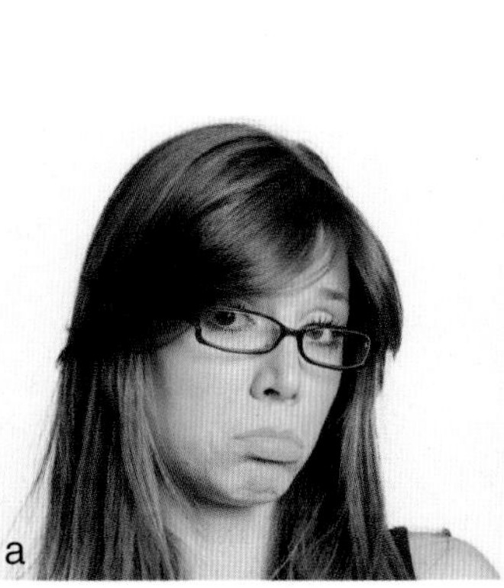

Frankfort plane
Plane parallel with floor

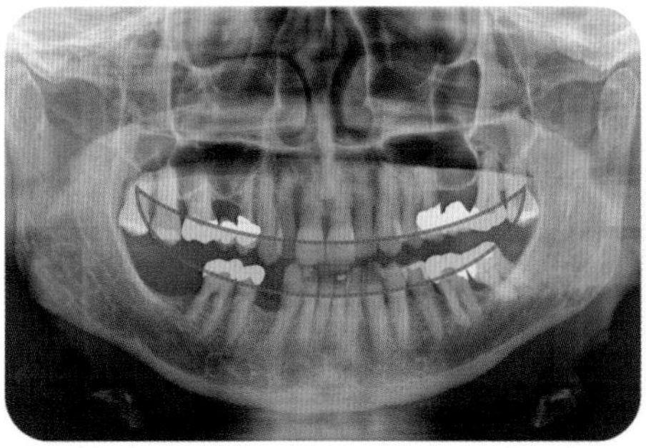

Reverse smile line
Chin tipped up

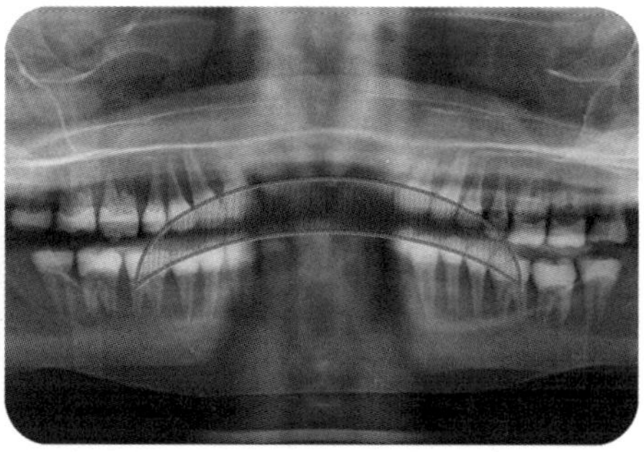

HELPFUL HINT

The Frankfort Plane—Tipped Down

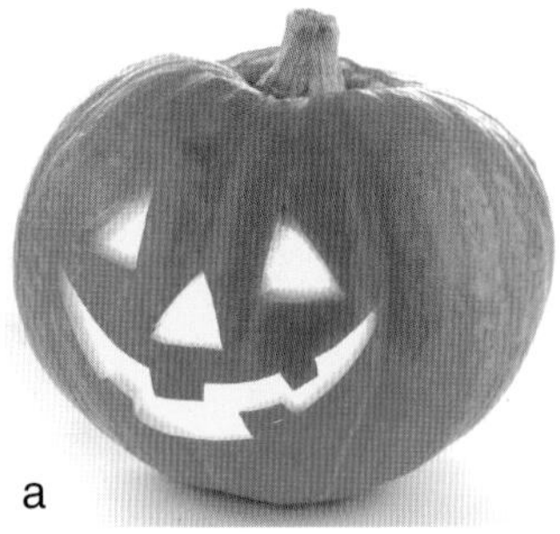

Frankfort plane
Plane parallel with floor

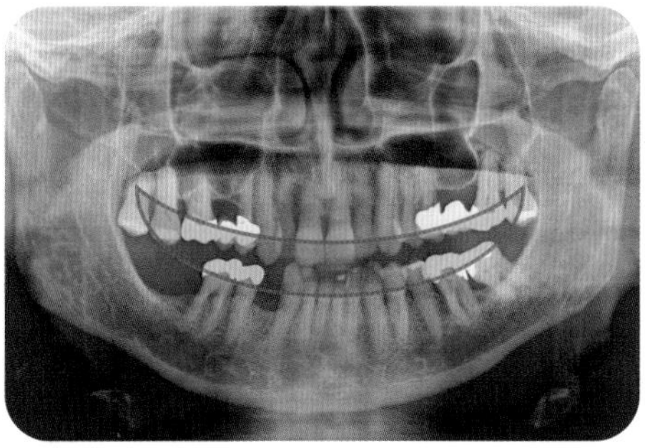

Exaggerated smile line
Chin tipped down

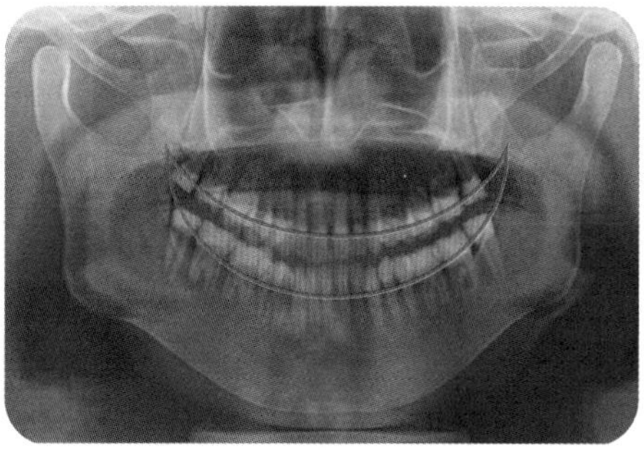

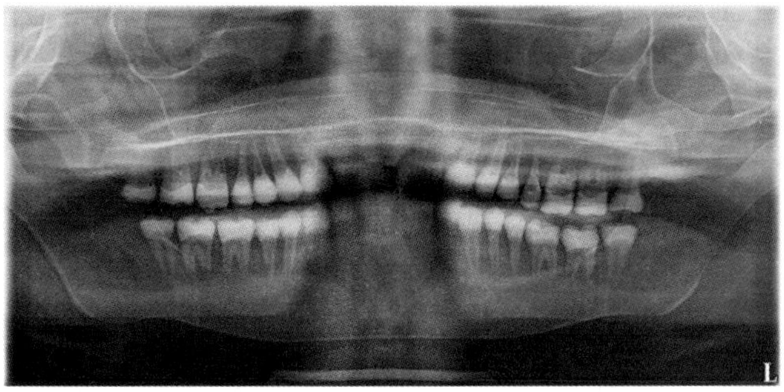

Fig 25-23 A "reverse smile line" is seen on a panoramic image when the patient's chin is tipped up. The condyles do not appear on the image.

on the bite-block or anterior to the focal trough (Figure 25-26), anterior teeth appear "narrow" and out of focus on the image (Figure 25-27). In addition, pronounced overlap of the premolars may be seen.

Solution. To prevent such an error, the dental radiographer must position the patient such that the anterior teeth are in an end-to-end position in the groove on the bite-block. The forehead support must then be adjusted to stabilize the patient's head position and prevent the patient from sliding forward on the bite-block.

Teeth Posterior to the Focal Trough.

Problem. If the patient's anterior teeth are not positioned in the focal trough, as indicated by the groove in the bite-block, the teeth appear blurred. If the patient's anterior teeth are aligned too far back on the bite-block or posterior to the focal trough (Figure 25-28), the teeth appear "widened" and out of focus on the image (Figure 25-29). Also, the roots of the anterior teeth may appear to be cut off.

Solution. To prevent such an error, the dental radiographer must position the patient such that the anterior teeth are in an end-to-end position in the groove on the bite-block.

Head Turned.

Problem. If the patient's head is turned slightly to one side and not centered on the bite-block (Figure 25-30), the structures on one side are closer to the receptor while the structures on the other side are farther away. As a result, the ramus and posterior teeth on one side of the image appear larger than those on the other side of the image. The side *farthest* from the receptor appears *magnified*, and the side *closest* to the receptor appears *smaller* (Figure 25-31). For example, if the patient's head is turned to the right, the teeth on the patient's right side are closer to the receptor. The teeth closest to the receptor demonstrate the least amount of magnification.

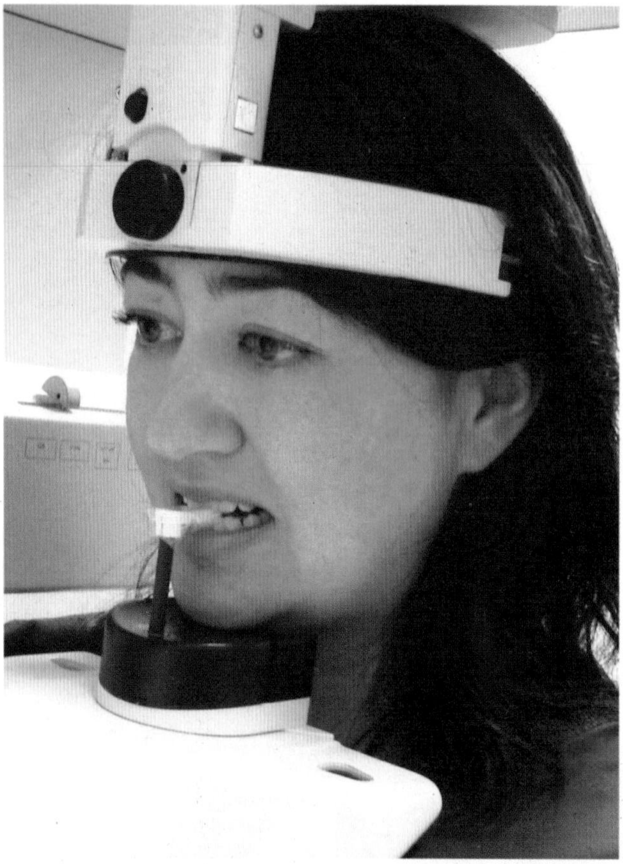

Fig 25-24 The patient's head is incorrectly positioned; the chin is tipped down.

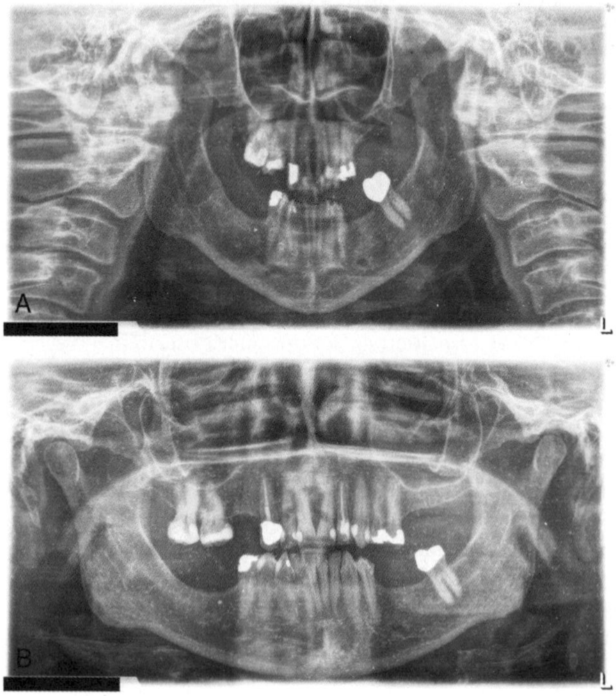

Fig 25-25 **A,** An "exaggerated smile line" is seen on a panoramic image when the patient's chin is tipped down. The anterior body of the mandible is widened vertically. **B,** Same patient when positioned correctly.

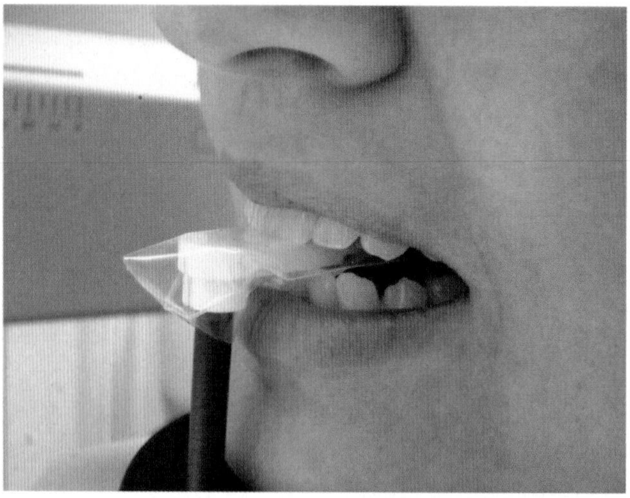

Fig 25-26 The patient is incorrectly positioned; the teeth have been placed too far forward on the bite-block.

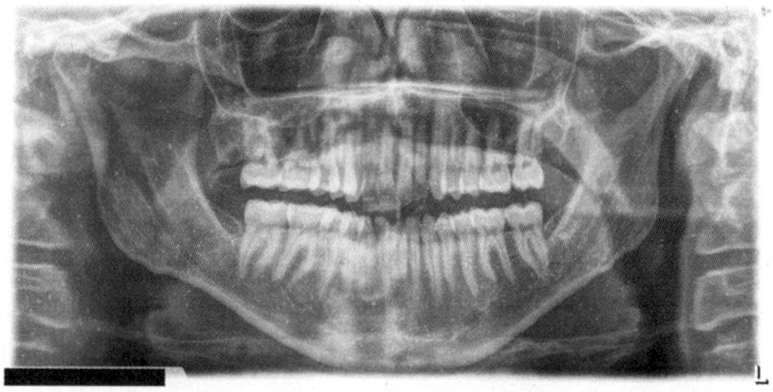

Fig 25-27 Anterior teeth appear narrowed and blurred on the panoramic image when the patient's teeth are positioned too far forward on the bite-block.

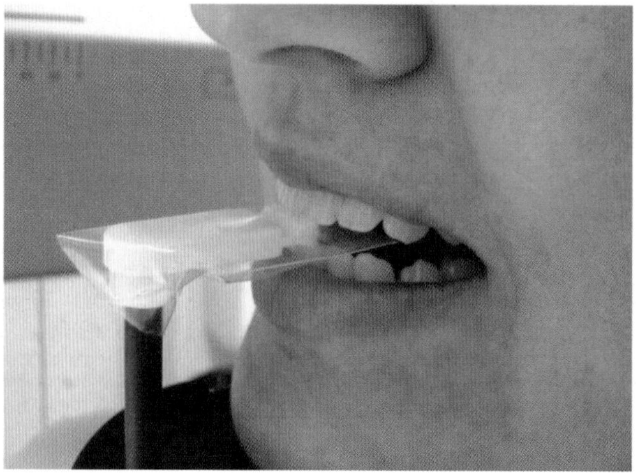

Fig 25-28 The patient is incorrectly positioned; the teeth have been placed too far back and not on the bite-block.

Solution. To prevent such an error, the dental radiographer must position the patient's head such that the midsagittal plane (imaginary plane that divides the face into right and left equal sides) is perpendicular to the floor while the midline is centered on the bite-stick. The

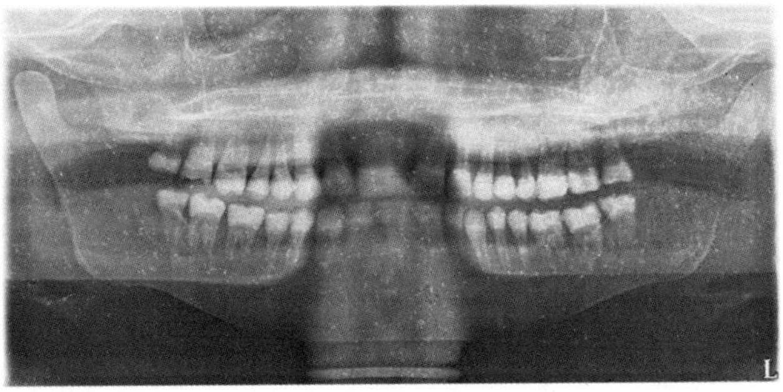

Fig 25-29 Anterior teeth appear widened and blurred on the panoramic image when the patient's teeth are positioned too far back on the bite-block.

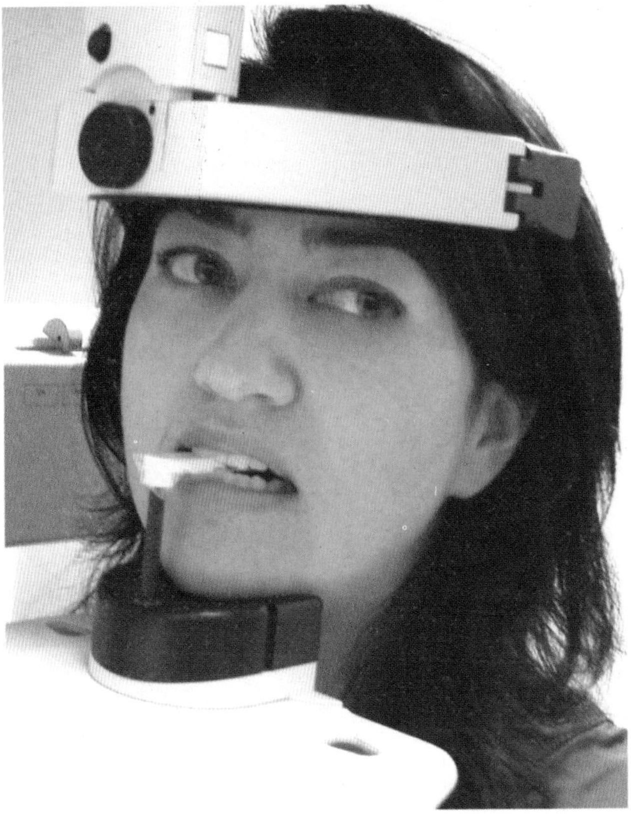

Fig 25-30 The patient is incorrectly positioned; the head is not centered.

lateral head supports must then be adjusted to stabilize the position of the patient's head.

Slumped Posture.

Problem. When the patient is slouched, slumped, or not standing with the shoulders back, the x-ray beam passes through more of the cervical spine because the beam is angled upward at a negative vertical angulation (−10 degrees). The cervical spine appears as a radiopacity in the center of the image and obscures diagnostic information (Figure 25-32).

Solution. To prevent such an error, the dental radiographer must instruct the patient to stand or sit "as tall as possible" with a straight back. An additional instruction to the patient may include "step forward slightly closer to the machine." This movement has the effect of straightening the cervical spine.

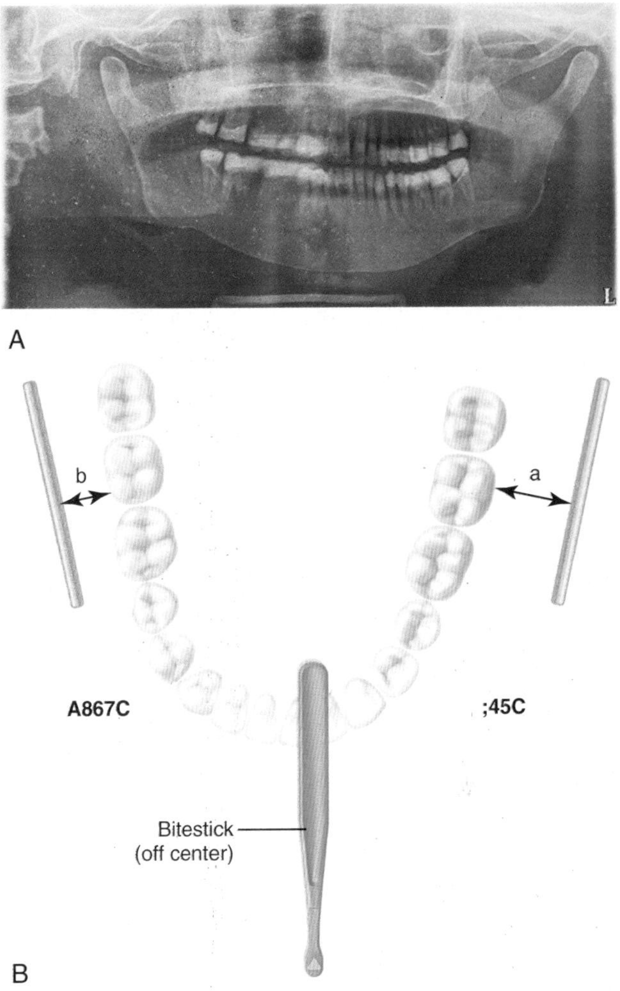

Fig 25-31 **A,** The patient's left ramus (the side farthest from the receptor) appears magnified on the panoramic image when the midsagittal plane is not aligned perpendicular to the floor. Notice that the posterior teeth on the left appear enlarged and have pronounced overlapped contacts. **B,** The diagram illustrates that if the head is turned to the right, then the teeth are closer to the receptor on that side.

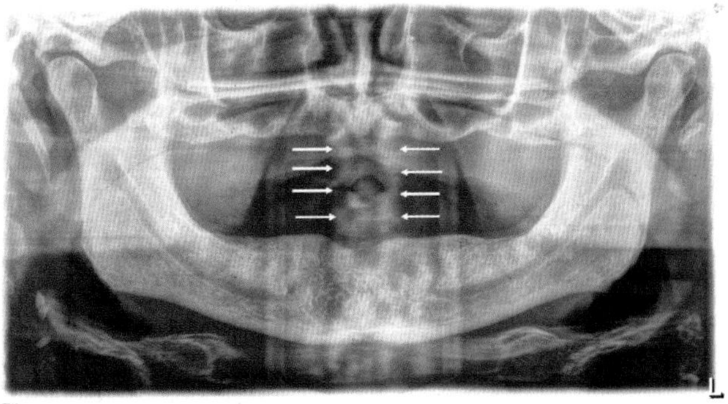

Fig 25-32 If the patient is not standing erect, superimposition of the cervical spine (arrows) may be seen at the center of the panoramic image.

Visit the Evolve site for interactive exercises on panoramic positioning errors.

For a summary of patient positioning errors and how each one affects areas of the panoramic image, see Table 25-1.

TABLE 25-1 Patient Positioning Errors and Affected Areas (See Box 25-1)

	Lips Open	Tongue Not on Palate	Chin Tipped Up	Chin Tipped Down	Anterior to Focal Trough	Posterior to Focal Trough	Head Turned	Slumped Posture
Area 1	anterior teeth obscured by radiolucent area where lips are parted	apices of maxillary anterior teeth obscured by radiolucent air space	apices of maxillary anterior teeth cut off reverse smile line seen	apices of mandibular anterior teeth cut off exaggerated smile line seen	anterior teeth appear narrow	anterior teeth appear wide	posterior teeth appear wide on one side and narrow on the other	anterior teeth obscured by radiopaque image of spine
Area 2					cervical spine superimposed over the ramus and condyles on both sides	ramus on each side appears large	ramus appears wide on side with wide teeth and narrow on other side	
Area 3		maxillary alveolar bone obscured by radiolucent air space	apices of maxillary teeth obscured by radiopaque band of hard palate			conchae are laterally distorted across maxillary sinus soft tissue of nose seen	conchae are laterally distorted across maxillary sinus on side with wide ramus	
Area 4				anterior body of mandible is widened vertically with overlapped hyoid bone				ghost image of spine obscures mid portion of mandible
Area 5			condyles seen near lateral edge of image or not visible	condyles seen near upper edge of image or cut off on both sides		condyles seen near lateral edge of image or not visible	earlobe seen on side with wide ramus	

ADVANTAGES AND DISADVANTAGES

As with all radiographic techniques, panoramic imaging has both advantages and disadvantages.

Advantages of Panoramic Imaging

1. *Field size.* The panoramic image covers the entire maxilla and mandible. More anatomic structures can be viewed on a panoramic image than with a complete mouth series (CMS). In addition, lesions and conditions of the jaws that may not be seen on intraoral images can be detected on a panoramic image.
2. *Simplicity.* Exposure of a panoramic receptor is relatively simple and requires minimal amounts of time and training for the dental radiographer.
3. *Patient cooperation.* The exposure of a panoramic image is more acceptable to the patient because no discomfort is involved. For example, children who cannot tolerate intraoral projections may find it easier to sit still during the exposure of a panoramic image.
4. *Minimal exposure.* A panoramic image involves only minimal radiation exposure of the patient.

Disadvantages of Panoramic Imaging

1. *Image quality.* The images seen on a panoramic image are not as sharp as images produced with intraoral projections. As a result, the panoramic image cannot be used to diagnose dental caries, periodontal disease, or periapical lesions.
2. *Focal trough limitations.* Objects of interest that are located outside the focal trough cannot be seen.
3. *Distortion.* Certain amounts of magnification, distortion, and overlapping are present on a panoramic image, even when proper technique is used.
4. *Equipment cost.* The cost of a panoramic x-ray unit is relatively high compared with the cost of an intraoral x-ray unit.

HELPFUL HINTS

For exposing panoramic receptors:

- **DO** cover the bite-block with a disposable plastic cover slip before positioning the patient.
- **DO** consider the patient size to choose the exposure factors (kilovoltage, milliamperage, time) according to the manufacturer's recommendations.
- **DO** briefly explain to the patient the imaging procedure that is about to be performed.
- **DO** place a lead apron *without* a thyroid collar on the patient and secure it.
- **DO** ask the patient to remove all dense objects from the head-and-neck area before positioning the patient.
- **DO** instruct the patient to stand or sit "as straight and tall as possible."
- **DO** instruct the patient to place his or her front teeth in the deep groove on the bite-block in an end-to-end position.
- **DO** position the midsagittal plane of the patient perpendicular to the floor.
- **DO** position the Frankfort plane of the patient parallel with the floor.
- **DO** instruct the patient to close the lips on the bite-block and to swallow once; then ask the patient to place the tongue against the roof of the mouth and to maintain that position during the exposure.
- **DO** instruct the patient to remain still during the exposure.

SUMMARY

- The panoramic image allows the dental professional to view a large area of the maxilla and the mandible on a single projection.
- Uses of the panoramic image include (1) evaluation of the dentition and surrounding structures; (2) evaluation of impacted teeth; (3) evaluation of eruption patterns and growth and development; (4) detection of diseases, lesions, and conditions of the jaws; (5) examination of extent of large lesions; and (6) evaluation of trauma.
- The panoramic image is typically used to supplement bite-wing and periapical images and is not a substitute for intraoral projections. The panoramic image should not be used to diagnose caries, periodontal disease, or periapical lesions.
- In panoramic imaging, both the receptor and the tubehead are connected and rotate simultaneously around the patient during exposure. Rotational centers allow the image layer to conform to the elliptical shape of the dental arches.
- The focal trough is a three-dimensional curved zone in which structures are clearly demonstrated on a panoramic image. Structures within the focal trough appear reasonably well defined, whereas structures outside the focal trough appear blurred.
- Special equipment, including the x-ray unit, the receptor, and—when using film—intensifying screens and a cassette, is necessary for the panoramic imaging procedure.
- Before preparing the patient for exposure of a panoramic projection, the following tasks must be completed: infection prevention procedures, equipment preparation, selection of the exposure factors, and adjustment of the panoramic x-ray machine according to patient height and proper alignment of movable parts.
- After preparing the equipment, the dental radiographer must prepare the patient by explaining the imaging procedure, placing the lead apron, and requesting that the patient remove all dense objects from the head-and-neck region.
- The patient must then be positioned according to the manufacturer's recommendations for the alignment of the spine, teeth, the midsagittal plane, the Frankfort plane, lips, and the tongue.
- The dental radiographer must be able to describe the features of a diagnostic panoramic image.
- The dental radiographer must be able to identify patient preparation and patient positioning errors and know the necessary steps to correct such errors.
- Advantages of panoramic imaging include field size, simplicity of use, patient cooperation, and minimal patient exposure to x-radiation.
- Disadvantages of panoramic imaging include image quality, limitations imposed by the focal trough, image distortion, and the high cost of equipment.

BIBLIOGRAPHY

Frommer HH, Stabulas-Savage JJ: Panoramic radiography. In Radiology for the dental professional, ed 9, St Louis, 2011, Mosby.

Johnson ON: Panoramic radiography. In Essentials of dental radiography for dental assistants and hygienists, ed 9, Upper Saddle River, NJ, 2011, Prentice Hall.

Langland OE, Langlais RP, Preece JW: Troubleshooting panoramic techniques. In Principles of dental imaging, ed 2, Philadelphia, 2002, Lippincott Williams & Wilkins.

Mallya SM, Lam EWN: Panoramic imaging. In White and Pharoah's Oral radiology: principles and interpretation, ed 8, St. Louis, 2019, Elsevier.

Miles DA, Van Dis ML, Jensen CW, et al: Panoramic imaging. In Radiographic imaging for the dental team, ed 4, Philadelphia, 2009, Saunders.

Miles DA, Van Dis ML, Razmus TF: Plain film extraoral radiographic techniques. In Basic principles of oral and maxillofacial radiology, Philadelphia, 1992, Saunders.

Olson SS: Auxiliary radiographic techniques. In Dental radiography laboratory manual, Philadelphia, 1995, Saunders.

QUIZ QUESTIONS

Multiple Choice

____ 1. Which describes a use of a panoramic image?
  a. evaluation of caries
  b. evaluation of periodontal disease
  c. evaluation of impacted molars
  d. evaluation of periapical disease

____ 2. The zone in which structures are clearly demonstrated on a panoramic image is termed the:
  a. focal trough
  b. rotation center
  c. ghost image
  d. midsagittal plane

____ 3. Rare earth intensifying screens are recommended in film-based panoramic imaging because:
  a. rare earth screens emit a blue light
  b. rare earth screens provide a more diagnostic image
  c. rare earth screens require less x-ray exposure for the patient
  d. the images convert faster in automatic processors

____ 4. A thyroid collar is not recommended in panoramic imaging because:
  a. it blocks the x-ray beam and obscures information
  b. there is a relatively low dose of radiation to the thyroid gland in panoramic imaging
  c. it is impossible to sterilize the thyroid collar
  d. all of the above

____ 5. Which imaginary plane passes from the bottom of the eye socket through the top of the ear canal?
   a. midsagittal
   b. Frankfort
   c. frontal
   d. axial

Matching

For questions 6 to 20, match the following types of procedures with the statements given below.

a. Panoramic imaging
b. Intraoral imaging
c. Both panoramic and intraoral imaging

____ **6.** The receptor and the tubehead rotate around the patient.
____ **7.** This type of image is used to examine the extent of large lesions.
____ **8.** The dental arches must be aligned to the focal trough.
____ **9.** The tubehead contains a filament used to produce electrons and a target used to produce x-rays.
____ **10.** The collimator is a lead plate with an opening in the shape of a narrow vertical slit.
____ **11.** The collimator is a lead plate with a small, round or rectangular opening.
____ **12.** The vertical angulation of the tubehead is variable.
____ **13.** A head positioner is used to position the patient's head.
____ **14.** A screen film is used.
____ **15.** A cassette holder with two intensifying screens is used.
____ **16.** The x-ray film must be loaded into a cassette in a darkroom under safelight conditions.
____ **17.** A lead apron with a thyroid collar must be placed on the patient.
____ **18.** Earrings and necklaces must be removed before exposure.
____ **19.** The midsagittal plane must be positioned perpendicular to the floor.
____ **20.** The vertebral column must be perfectly straight.

Essay

21. Discuss the equipment preparations necessary before exposure of a panoramic projection.
22. Discuss the patient preparations necessary before exposure of a panoramic projection.
23. Discuss the patient positioning steps necessary before exposure of a panoramic projection.
24. Give examples of Frankfort plane positioning errors, and discuss what steps can be taken to correct such errors.
25. Discuss the advantages and disadvantages of panoramic imaging.

Identify the Errors

26. Identify the cause of the large radiopaque area in Figure 25-33.
27. Identify the errors in Figure 25-34.
28. Identify the errors in Figure 25-35.
29. Identify the errors in Figure 25-36.
30. Identify the errors in Figure 25-37.
31. Identify the errors in Figure 25-38.
32. Identify why the right ramus appears wider than the left ramus in Figure 25-39.
33. Identify the errors in Figure 25-40.
34. Identify the errors in Figure 25-41.
35. Identify the errors in Figure 25-42.
36. Identify the errors in Figure 25-43.

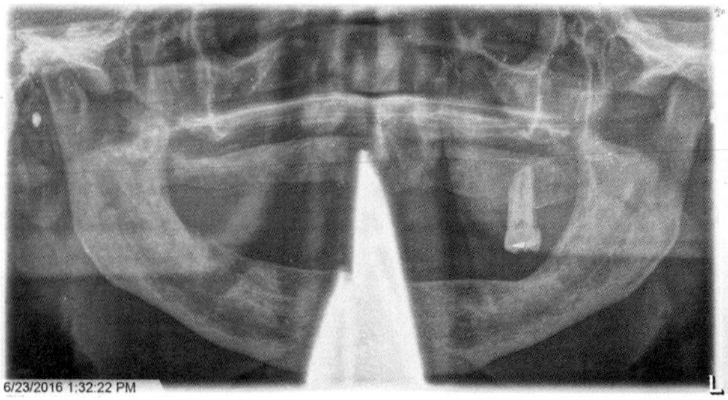

Fig 25-33

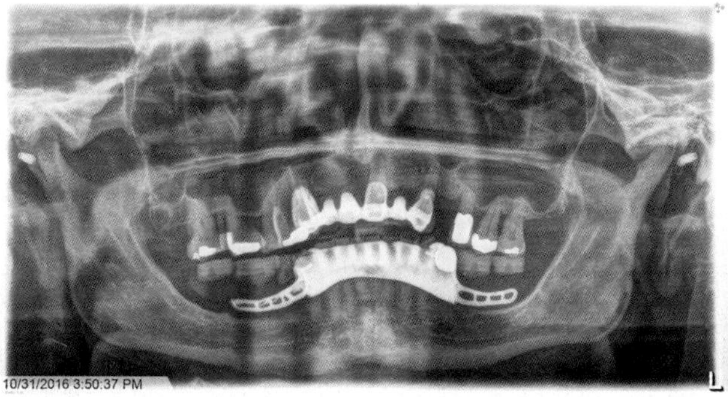

Fig 25-34

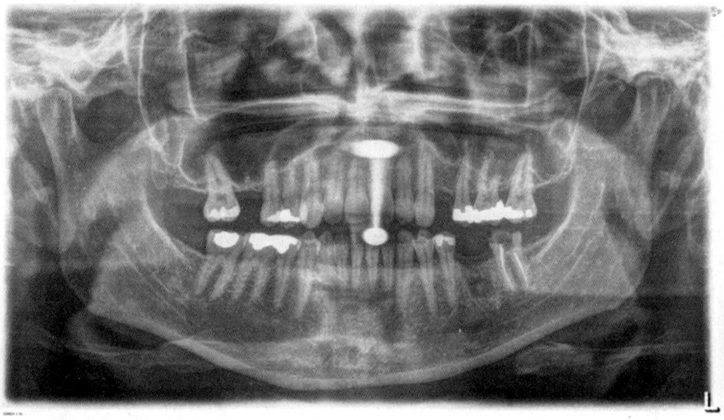

Fig 25-35

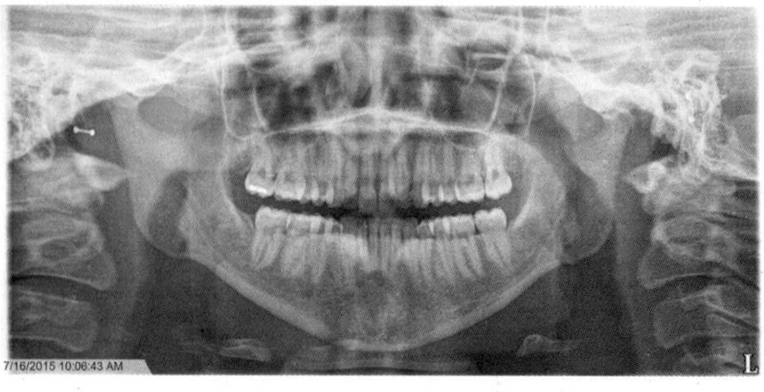

Fig 25-36

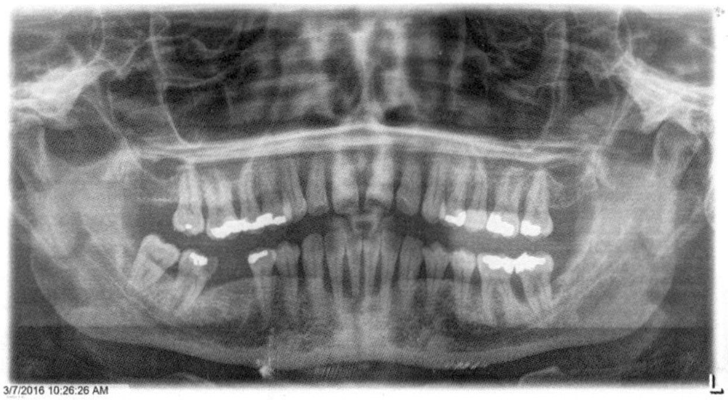

Fig 25-37

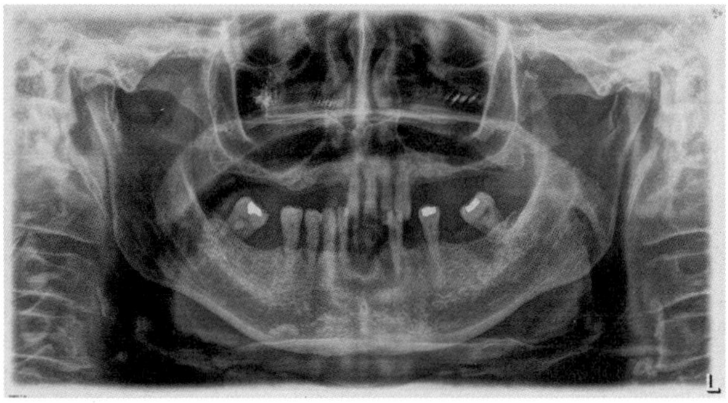

Fig 25-38

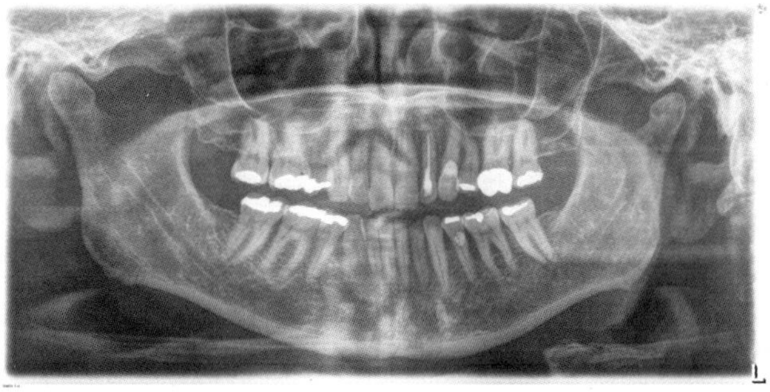

Fig 25-39

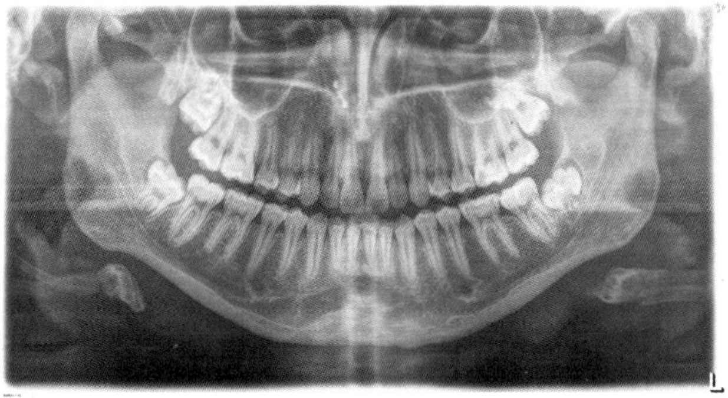

Fig 25-40

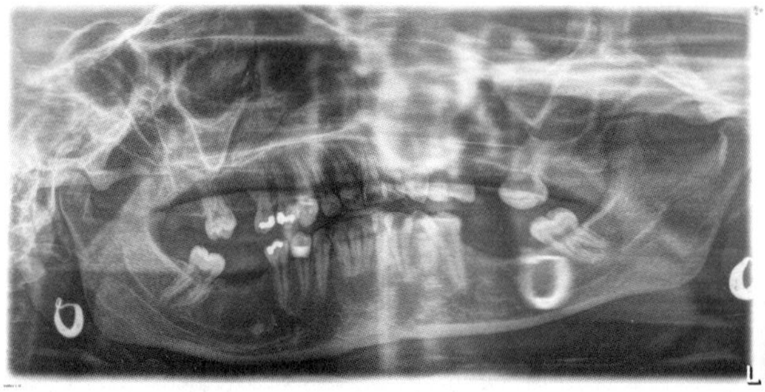

Fig 25-41

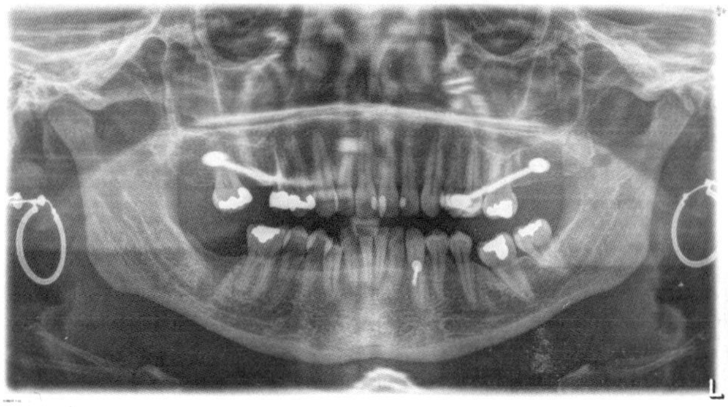

Fig 25-42

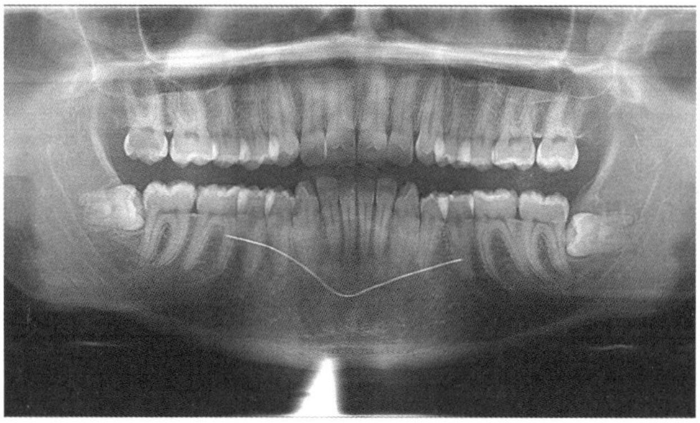

Fig 25-43 Courtesy Anthony Mecham DMD, Roseman University College of Dental Medicine, South Jordan, UT.

26

Extraoral Imaging

LEARNING OBJECTIVES

After completion of this chapter, the student will be able to do the following:

1. Define the key terms associated with extraoral imaging.
2. Describe the purpose and uses of extraoral imaging.
3. Describe the equipment used in extraoral imaging.
4. Detail the equipment and patient preparations necessary before exposing an extraoral projection.
5. Identify the purpose and describe the head position, the receptor placement, and the beam alignment for each of the following extraoral projections: lateral jaw projection—body of the mandible, lateral jaw projection—ramus of the mandible, lateral cephalometric projection, posteroanterior projection, Waters projection, submentovertex projection, reverse Towne projection, extraoral bite-wing images, and transcranial projection.

As discussed in Chapter 25, it is not always possible to obtain adequate diagnostic information from intraoral images alone. Jaw fractures, impacted teeth, and large lesions cannot be adequately examined on intraoral projections; in such cases, an extraoral image can be used to view a large area of the jaws and the skull.

In general dental practices, the panoramic image is one of the most popular extraoral projections. In dental specialty practices such as oral surgery and orthodontics, it is commonplace for additional extraoral projections to be used. Since the introduction of cone-beam computer tomography to dentistry, viewing anatomic structures in three dimensions may eliminate the need for the extraoral projections outlined in this chapter. Because many dental radiographers may not use the techniques detailed here, instructors using this text may choose to spend limited time on extraoral imaging, and this chapter may serve as a reference source if needed.

The purpose of this chapter is to present the basic concepts of extraoral imaging and describe the necessary patient and equipment preparations. In addition, this chapter introduces a number of extraoral projection techniques and describes receptor placement, patient positioning, and beam alignment for such projections.

BASIC CONCEPTS

As the term **extraoral** suggests, an extraoral receptor is one that is placed *outside the mouth* during x-ray exposure. **Extraoral imaging** is used to view large areas of the jaws or the skull. A variety of projections are used in extraoral imaging, and the choice of projection depends on what information is needed.

Purpose and Use

The extraoral image shows an overall view of the jaws and skull. The extraoral projection is typically used for the following purposes:

- To evaluate large areas of the skull and jaws
- To evaluate growth and development
- To evaluate impacted teeth
- To detect diseases, lesions, and conditions of the jaws
- To examine the extent of large lesions
- To evaluate trauma
- To evaluate the temporomandibular joint area

In some cases, an extraoral projection is indicated because the patient has swelling or discomfort and is unable to tolerate the placement of intraoral receptors. In other cases, an extraoral image may be a part of the records collection/information gathering process. An extraoral projection may be used alone or in conjunction with intraoral images. Like the panoramic projection, an extraoral image does not appear as defined or sharp as what is seen on an intraoral projection.

Equipment

X-Ray Units. A standard intraoral x-ray machine (see Chapter 7) may be used for some extraoral images (e.g., lateral jaw and transcranial projections). To aid in patient positioning and alignment of the x-ray beam, special head-positioning and beam-alignment devices can be added to the intraoral x-ray machine (Figure 26-1). Some panoramic x-ray units (see Chapter 25) may also be used for obtaining extraoral projections. In such cases, the panoramic x-ray tubehead is used in conjunction with a special extension arm and a device known as a **cephalostat**, or *craniostat* (Figure 26-2). The cephalostat includes a receptor holder and head positioner, which allows the dental radiographer to position both the receptor and the patient easily.

Image Receptors. Extraoral imaging may be digital or film-based; the dental radiographer must be familiar with both in order to work in a variety of dental practices. With digital imaging, the receptor is a sensor. In the technique section in this chapter, when the term *receptor* is used to refer to film-based imaging, it is referring to the cassette and its contents (screen film and intensifying screens).

Screen film is used for extraoral exposures. The screen film is sensitive to the light emitted from intensifying screens (see Chapter 9). The use of a screen film and intensifying screens minimizes the x-ray exposure necessary to produce a diagnostic image. As discussed in Chapters 9 and 25, some screen films are sensitive to green light (T-Mat), whereas others are sensitive to blue light (X-Omat DBF). Extraoral film sizes vary; the size most often used is 8×10 inch.

An occlusal receptor (size 4) may be used for some extraoral images (e.g., lateral jaw). In film-based extraoral imaging, the occlusal film is used as a **nonscreen film** and does not require the use of screens for exposure. As discussed in Chapter 9, a nonscreen film requires more exposure time than does a screen film. As a result, the occlusal film

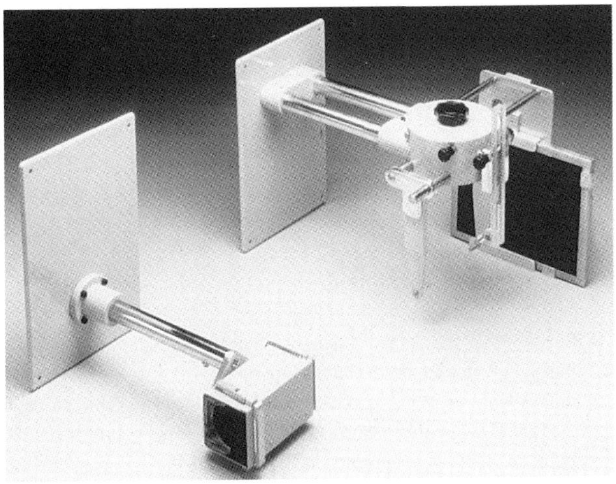

Fig 26-1 This unit can be used with most intraoral x-ray tubeheads. It is equipped with a collimator to allow accurate beam alignment and a head positioner to allow for proper patient positioning. (Courtesy Wehmer Corporation, Lombard, IL.)

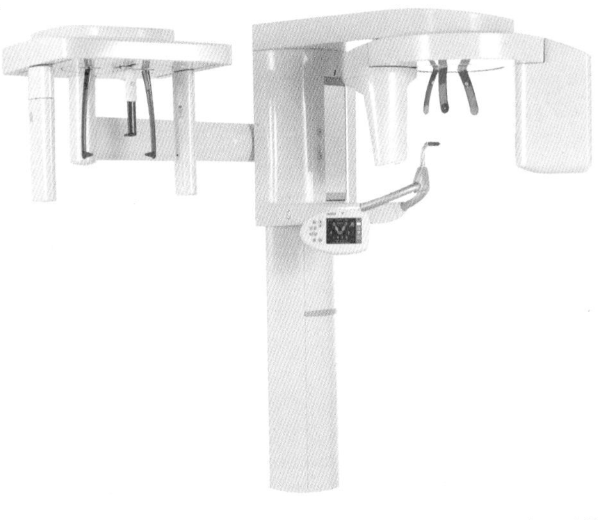

Fig 26-2 An extraoral imaging unit such as the Orthophos XG 5 contains a cephalostat for positioning the patient's head. (Courtesy Sirona USA, Charlotte, NC.)

used extraorally requires more radiation exposure than does a screen film. In addition, the occlusal film used extraorally does not cover as large an area as does a screen film.

Additional Equipment. In film-based extraoral imaging, additional equipment may include intensifying screens, a cassette, and a grid; these items are not used in digital imaging.

An intensifying screen is a device that converts x-ray energy into visible light; the light, in turn, exposes the screen film. As discussed in Chapters 9 and 25, calcium tungstate screens emit blue light, and rare earth screens emit green light. The screen film must be compatible with the light emitted from the screen; blue-sensitive film must be paired with screens that emit blue light, and green-sensitive film must be paired with screens that emit green light. Rare earth screens require less exposure than calcium tungstate screens and are recommended for film-based extraoral imaging. To minimize patient exposure, the fastest film and screen combination that provides a diagnostic image should be used.

HELPFUL HINT

Intensifying Screens

Calcium Tungstate Screens

- Emit **blue** light
- Used with **blue** sensitive film

Rare Earth Screens

- Emit **green** light
- Used with **green** sensitive film
- **More efficient**
- **Less x-ray exposure**

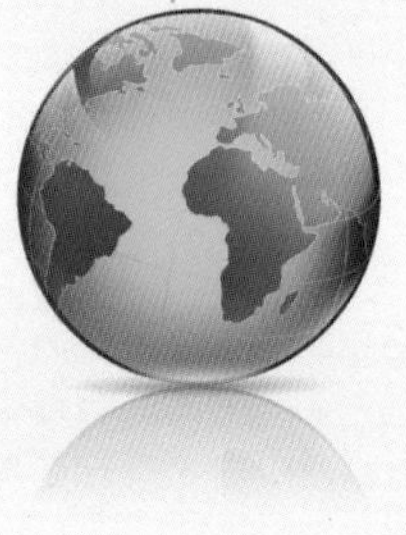

A cassette is used to hold the screen film in tight contact with the intensifying screens and to protect the film from exposure to light (see Chapter 9). Extraoral cassettes are rigid and are constructed of metal and plastic.

The front side of the cassette is typically constructed of plastic and permits the passage of the x-ray beam, whereas the back side is made of metal to reduce scatter radiation. The front side is also known as the "tube side," or the side that faces the x-ray beam. The front side of the cassette must always face the patient during exposure. The cassette must be labeled before exposure to orient the finished image; a metallic "R" or "L" can be used to identify the patient's right or left side. These metallic letters must always be placed on the front of the cassette.

In film-based imaging, a grid is a device that may be used to reduce the amount of scatter radiation that reaches an extraoral film during exposure. Scatter radiation causes film fog and reduces contrast. A grid can be used to decrease film fog and increase the contrast of the image.

A grid is composed of a series of thin lead strips embedded in a material (e.g., plastic) that permits the passage of the x-ray beam. The grid is placed between the patient's head and the film. During exposure, the grid permits the passage of the x-ray beam between the lead strips. When some of the x-rays interact with the patient's tissues, scatter radiation is produced; this scatter radiation is then directed at the grid and the film at an angle. As a result, scatter radiation is absorbed by the lead strips and does not reach the surface of the film to cause film fog (Figure 26-3). To compensate for the lead strips found in the grid, exposure time must be increased. Because of this increase in exposure time, a grid should be used only when improved image quality and high contrast are necessary.

Diagnostic Extraoral Image

A diagnostic extraoral image must demonstrate accurate anatomic features and proper density and contrast. The anatomic features vary depending on the extraoral projection. Proper density and contrast result from the use of correct exposure factors as recommended by the x-ray unit manufacturer.

STEP-BY-STEP PROCEDURES

Step-by-step procedures for the exposure of an extraoral projection include equipment preparation, patient preparation, and patient positioning. Before exposing an extraoral projection, infection prevention procedures (as described in Chapter 16) must be completed. If an extraoral x-ray unit with cephalostat is used, the ear rods must be disinfected between patients.

PROCEDURE 26-1 Equipment Preparation for Extraoral Imaging

1. Prepare receptor
   - If using a digital sensor, follow manufacturer recommendations.
   - If using screen film, load the extraoral cassette in the darkroom under safelight conditions.
   - Place one screen film between two intensifying screens, and securely close.
2. Choose exposure factors
   - Set exposure factors (kilovoltage, milliamperage, time) according to the manufacturer's recommendations.

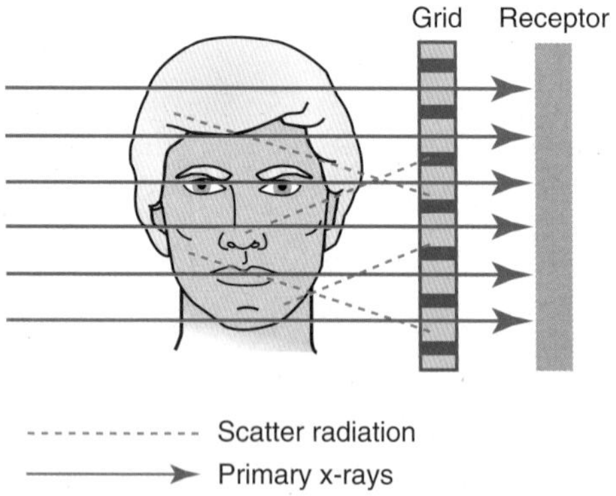

Fig 26-3 A grid decreases the amount of scatter radiation that reaches the extraoral receptor. (Courtesy Dr. Robert M. Jaynes, Columbus, OH.)

Equipment Preparation

The dental radiographer must prepare the equipment *before* preparing a patient for the exposure of an extraoral projection (Procedure 26-1). The equipment preparation varies depending on the receptor used (digital sensor or film) and the specific extraoral x-ray unit. The dental radiographer must be familiar with the manufacturer's specific directions for equipment preparation found in the instruction manual.

Patient Preparation

After preparing the equipment, the dental radiographer must prepare the patient for the procedure (Procedure 26-2). Patient preparation is the same for digital and film-based extraoral imaging.

Patient Positioning

Patient positioning varies with each extraoral projection and is discussed in the section of this chapter on specific extraoral projection techniques.

EXTRAORAL PROJECTION TECHNIQUES

A variety of projection techniques are used in extraoral imaging (Table 26-1). The purpose, receptor placement, head position, beam alignment, and exposure factors differ for each projection used. Extraoral projection techniques are classified by the area of interest and include:

- Lateral jaw imaging
- Skull imaging
- Extraoral bite-wing imaging
- Temporomandibular joint imaging

PROCEDURE 26-2 Patient Preparation for Extraoral Imaging

1. Explain imaging procedure
   - Briefly explain the imaging procedure to the patient.
2. Place lead apron
   - Place and secure a lead apron without a thyroid collar on the patient.
   - Place the lead apron low around the neck so that it does not block the x-ray beam.
   - Use a double-sided lead apron to protect the patient (see Chapter 25).
3. Remove all objects
   - Request that the patient remove all objects from the head-and-neck region that may interfere with the procedure.
   - Items to remove include eyeglasses, earrings, facial and intraoral piercings, necklaces, napkin chains, hearing aids, hairpins, barrettes, and any intraoral prostheses (complete and partial dentures).

Lateral Jaw Imaging

Lateral jaw imaging is used to examine the posterior region of the mandible and is valuable for use in children, in patients with limited jaw opening resulting from a fracture or swelling, and in patients who have difficulty stabilizing or tolerating intraoral receptor placement. Although lateral jaw imaging is useful, it is important to note that the panoramic image is preferred because more diagnostic information is obtained.

As the term *lateral jaw imaging* indicates, the receptor in this extraoral projection is positioned lateral to the jaw during exposure. Lateral jaw imaging does not require the use of a special x-ray unit; a standard intraoral x-ray machine can be used. The following two techniques are used with lateral jaw projection:

- Body of mandible
- Ramus of mandible

Body of Mandible.

Purpose. The purpose of the **lateral jaw projection—body of mandible** is to evaluate impacted teeth, fractures, and lesions located in the body of the mandible. This projection demonstrates the mandibular premolar and molar regions and the inferior border of the mandible (Figure 26-4).

Receptor placement. The receptor is placed flat against the patient's cheek and is centered over the body of the mandible. The receptor must also be positioned parallel with the body of the mandible. The patient must hold the receptor in position, with the thumb placed under the edge and the palm against the outer surface.

Head position. The head is tipped approximately 15 degrees toward the side being imaged. The chin is extended and elevated slightly.

Beam alignment. The central ray is directed to a point just below the inferior border of the mandible on the side *opposite* the receptor. The beam is directed upward (−15 to −20 degrees) and centered on the body of the mandible. The beam must be directed perpendicular to the receptor.

Exposure factors. Exposure factors for this lateral jaw projection vary with the receptor and equipment used.

Ramus of Mandible.

Purpose. The purpose of the **lateral jaw projection—ramus of mandible** is to evaluate impacted third molars, large lesions, and fractures that extend into the ramus of the mandible. This projection demonstrates a view of the ramus from the angle of the mandible to the condyle (Figure 26-5).

TABLE 26-1 Extraoral Projection Techniques

Projection	Receptor Placement	Head Position	X-Ray Beam Point of Entry
Lateral jaw, body (mandible)	Flat against cheek Centered over body of mandible	Tipped 15 degrees toward side being imaged Chin extended and elevated	Below inferior border of mandible Vertical angulation −15 to −20 degrees ⊥ to horizontal plane of receptor
Lateral jaw, ramus (mandible)	Flat against cheek Centered over ramus of mandible	Tipped 15 degrees toward side being imaged Chin extended and elevated	Posterior to third molar area Vertical angulation −15 to −20 degrees ⊥ to horizontal plane of receptor
Lateral cephalometric	⊥ to floor Long axis horizontal	Left side near receptor MSP ⊥ to floor FP || to floor	Centered over receptor and ⊥ to receptor
Posteroanterior	⊥ to floor Long axis vertical	Forehead and nose touch receptor MSP ⊥ to floor FP || to floor	Centered over receptor and ⊥ to receptor
Waters	⊥ to floor Long axis vertical	Chin touches receptor Tip of nose 1-2 inches from receptor MSP ⊥ to floor	Centered over receptor and ⊥ to receptor
Submentovertex	⊥ to floor Long axis vertical	Head tipped back Top of head touches receptor MSP and FP ⊥ to floor	Centered over receptor and ⊥ to receptor
Reverse Towne	⊥ to floor Long axis vertical	Head tipped down Mouth open Top of forehead touches receptor MSP ⊥ to floor	Centered over receptor and ⊥ to receptor
Transcranial	Flat against ear Centered over TMJ	MSP ⊥ to floor	2 inches above and 0.5 inch below the ear canal opening Vertical angulation +25 degrees Horizontal angulation 20 degrees

FP, Frankfort plane; *MSP*, midsagittal plane; *TMJ*, temporomandibular joint; ⊥, perpendicular; ||, parallel.

Receptor placement. The receptor is placed flat against the patient's cheek and is centered over the ramus of the mandible. The receptor is also positioned parallel with the ramus of the mandible. The patient must hold the receptor in position, with the thumb placed under the edge and the palm placed against the outer surface.

Head position. The head is tipped approximately 15 degrees toward the side being imaged. The chin is extended and elevated slightly.

Beam alignment. The central ray is directed to a point posterior to the third molar region on the side *opposite* the receptor. The beam is directed upward (−15 to −20 degrees) and centered on the ramus of the mandible. The beam must be directed perpendicular to the receptor.

Exposure factors. Exposure factors for this lateral jaw projection vary with the receptor and equipment used.

Skull Imaging. Skull imaging is used to examine the bones of the face and skull and is most often used in oral surgery and orthodontics. Most skull projections require the use of an extraoral x-ray unit and a cephalostat.

Images of the skull may be difficult to interpret because of the numerous anatomic structures that exist in a very small area; these structures often appear superimposed over each other. In many cases, multiple exposures may be necessary to obtain a clear view of the area in question. The most common skull images and their uses are listed in Table 26-2.

Lateral Cephalometric Projection.

Purpose. The purpose of the lateral cephalometric projection is to evaluate facial growth and development, trauma, and disease and developmental abnormalities. This projection demonstrates the bones of the face and skull, as well as the soft tissue profile of the face (Figure 26-6). In film-based imaging, the soft tissue outline of the face is more readily seen when a filter is used. A filter is placed at the x-ray source or between the patient and the receptor and serves to remove some of the x-rays that pass through the soft tissue of the face, thus enhancing the image of the soft tissue profile of the face.

Receptor placement. The receptor is placed perpendicular to the floor in a receptor-holding device. The long axis of the receptor is positioned *horizontally*.

Head position. The left side of the patient's head is positioned adjacent to the receptor. The midsagittal plane (an imaginary plane that divides the face in half) must be aligned perpendicular to the floor and parallel to the receptor. The Frankfort plane (a plane extending from the bottom of the eye socket to the top of the ear canal) is aligned parallel to the floor. The head is centered over the receptor.

Beam alignment. The central ray is directed through the center of the receptor and perpendicular to the receptor.

Exposure factors. Exposure factors for the lateral cephalometric projection vary with the receptor and equipment used.

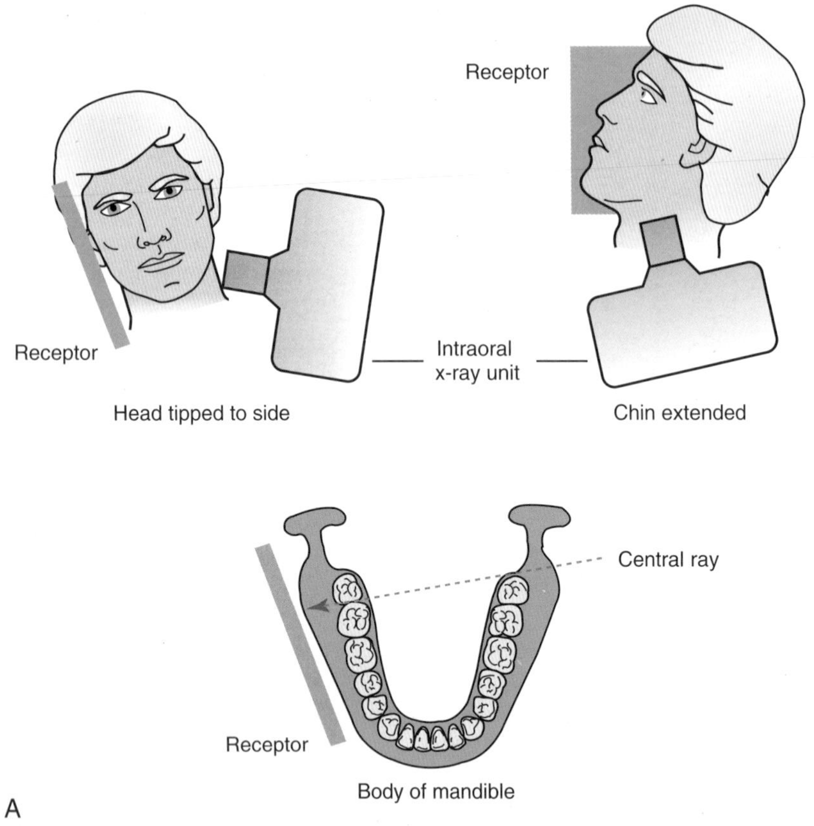

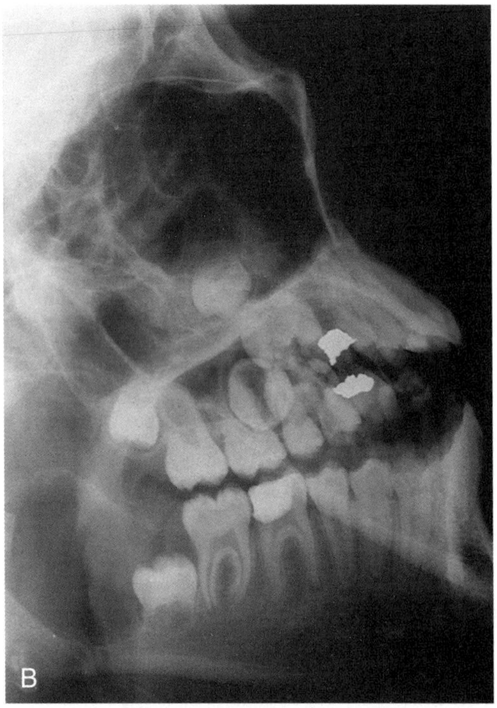

Fig 26-4 **A,** For the lateral jaw projection of the body of the mandible, proper patient positioning and receptor positioning are shown as viewed from the front and side of the patient. **B,** Example of lateral jaw image—body of mandible. (**A,** Courtesy Dr. Robert M. Jaynes, Columbus, OH. **B,** From Miles: Radiographic imaging for the dental team, ed 4, St Louis, 2009, Saunders.)

TABLE 26-2 Skull Imaging

Projection	Use
Lateral cephalometric	To evaluate **facial growth and development**, trauma, disease and developmental abnormalities; shows **soft tissue profile**
Posteroanterior	To evaluate facial growth and development, **trauma**, disease and developmental abnormalities; shows sinuses, nasal cavity, and orbits
Waters	To evaluate the **maxillary sinus area;** shows sinuses, nasal cavity, and orbits
Submentovertex	To identify the **position of the condyles**, demonstrate the base of the skull, and evaluate **fractures of the zygomatic arch**
Reverse Towne	To identify **fractures of the condylar neck and ramus**
Temporomandibular joint (TMJ)	To evaluate the **TMJ area**

Posteroanterior Projection.

Purpose. The purpose of the posteroanterior projection is to evaluate facial growth and development, trauma, and disease and developmental abnormalities. This projection also demonstrates the frontal and ethmoid sinuses, the orbits, and the nasal cavity (Figure 26-7).

Receptor placement. The receptor is positioned perpendicular to the floor in a receptor-holding device. The long axis of the receptor is positioned *vertically*.

Head position. The patient faces the receptor; the forehead and nose both touch the receptor. The midsagittal plane is aligned perpendicular to the floor, and the Frankfort plane is aligned parallel to the floor. The head is centered over the receptor.

Beam alignment. The central ray is directed through the center of the head and perpendicular to the receptor.

Exposure factors. Exposure factors for the posteroanterior projection vary with the receptor and equipment used.

Waters Projection.

Purpose. The purpose of the Waters projection is to evaluate the maxillary sinus area. This projection also demonstrates the frontal and ethmoid sinuses, the orbits, and the nasal cavity (Figure 26-8).

Receptor placement. The receptor is positioned perpendicular to the floor in a receptor-holding device. The long axis of the receptor is positioned *vertically*.

Head position. The patient faces the receptor and elevates the chin; the chin touches the receptor, and the tip of the nose is positioned 0.5 to 1 inch away from the receptor. The midsagittal plane must be aligned perpendicular to the floor, and the head is centered over the receptor.

Beam alignment. The central ray is directed through the center of the head and perpendicular to the receptor.

Exposure factors. Exposure factors for the Waters projection vary with the receptor and equipment used.

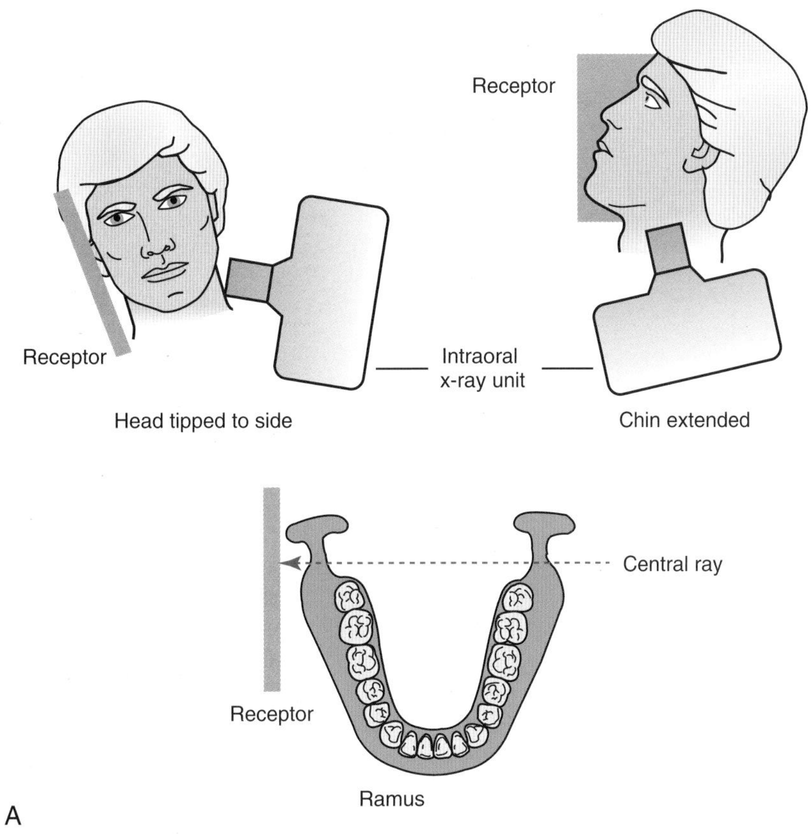

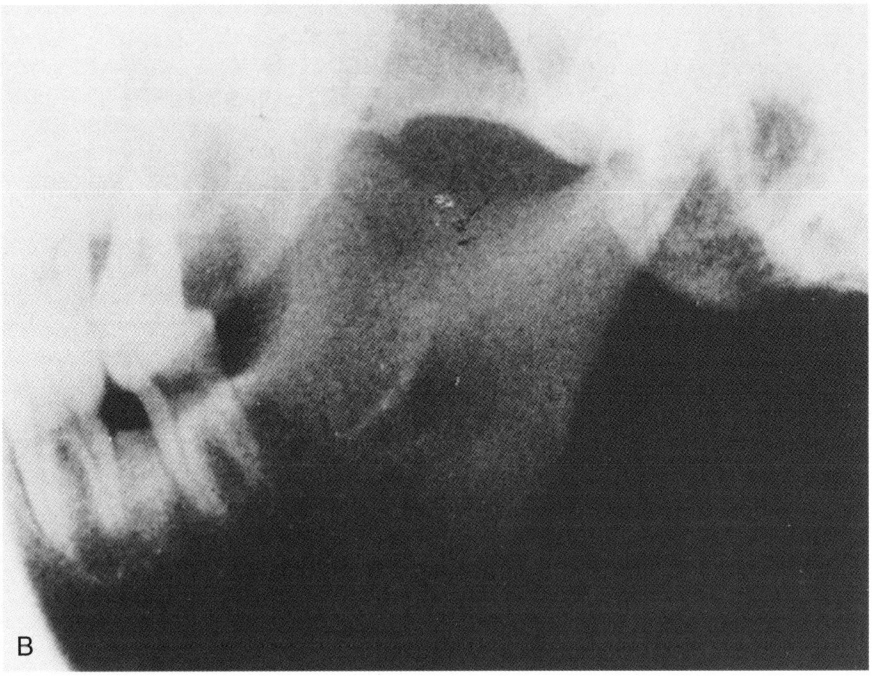

Fig 26-5 A, For the lateral jaw projection of the ramus of the mandible, proper patient positioning and receptor positioning are shown as viewed from the front and side of the patient. B, Example of lateral jaw image—ramus of mandible. (A and B, Courtesy Dr. Robert M. Jaynes, Columbus, OH.)

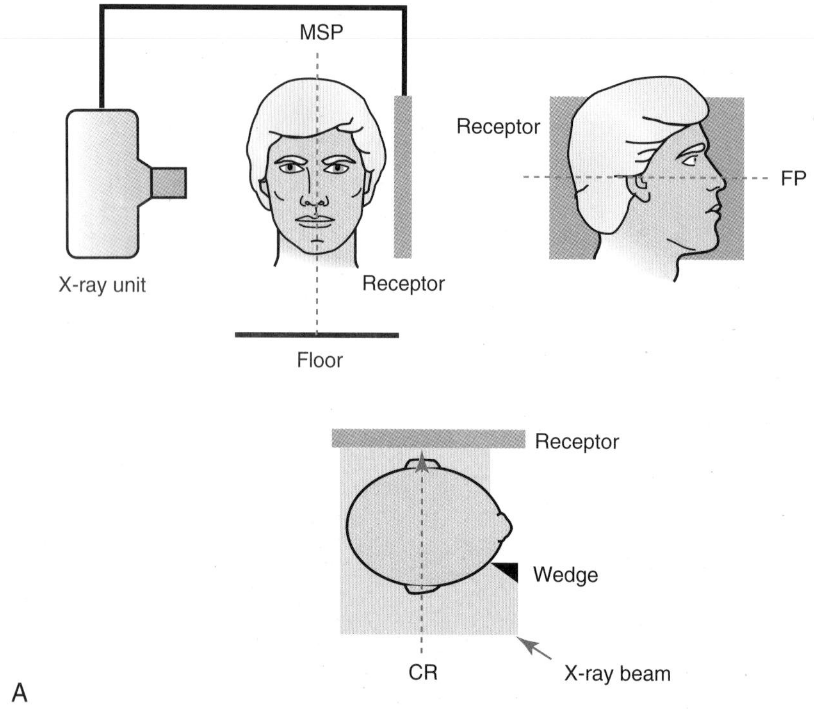

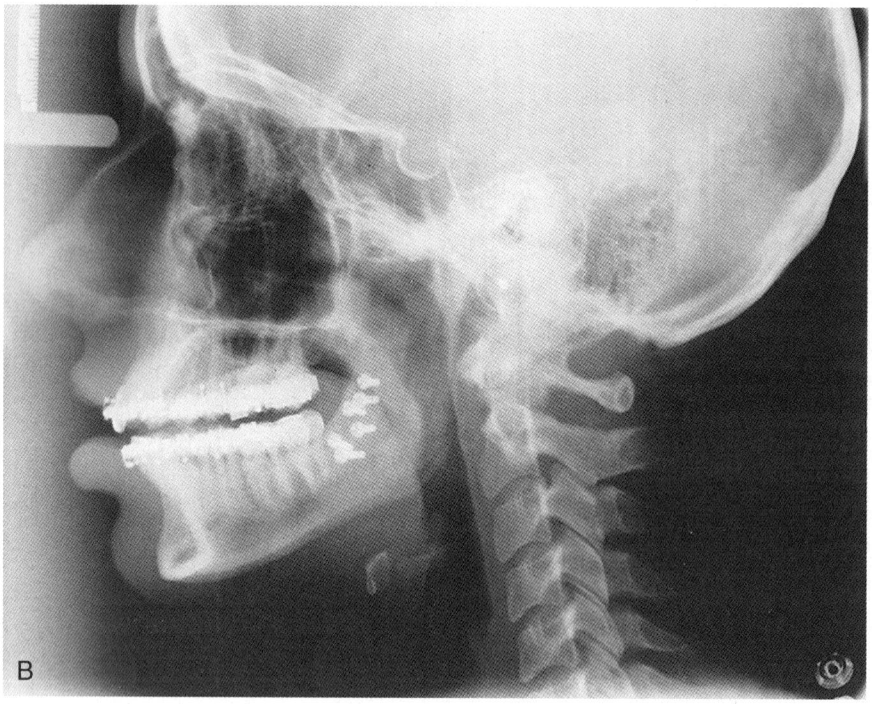

Fig 26-6 **A,** For the lateral cephalometric projection, proper patient positioning and receptor positioning are shown as viewed from the front, side, and top of the patient. *CR*, central ray; *FP*, Frankfort plane; *MSP*, Midsagittal plane. **B,** Example of lateral cephalometric image. (**A** and **B,** Courtesy Dr. Robert M. Jaynes, Columbus, OH.)

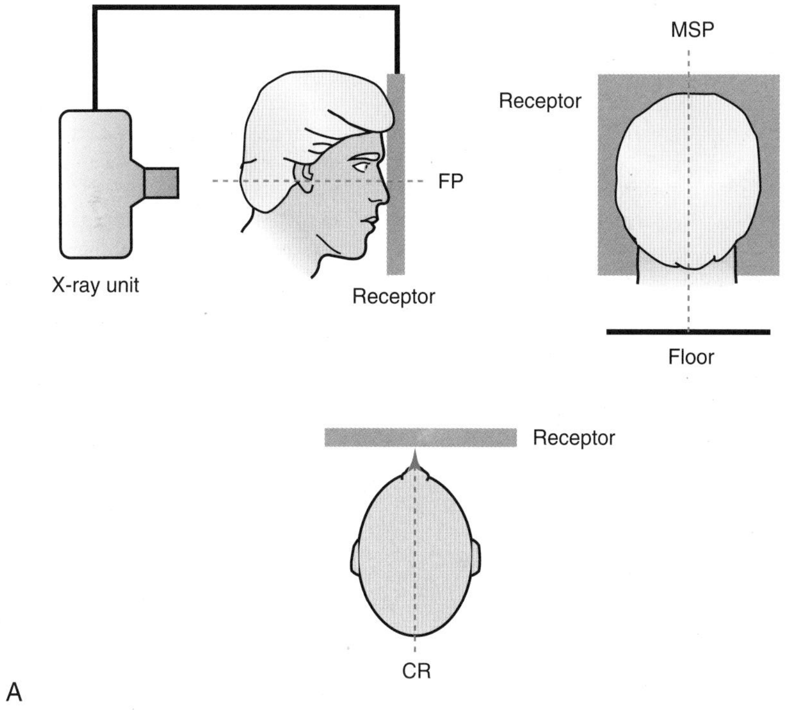

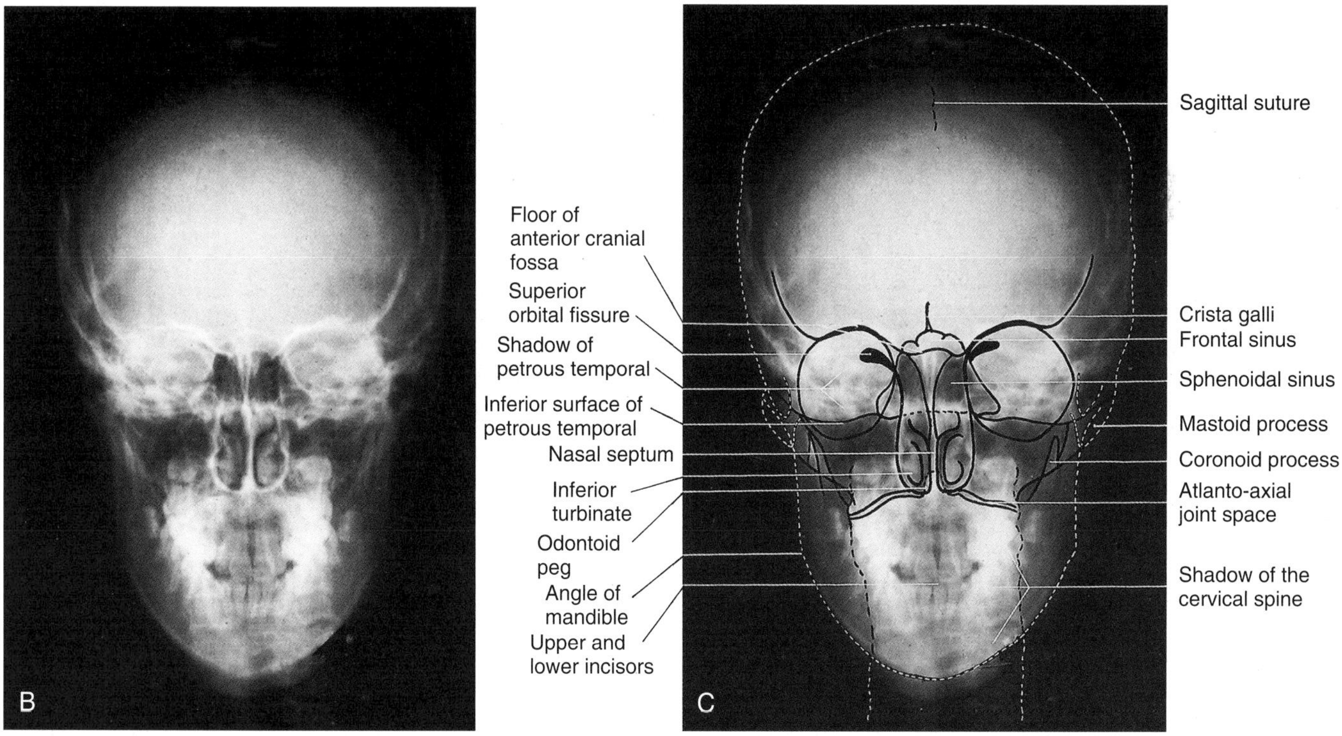

Fig 26-7 A, For the posteroanterior skull projection, proper patient positioning and receptor positioning are shown as viewed from the side, back, and top of the patient. *MSP*, Midsagittal plane; *FP*, Frankfort plane; *CR*, central ray. **B,** Example of a posteroanterior skull image. **C,** Anatomic landmarks identified in the posteroanterior image. (**A,** Courtesy Dr. Robert M. Jaynes, Columbus, OH. **B** and **C,** From Whaites and Drage: Essentials of dental radiography and radiology, ed 5, London, 2013, Churchill Livingstone.)

Submentovertex Projection.

Purpose. The purpose of the submentovertex projection is to identify the position of the condyles, demonstrate the base of the skull, and evaluate fractures of the zygomatic arch. This projection also demonstrates the sphenoid and ethmoid sinuses and the lateral wall of the maxillary sinus (Figure 26-9).

Receptor placement. The receptor is positioned perpendicular to the floor in a receptor-holding device. The long axis of the receptor is positioned *vertically*.

Head position. The patient's head and neck are tipped back as far as possible; the vertex (top) of the skull touches the receptor. Both the midsagittal plane and the Frankfort plane are aligned perpendicular to the floor. The head is centered on the receptor.

Beam alignment. The central ray is directed through the center of the head and perpendicular to the receptor.

Exposure factors. Exposure factors for this projection vary with the receptor and equipment used. If the zygomatic arch is the area of interest, the exposure time is reduced to approximately one-third the normal exposure time for a submentovertex projection.

Reverse Towne Projection.

Purpose. The purpose of the reverse Towne projection is to identify fractures of the condylar neck and ramus area (Figure 26-10).

Receptor placement. The receptor is positioned perpendicular to the floor in a receptor-holding device. The long axis of the receptor is positioned *vertically*.

Head position. The patient faces the receptor, with the head tipped down and the mouth open as wide as possible; the chin rests on the chest, and the top of the forehead touches the receptor. The midsagittal plane must be aligned perpendicular to the floor, and the head is centered on the receptor.

Beam alignment. The central ray is directed through the center of the head and perpendicular to the receptor.

Exposure factors. Exposure factors for the reverse Towne projection varies with the receptor and equipment used.

Extraoral Bite-wing Imaging. As discussed in Chapter 21, bite-wing images reveal the crowns of the maxillary and mandibular teeth, interproximal regions and crestal bone on one image. The bite-wing image is primarily used for detection of dental caries. Bite-wing images are traditionally acquired from intraoral x-ray machines. Currently, manufacturers of panoramic x-ray equipment have developed machines that not only obtain panoramic images but extraoral bite-wings as well.

Extraoral bite-wing images are anatomically accurate and provide a great deal of information with each scan (Figure 26-11). The extraoral bite-wing is a useful alternative for the patient who experiences discomfort with intraoral exposures, therefore reducing retakes. This image is also helpful for children or other patients with special needs, such as a gag reflex, large tori, or a small mouth (Figure 26-12).

Purpose. The purpose of the extraoral bite-wing (also referred to as the *panoramic bite-wing*) is to provide diagnostic information about the maxillary and mandibular teeth, the interproximal regions, the periapical bone, and surrounding structures (Figure 26-13). The extraoral bite-wing image is similar to the traditional bite-wing image, but a larger view of dental anatomic structures is revealed. Therefore one exposure per side is sufficient to cover the entire right or left side of the patient.

Receptor placement. The receptor is placed according to manufacturer's recommendations for panoramic imaging.

Head position. The head is positioned with the Frankfort plane parallel to the floor, the midsagittal plane perpendicular to the floor, and the anterior teeth on the bite stick, placing the teeth into the focal trough. Instruct the patient to stand straight and hold still during the entire exposure. As with most extraoral imaging procedures, all removable items in the head and neck region (such as eyeglasses, jewelry, intraoral prostheses) must be removed before exposure.

Beam alignment. The beam alignment is dependent on the panoramic machine.

Exposure factors. Exposure factors for the extraoral bite-wing vary with the receptor and equipment used. Adjustments can be made for children, teenagers and adults, as well as jaw size. Some exposure times may be shorter than panoramic imaging as the scan time is quick.

It should be noted that errors seen with panoramic imaging may also be seen when exposing extraoral bite-wing images. These errors include patient movement, ghost images, Frankfort and midsagittal plane errors, and errors with the focal trough.

Temporomandibular Joint Imaging. The temporomandibular joint (TMJ) is a highly specialized joint that allows for the movement of the mandible. As the term *temporomandibular* indicates, this joint includes the temporal bone and the mandible. The glenoid fossa and the articular eminence of the temporal bone, the condyle of the mandible, and the articular disk between the bones make up the TMJ area. This area can be very difficult to examine on an image because of multiple adjacent bony structures. Imaging of the TMJ area has improved and continues to evolve with the advancement of imaging technologies such as computed tomography (CT) imaging, magnetic resonance (MR) imaging, and cone beam imaging (Chapter 27). Digital and film-based imaging cannot be used to examine the articular disk and other soft tissue areas of the TMJ; instead, a specialized imaging technique (e.g., MR imaging [MRI]) must be used. Digital and film-based imaging, however, can be used to show bone and the relationship of the joint components. For example, changes in bone (e.g., erosions, bony deposits) can be seen on TMJ images. The following two extraoral techniques may be used in TMJ imaging:

- Transcranial projection
- Temporomandibular joint tomography

Transcranial Projection.

Purpose. The purpose of the transcranial projection is to evaluate the superior surface of the condyle and the articular eminence (Figure 26-14). This projection can also be used to evaluate movement of the condyle when the mouth is opened and to compare the joint spaces (right versus left).

Receptor placement. The receptor is placed flat against the patient's ear and is centered over the TMJ.

Head position. The midsagittal plane must be aligned perpendicular to the floor and parallel to the receptor.

Beam alignment. The central ray is directed toward a point 2 inches above and 0.5 inch behind the opening of the ear canal. The beam is directed downward (a vertical angulation of +25 degrees) and forward and is centered on the TMJ that is being imaged.

Exposure factors. Exposure factors for the transcranial projection vary with the receptor and equipment used.

Equipment. The intraoral x-ray unit can be used in the exposure of a transcranial projection. Special positioning devices can be used to coordinate the alignment of the receptor, the patient's head, and the beam to obtain an accurate transcranial image. Such devices are also used to reproduce the same patient positioning in subsequent exposures, thereby permitting comparison of images.

Temporomandibular Joint Tomography. The technique of temporomandibular joint tomography is used to examine the TMJ. *Tomography*, as defined in Chapter 25, is a technique used to show

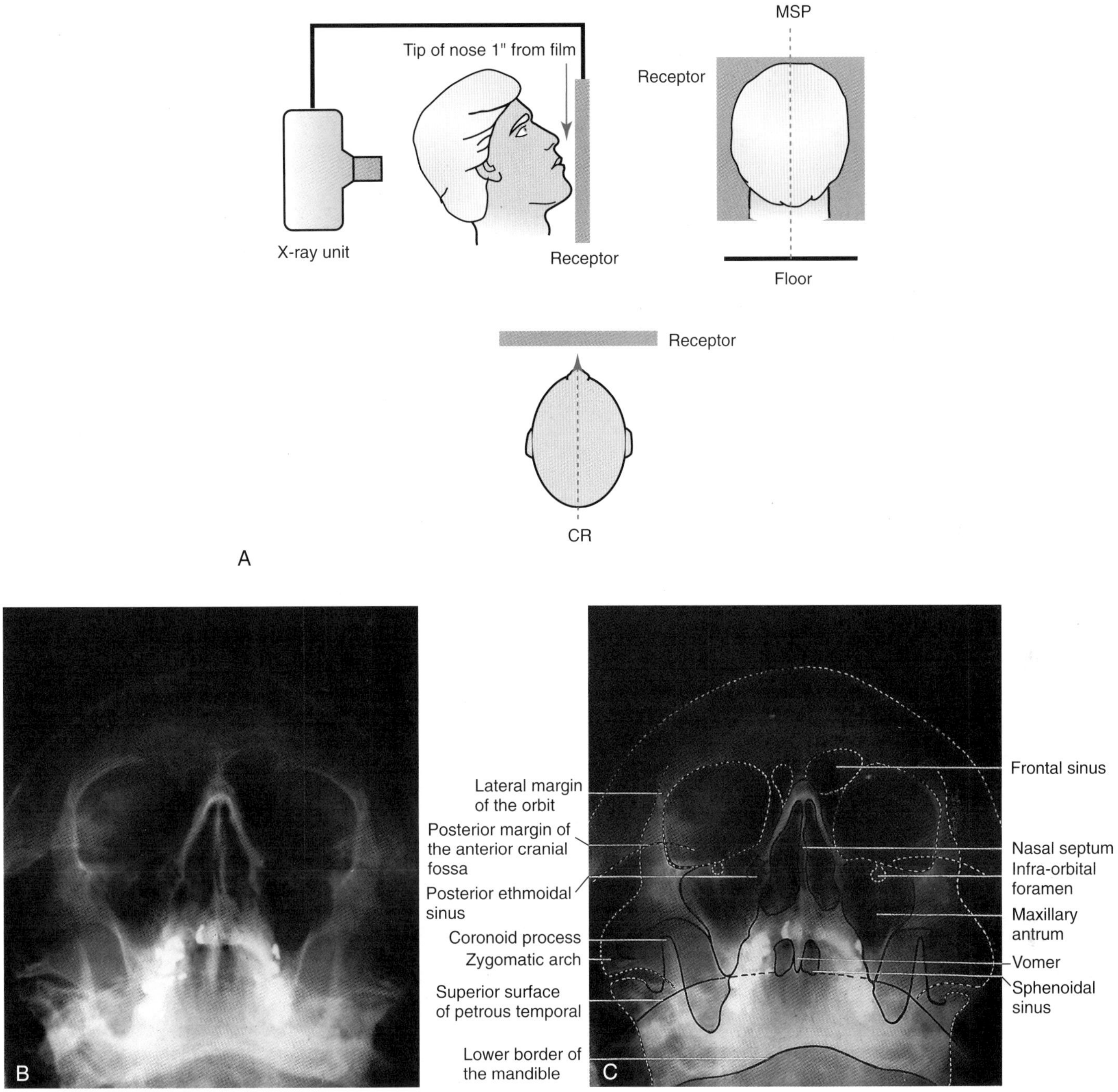

Fig 26-8 **A,** For the Waters projection, proper patient positioning and receptor positioning are shown as viewed from the side, back, and top of the patient. *MSP*, Midsagittal plane; *CR*, central ray. **B,** Example of a Waters view skull image. **C,** Anatomic landmarks identified in the Waters view image. (**A,** Courtesy Dr. Robert M. Jaynes, Columbus, OH. **B** and **C,** From Whaites and Drage: Essentials of dental radiography and radiology, ed 5, London, 2013, Churchill Livingstone.)

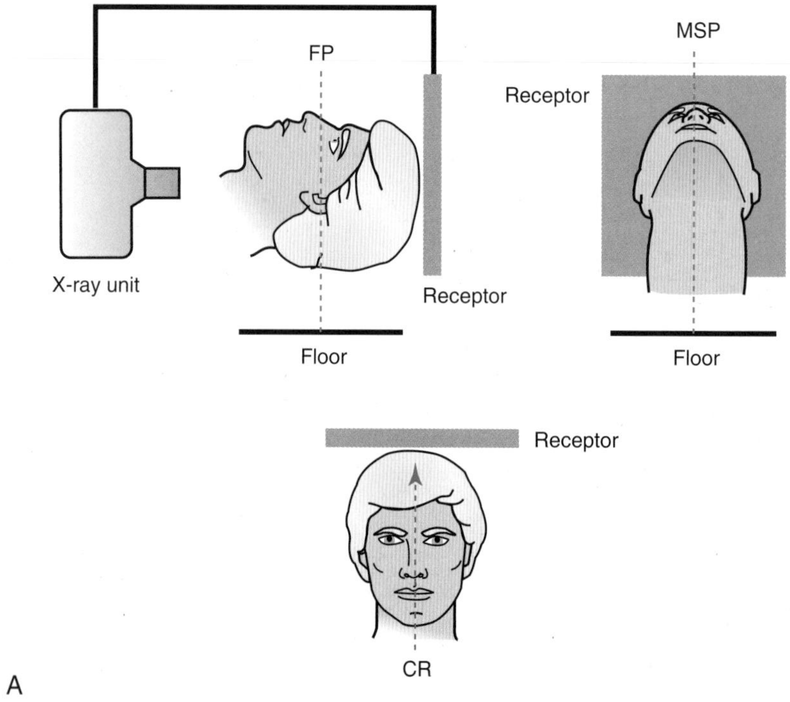

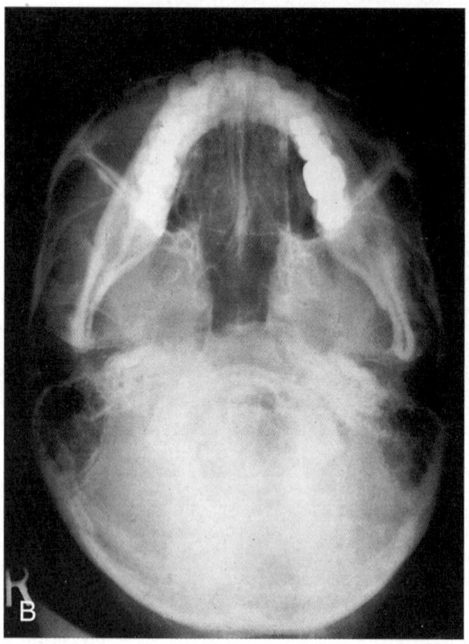

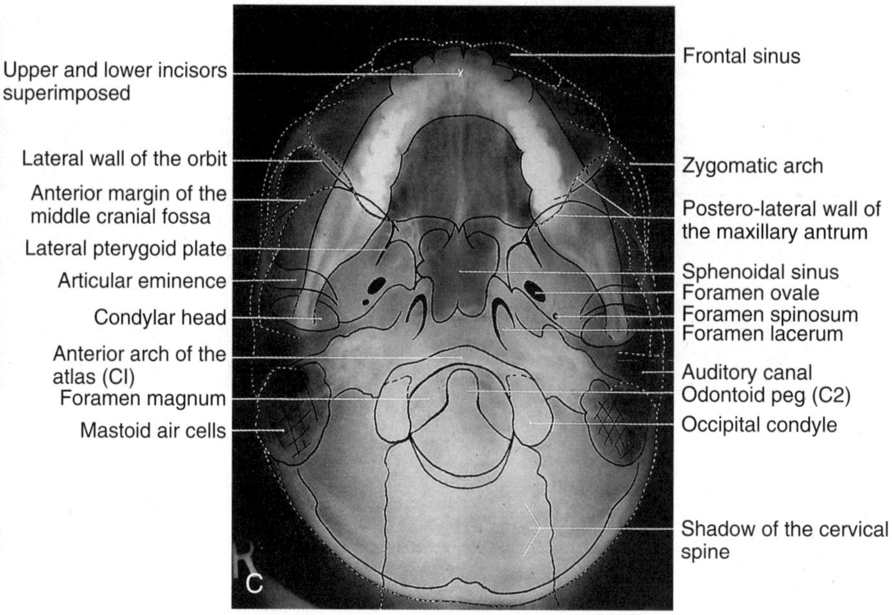

Fig 26-9 **A,** For the submentovertex projection, proper patient positioning and receptor positioning are shown as viewed from the side, front, and top of the patient. *CR*, central ray; *FP*, Frankfort plane; *MSP*, Midsagittal plane. **B,** Example of a submentovertex image. **C,** Anatomic landmarks identified in the submentovertex image. (**A,** Courtesy Dr. Robert M. Jaynes, Columbus, OH. **B** and **C,** From Whaites and Drage: Essentials of dental radiography and radiology, ed 5, London, 2013, Churchill Livingstone.)

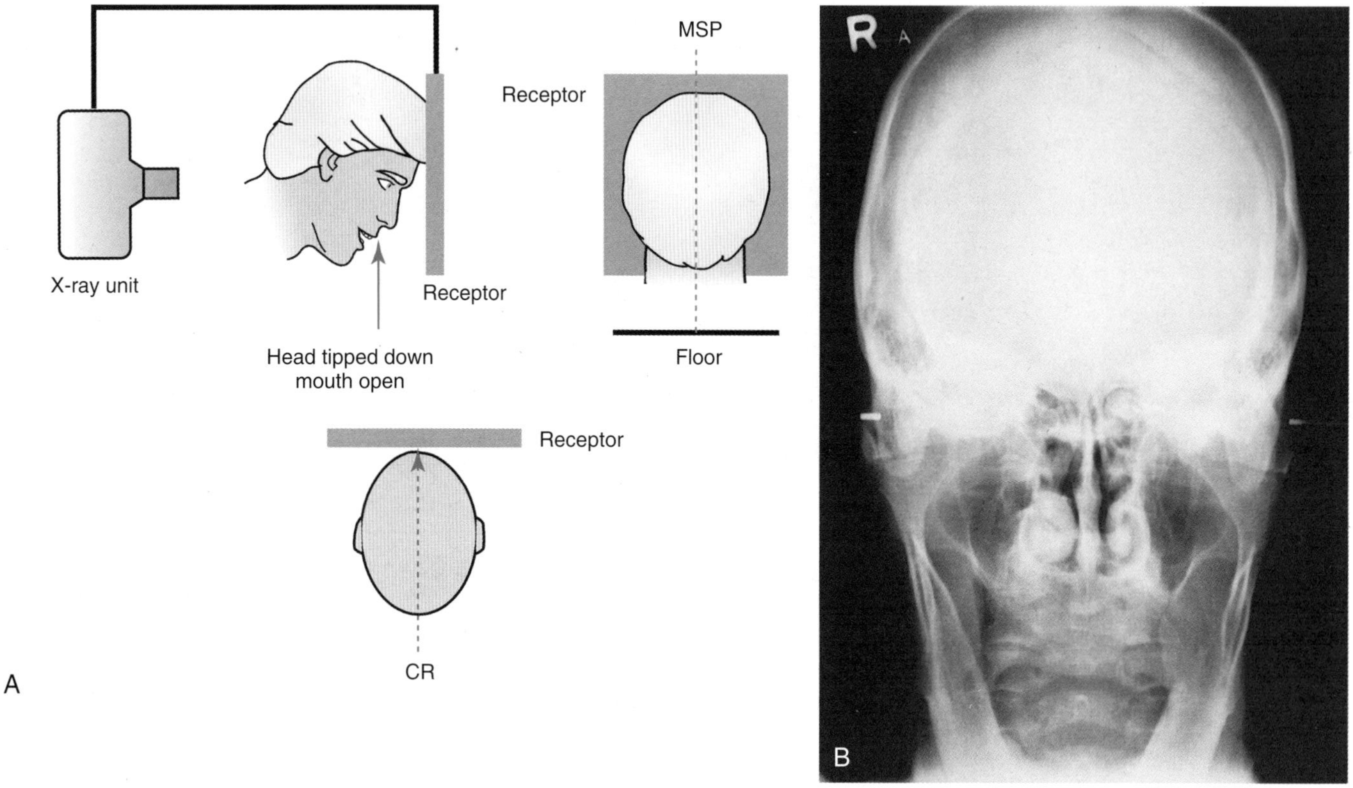

Fig 26-10 **A,** For the reverse Towne projection, proper patient positioning and receptor positioning are shown as viewed from the side, back, and top of the patient. *MSP*, midsagittal plane; *CR*, central ray. **B,** Example of a reverse Towne image. (**A** and **B,** Courtesy Dr. Robert M. Jaynes, Columbus, OH.)

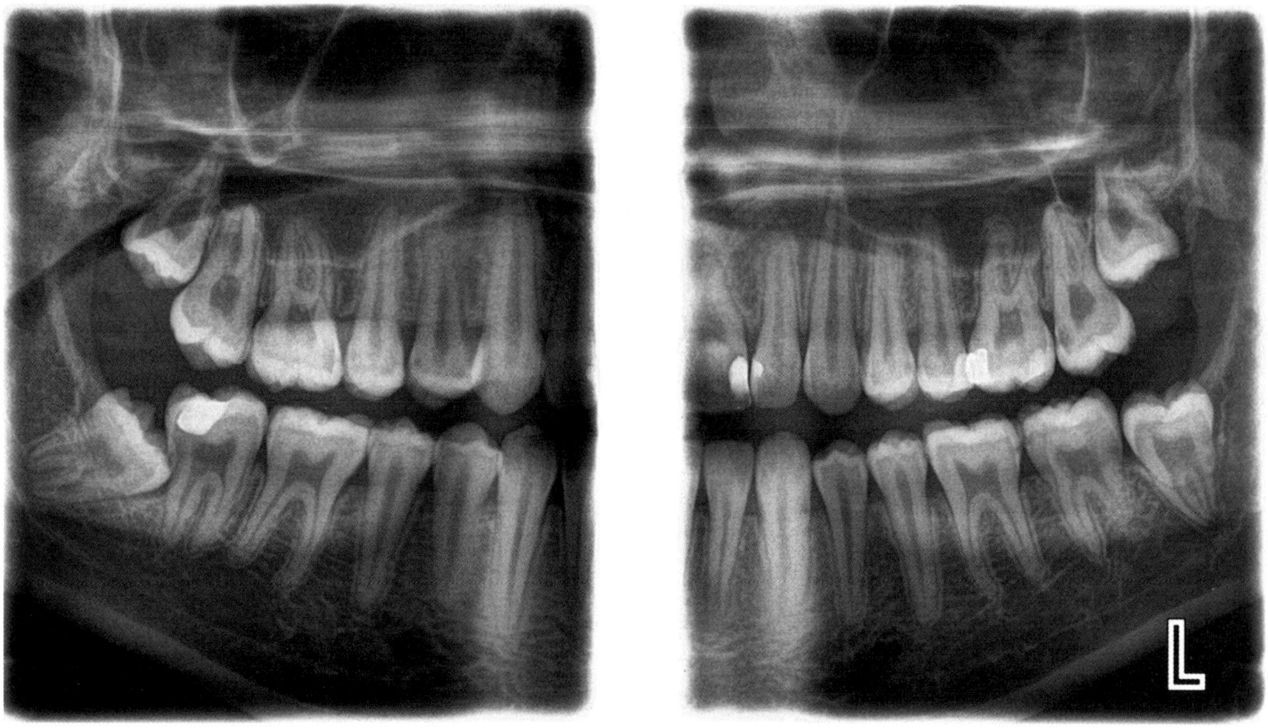

Fig 26-11 Interproximal caries are visible on the extraoral bite-wing images. (Courtesy Planmeca, Hoffman Estates, IL.)

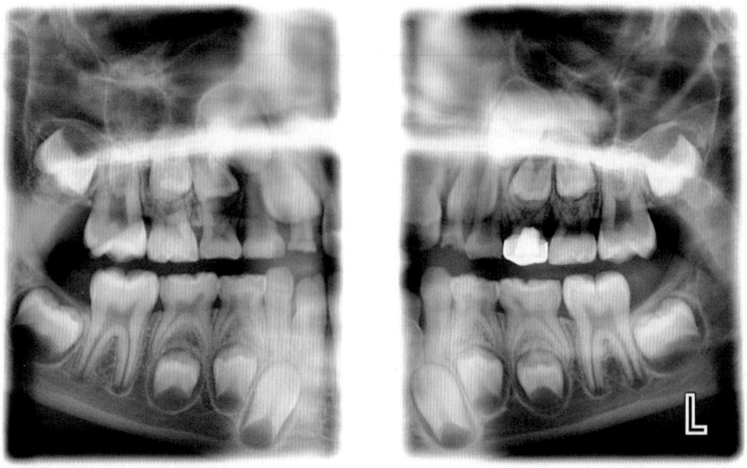

Fig 26-12 Pediatric extraoral bite-wing images. (Courtesy Planmeca, Hoffman Estates, IL.)

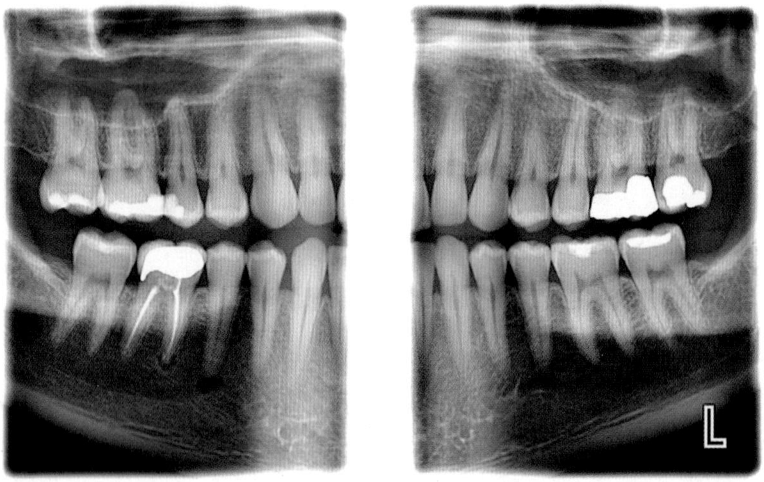

Fig 26-13 Extraoral bite-wing images. (Courtesy Planmeca, Hoffman Estates, IL.)

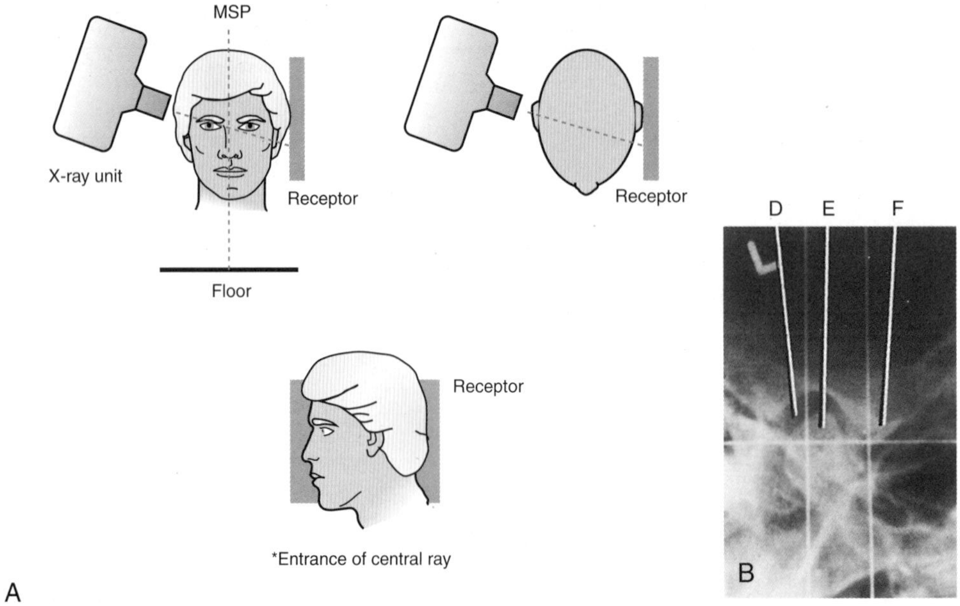

Fig 26-14 **A,** For the transcranial projection, proper patient positioning and receptor positioning are shown as viewed from the front, top, and side of the patient. *MSP*, midsagittal plane. **B,** Transcranial view of temporomandibular joint in the rest position. *D*, Glenoid fossa; *E*, head of mandibular condyle; *F*, articular eminence. (**A,** Courtesy Dr. Robert M. Jaynes, Columbus, OH. **B,** From Kasle MJ: An atlas of dental radiographic anatomy, ed 4, Philadelphia, 1994, Saunders.)

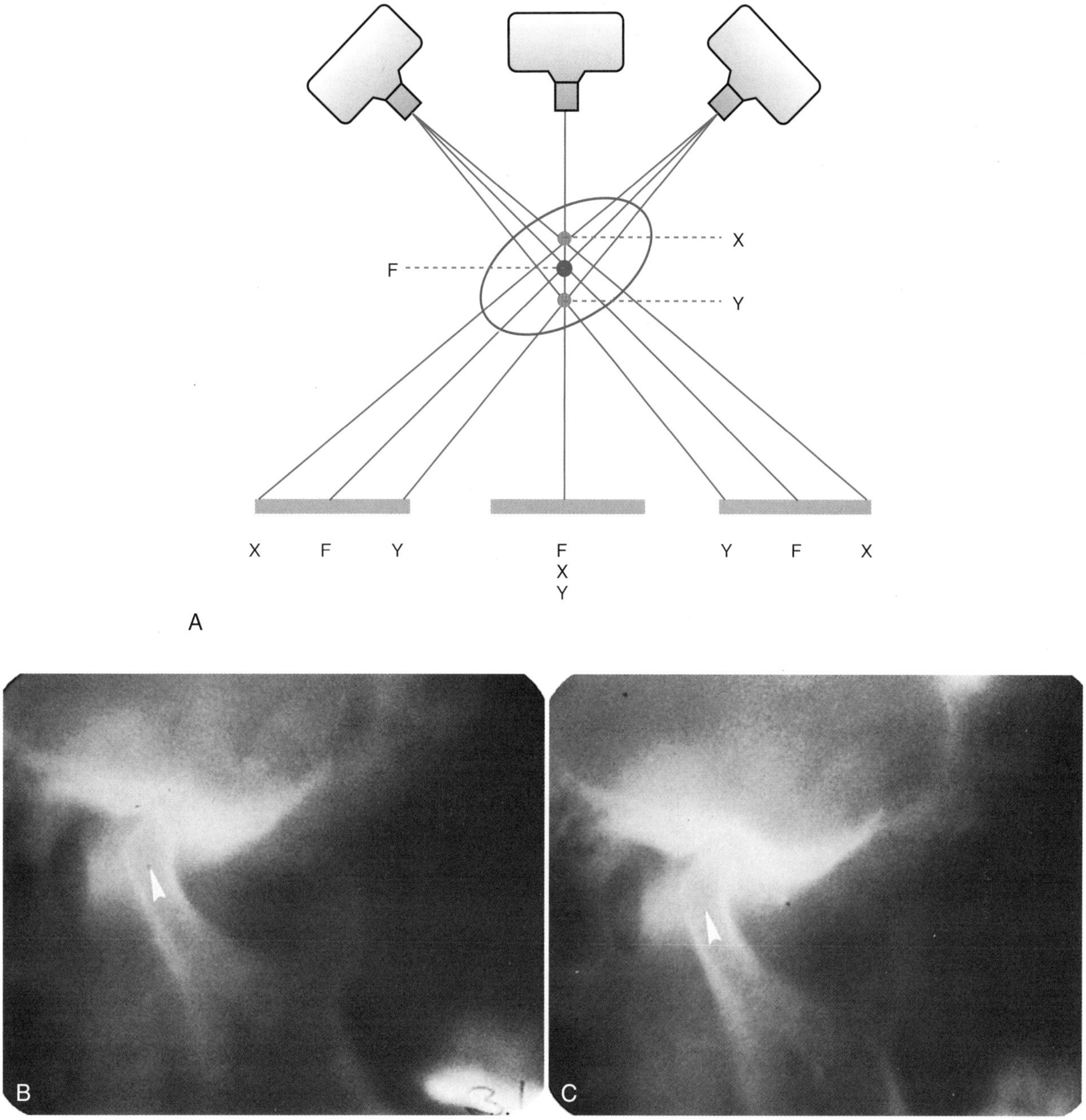

Fig 26-15 **A,** As the tubehead and the receptor move in opposite directions around the patient, objects in the image layer (*F*) appear sharp on the image. Objects on either side of the image layer (*X, Y*) are blurred. **B** and **C,** Corrected axis tomograms showing decreased joint space and posterior positioning of the left condyle (*arrowheads*) caused by the anteriorly placed meniscus. (**A,** Courtesy Dr. Robert M. Jaynes, Columbus, OH. **B** and **C,** From Kasle MJ: An atlas of dental radiographic anatomy, ed 4, Philadelphia, 1994, Saunders.)

structures located within a selected plane of tissue while blurring structures outside the selected plane. In TMJ tomography, this is accomplished by moving the receptor and x-ray tubehead in opposite directions around a fixed rotation point. The location of this rotation point determines what plane of the head will be imaged (Figure 26-15).

TMJ tomography provides imaging of the bony components of the TMJ. As a result, the condyle, the articular eminence, and the glenoid fossa can all be examined on an image known as the tomogram. In addition, the tomogram can be used to estimate joint space and evaluate the extent of movement of the condyle when the mouth is open.

As imaging modalities have improved (CT imaging, MR imaging, and cone-beam computed tomography), superior contrast resolution is possible and the use of film-based tomography for TMJ evaluation has decreased. Further discussion of the specifics of TMJ tomography is beyond the scope of this text.

SUMMARY

- The extraoral receptor is placed outside the mouth during x-ray exposure.
- Uses of extraoral projections include (1) evaluation of large areas of skull and jaws; (2) evaluation of growth and development; (3) evaluation of impacted teeth; (4) detection of diseases, lesions, and conditions of the jaws; (5) examination of the extent of large lesions; (6) evaluation of trauma; and (7) evaluation of the TMJ area.
- Special equipment, including the x-ray unit and receptor (digital sensor or screen film), is necessary for extraoral imaging; in film-based extraoral imaging, intensifying screens and cassette are also needed.
- Prior to exposure of an extraoral projection, the receptor must be prepared, infection prevention procedures completed, and exposure factors selected.
- After preparing the equipment, the dental radiographer must explain the imaging procedures to the patient, place the lead apron, and request that the patient remove all dense objects from the head-and-neck region.
- A variety of projection techniques are used in extraoral imaging; the choice of projection depends on what information is needed.

BIBLIOGRAPHY

Danforth RA, Dus I, Mah J: 3-D volume imaging for dentistry: a new dimension, J Calif Dent Assoc 31(11):817, 2003.

Frommer HH, Stabulas-Savage JJ: Extraoral techniques. In Radiology for the dental professional, ed 9, St Louis, 2011, Mosby.

Johnson ON: Extraoral radiography. In Essentials of dental radiography for dental assistants and hygienists, ed 9, Upper Saddle River, NJ, 2011, Prentice Hall.

Mallya SM, Lam EWN: Cephalometric and Skull Imaging. In White and Pharoah's Oral radiology: principles and interpretation, ed 8, St. Louis, 2019, Elsevier.

Miles DA, Van Dis ML, Jensen CW, et al: Extraoral radiography. In Radiographic imaging for dental auxiliaries, ed 4, St Louis, 2009, Saunders.

Miles DA, Van Dis ML, Razmus TF: Plain film extraoral radiographic techniques. In Basic principles of oral and maxillofacial radiology, Philadelphia, 1992, Saunders.

Olson SS: Auxiliary radiographic techniques. In Dental radiography laboratory manual, Philadelphia, 1995, Saunders.

QUIZ QUESTIONS

Essay

Describe the head position, receptor placement, and beam alignment for each of the following extraoral images:

1. Lateral jaw projection—body of mandible
2. Lateral jaw projection—ramus of mandible
3. Lateral cephalometric projection
4. Posteroanterior projection
5. Waters projection
6. Submentovertex projection
7. Reverse Towne projection
8. Extraoral bite-wing projection
9. Transcranial projection

Multiple Choice

_____ 10. Which projection is best for the examination of the maxillary sinus?
- **a.** lateral jaw
- **b.** reverse Towne
- **c.** Waters
- **d.** submentovertex

_____ 11. Which projection is best for the examination of fractures of the zygomatic arch?
- **a.** submentovertex
- **b.** reverse Towne
- **c.** Waters
- **d.** lateral cephalometric

_____ 12. Which projection is best for examination of fractures of the condylar neck?
- **a.** submentovertex
- **b.** Waters
- **c.** lateral cephalometric
- **d.** reverse Towne

_____ 13. Which projection is best for the examination of the soft tissue profile of the face?
- **a.** transcranial
- **b.** lateral cephalometric
- **c.** reverse Towne
- **d.** posteroanterior

_____ 14. Which projection is best for the examination of the condyle and articular eminence?
- **a.** transcranial
- **b.** posteroanterior
- **c.** Waters
- **d.** submentovertex

_____ 15. Which projection is best for the examination of fractures of the mandibular body?
- **a.** lateral cephalometric
- **b.** submentovertex
- **c.** lateral jaw
- **d.** transcranial

_____ 16. Which projection is best for the examination of a large lesion in the ramus?
- **a.** posteroanterior
- **b.** Waters
- **c.** lateral cephalometric
- **d.** lateral jaw

IDENTIFICATION

17. Identify the patient positioning error seen in the extraoral bite-wing images in Figure 26-16 A, B and C.

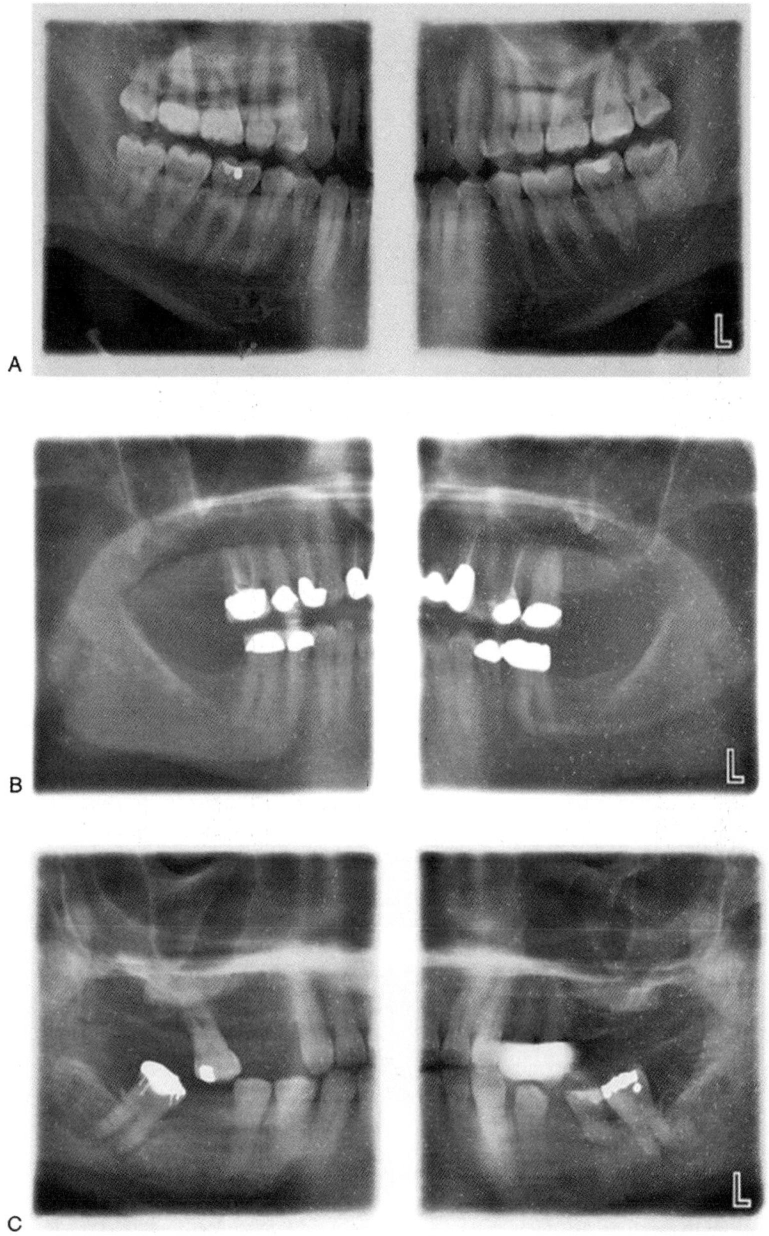

Fig 26-16 A, B, C (Courtesy Planmeca, Hoffman Estates, IL.)

27

Three-Dimensional Digital Imaging

LEARNING OBJECTIVES

After completion of this chapter, the student will be able to do the following:

1. Define the key terms associated with three-dimensional digital imaging.
2. Describe the fundamentals of three-dimensional digital imaging.
3. Describe the training needed and equipment used in three-dimensional digital imaging.
4. Discuss the common uses of three-dimensional digital imaging.
5. Detail the equipment and patient preparation necessary before exposure to x-radiation using three-dimensional digital imaging.
6. Identify advantages and disadvantages of three-dimensional digital imaging.

All of the images discussed in the previous chapters of this text have been two-dimensional. Dental imaging is no longer limited to two dimensions; three-dimensional imaging is now available. In 1999 a technology termed cone-beam computed tomography (CBCT) was introduced that allows for the viewing of structures in the oral-maxillofacial complex in three dimensions. The adoption of three-dimensional digital imaging in dentistry has expanded since that time as the result of numerous technical improvements and commercial marketing. CBCT has become a desired technology because of the accurate and detailed information it provides. As discussed in previous chapters, magnification, distortion, and overlap of anatomy minimize the diagnostic quality of dental images. These geometric characteristics limit the accurate interpretation of traditional two-dimensional images (Figure 27-1). The dental practitioner, therefore, may not have the ability to evaluate pathology (e.g., bony and soft tissue), distances to critical anatomic landmarks (e.g., maxillary sinus, mandibular canal), locations of impacted teeth, eruption patterns, or other concerns of the oral and maxillofacial complex. Three-dimensional imaging provides more detailed information, allowing for a more accurate interpretation.

The purpose of this chapter is to discuss the basic concepts, indications for use, training needed, equipment used, and the advantages and disadvantages of three-dimensional digital imaging. The dental radiographer must have a basic understanding of three-dimensional digital imaging.

BASIC CONCEPTS

Terminology

Cone-beam computed tomography (CBCT): Term used to describe computer-assisted digital imaging in dentistry; this imaging technique uses a cone-shaped x-ray beam to acquire information and present it in three dimensions.

Cone-beam volume tomography (CBVT): Term used to describe computer-assisted digital imaging in dentistry, used interchangeably with *cone-beam volume imaging (CBVI)*; these terms are used to differentiate this procedure from medical computed tomography (CT).

DICOM data: The universal format for handling, storing, and transmitting three-dimensional images; the acronym refers to *Digital Imaging and Communications in Medicine.*

Field of view (FOV): The area that can be captured when performing imaging procedures.

Multiplanar reconstruction (MPR): The reconstruction of raw data into images when imported into viewing software to create three anatomic planes of the body.

Plane, axial: A horizontal plane that divides the body into superior and inferior parts; runs parallel to the ground.

Plane, coronal: A vertical plane that divides the body into anterior and posterior sides; runs perpendicular to the ground.

Plane, sagittal: A vertical plane that divides the body into right and left sides; runs perpendicular to the ground. A midsagittal plane describes a plane that runs through the midline of the body.

Resolution, contrast: The number of gray-scale colors available for each pixel in the image.

Resolution, spatial: A measurement of pixel size in multiplanar reconstruction.

Three-dimensional digital imaging: An image that demonstrates the anatomy in three dimensions.

Three-dimensional volume rendering: A three-dimensional shape that is created from two-dimensional images.

Voxel: The smallest element of a three-dimensional image; also referred to as *volume element* or *three-dimensional pixel.*

Fundamentals

For years, three-dimensional imaging was primarily used in medicine. Today, manufacturers of CBCT units have developed three-dimensional imaging specifically to evaluate the oral and maxillofacial complex. CBCT is so named because it uses a cone-shaped x-ray beam to acquire three-dimensional information (Figure 27-2). The source of radiation in CBCT machines rotates around the head of the patient, as in panoramic imaging.

With CBCT imaging, the region of interest of the patient anatomy is termed the field of view (FOV). In a single scan, the source of radiation and the digital sensor rotate around the patient and acquire multiple images of the FOV. The smallest FOV is used to obtain the necessary diagnostic information from the appropriate area of anatomy. For diagnostic purposes, manufacturers of CBCT units provide settings for a variety of FOV sizes to accommodate the region of interest (Figure 27-3).

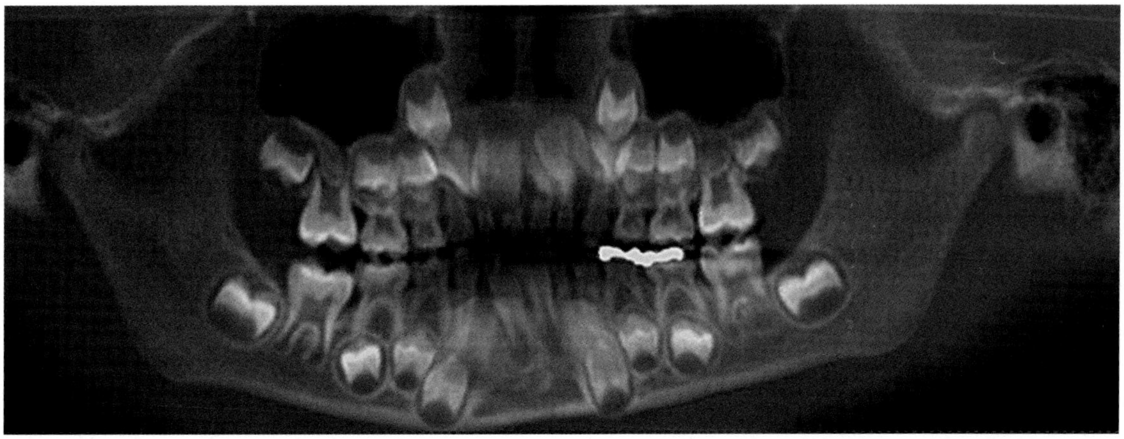

Fig 27-1 Panoramic image revealing mixed dentition of a 6-year-old child. It is difficult to determine the eruption pattern of permanent teeth, especially in the anterior maxilla. (Courtesy Carolina OMF Imaging, W. Bruce Howerton Jr., DDS, MS, Franklinton, NC.)

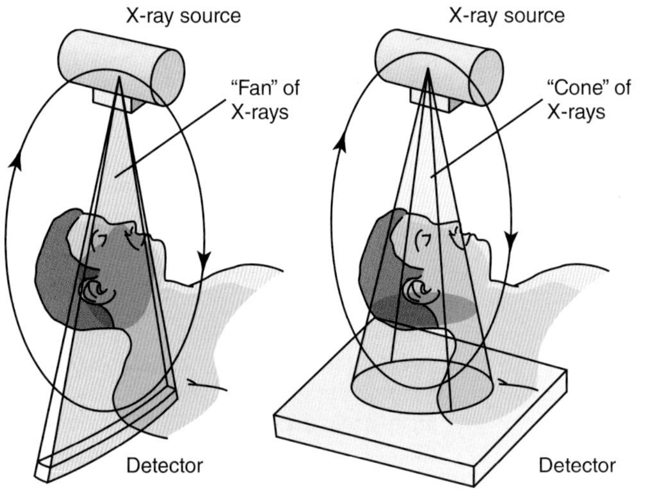

Fig 27-2 Cone-shaped beam used in cone-beam computed tomography (CBCT).

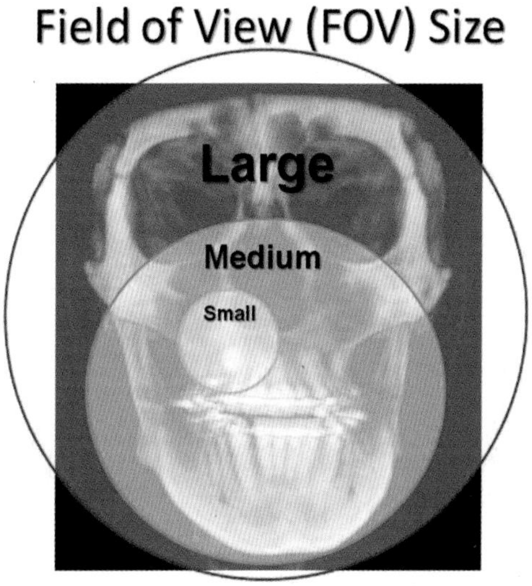

Fig 27-3 Examples of various sizes of the field of view.

As the divergent rays exit the machine, some radiation is attenuated by the patient, and some of the radiation passes through the patient and is received by a digital receptor. The information that the receptor receives is termed *raw data*. The data is reconstructed and imported into viewing software to observe anatomic features of the teeth, oral and maxillofacial region, ears, nose, and throat. In contrast to producing a single intraoral image, as in two-dimensional imaging, raw data is three-dimensional in volume and undergoes reconstruction, forming a "stack" of axial images termed *DICOM images*.

DICOM images are imported into the viewing software that allows the dental practitioner to see the FOV in three dimensions. Once the images are imported, the data is viewed in three planes: axial (X), coronal (Y), and sagittal (Z) (Figure 27-4).

- The axial plane is a horizontal plane that divides the anatomic features within the FOV into superior and inferior slices (Figure 27-5).
- The coronal plane is a vertical plane that divides the anatomic features within the FOV into anterior and posterior slices (Figure 27-6).
- The sagittal plane is also a vertical plane that divides the anatomic features within the FOV into right and left slices (Figure 27-7).

When viewed together, axial, coronal, and sagittal images are referred to as multiplanar reconstructed images (MPR images).

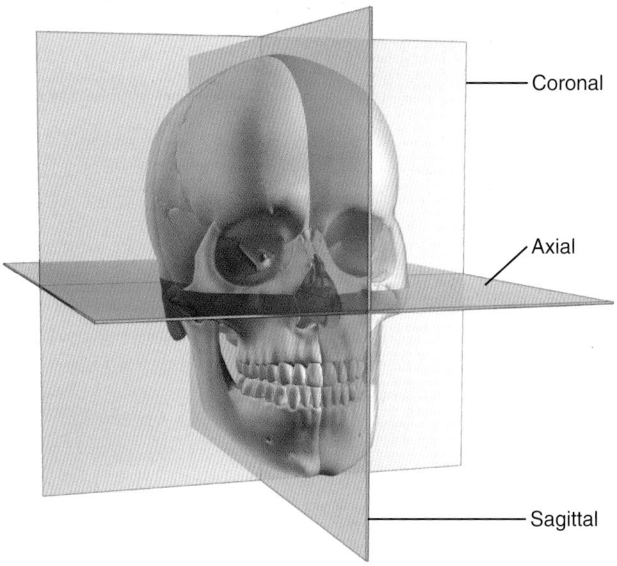

Fig 27-4 An illustration of the three planes: axial (or transverse) (X), coronal (Y), and sagittal (Z).

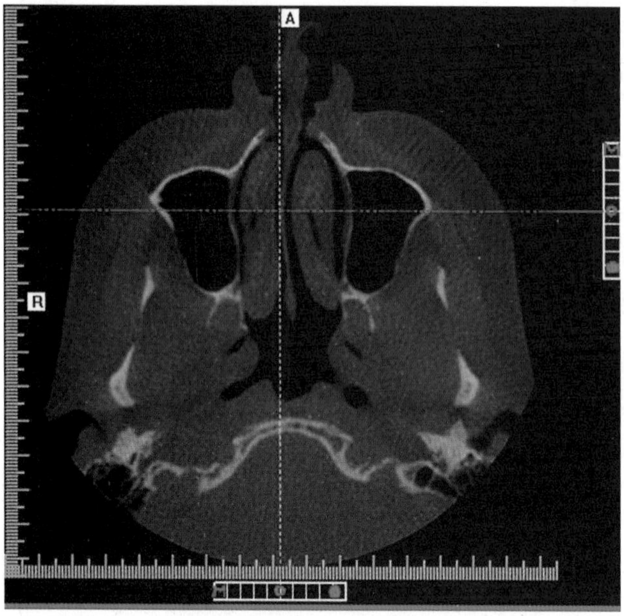

Fig 27-5 An axial image. (Courtesy Carolina OMF Imaging, W. Bruce Howerton Jr., DDS, MS, Franklinton, NC.)

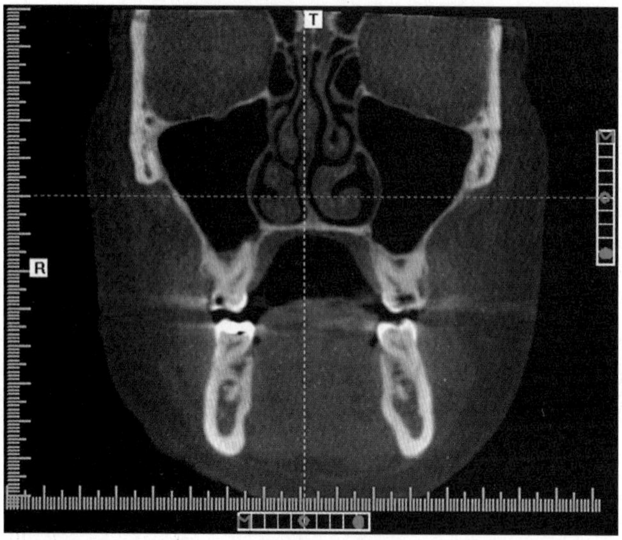

Fig 27-6 A coronal image. (Courtesy Carolina OMF Imaging, W. Bruce Howerton Jr., DDS, MS, Franklinton, NC.)

Anatomic features within the FOV provide accurate dimensional measurements of the patient with a 1 : 1 ratio relationship. One of the advantages of using DICOM data is that images can be shared among dental professionals, imaging centers, and referring physicians. The volume of data produced is similar to medical CT, but CBCT uses much less radiation to acquire the images.

Training

Most dentists who use the CBCT imaging techniques do not have the formal training that is required to interpret data on anatomic areas beyond the maxilla and the mandible. The American Academy of Oral and Maxillofacial Radiology (AAOMR) recommends that CBCT images be interpreted only by a board-certified oral and maxillofacial radiologist, or by a dentist with adequate training and/or experience.

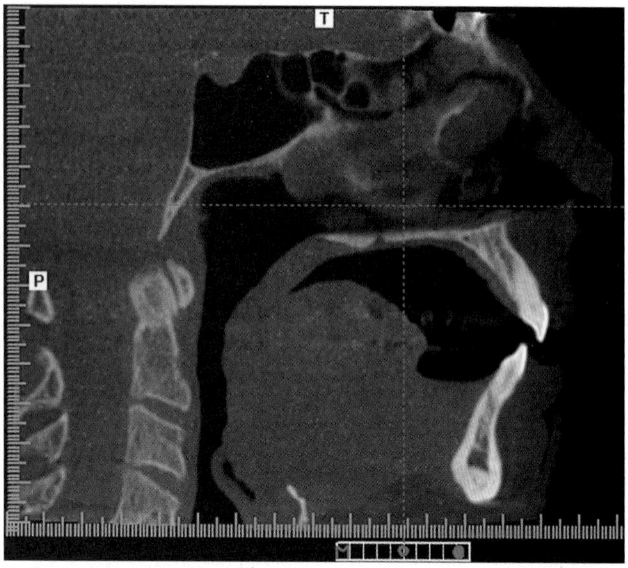

Fig 27-7 A sagittal image. (Courtesy Carolina OMF Imaging, W. Bruce Howerton Jr., DDS, MS, Franklinton, NC.)

The Intersocietal Accreditation Commission (IAC) is a nonprofit organization that has developed standards applicable to the minimal requirements for optimum patient care when using dental computed tomography. The company mission statement includes programs for accreditation dedicated to ensure quality patient care. To receive accreditation from this organization, a dentist must satisfactorily pass peer review processes and other requirements outlined by the IAC. The IAC logo seen in a dental office assures the patient that the CBCT machine is operating correctly, the dentist and staff members are using the technology appropriately, and the data is being read comprehensively.

Equipment

The use of specialized equipment is necessary for three-dimensional digital imaging. The essential components for this type of imaging system include a CBCT machine, a computer, and viewing software.

CBCT Machine. Prior to installation of a CBCT unit, a radiation physicist is contacted to evaluate the proper physical space in the dental office to house a CBCT machine. Before a CBCT machine can be operational, the dentist must comply with state and local regulations concerning the use of this equipment. This includes following guidelines to ensure a safe environment for staff and patients in relation to CBCT units and the use of ionizing radiation.

Appropriate training of the dentist and staff members to acquire proper data can be validated periodically by the IAC. These tests not only confirm that consistent CBCT scans are being exposed, but also assure the patient population that the technology is being used in the proper manner.

The CBCT machine is comparable in size and appearance to a panoramic machine. With the CBCT machine, the patient sits, stands, or is placed in a supine position during the scanning process. In a single rotation, the source of radiation and the receptor capture the FOV. The radiation that exits the patient is received by a solid-state flat panel detector and becomes the raw data that is sent to the computer. Scan times vary between 7 and 30 seconds; shorter scan times are desirable to eliminate artifacts created by patient movement. Factors that can be altered when scanning the patient are FOV size and resolution.

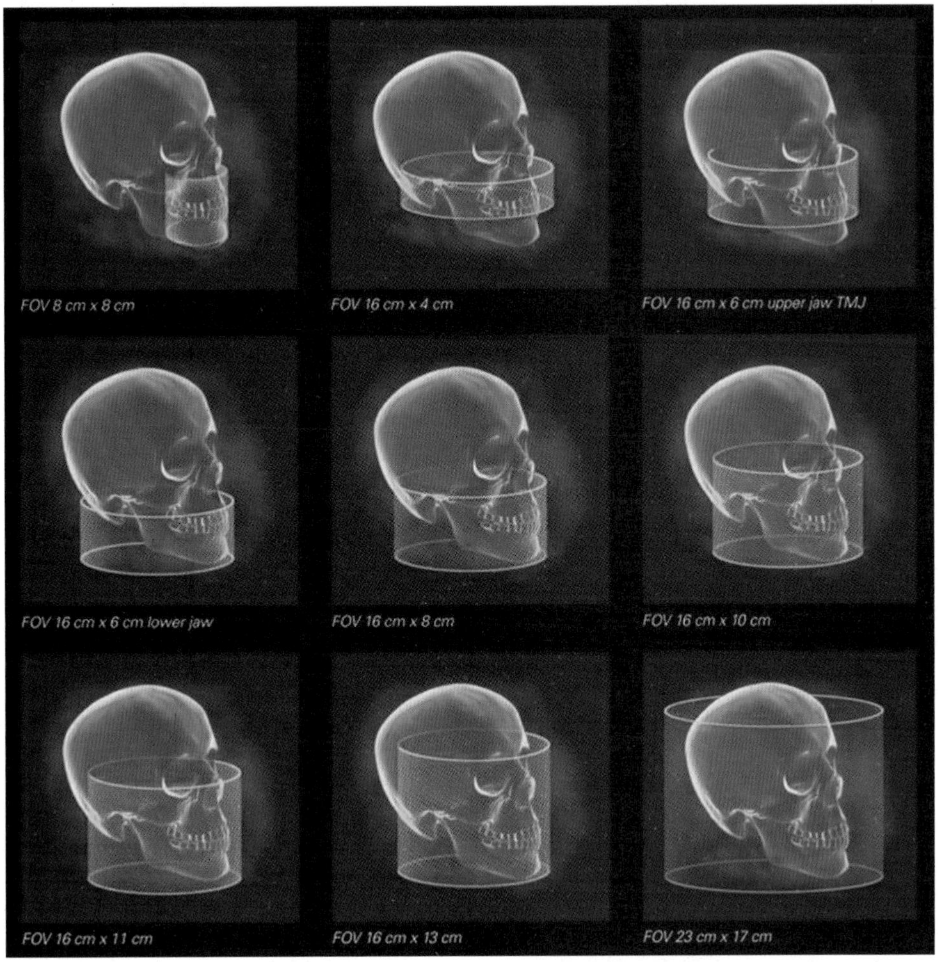

Fig 27-8 An illustrative guide demonstrates the various sizes that the operator can select based on the region of interest. (Courtesy KaVo Imaging, Brea, CA.)

Contrast resolution refers to the number of gray scales available, and spatial resolution is the measurement, in millimeters, of the size of pixels in the MPR images. *Spatial resolution* also refers to the measurement of three-dimensional pixels, termed voxels, in the volume of data. Choosing the appropriate FOV and the resolution is dependent on the region of interest and the reason for the scan—for example, dental implant placement, temporomandibular joint examination, or pathology review (Figure 27-8).

The number of manufacturers producing CBCT units for dental use continues to grow rapidly. Figure 27-9 displays examples of several CBCT machines.

Computer. A computer connected to the CBCT machine accepts raw data and reconstructs the data into a stack of axial images (DICOM images). The computer has separate proprietary viewing software to import DICOM images. The reason for exposing the scan dictates the proper region of interest, and therefore determines the FOV and correct spatial resolution.

Viewing Software. The viewing software allows the dental practitioner to view axial, coronal, and sagittal images, select the region of interest such as a presurgical dental implant site or the location of an impacted canine, and scroll through these images on a computer monitor to create three-dimensional information. This information assists the dentist or physician in diagnosis and treatment planning (Figure 27-10). Each CBCT machine has its proprietary viewing software, but many third-party DICOM viewing software packages are available with additional features (Figure 27-11).

Common Uses

CBCT examinations should be performed only when necessary to provide information that cannot be provided using other imaging modalities. As detailed in a recent advisory statement from the American Dental Association Council on Scientific Affairs, a CBCT examination should be prescribed by a dentist who has appropriate training and education in CBCT imaging, including an understanding of the significance of CBCT selection and imaging findings. Dental practitioners should prescribe CBCT imaging only when the diagnostic yield is expected to benefit patient care, enhance patient safety, or significantly improve clinical outcomes.

CBCT imaging applications greatly improve interpretation, diagnosis, and treatment planning in many aspects of dental care. Some of the common uses of three-dimensional imaging include the following:

- Implant placement (Figure 27-12)
- Extraction or exposure of impacted teeth (Figure 27-13)
- Definition of anatomic structures, such as inferior alveolar nerve and mental foramen location (Figure 27-14)
- Endodontic assessment (Figure 27-15)

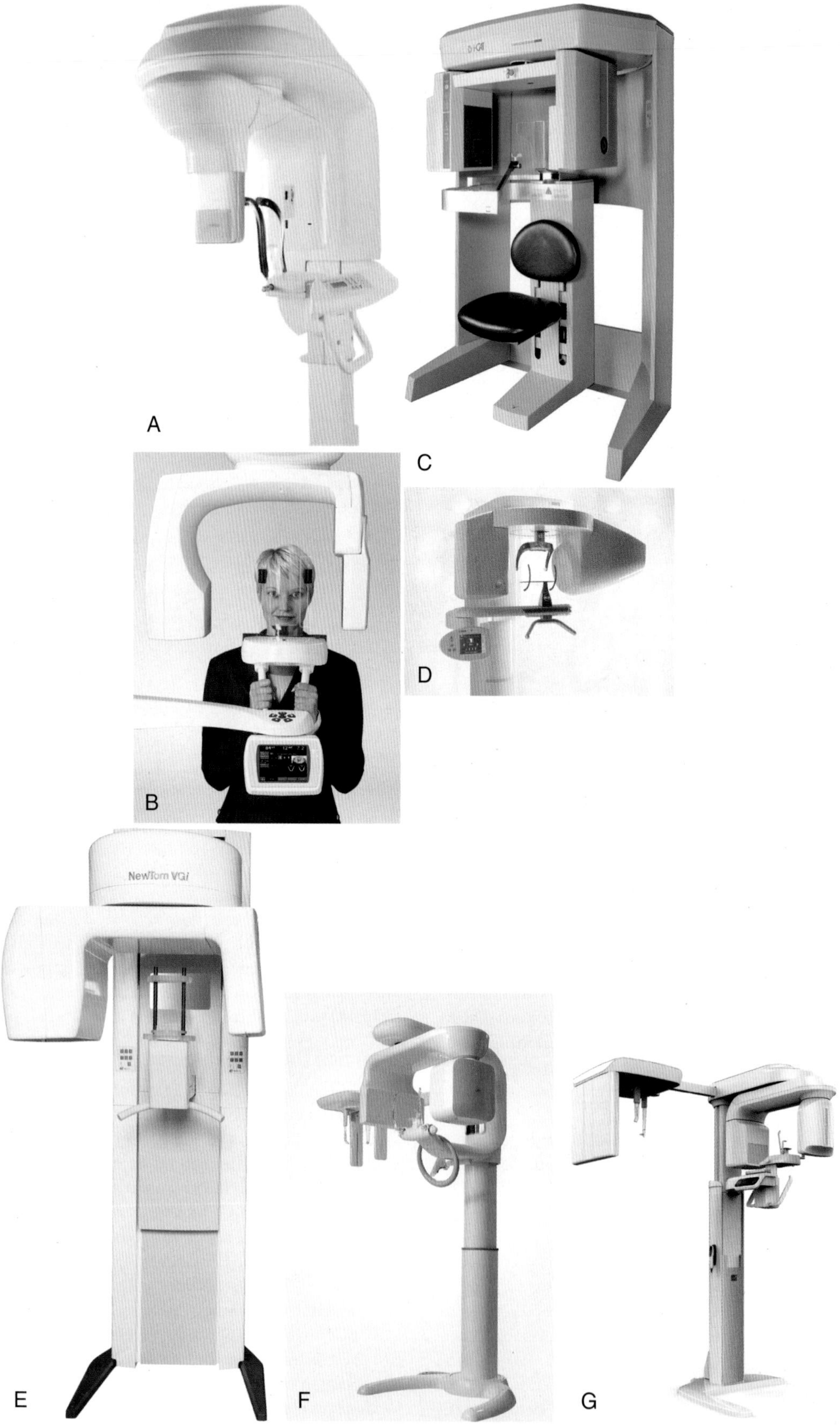

Fig 27-9 Examples of cone-beam computed tomography (CBCT) machines. **A,** Carestream 9300 3D Extraoral Imaging System. **B,** Planmeca ProMax 3D. **C,** Next Generation i-CAT Imaging System. **D,** GALILEOS 3D Cone Beam Scanner. **E,** NewTom VG*i*. **F,** Rayscan α Expert 3D. **G,** VATECH America PaX-i3D.

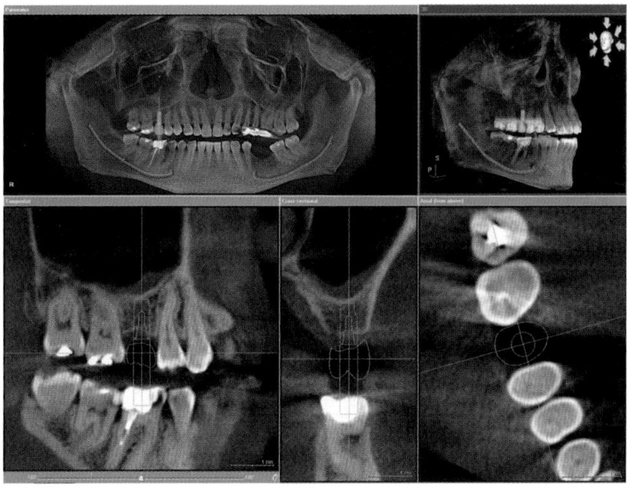

Fig 27-10 The diagnostic capabilities of three-dimensional cone-beam imaging viewed in this example of implant placement for tooth #3. (Courtesy Sirona Dental System, Charlotte, NC.)

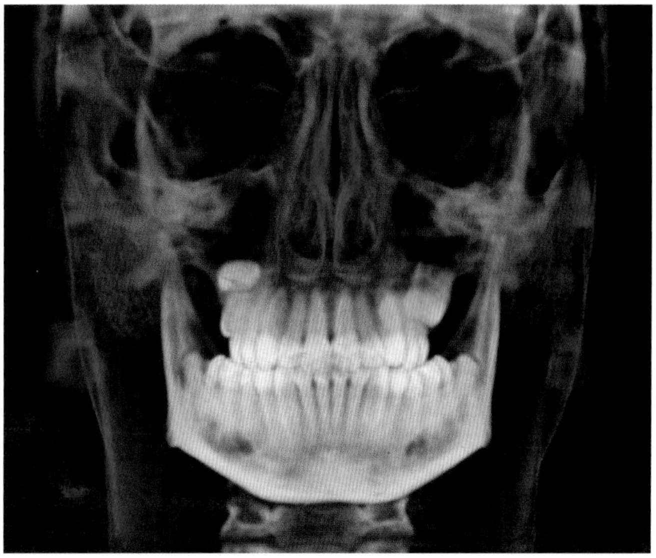

Fig 27-11 Software tools illustrate the maxilla and mandible in three dimensions while allowing the dental professional to select appropriate treatment plans for a variety of procedures. (Courtesy KaVo Imaging, Brea, CA.)

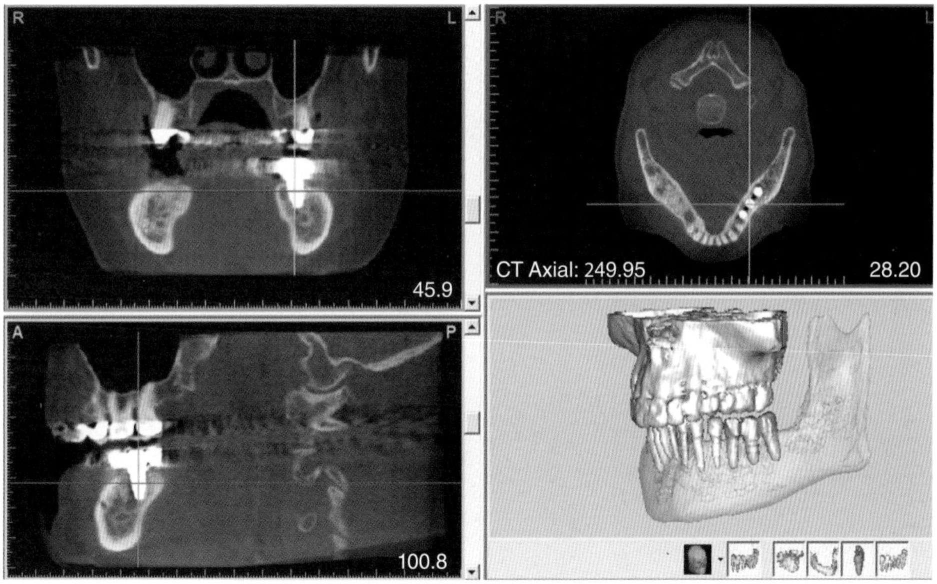

Fig 27-12 An implant placed in the mandible to replace tooth #19 viewed from coronal, axial, and sagittal planes to ensure secure placement in bone. (Courtesy Carolina OMF Imaging, W. Bruce Howerton Jr., DDS, MS, Franklinton, NC.)

- Airway and sinus analysis (Figure 27-16)
- Evaluation of temporomandibular joint (TMJ) disorders (Figure 27-17)
- Orthodontic evaluation (Figure 27-18)
- Evaluation of lesions and abnormalities (Figure 27-19)
- Trauma evaluation

As seen in Figures 27-12 through Figure 27-19, CBCT is revolutionizing the practice of dentistry. Interpretation of CBCT images requires training so that the dental practitioner can recognize findings outside the region of interest, specifically outside the maxilla and the mandible. Such regions include the cerebral hemispheres or areas lateral to the oropharynx (for hard tissue calcifications) and the paranasal sinuses. These regions are not typically evaluated on a routine basis, although they are clearly visible with three-dimensional imaging. Each CBCT image requires interpretation and must be completed and documented in the patient record. Failure to interpret CBCT images may result in poor treatment outcomes for the dental provider and, more importantly, negative consequences for patients.

STEP-BY-STEP PROCEDURES

Patient Preparation. Depending on manufacturer guidelines, patients may be asked to sit or stand or be placed in the supine

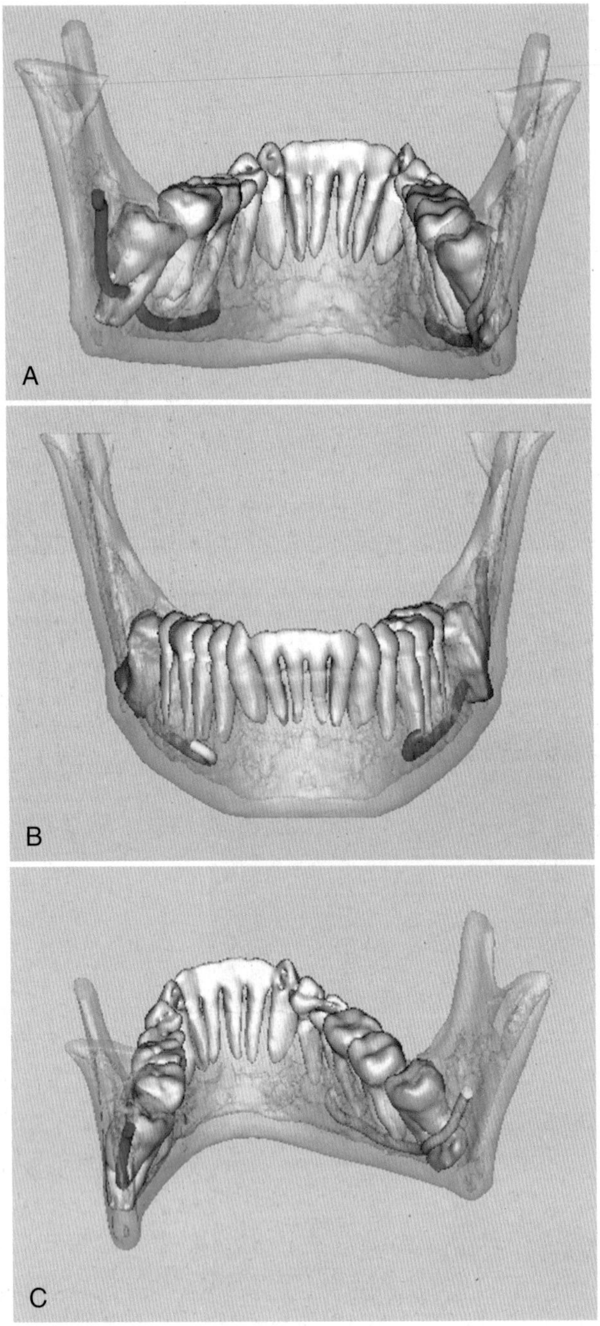

Fig 27-13 **A,** Impacted mandibular third molars (tooth #17 in green; tooth #32 in pink). Note the roots of #17 surrounding the mandibular canal. **B,** Teeth #17 and #32 positioned facial to the mandibular canal. **C,** Transparent mandible allowing full view of the location of the mandibular canals. (Courtesy Carolina OMF Imaging, W. Bruce Howerton Jr., Franklinton, NC.)

position during radiation exposure. Instructions given to the patient before the imaging procedure include requesting the removal of all metallic items in the head-and-neck region, including jewelry, eyeglasses, and removable dental appliances. In certain instances, an intraoral guide may be placed in the patient's mouth during the scanning process. Referring specialists may also request that the scan be performed with the patient keeping the upper and lower teeth slightly apart, which requires a cotton roll, gauze square, or bite registration material to be placed between the maxillary and mandibular anterior teeth.

Patient Positioning. As with all imaging procedures, the patient is instructed to remain very still during the exposure of three-dimensional images. As mentioned earlier, scan times vary from 7 to 30 seconds. Ergonomic head and chin supports have been designed for improved patient comfort. Manufacturers may install laser lights to help with proper alignment of clinical structures and to ensure correct anatomic positioning. As with most extraoral imaging procedures, patients have an open and comfortable view of the surrounding area (Figure 27-20).

ADVANTAGES AND DISADVANTAGES

Advantages of Three-Dimensional Digital Imaging

1. *Lower radiation dose.* Compared with traditional medical CT scans, CBCT imaging involves a lower radiation dose to the patient. Studies have found the effective dose estimates for a dental CBCT scan to be comparable with three or four full-mouth series of intraoral images.
2. *Brief scanning time.* With some machines, cone-beam data can be acquired with a quick 8- to 10-second scan. This short exposure time decreases the chance for motion artifacts to occur and encourages a high level of patient cooperation.
3. *Anatomically accurate images.* CBCT eliminates the superimposition of structures, and the magnification of measurements does not occur. Cone-beam data provides an accurate measurement of anatomic structures with a 1 : 1 ratio relationship (Figure 27-21).
4. *Ability to save and easily transport images.* Three-dimensional images can be saved and shared digitally in a .jpg (*Joint Photographic Experts Group*) or .bmp (*bitmap*) format and then viewed online, placed on a compact disc, or printed on paper or film. The images can also be shared electronically.

Disadvantages of Three-Dimensional Digital Imaging

1. *Patient movement and artifacts.* Motion artifact occurs when a patient moves during the imaging procedure and is one of the most common reasons for image degradation. This type of artifact may occur with both two-dimensional and three-dimensional imaging. CBCT machines are equipped with devices to stabilize the patient's head and neck, and the patient should also be instructed prior to the procedure to remain still during exposure. Radiation is stopped and may not reach the receptor when it interacts with an area of high attenuation, such as a metal crown, bridge, or large amalgam restoration. Streak artifacts from these types of metallic restorations may eliminate or obscure the surrounding anatomy (Figure 27-22).
2. *Size of the FOV.* If the FOV is small, findings or pathology in other regions of the oral and maxillofacial area may be missed. The FOV should include not only the region of interest but also anatomic features related to the region of interest. For example, a patient presents with pain in a maxillary molar tooth. To appropriately diagnose this condition, the FOV should include the maxillary posterior teeth, the temporomandibular joint complex, the auditory complex, and the paranasal sinuses.

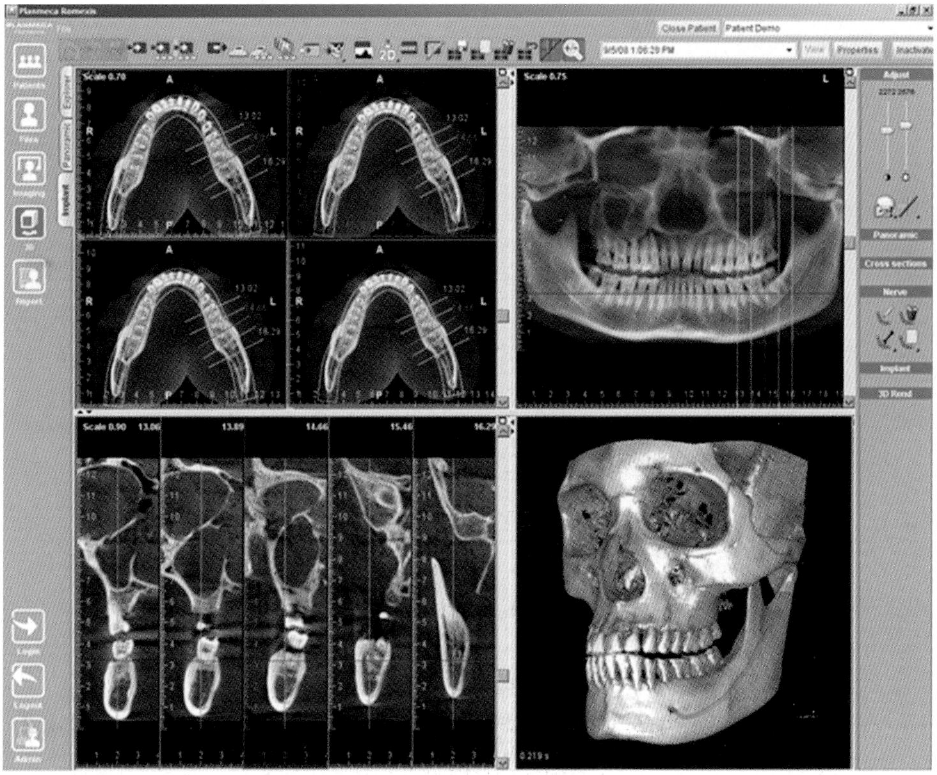

Fig 27-14 Planmeca Romexis 3D Explorer, the 3D image acquisition software for Planmeca ProMax 3D, which enables flexible viewing in all three relevant projections: axial, coronal, and sagittal. A rendered three-dimensional view provides a realistic overview of the anatomy, highlighting the mandibular canal in red. (Courtesy Planmeca Oy, Helsinki, Finland.)

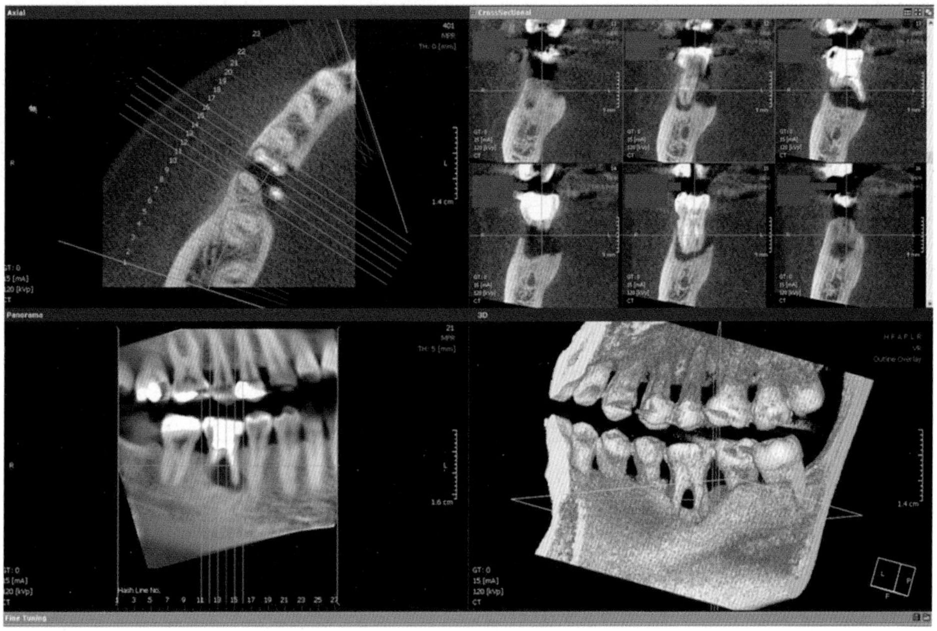

Fig 27-15 Inflammation and resulting bone loss surrounding a tooth with prior endodontic therapy. Multiple views, including a three-dimensional image, reveal the extent of bone loss.

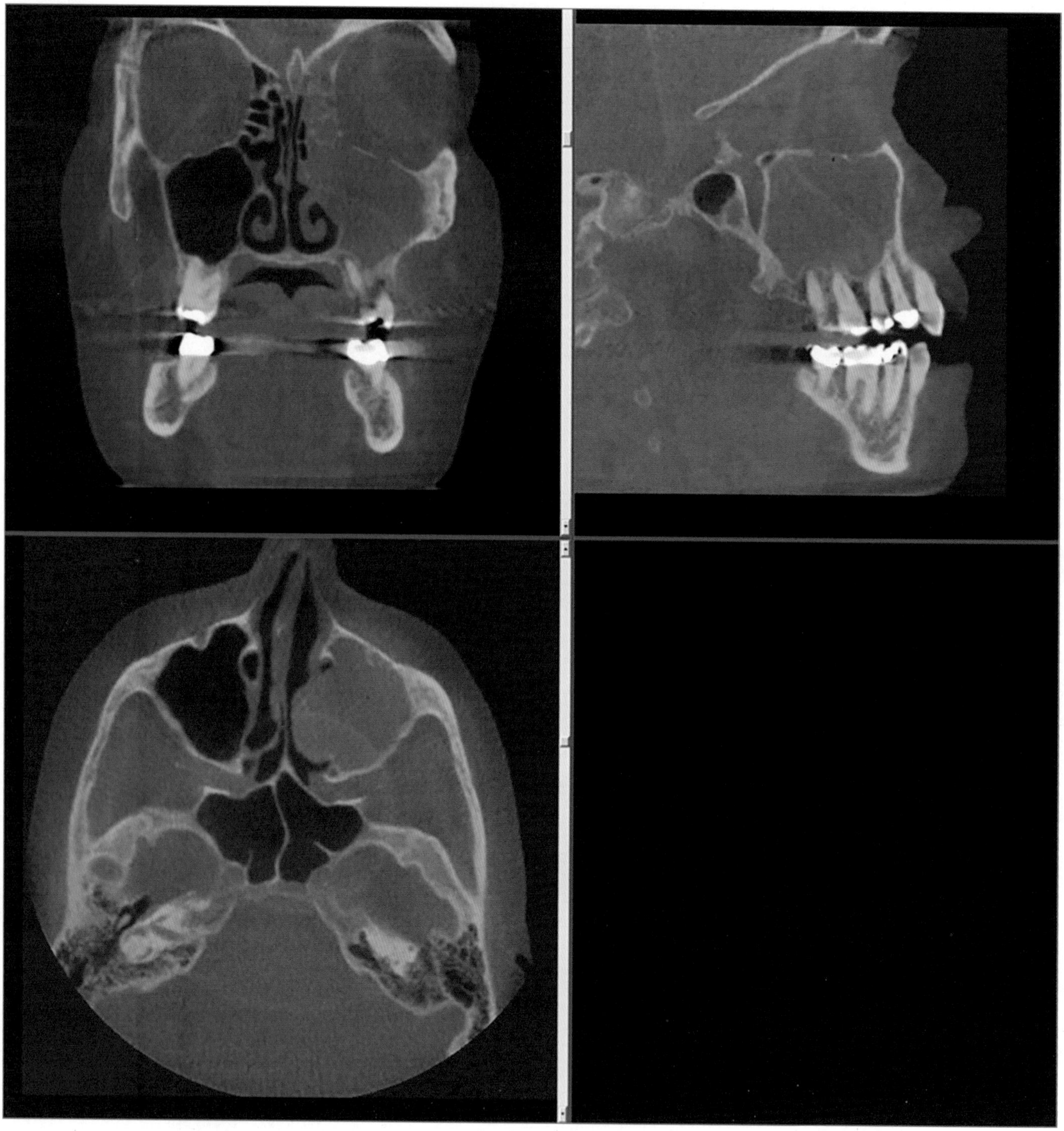

Fig 27-16 Coronal, sagittal, and axial images demonstrate opacification of the left frontal, ethmoid, and maxillary sinuses. (Courtesy Carolina OMF Imaging, W. Bruce Howerton Jr., DDS, MS, Franklinton, NC.)

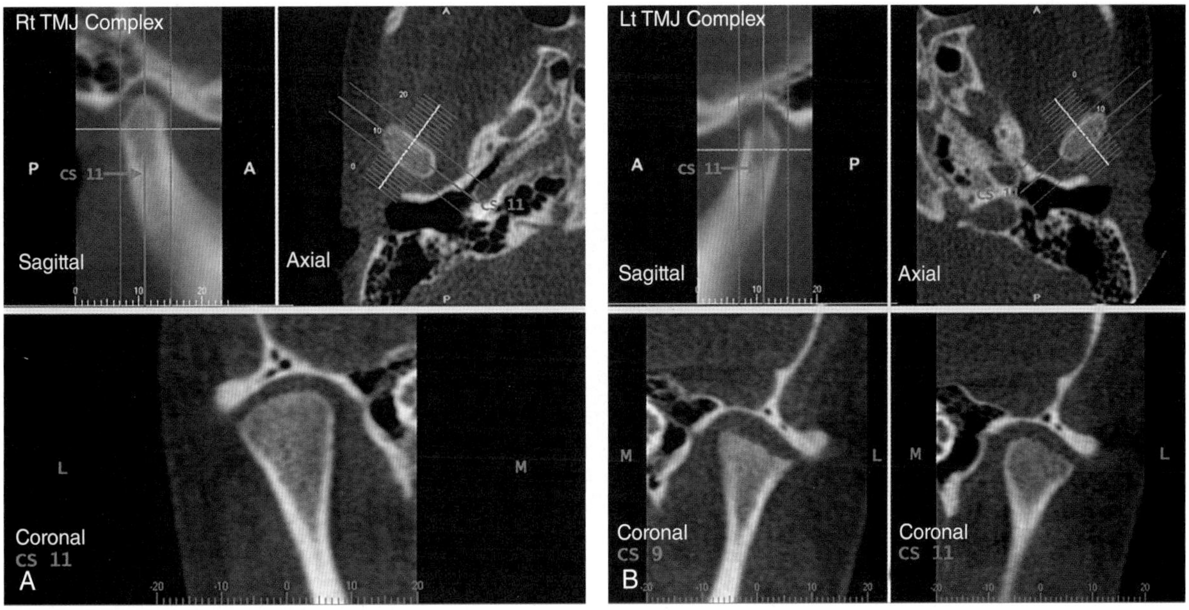

Fig 27-17 **A,** Coronal image demonstrating normal appearance of the right condyle. **B,** Coronal image on the left revealing erosion of the superior border of the mandibular condyle. (Courtesy Carolina OMF Imaging, W. Bruce Howerton Jr., DDS, MS, Franklinton, NC.)

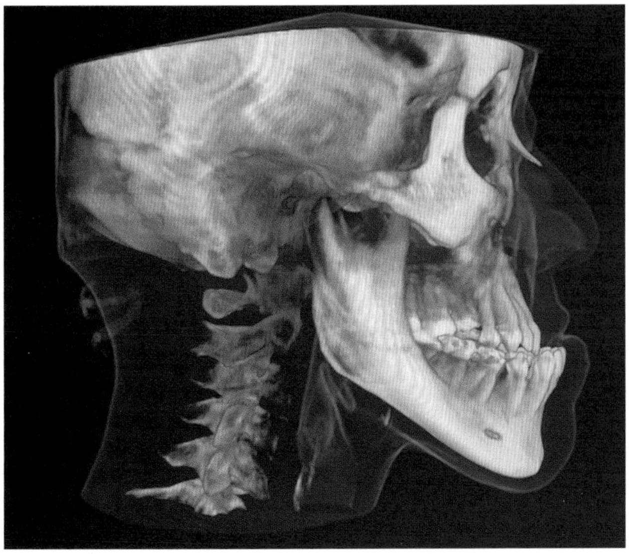

Fig 27-18 The Carestream 9500 3D System provides a large FOV and thus enables the orthodontist to make a comprehensive dental and skeletal assessment of the patient before the beginning of treatment. (Courtesy Carestream Health, Inc., Rochester, NY.)

3. *Cost of equipment; training needed for imaging software.* The cost of the setup of CBCT equipment may be prohibitive for many dental offices. CBCT machines range in cost from $80,000 to $175,000. Because this technology has been accessible for more than 20 years now, previously owned machines are available for purchase. In addition, becoming fully acquainted with the imaging software and correctly using DICOM data require time and dedication to learn the skills needed to create accurate three-dimensional volume images.
4. *Lack of training in interpretation of image data on areas outside the maxilla and the mandible.* Many dental professionals who incorporate this technology into their practices have not had the training required to interpret data on anatomic areas beyond the maxilla and the mandible. The AAOMR recommends that CBCT and implant imaging be interpreted only by a board-certified oral and maxillofacial radiologist or a dentist with adequate training and/or experience. The ADA suggests that the CBCT image be evaluated by a dentist with appropriate training and education in CBCT interpretation.

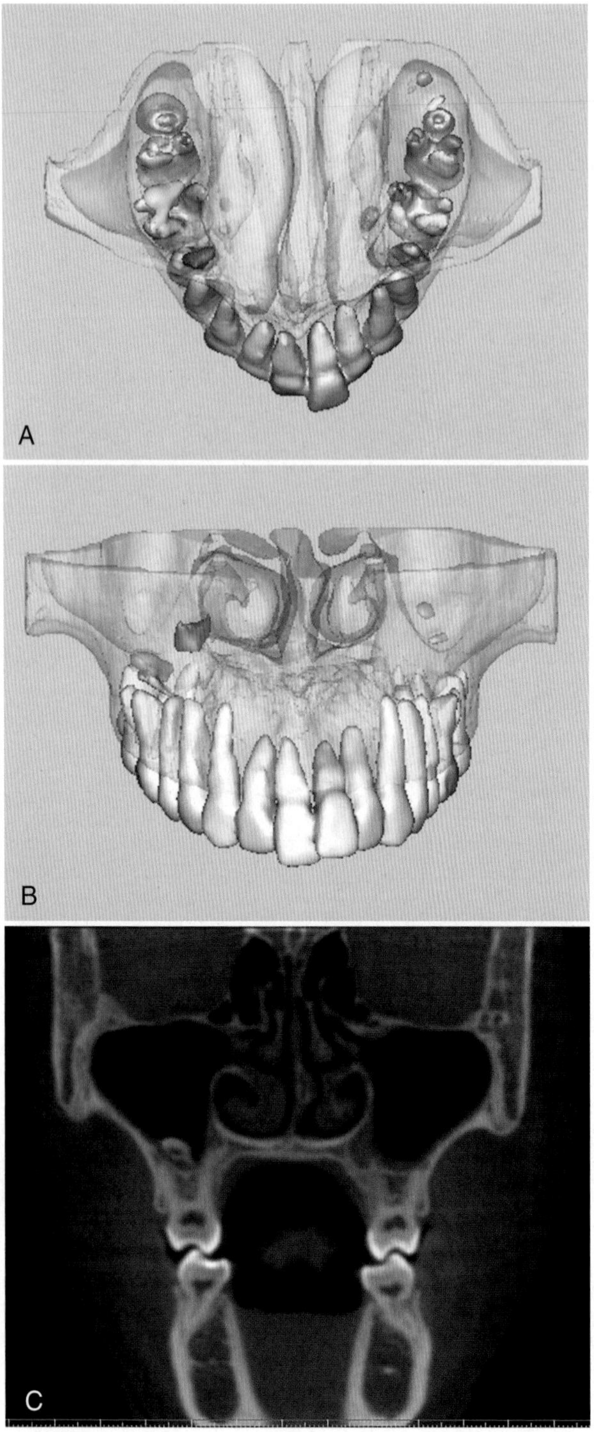

Fig 27-19 **A,** Imaging software that allows visualization of maxillary teeth through the maxilla. **B,** Unknown objects (in green, red, yellow, turquoise, and violet) noted in the sinus near maxillary posterior teeth. A differential diagnosis included multiple osteomas. **C,** Coronal image revealing the location of the larger osteoma. (Courtesy Carolina OMF Imaging, W. Bruce Howerton Jr., DDS, MS, Franklinton, NC.)

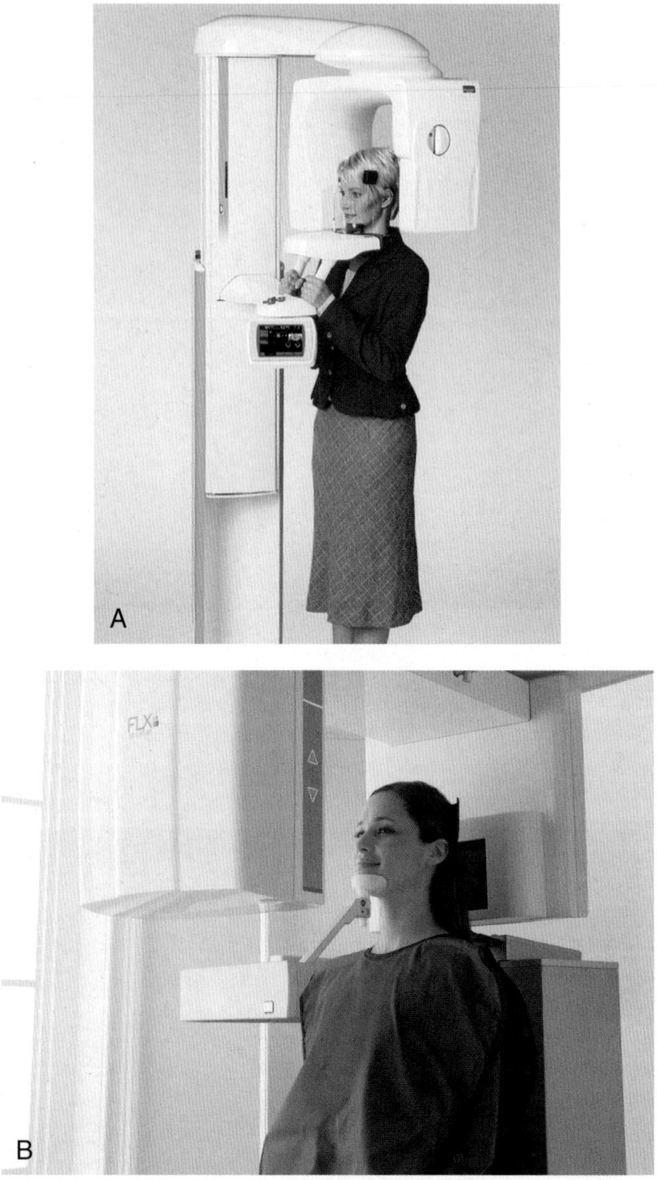

Fig 27-20 **A,** The Planmeca ProMax 3D imaging system, which offers a comfortable and open view of the surroundings to the patient. (Courtesy Planmeca Oy, Helsinki, Finland.) **B,** The i-CAT Flex imaging system allows the patient to be seated comfortably during the scanning process. (Courtesy KaVo Imaging, Brea, CA.)

SUMMARY

- Three-dimensional imaging provides the dental professional with a more complete interpretive image than does traditional dental imaging, which can provide only two dimensions.
- Three-dimensional imaging serves a number of diagnostic purposes for dental practitioners.
- Anatomic structures of the reconstructed volume of data provide accurate dimensional measurements of the patient with a 1:1 ratio relationship (Figure 27-23).
- The essential components for three-dimensional imaging include a CBCT machine, a computer, and various types of viewing software.

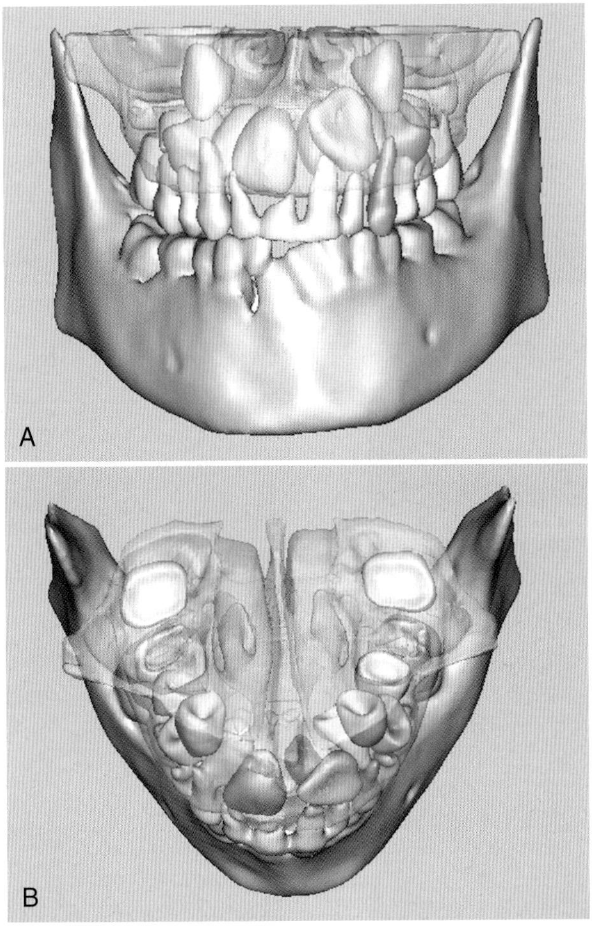

Fig 27-21 (Refer to the panoramic image in Figure 27-1.) **A,** Through the use of three-dimensional imaging and viewing software, the transparent maxilla reveals an inverted tooth #9 (shaded green) as well as a supernumerary tooth (shaded purple). **B,** The exact location of teeth in the anterior maxilla visualized from a superior view (looking down on the roots of the teeth). (Courtesy Carolina OMF Imaging, W. Bruce Howerton Jr., DDS, MS, Franklinton, NC.)

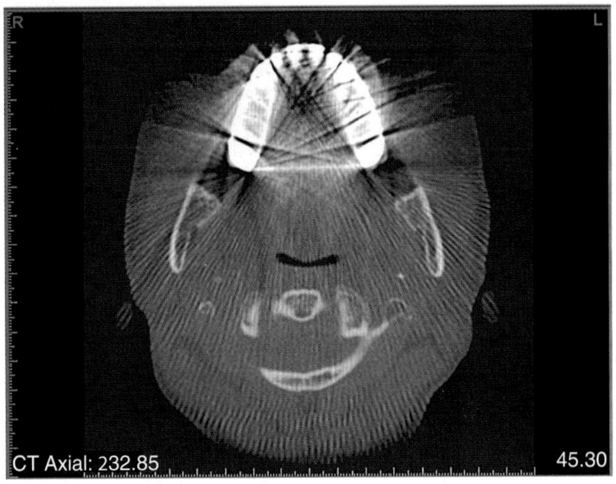

Fig 27-22 Streak artifacts demonstrated in this axial image of a patient with many full-coverage restorations. (Courtesy Carolina OMF Imaging, W. Bruce Howerton Jr., DDS, MS, Franklinton, NC.)

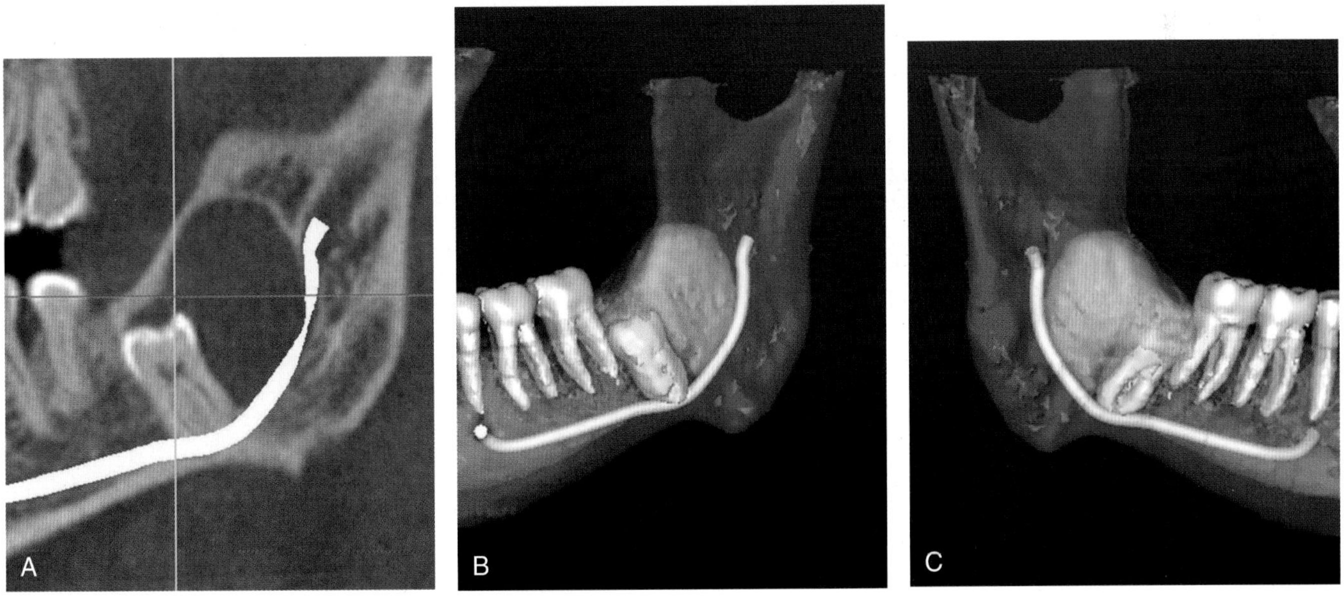

Fig 27-23 **A,** This sagittal view demonstrates the presence of a large radiolucent lesion associated with tooth #17. **B,** With the use of viewing software, a three-dimensional volume rendering is created to illustrate the exact size and location of a dentigerous cyst. **C,** The transparent mandible allows the dental professional to view the borders of the cyst as well as the proximity to the mandibular canal. (Courtesy Carolina OMF Imaging, W. Bruce Howerton Jr., DDS, MS, Franklinton, NC.)

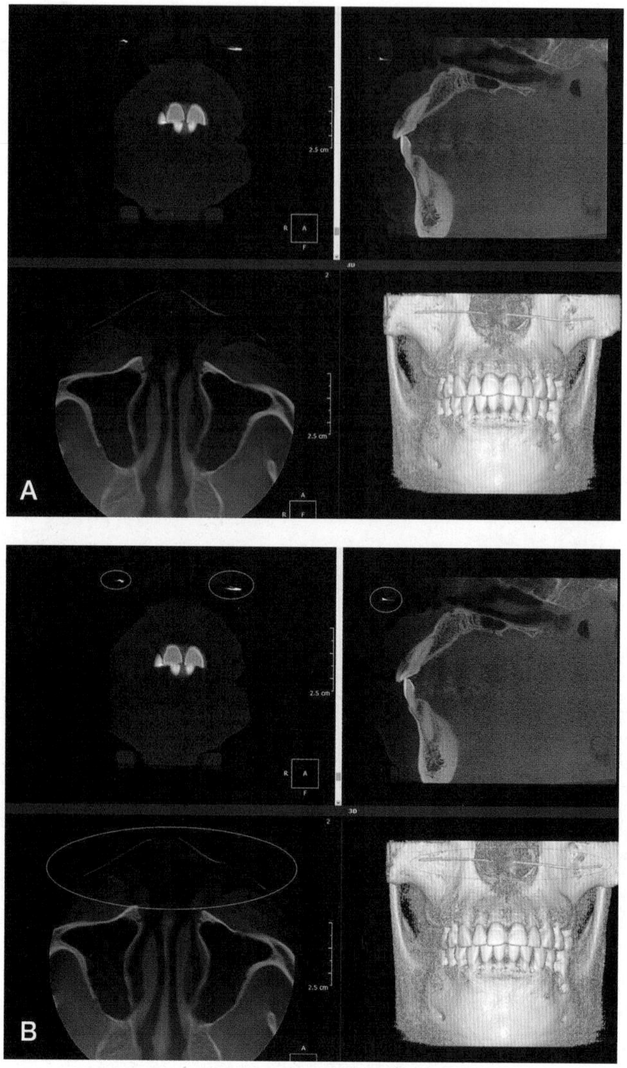

Fig 27-24 A, B (Courtesy Carolina OMF Imaging, W. Bruce Howerton Jr., DDS, MS, Franklinton, NC.)

- The advantages of three-dimensional imaging include a lower dose of radiation to the patient, a brief scanning time, anatomically accurate images, and ability to easily save and transport the images.
- The disadvantages of three-dimensional imaging include patient movement artifacts, limited FOV size, cost of equipment, and lack of training in interpretation of image data on areas outside of the maxilla and the mandible.

BIBLIOGRAPHY

American Dental Association Council on Scientific Affairs: The use of cone-beam computed tomography in dentistry, J Am Dent Assoc 143:899, 2012.

Danforth RA, Miles DA: Cone beam volume imaging: 3D applications for dentistry, Ir Dent 10(9):14, 2007.

Howerton WB, Mora MA: Advancements in digital imaging: what is new and on the horizon? J Am Dent Assoc 139:20S, 2008.

Intersocietal Accreditation Commission, www.intersocietal.org.

Ludlow JB, Davies-Ludlow LE, Brooks SL, et al: Dosimetry of 3 CBCT devices for oral and maxillofacial radiology: CB Mercuray, NewTom 3G and i-CAT, Dentomaxillofac Radiol 35:219, 2006.

Ludlow JB, Davies-Ludlow LE, White SC: Patient risk related to common dental radiographic examinations, J Am Dent Assoc 139:1237, 2008.

Mallya SM, Lam EWN: Cone beam computed tomography: volume acquisition. In White and Pharoah's Oral radiology: principles and interpretation, ed 8, St. Louis, 2019, Elsevier.

Mallya SM, Lam EWN: Cone beam computed tomography: volume preparation. In White and Pharoah's Oral radiology: principles and interpretation, ed 8, St. Louis, 2019, Elsevier.

Roberts JA, Drage NA, Davies J, et al: Effective dose from cone beam CT examinations in dentistry, Br J Radiol 82:35, 2009.

Tyndall DA, et al: Position statement of the American Academy of Oral and Maxillofacial Radiology on selection criteria for the use of radiology in dental implantology with emphasis on cone beam computed tomography, Oral Surg Oral Med Oral Pathol Oral Radiol Endod 113:817, 2012.

White SC, Heslop EW, Hollender LG, et al: American Academy of Oral and Maxillofacial Radiology, ad hoc Committee on Parameters of Care: Parameters of radiologic care: an official report of the American Academy of Oral and Maxillofacial Radiology, Oral Surg Oral Med Oral Pathol Oral Radiol Endod 91(5):498, 2001.

QUIZ QUESTIONS

Matching

For questions 1 to 10, match each term with its corresponding definition.

a. cone-beam computed tomography
b. DICOM data
c. field of view
d. multiplanar reconstruction (MPR)
e. coronal plane
f. sagittal plane
g. contrast resolution
h. spatial resolution
i. voxel
j. three-dimensional volume rendering

____ **1.** The universal format for handling, storing, and transmitting three-dimensional images.

____ **2.** The smallest element of a three-dimensional image.

____ **3.** A measurement of pixel size in multiplanar reconstruction.

____ **4.** A vertical plane that divides the body into right and left sides; runs perpendicular to the ground.

____ **5.** The reconstruction of raw data into images when imported into viewing software to create three anatomic planes of the body.

____ **6.** The area that can be captured when performing imaging procedures.

____ **7.** Term used to describe computer-assisted digital imaging in dentistry; this imaging technique uses a cone-shaped x-ray beam to acquire information and present it in three dimensions.

____ **8.** A vertical plane that divides the body into anterior and posterior sides; runs perpendicular to the ground.

____ **9.** The number of gray-scale colors available to be chosen for each pixel in the image.

____ **10.** A three-dimensional shape that is created from two-dimensional images.

TRUE OR FALSE

____ **11.** Compared with traditional computed tomography (CT) procedures, cone-beam imaging provides a higher radiation dose for the patient.

____ **12.** A short exposure time decreases the chances for motion artifacts to occur and encourages a high level of patient cooperation.

____ **13.** If the field of view is small, findings or pathology in other regions of the oral and maxillofacial complex may be missed.

____ **14.** Cone-beam data has a 2:1 relationship with the anatomy.

____ **15.** A disadvantage of use of cone-beam data is that many dental professionals who incorporate CBCT into their practices have not had the training required to interpret anatomy beyond the maxilla and mandible.

____ **16.** Three-dimensional imaging provides an in-depth image that gives dental professionals a more complete interpretive image than with two-dimensional scans of traditional imaging.

____ **17.** Three-dimensional imaging serves a number of diagnostic purposes for dental practitioners.

MULTIPLE CHOICE

18. An area of high attenuation that could stop radiation from reaching the receptor could include which restoration(s)?
a. metal crown
b. bridge
c. large amalgam restoration
d. all of the above

19. Which is/are advantage(s) of CBCT imaging?
a. images can be saved digitally in a .jpg or .bmp format
b. images can be placed on a compact disc
c. images can be emailed to referring dentists
d. all of the above

20. The fact that the cone-beam data has a 1:1 relationship with the anatomy means that:
a. anatomically accurate images are produced
b. magnification of measurements does not occur
c. CBCT eliminates the superimposition of structures
d. all of the above

ESSAY

21. Name some of the common uses of three-dimensional imaging.

22. Why is it important for the dental professional who interprets a CBCT scan to be a board-certified oral and maxillofacial radiologist or a dentist with adequate training or experience?

23. Prior to performing CBCT, what instructions should be given to the patient?

24. Name the essential specialized equipment necessary for three-dimensional digital imaging.

IDENTIFICATION

25. Identify the object outlined with circles in Figure 27-24B.

28

Normal Anatomy: Intraoral Images

LEARNING OBJECTIVES

After completion of this chapter, the student will be able to do the following:

1. Define the key terms associated with normal anatomy on intraoral images.
2. State the difference between cortical and cancellous bone.
3. Define and discuss the general terms that describe prominences, spaces, and depressions in bone.
4. In relation to normal anatomic landmarks of the maxilla on a human skull:
   - Identify and describe the normal anatomic landmarks of the maxilla on a human skull.
   - Identify and describe the normal anatomic landmarks of the maxilla as viewed on dental images.
   - Identify each normal landmark of the maxilla as either radiolucent or radiopaque as viewed on dental images.
5. In relation to normal anatomic landmarks of the mandible on a human skull:
   - Identify and describe the normal anatomic landmarks of the mandible on a human skull.
   - Identify and describe the normal anatomic landmarks of the mandible as viewed on dental images.
   - Identify each normal landmark of the mandible as either radiolucent or radiopaque as viewed on dental images.
6. Identify and describe the appearance of normal tooth anatomy and supporting structures as viewed on dental images; identify each normal tooth structure as radiolucent or radiopaque as viewed on dental images.
7. Identify the primary teeth and eruption patterns of the permanent teeth as viewed on dental images.

The dental radiographer must be able to recognize the normal anatomic landmarks viewed on intraoral images. Recognition of such normal anatomic landmarks enables the radiographer to accurately mount and interpret intraoral images. Without a working knowledge of normal anatomy, the dental radiographer may incorrectly mount dental images or mistake normal anatomic structures for pathologic conditions. Although some manufacturers of digital imaging equipment allow for automated mounting of exposed images, it is still the responsibility of the dental radiographer to verify that the images are placed in correct anatomic order.

Before normal anatomic landmarks can be identified, the dental radiographer must have a thorough knowledge of the anatomy of the maxilla and the mandible. Each normal anatomic landmark seen on intraoral images corresponds to what is seen on the human skull. If the dental radiographer can identify the anatomic landmarks of the maxilla and the mandible on the human skull, the same normal anatomic landmarks can be identified on a dental image.

The purpose of this chapter is to review the normal anatomy of the maxilla and the mandible on the skull and to describe the normal anatomic landmarks as viewed on intraoral images. A review of tooth anatomy and supporting structures, as well as an overview of the primary and mixed dentitions with eruption sequences, is also included.

DEFINITIONS OF GENERAL TERMS

A number of general terms are used to describe the anatomy of the skull. Terms describing types of bone, bony prominences, and bony spaces and depressions can be used to characterize areas of the maxilla and the mandible normally seen on dental images. The dental radiographer can use these general terms to describe what is viewed on intraoral images.

Types of Bone

The composition of bone in the human body can be described as either *cortical* or *cancellous*.

Cortical Bone. The term cortical is derived from the Latin word *cortex* and means "outer layer." Cortical bone, also referred to as *compact bone*, is the dense outer layer of bone (Figure 28-1). Cortical bone resists the passage of the x-ray beam and appears radiopaque on a dental image. The inferior border of the mandible is composed of cortical bone and appears radiopaque (Figure 28-2).

Cancellous Bone. The term cancellous is also derived from Latin and means "arranged like a lattice." Cancellous bone is the soft, spongy bone located between two layers of dense cortical bone (see Figure 28-1). Cancellous bone is composed of numerous bony trabeculae that form

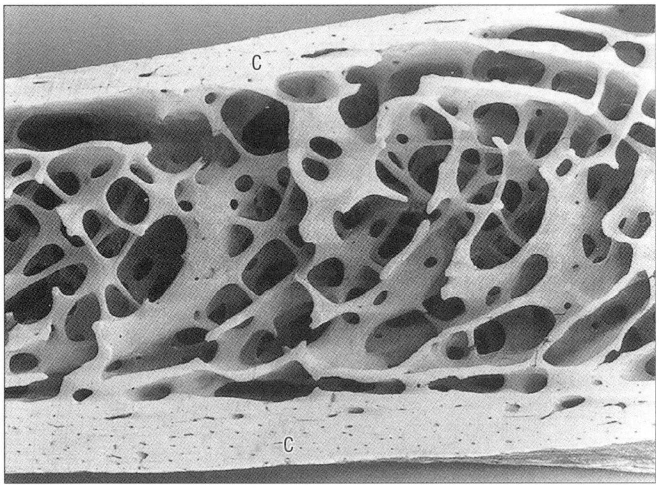

Fig 28-1 Cortical bone and cancellous bone. (From Standrings: Gray's anatomy, ed 40, London, 2009, Churchill Livingstone.)

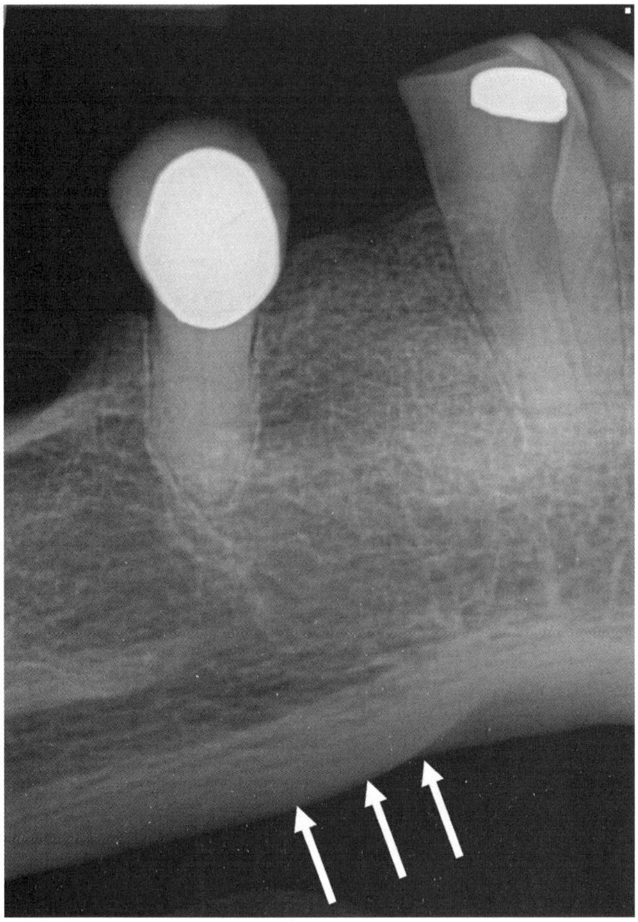

Fig 28-2 Cortical bone appears highly radiopaque on a dental image.

a lattice-like network of intercommunicating spaces filled with bone marrow. The trabeculae, actual pieces of bone, resist the passage of the x-ray beam and appear radiopaque; in contrast, the marrow spaces permit the passage of the x-ray beam and appear radiolucent. The

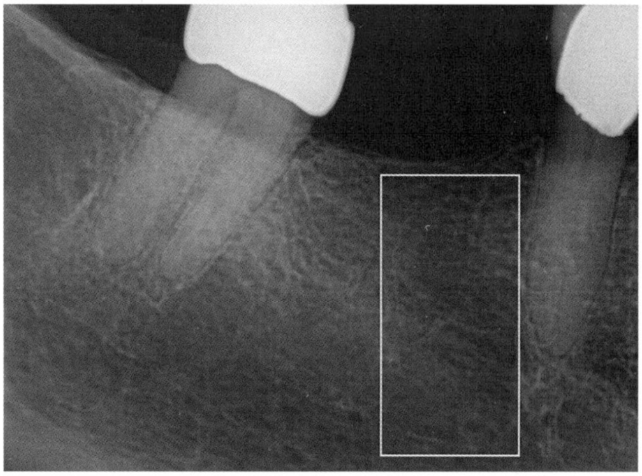

Fig 28-3 Cancellous bone appears predominantly radiolucent.

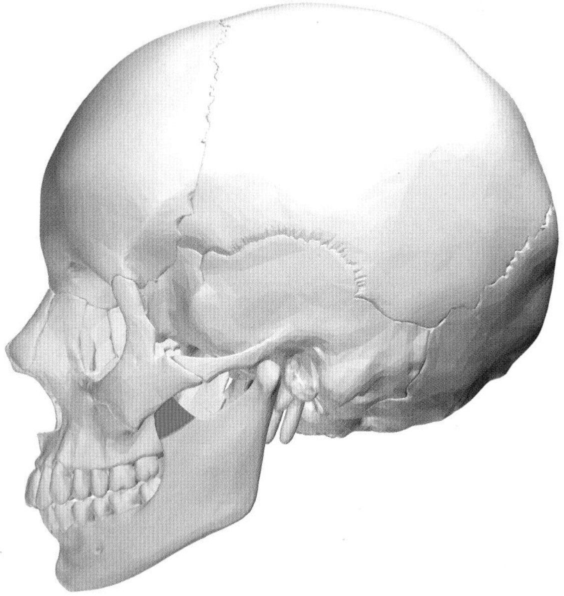

Fig 28-4 Coronoid process of mandible indicated in red. (Image created from BodyParts3D, ©The Database Center for Life Science licensed under CC Attribution-Share Alike 2.1 Japan [http://creativecommons.org/licenses/by-sa/2.1/jp/legalcode] / User: Was a bee / Wikimedia Commons / https://commons.wikimedia.org/wiki/File:Coronoid_process_of_mandible_-_lateral_view.png.)

larger the trabeculations, the more radiolucent the area of cancellous bone appears. Cancellous bone appears predominantly radiolucent (Figure 28-3).

Prominences of Bone

Prominences of bone are composed of dense cortical bone and appear radiopaque on dental images. Five terms can be used to describe the bony prominences seen in maxillary and mandibular periapical images, as follows:

Process: A marked prominence or projection of bone; an example is the coronoid process of the mandible (Figure 28-4).

Ridge: A linear prominence or projection of bone; an example is the external oblique ridge of the mandible (Figure 28-5).

Spine: A sharp, thorn-like projection of bone; an example is the anterior nasal spine of the maxilla (Figure 28-6).

Tubercle: A small bump or nodule of bone; an example is the mental tubercles of the mandible (Figure 28-7).

Tuberosity: A rounded prominence of bone; an example is the maxillary tuberosity (Figure 28-8).

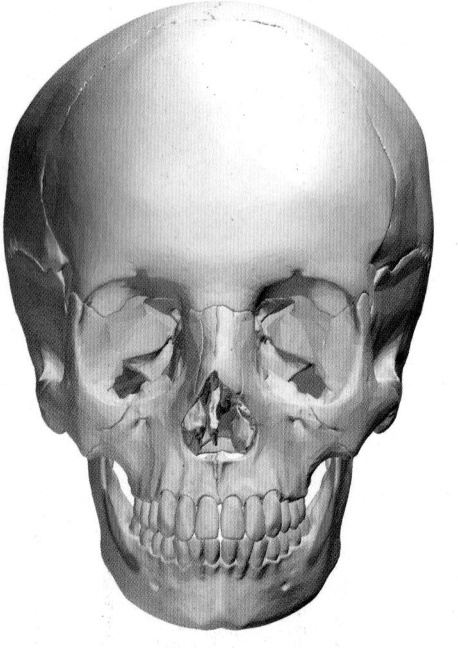

Fig 28-5 External oblique ridge indicated in red. (Image created from BodyParts3D, ©The Database Center for Life Science licensed under CC Attribution-Share Alike 2.1 Japan [http://creativecommons.org/licenses/by-sa/2.1/jp/legalcode] / User: Was a bee / Wikimedia Commons / https://commons.wikimedia.org/wiki/File:External_oblique_line_of_mandible_-_skull_-_anterior_view.png.)

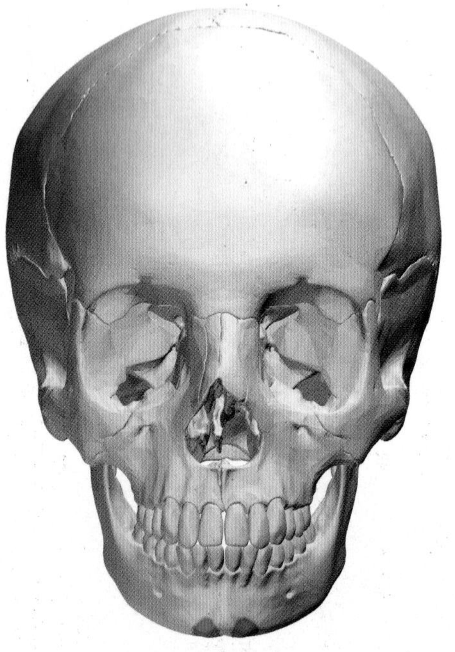

Fig 28-7 Mental tubercles indicated in red. (Image created from BodyParts3D, ©The Database Center for Life Science licensed under CC Attribution-Share Alike 2.1 Japan [http://creativecommons.org/licenses/by-sa/2.1/jp/legalcode] / User: Was a bee / Wikimedia Commons / https://commons.wikimedia.org/wiki/File:Mental_tubercle_-_skull_-_anterior_view01.png.)

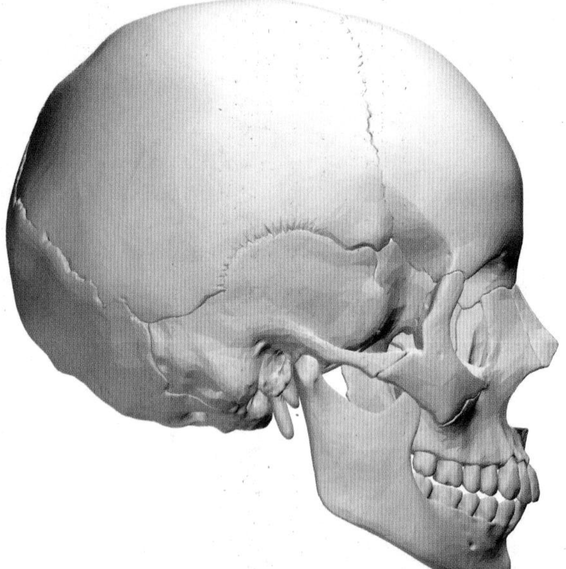

Fig 28-6 Anterior nasal spine indicated in red. (Image created from BodyParts3D, ©The Database Center for Life Science licensed under CC Attribution-Share Alike 2.1 Japan [http://creativecommons.org/licenses/by-sa/2.1/jp/legalcode] / User: Was a bee / Wikimedia Commons / https://commons.wikimedia.org/wiki/File:Anterior_nasal_spine_of_maxilla_-_skull_-_lateral_view.png.)

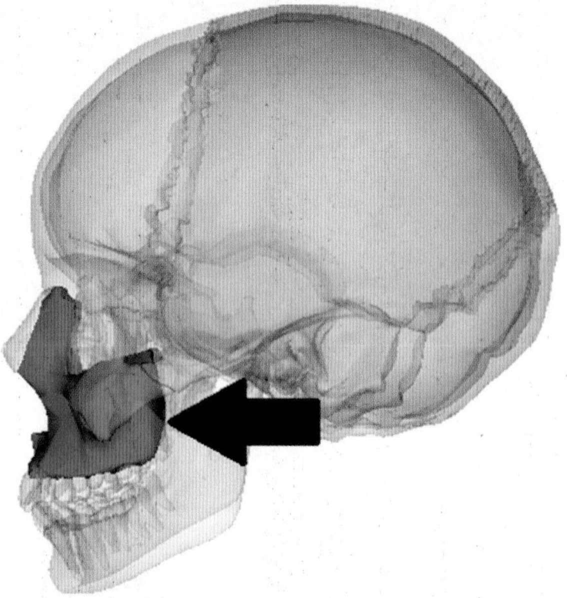

Fig 28-8 Maxillary tuberosity (arrow). (Image created from BodyParts3D, © The Database Center for Life Science licensed under CC Attribution-Share Alike 2.1 Japan [http://creativecommons.org/licenses/by-sa/2.1/jp/legalcode] / Modified from User: Was a bee / Wikimedia Commons / https://commons.wikimedia.org/wiki/File:Maxilla_image.png.)

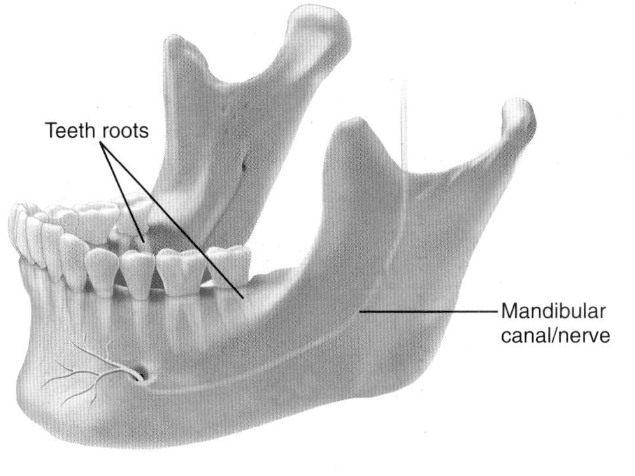

Fig 28-9 Mandibular canal.

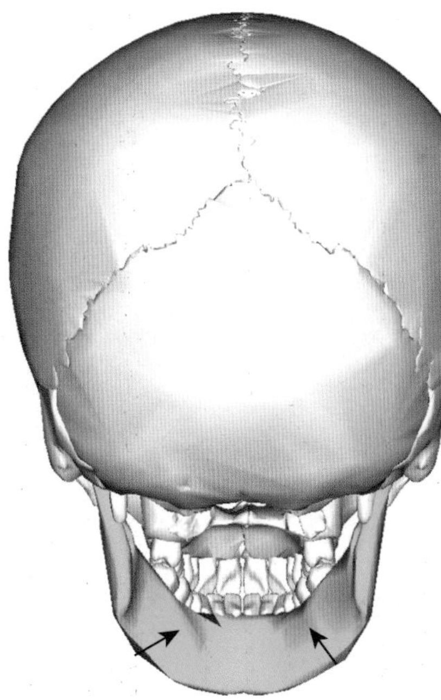

Fig 28-11 Submandibular fossa (arrows). (Image created from BodyParts3D, © The Database Center for Life Science licensed under CC Attribution-Share Alike 2.1 Japan [http://creativecommons.org/licenses/by-sa/2.1/jp/legalcode] / User: Was a bee / Wikimedia Commons / https://commons.wikimedia.org/wiki/File:Mandible_posterior.png.)

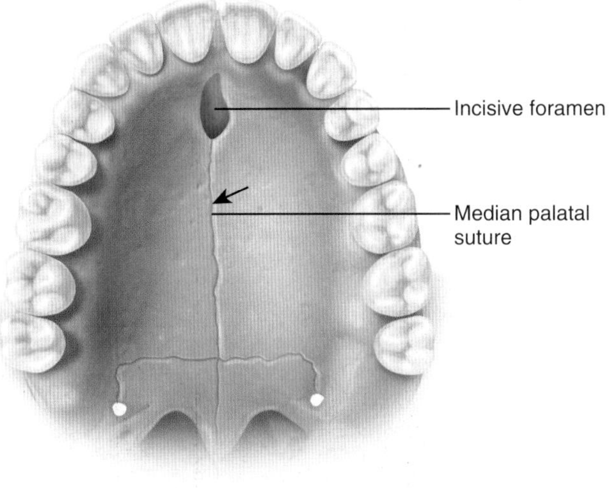

Fig 28-10 Incisive foramen indicated in green and median palatal suture.

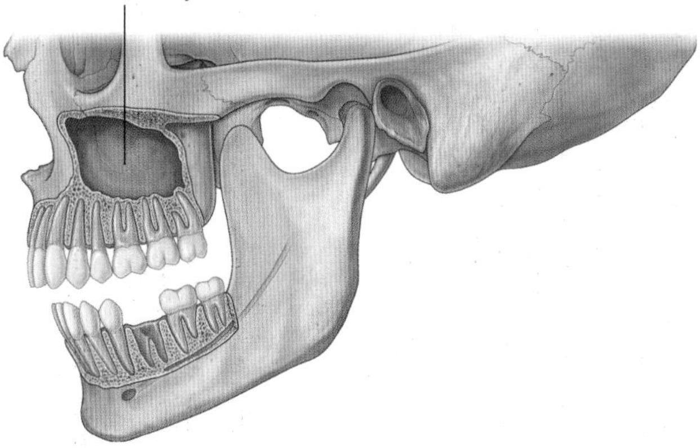

Fig 28-12 Maxillary sinus. (From Drake RL, et al: Gray's atlas of anatomy, Philadelphia, 2008, Churchill Livingstone.)

Spaces and Depressions in Bone

Spaces and depressions in bone do not resist the passage of the x-ray beam and appear radiolucent on dental images. Four terms can be used to describe the spaces and depressions in bone viewed in maxillary and mandibular periapical images, as follows:

Canal: A tubelike passageway through bone that contains nerves and blood vessels; an example is the mandibular canal (Figure 28-9).

Foramen: An opening or hole in bone that permits the passage of nerves and blood vessels; an example is the incisive foramen of the maxilla (Figure 28-10).

Fossa: A broad, shallow, scooped-out or depressed area of bone; an example is the submandibular fossa of the mandible (Figure 28-11).

Sinus: A hollow space, cavity, or recess in bone; an example is the maxillary sinus (Figure 28-12).

Miscellaneous Terms

Two other general terms can be used to describe normal landmarks viewed on a dental image, as follows:

Septum: A bony wall or partition that divides two spaces or cavities. A septum may be present within the space of a fossa or sinus. A bony septum appears radiopaque, in contrast to a space or cavity, which appears radiolucent. An example is the nasal septum (Figure 28-13).

Suture: An immovable joint that represents a line of union between adjoining bones of the skull. Sutures are found only in the skull. On dental images, a suture appears as a thin radiolucent line. An example is the median palatine suture of the maxilla (see Figure 28-10).

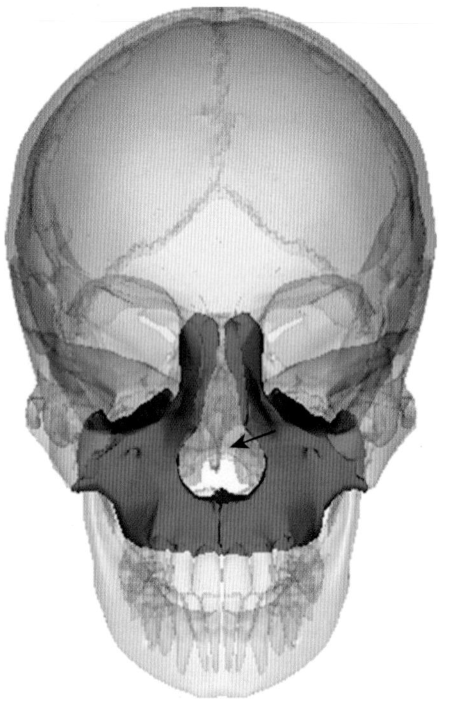

Fig 28-13 The nasal septum (arrow) divides the nasal cavity. Paired maxilla bones are indicated in red. (Image created from BodyParts3D, © The Database Center for Life Science licensed under CC Attribution-Share Alike 2.1 Japan [http://creativecommons.org/licenses/by-sa/2.1/jp/legalcode] / Modified from User: Was a bee / Wikimedia Commons / https://commons.wikimedia.org/wiki/File:Maxilla_image.png.)

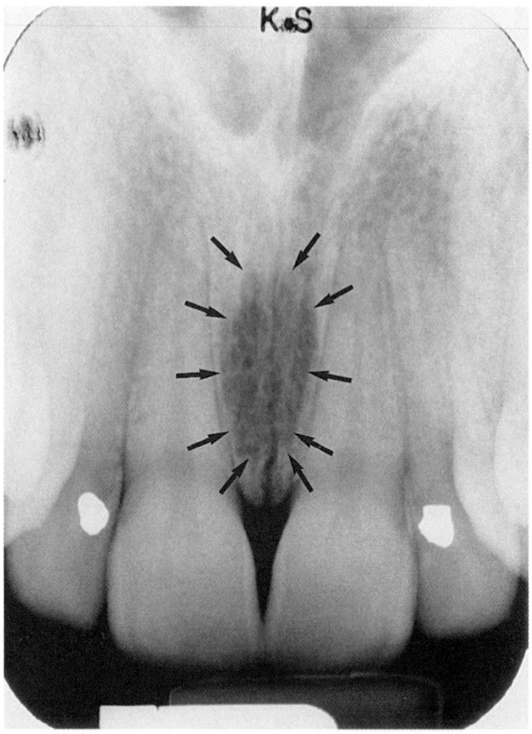

Fig 28-14 The incisive foramen appears radiolucent. (From Haring JI, Lind LJ: Radiographic interpretation for the dental hygienist, Philadelphia, 1993, Saunders.)

NORMAL ANATOMIC LANDMARKS

Bony Landmarks of the Maxilla

The upper jaw is composed of two paired bones, the *maxillae* (see Figure 28-13). The paired maxillae meet at the midline of the face and are often referred to as a *single bone*, the maxilla. The maxilla has been described as the architectural cornerstone of the face. All the bones of the face, with the exception of the mandible, articulate with the maxilla. The maxilla forms the floor of the orbit of the eyes, the sides and floor of the nasal cavities, and the hard palate. The lower border of the maxilla supports maxillary teeth. This section describes the bony landmarks of the maxilla and how each one is viewed on an intraoral image.

Incisive Foramen.

Description. The incisive foramen (also known as the *nasopalatine foramen*) is an opening or hole in the bone located at the midline of the anterior portion of the hard palate directly posterior to the maxillary central incisors (see Figure 28-10). The nasopalatine nerve exits the maxilla through the incisive foramen.

Appearance. On an anterior maxillary periapical image, the incisive foramen appears as a small, ovoid or round radiolucent area located between the roots of the maxillary central incisors (Figure 28-14).

Superior Foramina of Incisive Canal.

Description. The superior foramina of the incisive canal are two tiny openings or holes in bone that are located on the floor of the nasal cavity (*foramina* is the plural of *foramen*) (Figure 28-15). The superior foramina are the openings of two small canals that extend downward and medially from the floor of the nasal cavity. These two small canals join together to form the incisive canal and share a common exit, the *incisive foramen.* The nasopalatine nerve enters the maxilla through the superior foramina, travels through the incisive canal, and exits at the incisive foramen.

Appearance. On an anterior maxillary periapical image, the superior foramina appear as two small, round radiolucencies located superior to the apices of the maxillary central incisors (Figure 28-16).

Median Palatal Suture.

Description. The median palatal suture is the immovable joint between the two palatine processes of the maxilla. (The palatine processes of the maxilla form the major portion of the hard palate.) The median palatal suture extends from the alveolar bone between the maxillary central incisors to the posterior hard palate (see Figure 28-10).

Appearance. On an anterior maxillary periapical image, the median palatal suture appears as a thin radiolucent line between the maxillary central incisors (Figure 28-17). The median palatal suture is bounded on both sides by dense cortical bone that appears radiopaque. As the median palatal suture fuses with age, it may become less distinct on a dental image.

Lateral Fossa.

Description. The lateral fossa (also known as the *canine fossa*) is a smooth, depressed area of the maxilla located just inferior and medial to the infraorbital foramen between maxillary canine and lateral incisors (Figure 28-18).

Appearance. On an anterior maxillary periapical image, the lateral fossa appears as a radiolucent area between the maxillary canine and lateral incisor (Figure 28-19). In some periapical images, the lateral fossa may appear as a distinct radiolucency; in others, it may appear to be absent. The appearance of the lateral fossa varies depending on the anatomy of the individual.

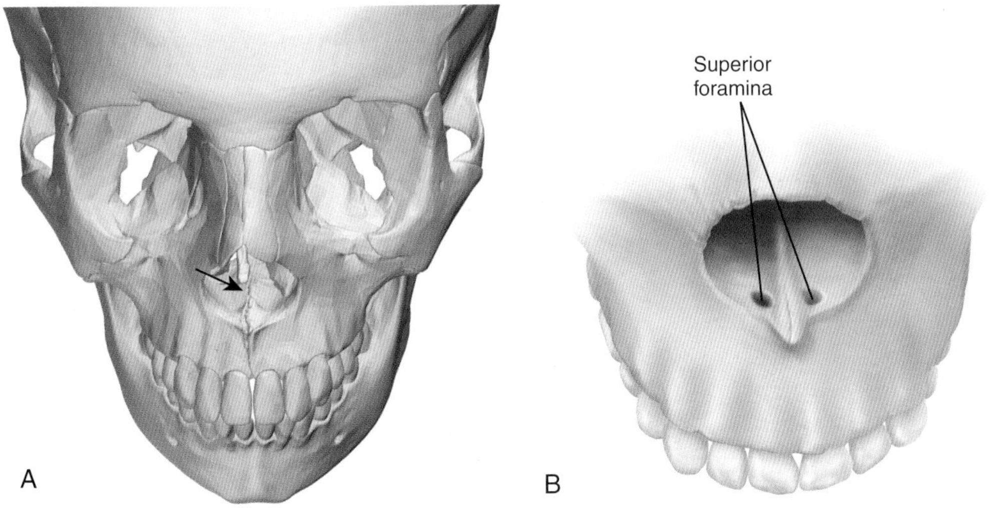

Fig 28-15 A, The superior foramina of the incisive canal are located on the anterior floor of the nasal cavity. (Images created from BodyParts3D, ©The Database Center for Life Science licensed under CC Attribution-Share Alike 2.1 Japan [http://creativecommons.org/licenses/by-sa/2.1/jp/legalcode] / Modified from User: Was a bee / Wikimedia Commons / https://commons.wikimedia.org/wiki/File:Sagittal_suture_-_skull_-_anterior_view02.png.) B, The superior foramina.

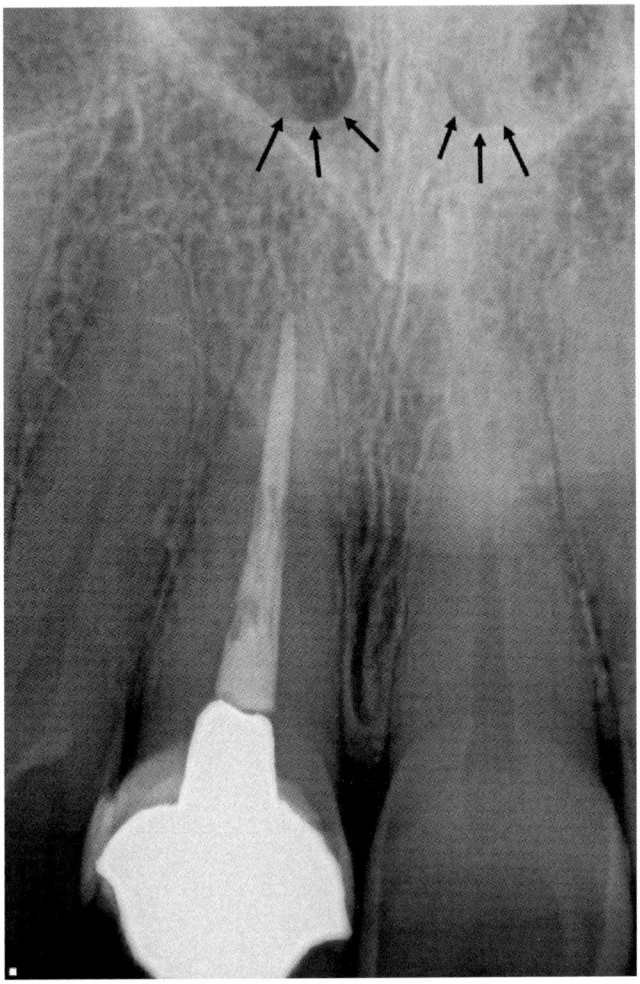

Fig 28-16 The superior foramina of the incisive canal appear as two small, round radiolucencies.

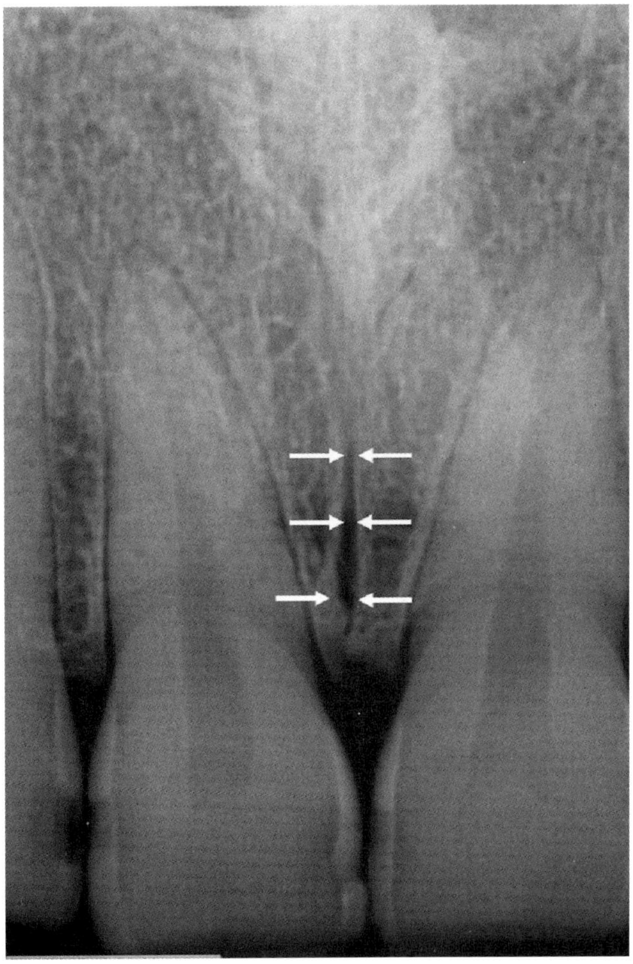

Fig 28-17 The median palatal suture appears as a thin radiolucent line.

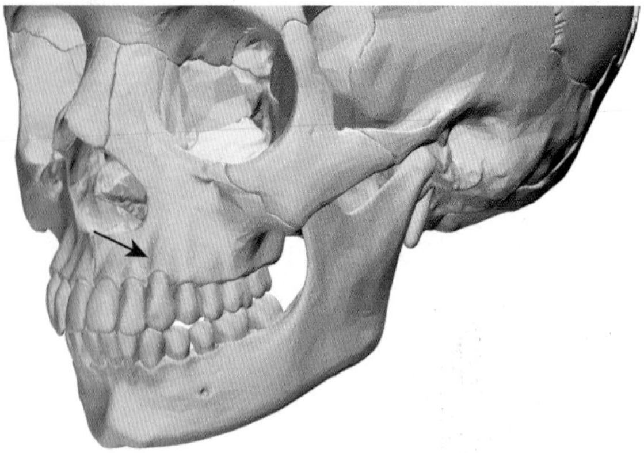

Fig 28-18 Lateral fossa. (Image created from BodyParts3D, © The Database Center for Life Science licensed under CC Attribution-Share Alike 2.1 Japan [http://creativecommons.org/licenses/by-sa/2.1/jp/legalcode] / Modified from User: Was a bee / Wikimedia Commons / https://commons.wikimedia.org/wiki/File:Coronal_suture_-_skull_-_anterior_view03.png.)

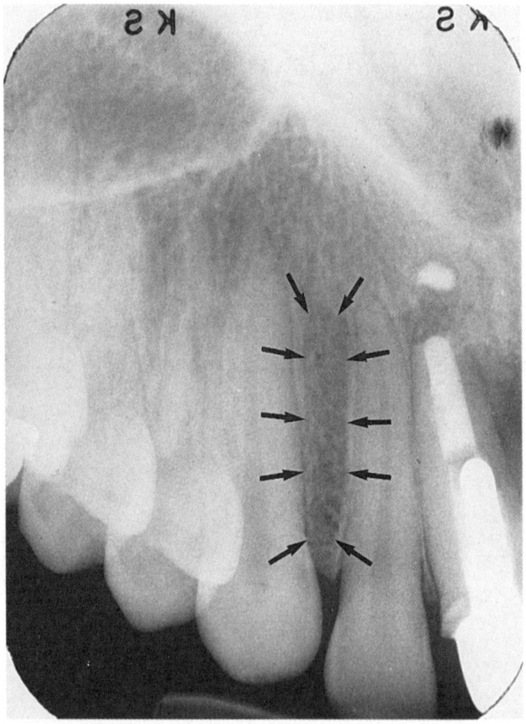

Fig 28-19 The lateral fossa appears as a radiolucent area between the lateral incisor and the canine. (Photo Courtesy Allyson Bowcutt.)

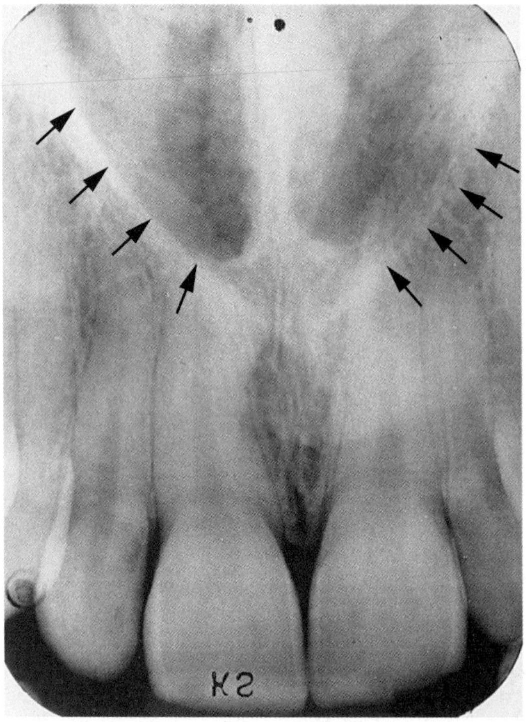

Fig 28-20 The nasal cavity appears as a large radiolucent area above the maxillary incisors. (From Haring JI, Lind LJ: Radiographic interpretation for the dental hygienist, Philadelphia, 1993, Saunders.)

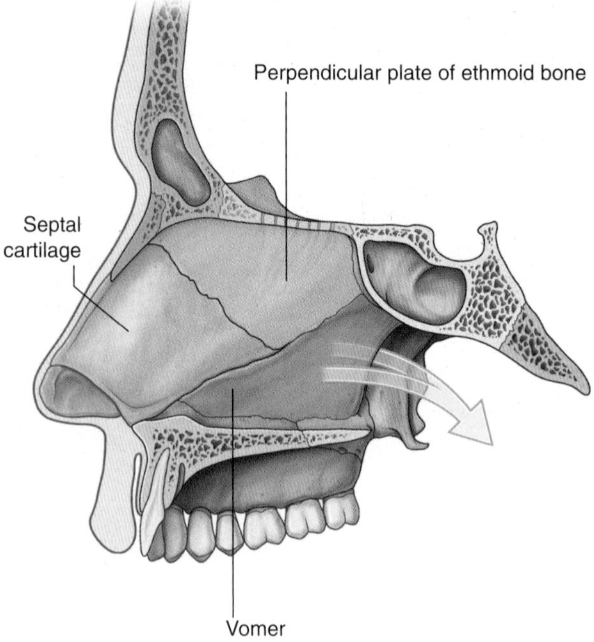

Fig 28-21 The nasal septum is made up of the perpendicular plate of the ethmoid bone, the vomer, and cartilage. (From Drake, RL: Gray's anatomy for students, ed 3, London, 2015, Churchill Livingstone.)

Nasal Cavity.

Description. The nasal cavity (also known as the *nasal fossa*) is a pear-shaped compartment of bone located superior to the maxilla (see Figure 28-13). The inferior portion, or floor, of the nasal cavity is formed by the palatal processes of the maxilla and the horizontal portions of palatine bones. The lateral walls of the nasal cavity are formed by the ethmoid bone and the maxillae. The nasal cavity is divided by a bony partition, or wall, called the *nasal septum*.

Appearance. On an anterior maxillary periapical image, the nasal cavity appears as a large, radiolucent area superior to the maxillary incisors (Figure 28-20).

Nasal Septum.

Description. The nasal septum is a vertical bony wall or partition that divides the nasal cavity into the right and left nasal fossae (*fossae* is the plural of *fossa*) (see Figure 28-13). The nasal septum is formed by cartilage and two bones—the vomer and a portion of the ethmoid bone (Figure 28-21).

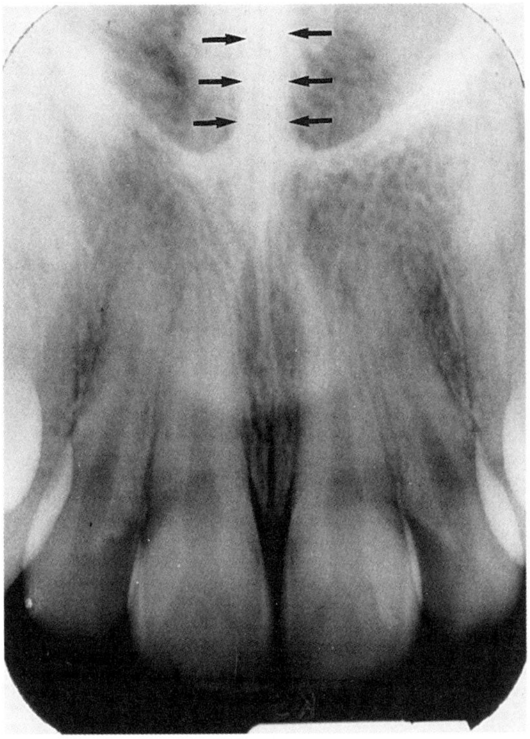

Fig 28-22 The nasal septum appears as a radiopaque partition that divides the nasal cavity. (From Haring JI, Lind LJ: Radiographic interpretation for the dental hygienist, Philadelphia, 1993, Saunders.)

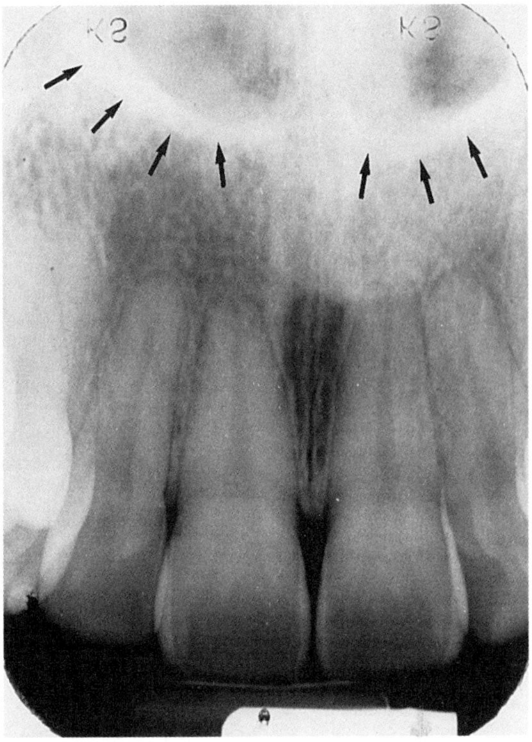

Fig 28-23 The floor of the nasal cavity appears as a radiopaque band. (From Haring JI, Lind LJ: Radiographic interpretation for the dental hygienist, Philadelphia, 1993, Saunders.)

Appearance. On an anterior maxillary periapical image, the nasal septum appears as a vertical radiopaque partition that divides the nasal cavity (Figure 28-22). The nasal septum may be superimposed over the median palatal suture.

Floor of Nasal Cavity.

Description. The floor of the nasal cavity is a bony wall formed by the palatal processes of the maxilla and the horizontal portions of palatine bones (see Figure 28-15). The floor is composed of dense cortical bone and defines the inferior border of the nasal cavity.

Appearance. On an anterior maxillary periapical image, the floor of the nasal cavity appears as a dense radiopaque band of bone superior to the maxillary incisors (Figure 28-23).

Anterior Nasal Spine.

Description. The anterior nasal spine is a sharp projection of the maxilla located at the anterior and inferior portion of the nasal cavity (see Figure 28-6).

Appearance. On an anterior maxillary periapical image, the anterior nasal spine appears as a V-shaped radiopaque area located at the intersection of the floor of the nasal cavity and the nasal septum (Figure 28-24).

Inferior Nasal Conchae.

Description. The inferior nasal conchae are wafer-thin, curved plates of bone that extend from the lateral walls of the nasal cavity (Figure 28-25). Inferior nasal conchae are seen in the lower lateral portions of the nasal cavity. The term *concha* is derived from Latin and means "shell shaped" or "scroll shaped."

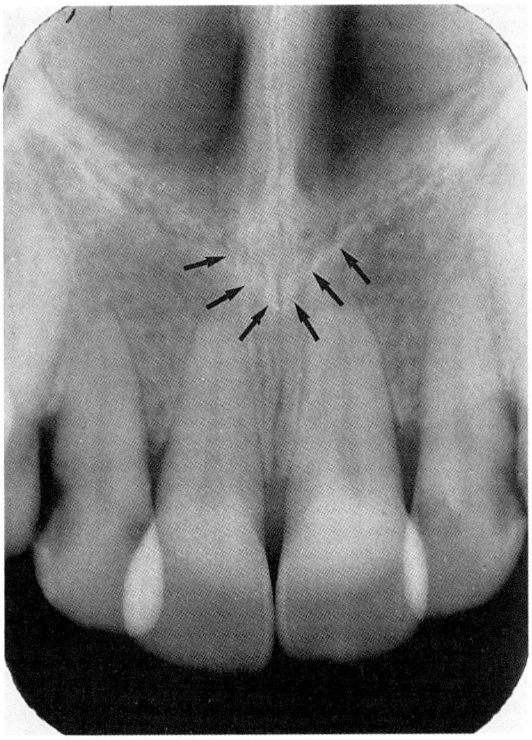

Fig 28-24 The anterior nasal spine appears as a V-shaped radiopacity at the midline of the floor of the nasal cavity. (From Haring JI, Lind LJ: Radiographic interpretation for the dental hygienist, Philadelphia, 1993, Saunders.)

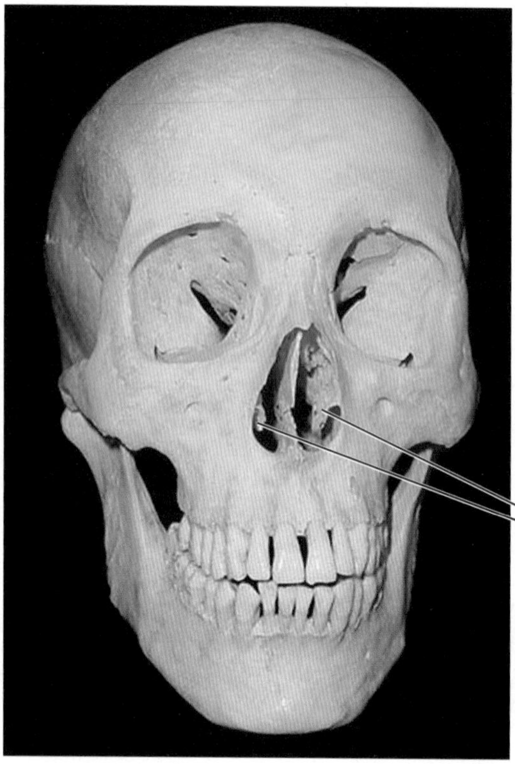

Fig 28-25 Inferior nasal conchae. (From Fehrenbach M, Herring S: Illustrated anatomy of the head and neck, ed 4, Philadelphia, 2011, Saunders.)

Appearance. On an anterior maxillary periapical image, the inferior nasal conchae appear as diffuse radiopaque masses or projections within the nasal cavity (Figure 28-26).

Maxillary Sinus.

Description. The maxillary sinuses are paired cavities or compartments of bone located within the maxilla (Figure 28-27). Maxillary sinuses are located superior to maxillary premolar and molar teeth. Rarely does the maxillary sinus extend anteriorly beyond the canines. At birth, the maxillary sinus is the size of a small pea. With growth, the maxillary sinus expands and eventually occupies a large portion of the maxilla. The maxillary sinus may extend to include interdental bone, molar furcation areas, or the maxillary tuberosity region.

Appearance. On a posterior maxillary periapical image, the maxillary sinus appears as a radiolucent area located superior to the apices of maxillary premolars and molars (Figure 28-28). The floor of the maxillary sinus is composed of dense cortical bone and appears as a radiopaque line.

Septa Within Maxillary Sinus.

Description. Bony septa (*septa* is the plural of *septum*) may be seen within the maxillary sinus. Septa are bony walls or partitions that appear to divide the maxillary sinus into compartments.

Appearance. On a posterior maxillary periapical image, the septa appear as radiopaque lines within the maxillary sinus (Figure 28-29). In some periapical images, the septa appear as distinct radiopaque lines; in others, no septa are seen. The presence and number of bony septa within a maxillary sinus vary depending on the anatomy of the individual.

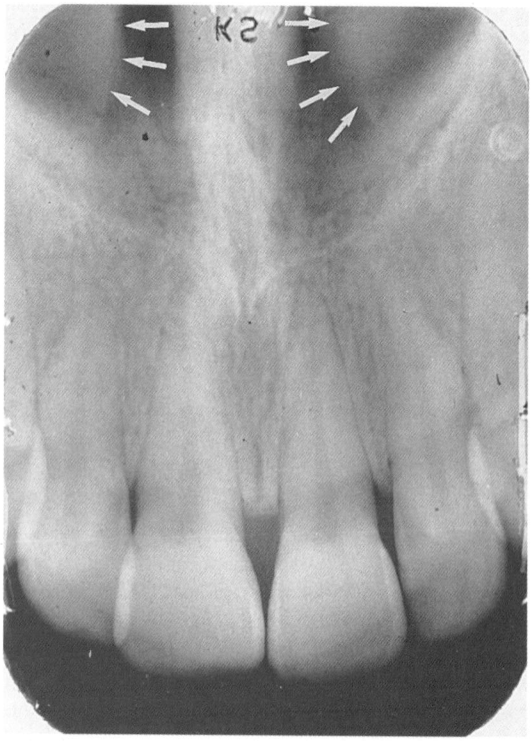

Fig 28-26 The inferior nasal conchae appear as diffuse radiopacities within the nasal cavity. (From Haring JI, Lind LJ: Radiographic interpretation for the dental hygienist, Philadelphia, 1993, Saunders.)

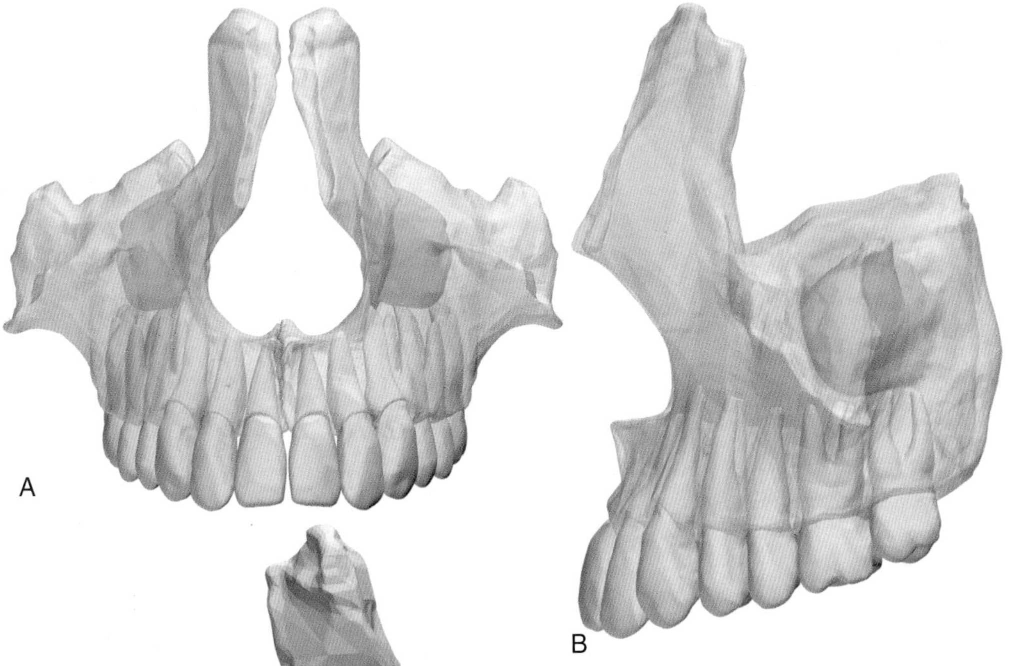

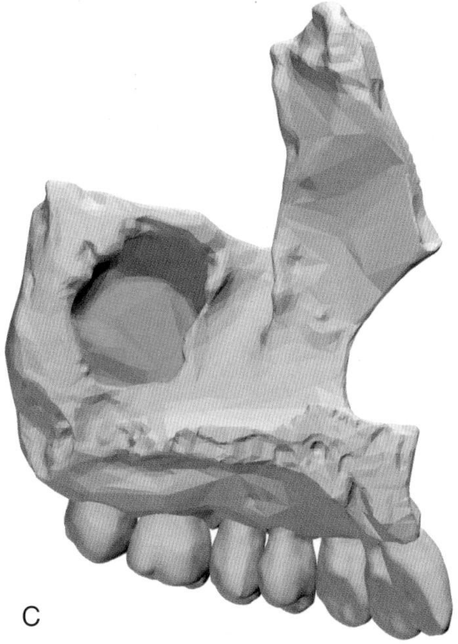

Fig 28-27 **A,** Maxillary sinus, anterior view. **B,** Maxillary sinus, lateral view. **C,** Maxillary sinus, medial view. (Images created from BodyParts3D, © The Database Center for Life Science licensed under CC Attribution-Share Alike 2.1 Japan [http://creativecommons.org/licenses/by-sa/2.1/jp/legalcode] / User: Was a bee / Wikimedia Commons / **A,** https://commons.wikimedia.org/wiki/File:Maxillary_sinus_-_posterior_view.png. **B,** https://commons.wikimedia.org/wiki/File:Maxillary_sinus_-_lateral_view.png. **C,** https://commons.wikimedia.org/wiki/File:Maxillary_sinus_-_medial_view.png.)

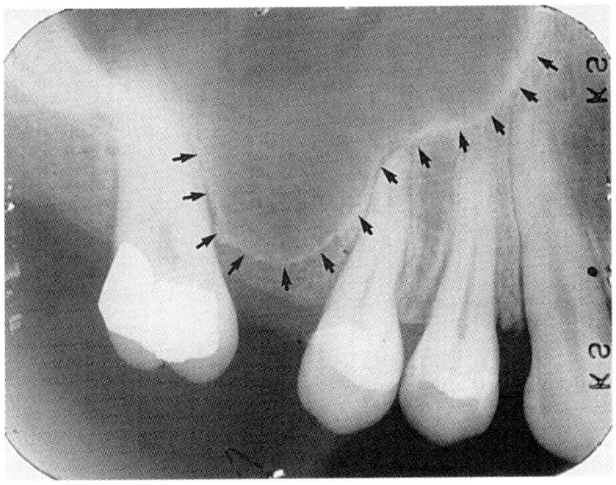

Fig 28-28 The maxillary sinus appears as a radiolucent area above the maxillary posterior teeth. (From Haring JI, Lind LJ: Radiographic interpretation for the dental hygienist, Philadelphia, 1993, Saunders.)

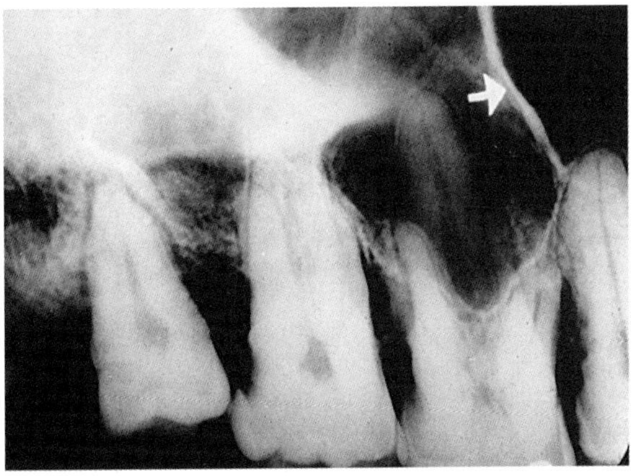

Fig 28-29 Septa within the maxillary sinus appear as radiopaque lines. (From Haring JI, Lind LJ: Radiographic interpretation for the dental hygienist, Philadelphia, 1993, Saunders.)

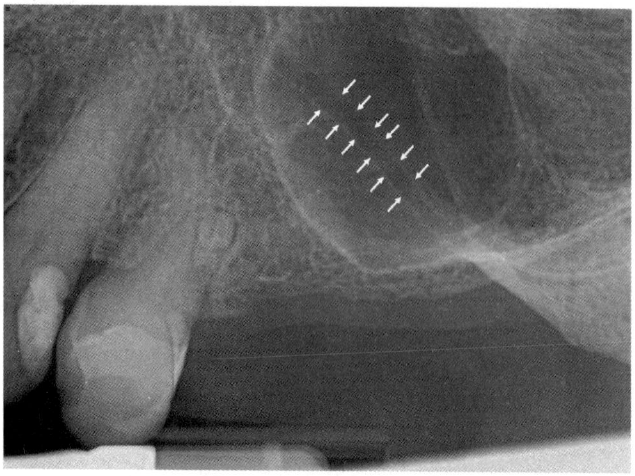

Fig 28-30 Nutrient canals appear as narrow radiolucent bands.

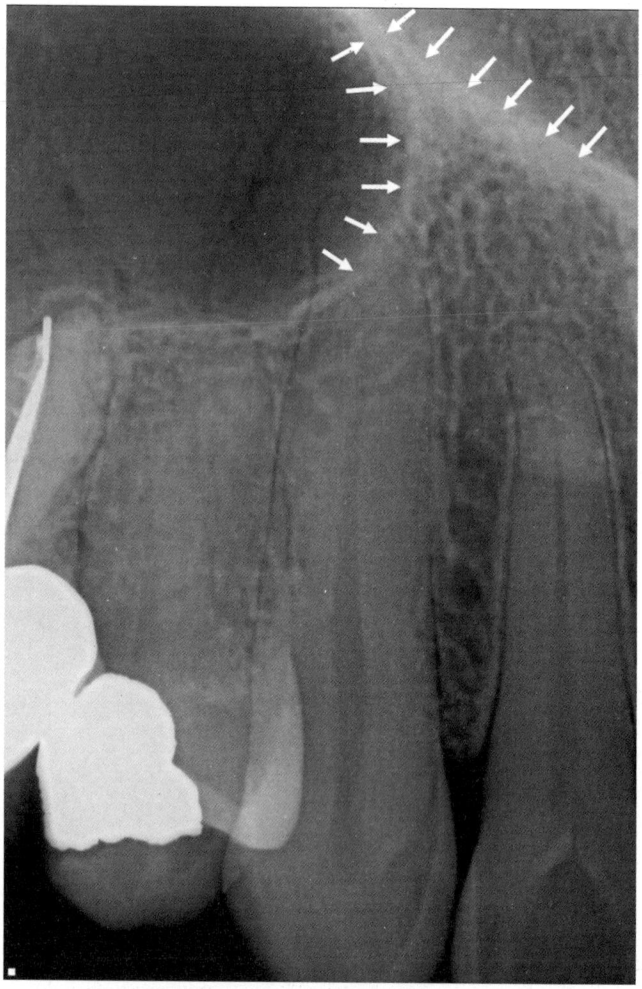

Fig 28-31 The inverted Y appears as a radiopaque upside-down Y.

Nutrient Canals Within Maxillary Sinus.

Description. Nutrient canals may be seen within maxillary sinuses. Nutrient canals are tiny, tubelike passageways through bone, which contain blood vessels and nerves that supply maxillary teeth and interdental areas.

Appearance. On a posterior maxillary periapical image, a nutrient canal appears as a narrow radiolucent band bounded by two thin radiopaque lines (Figure 28-30). The radiopaque lines represent the cortical bone that makes up the walls of the canal.

Inverted Y.

Description. The term inverted Y refers to the intersection of the maxillary sinus and the nasal cavity as viewed on a dental image.

Appearance. On a maxillary canine periapical image, the inverted Y appears as a radiopaque upside-down Y formed by the intersection of the lateral wall of the nasal fossa and the anterior border of the maxillary sinus (Figure 28-31). The lateral wall of the nasal cavity and the anterior border of the maxillary sinus are both composed of dense cortical bone and appear as a radiopaque line or band. The inverted Y is located superior to the maxillary canine.

Maxillary Tuberosity.

Description. The maxillary tuberosity is a rounded prominence of bone that extends posterior to the third molar region (see Figure 28-8). Blood vessels and nerves enter the maxilla in this region and supply posterior teeth.

Appearance. On a posterior maxillary periapical image, the maxillary tuberosity appears as a radiopaque bulge distal to the third molar region (Figure 28-32).

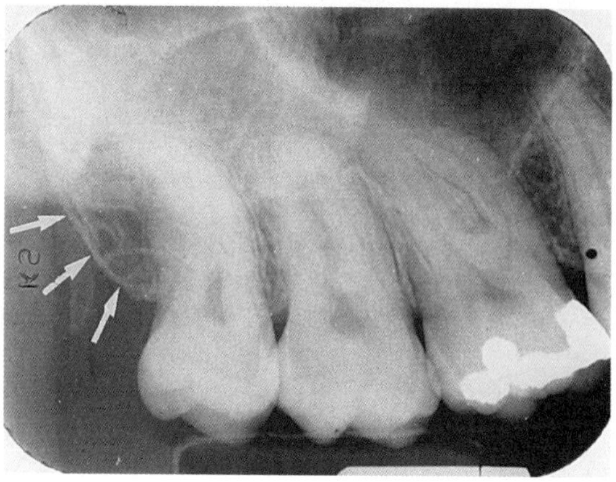

Fig 28-32 The maxillary tuberosity appears as a radiopaque bulge distal to the third molar region. (From Haring JI, Lind LJ: Radiographic interpretation for the dental hygienist, Philadelphia, 1993, Saunders.)

Hamulus.

Description. The hamulus (also known as the *hamular process*) is a small, hooklike projection of bone extending from the medial pterygoid plate of the sphenoid bone (Figure 28-33). The hamulus is located posterior to the maxillary tuberosity region.

Appearance. On a posterior maxillary periapical image, the hamulus appears as a radiopaque hook-like projection posterior to the maxillary tuberosity area (Figure 28-34). The image appearance of the hamulus varies in length, shape, and density.

Zygomatic Process of the Maxilla.

Description. The zygomatic process of the maxilla is a bony projection of the maxilla that articulates with the zygoma, or malar bone (Figure 28-35). The zygomatic process of the maxilla is composed of dense cortical bone.

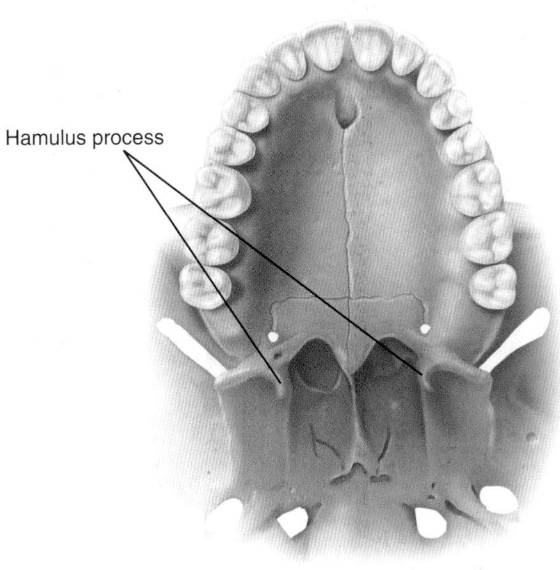

Fig 28-33 Inferior view of the hamular processes.

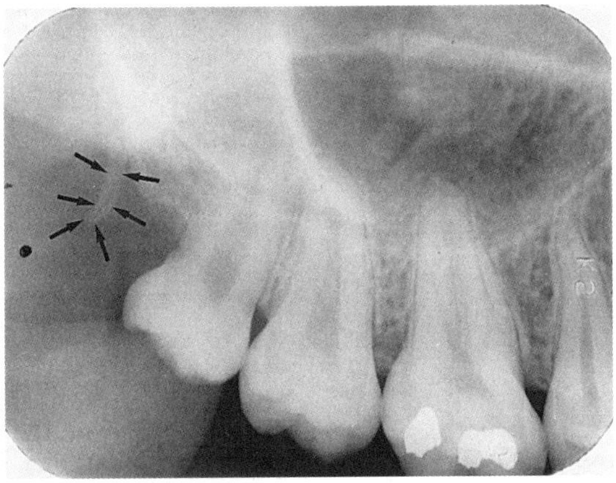

Fig 28-34 The hamulus appears as a hook-like radiopacity distal to the maxillary tuberosity area. (From Haring JI, Lind LJ: Radiographic interpretation for the dental hygienist, Philadelphia, 1993, Saunders.)

Appearance. On a posterior maxillary periapical image, the zygomatic process of the maxilla appears as a J-shaped or U-shaped radiopacity located superior to the maxillary first molar region (Figure 28-36).

Zygoma.

Description. The **zygoma**, or *cheekbone* (also referred to as the *malar bone* or *zygomatic bone*), articulates with the zygomatic process of the maxilla (Figure 28-37). The zygoma is composed of dense cortical bone.

Appearance. On a posterior maxillary periapical image, the zygoma appears as a diffuse radiopaque band extending posteriorly from the zygomatic process of the maxilla (Figure 28-38).

Bony Landmarks of the Mandible

The term **mandible** comes from Latin *mandibula*, meaning "jaw bone." The mandible is the horseshoe-shaped bone that forms the lower jaw.

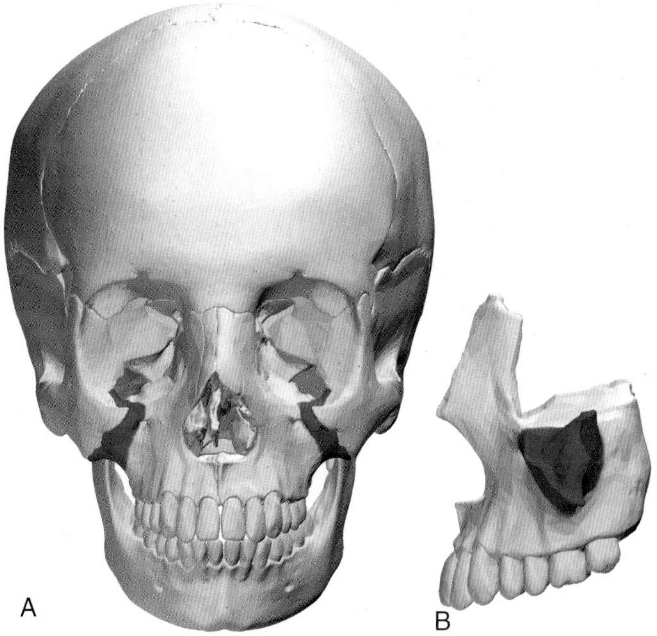

Fig 28-35 **A**, Zygomatic process of the maxilla, anterior view. **B**, Zygomatic process of the maxilla, lateral view with zygoma removed. Notice the U-shaped area of dense cortical bone. (Images created from BodyParts3D, © The Database Center for Life Science licensed under CC Attribution-Share Alike 2.1 Japan [http://creativecommons.org/licenses/by-sa/2.1/jp/legalcode] / User: Was a bee / Wikimedia Commons / **A**, https://commons.wikimedia.org/wiki/File:Zygomatic_process_of_maxilla_-_skull_-_anterior_view.png. **B**, https://commons.wikimedia.org/wiki/File:Zygomatic_process_of_maxilla_-_close_up_-_lateral_view.png.)

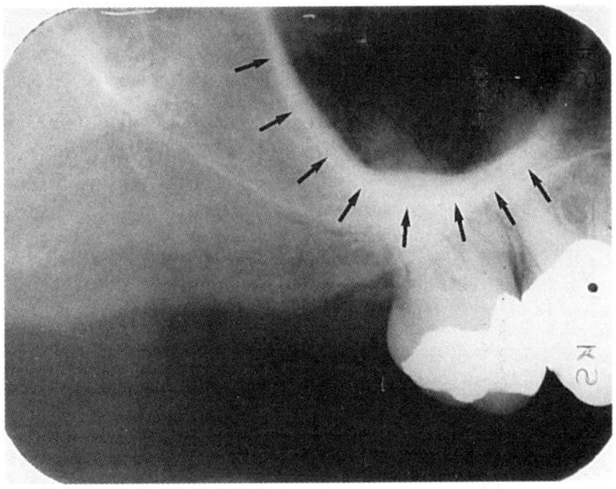

Fig 28-36 The zygomatic process of the maxilla appears as a J-shaped or U-shaped radiopacity superior to the maxillary molars. (From Haring JI, Lind LJ: Radiographic interpretation for the dental hygienist, Philadelphia, 1993, Saunders.)

It is the largest and strongest bone of the face. The mandible is a single bone that is divided into the following sections:

Ramus. The ramus is the vertical portion of the mandible that is found posterior to the third molar (Figure 28-39). The mandible has two rami (*rami* is the plural of *ramus*), one on each side.

Body of the mandible. The body of the mandible is the horizontal, U-shaped portion that extends from ramus to ramus (Figure 28-40).

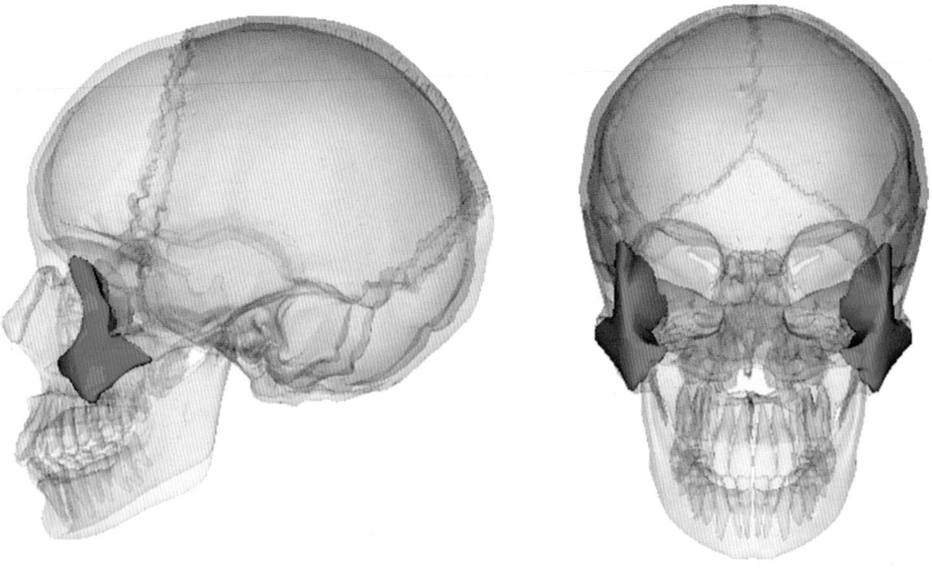

Fig 28-37 The zygoma, lateral and anterior views. (Images created from BodyParts3D, © The Database Center for Life Science licensed under CC Attribution-Share Alike 2.1 Japan [http://creativecommons.org/licenses/by-sa/2.1/jp/legalcode] / User: Was a bee / Wikimedia Commons / https://commons.wikimedia.org/wiki/File:Zygomatic_bone.png.)

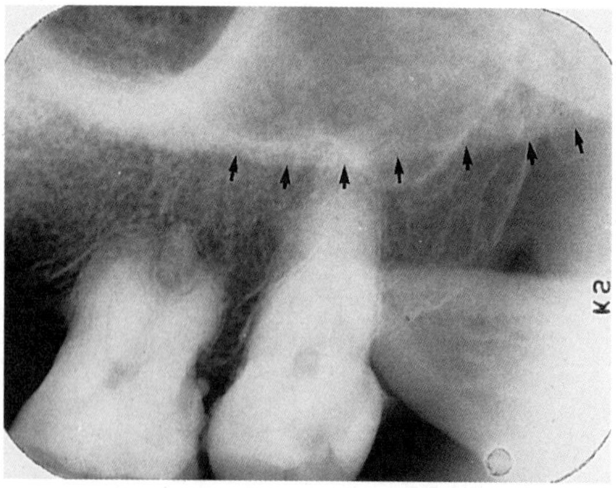

Fig 28-38 The zygoma appears as a diffuse radiopaque band that extends distally from the zygomatic process of the maxilla. (From Haring JI, Lind LJ: Radiographic interpretation for the dental hygienist, Philadelphia, 1993, Saunders.)

Angle of the mandible. The angle of the mandible is the corner portion formed by the junction of the posterior and lower borders of the ramus (Figure 28-41).

Alveolar process. The alveolar process is the portion of the mandible that encases and supports teeth (Figure 28-42).

This section describes the bony landmarks of the mandible and how each one is viewed on an intraoral image.

Genial Tubercles.

Description. Genial tubercles are tiny bumps of bone that serve as attachment sites for the genioglossus and geniohyoid muscles (Figure 28-43). Genial tubercles are located on the lingual aspect of the mandible.

Appearance. On a mandibular periapical image, genial tubercles appear as a ring-shaped radiopacity inferior to the apices of the mandibular incisors (Figure 28-44).

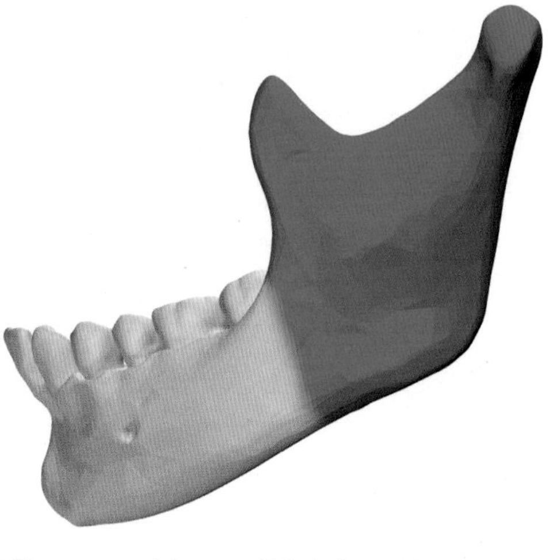

Fig 28-39 The ramus of the mandible indicated in red. (Image created from BodyParts3D, © The Database Center for Life Science licensed under CC Attribution-Share Alike 2.1 Japan [http://creativecommons.org/licenses/by-sa/2.1/jp/legalcode] / User: Was a bee / Wikimedia Commons / https://commons.wikimedia.org/wiki/File:Ramus_of_the_mandible_-_close_up_-_lateral_view.png.)

Lingual Foramen.

Description. The lingual foramen is a tiny opening or hole in bone located on the internal surface of the mandible (Figure 28-45). The lingual foramen is located near the midline and is surrounded by genial tubercles.

Appearance. On a mandibular periapical image, the lingual foramen appears as a small, radiolucent dot located inferior to the apices of the mandibular incisors (Figure 28-46). The lingual foramen is surrounded by genial tubercles, which appear as a radiopaque ring.

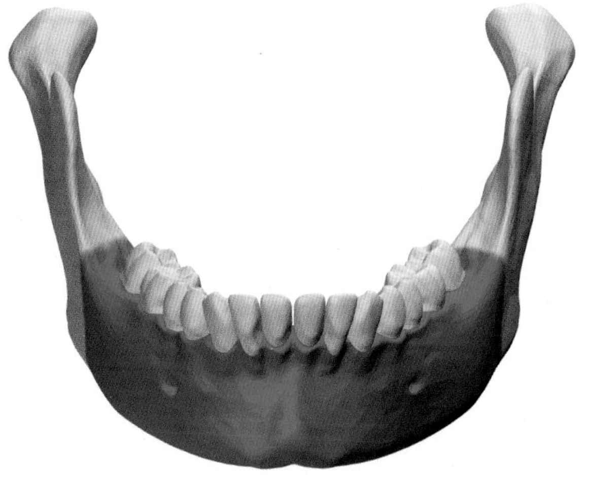

Fig 28-40 The body of the mandible indicated in red. (Image created from BodyParts3D, © The Database Center for Life Science licensed under CC Attribution-Share Alike 2.1 Japan [http://creativecommons.org/licenses/by-sa/2.1/jp/legalcode] / User: Was a bee / Wikimedia Commons / https://commons.wikimedia.org/wiki/File:Body_of_mandible_-_close_up_-_anterior_view.png.)

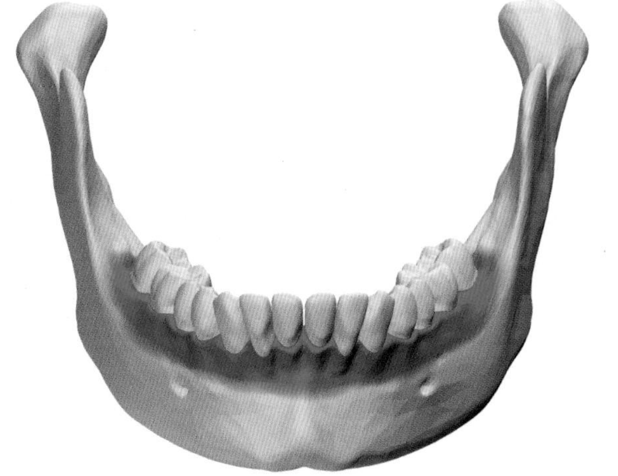

Fig 28-42 The alveolar process indicated in red. (Image created from BodyParts3D, © The Database Center for Life Science licensed under CC Attribution-Share Alike 2.1 Japan [http://creativecommons.org/licenses/by-sa/2.1/jp/legalcode] / User: Was a bee / Wikimedia Commons / https://commons.wikimedia.org/wiki/File:Alveolar_part_of_mandible_-_close_up-_anterior_view.png.)

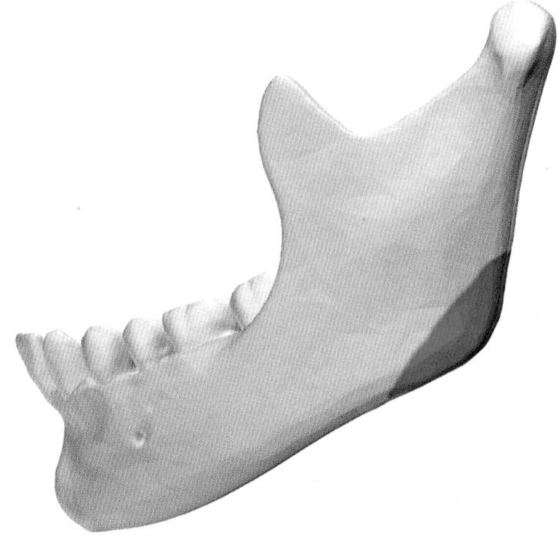

Fig 28-41 The angle of the mandible indicated in red. (Image created from BodyParts3D, © The Database Center for Life Science licensed under CC Attribution-Share Alike 2.1 Japan [http://creativecommons.org/licenses/by-sa/2.1/jp/legalcode] / User: Was a bee / Wikimedia Commons / https://commons.wikimedia.org/wiki/File:Mandibular_angle_-_close-up_-_lateral_view.png.)

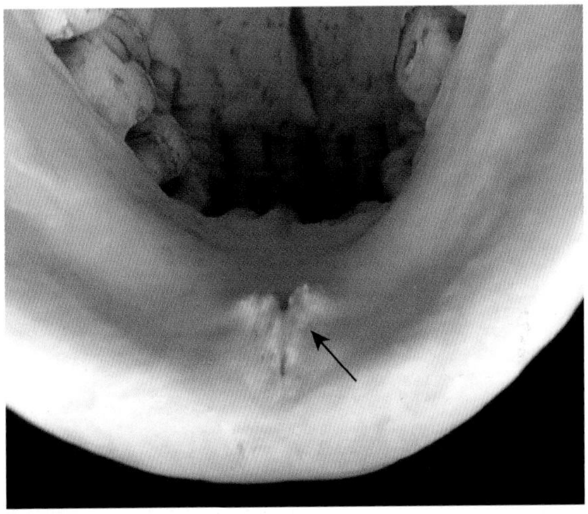

Fig 28-43 The genial tubercles.

Nutrient Canals.

Description. As described earlier, nutrient canals are tubelike passageways through bone that contain nerves and blood vessels that supply teeth. Interdental nutrient canals are most often seen in the anterior mandible, a region that typically has thin bone.

Appearance. On a mandibular periapical image, nutrient canals appear as vertical radiolucent bands (Figure 28-47). On a dental image, nutrient canals are readily seen in areas of thin bone. In the edentulous mandible, nutrient canals may appear more prominent.

Mental Ridge.

Description. The mental ridge is a linear prominence of cortical bone located on the external surface of the anterior portion of the mandible (Figure 28-48). The mental ridge extends from the premolar region to the midline and slopes slightly upward.

Appearance. On a mandibular periapical image, the mental ridge appears as a thick radiopaque band that extends from the premolar region to the incisor region (Figure 28-49). On a dental image, the mental ridge often appears superimposed over mandibular anterior teeth.

Mental Fossa.

Description. The mental fossa is a scooped-out, depressed area of bone located on the external surface of the anterior mandible (see Figure 28-48). The mental fossa is located above the mental ridge in the mandibular incisor region.

Appearance. On a mandibular periapical image, the mental fossa appears as a radiolucent area above the mental ridge (Figure 28-50). On a dental image, the appearance of the mental fossa varies and is determined by the thickness of the bone in the anterior region of the mandible.

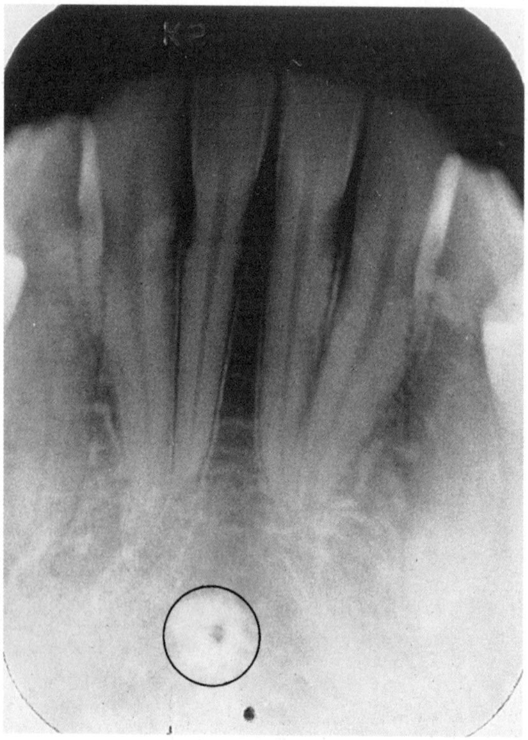

Fig 28-44 Genial tubercles appear as a ring-shaped radiopacity. (From Haring JI, Lind LJ: Radiographic interpretation for the dental hygienist, Philadelphia, 1993, Saunders.)

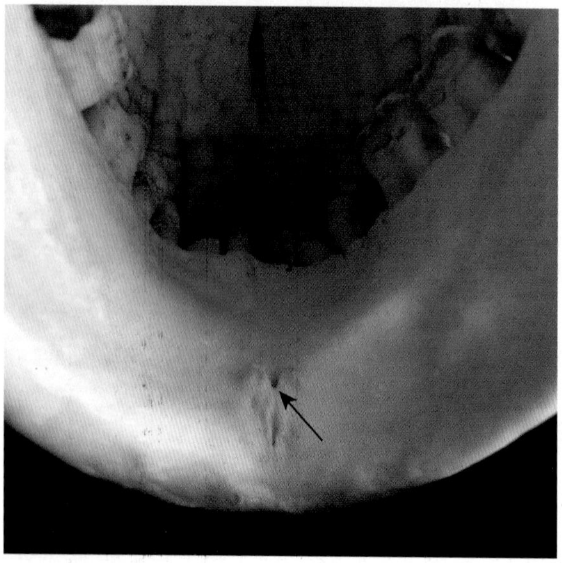

Fig 28-45 The lingual foramen.

Mental Foramen.

Description. The mental foramen is an opening or hole in bone located on the external surface of the mandible in the region of the mandibular premolars (Figure 28-51). Blood vessels and nerves that supply the lower lip exit through the mental foramen.

Appearance. On a mandibular periapical image, the mental foramen appears as a small, ovoid or round radiolucent area located in the apical region of the mandibular premolars (Figure 28-52). The mental foramen may be misdiagnosed as a periapical lesion (periapical cyst, granuloma, or abscess) because of its apical location.

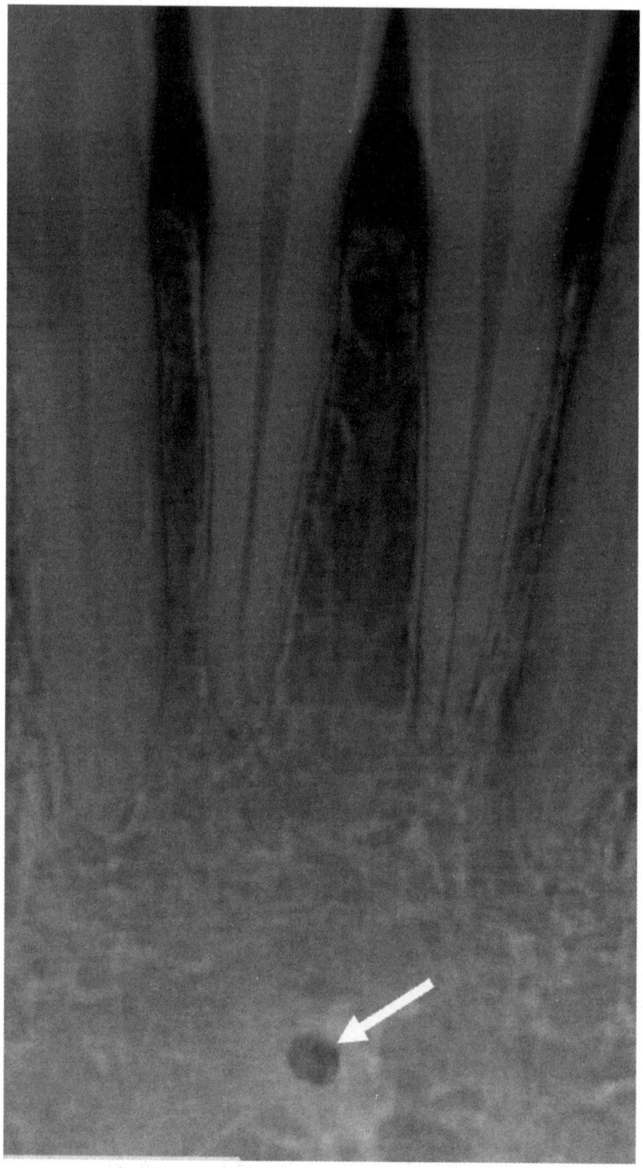

Fig 28-46 The lingual foramen appears as a small, radiolucent dot.

Mandibular Canal.

Description. The mandibular canal is a tubelike passageway through bone that travels the length of the mandible (Figure 28-53). The mandibular canal extends from the mandibular foramen to the mental foramen and houses the inferior alveolar nerve and blood vessels.

Appearance. On a mandibular periapical image, the mandibular canal appears as a radiolucent band (Figure 28-54). Two thin radiopaque lines that represent the cortical walls of the canal outline the mandibular canal. The mandibular canal appears below or superimposed over the apices of the mandibular molar teeth.

Mylohyoid Ridge.

Description. The mylohyoid ridge (also known as the internal oblique ridge) is a linear prominence of bone located on the internal

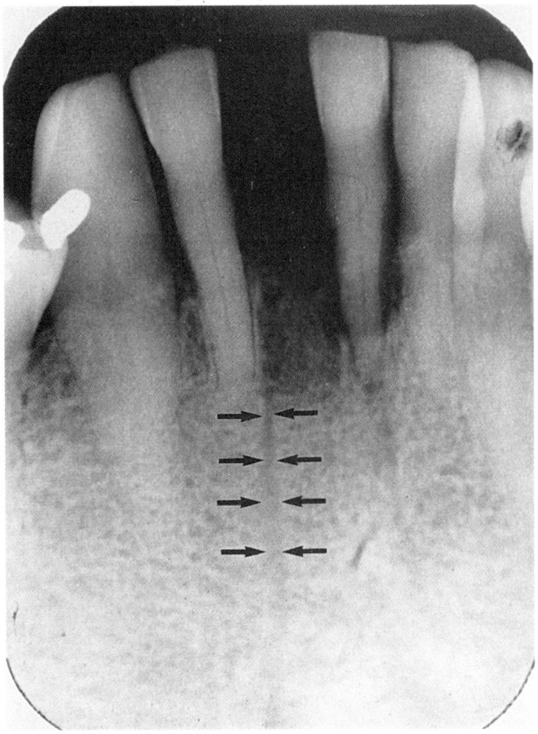

Fig 28-47 Nutrient canals appear as thin radiolucent bands. (From Haring JI, Lind LJ: Radiographic interpretation for the dental hygienist, Philadelphia, 1993, Saunders.)

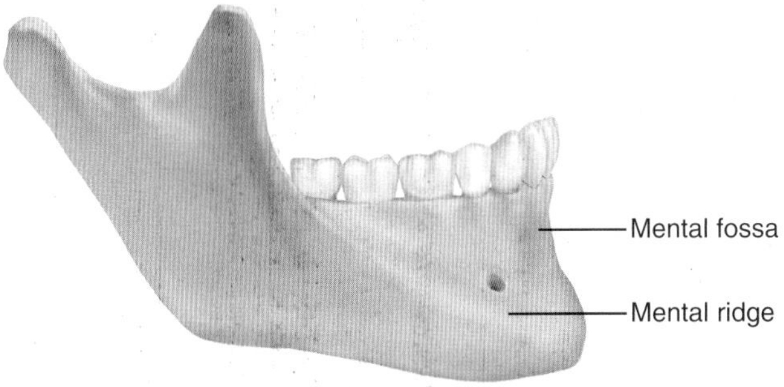

Fig 28-48 The mental ridge and mental fossa.

surface of the mandible (Figure 28-55). The mylohyoid ridge extends from the third molar region downward and forward to the second premolar area. The mylohyoid ridge serves as an attachment site for a muscle of the same name.

Appearance. On a mandibular periapical image, the mylohyoid ridge appears as a dense radiopaque band that extends downward and forward from the third molar region at the level of the apices of the posterior teeth (Figure 28-56). The mylohyoid ridge usually appears most prominently in the molar region and may be superimposed over the roots of the mandibular teeth.

External Oblique Ridge.

Description. The external oblique ridge (also known as the *external oblique line*) is a linear prominence of bone located on the external surface of the body of the mandible (Figure 28-57). The anterior border of the ramus ends in the external oblique ridge.

Appearance. On a mandibular molar periapical image, the external oblique ridge appears as a radiopaque band extending downward

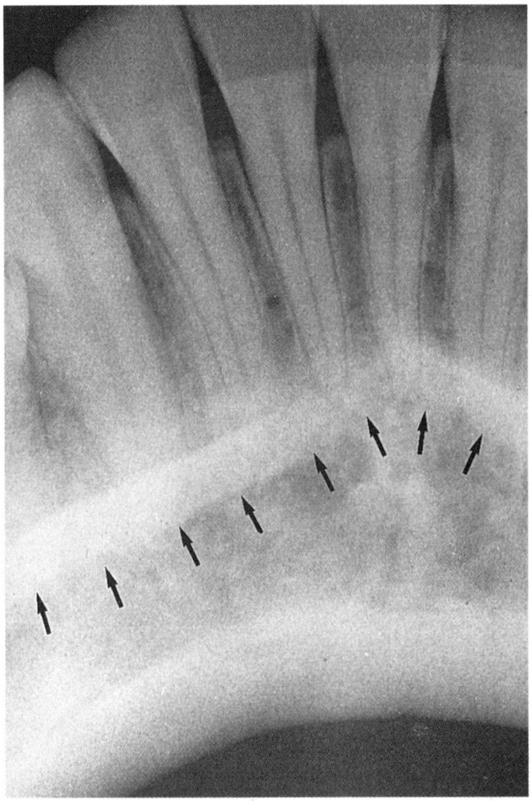

Fig 28-49 The mental ridge appears as a radiopaque band in the premolar and incisor region. (From Haring JI, Lind LJ: Radiographic interpretation for the dental hygienist, Philadelphia, 1993, Saunders.)

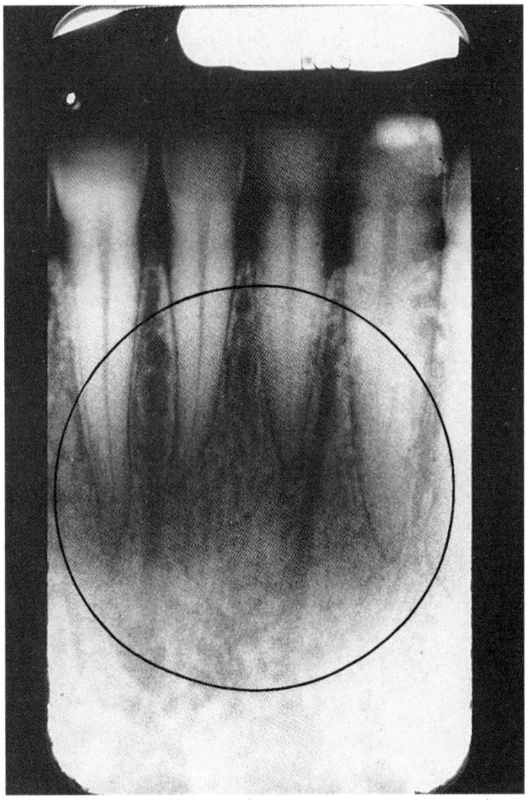

Fig 28-50 The mental fossa appears as a radiolucent area above the mental ridge. (From Haring JI, Lind LJ: Radiographic interpretation for the dental hygienist, Philadelphia, 1993, Saunders.)

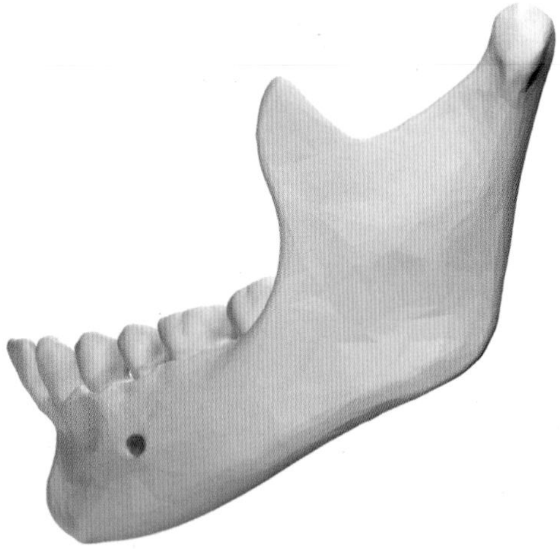

Fig 28-51 The mental foramen indicated in red. (Image created from BodyParts3D, © The Database Center for Life Science licensed under CC Attribution-Share Alike 2.1 Japan [http://creativecommons.org/licenses/by-sa/2.1/jp/legalcode] / User: Was a bee / Wikimedia Commons / https://commons.wikimedia.org/wiki/File:Mental_foramen_-_close_up_-_lateral_view.png.)

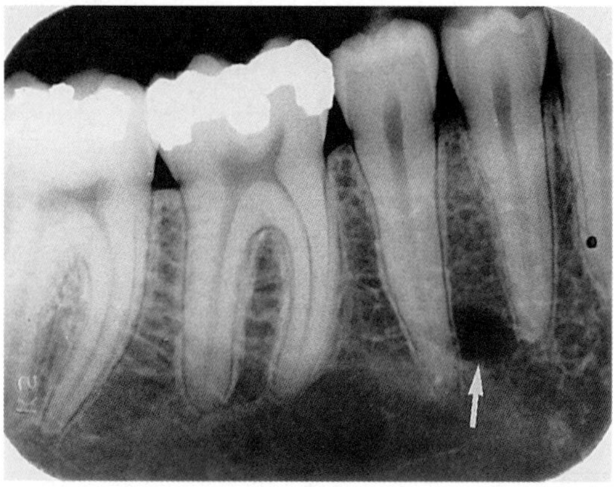

Fig 28-52 The mental foramen appears as a radiolucency in the mandibular premolar region. (From Haring JI, Lind LJ: Radiographic interpretation for the dental hygienist, Philadelphia, 1993, Saunders.)

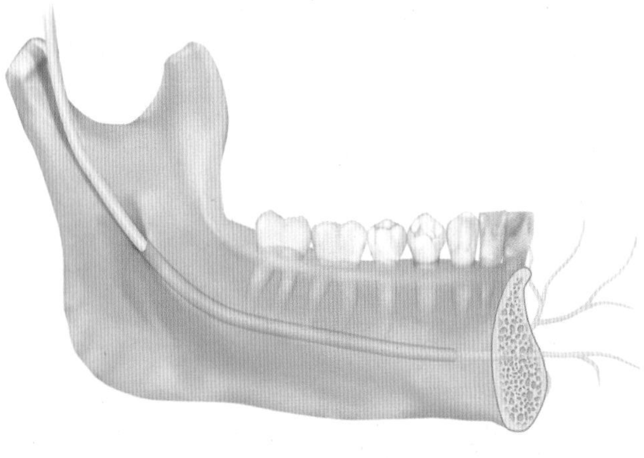

Fig 28-53 The mandibular canal.

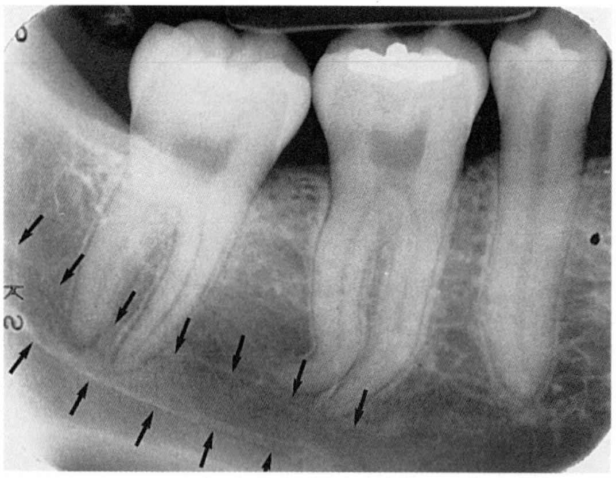

Fig 28-54 The mandibular canal appears as a radiolucent band outlined by two thin radiopaque lines. (From Haring JI, Lind LJ: Radiographic interpretation for the dental hygienist, Philadelphia, 1993, Saunders.)

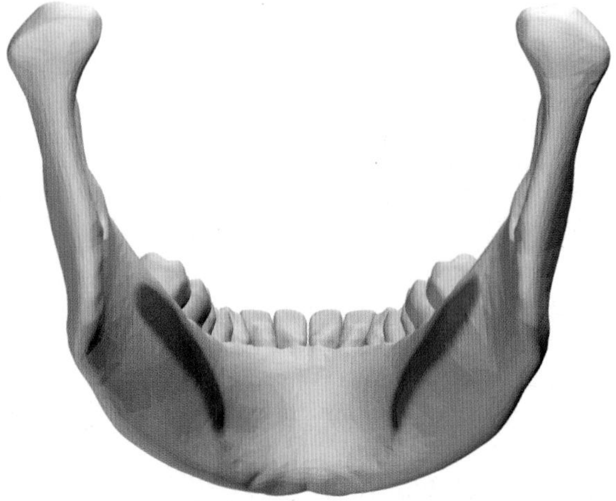

Fig 28-55 A posterior view of the ramus with the mylohyoid ridge indicated in red. (Image created from BodyParts3D, ©The Database Center for Life Science licensed under CC Attribution-Share Alike 2.1 Japan [http://creativecommons.org/licenses/by-sa/2.1/jp/legalcode] / User: Was a bee / Wikimedia Commons / https://commons.wikimedia.org/wiki/File:Mylohyoid_line_-_close_up_-_posterior_view.png.)

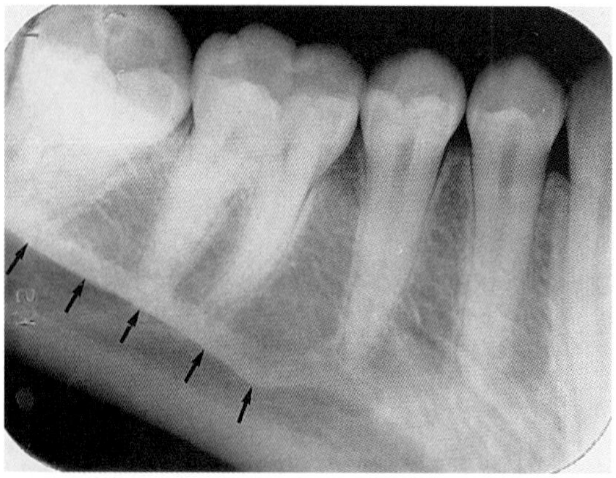

Fig 28-56 The mylohyoid ridge appears as a radiopaque band in the mandibular molar region. (From Haring JI, Lind LJ: Radiographic interpretation for the dental hygienist, Philadelphia, 1993, Saunders.)

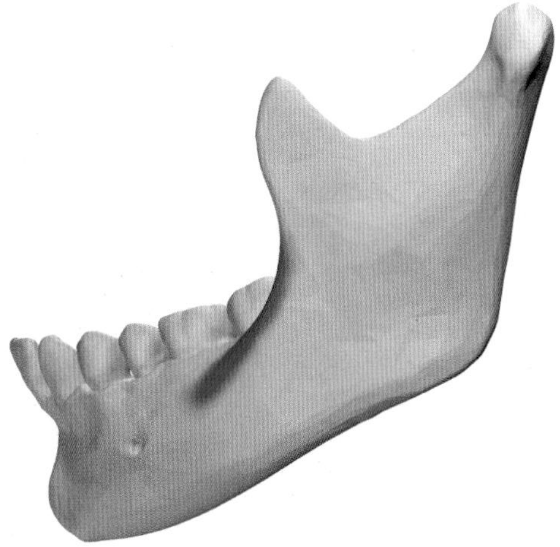

Fig 28-57 A lateral view of the mandible with the external oblique ridge indicated in red. (Image created from BodyParts3D, © The Database Center for Life Science licensed under CC Attribution-Share Alike 2.1 Japan [http://creativecommons.org/licenses/by-sa/2.1/jp/legalcode] / User: Was a bee / Wikimedia Commons / https://commons.wikimedia.org/wiki/File:External_oblique_line_of_mandible_-_close_up_-_lateral_view.png.)

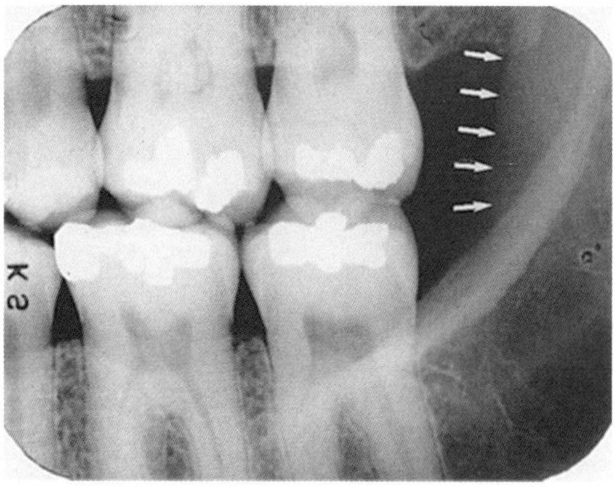

Fig 28-59 The descending ramus of the mandible appears as a vertical radiopaque band. (From Haring JI, Lind LJ: Radiographic interpretation for the dental hygienist, Philadelphia, 1993, Saunders.)

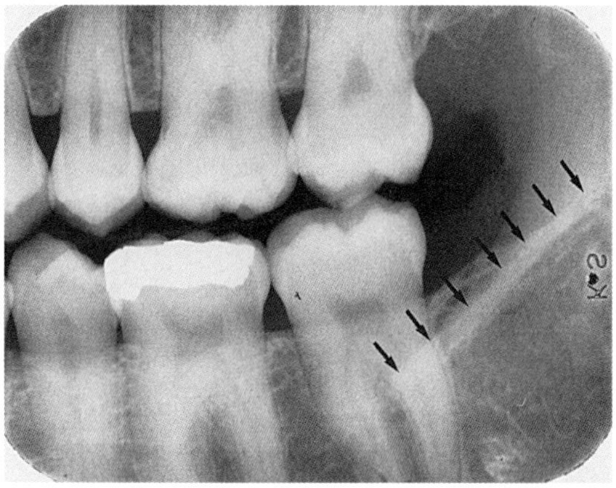

Fig 28-58 The external oblique ridge appears as a radiopaque band. (From Haring JI, Lind LJ: Radiographic interpretation for the dental hygienist, Philadelphia, 1993, Saunders.)

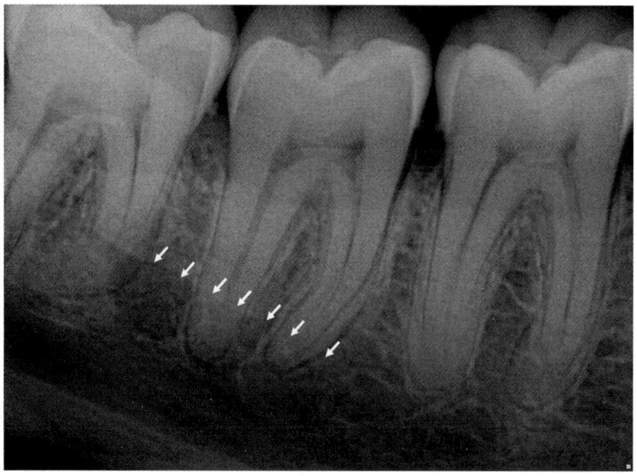

Fig 28-60 The submandibular fossa appears as a radiolucent area inferior to the mylohyoid ridge.

and forward from the anterior border of the ramus of the mandible (Figure 28-58). The external oblique ridge typically ends in the mandibular third molar region. Both the internal and external oblique ridges may also be viewed on molar bite-wing images.

Anterior Border of the Ramus.

Description. The anterior border of the ramus extends vertically downward from the coronoid process to the external oblique ridge.

Appearance. On a molar bite-wing image, the descending ramus of the mandible may be seen as a slightly radiopaque vertical band posterior to the maxillary and mandibular molars (Figure 28-59).

Submandibular Fossa.

Description. The submandibular fossa (also known as the *mandibular fossa* or *submaxillary fossa*) is a scooped-out, depressed area of bone located on the internal surface of the mandible inferior to the mylohyoid ridge (see Figure 28-11). The submandibular salivary gland is found in the submandibular fossa.

Appearance. On a mandibular periapical image, the submandibular fossa appears as a radiolucent area in the molar region below the mylohyoid ridge (Figure 28-60). Few bony trabeculae are usually seen in the region of the submandibular fossa. On some periapical images, the submandibular fossa may appear as a distinct radiolucency; in others, it may be slightly more radiolucent than the adjacent bone.

Coronoid Process.

Description. The coronoid process is a marked prominence of bone on the anterior ramus of the mandible (Figure 28-61). The coronoid process serves as an attachment site for one of the muscles of mastication.

Appearance. The coronoid process is *not* seen on a mandibular periapical image but may appear on a maxillary molar periapical image. The coronoid process appears as a triangular radiopacity superimposed over, or inferior to, the maxillary tuberosity region (Figure 28-62).

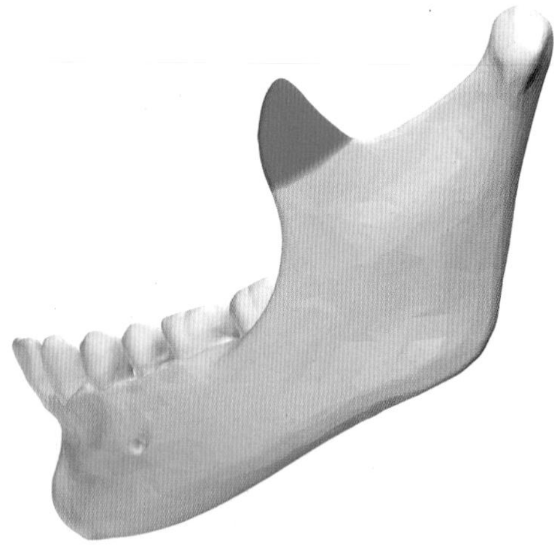

Fig 28-61 The coronoid process indicated in red. (Image created from BodyParts3D, ©The Database Center for Life Science licensed under CC Attribution-Share Alike 2.1 Japan [http://creativecommons.org/licenses/by-sa/2.1/jp/legalcode] / User: Was a bee / Wikimedia Commons / https://commons.wikimedia.org/wiki/File:Coronoid_process_of_mandible_-_close_up_-_lateral_view.png.)

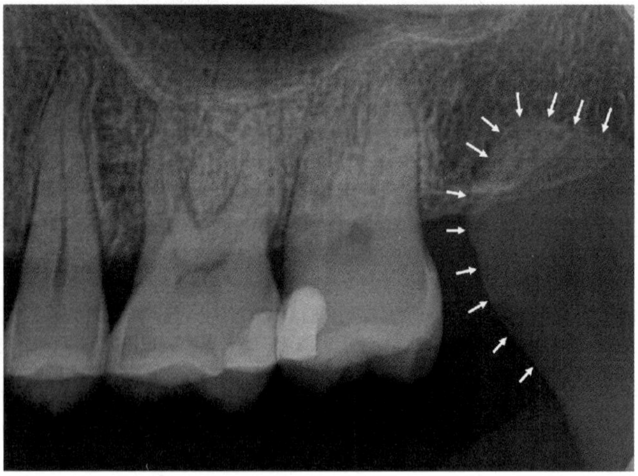

Fig 28-62 The coronoid process appears as a triangular radiopacity.

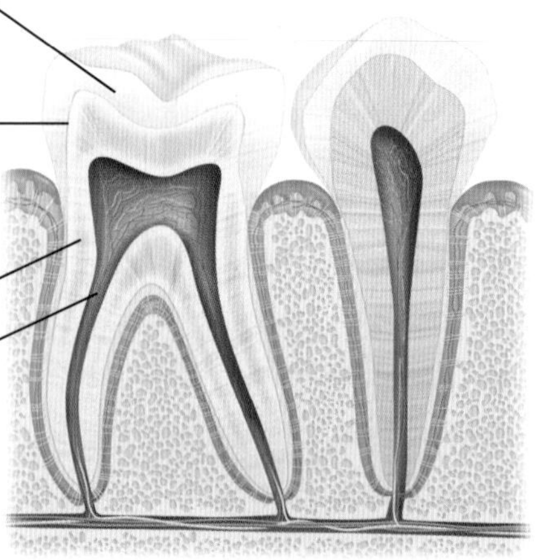

Fig 28-63 Tooth structures: enamel, dentin, dentino-enamel junction, and pulp cavity.

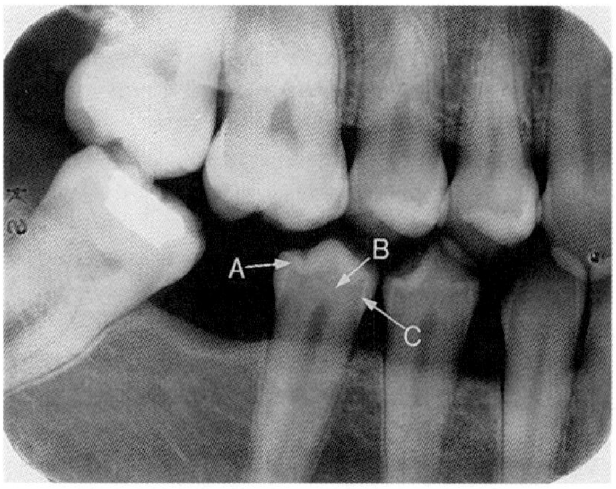

Fig 28-64 Tooth structures. A, enamel; B, dentin; C, dentino-enamel junction. (From Haring JI, Lind LJ: Radiographic interpretation for the dental hygienist, Philadelphia, 1993, Saunders.)

NORMAL TOOTH ANATOMY

Tooth Structure

Tooth structures that can be viewed on dental images include the following: enamel, dentin, the dentino-enamel junction, and the pulp cavity (Figure 28-63).

Enamel. Enamel is the densest structure found in the human body. Enamel is the outermost radiopaque layer of the crown of a tooth (Figure 28-64).

Dentin. Dentin is found beneath the enamel layer of a tooth and surrounds the pulp cavity (see Figure 28-64). Dentin appears radiopaque and makes up the majority of the tooth structure. Dentin is not as radiopaque as enamel.

Dentino-Enamel Junction. The dentino-enamel junction (DEJ) is the junction between the dentin and the enamel of a tooth. The DEJ appears as a line where the enamel (very radiopaque) meets the dentin (less radiopaque) (see Figure 28-64).

Pulp Cavity. The pulp cavity consists of a pulp chamber and pulp canals. It contains blood vessels, nerves, and lymphatics and appears relatively radiolucent on a dental image (Figure 28-65). When viewed on a dental image, the pulp cavity is generally larger in children than in adults because it decreases in size with age as a result of the formation of secondary dentin. The size and shape of the pulp cavity vary with each tooth.

Supporting Structures

The *alveolar process*, or alveolar bone, serves as the supporting structure for teeth. The alveolar bone is the bone of the maxilla and the mandible that supports and encases the roots of teeth (Figure 28-66). Alveolar bone is composed of dense cortical bone and cancellous bone.

Anatomy of Alveolar Bone. The anatomic landmarks of the alveolar process include the lamina dura, the alveolar crest, and the periodontal ligament space (Figure 28-67).

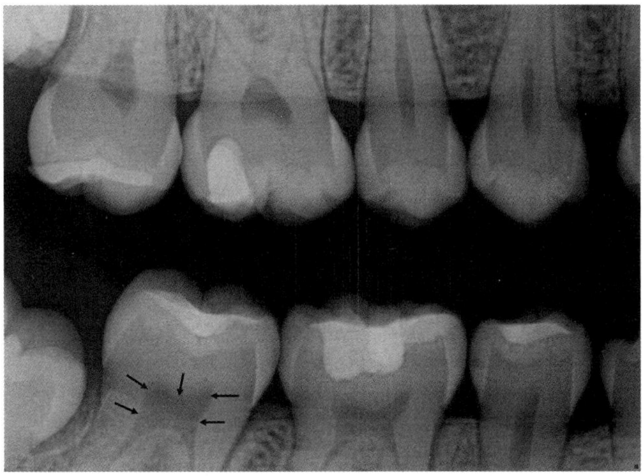

Fig 28-65 The pulp cavity.

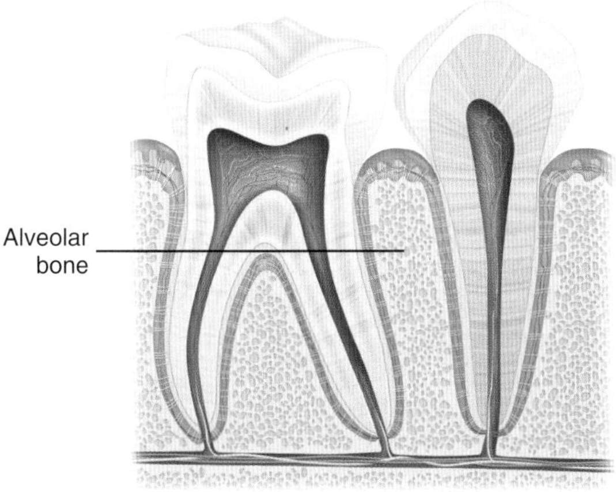

Fig 28-66 Alveolar bone.

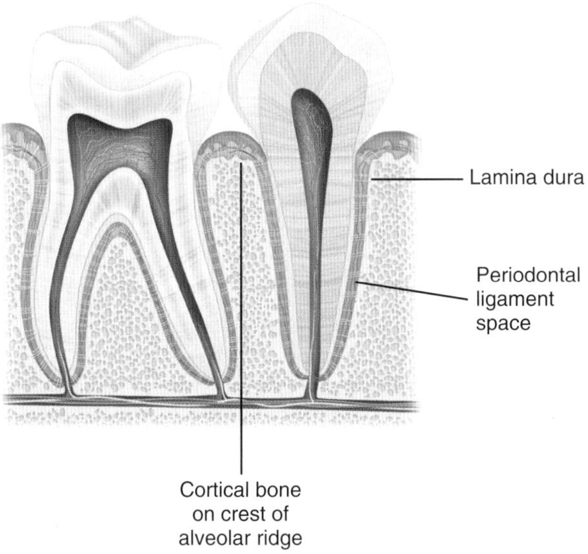

Fig 28-67 The alveolar process: lamina dura, alveolar crest, and periodontal ligament space.

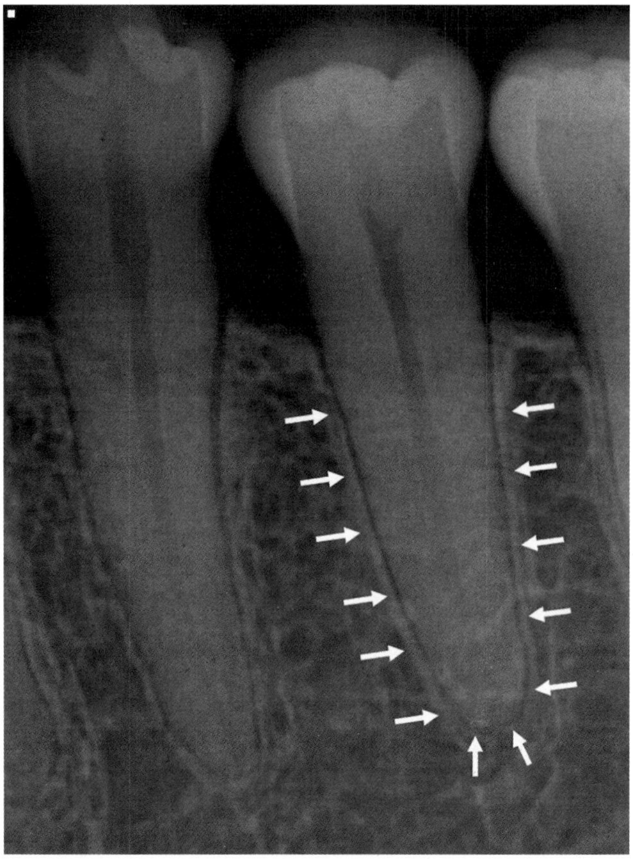

Fig 28-68 The lamina dura appears as a dense, thin radiopaque line around the root of a tooth.

Lamina Dura.

Description. The lamina dura is the wall of the tooth socket that surrounds the root of a tooth. The lamina dura is made up of dense cortical bone.

Appearance. On a dental image, the lamina dura appears as a dense radiopaque line that surrounds the root of a tooth (Figure 28-68).

Alveolar Crest.

Description. The alveolar crest is the most coronal portion of alveolar bone found between teeth. The alveolar crest is made up of dense cortical bone and is continuous with the lamina dura.

Appearance. On a dental image, the alveolar crest appears radiopaque and is typically located 1.5 to 2.0 mm below the junction of the crown and the root surfaces (the cemento-enamel junction) (Figure 28-69).

Periodontal Ligament Space.

Description. The periodontal ligament space (PDL space) is the space between the root of the tooth and the lamina dura. The PDL space contains connective tissue fibers, blood vessels, and lymphatics.

Appearance. On a dental image, the PDL space appears as a thin radiolucent line around the root of a tooth. In the healthy periodontium, the PDL space appears as a continuous radiolucent line of uniform thickness (Figure 28-70).

Shape and Density of Alveolar Bone. Alveolar bone located between the roots of teeth varies in shape and density.

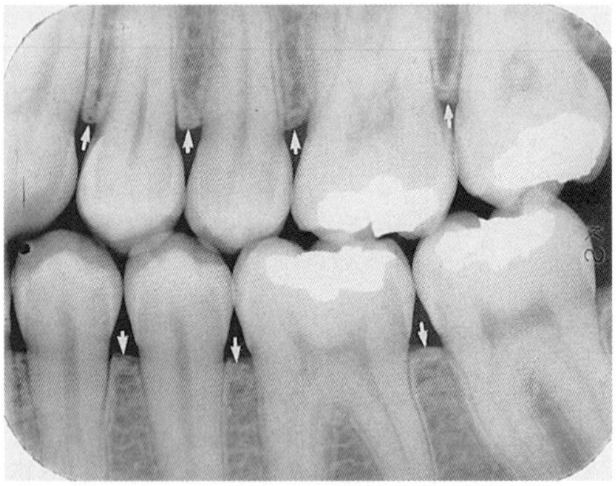

Fig 28-69 The alveolar crest typically appears 1.5 to 2.0 mm below the cemento-enamel junction. (From Haring JI, Lind LJ: Radiographic interpretation for the dental hygienist, Philadelphia, 1993, Saunders.)

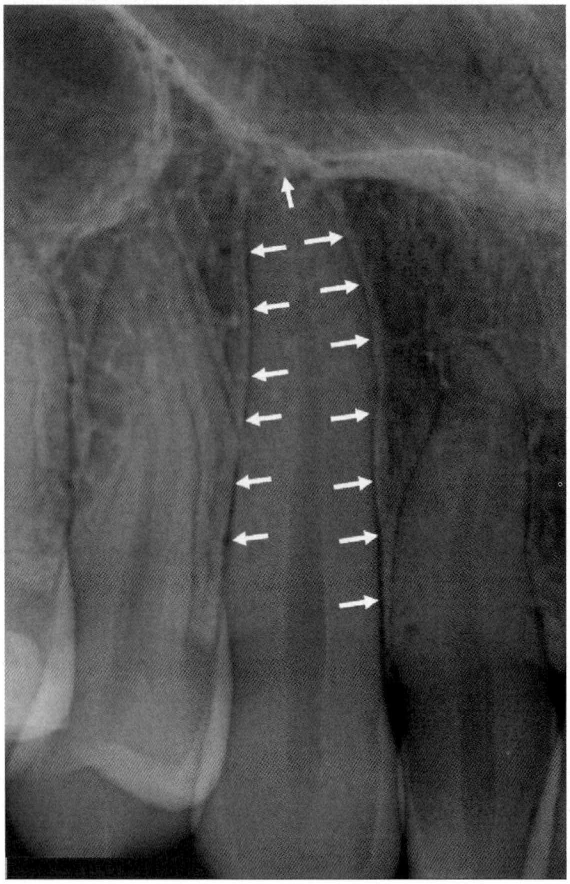

Fig 28-70 The periodontal ligament space appears as a thin radiolucent line around the root of the tooth.

Anterior region. Healthy alveolar crest located in the anterior region appears pointed and sharp between teeth (Figure 28-71). The alveolar crest appears as a dense radiopaque line in the anterior region.

Posterior region. Healthy alveolar crest located in the posterior region appears flat and smooth between teeth (Figure 28-72). The alveolar crest located in the posterior region tends to appear less dense and less radiopaque than the alveolar crest seen in the anterior region.

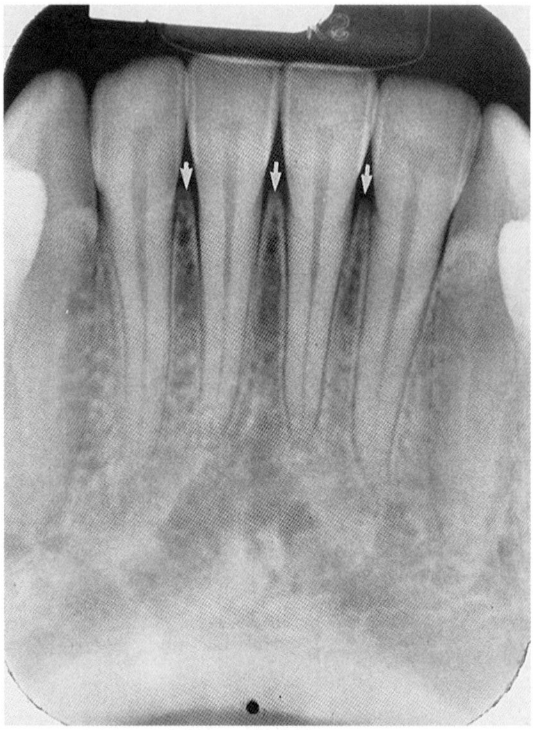

Fig 28-71 The anterior alveolar crest normally appears pointed and sharp. (From Haring JI, Lind LJ: Radiographic interpretation for the dental hygienist, Philadelphia, 1993, Saunders.)

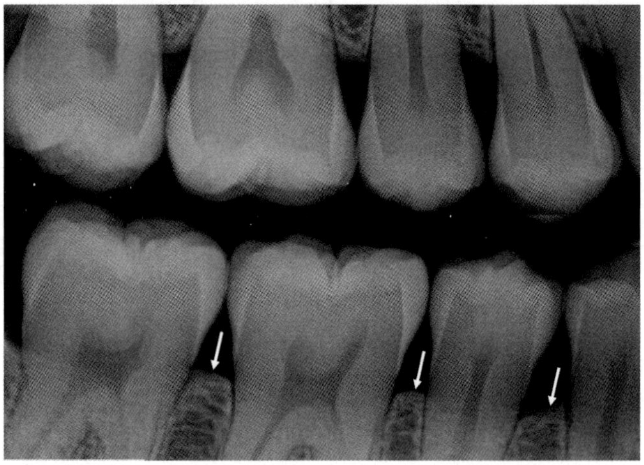

Fig 28-72 The posterior alveolar crest normally appears flat and smooth.

PRIMARY AND MIXED DENTITIONS

The central focus of this chapter on normal anatomy has been the adult dentition. In order for the dental radiographer to be confident in recognizing normal anatomy in children, a review of the primary and mixed dentitions is included.

Primary Dentition

Primary teeth begin to erupt at the age of 6 months. By the age of 3, all 20 primary teeth should be erupted and functioning. The **primary dentition** (also known as *deciduous dentition*) is comprised of

10 maxillary and 10 mandibular teeth. Although these teeth are eventually shed and replaced by the permanent dentition, the primary teeth play an integral role in the formation of the mandible and maxilla, as well as in the proper alignment, spacing, and occlusion of the permanent teeth.

An imaging examination of a child with a primary dentition is a common occurrence in dental practices. The anterior primary teeth include central incisors, lateral incisors, and canines. The posterior primary teeth include first molars and second molars. It is important to note that primary dentition does *not* include premolars or third molars. The Universal Numbering System for the primary dentition is based on the letters of the alphabet, from A to T (Figure 28-73). In a child under the age of 6, a bite-wing examination of the primary teeth includes the canines and the first and second molars (Figure 28-74).

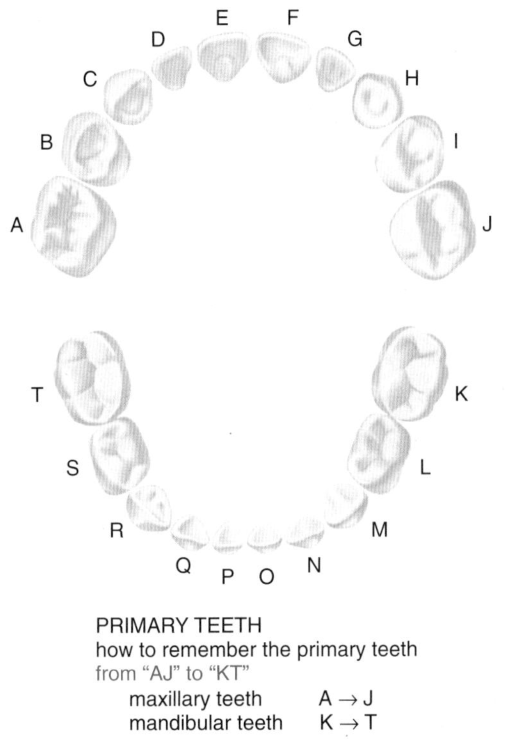

Fig 28-73 An illustration of the 20 teeth of the primary dentition labeled with the Universal Numbering System (A through T).

In a slightly older child, the bite-wing image includes the erupting first molars (Figure 28-75).

Some of the differences between primary and permanent teeth are obvious clinically; primary teeth are smaller and appear whiter than permanent teeth. On dental images, other differences can be noted. The roots of primary teeth flare apically to allow room in

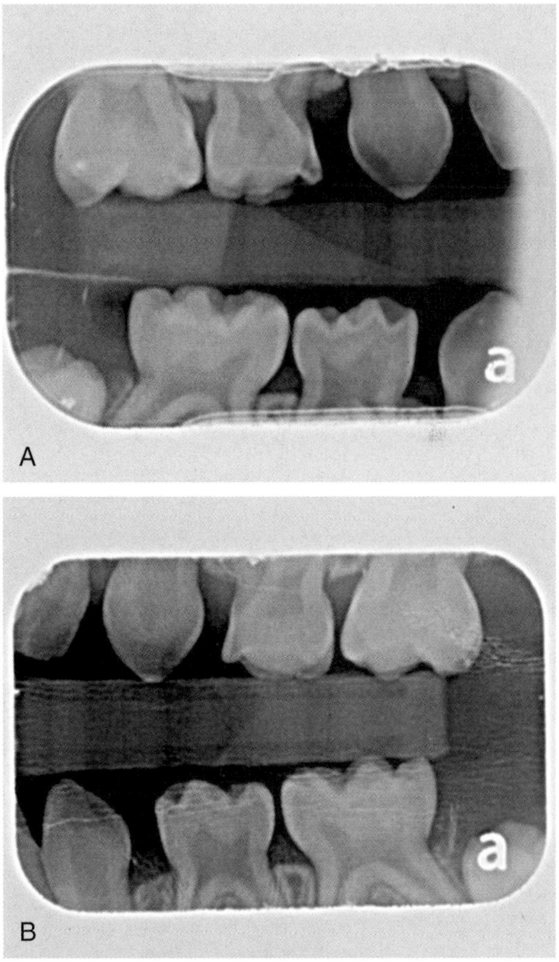

Fig 28-74 Two bite-wing images of a child with a primary dentition. Notice the large pulp chambers and spacing between teeth. (Courtesy Cary Pediatric Dentistry, Cary, NC.)

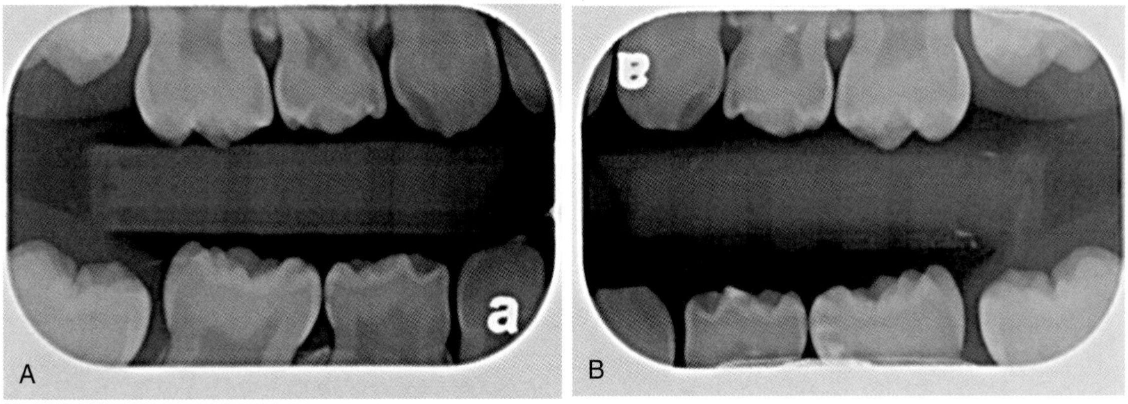

Fig 28-75 Two bite-wing images of a child with a primary dentition. Permanent teeth #3, 14, 19, and 30 are beginning to erupt. (Courtesy Cary Pediatric Dentistry, Cary, NC.)

between for the developing permanent crowns to form. The pulp chambers of primary teeth are larger compared with permanent teeth (Figure 28-76).

Mixed Dentition

Between the ages of 6 and 12, a mixed dentition that includes both primary and permanent teeth is seen in the oral cavity. The mixed or transitional dentition stage starts when the first permanent molar appears in the mouth at the age of 5 or 6 and lasts until the last primary tooth is lost, around the age of 12. The mixed dentition period can produce a variety of dental concerns, including malocclusion, crowding, spacing issues, and temporomandibular joint dysfunction, as well as an increase in plaque levels and gingivitis resulting from the difficulties of brushing loose or malpositioned teeth (Figure 28-77).

The periapical, bite-wing, and occlusal imaging techniques can be used to examine the primary and mixed dentitions (Figure 28-78). Problems such as lack of patient cooperation and the stimulation of the gag reflex may result in less than ideal intraoral images (see Chapter 24). With some children, it may not be possible to obtain diagnostic intraoral images. In such instances, extraoral imaging may be required to obtain diagnostic information. Extraoral images such as the panoramic or images produced with CBCT (Cone-Beam Computed Tomography) may be needed to obtain diagnostic information during this transitional dentition stage (Figure 28-79).

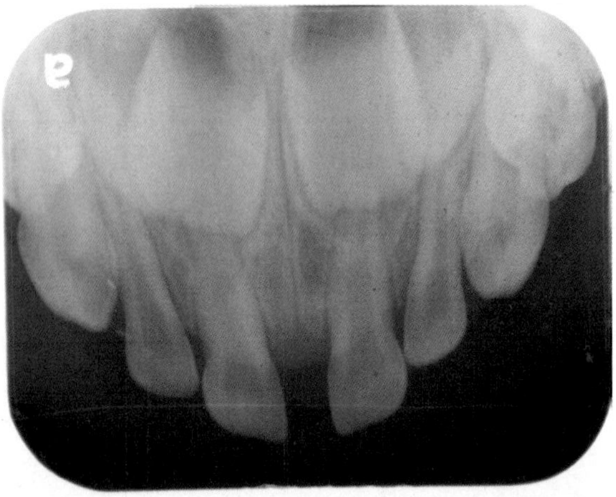

Fig 28-76 A maxillary occlusal image of a young child reveals the anterior primary teeth with developing permanent anterior teeth #7-10 still unerupted. Note the larger pulp chambers in the primary dentition. (Courtesy Cary Pediatric Dentistry, Cary, NC.)

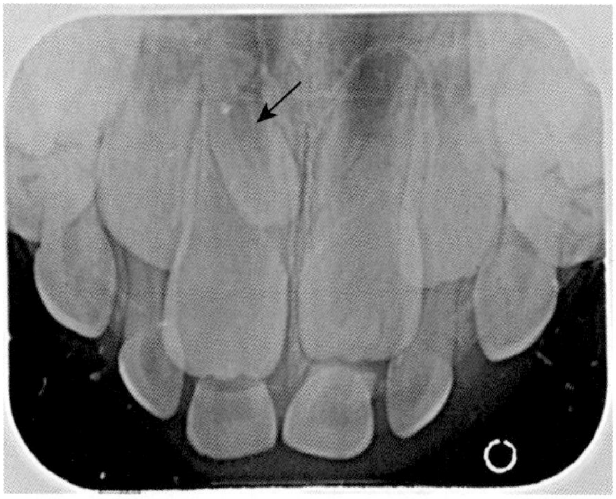

Fig 28-78 A maxillary occlusal image reveals teeth #E and F nearing exfoliation, with teeth #8 and 9 ready to erupt. Note the small supernumerary (extra) tooth near the midline (*arrow*).

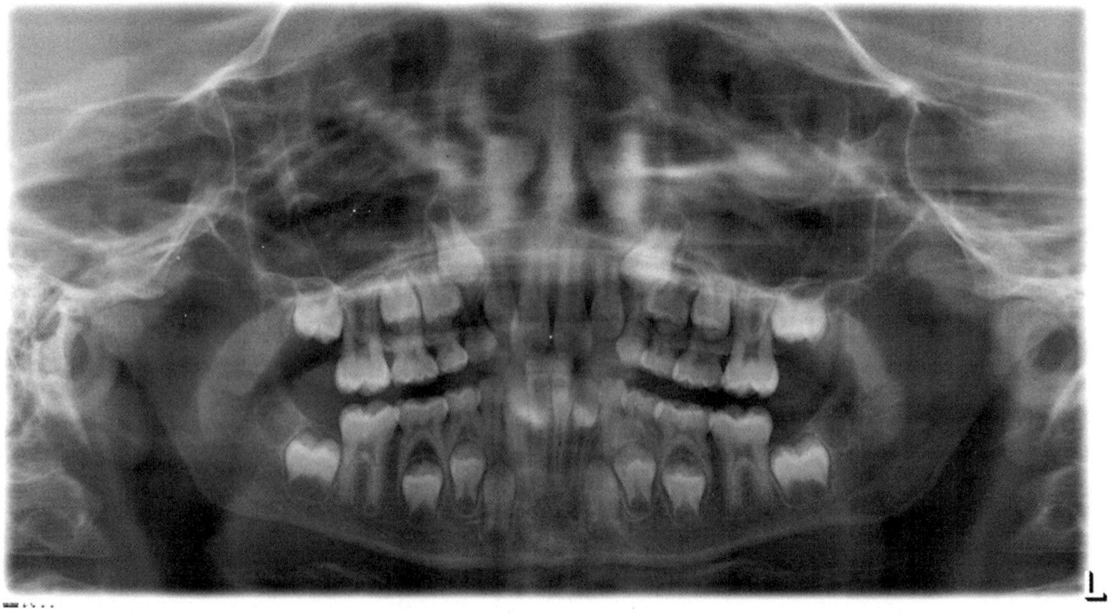

Fig 28-77 A panoramic image of a 9-year-old patient reveals a mixed dentition. (Courtesy Cary Pediatric Dentistry, Cary, NC.)

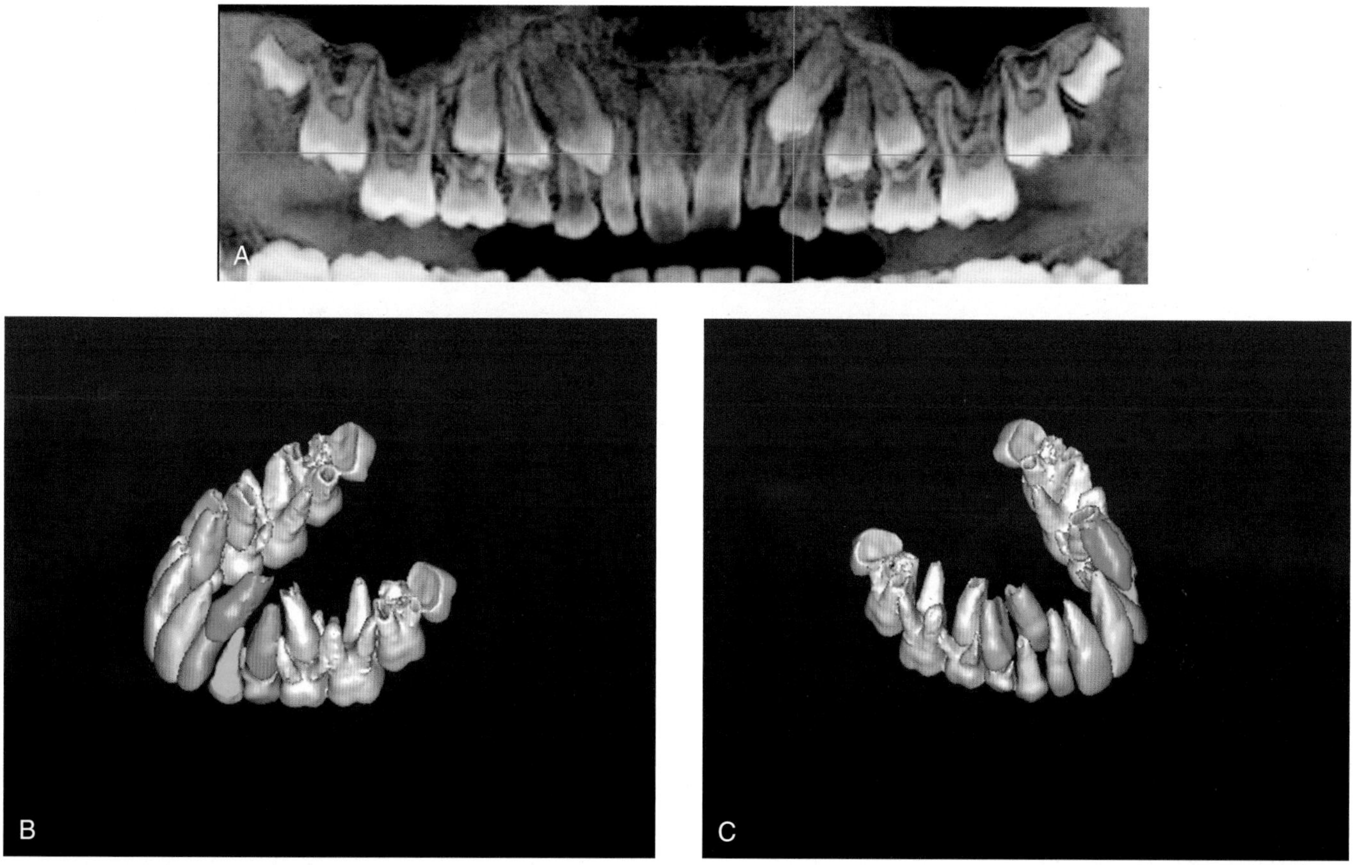

Fig 28-79 A, A section of a panoramic image reveals a patient with a mixed dentition. Primary teeth A, B, C, H, I, and J are present in the oral cavity, along with permanent teeth #3, 7, 8, 9, 10, and 14. Teeth #1, 2, 15, and 16 have not yet erupted. B, C, Images produced with cone-beam computer tomography and viewing software show the exact location of the developing permanent teeth. (Courtesy Carolina OMF Imaging, W. Bruce Howerton, Jr., DDS, MS, Franklinton, NC.)

SUMMARY

- The dental radiographer must have a thorough knowledge of the anatomy of the maxilla and the mandible; each normal anatomic landmark seen on an intraoral image corresponds to one seen on the human skull.
- Knowledge of the anatomy of the maxilla and the mandible found on the human skull enables the dental radiographer to identify the normal anatomy that is found on intraoral images.
- Recognition of normal anatomic landmarks enables the dental radiographer to distinguish between maxillary and mandibular periapical exposures and accurately mount intraoral dental images.
- Recognition of normal anatomic landmarks is also necessary for the accurate interpretation of dental images.
- Knowledge of the normal anatomy seen on intraoral images is essential before the dental radiographer can begin to recognize abnormalities (e.g., diseases, lesions).
- Recognition of normal anatomy in the child patient is needed for the accurate interpretation of images involving the primary and mixed dentitions.

BIBLIOGRAPHY

Frommer HH, Savage-Stabulas JJ: Film mounting and radiographic anatomy. In Radiology for the dental professional, ed 9, St Louis, 2011, Mosby.

Haring JI, Lind LJ: Normal anatomy (periapical films). In Radiographic interpretation for the dental hygienist, Philadelphia, 1993, Saunders.

Mallya SM, Lam EWN: Radiographic anatomy. In White and Pharoah's Oral radiology: principles and interpretation, ed 8, St. Louis, 2019, Elsevier.

Miles DA, Van Dis ML, Jensen CW, et al: Normal anatomy and film mounting. In Radiographic imaging for dental auxiliaries, ed 3, St Louis, 2009, Saunders.

QUIZ QUESTIONS

Matching

Match the following terms with the proper definitions:

Hole or opening in bone
Broad, shallow depression in bone
Cavity, recess, or hollow space in bone
Passageway through bone
Spongelike bone
Bony partition that separates two spaces
Immovable joint between bones
Hard or compact bone

_____ 1. Fossa
_____ 2. Canal
_____ 3. Foramen
_____ 4. Sinus
_____ 5. Septum
_____ 6. Suture
_____ 7. Cortical
_____ 8. Cancellous

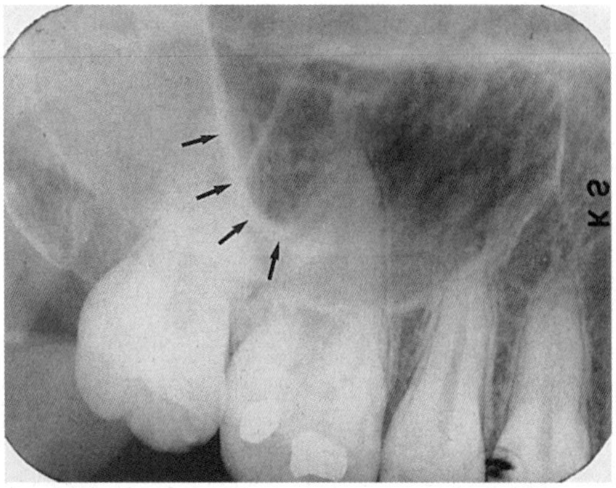

Fig 28-80

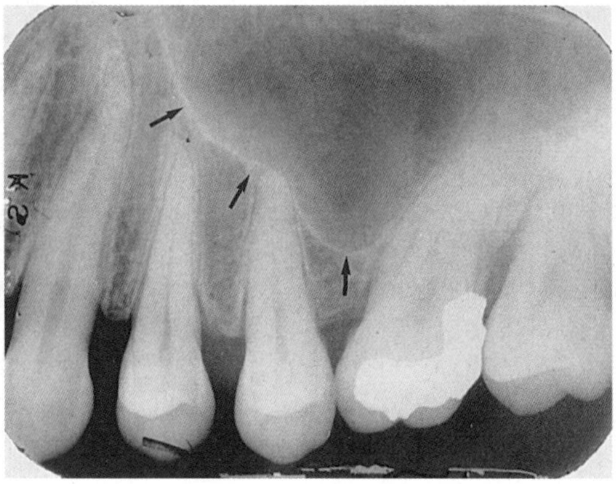

Fig 28-81

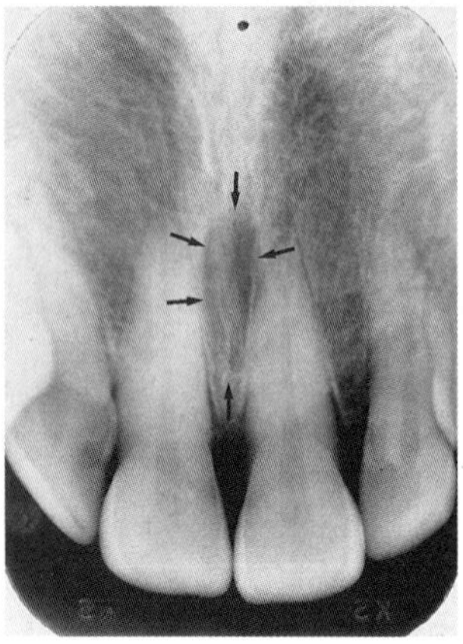

Fig 28-82

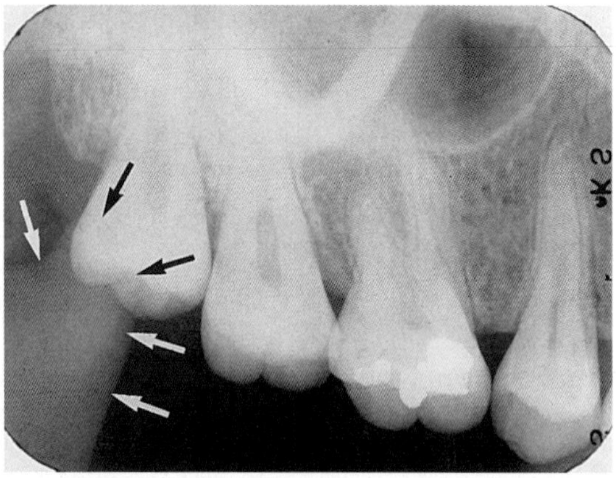

Fig 28-83

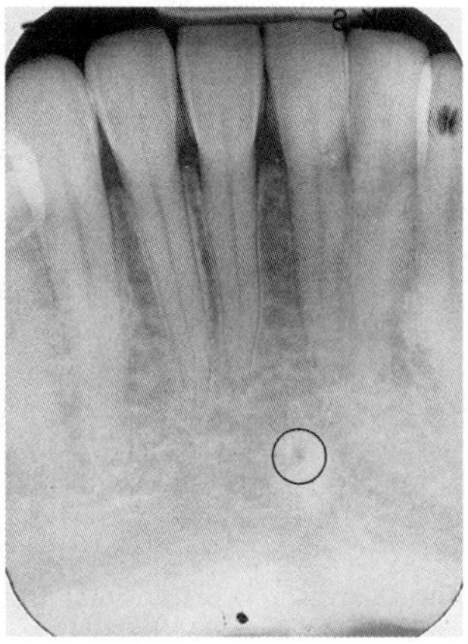

Fig 28-84

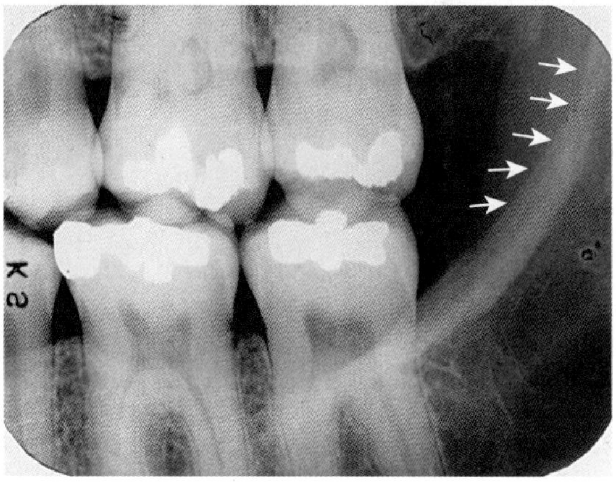

Fig 28-85 (From Haring JI, Lind LJ: Radiographic interpretation for the dental hygienist, Philadelphia, 1993, Saunders.)

Identification

For questions 9 to 16, refer to Figures 28-80 through 28-87. Identify the normal anatomic landmarks indicated by arrows (or circle) as required.

9. Identify the normal anatomic landmark shown in Figure 28-80.
10. Identify the normal anatomic landmark shown in Figure 28-81.
11. Identify the normal anatomic landmark shown in Figure 28-82.
12. Identify the normal anatomic landmark shown in Figure 28-83.
13. Identify the normal anatomic landmark shown in Figure 28-84.
14. Identify the normal anatomic landmark shown in Figure 28-85.
15. Identify the normal anatomic landmark shown in Figure 28-86.
16. Identify the normal anatomic landmark shown in Figure 28-87.

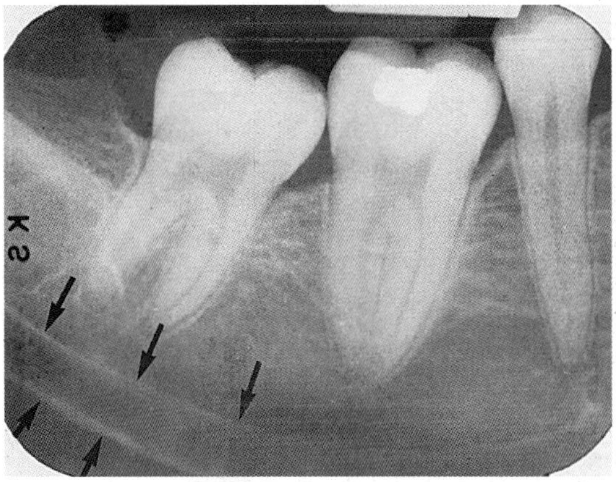

Fig 28-86

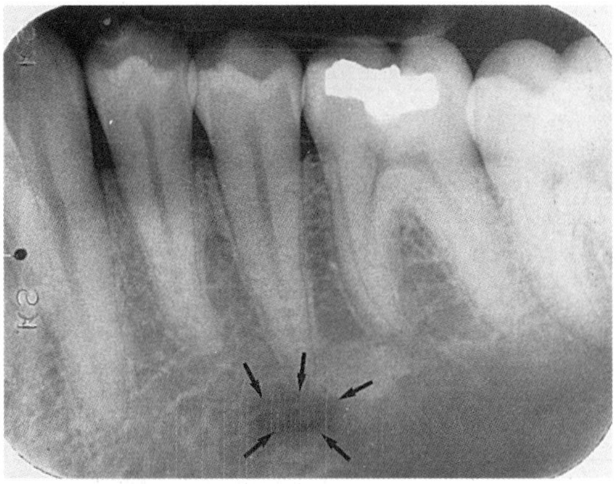

Fig 28-87

Interpretation

17. From the information seen in this panoramic image, list the primary teeth that are present in the oral cavity (Figure 28-88).

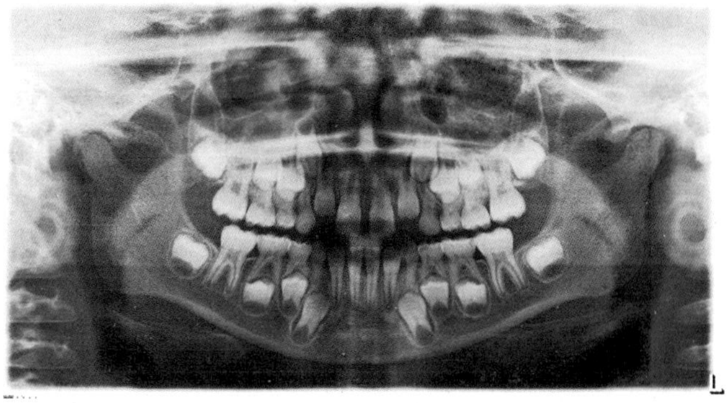

Fig 28-88 (Courtesy Cary Pediatric Dentistry, Cary, NC.)

29

Normal Anatomy: Panoramic Images

LEARNING OBJECTIVES

After completion of this chapter, the student will be able to do the following:

1. Define the key terms associated with normal anatomy on panoramic images.
2. Identify and describe the bony landmarks of the maxilla and surrounding structures as viewed on the panoramic image.
3. Identify and describe the bony landmarks of the mandible and surrounding structures as viewed on the panoramic image.
4. Identify air spaces as viewed on the panoramic image.
5. Identify soft tissues as viewed on the panoramic image.

A panoramic image allows the dental professional to view large areas of the mandible and the maxilla on a single projection. The dental professional must be able to recognize normal anatomic landmarks on intraoral images and normal anatomic structures viewed on panoramic images. The recognition of landmarks enables the dental professional to interpret panoramic images accurately. Without a working knowledge of anatomy, normal anatomic structures may be mistaken for artifacts and pathologic conditions.

To interpret the panoramic image and identify normal anatomic landmarks, the dental professional must have thorough knowledge of the anatomy of the maxilla and the mandible. Each normal anatomic landmark seen on a panoramic image corresponds to what is seen on the human skull. If the dental professional is familiar with the anatomy of the human skull, normal anatomy viewed on a panoramic image may be easily identified.

The purpose of this chapter is to describe the normal anatomy of the maxilla and the mandible as viewed on a panoramic image. In addition to the normal anatomic landmarks, air space images and soft tissue images are also described in this chapter.

NORMAL ANATOMIC LANDMARKS

Bony Landmarks of Maxilla and Surrounding Structures

The maxilla forms the floor of the orbit of the eyes, the sides and floor of the nasal cavity, and the hard palate. The lower border of the maxilla supports maxillary teeth. This section reviews the bony landmarks of the maxilla and surrounding structures that can be viewed on a panoramic image.

Each of the following bony landmarks of the maxilla and surrounding structures is identified on Figure 29-1.

Mastoid Process

Description. The mastoid process is a marked prominence of bone located posterior and inferior to the temporomandibular joint (TMJ). The mastoid process is part of the temporal bone.

Appearance. The mastoid process appears as a large rounded *radiopacity* located posterior and inferior to the TMJ area. The mastoid process is *not* seen on intraoral images.

Styloid Process

Description. The term *styloid* is derived from Greek *stylos* meaning long and tapered, like a pen or stylus. The styloid process is a long, pointed, and sharp projection of bone that extends downward from the inferior surface of the temporal bone. The styloid process is located anterior to the mastoid process.

Appearance. The styloid process appears as a long *radiopaque* spine that extends from the temporal bone anterior to the mastoid process. The styloid process is *not* seen on intraoral images.

External Auditory Meatus

Description. The external auditory meatus (also known as the *external acoustic meatus*) is a hole, or opening, in the temporal bone located superior and anterior to the mastoid process.

Appearance. The external auditory meatus appears as a round or ovoid *radiolucency* anterior and superior to the mastoid process. The external auditory meatus is *not* seen on intraoral images.

Glenoid Fossa

Description. The glenoid fossa is a concave, depressed area of the temporal bone. The mandibular condyle rests in the glenoid fossa when the teeth are in maximum intercuspation, meaning that the teeth are clenched together. The glenoid fossa is located anterior to the mastoid process and the external auditory meatus.

Appearance. The glenoid fossa appears as a concave *radiopacity* superior to the mandibular condyle. The glenoid fossa is *not* seen on intraoral images.

Articular Eminence

Description. The articular eminence (also known as the *articular tubercle*) is a rounded projection of the temporal bone located anterior to the glenoid fossa.

Appearance. The articular eminence appears as a rounded *radiopaque* projection of the bone located anterior to the glenoid fossa. The articular eminence is *not* seen on intraoral images.

Lateral Pterygoid Plate

Description. The lateral pterygoid plate is a thin, wing-shaped bony extension of the sphenoid bone located distal to the maxillary tuberosity region.

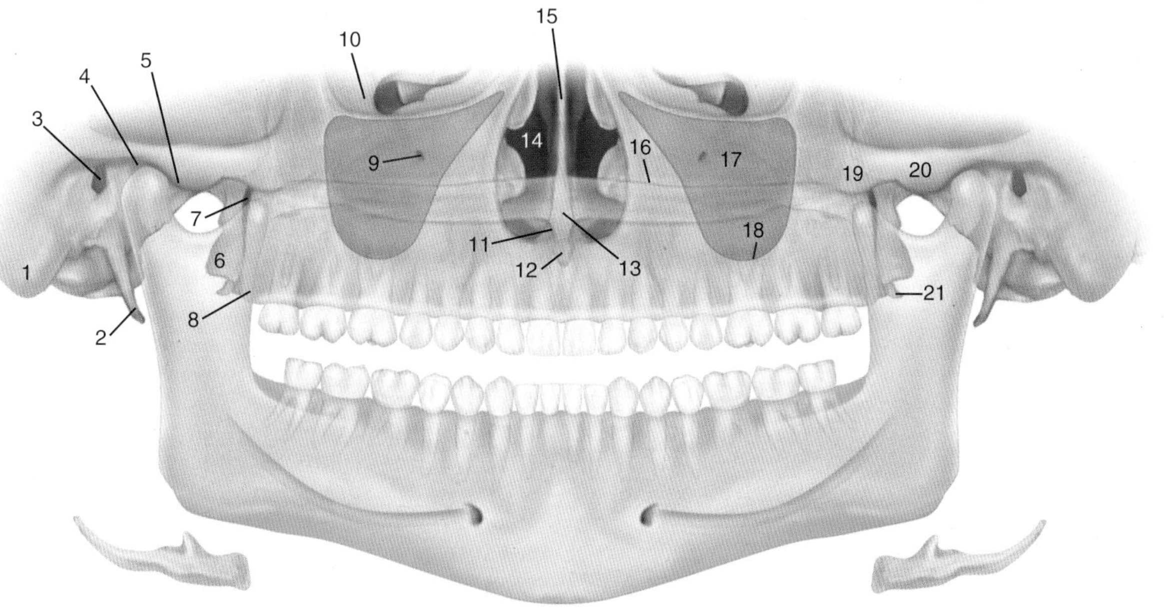

Fig 29-1 Normal anatomic landmarks of the maxilla and surrounding structures: **1**, mastoid process; **2**, styloid process; **3**, external auditory meatus; **4**, glenoid fossa; **5**, articular eminence; **6**, lateral pterygoid plate; **7**, pterygomaxillary fissure; **8**, maxillary tuberosity; **9**, infraorbital foramen; **10**, orbit; **11**, incisive canal; **12**, incisive foramen; **13**, anterior nasal spine; **14**, nasal cavity and conchae; **15**, nasal septum; **16**, hard palate; **17**, maxillary sinus; **18**, floor of maxillary sinus; **19**, zygomatic process of maxilla; **20**, zygomatic arch; **21**, hamulus. (Modified from Dental Auxiliary Education Projects: Normal radiographic landmarks, New York, Teachers College Press, ©1982 by Teachers College, Columbia University. All rights reserved.)

Appearance. The lateral pterygoid plate appears as a *radiopaque* projection of bone distal to the maxillary tuberosity region. The lateral pterygoid plate is *not* seen on intraoral images.

Pterygomaxillary Fissure

Description. The **pterygomaxillary fissure** is a narrow space that separates the lateral pterygoid plate and the maxilla.

Appearance. The pterygomaxillary fissure appears as a *radiolucent* area between the lateral pterygoid plate and the maxilla. This radiolucent area has the shape of an elongated and inverted teardrop that is outlined anteriorly by the posterior border of the maxillary sinus and posteriorly by the lateral pterygoid plate. The zygoma is often superimposed on this region and obscures the pterygomaxillary fissure. The pterygomaxillary fissure is *not* seen on intraoral images.

Maxillary Tuberosity

Description. The **maxillary tuberosity** is a rounded prominence of bone that extends posterior to the third molar region.

Appearance. The maxillary tuberosity appears as a *radiopaque* bulge distal to the third molar region. The maxillary tuberosity may also be viewed on intraoral images.

Infraorbital Foramen

Description. The **infraorbital foramen** is a hole, or opening, in bone inferior to the border of the orbit.

Appearance. The infraorbital foramen appears as a round or ovoid *radiolucency* inferior to the orbit. The infraorbital foramen may be superimposed over the maxillary sinus. The infraorbital foramen is *not* seen on intraoral images.

Orbit

Description. The **orbit** is the bony cavity that contains the eyeball.

Appearance. The orbit appears as a round *radiolucent* compartment with radiopaque borders located superior to the maxillary sinuses. On most panoramic images, only the inferior border of the orbit is visible, where it appears as a radiopaque line. The orbit is *not* seen on intraoral images.

Incisive Canal

Description. The **incisive canal** (also known as the *nasopalatine canal*) is a passageway through bone that extends from the superior foramina of the incisive canal (located on the floor of the nasal cavity) to the incisive foramen (located on the anterior hard palate).

Appearance. The incisive canal appears as a tubelike *radiolucent* area with radiopaque borders. The incisive canal is located between the maxillary central incisors. The incisive canal may also be viewed on intraoral images.

Incisive Foramen

Description. The **incisive foramen** (also known as the *nasopalatine foramen*) is an opening, or hole, in bone that is located at the midline of the anterior portion of the hard palate directly posterior to the maxillary central incisors.

Appearance. The incisive foramen appears as a small, ovoid or round *radiolucency* located between the roots of the maxillary central incisors. The incisive foramen may also be viewed on intraoral images.

Anterior Nasal Spine

Description. The **anterior nasal spine** is a sharp bony projection of the maxilla located at the anterior-inferior portion of the nasal cavity.

Appearance. The anterior nasal spine appears as a V-shaped *radiopaque* area located at the intersection of the floor of the nasal cavity and the nasal septum. The anterior nasal spine may also be viewed on intraoral images.

Nasal Cavity

Description. The **nasal cavity** (also known as the *nasal fossa*) is a pear-shaped compartment of bone located superior to the maxilla.

Appearance. The nasal cavity appears as a large *radiolucent* area superior to the maxillary incisors. The nasal cavity may also be viewed on intraoral images.

Nasal Septum

Description. The nasal septum is a vertical bony wall or partition that divides the nasal cavity into the right and left nasal fossae.

Appearance. The nasal septum appears as a vertical *radiopaque* partition that divides the nasal cavity. The nasal septum may not always appear straight or symmetric. The nasal septum may also be viewed on intraoral images.

Hard Palate

Description. The hard palate is the bony wall that separates the nasal cavity from the oral cavity.

Appearance. The hard palate appears as a horizontal *radiopaque* band superior to the apices of maxillary teeth. The hard palate may also be viewed on intraoral images.

Maxillary Sinus and Floor of Maxillary Sinus

Description. The maxillary sinuses are paired cavities or compartments of bone that are located within the maxilla, superior to maxillary posterior teeth.

Appearance. The maxillary sinuses appear as paired *radiolucent* areas located superior to the apices of maxillary premolars and molars. The floor of the maxillary sinus is composed of dense cortical bone and appears as a *radiopaque* line. The maxillary sinus and the floor of the maxillary sinus may also be viewed on intraoral images.

Zygomatic Process of Maxilla

Description. The zygomatic process of the maxilla is a bony projection of the maxilla that articulates with the zygoma, or cheekbone.

Appearance. The zygomatic process of the maxilla appears as a J- or U-shaped *radiopacity* located superior to the maxillary first molar region. The zygomatic process of the maxilla may also be viewed on intraoral images.

Zygoma

Description. The zygoma (also known as the *malar bone* or *zygomatic bone*) is the cheekbone, and it articulates with the zygomatic process of the maxilla.

Appearance. The zygoma appears as a diffuse *radiopaque* band that extends posteriorly from the zygomatic process of the maxilla. The zygoma may also be viewed on intraoral images.

Hamulus

Description. The term *hamulus* is derived from Latin *hamus* meaning hook. The hamulus (also known as the *hamular process*) is a small, hook-like projection of bone that extends from the medial pterygoid plate of the sphenoid bone. The hamulus is located posterior to the maxillary tuberosity.

Appearance. The hamulus appears as a *radiopaque* hook-like projection posterior to the maxillary tuberosity area. The hamulus may also be viewed on intraoral images.

Figures 29-2, 29-3, and 29-4 illustrate the normal anatomic landmarks of the maxilla and surrounding structures that can be viewed on a panoramic image.

Bony Landmarks of Mandible and Surrounding Structures

This section reviews the bony landmarks of the mandible and surrounding structures that can be viewed on a panoramic image.

The mandible can be divided into sections (Figure 29-6). The base or body of the mandible is the curved, horizontal section. The ramus consists of the two vertical sections of the mandible. The junction of the body and the ramus is referred to as the angle of the mandible.

Each of the following bony landmarks of the mandible and surrounding structures is identified on Figure 29-5.

Mandibular Condyle

Description. The mandibular condyle is a rounded projection of bone extending from the posterior superior border of the ramus of the mandible. The mandibular condyle rests in the glenoid fossa of the temporal bone.

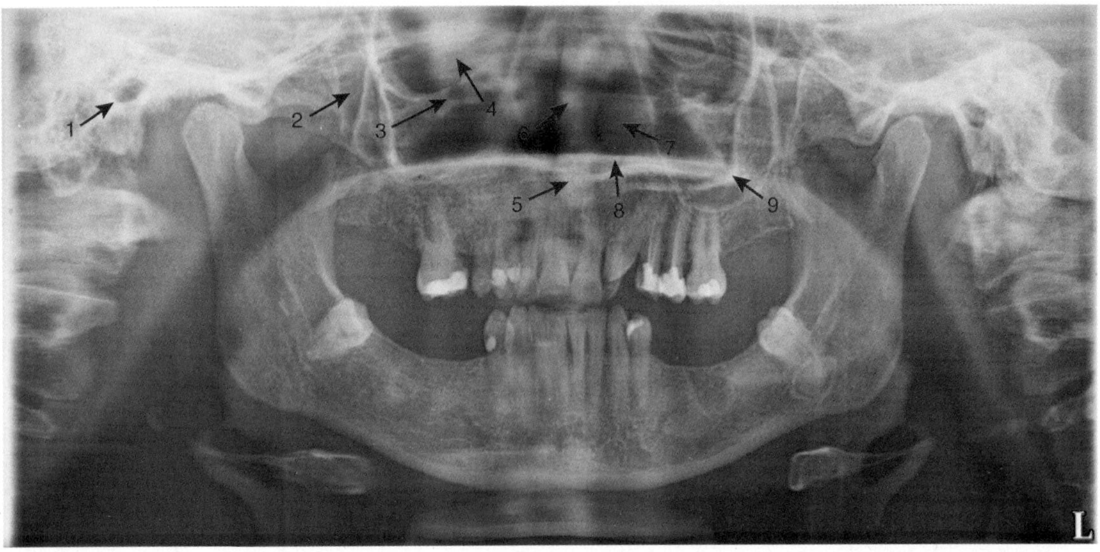

Fig 29-2 Normal anatomic landmarks of the maxilla and surrounding structures seen on a panoramic image:**1**, external auditory meatus; **2**, pterygomaxillary fissure; **3**, infraorbital foramen; **4**, orbit; **5**, anterior nasal spine; **6**, nasal septum; **7**, nasal conchae; **8**, hard palate; **9**, zygomatic process of maxilla.

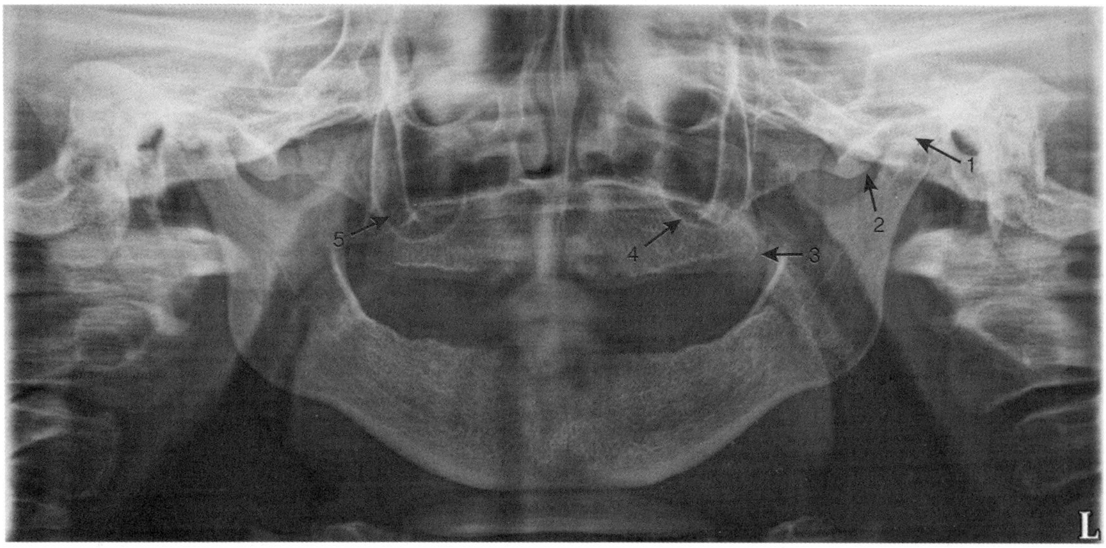

Fig 29-3 Normal anatomic landmarks of the maxilla and surrounding structures seen on a panoramic image:**1**, glenoid fossa; **2**, articular eminence; **3**, maxillary tuberosity; **4**, maxillary sinus; **5**, zygoma.

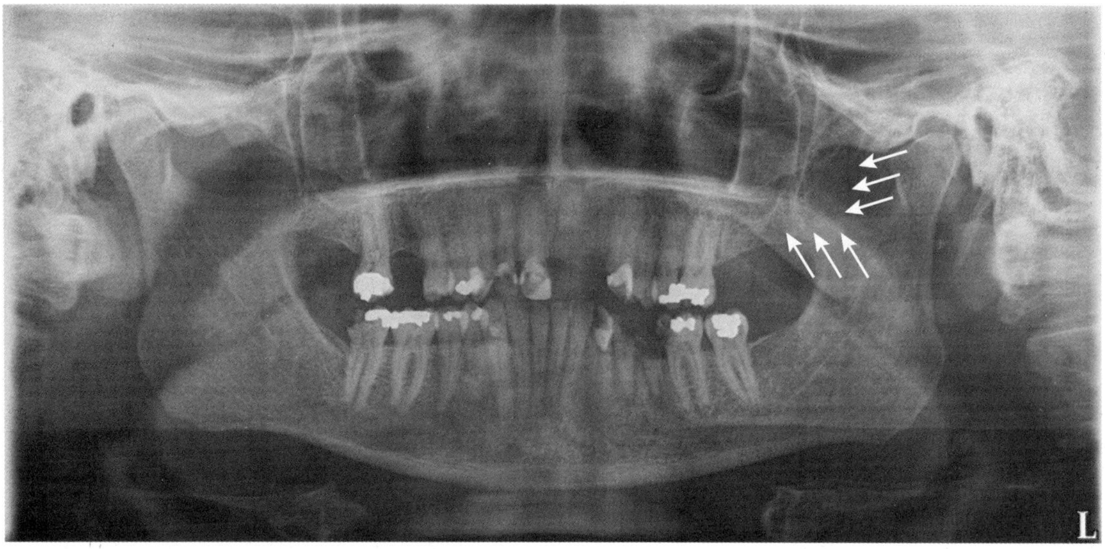

Fig 29-4 Lateral pterygoid plate.

Appearance. The mandibular condyle appears as a bony, rounded *radiopaque* projection extending from the posterior border of the ramus of the mandible. The condyle varies in shape and size and is dependent on the anatomy and positioning of the patient. The mandibular condyle is *not* seen on intraoral images.

Sigmoid Notch

Description. The sigmoid notch (also known as the *mandibular notch*) is a curved depression located between the mandibular condyle and the coronoid process of the mandible.

Appearance. The sigmoid notch appears as a *radiopaque* curved depression located between the mandibular condyle and the coronoid process on the superior border of the ramus. The sigmoid notch is *not* seen on intraoral images.

Coronoid Process

Description. The coronoid process is a thin prominence of bone that is shaped like a crow's beak and is found on the anterior-superior ramus of the mandible.

Appearance. The coronoid process appears as a triangular *radiopacity* posterior to the maxillary tuberosity region. In some instances, the coronoid process may be seen on a maxillary molar periapical image.

Mandibular Foramen

Description. The mandibular foramen is a round or ovoid hole in bone on the lingual aspect of the ramus of the mandible.

Appearance. The mandibular foramen appears as a round or ovoid *radiolucency* centered within the ramus of the mandible. The mandibular foramen is *not* seen on intraoral images.

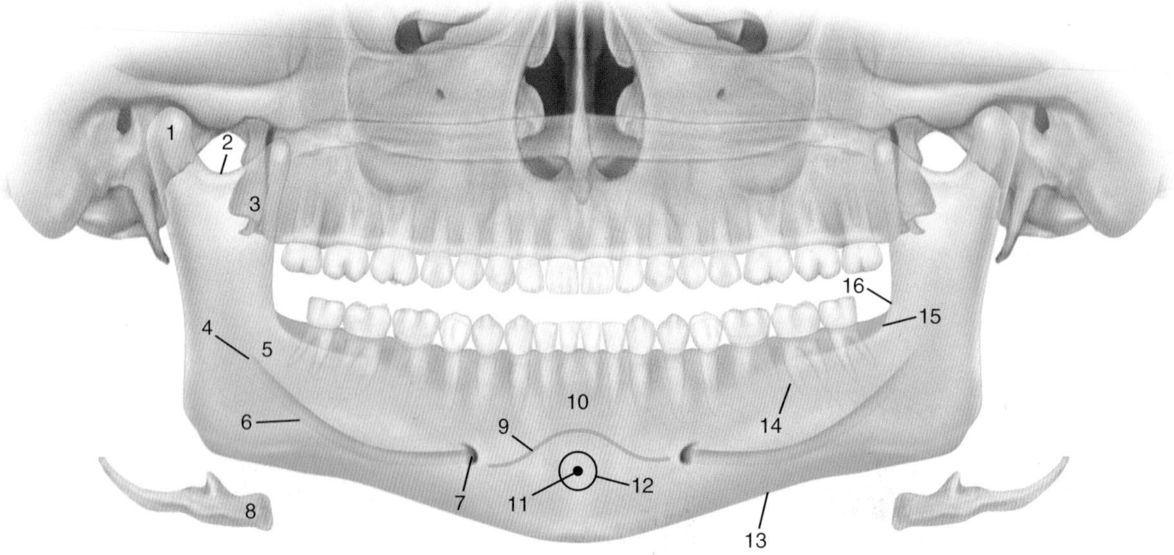

Fig 29-5 Normal anatomic landmarks of the mandible and surrounding structures:**1**, condyle; **2**, sigmoid notch; **3**, coronoid process; **4**, mandibular foramen; **5**, lingula; **6**, mandibular canal; **7**, mental foramen; **8**, hyoid bone; **9**, mental ridge; **10**, mental fossa; **11**, lingual foramen; **12**, genial tubercles; **13**, inferior border of mandible; **14**, mylohyoid ridge; **15**, internal oblique ridge; **16**, external oblique ridge. (Modified from Dental Auxiliary Education Project: Normal radiographic landmarks, New York, Teachers College Press, ©1982 by Teachers College, Columbia University. All rights reserved.)

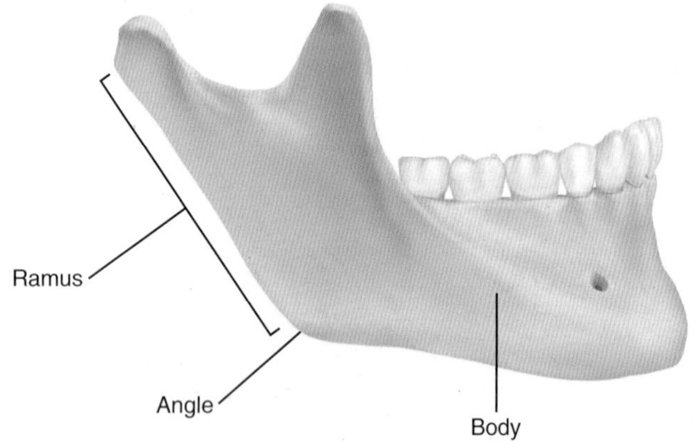

Fig 29-6 The sections of the mandible include the ramus, angle, and body.

Lingula

Description. The term *lingula* is derived from Latin *lingua* meaning tongue. The lingula is a small, tongue-shaped projection of bone seen adjacent to the mandibular foramen.

Appearance. The lingula appears as an indistinct *radiopacity* anterior to the mandibular foramen. The lingula is *not* seen on intraoral images.

Mandibular Canal

Description. The mandibular canal is a tubelike passageway through bone that travels within the body or length of the mandible. The mandibular canal extends from the mandibular foramen to the mental foramen and houses the inferior alveolar nerve and blood vessels.

Appearance. The mandibular canal appears as a *radiolucent* band outlined by two thin radiopaque lines representing the cortical walls of the canal. The mandibular canal may also be viewed on intraoral images.

Mental Foramen

Description. The mental foramen is an opening or hole in bone located on the external surface of the mandible in the region of the mandibular premolars.

Appearance. The mental foramen appears as a small, ovoid or round *radiolucency* located in the apical region of the mandibular premolars. The mental foramen may also be viewed on intraoral images.

Hyoid Bone

Description. The term *hyoid* is derived from Greek *hyoeides* meaning shaped like the letter upsilon (ϒ). The hyoid bone is a horseshoe-shaped bone that lies below the mandible, between the chin and thyroid cartilage. Ligaments and muscles located inferior to the mandible support the hyoid bone.

Appearance. The hyoid bone appears as a "floating" curved radiopacity at or below the inferior border of the body of the mandible. Depending on patient positioning, the hyoid bone may not be visible at all, or may be superimposed over the body of the mandible. The hyoid bone is located at the midline and, as a result, appears as a double image (see Chapter 25) and is viewed on both the right and left sides of the panoramic image. The hyoid bone is *not* seen on intraoral images.

Mental Ridge

Description. The mental ridge is a linear prominence of cortical bone located on the external surface of the anterior portion of the mandible that extends from the premolar region to the midline.

Appearance. The mental ridge appears as a thick *radiopaque* band that extends from the mandibular premolar region to the incisor region. The mental ridge may also be viewed on intraoral images.

Mental Fossa

Description. The mental fossa is a scooped-out depressed area of bone located on the external surface of the anterior mandible above the mental ridge in the mandibular incisor region.

Appearance. The mental fossa appears as a *radiolucent* area above the mental ridge. The mental fossa may also be viewed on intraoral images.

Lingual Foramen

Description. The lingual foramen is a tiny opening, or hole, in bone located on the internal surface of the mandible near the midline.

Appearance. The lingual foramen appears as a small *radiolucent* dot located inferior to the apices of the mandibular incisors. The lingual foramen may also be viewed on intraoral images.

Genial Tubercles

Description. The genial tubercles are tiny bumps of bone that are located on the lingual aspect of the mandible.

Appearance. The genial tubercles appear as a ring-shaped *radiopacity* surrounding the lingual foramen. The genial tubercles may also be viewed on intraoral images.

Inferior Border of Mandible

Description. The inferior border of the mandible is a thick, linear prominence of cortical bone that defines the lower border of the mandible.

Appearance. The inferior border of the mandible appears as a dense *radiopaque* band that outlines the lower border of the mandible. The inferior border of the mandible may also be viewed on intraoral images.

Mylohyoid Ridge

Description. The mylohyoid ridge is a linear prominence of bone located on the internal surface of the mandible that extends from the third molar region downward and forward toward the apical area of the premolars.

Appearance. The mylohyoid ridge appears as a dense *radiopaque* band that extends from the third molar area downward and forward toward the apical areas of the premolars. The mylohyoid ridge may also be viewed on intraoral images.

Internal Oblique Ridge

Description. The internal oblique ridge is a linear prominence of bone located on the internal surface of the mandible that extends downward and forward from the ramus.

Appearance. The internal oblique ridge appears as a dense *radiopaque* band that extends downward and forward from the ramus. The internal oblique ridge may also be viewed on intraoral images.

External Oblique Ridge

Description. The external oblique ridge is a linear prominence of bone located on the external surface of the mandible that extends downward and forward from the ramus to the molar region.

Appearance. On a panoramic image, the external oblique ridge appears as a dense *radiopaque* band that extends downward and forward from the ramus to the molar region. The external oblique ridge may also be viewed on intraoral images.

Angle of the Mandible

Description. The angle of the mandible is the angle formed where the horizontal lower edge of the body meets the perpendicular posterior edge of the ramus.

Appearance. On a panoramic image, the angle of the mandible appears *radiopaque* where the ramus joins the body of the mandible. The angle of the mandible is *not* visible on intraoral images.

Figures 29-7, 29-8, and 29-9 illustrate the normal anatomic landmarks of the mandible and surrounding structures that can be viewed on a panoramic image.

AIR SPACES SEEN ON PANORAMIC IMAGES

An air space image appears radiolucent. This section reviews air spaces that can be seen on a panoramic image.

These air spaces are not viewed on intraoral images. Each of the following air space images is identified on Figure 29-10.

Palatoglossal Air Space

Description. The term palatoglossal air space refers to the air space between the palate (*palato*) and the tongue (*glossal*).

Appearance. The palatoglossal air space appears as a horizontal well-defined *radiolucent* band located superior to the apices of maxillary teeth.

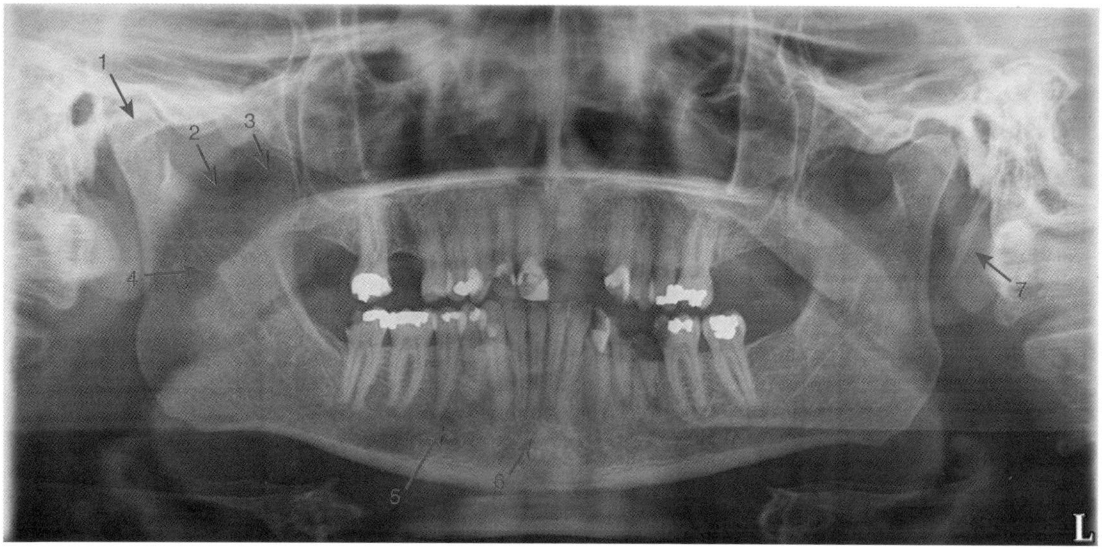

Fig 29-7 Normal anatomic landmarks of the mandible and surrounding structures seen on a panoramic image: **1,** condyle; **2,** sigmoid notch; **3,** coronoid process; **4,** mandibular foramen; **5,** mental foramen; **6,** genial tubercles; **7,** styloid process.

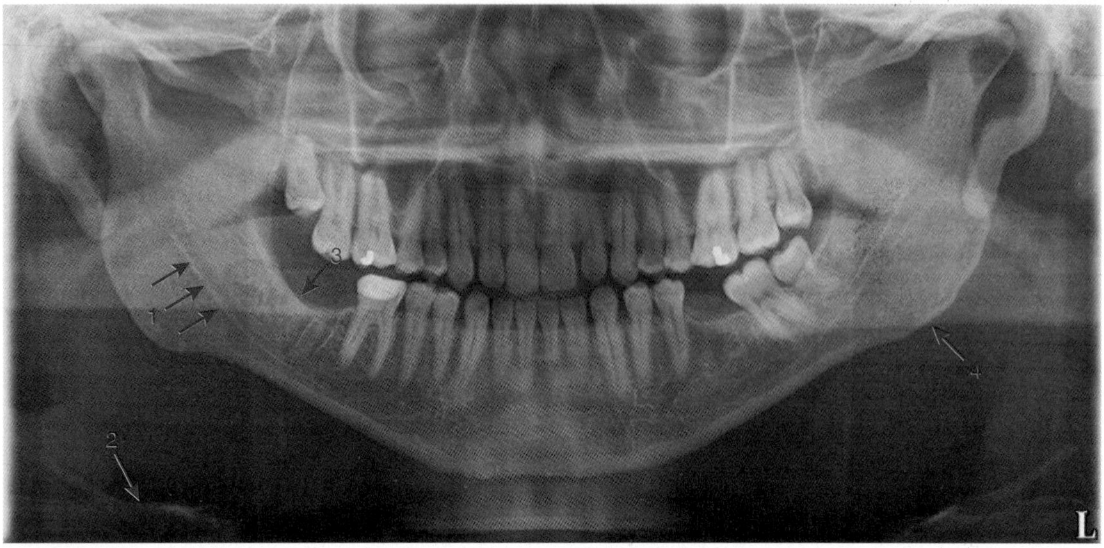

Fig 29-8 Normal anatomic landmarks of the mandible and surrounding structures seen on a panoramic image: **1**, mandibular canal; **2**, hyoid; **3**, internal oblique ridge; **4**, angle of mandible.

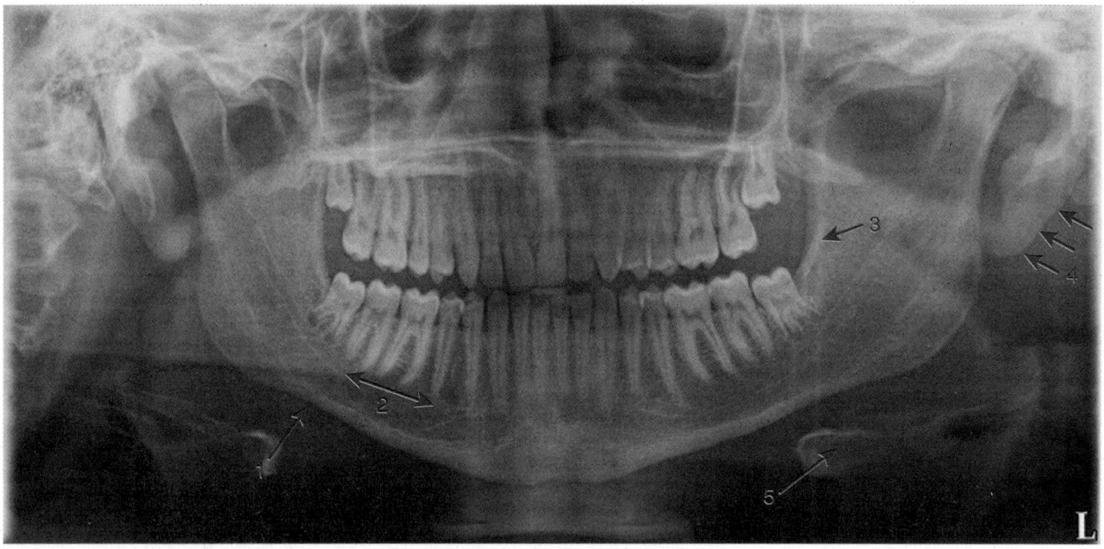

Fig 29-9 Normal anatomic landmarks of the mandible and surrounding structures as seen on a panoramic image: **1**, inferior border of mandible; **2**, submandibular fossa; **3**, external oblique ridge; **4**, soft tissue of ear; **5**, hyoid bone.

Nasopharyngeal Air Space

Description. The term nasopharyngeal air space refers to the air space in the pharynx (*pharyngeal*) that is located posterior to the nasal cavity (*naso*).

Appearance. The nasopharyngeal air space appears as a diagonal *radiolucent* band located superior to the radiopaque shadow of the soft palate and the uvula.

Glossopharyngeal Air Space

Description. The term glossopharyngeal air space refers to the air space in the pharynx (*pharyngeal*) that is located posterior to the tongue (*glosso*) and the oral cavity.

Appearance. The glossopharyngeal air space appears as a vertical *radiolucent* band superimposed over the ramus of the mandible. The glossopharyngeal air space is continuous with both the nasopharyngeal air space and the palatoglossal air space.

Figure 29-11 illustrates air spaces that can be viewed on a panoramic image.

SOFT TISSUES SEEN ON PANORAMIC IMAGES

A soft tissue image appears as a faint radiopacity. This section describes soft tissues that can be seen on a panoramic image. Each of the following soft tissues is labeled on Figure 29-12.

Tongue The tongue is a movable muscular organ attached to the floor of the mouth. The tongue appears as a faint dom-e-shaped *radiopaque* area superimposed over maxillary posterior teeth. The tongue is *not* seen on intraoral images.

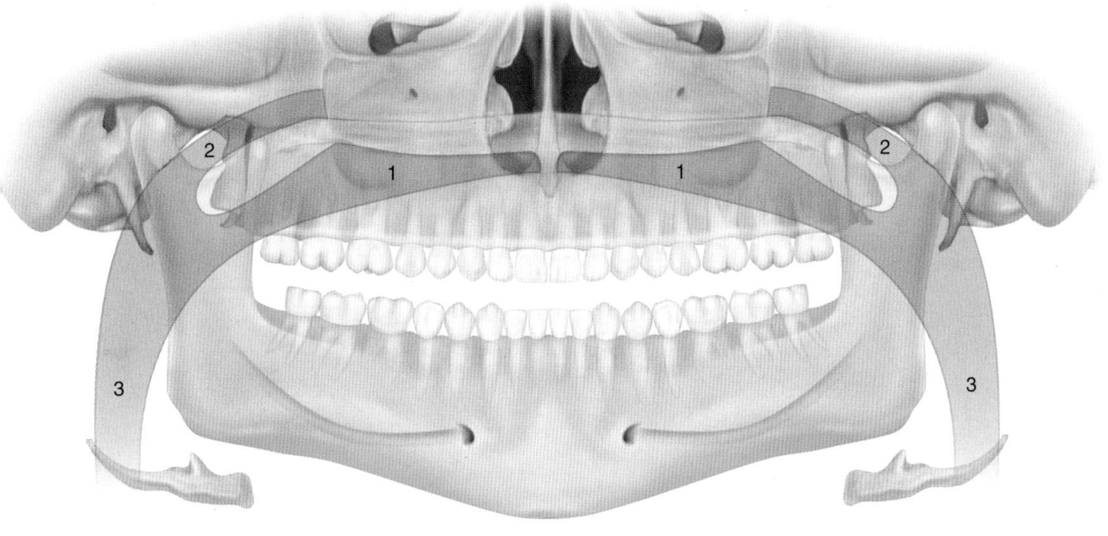

Fig 29-10 Air spaces seen on panoramic image:1, palatoglossal air space; 2, nasopharyngeal air space; 3, glossopharyngeal air space. (Modified from Dental Auxiliary Education Project: Normal radiographic landmarks, New York, Teachers College Press, ©1982 by Teachers College, Columbia University. All rights reserved.)

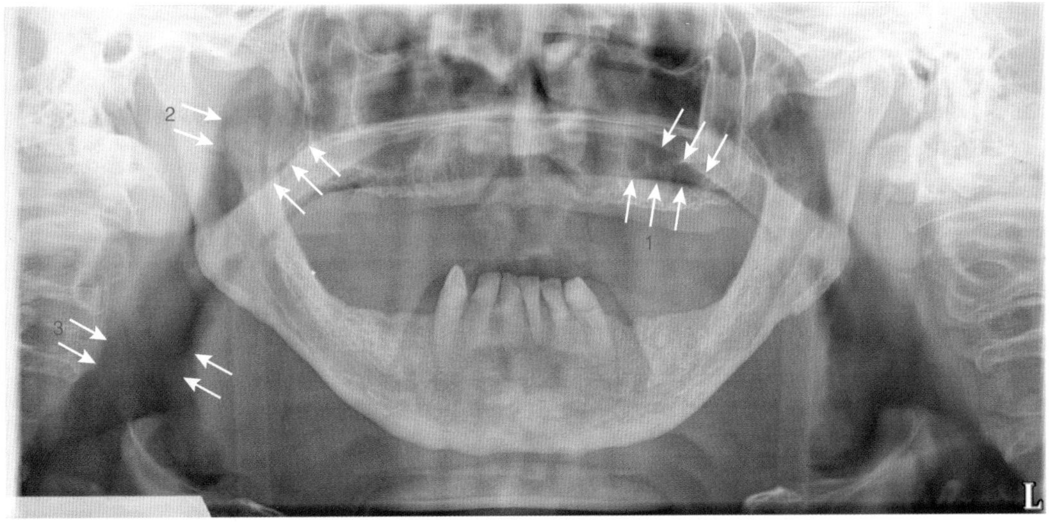

Fig 29-11 Air spaces seen on panoramic image:1, palatoglossal air space; 2, nasopharyngeal air space; 3, glossopharyngeal air space.

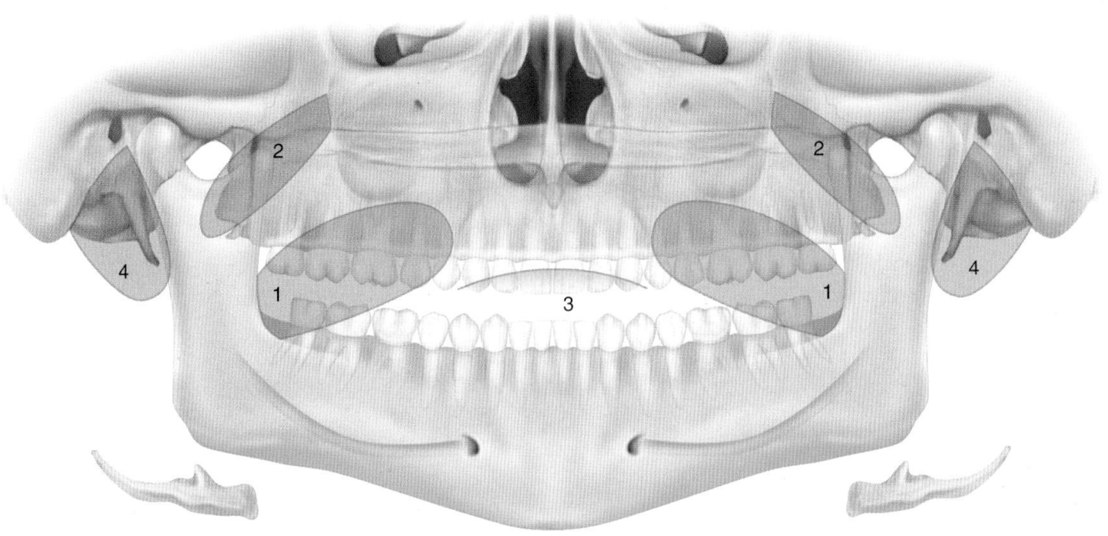

Fig 29-12 Soft tissues seen on panoramic image: 1, tongue; 2, soft palate and uvula; 3, lipline; 4, ear. (Modified from Dental Auxiliary Education Project: Normal radiographic landmarks, New York, Teachers College Press, ©1982 by Teachers College, Columbia University. All rights reserved.)

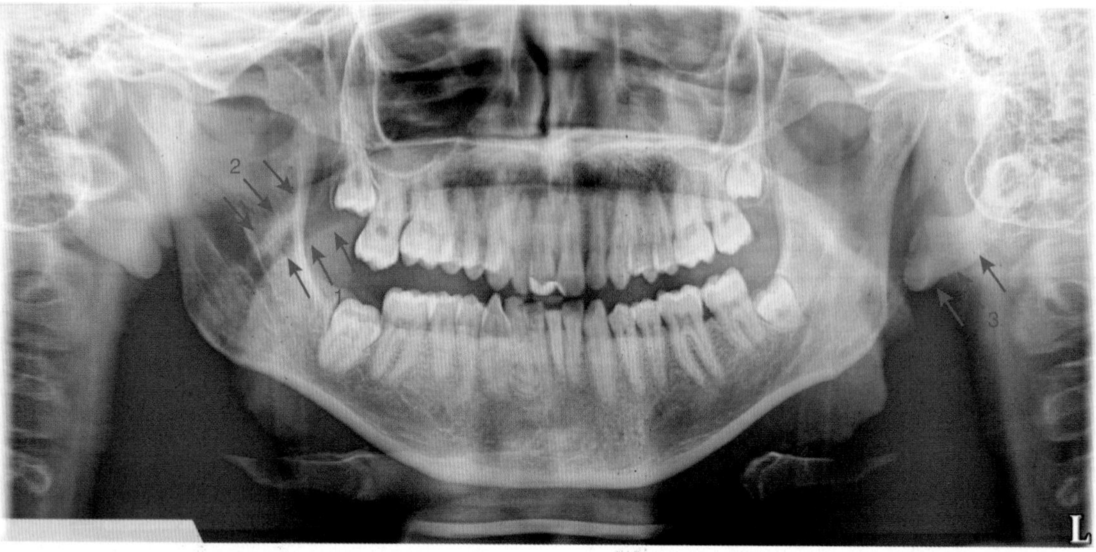

Fig 29-13 Soft tissues seen on panoramic image: **1**, tongue; **2**, soft palate and uvula; **3**, ear.

Soft Palate and Uvula The soft palate and the uvula form a muscular curtain that separates the oral cavity from the nasal cavity. The soft palate and the uvula appear as a faint diagonal *radiopaque* area that projects posteriorly and inferiorly from the maxillary tuberosity region. The soft palate and uvula are *not* seen on intraoral images.

Lipline The lipline is formed by the positioning of the patient's lips. On a panoramic image, the lipline is seen in the region of anterior teeth. Areas of teeth not covered by the lips appear more *radiolucent;* areas covered by the lips appear more *radiopaque.* The lipline may also be viewed on intraoral images.

Ear The visible outer ear is composed of cartilage with a thin covering of connective tissue and skin. It appears as a *radiopaque* shadow that projects anteriorly and inferiorly from the mastoid process. The ear is seen superimposed over the styloid process. The ear is *not* seen on intraoral images.

Figure 29-13 illustrates soft tissues that can be seen on a panoramic image.

SUMMARY

- The panoramic image allows the dental professional to view a large area of the maxilla and the mandible on a single projection.
- Knowledge of normal anatomic landmarks is necessary to interpret panoramic images; each normal anatomic landmark seen on a panoramic image corresponds to that seen on a human skull.
- Knowledge of the anatomy of the maxilla, the mandible, and adjacent bones as viewed on the human skull enables the dental radiographer to identify normal anatomy seen on a panoramic image.
- Knowledge of air spaces and soft tissues is necessary to interpret panoramic images.
- All anatomic landmarks, air spaces, and soft tissues viewed on a panoramic image are described in this chapter.

BIBLIOGRAPHY

Haring JI, Lind LJ: Normal anatomy (panoramic films). In Radiographic interpretation for the dental hygienist, Philadelphia, 1993, Saunders.

Mallya SM, Lam EWN: Panoramic imaging. In White and Pharoah's Oral radiology: principles and interpretation, ed 8, St. Louis, 2019, Elsevier.

QUIZ QUESTIONS

Identification

____ 1. Identify the normal anatomic landmarks labeled 1 to 15 in Figure 29-14.
____ 2. Identify the normal anatomic landmarks labeled 1 to 16 in Figure 29-15.
____ 3. In Figure 29-16:
Identify the faint radiopacity labeled A.
Identify the radiolucent band labeled B.
Identify the radiolucent band labeled C.

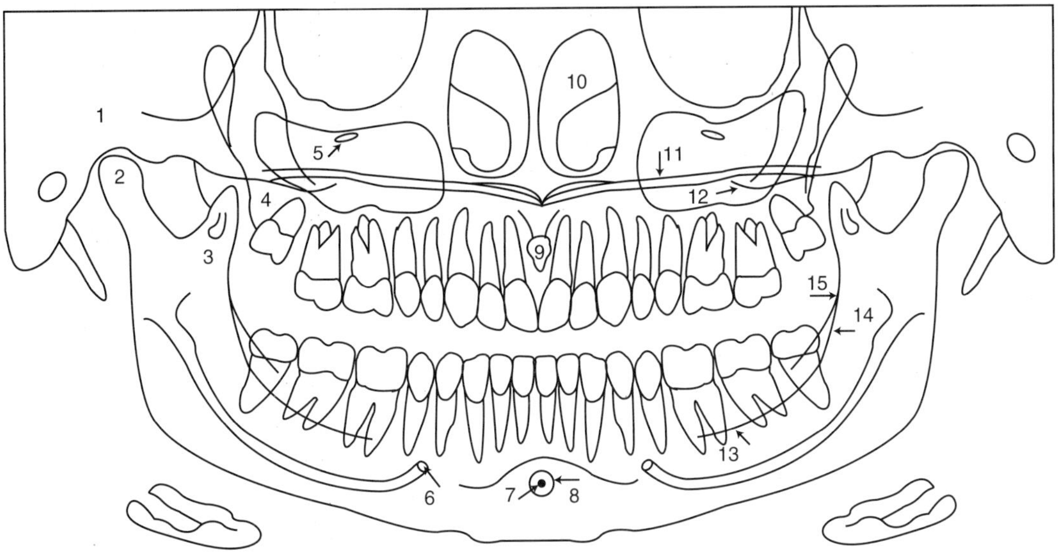

Fig 29-14 From Haring JI, Lind LJ: Radiographic interpretation for the dental hygienist, Philadelphia, 1993, Saunders.

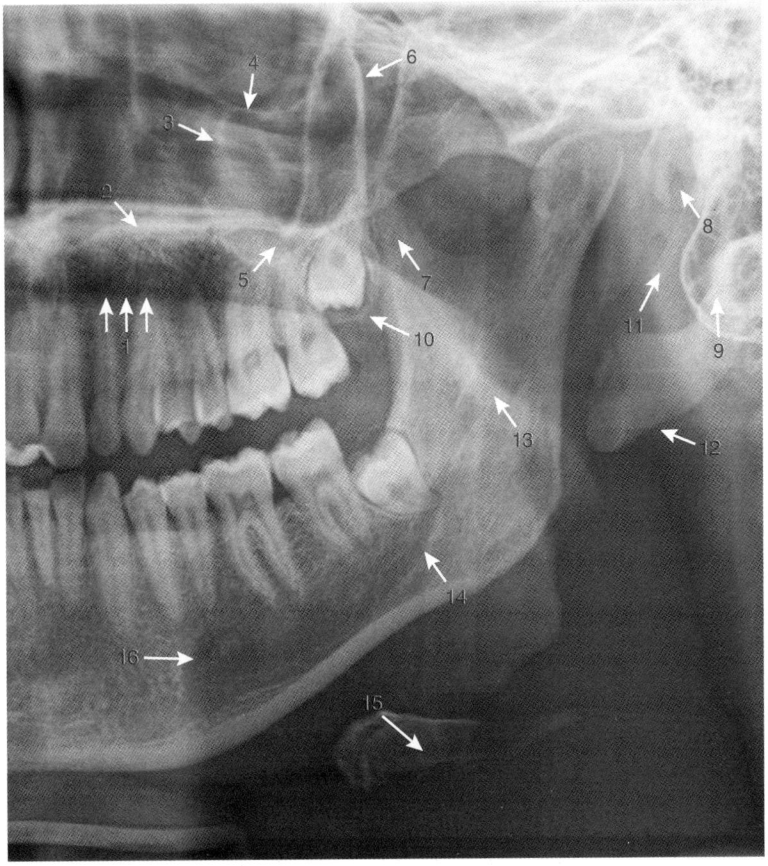

Fig 29-15

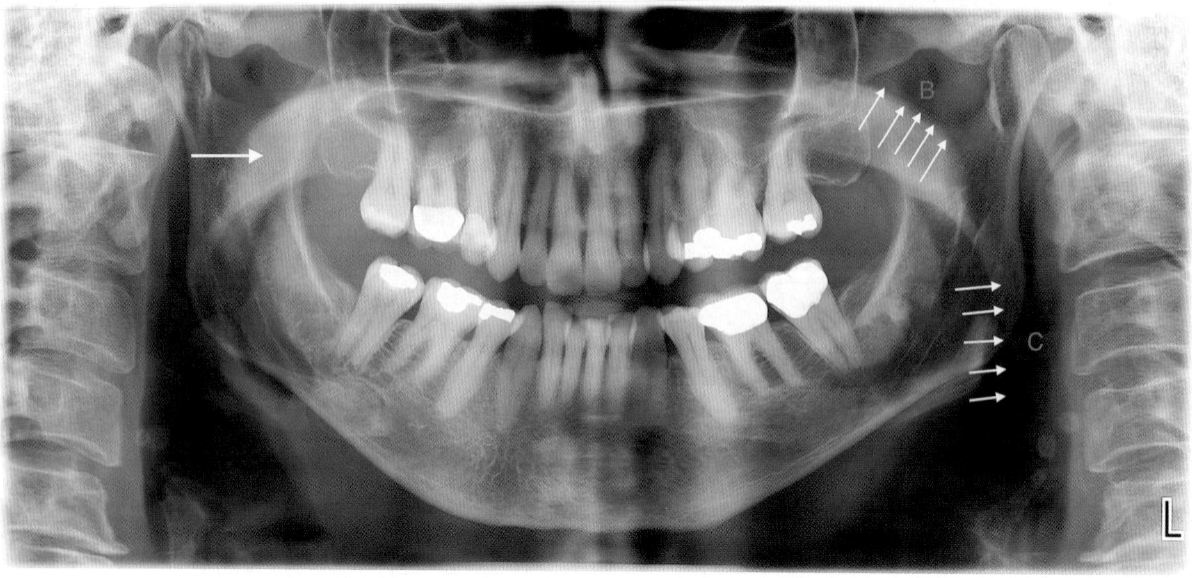

Fig 29-16

30 Introduction to Image Interpretation

LEARNING OBJECTIVES

After completion of this chapter, the student will be able to do the following:

1. Define the key terms associated with interpreting images.
2. Summarize the importance of the interpretation of images.
3. Describe who is able to interpret images by defining the roles of the dentist and the dental auxiliary in the interpretation of dental images.
4. Discuss the difference between interpretation and diagnosis.
5. Describe when and where dental images are interpreted.
6. Discuss the sequence for interpreting images.
7. Describe how interpretation is documented.
8. Describe how interpretation can be used to educate the dental patient about the importance and use of dental images.

Image interpretation is an essential part of the diagnostic process. The ability to evaluate and recognize what is revealed by a dental image enables the dental professional to play a vital role in the detection of those diseases, lesions, and conditions of jaws that cannot be identified clinically. The chapters in this part of the text present an overview of interpretation topics. Detailed information on interpretation is beyond the scope of this text.

The purpose of this chapter is to present the basic concepts of image interpretation and to review interpretation guidelines.

BASIC CONCEPTS

An explanation of what is viewed on a dental image, or interpretation, is an important component of patient care. Before the dental radiographer can inspect dental images adequately, a thorough understanding of the terminology and importance of interpretation is necessary.

Interpretation Terminology

Before discussion of the principles of interpretation, an explanation of basic terms is provided below:

Interpret: To offer an explanation.

Interpretation: An explanation.

Image interpretation: An explanation of what is viewed on a dental image; the ability to read what is revealed by a dental image.

Diagnosis: The identification of a disease by examination or analysis. In the dental setting, the dentist is responsible for establishing a diagnosis.

Importance of Interpretation

In addition to understanding the importance of dental images, the dental radiographer must also understand the importance of interpretation. As described in Chapter 12, dental images are essential for diagnostic purposes. *All* dental images must be carefully reviewed and interpreted. A great deal of information about teeth and supporting bone is obtained from interpretation. Consequently, image interpretation is of paramount importance to the dental professional. Dental images document a patient's condition at a specific point in time and allow the dental professional to gather information about diseases, lesions, and conditions of teeth and jaws that cannot be identified clinically. Image interpretation enables the dental professional to play a vital role in their detection.

GUIDELINES

The dental radiographer must know who can interpret dental images, the difference between interpretation and diagnosis, when and where images are interpreted, and how to use interpretation to educate the dental patient.

Who Interprets Images?

Training is necessary to interpret dental images. Any dental professional with training in interpretation can examine images. Both the dentist and the dental hygienist are trained to interpret dental images; dental and dental hygiene curricula include instruction in image interpretation. The dental assistant, however, may or may not be trained in the interpretation of dental images. The amount and scope of training in dental imaging dictate whether the dental assistant can perform image interpretation.

The dental radiographer plays an important role in the preliminary interpretation of dental images. The dental radiographer acts as an additional pair of eyes examining the images and can direct the attention of the dentist to any areas of question or concern. To interpret images, the dental radiographer must be confident in the identification and recognition of the following:

- Normal anatomy (see Chapters 28 and 29)
- Dental restorations, dental materials, and foreign objects (see Chapter 32)
- Dental caries (see Chapter 33)
- Periodontal disease (see Chapter 34)
- Trauma, pulpal lesions, and periapical lesions (see Chapter 35)
- Lesions of bone and bone anomalies
- Common artifacts and errors

Interpretation versus Diagnosis

In the dental setting, the terms *interpretation* and *diagnosis* are often confused; it is important to note that these terms have very different meanings and should not be used synonymously. *Interpretation* refers to an explanation of what is viewed on a dental image, whereas *diagnosis* refers to the identification of disease by examination or analysis. In dentistry, a diagnosis is made by the dentist after a thorough review of the medical history, dental history, clinical examination, imaging examination, and clinical or laboratory tests.

Although any dental professional with training in interpretation may examine dental images, the final interpretation and diagnosis are the responsibilities of the dentist. Dental hygienists and assistants are restricted by law from rendering a diagnosis.

When and Where Are Images Interpreted?

It is essential to remember that dental images are prescribed and obtained to benefit the patient. To benefit the patient optimally, dental images must be exposed at the beginning of the dental appointment, mounted, interpreted, and then used for diagnostic, therapeutic, and educational purposes. Ideally, dental images should be reviewed and interpreted immediately after placement in the computer software, or in a mount, and in the presence of the patient. If any suspicious or questionable areas are seen on the images, the patient can be examined by the dentist or dental hygienist to obtain additional information or to confirm the suspected problem. When the patient is not present during the interpretation of dental images, much needed clinical information is unavailable.

Digital images are typically viewed by the dental professional on a computer monitor in the operatory (Figure 30-1). Mounted dental radiographs are usually examined on the viewbox in the operatory and are best interpreted in a room with dimmed lighting, as described in Chapter 11.

What Is the Sequence for Interpreting Images?

As described in Chapter 11, all mounted images must be viewed in a sequential order. The dental radiographer must have an established viewing sequence to prevent errors in interpretation. To interpret a complete mouth series (CMS), a *recommended viewing sequence* is as follows:

1. Begin with maxillary periapical images—view tooth #1 on the upper left side of the mount, move horizontally to the maxillary right, and finish with tooth #16.
2. Move to the mandibular right and continue with mandibular periapical images—begin with tooth #17, move across to the mandibular left, and finish with tooth #32.
3. Move up to the bite-wings, and view the bite-wings from your left to right, similar to facing the patient.

The dental radiographer may use this recommended viewing sequence to examine intraoral images for each of the following:

- Unerupted, missing, and impacted teeth
- Dental caries and the size and shape of the pulp cavities
- Bony changes, the level of alveolar bone, and calculus
- Roots and periapical areas
- All areas not previously examined (e.g., remaining areas of the jaws, sinuses)

As part of a thorough interpretation, multiple examinations of dental images are necessary to check for all the problems just listed. For example, the dental radiographer should first view the images quickly for evidence of unerupted or impacted teeth. Next, the examination sequence should be repeated for caries, pulp size, and pulp shape. The sequence must be repeated as many times as necessary to evaluate all surfaces of teeth and supporting structures for evidence of disease and abnormalities. An example of an interpretation checklist that can be used in training the dental radiographer appears in Figure 30-2. When learning interpretation skills, a checklist can be used to provide the student with an organized format to gather essential information that is needed prior to diagnosis and treatment planning, a defined process to follow that serves as a roadmap for consistency, a step-by-step list of what to examine on dental images, and a list of findings to verify clinically.

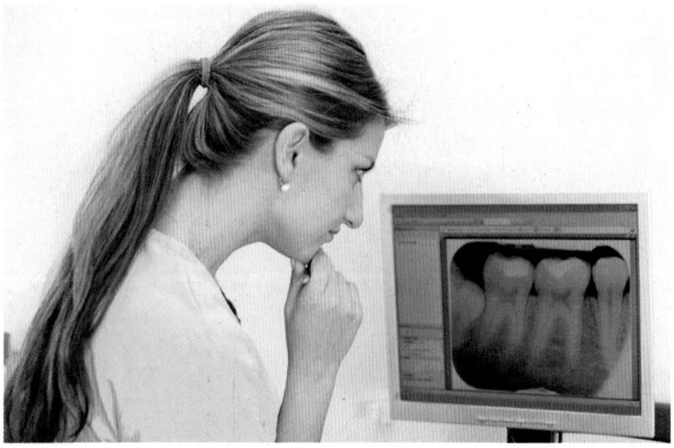

Fig 30-1 Digital images are typically viewed by the dental professional on a computer monitor in the operatory. (Copyright Vitapix/istock.com).

How Is Interpretation Documented?

All dental images must be reviewed and interpreted. The interpretation must be documented in the patient record and include the following:

- Date of exposure
- Number and type of images
- Evaluation of diagnostic quality
- List of limiting factors, retakes, or additional images needed
- Description of teeth—indicate impactions, number anomalies, crown anomalies, defective restorations, caries, calculus, pulpal changes, root abnormalities, and other miscellaneous features
- Description of bone and supporting structures of the teeth—indicate periapical radiolucencies and radiopacities, bone loss, changes in crestal lamina dura and radicular lamina dura, changes in periodontal ligament space, any furcation involvement, interdental trabecular pattern of bone, any lesions of bone, or bone anomalies
- Description of artifacts
- Indication of any areas that require additional imaging or clinic evaluation/confirmation

An example of how to document the interpretation of dental images in the patient record appears in Figure 30-3.

Interpretation and Patient Education

Interpretation of dental images can be used as an educational tool in the professional setting. In addition to providing a preliminary interpretation, the dental radiographer can educate the patient by identifying and discussing what is normally found on a dental image. Then the dentist can focus on specific problems or areas of concern. In this manner, all members of the dental team can work together using interpretation to educate patients about the importance and use of dental images.

Dental Image Interpretation Checklist

Images	# of Images ___ BW ___ PA ___ PAN		Date Images Exposed ___ / ___ /___
Diagnostic Quality	☐No ☐Yes	Additional Images Needed	☐No ☐Yes
Retakes	☐No ☐Yes	Limiting Factors	☐No ☐Yes *List factors*
Teeth			
Impacted Teeth	☐No ☐Yes ☐N/A*	Pulp Cavity Features ☐N/A*	☐Normal ☐Pulp stones ☐Sclerotic ☐Resorption ☐Obliterated ☐Previous RCT ☐Other
Number Anomalies supernumerary teeth/ congenitally missing teeth	☐No ☐Yes ☐N/A*		
Crown Anomalies size/shape defects	☐No ☐Yes ☐N/A*	Root Features ☐N/A*	☐Normal ☐Short or long ☐Root tips ☐Extra roots ☐Root fracture ☐Dilacerations ☐Resorption ☐Hypercementosis
Defective Restorations overhang/open contacts	☐No ☐Yes ☐N/A*		
Caries suspicious areas to be evaluated clinically	☐No ☐Yes ☐N/A*	Miscellaneous Features ☐N/A*	☐None ☐Attrition ☐Implants ☐Abrasion ☐Other ☐Trauma
Calculus	☐No ☐Yes ☐N/A*		
Bone			
Periapical Area radiolucency	☐No ☐Yes ☐N/A*	Lamina Dura Crestal ☐N/A*	☐Intact ☐Fuzzy, indistinct ☐Notched
Periapical Area radiopacity	☐No ☐Yes ☐N/A*	Lamina Dura Radicular ☐N/A*	☐Normal ☐Thickened ☐Absent
Bone Loss percent and pattern *see periodontal charting*	☐No bone loss ☐N/A* ☐≤ 20% *slight* *L or G* ☐21-49% *moderate* *L or G* ☐≥ 50% *severe* *L or G* ☐Horizontal ☐Vertical	PDL Space ☐N/A*	☐Normal ☐Widened ☐Obliterated
		Furcation Involvement ☐N/A*	☐None ☐Wide pdl in furcation *See periodontal charting* ☐≤ 3 furcations ☐≥ 4 furcations
		Interdental Trabeculations ☐N/A*	☐Normal ☐↑Density ☐↓Density
Bone Anomalies non-tooth related lesions	☐No ☐Yes ☐N/A*	Other: ________ ☐N/A*	*N/A *Cannot be determined from images reviewed; additional images needed*
Artifacts	☐No ☐Yes		

Fig 30-2 An example of an interpretation checklist. (Courtesy Dr. Joen M. Iannucci, Professor of Clinical Dentistry, The Ohio State University, Columbus, OH.)

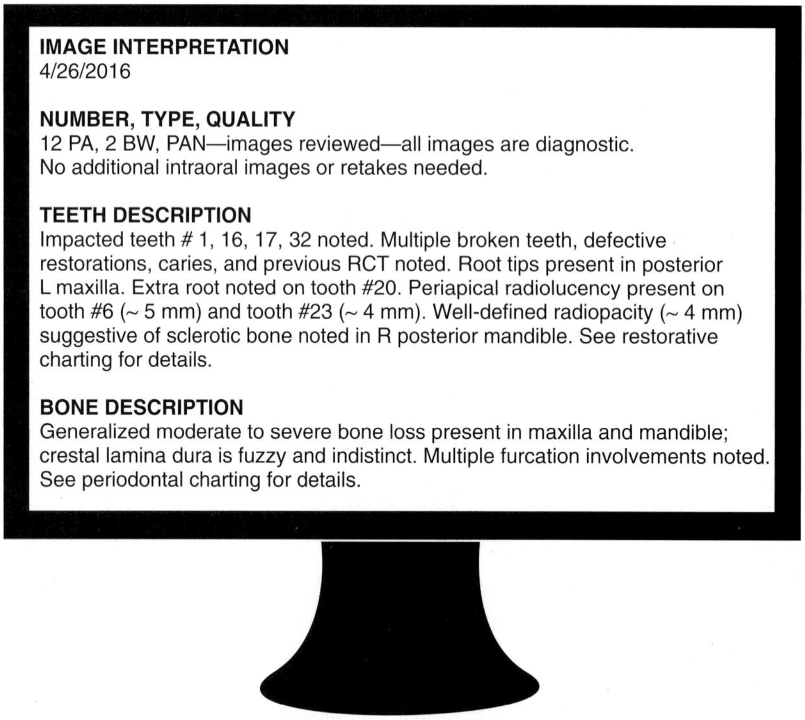

Fig 30-3 Example of image interpretation documentation.

SUMMARY

- Image interpretation is an explanation of what is viewed on a dental image, or the ability to read what is revealed by a dental image.
- Image interpretation is an important component of patient care and enables the dental professional to detect diseases, lesions, and conditions that cannot be identified clinically.
- Any dental professional with training in interpretation can examine images. To interpret dental images, the dental radiographer must be confident in the identification and recognition of normal anatomy; restorations, dental materials, and foreign objects; dental caries; periodontal disease; traumatic injuries; and periapical lesions.
- Although any dental professional with training in interpretation may examine dental images, the final interpretation and diagnosis are the responsibilities of the dentist.
- Dental auxiliaries are restricted by law from providing a diagnosis but can facilitate patient care by performing a preliminary image interpretation.
- Whenever possible, a dental imaging examination should take place at the beginning of the appointment, and dental images should be interpreted with the patient present.
- All dental image interpretation must be documented in the patient record.
- The dental professional can use interpretation to educate patients about the importance and use of dental images.

BIBLIOGRAPHY

Haring JI, Lind LJ: The importance of dental radiographs and interpretation. In Radiographic interpretation for the dental hygienist, Philadelphia, 1993, Saunders.

Johnson ON, Thomson EM: Preliminary interpretation of the radiographs. In Essentials of dental radiography for dental assistants and hygienists, ed 9, Upper Saddle River, NJ, 2011, Prentice Hall.

Mallya SM, Lam EWN: Principles of radiographic interpretation. In White and Pharoah's Oral radiology: principles and interpretation, ed 8, St. Louis, 2019, Elsevier.

Miles DA, Van Dis ML, Williamson GF, et al: Interpretation: normal versus abnormal and common radiographic presentation of lesions. In Radiographic imaging for the dental team, ed 4, St Louis, 2009, Saunders.

QUIZ QUESTIONS

Essay

1. Summarize the importance of image interpretation.
2. Define the roles of each member of the dental team in the interpretation of dental images.
3. Discuss the difference between interpretation and diagnosis.
4. List the members of the dental team who may interpret dental images.
5. Describe when and where dental images are interpreted.
6. Describe how interpretation can be used to educate the patient about the importance and use of dental images.

True or False

____ 7. All images must be carefully reviewed and interpreted.

____ 8. Any dental professional with training in interpretation can examine images.

____ 9. The amount and scope of training received dictate whether the dental assistant can perform image interpretation.

____ 10. The terms *interpretation* and *diagnosis* can be used synonymously.

____ 11. Any dental professional can provide a diagnosis.

____ 12. Dental images should not be interpreted in the presence of the patient.

____ 13. No specific guidelines exist regarding when and where dental images should be interpreted.

____ 14. The dental radiographer can educate the patient by identifying and discussing what is normally found on a dental image.

____ 15. All members of the dental team can work together using interpretation to educate patients about the importance and use of dental images.

31

Descriptive Terminology

LEARNING OBJECTIVES

After completion of this chapter, the student will be able to do the following:

1. Define descriptive terminology, describe why the dental professional should use descriptive terms, and differentiate between descriptive terminology and diagnosis.
2. Compare and contrast the terms *radiolucent* and *radiopaque*.
3. In relation to how to describe radiolucent lesions:
   - Identify radiolucent lesions on a dental image in terms of appearance, location, and size.
   - Define and discuss the terms *unilocular* and *multilocular*.
   - Define and discuss the terms *periapical, inter-radicular, edentulous zone, pericoronal*, and *alveolar bone loss* in relation to radiolucent lesions.
4. In relation to how to describe radiopaque lesions:
   - Identify radiopaque lesions on a dental image in terms of appearance, location, and size.
   - Define and discuss the terms *focal opacity, target lesion, multifocal confluent pattern, irregular/ill-defined opacity, ground glass opacity, mixed lucent-opaque lesion*, and *soft tissue opacity*.
   - Define and discuss the terms *periapical, inter-radicular, edentulous zone*, and *pericoronal* in relation to radiopaque lesions.

Interpretation, as defined in Chapter 30, is the ability to read what is revealed by a dental image. To interpret dental images, the dental professional must be able to describe what is observed in accurate and succinct terms. A working knowledge of *descriptive terminology* is important for communication and documentation and is essential in interpretation.

DEFINITION AND USES

What Is Descriptive Terminology?

In dental imaging, a number of different terms can be used to describe the appearance, location, and size of a lesion; these terms represent what is called *descriptive terminology*. This information should be documented for all lesions viewed on dental images.

Why Use Descriptive Terminology?

Descriptive terminology allows dental professionals to intelligently describe and discuss what is seen on dental images and to communicate using a common language. Communication among dental professionals about dental image findings takes place each time a case is discussed or when a patient is referred to a specialist for evaluation. The use of descriptive terminology reduces the chance for miscommunication among dental professionals.

Descriptive terminology also allows the dental professional to document what is seen on a dental image in the patient record in terms of appearance, location, and size. Documentation of what is viewed on dental images is essential for legal purposes. A written description of what is viewed indicates that a qualified dental professional interpreted the dental image. If a notation of interpretation is not included in the patient record, no legal documentation exists that the dental images were reviewed.

Descriptive Terminology versus Diagnosis

Is describing a lesion the same as making a diagnosis? Descriptive terminology allows the dental professional to describe what is seen on a dental image *without* implying a diagnosis. A **diagnosis** is the identification of disease by examination or analysis. It is important to note that it is extremely difficult, if not impossible, to establish a diagnosis from a dental image alone. An evaluation and analysis of the patient's medical and dental histories, clinical findings, signs and symptoms, laboratory tests, and biopsy results allow the dentist to make a definitive diagnosis.

REVIEW OF BASIC TERMS

The use of descriptive terminology requires that the dental professional have a solid understanding of basic terms including *radiolucent* and *radiopaque*. In addition, an understanding of how to describe lesions viewed on dental images using the appropriate terms is essential.

Radiolucent versus Radiopaque

The terms *radiolucent* and *radiopaque* are used to describe the appearances of all the structures seen on a dental image. A dental image appears radiolucent (black or dark) where the tissues are soft or thin, and it appears radiopaque (white or light) where the tissues are thick or dense. Most structures do not exhibit uniform thickness and therefore appear gray instead of black or white.

Radiolucent refers to that portion of a processed dental image that is dark or black. Radiolucent structures lack density and permit the passage of the x-ray beam with little or no resistance.

Dental caries appears radiolucent because the area of a tooth with dental caries is less dense than surrounding structures and therefore readily permits the passage of the x-ray beam (Figure 31-1). Consequently, most of the energy of the x-ray beam freely passes through the area of dental caries to the recording surface of the receptor, resulting in a dark or radiolucent area on the dental image (Figure 31-2). Other radiolucent structures include air spaces, the dental pulp cavity, and the periodontal ligament space.

Radiopaque refers to that portion of a dental image that appears light or white. Radiopaque structures are dense and absorb or resist the passage of the x-ray beam.

A metallic restoration appears radiopaque because it is very dense and absorbs the radiation (Figure 31-3). As a result, very little, if any, radiation reaches the surface of the receptor, which results in a white or radiopaque area on the dental image (see Figure 31-2). Examples of other radiopaque structures include amalgam, enamel, dentin, and bone.

How to Describe Lesions

In order to properly document a lesion seen on a dental image, the lesion must be described in terms of appearance, location, and size. As detailed in the next portion of this chapter, specific terms are used to describe the appearance of a radiolucent lesion versus the appearance of a radiopaque lesion. In contrast, the terms related to location of a lesion may describe *either* a radiolucent or a radiopaque lesion, with the exception of alveolar bone loss. In regard to the size of lesions, the preferred unit of measurement is the millimeter or centimeter.

Terms Used to Describe Radiolucent Lesions

A lesion that appears radiolucent permits the passage of the x-ray beam and represents destruction of bone or a space-occupying entity within the bones of the jaws. A radiolucent lesion must be described in the patient record using appropriate terminology for appearance, location, and size.

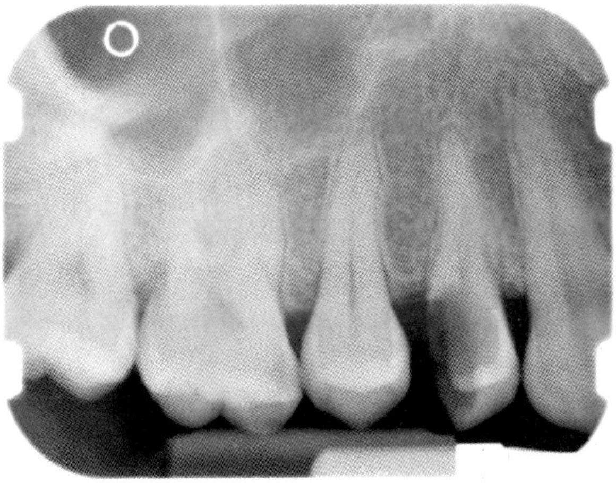

Fig 31-1 Dental caries appears radiolucent on a dental image.

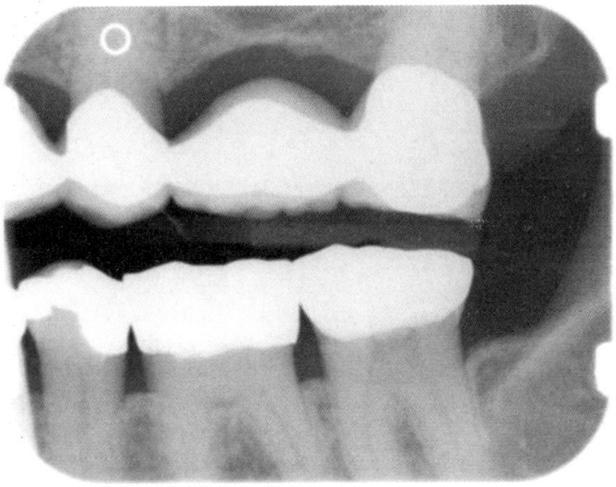

Fig 31-3 Two gold crowns on the mandibular molars appear radiopaque on a dental image.

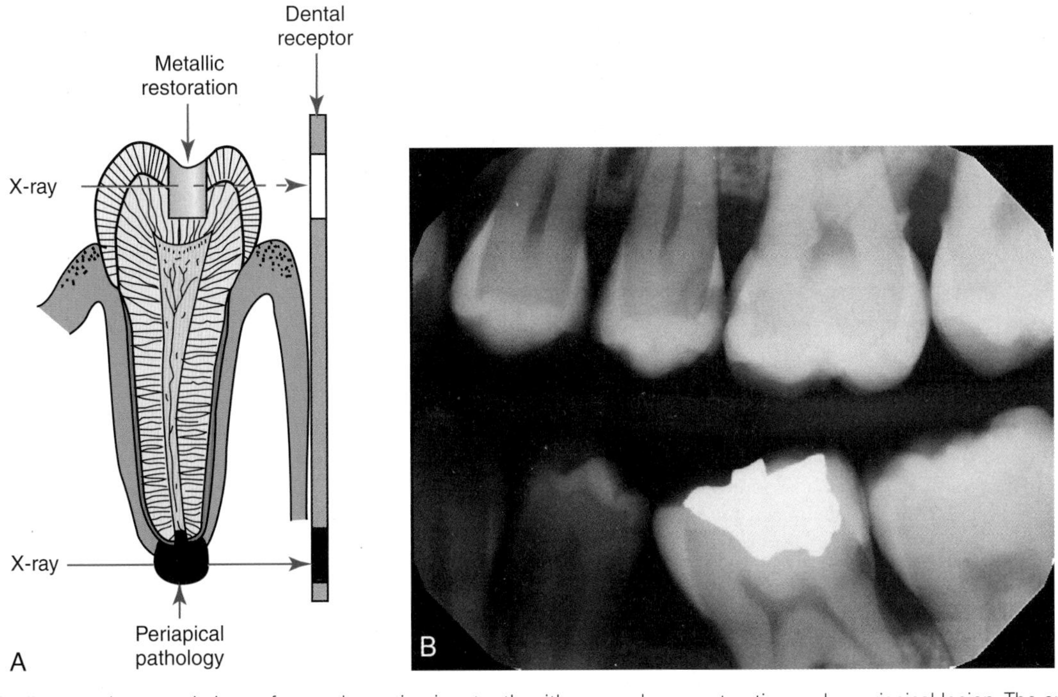

Fig 31-2 **A,** This diagram shows variations of x-ray absorption in a tooth with an amalgam restoration and a periapical lesion. The amalgam restoration absorbs the x-ray beam. The x-ray beam does not reach the receptor surface, and a white or radiopaque area results. The lesion at the apex of the tooth lacks density and is easily penetrated by the x-ray beam. The beam reaches the receptor and results in a dark or radiolucent area. **B,** Interproximal dental caries is penetrated by the x-ray beam and lack density, resulting in a radiolucency in the tooth structures. The amalgam restoration prevents the x-ray beam from reaching the receptor, and a radiopaque area results.

BOX 31-1 Radiolucent Lesions of the Jaws

Unilocular Radiolucencies
- Periapical cyst
- Periapical granuloma
- Periapical abscess
- Periapical cemental dysplasia*†
- Incisive canal cyst
- Traumatic bone cyst
- Residual bone cyst
- Lateral periodontal cyst
- Odontogenic keratocyst*
- Primordial cyst
- Osteoporotic bone marrow defect
- Dentigerous cyst
- Static bone cyst
- Ameloblastoma*
- Adenomatoid odontogenic tumor†
- Calcifying epithelial odontogenic tumor*†
- Ameloblastic fibroma*
- Central giant cell granuloma*
- Central neurogenic neoplasms
- Ameloblastic fibroma*
- Calcifying epithelial odontogenic tumor*†

Multilocular Radiolucencies
- Odontogenic keratocyst*
- Ameloblastoma*
- Central giant cell granuloma*
- Botryoid odontogenic cyst
- Aneurysmal bone cyst
- Cherubism*
- Hyperparathyroidism
- Myxoma

"Moth-Eaten" Radiolucencies
- Osteomyelitis
- Metastatic carcinoma†
- Osteosarcoma*†
- Chondrosarcoma*†
- Ewing's sarcoma
- Lymphoma
- Burkitt's lymphoma
- Fibrosarcoma
- Multiple myeloma*

Widened Periodontal Ligament Space
- Scleroderma
- Osteosarcoma*
- Periodontal inflammation
- Endodontic inflammation

Multifocal Radiolucencies
- Basal cell nevus syndrome
- Histiocytosis X
- Multiple myeloma*
- Cherubism*†
- Periapical cemental dysplasia*†

*Indicates that the lesion may exhibit more than one radiolucent appearance.
†Indicates that the lesion may also appear with a radiopaque component.

Appearance. The appearance of most radiolucent lesions can be classified as either *unilocular* or *multilocular*. Other radiolucent classifications include a "moth-eaten" pattern, a widened periodontal ligament space, or a multifocal pattern. Box 31-1 lists examples of radiolucent lesions in each of these categories.

Unilocular radiolucent lesions. The term *unilocular* is derived from two Latin words, *uni* ("one") and *loculus* ("small space" or "compartment"), and refers to a radiolucent lesion that exhibits one compartment. Unilocular lesions tend to be small and nonexpansile and have borders that may appear corticated or noncorticated on the dental image.

Unilocular lesion—corticated borders. The term *corticated* comes from the Latin *cortex* ("an outer layer") and refers to the outer layer or border of a radiolucent lesion. A unilocular radiolucent lesion with corticated borders exhibits a thin, well-demarcated radiopaque rim of bone at the periphery (Figure 31-4). A unilocular corticated lesion is usually indicative of a benign, slow-growing process.

Unilocular lesion—noncorticated borders. A unilocular lesion with noncorticated borders does *not* exhibit a thin radiopaque rim of bone at the periphery (Figure 31-5). Instead, the periphery of a unilocular noncorticated lesion appears fuzzy or poorly defined. A radiolucency with ill-defined or irregular margins may represent either a benign or malignant process.

Multilocular radiolucent lesions. The term multilocular refers to a lesion that exhibits multiple radiolucent compartments that resemble soap bubbles (Figure 31-6). A multilocular lesion with multiple compartments is typically larger than a unilocular lesion with one compartment. Such a lesion typically exhibits well-defined, corticated margins. A multilocular radiolucent lesion is frequently large and expansile and tends to displace the buccal and lingual plates of bone.

Multilocular lesions are typically benign lesions with aggressive growth potential. As a general rule, most multilocular lesions represent a reactive or neoplastic process. The odontogenic keratocyst, ameloblastoma, and the central giant cell granuloma are examples of multilocular radiolucencies viewed on dental images.

Location. In addition to appearance, radiolucent lesions can also be described in terms of location. The location of a lesion is important for communication and documentation purposes. A radiolucent lesion may appear in a *periapical, inter-radicular, edentulous*, or *pericoronal* location. A radiolucent lesion may also appear as *alveolar bone loss*. Box 31-2 lists examples of radiolucent lesions and common locations.

Periapical location. The term periapical refers to the area around the apex of a tooth (Figure 31-7). It is derived from the Greek word *peri* ("around") and the Latin word *apex*, referring, in this case, to the terminal end of a tooth root. An example of a common periapical radiolucency is a periapical cyst seen secondary to pulpal necrosis.

Inter-radicular location. The term inter-radicular refers to the area between the roots of adjacent teeth (Figure 31-8). The term *inter* is Latin for "between," and *radicular* means "pertaining to a root." An example of a radiolucent lesion found in an inter-radicular location is the lateral periodontal cyst. Figure 31-9 reveals a unilocular, corticated lesion in the inter-radicular *and* periapical locations.

Edentulous zone. Edentulous zone refers to an area without teeth. (Figure 31-10). (*Edentulous* means "without teeth.") A variety of radiolucent lesions may occur in an edentulous zone.

Pericoronal location. The term pericoronal refers to the area around the crown of an impacted tooth (Figure 31-11). It is derived from the Greek word *peri* ("around,") and *corona* is Latin for "crown." A dentigerous cyst is an example of a radiolucent lesion seen in a pericoronal location.

Alveolar bone loss. Alveolar bone loss refers to loss of maxillary or mandibular bone that surrounds and supports the teeth (Figure 31-12). Alveolar bone loss appears radiolucent. Alveolar bone loss is seen not only with periodontal disease but also with systemic illnesses, such as diabetes, histiocytosis X, and leukemia. Malignant neoplasms may also cause alveolar bone loss.

Size. Radiolucent lesions viewed on a dental image can vary in size from several millimeters to several centimeters in diameter. Often the size of a lesion dictates the type of treatment necessary. Documentation of the size of a lesion is important for treatment considerations as well as for future comparisons. Radiolucent lesions can be easily measured on a dental image with a millimeter ruler. Figure 31-13 illustrates some common items and their respective sizes in millimeters for comparison purposes.

Terms Used to Describe Radiopaque Lesions

A lesion that appears radiopaque resists the passage of the x-ray beam and represents a thickness of mineralized tissue. A radiopaque lesion must be described in the patient record using appropriate terminology for appearance, location, and size.

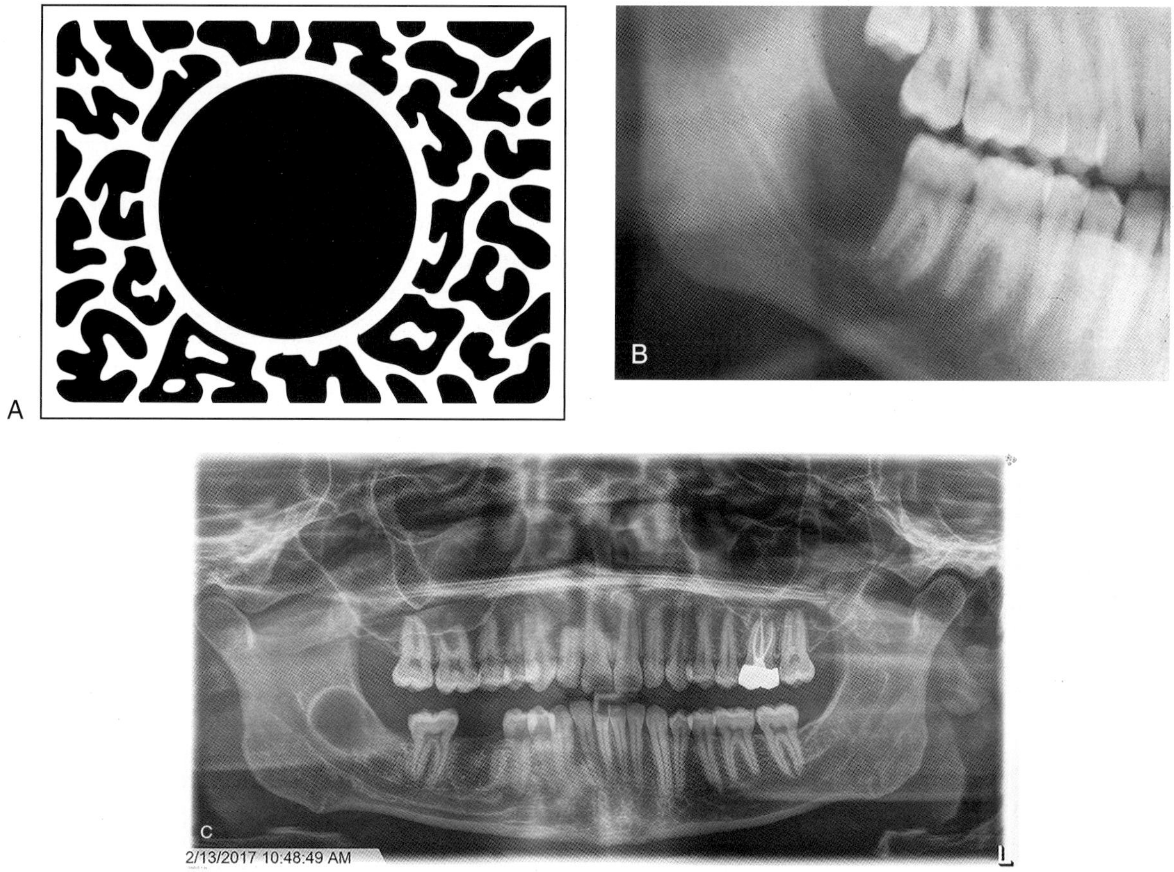

Fig 31-4 A, Unilocular radiolucent lesion with corticated borders. (Modified from Eversole LR: Clinical outline of oral pathology: diagnosis and treatment, ed 2, Philadelphia, 1984, Lea & Febiger.) B, Unilocular radiolucent lesion with corticated borders distal to tooth #31. C, Unilocular radiolucent lesion with corticated borders in the right ramus of the mandible.

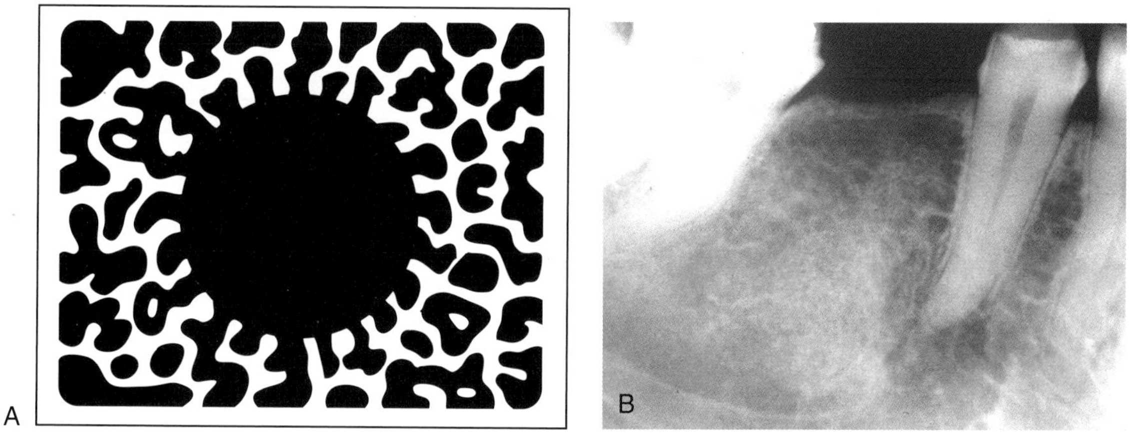

Fig 31-5 A, Unilocular radiolucent lesion with noncorticated borders. (Modified from Eversole LR: Clinical outline of oral pathology: diagnosis and treatment, ed 2, Philadelphia, 1984, Lea & Febiger.) B, Unilocular radiolucent lesion with noncorticated borders at the apex of tooth #29.

Appearance. The appearance of a radiopaque lesion can be described using one of the following terms: focal opacity, target lesion, multifocal confluent, irregular, ground glass, or mixed lucent-opaque. Radiopaque lesions occur not only in bone but in soft tissue as well. A radiopaque lesion located in soft tissue can be described as a soft tissue radiopacity. Box 31-3 lists examples of radiopaque lesions of the jaws.

Focal opacity. The term **focal opacity** refers to a well-defined, localized radiopaque lesion on a dental image (Figure 31-14). Condensing osteitis is an example of a radiopaque lesion that can be described as a focal opacity.

Target lesion. The term **target lesion** refers to a well-defined, localized radiopaque area surrounded by a uniform radiolucent halo (Figure 31-15). A benign cementoblastoma is an example of a radiopacity described as a target lesion.

Multifocal confluent pattern. A **multifocal confluent** radiopaque pattern can be described as multiple radiopacities that appear to overlap

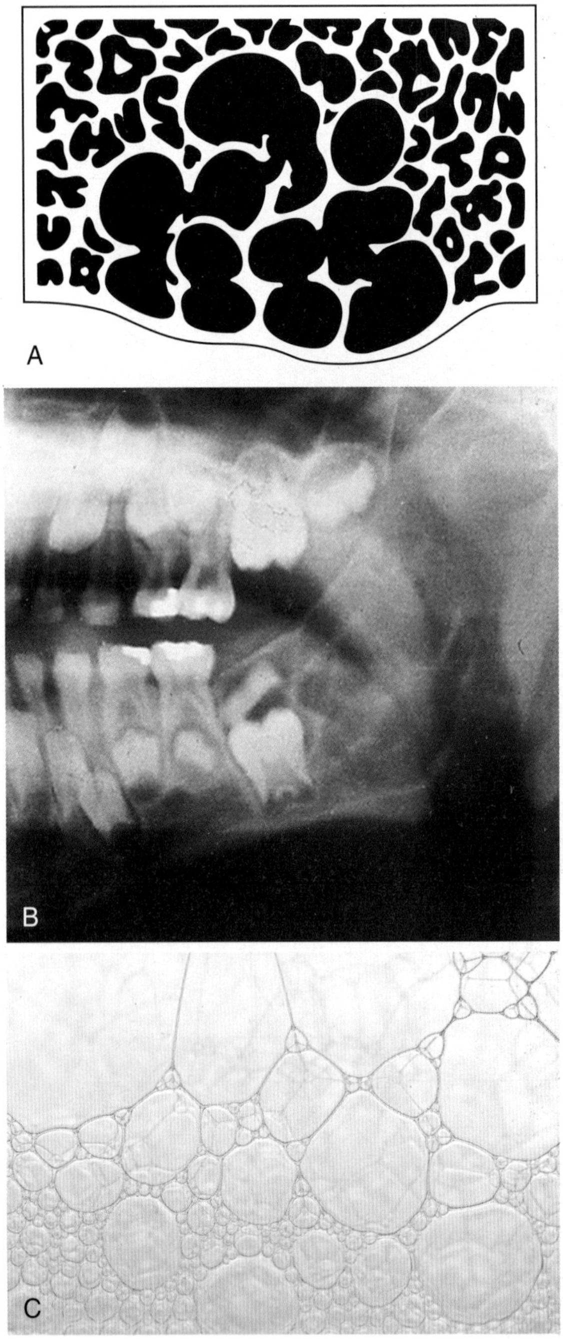

Fig 31-6 **A,** Multilocular radiolucent lesion. (Modified from Eversole LR: Clinical outline of oral pathology: diagnosis and treatment, ed 2, Philadelphia, 1984, Lea & Febiger.) **B,** Multilocular expansile lesion in the ramus of the mandible. **C,** A multilocular lesion has a soap bubble–like appearance.

or flow together (Figure 31-16). Diseases such as osteitis deformans and florid osseous dysplasia exhibit a multifocal confluent radiopaque pattern. Multifocal confluent radiopacities that involve multiple quadrants of the jaws usually represent benign fibro-osseous disorders.

Irregular/ill-defined opacity. A radiopacity may exhibit an *irregular, poorly defined* pattern (Figure 31-17). Irregular radiopacities may represent a malignant condition. Examples of irregular, ill-defined radiopaque lesions include osteosarcoma and chondrosarcoma.

BOX 31-2 Locations of Radiolucent Lesions

Periapical Radiolucencies
- Periapical cyst
- Periapical granuloma
- Periapical abscess
- Periapical cemento-osseous dysplasia*†
- Incisive canal cyst
- Traumatic bone cyst*
- Residual cyst*
- Odontogenic keratocyst*
- Central giant cell granuloma

Inter-radicular Radiolucencies
- Lateral periodontal cyst
- Residual cyst*
- Odontogenic keratocyst*
- Primordial cyst*
- Traumatic bone cyst*
- Botryoid odontogenic cyst

Edentulous Zone
- Periapical cyst‡
- Periapical granuloma‡
- Periapical abscess‡
- Periapical cemental dysplasia*†‡
- Incisive canal cyst‡
- Residual cyst‡
- Odontogenic keratocyst*
- Central giant cell granuloma*
- Primordial cyst*
- Ameloblastoma*
- Calcifying epithelial odontogenic tumor*†
- Static bone cyst

Pericoronal Radiolucencies
- Dentigerous cyst
- Odontogenic keratocyst*
- Ameloblastoma*
- Adenomatoid odontogenic tumor†
- Calcifying epithelial odontogenic tumor*†

Alveolar Bone Loss
- Periodontitis
- Histiocytosis X
- Cyclic neutropenia
- Leukemia

No Specific Location
- Multiple myeloma
- Cherubism
- Myxoma
- Osteosarcoma†
- Osteomyelitis
- Metastatic carcinoma†
- Chondrosarcoma†
- Ewing's sarcoma
- Lymphoma
- Burkitt's lymphoma
- Fibrosarcoma
- Multiple myeloma
- Osteoporotic bone marrow defect
- Ameloblastic fibroma
- Aneurysmal bone cyst
- Hyperparathyroidism

*Indicates that the lesion may exhibit more than one radiolucent appearance.

†Indicates that the lesion may also appear with a radiopaque component.

‡Indicates that this location is possible, after extraction of a related tooth.

Ground glass opacity. A ground glass appearance of bone can be described as a granular or pebbled radiopacity that resembles pulverized glass (Figure 31-18). A ground glass radiopacity is often said to resemble the texture of an orange peel. Diseases such as fibrous dysplasia, osteitis deformans, and osteopetrosis may exhibit a ground glass or orange-peel appearance.

Mixed lucent-opaque lesion. A mixed lucent-opaque lesion exhibits both radiopaque and radiolucent components (Figure 31-19). Mixed lucent-opaque lesions often represent calcifying tumors. Many such tumors appear as a radiolucent area with central opaque flecks or calcifications. An example of a mixed lucent-opaque lesion is a compound odontoma.

Soft tissue opacity. A soft tissue opacity appears as a well-defined, radiopaque area located in soft tissue (Figure 31-20). A *sialolith* (salivary stone) or a calcified lymph node is an example of a soft tissue opacity.

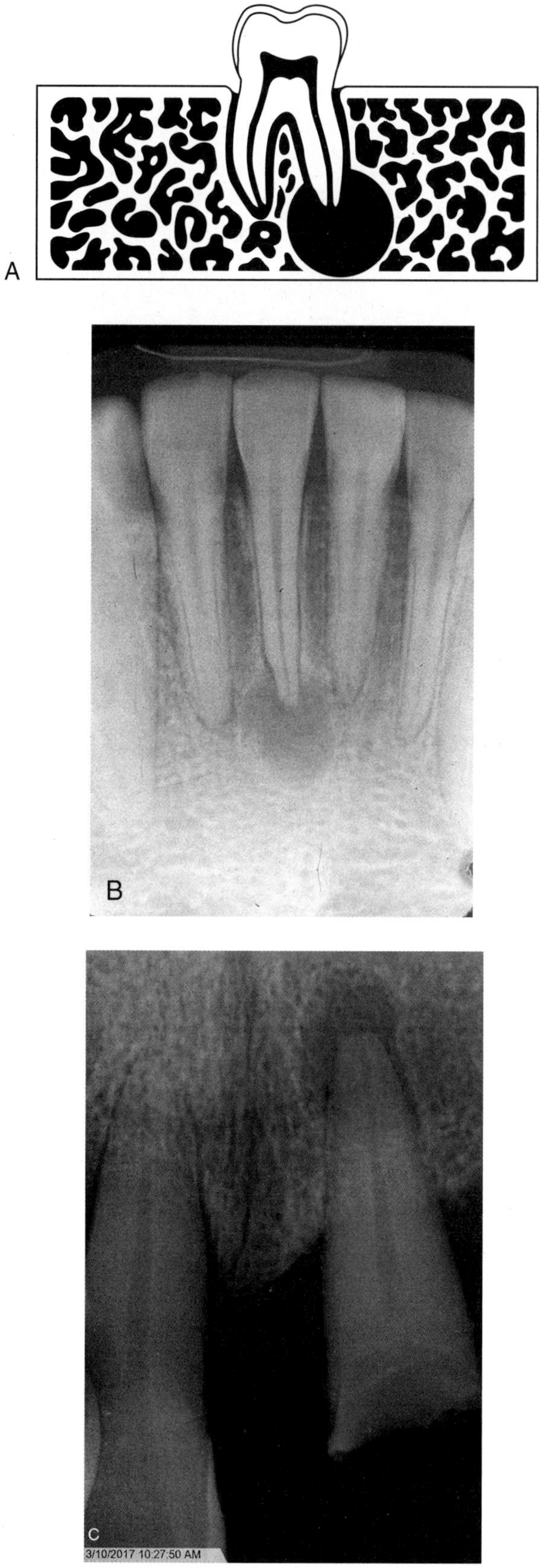

Fig 31-7 A, Unilocular corticated radiolucent lesion in periapical location. (Modified from Eversole LR: Clinical outline of oral pathology: diagnosis and treatment, ed 2, Philadelphia, 1984, Lea & Febiger.) B, Unilocular corticated radiolucent lesion at the apex of tooth #25. C, Unilocular corticated radiolucent lesion at the apex of tooth #9.

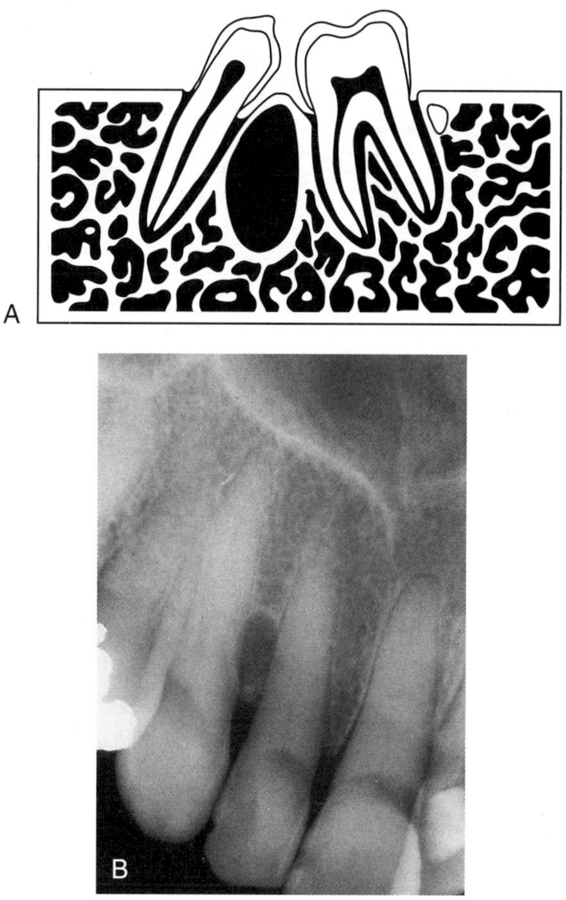

Fig 31-8 A, Unilocular corticated radiolucent lesion in inter-radicular location. (Modified from Eversole LR: Clinical outline of oral pathology: diagnosis and treatment, ed 2, Philadelphia, 1984, Lea & Febiger.) B, Unilocular corticated radiolucent lesion in inter-radicular location between teeth #6 and #7.

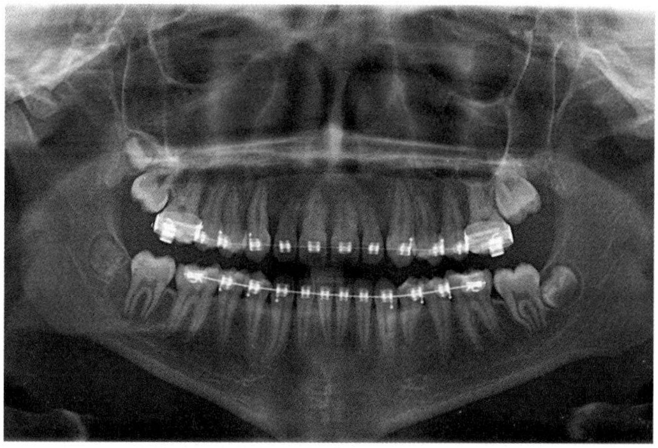

Fig 31-9 A unilocular corticated radiolucent lesion is found in the periapical location and the inter-radicular location, including the mesial and distal roots and furcation of tooth #31. The lesion has prevented the mesial movement of tooth #32, pushing tooth #32 posteriorly. (Courtesy Carolina OMF Imaging, W. Bruce Howerton, Jr., DDS, MS, Franklinton, NC.)

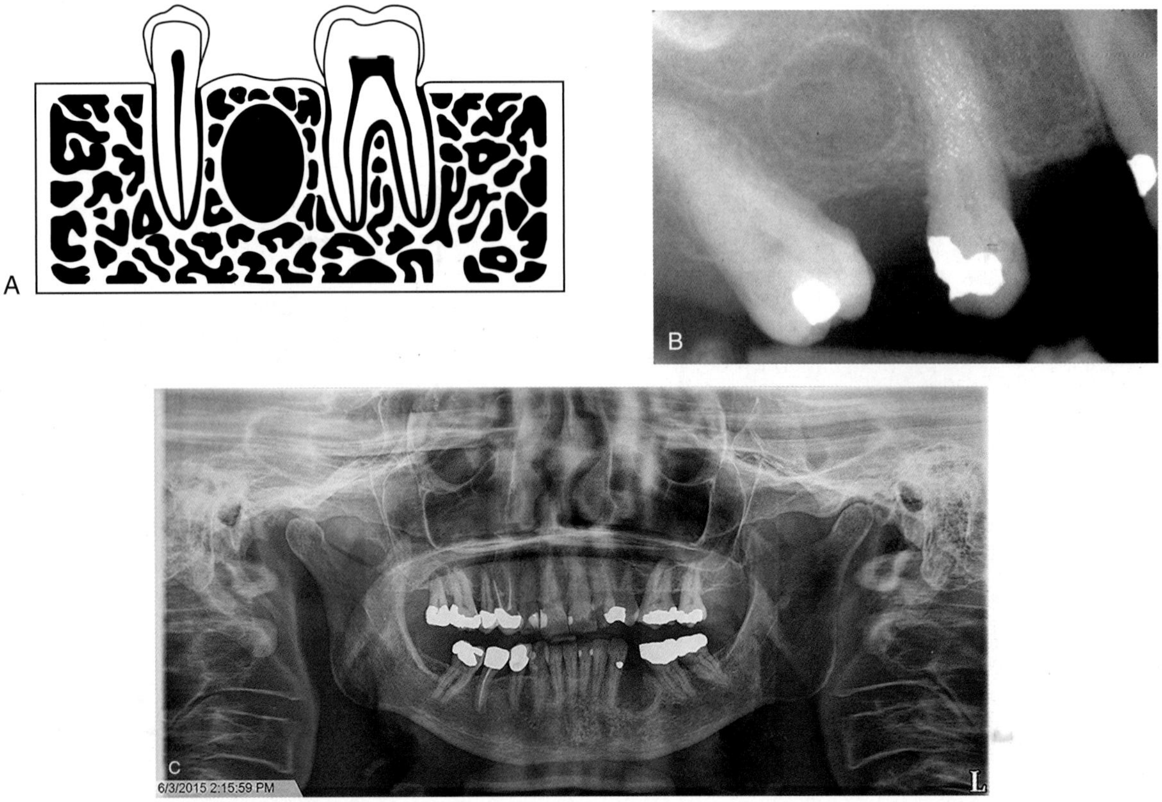

Fig 31-10 **A,** Unilocular corticated radiolucent lesion in edentulous zone. (Modified from Eversole LR: Clinical outline of oral pathology: diagnosis and treatment, ed 2, Philadelphia, 1984, Lea & Febiger.) **B,** Unilocular corticated radiolucent lesion in edentulous zone between teeth #2 and #4. **C,** Unilocular corticated radiolucent lesion in edentulous zone between teeth #19 and #22.

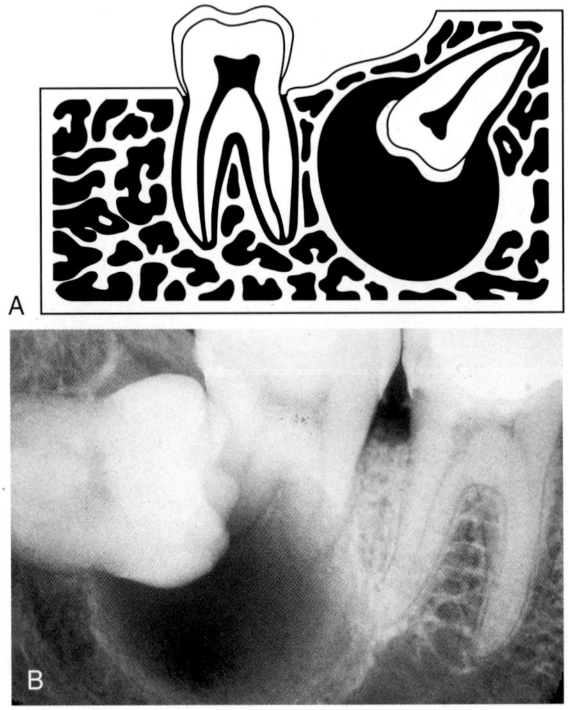

Fig 31-11 **A,** Unilocular corticated radiolucent lesion located in pericoronal location. (Modified from Eversole LR: Clinical outline of oral pathology: diagnosis and treatment, ed 2, Philadelphia, 1984, Lea & Febiger.) **B,** Unilocular corticated radiolucent lesion located in pericoronal location around impacted tooth #32.

Location. As with radiolucent lesions, radiopaque lesions can also be described in terms of location. The location of a lesion is important for communication and documentation purposes. Radiopaque lesions may appear in the same locations as radiolucent lesions: in periapical, inter-radicular, edentulous, or pericoronal locations. Box 31-4 lists examples of radiopaque lesions and common locations.

Periapical location. The term periapical refers to the area around the apex of a tooth (Figure 31-21). An example of a periapical radiopacity is benign cementoblastoma.

Inter-radicular location. The term inter-radicular refers to the area between the roots of adjacent teeth (Figure 31-22). An example of a radiopaque lesion found in an inter-radicular location is sclerotic bone.

Edentulous zone. The term edentulous zone refers to an area without teeth; an example of a radiopaque lesion in an edentulous zone is complex odontoma (Figure 31-23). A variety of radiopaque lesions may occur in an edentulous zone.

Pericoronal location. The term pericoronal refers to the area around the crown of an impacted tooth (Figure 31-24). An adenomatoid odontogenic tumor is an example of a mixed lucent-opaque lesion seen in a pericoronal location.

Size. Radiopaque lesions can vary in size from several millimeters to several centimeters in diameter and can be easily measured on a dental image with a ruler. Documentation of the size of a lesion is important for treatment decisions and for comparative purposes.

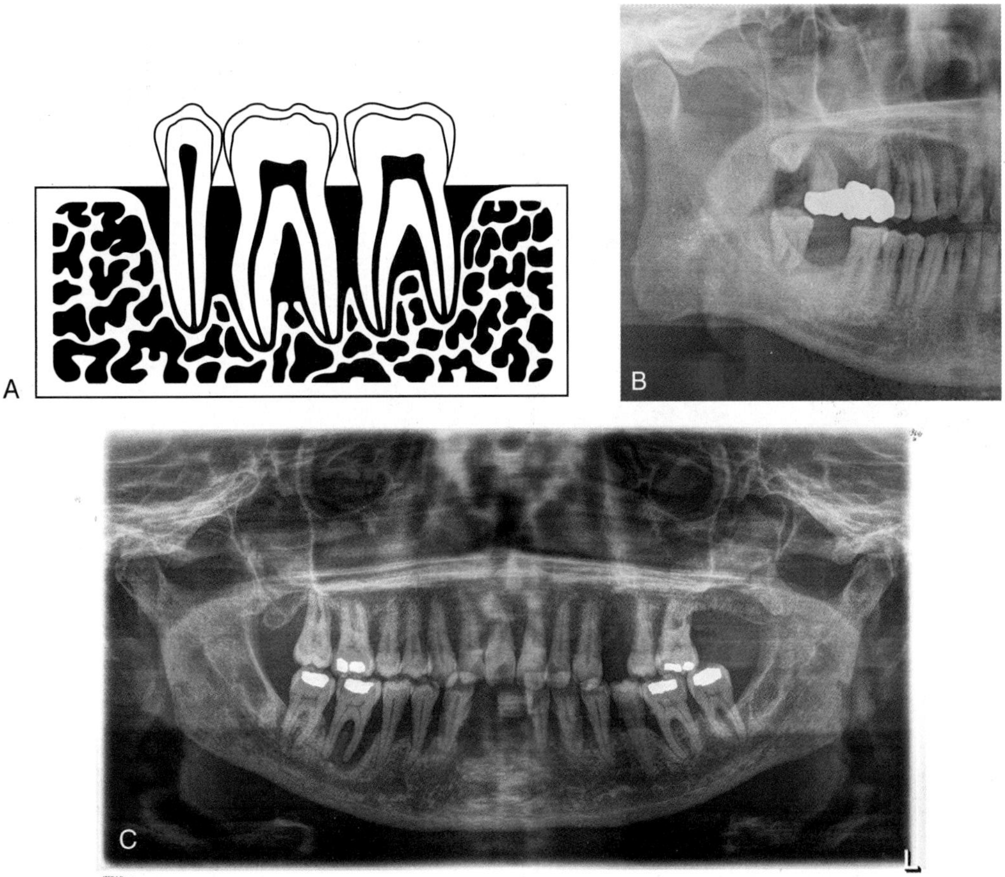

Fig 31-12 A, Radiolucent area caused by alveolar bone loss. (Modified from Eversole LR: Clinical outline of oral pathology: diagnosis and treatment, ed 2, Philadelphia, 1984, Lea & Febiger.) B, Extreme alveolar bone loss. C, Extreme alveolar bone loss visible in four quadrants.

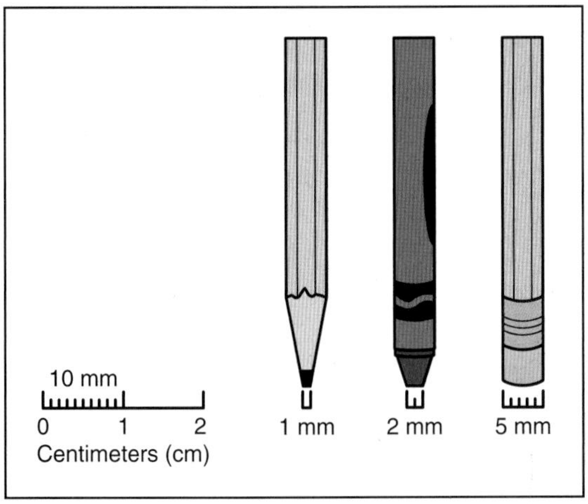

Fig 31-13 The tip of a pencil is approximately 1 mm in diameter, and the end of a pencil eraser is approximately 5 millimeters in diameter.

BOX 31-3 Radiopaque Lesions of the Jaws

Focal Opacities
- Periapical cemento-osseous dysplasia*
- Condensing osteitis
- Sclerotic bone

Target Lesions
- Benign cementoblastoma
- Complex odontoma

Multifocal Confluent Radiopacities
- Osteitis deformans
- Florid osseous dysplasia
- Gardner's syndrome

Mixed Lucent-Opaque Lesions
- Adenomatoid odontogenic tumor
- Calcifying epithelial odontogenic tumor
- Ameloblastic fibroma
- Ameloblastic fibro-odontoma
- Compound odontoma
- Ossifying/cementifying fibroma
- Periapical cemental dysplasia
- Calcifying and keratinizing epithelial odontogenic cyst

Irregular Radiopacities
- Osteosarcoma*
- Chondrosarcoma*
- Metastatic carcinoma*

Soft Tissue Radiopacities
- Sialolithiasis
- Calcified lymph nodes
- Foreign bodies
- Myositis ossificans

Ground Glass Radiopacities
- Fibrous dysplasia
- Osteitis deformans
- Osteopetrosis
- Hyperparathyroidism

*Indicates that the lesion may also appear with a radiolucent component.

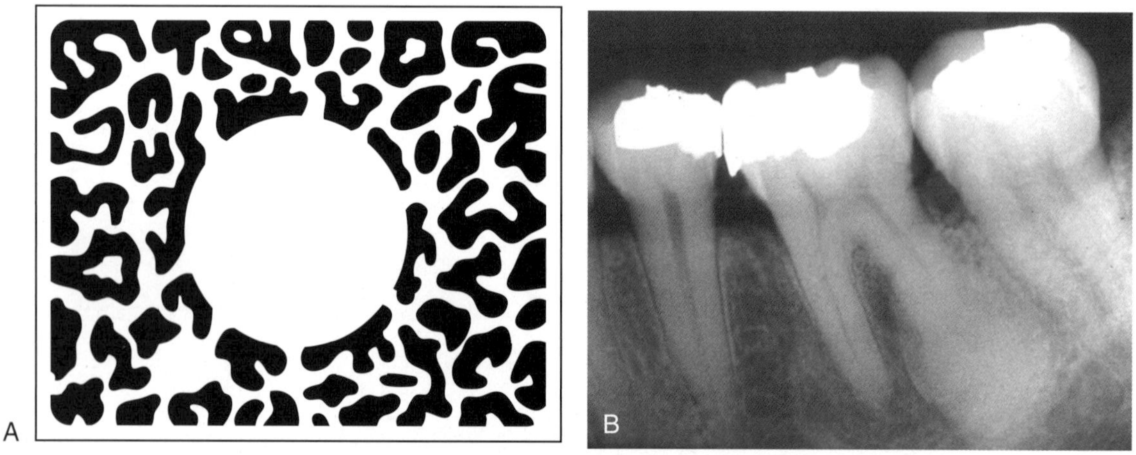

Fig 31-14 **A,** Focal opacity. (Modified from Eversole LR: Clinical outline of oral pathology: diagnosis and treatment, ed 2, Philadelphia, 1984, Lea & Febiger.) **B,** Focal opacity surrounding the distal root of tooth #19.

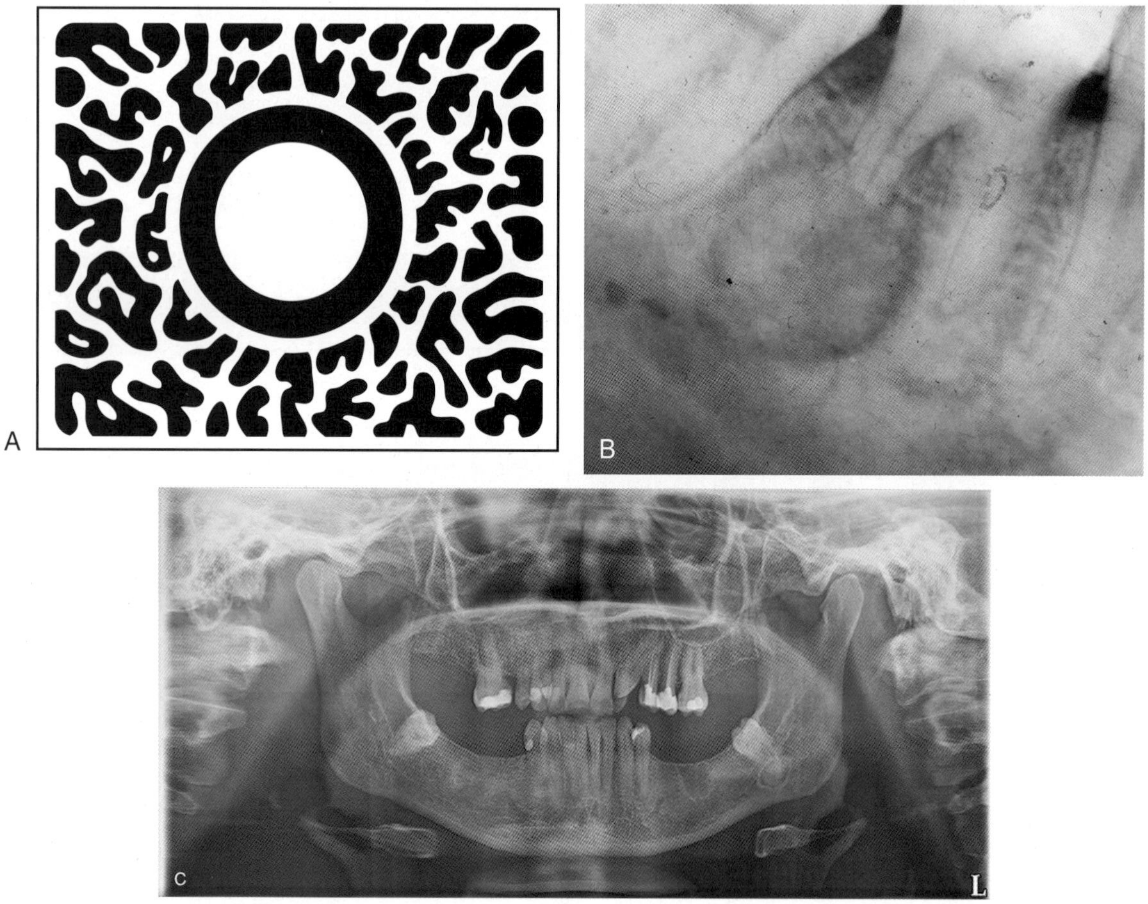

Fig 31-15 **A,** Target lesion. (Modified from Eversole LR: Clinical outline of oral pathology: diagnosis and treatment, ed 2, Philadelphia, 1984, Lea & Febiger.) **B,** Target lesion around the distal root of tooth #30. **C,** Target lesion surrounding the roots of tooth #17.

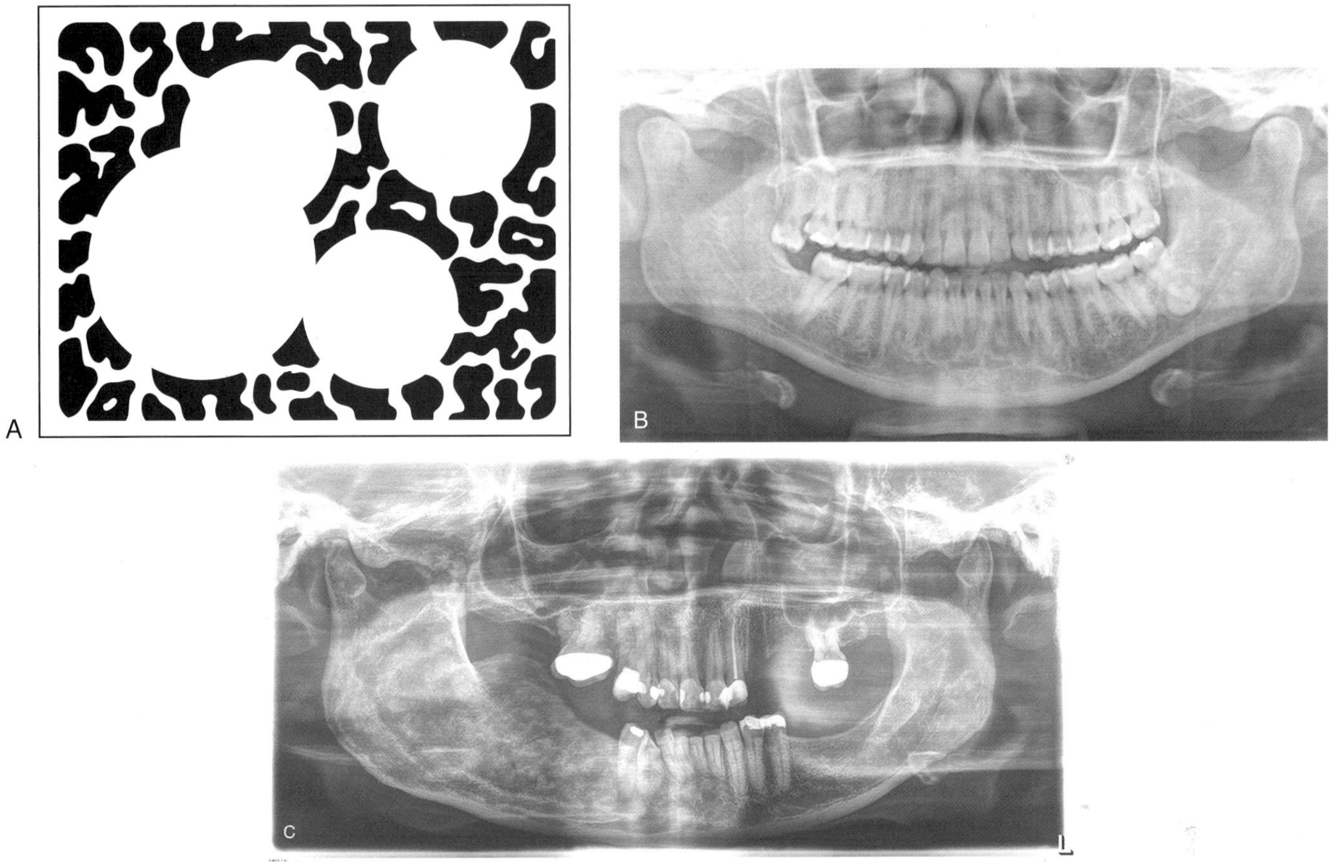

Fig 31-16 **A,** Multifocal confluent radiopacity. (Modified from Eversole LR: Clinical outline of oral pathology: diagnosis and treatment, ed 2, Philadelphia, 1984, Lea & Febiger.) **B,** Multifocal confluent radiopacities of the mandible. **C,** Multifocal confluent radiopacities of the right ramus and adjacent mandibular alveolar bone.

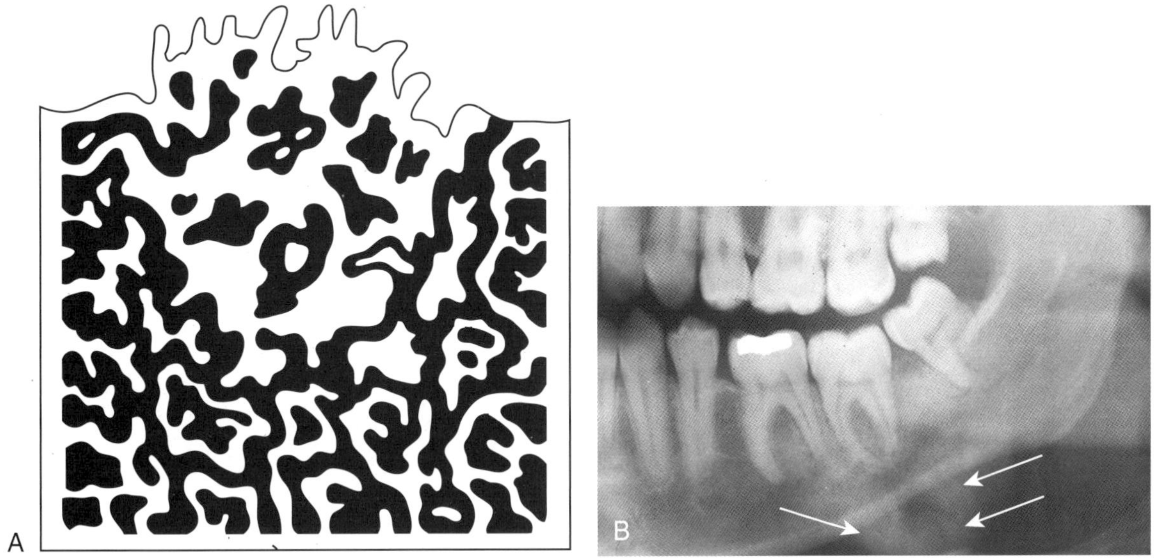

Fig 31-17 **A,** Irregular, ill-defined radiopaque pattern. (Modified from Eversole LR: Clinical outline of oral pathology: diagnosis and treatment, ed 2, Philadelphia, 1984, Lea & Febiger.) **B,** Irregular, ill-defined radiopacity of the mandible.

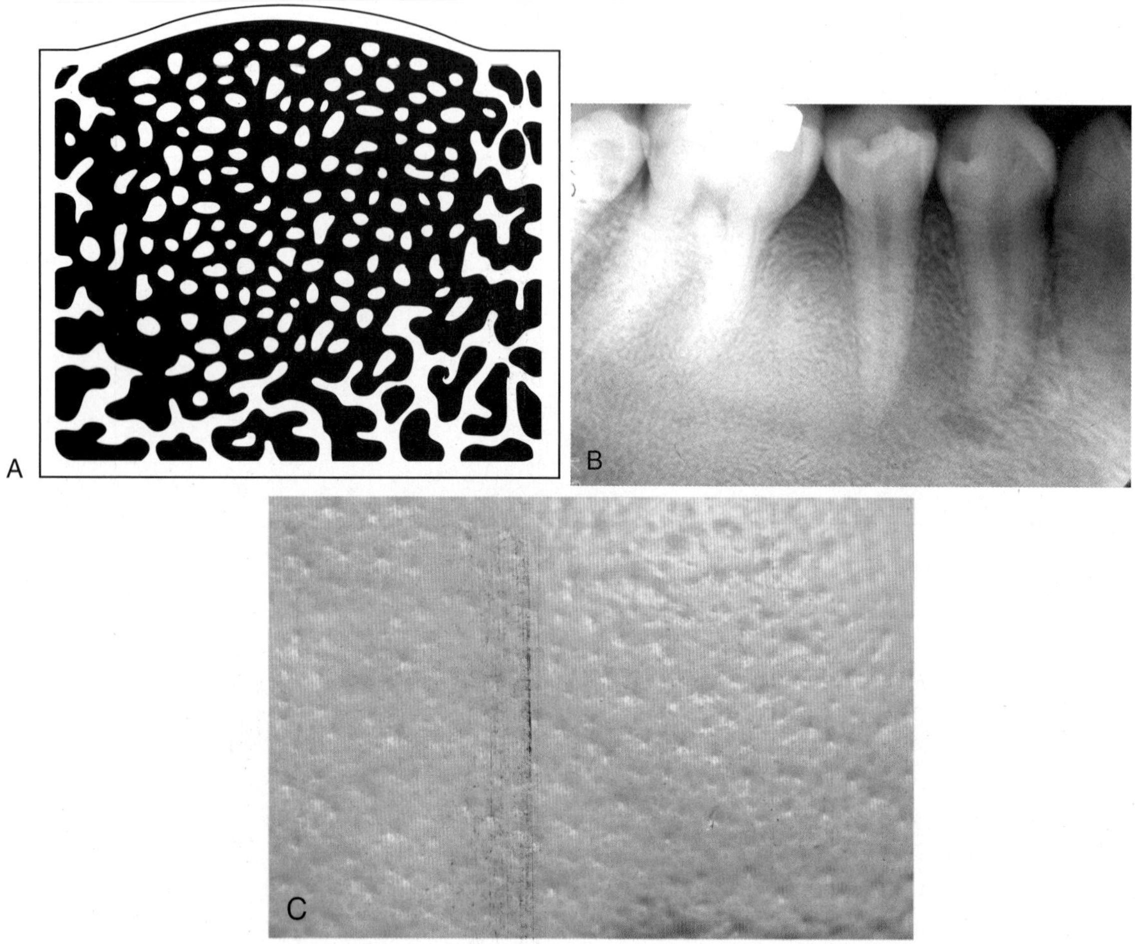

Fig 31-18 **A,** Ground glass radiopacity. (Modified from Eversole LR: Clinical outline of oral pathology: diagnosis and treatment, ed 2, Philadelphia, 1984, Lea & Febiger.) **B,** Ground glass appearance of bone. **C,** The ground glass appearance resembles the texture of an orange peel.

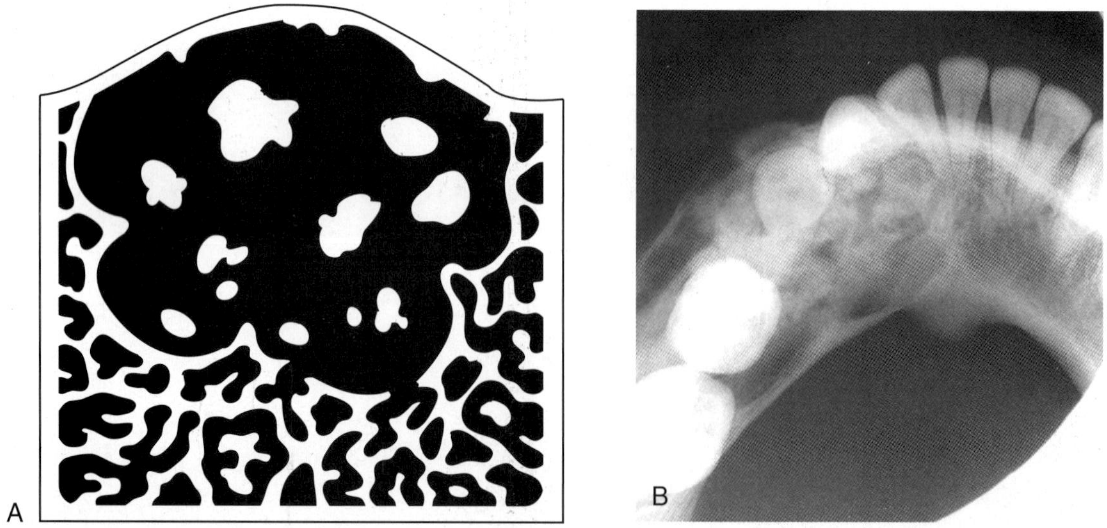

Fig 31-19 **A,** Mixed lucent-opaque lesion. (Modified from Eversole LR: Clinical outline of oral pathology: diagnosis and treatment, ed 2, Philadelphia, 1984, Lea & Febiger.) **B,** A mixed lucent-opaque lesion of the mandible. **C,** A sectioned panoramic image reveals that tooth #22 is possibly impacted and primary tooth #M is retained. (Courtesy Carolina OMF Imaging, W. Bruce Howerton, Jr., DDS, MS, Franklinton, NC.) **D,** CBCT (cone-beam computed tomography) data reveals a compound odontoma preventing the eruption of tooth #22. This region demonstrates radiographic signs of mixed attenuation (radiolucent and radiopaque components). (Courtesy Carolina OMF Imaging, W. Bruce Howerton, Jr., DDS, MS, Franklinton, NC.)

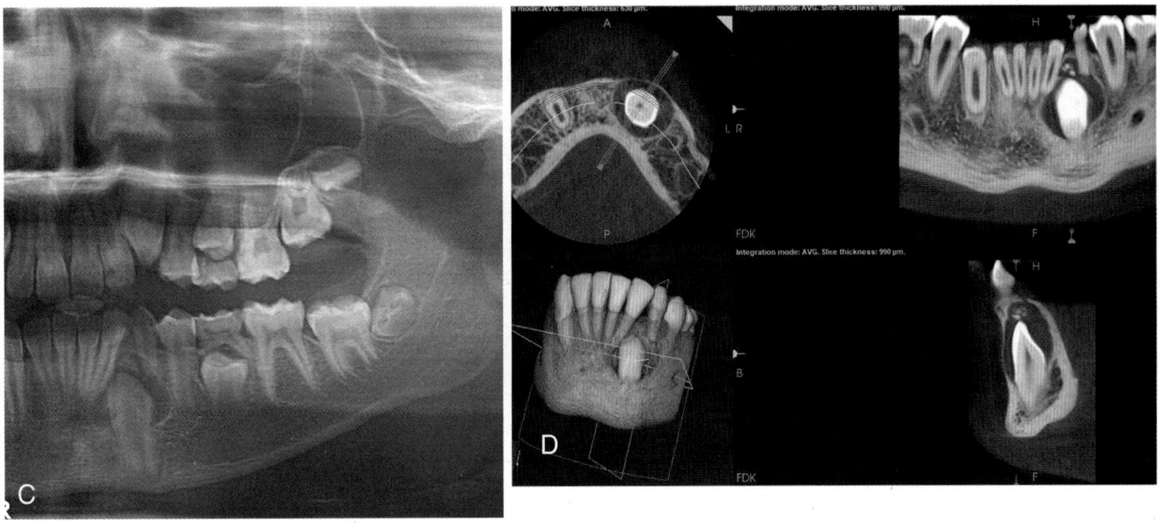

Fig 31-19 (*Continued*)

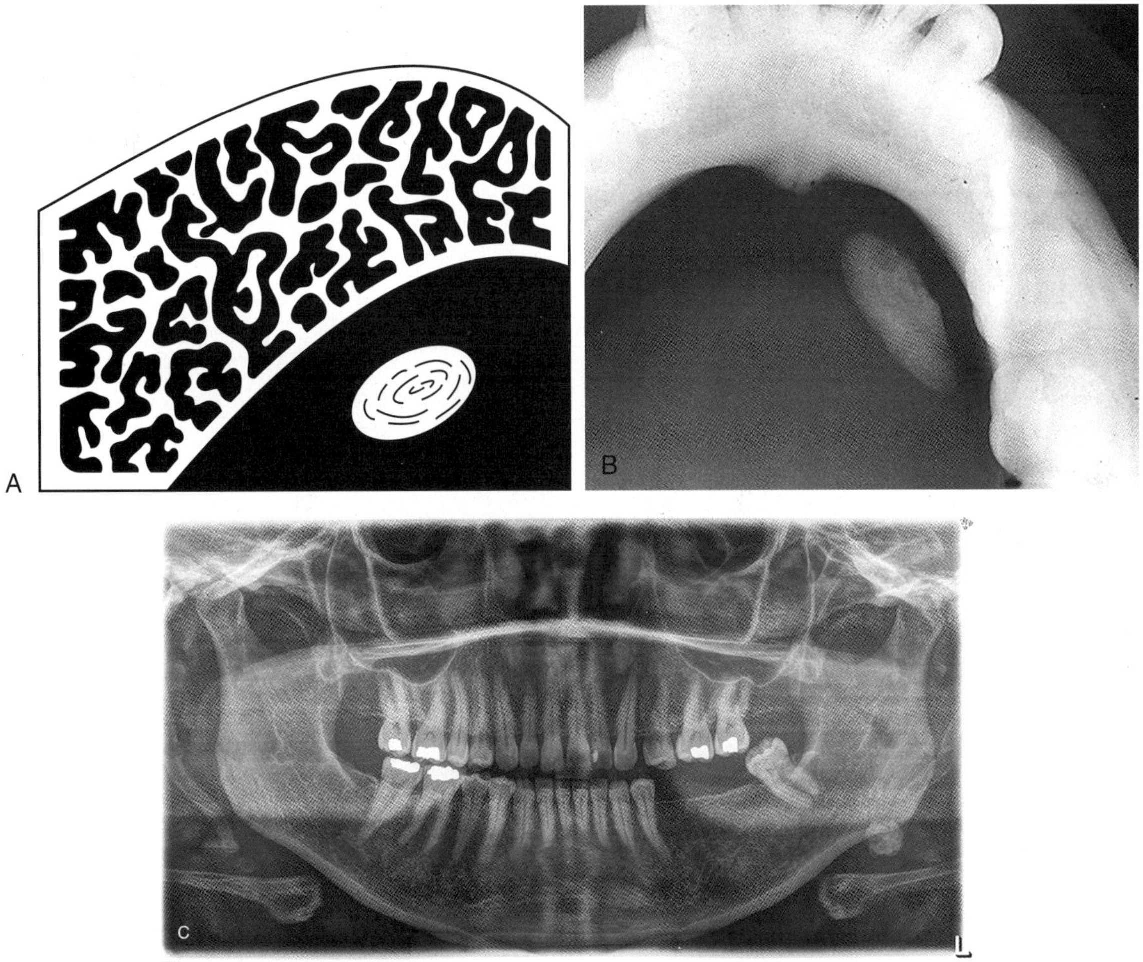

Fig 31-20 A, Soft tissue opacity. (Modified from Eversole LR: Clinical outline of oral pathology: diagnosis and treatment, ed 2, Philadelphia, 1984, Lea & Febiger.) B, A large ovoid soft tissue radiopacity. C, A soft tissue radiopacity is superimposed over the mandibular left ramus, above the hyoid bone.

BOX 31-4 Locations of Radiopaque Lesions

Periapical Radiopacities
- Periapical cemento-osseous dysplasia*
- Condensing osteitis
- Benign cementoblastoma

Inter-radicular Radiopacities
- Sclerotic bone
- Calcifying and keratinizing epithelial odontogenic cyst*
- Adenomatoid odontogenic tumor*†
- Compound odontoma†
- Ossifying/cementifying fibroma*

Edentulous Zone
- Complex odontoma
- Calcifying epithelial odontogenic tumor*†
- Ossifying/cementifying fibroma*†

Pericoronal Radiopacities
- Adenomatoid odontogenic tumor*†
- Calcifying epithelial odontogenic tumor*†
- Ameloblastic fibro-odontoma
- Compound odontoma†

Multifocal Radiopacities
- Osteitis deformans
- Florid osseous dysplasia
- Gardner's syndrome
- Fibrous dysplasia
- Osteopetrosis

No Specific Location
- Osteosarcoma*
- Chondrosarcoma*
- Metastatic carcinoma*

*Indicates that the lesion may also appear with a radiolucent component.
†Indicates that the lesion may exhibit more than one location.

A
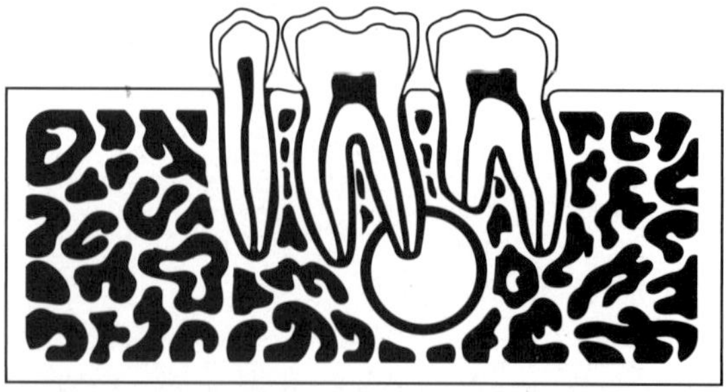

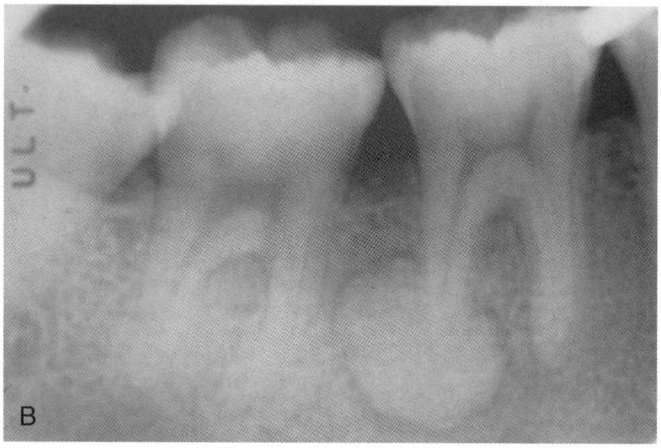
B

Fig 31-21 **A,** Radiopaque target lesion in a periapical location. (Modified from Eversole LR: Clinical outline of oral pathology: diagnosis and treatment, ed 2, Philadelphia, 1984, Lea & Febiger.) **B,** A radiopaque target lesion around the distal root of tooth #30. (From Neville BW, Damm DD, Allen CM, et al: Oral and maxillofacial pathology, ed 3, 2009, Saunders Elsevier.)

A
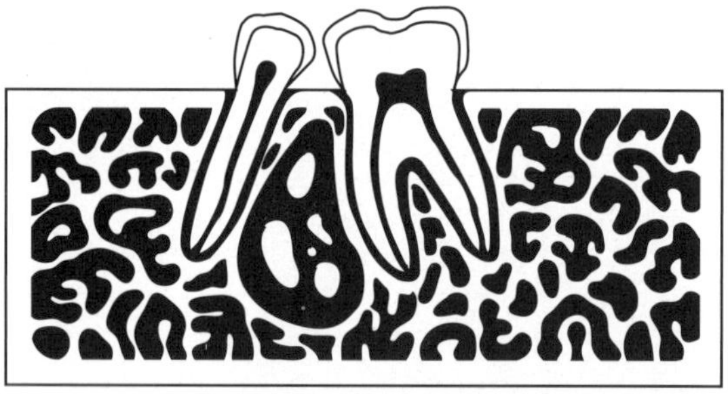

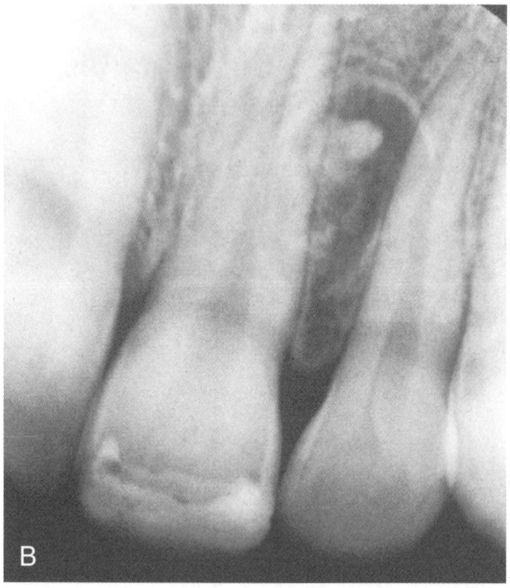
B

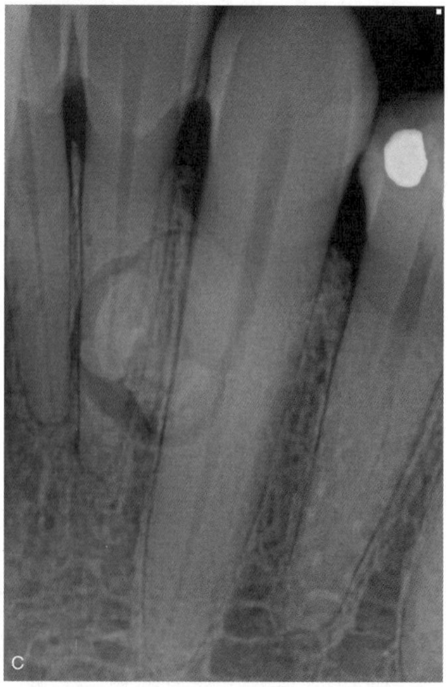
C

Fig 31-22 **A,** Mixed lucent-opaque lesion in inter-radicular location. (Modified from Eversole LR: Clinical outline of oral pathology: diagnosis and treatment, ed 2, Philadelphia, 1984, Lea & Febiger.) **B,** A mixed lucent-opaque target lesion in the inter-radicular location between teeth #9 and #10. (From Neville BW, Damm DD, Allen CM, et al: Oral and maxillofacial pathology, ed 3, 2009, Saunders Elsevier.) **C,** A mixed lucent-opaque target lesion in the inter-radicular location between teeth #22 and #23.

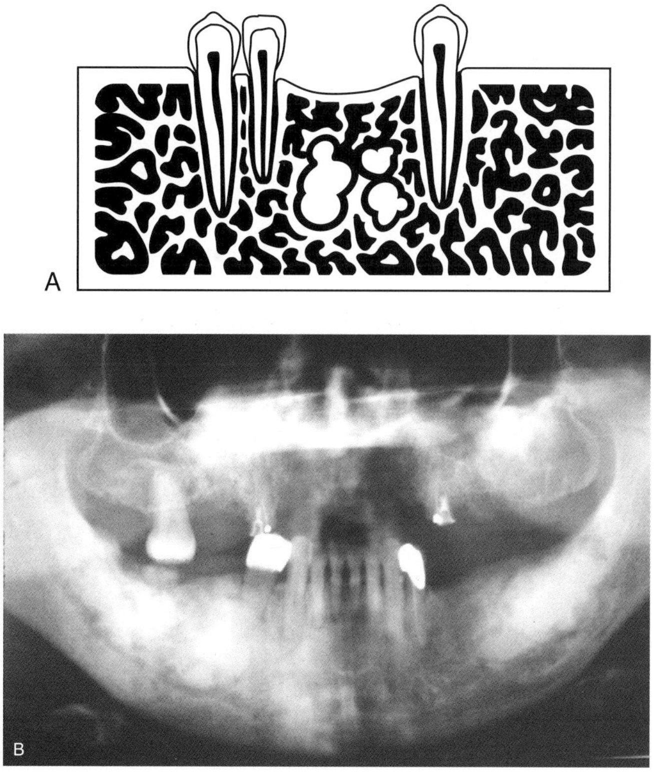

Fig 31-23 A, Multifocal confluent radiopacities in edentulous zone. (Modified from Eversole LR: Clinical outline of oral pathology: diagnosis and treatment, ed 2, Philadelphia, 1984, Lea & Febiger.) B, Multifocal confluent radiopacities in edentulous areas of the mandible. (From Neville BW, Damm DD, Allen CM, et al: Oral and maxillofacial pathology, ed 3, 2009, Saunders Elsevier.)

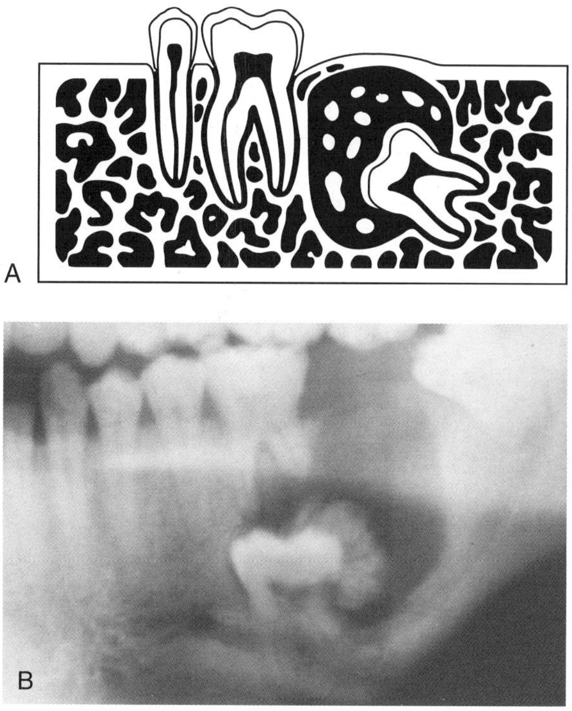

Fig 31-24 A, Mixed lucent-opaque lesion in pericoronal location. (Modified from Eversole LR: Clinical outline of oral pathology: diagnosis and treatment, ed 2, Philadelphia, 1984, Lea & Febiger.) B, Mixed lucent-opaque lesion around impacted tooth #18. (From Neville BW, Damm DD, Allen CM, et al: Oral and maxillofacial pathology, ed 3, 2009, Saunders Elsevier.)

SUMMARY

- To interpret dental images, the dental professional must be able to accurately describe what is seen.
- The use of descriptive terminology allows the dental professional to intelligently describe and discuss what is seen on a dental image.
- Descriptive terminology is important for communication and documentation purposes.
- To communicate with other professionals and patients, the dental professional must be familiar with the basic terminology used in dental imaging.
- The term *radiolucent* describes areas of a dental image that appear dark or black. Radiolucent structures lack density and permit the passage of the x-ray beam. Air spaces and soft tissues appear radiolucent.
- The term *radiopaque* describes areas of a dental image that appear light or white. Radiopaque structures are dense and resist the passage of the x-ray beam. Enamel, dentin, and bone appear radiopaque.
- All lesions viewed on a dental image should be documented and described in terms of appearance, location, and size.
- To play an important role in the interpretation of dental images, dental professionals must have a working knowledge of key terms to be able to describe the appearance, location, and size of radiolucent and radiopaque lesions.

BIBLIOGRAPHY

Eversole LR: Radiolucent lesions of the jaws. In Clinical outline of oral pathology: diagnosis and treatment, ed 3, Philadelphia, 1992, Lea & Febiger.

Eversole LR: Radiopaque lesions of the jaws. In Clinical outline of oral pathology: diagnosis and treatment, ed 3, Philadelphia, 1992, Lea & Febiger.

Mallya SM, Lam EWN: Benign tumors and neoplasms. In White and Pharoah's Oral radiology: principles and interpretation, ed 8, St. Louis, 2019, Elsevier.

Mallya SM, Lam EWN: Cysts. In White and Pharoah's Oral radiology: principles and interpretation, ed 8, St. Louis, 2019, Elsevier.

Mallya SM, Lam EWN: Diseases affecting the structure of bone. In White and Pharoah's Oral radiology: principles and interpretation, ed 8, St. Louis, 2019, Elsevier.

Neville BW, Damm DD, Allen CM, et al: Oral and maxillofacial pathology, ed 3, 2009, Saunders Elsevier.

Rubar JS: Survey of dental radiographic terms, Oral Surg Oral Med Oral Pathol 69:530, 1990.

Wood NK, Goaz PW: Generalized radiopacities. In Differential diagnosis of oral lesions, ed 5, St Louis, 1997, Mosby.
Wood NK, Goaz PW: Multilocular radiolucencies. In Differential diagnosis of oral lesions, ed 5, St Louis, 1997, Mosby.
Wood NK, Goaz PW: Periapical radiolucencies. In Differential diagnosis of oral lesions, ed 5, St Louis, 1997, Mosby.
Wood NK, Goaz PW: Periapical radiopacities. In Differential diagnosis of oral lesions, ed 5, St Louis, 1997, Mosby.
Wood NK, Goaz PW: Pericoronal radiolucencies. In Differential diagnosis of oral lesions, ed 5, St Louis, 1997, Mosby.

QUIZ QUESTIONS

Short Answer

1. Describe the lesion illustrated in Figure 31-25 in terms of the following:
   a. Appearance: ______
   b. Location: ______
   c. Size: ______
2. Describe the lesion illustrated in Figure 31-26 in terms of the following:
   a. Appearance: ______
   b. Location: ______
   c. Size: ______
3. Describe the lesion illustrated in Figure 31-27 in terms of the following:
   a. Appearance: ______
   b. Location: ______
   c. Size: ______
4. Describe the lesion illustrated in Figure 31-28 in terms of the following:
   a. Appearance: ______
   b. Location: ______
   c. Size: ______
5. Describe the lesion illustrated in Figure 31-29 in terms of the following:
   a. Appearance: ______
   b. Location: ______
   c. Size: ______
6. Describe the lesion illustrated in Figure 31-30 in terms of the following:
   a. Appearance: ______
   b. Location: ______
   c. Size: ______

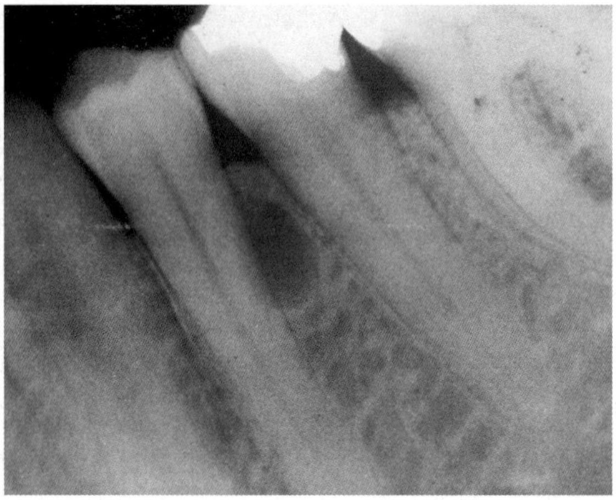

Fig 31-25

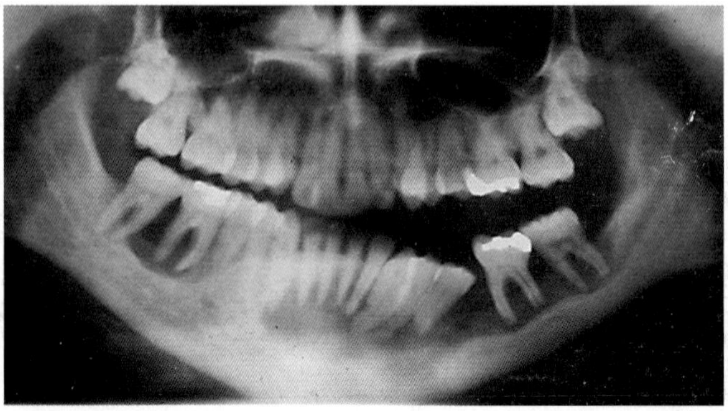

Fig 31-26

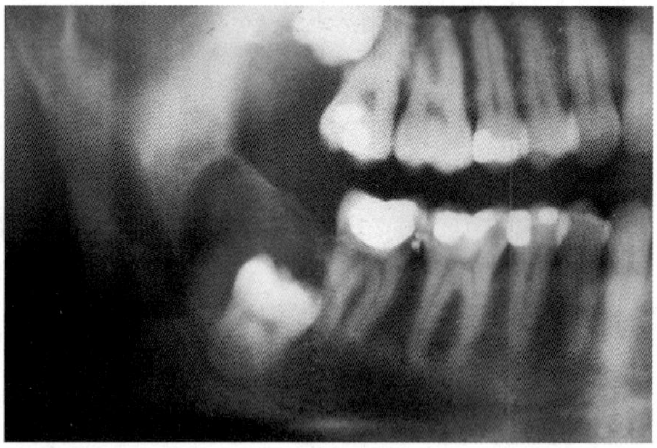

Fig 31-27

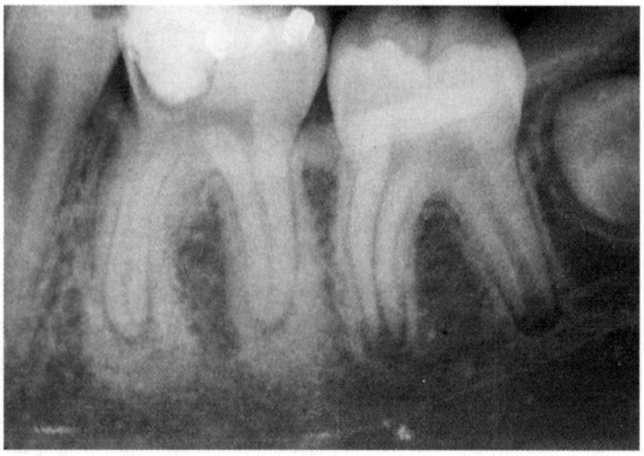

Fig 31-28

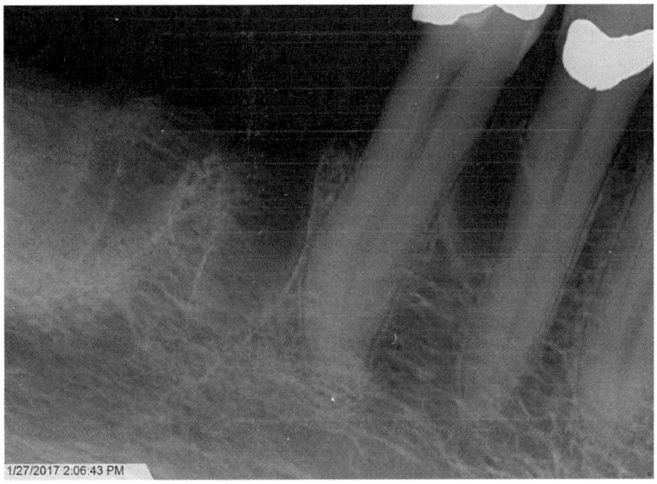

Fig 31-29

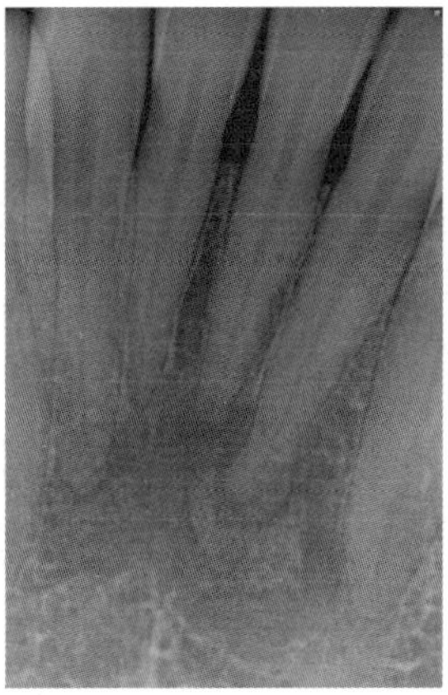

Fig 31-30

Matching

Match the following terms with the proper definitions:

a. Location of a lesion surrounding the crown of an impacted tooth.
b. Location of a lesion between the roots of adjacent teeth.
c. Location of a lesion surrounding the apex of a tooth.
d. Descriptive term for a radiopaque lesion that resembles an orange peel.
e. Descriptive term for structures that are dense and absorb or resist the passage of the x-ray beam.
f. Descriptive term for the periphery of a lesion surrounded by dense cortical bone.
g. Descriptive term for a radiopaque lesion that exhibits a well-demarcated localized area with a surrounding radiolucent ring.
h. Descriptive term for structures that lack density and permit the passage of the x-ray beam with little or no resistance.

_____ 7. Ground glass
_____ 8. Inter-radicular
_____ 9. Radiopaque
_____ 10. Pericoronal
_____ 11. Corticated
_____ 12. Target lesion
_____ 13. Periapical
_____ 14. Radiolucent

32

Identification of Restorations, Dental Materials, and Foreign Objects

LEARNING OBJECTIVES

After completion of this chapter, the student will be able to do the following:

1. Define the key terms associated with identifying restorations, materials, and foreign objects on dental images.
2. Discuss the importance of interpreting dental images while the patient is present.
3. On dental images, identify and describe the appearance of the following restorations: amalgam, gold, stainless steel and chrome, post and core, porcelain, porcelain-fused-to-metal, composite, and acrylic.
4. On dental images, identify and describe the appearance of the following: base materials, metallic pins, gutta percha, silver points, complete dentures, removable partial dentures, orthodontic bands, brackets and wires, fixed orthodontic retainers, dental implants, bone grafts, suture wires, metal splints and plates, bone screws, and stabilizing arches.
5. On dental images, identify and describe the appearance of the following: earrings, necklaces, nose jewelry, oral piercings, eyeglasses, patient napkin chains, hearing aids, shrapnel, and other miscellaneous objects.

Dental images are an important diagnostic tool that enables the practitioner to view dental restorations and dental materials. Dental images are also useful in identifying and locating foreign objects. Some restorations, dental materials, and foreign objects are easily identified on dental images; others are not. On dental images, the appearances of restorations, dental materials, and foreign objects vary, depending on the thickness of the material, density, and atomic number. Some may be identified by the degree of radiopacity present, outline, contour, or size; others require additional clinical information.

The dental professional should interpret all dental images while the patient is present. If questions arise as to what is seen on a dental image concerning dental restorations, dental materials, or foreign objects, clinical examination of the patient can be done to obtain additional information or to verify what is seen. When dental images are interpreted without the patient present, some important clinical information is not available.

The purpose of this chapter is to review common dental restorations, dental materials, and foreign objects viewed on dental images.

IDENTIFICATION OF RESTORATIONS

A variety of common restorative materials, including amalgam, gold, stainless steel, porcelain, composite, and acrylic, can be identified on dental images.

Metallic restorations (e.g., amalgam, gold) absorb x-rays, and as a result, very little (if any) radiation comes in contact with the receptor. Consequently, that area of the receptor remains unexposed, and the metallic restorations appear completely radiopaque (light or white) on a dental image. To illustrate this concept, place a processed film with a metallic restoration on a printed page. The underlying print can be easily read through the radiopaque area on the film (Figure 32-1).

Nonmetallic restorations (e.g., porcelain, composite, acrylic) may vary in appearance, from radiolucent (dark or black) to slightly radiopaque, depending on the density of the material. Of the nonmetallic restorations, porcelain is the most dense and least radiolucent, and acrylic is the least dense and most radiolucent.

Amalgam Restorations

Amalgam is the one of the most common restorative material used in dentistry. This mixture of mercury, silver, tin, and copper is a durable and inexpensive filling material. Amalgam absorbs the x-ray beam and prevents x-rays from reaching the receptor; consequently, amalgam appears completely radiopaque on a dental image. Amalgam may be seen in a variety of shapes, sizes, and locations on a dental image.

One-Surface and Multi-Surface Amalgam Restorations. One-surface amalgam restorations appear as distinct, small, round or ovoid radiopacities (Figures 32-2 and 32-3). One-surface amalgams may be seen on the buccal, lingual, or occlusal surfaces of teeth. Larger two-surface and multi-surface amalgam restorations also appear radiopaque and are characterized by their irregular outlines or borders (Figures 32-4 and 32-5). Multi-surface amalgam restorations may involve any tooth surface.

Amalgam Overhangs. Amalgam overhangs are extensions of amalgam seen beyond the crown portion of a tooth in the interproximal region. An amalgam overhang results from improper band placement around a tooth before condensing the amalgam restoration. Amalgam overhangs can be easily visualized on a dental image and appear radiopaque (Figures 32-6 and 32-7). An amalgam overhang disrupts the natural cleansing contours of the tooth, traps food and plaque, and contributes to bone loss. To prevent destruction of interproximal bone, amalgam overhangs must be removed and replaced with a restoration of better contour.

Amalgam Fragments. Fragments of amalgam may be inadvertently embedded in adjacent soft tissue during restoration of a tooth. Amalgam fragments or scraps vary in size and shape and appear as dense radiopacities with irregular borders on a dental image (Figures 32-8 and 32-9). Amalgam fragments may be seen in any location where soft tissue is present. If amalgam fragments are displaced into soft tissue during the placement or removal of an amalgam restoration or during the extraction of a tooth with an amalgam restoration present, a permanent area of pigmentation, known as an *amalgam tattoo*, may occur (Figure 32-10).

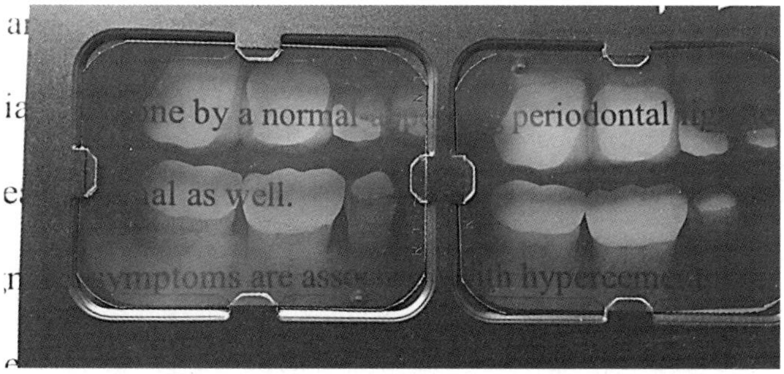

Fig 32-1 When a radiograph with a metallic restoration is placed on a printed page, the print can be easily seen.

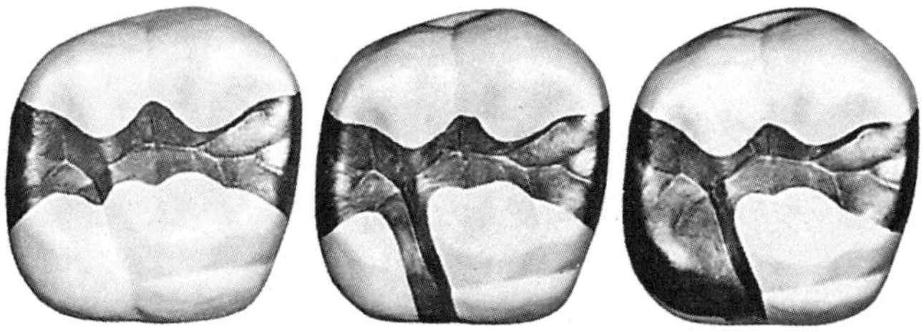

Fig 32-4 Example of multi-surface amalgam restorations. (From Heymann HO, Swift EJ, Ritter AV: Sturdevant's art and science of operative dentistry, ed 6, St Louis, 2013, Mosby.)

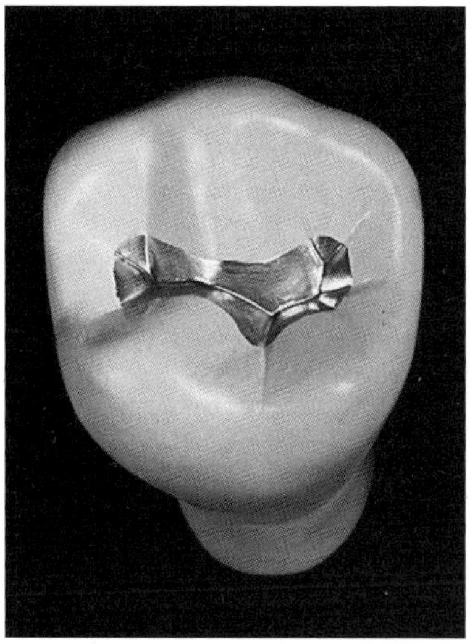

Fig 32-2 A one-surface occlusal amalgam. (From Heymann HO, Swift EJ, Ritter AV: Sturdevant's art and science of operative dentistry, ed 6, St Louis, 2013, Mosby.)

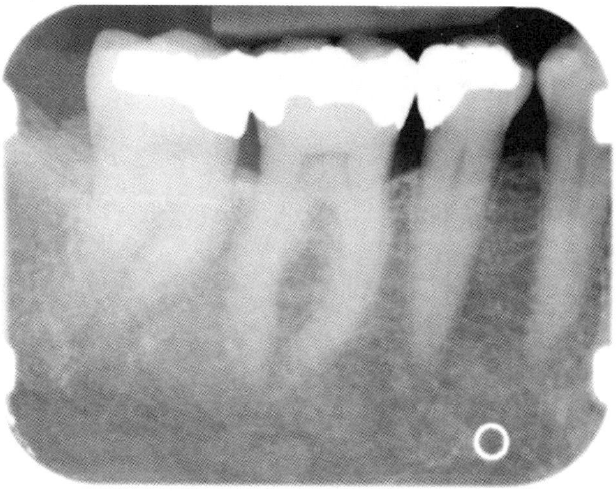

Fig 32-5 Three multi-surface amalgam restorations. Note the irregular outlines.

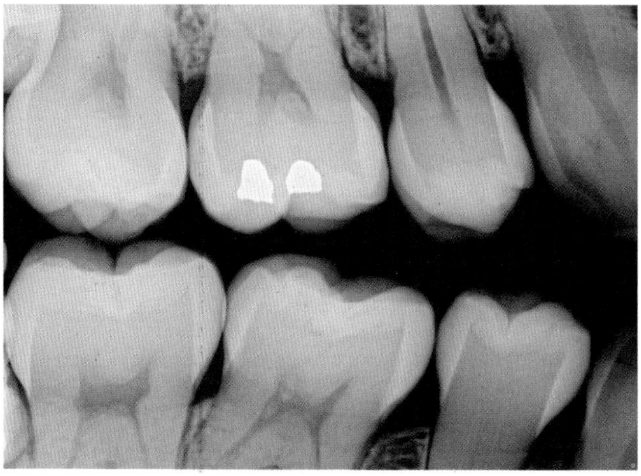

Fig 32-3 Two pit amalgams are seen in a maxillary first molar.

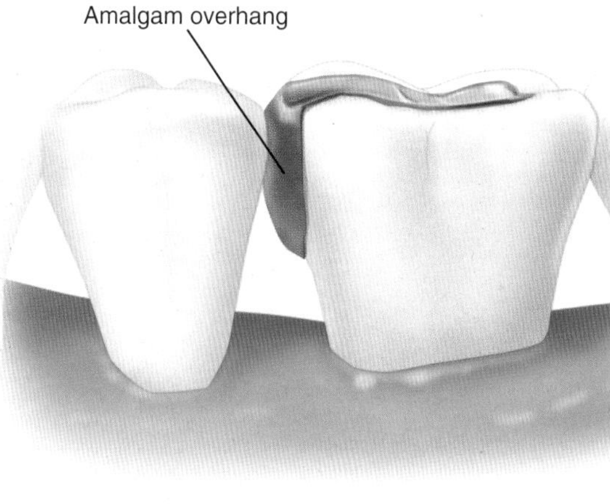

Fig 32-6 Amalgam overhang.

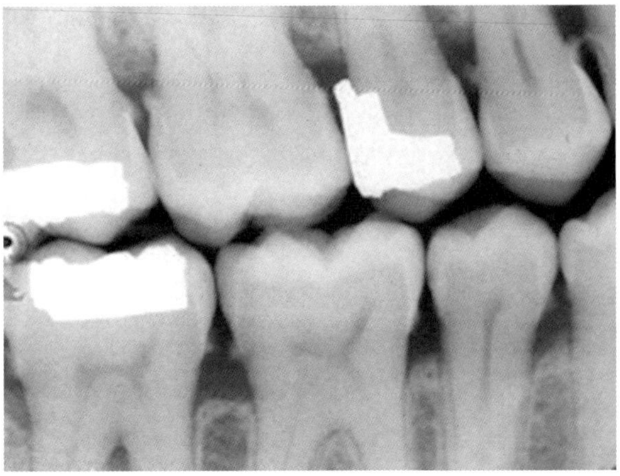

Fig 32-7 Amalgam overhang seen on the maxillary second premolar.

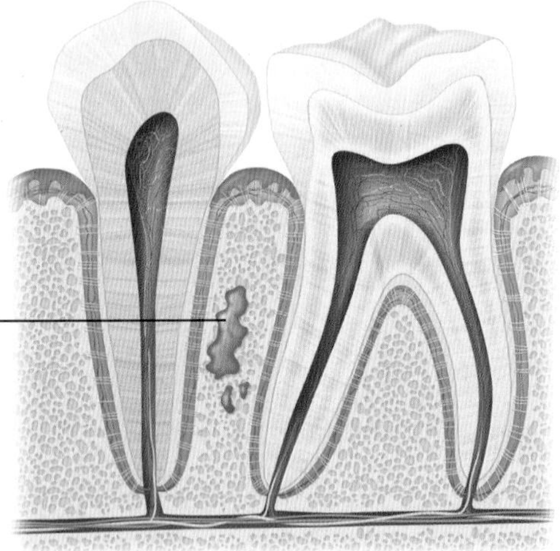

Fig 32-8 Amalgam fragments.

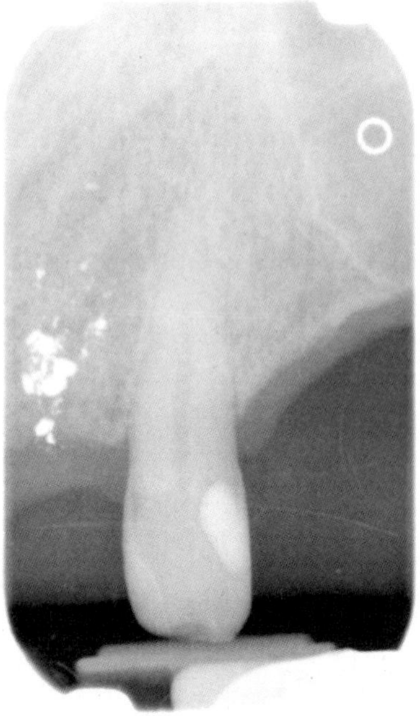

Fig 32-9 Amalgam fragment seen in soft tissue near the maxillary canine.

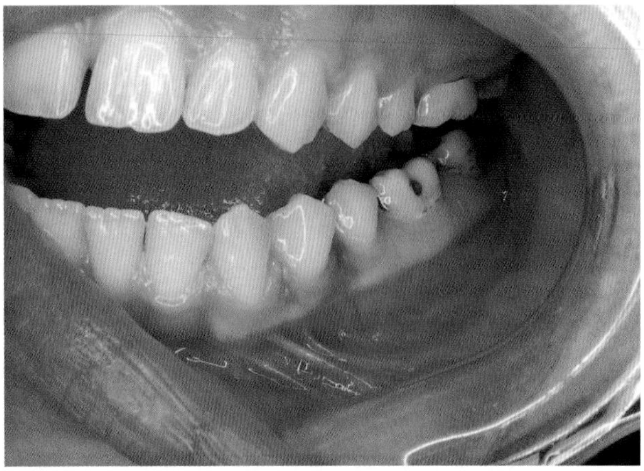

Fig 32-10 Amalgam tattoo seen by the bluish pigmentation of the gingiva. (From Ibsen OAC, Phelan JA: Oral pathology for the dental hygienist, ed 5, St. Louis, 2009, Saunders.)

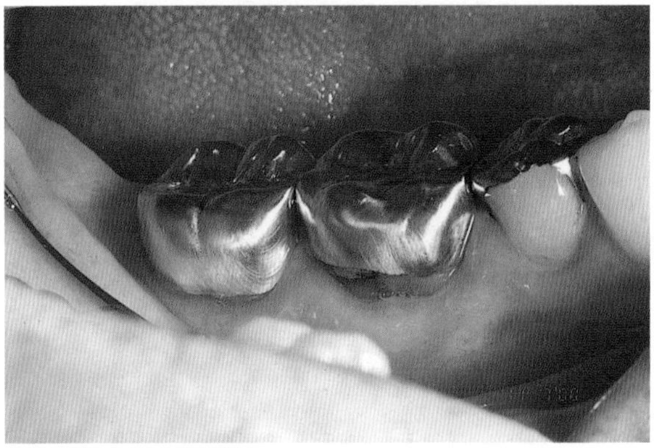

Fig 32-11 Gold crown. (From Hatrick CD, Eakle SW: Dental materials: clinical applications for dental assistants and dental hygienists, ed 3, St. Louis, 2015, Saunders.)

Gold Restorations

It is not always possible to differentiate one metallic restoration from another on a dental image; however, an educated guess is often possible if the shape and size of the restoration are considered. Both gold and amalgam appear equally radiopaque on a dental image. A large radiopaque restoration with smooth borders is most likely gold. Gold restorations appear completely radiopaque and, unlike amalgam restorations, exhibit a smooth marginal outline (Figures 32-11 and 32-12). If dental images are interpreted with the patient present, oral examination will verify whether the restorative material is gold or amalgam.

Gold Crowns and Bridges. Gold crowns and bridges appear as large radiopaque restorations with smooth contours and regular borders (Figure 32-13). Similarly, gold inlay and onlay restorations exhibit marginal outlines that appear smooth and regular (Figures 32-14 and 32-15).

Gold Foil Restorations. One-surface gold foil restorations appear as small round radiopacities on a dental image and are indistinguishable from one-surface amalgam restorations. A two-surface gold foil restoration may appear similar to a gold inlay, with smooth, regular marginal outlines, or may exhibit slightly irregular margins and resemble a two-surface amalgam.

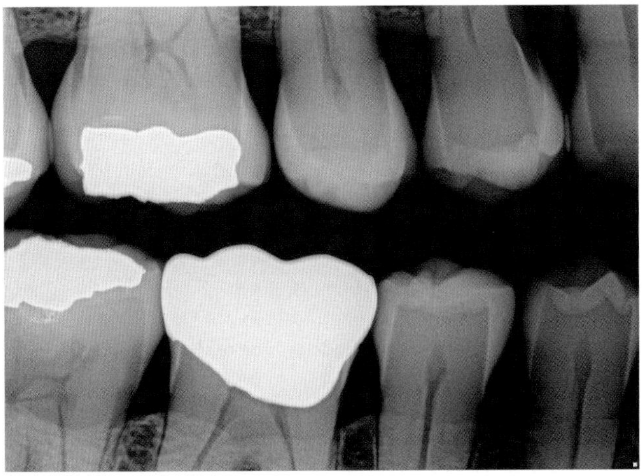

Fig 32-12 A gold crown seen on the mandibular first molar. Note the smooth outline and contour.

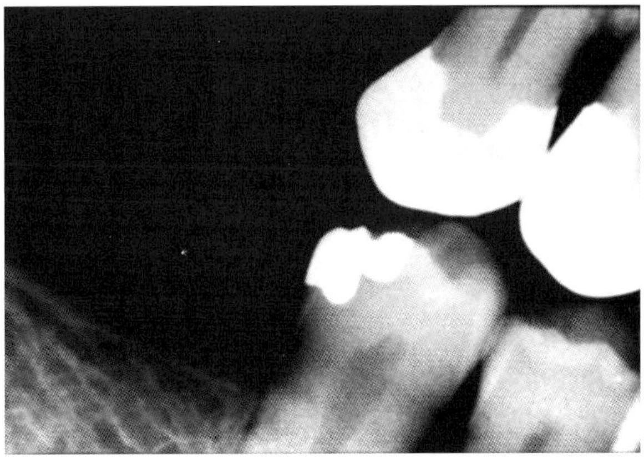

Fig 32-15 Gold onlays seen on maxillary premolars. Note the distinct outline and contours.

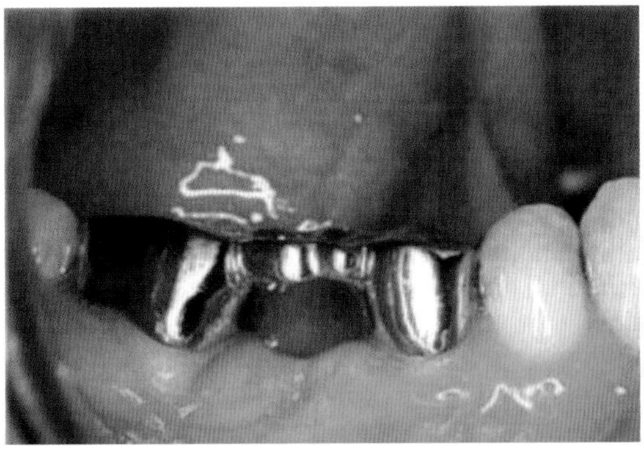

Fig 32-13 Gold bridge. (From Barclay CW, Walmsley D: Colour guide: fixed and removable prosthodontics, ed 2, St. Louis, 1998, Churchill Livingstone.)

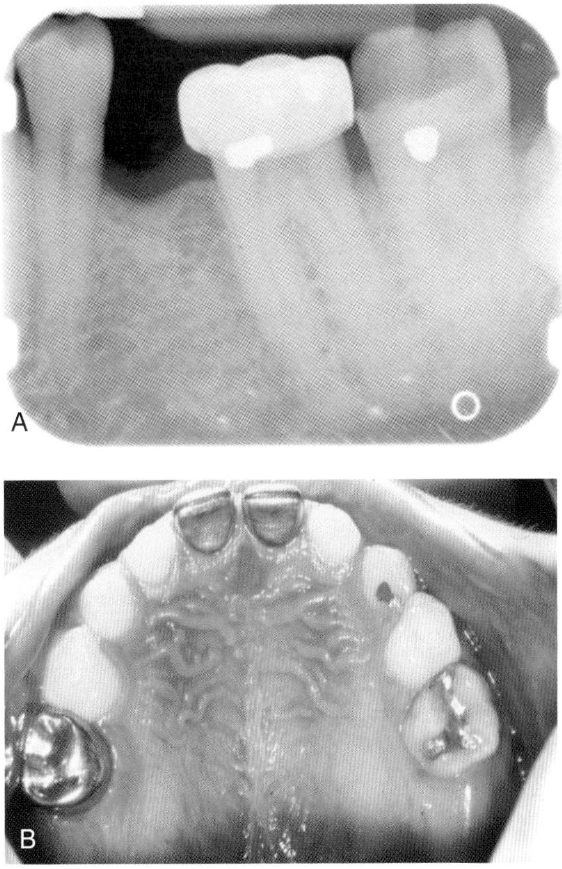

Fig 32-16 A, Stainless steel crown seen on the mandibular first molar. B, Stainless steel crown—notice the prefabricated appearance. (From Casamassimo: Pediatric dentistry: infancy through adolescence, ed 5, Saunders, 2012.)

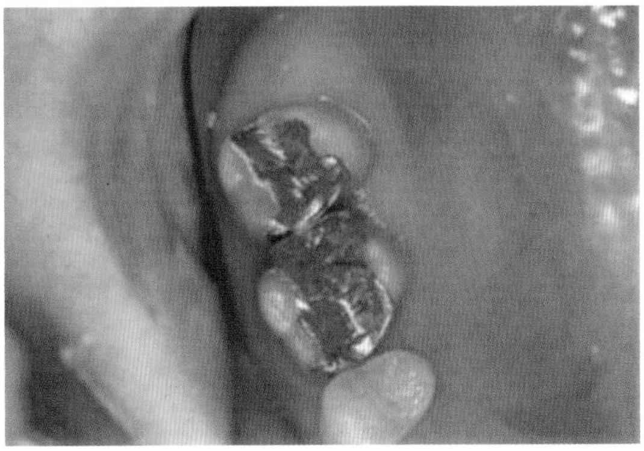

Fig 32-14 Gold inlay. (From Barclay CW, Walmsley D: Colour guide: fixed and removable prosthodontics, ed 2, St. Louis, 1998, Churchill Livingstone.)

Stainless Steel and Chrome Crown Restorations

Stainless steel and chrome crown restorations are prefabricated and usually used as interim or temporary restorations. These crowns are thin and do not absorb dental x-rays to the extent that amalgam, gold, and other cast metals do. As a result, both stainless steel and chrome crowns appear radiopaque, although not as densely radiopaque as amalgam or gold.

Because stainless steel and chrome crowns are prefabricated, the outlines and margins appear very smooth and regular. Often these crowns are not contoured properly to the cervical portion of the tooth and thus do not appear to fit the tooth well (Figure 32-16).

Restorations that are not contoured with the shape of the tooth may cause periodontal problems ranging from food impaction to gingival bleeding or possible bone loss. Because stainless steel and chrome crowns are thin, some areas may appear "see-through" on the dental image (Figures 32-17 and 32-18).

Post and Core Restorations

Post and core restorations can be seen in teeth treated with endodontic therapy. The post and core restoration is cast metal and appears as radiopaque as amalgam or gold. Post and core restorations appear radiopaque on a dental image. The core portion of the restoration resembles the prepared portion of a tooth crown, and the post portion extends into the pulp canal (Figure 32-19).

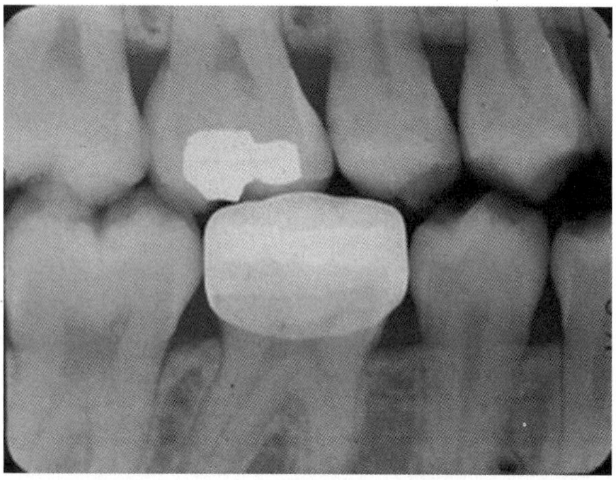

Fig 32-17 Stainless steel crown seen on the mandibular first molar. Note the area that appears "see-through."

Porcelain Restorations

A porcelain restoration appears radiopaque on a dental image. Unlike metallic restorations, which appear completely radiopaque, porcelain restorations are slightly radiopaque and resemble the radiodensity of dentin.

All-Porcelain Crowns and Bridges. All-porcelain crowns and bridges appear slightly radiopaque on a dental image (Figures 32-20 and 32-21). A thin radiopaque line outlining the prepared tooth may be evident through the slightly radiopaque porcelain crown (Figures 32-20 and 32-22). This thin line represents cement or other dental adhesive material used to adhere the crown to the tooth. The radiodensity of an all-porcelain bridge appears identical to that of the all-porcelain crown.

Porcelain-Fused-to-Metal Crowns. When viewed on a dental image, a porcelain-fused-to-metal crown has two components. The metal component appears *completely* radiopaque, and the porcelain component appears *slightly* radiopaque (Figures 32-23 and 32-24). The radiodensities of a porcelain-fused-to-metal bridge appear identical to those seen in the porcelain-fused-to-metal crown (Figure 32-25).

Composite Restorations

When viewed on a dental image, a composite restoration may vary in appearance from radiolucent to slightly radiopaque, depending on the composition of the composite material (Figures 32-26 and 32-27). Some manufacturers of composite materials add radiopaque particles to their products to help the viewer differentiate a composite restoration from dental caries (which appears radiolucent) on a dental image.

To determine whether a radiolucent area represents a composite restoration or caries, a careful visual and digital examination of the tooth in question enables the clinician to distinguish between the two.

Acrylic Restorations

Acrylic resin restorations are often used as an interim or temporary crown or filling. Of all the nonmetallic restorations, acrylic is the least dense and appears slightly radiopaque on a dental image.

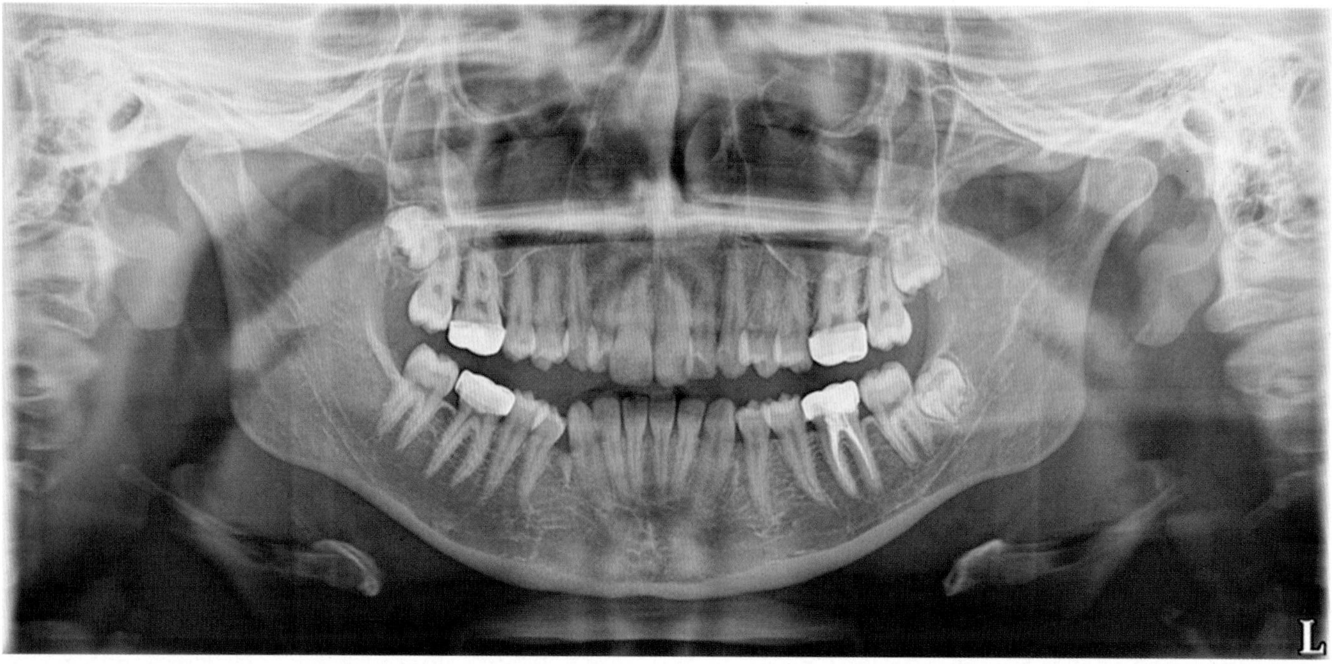

Fig 32-18 Stainless steel crowns visible on four permanent first molars.

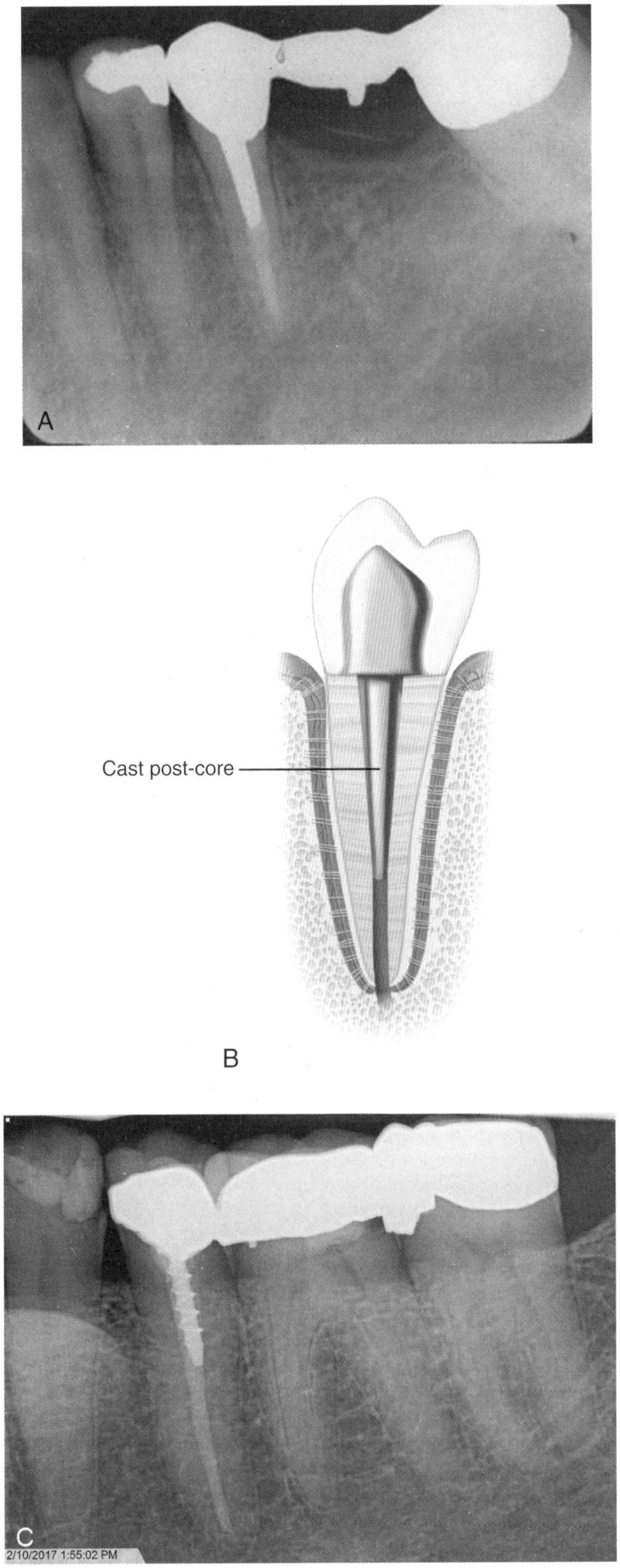

Fig 32-19 A, Post and core restoration seen on the mandibular second premolar. B, Diagram of post and core. C, Post and core restoration seen on the mandibular second premolar. The screw-shaped post extends into the pulp canal that has been treated with gutta percha.

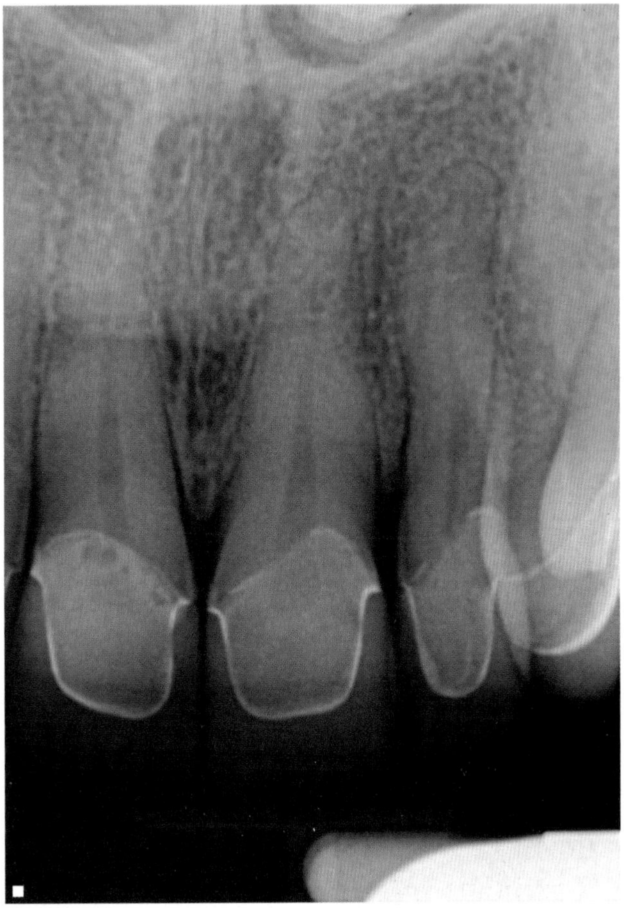

Fig 32-20 All-porcelain crowns seen in the anterior maxilla. Note the outlines of the teeth preparation covered with radiopaque cement.

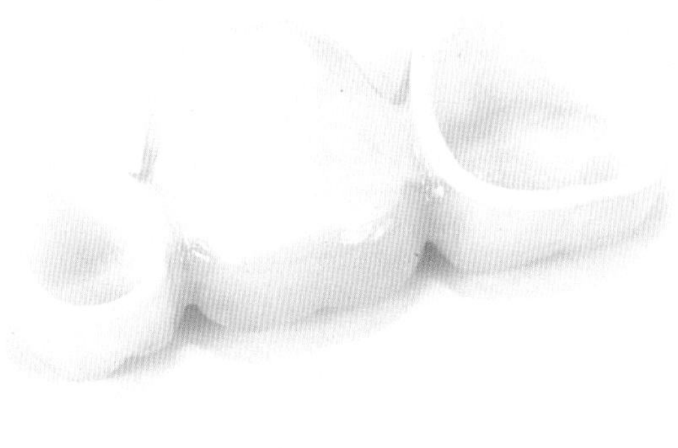

Fig 32-21 Porcelain bridge. (Copyright Hattanas Kumchai/iStock.com.)

IDENTIFICATION OF MATERIALS USED

A number of materials are used in dentistry for a variety of reasons, each specific to the specialty that requires the material. Practitioners in restorative dentistry, endodontics, prosthodontics, orthodontics, and oral surgery all use materials that can be identified on dental images.

Materials Used in Restorative Dentistry

Base Materials. Base materials, which include zinc phosphate cement and zinc oxide–eugenol paste, are used as cavity liners to protect

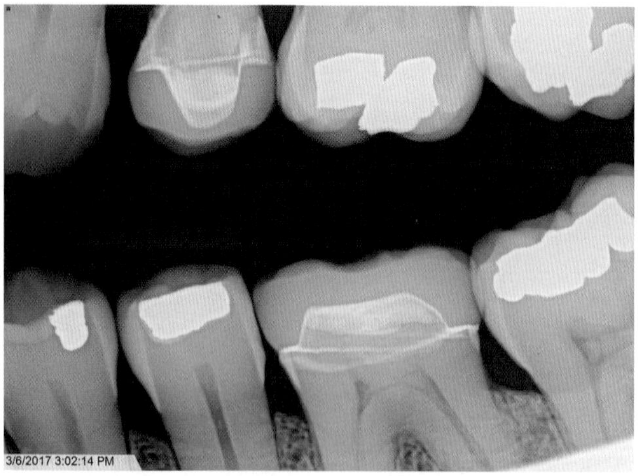

Fig 32-22 Porcelain crowns seen on the maxillary second premolar and the mandibular first molar on this bite-wing image.

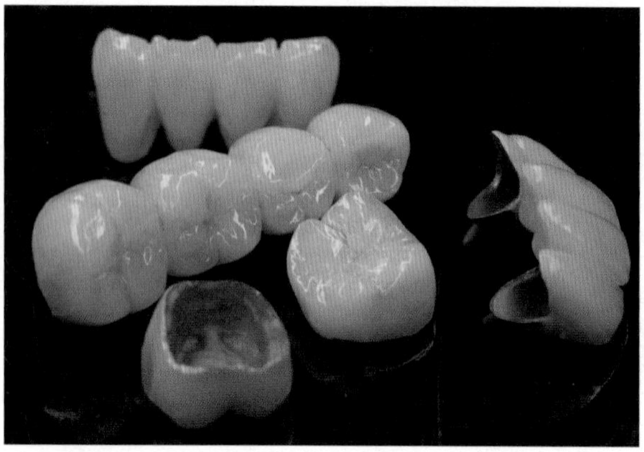

Fig 32-23 Porcelain-fused-to-metal crowns and bridges. (Courtesy W. Veneer Center, New York, NY.)

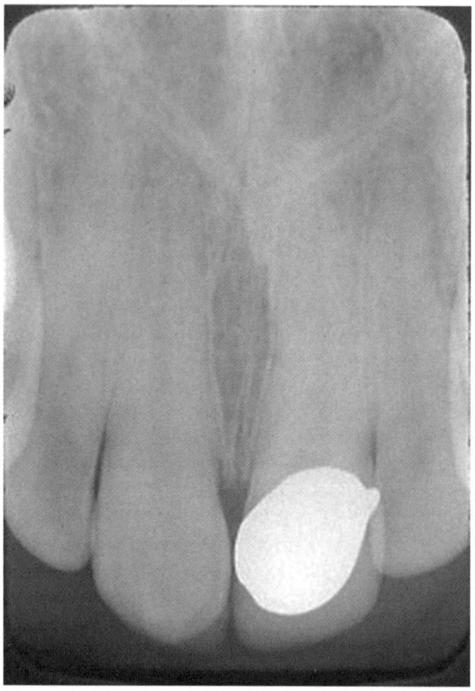

Fig 32-24 Porcelain-fused-to-metal crown seen on the maxillary central incisor.

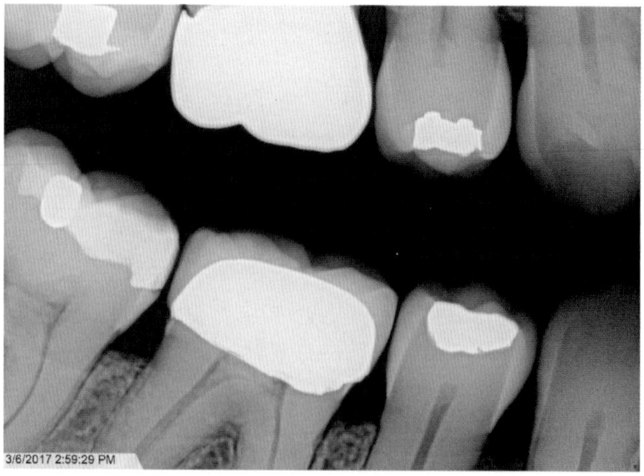

Fig 32-25 Porcelain-fused-to-metal crown seen on the mandibular first molar.

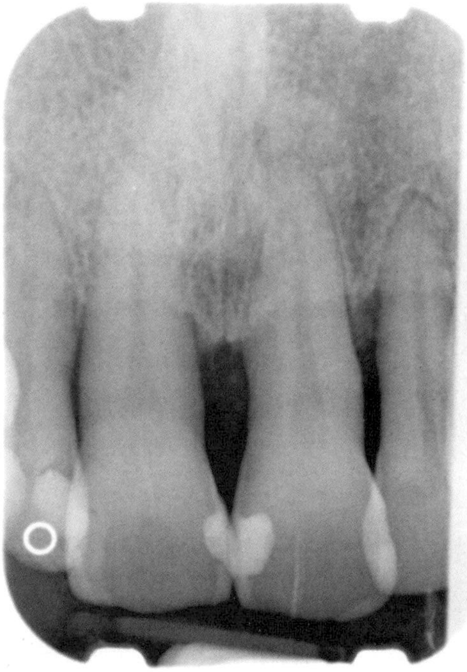

Fig 32-26 Composite restorations seen on maxillary anterior teeth.

the pulp of the tooth. Base materials are placed on the floor of a cavity preparation. A restorative material, such as amalgam, is then placed over the base material. A base material appears radiopaque. Compared with amalgam, the base material appears less radiopaque (Figure 32-28).

Metallic Pins. Metallic pins, used to enhance the retention of amalgam or composite, appear as cylindrical or screw-shaped radiopacities on a dental image (Figures 32-29 and 32-30).

Materials Used in Endodontics

Gutta Percha. Gutta percha is a rubberlike material used in endodontic therapy to fill the canals of the pulp. Gutta percha appears radiopaque, similar in density to that of base materials (Figure 32-31). Compared with metallic restorations, gutta percha appears less radiopaque.

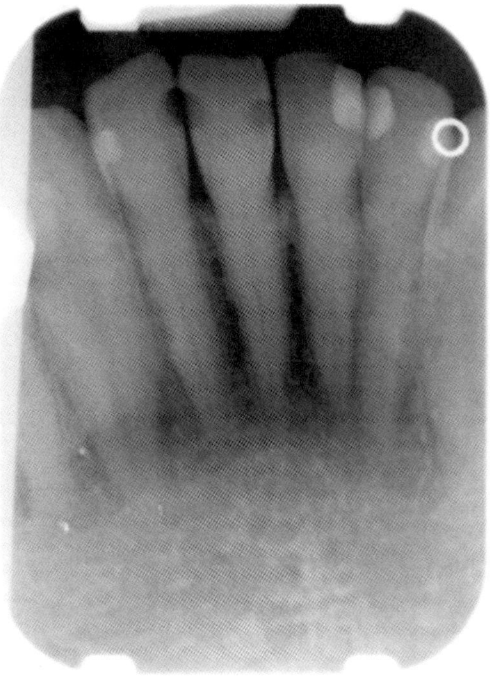

Fig 32-27 Composite restorations seen on mandibular anterior teeth. Note the radiolucent and radiopaque appearance of these restorations.

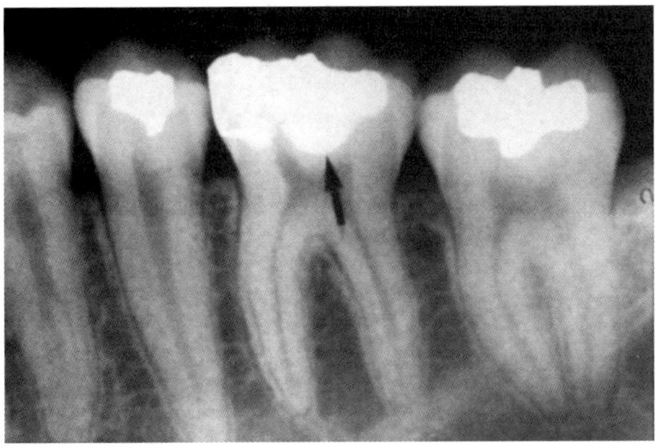

Fig 32-28 Base material seen under an amalgam restoration on a mandibular first molar.

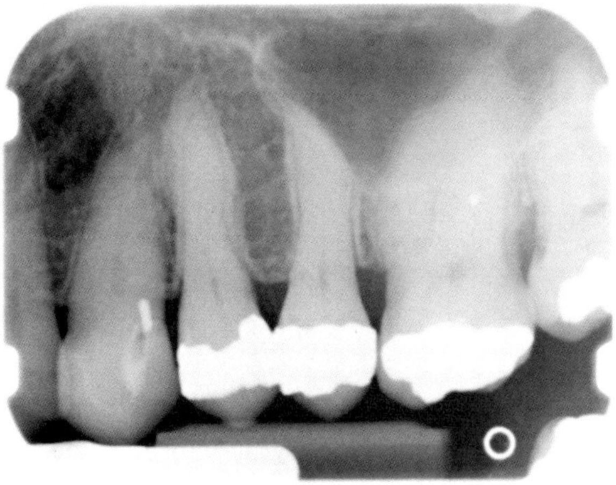

Fig 32-29 Metallic pin enhancing the retention capability of the composite restoration seen in this maxillary canine.

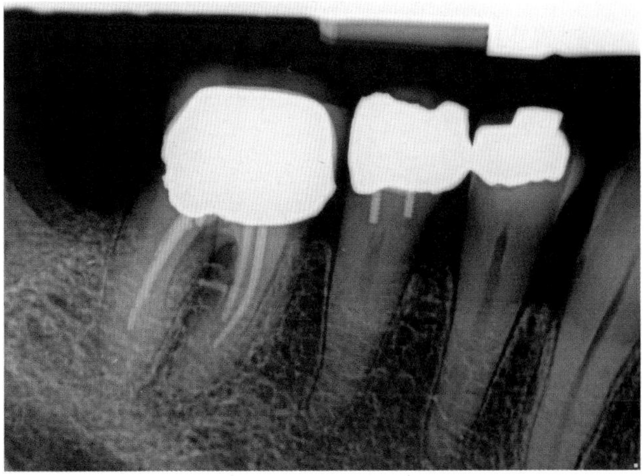

Fig 32-30 Metallic pins used to give strength to the restoration on the mandibular second premolar.

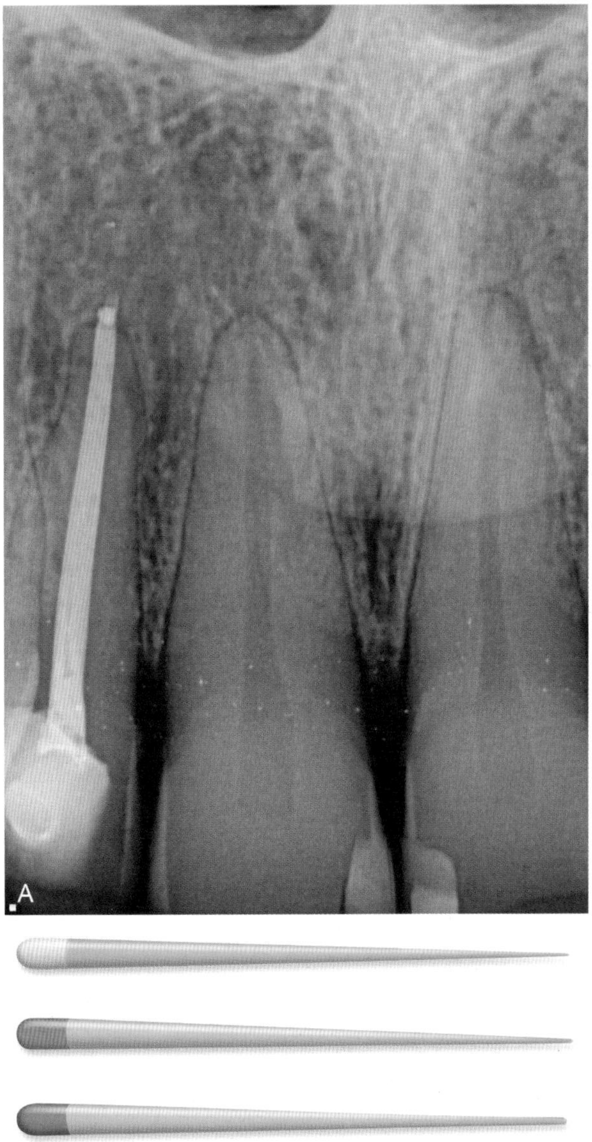

Fig 32-31 A, Gutta percha seen in the pulp canal of a maxillary lateral incisor. B, Gutta percha points. (Courtesy Dentsply Tulsa Dental Specialties, Tulsa, OK.)

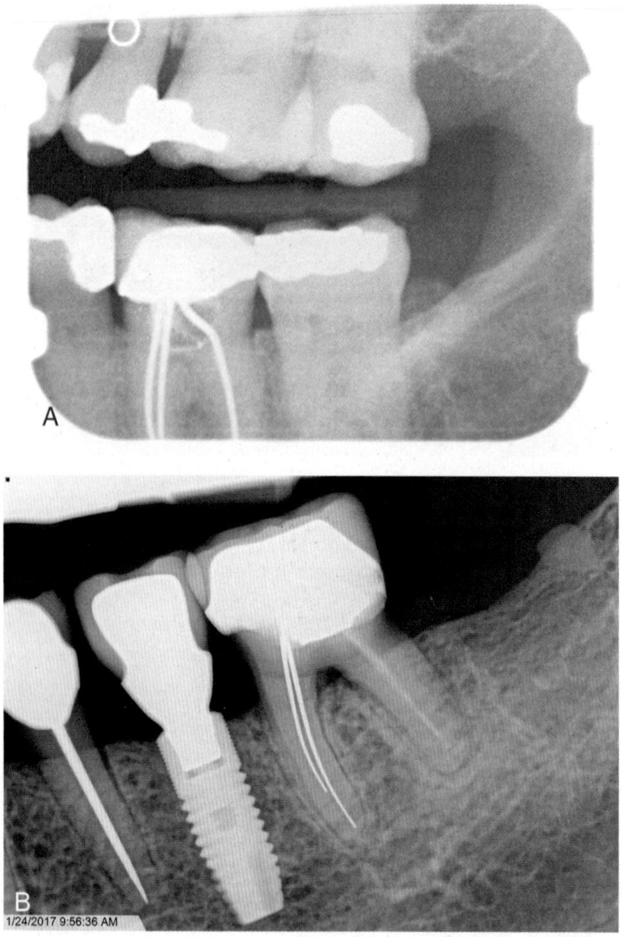

Fig 32-32 A, Silver point seen in the pulp canal underneath a porcelain-fused-to-metal crown on the mandibular first molar. B, Silver points seen in the mandibular first premolar and the mesial root of the mandibular first molar.

Silver Points. Silver points are also used in endodontic therapy to fill the canals of the pulp. Silver points appear highly radiopaque, similar to other metallic materials. Silver points appear more radiopaque than gutta percha (Fig. 32-32).

Materials Used in Prosthodontics

Complete and removable partial dentures may be occasionally observed on dental images. The appearances of complete and removable partial dentures vary, depending on the base materials and type of denture teeth used. Patients should be instructed to remove all complete and partial dentures before dental images are exposed. If not removed, complete and partial dentures may obscure important information concerning adjacent teeth and underlying bone.

Occasionally the decision is made to keep a denture in place during imaging procedures. For example, a patient who wears a maxillary denture and has natural mandibular teeth may be instructed to keep the denture in place during exposure of periapical images of the mandibular teeth. The denture acts to stabilize the bite-block used with the beam alignment devices and thus provide more diagnostic images.

Complete Dentures. A complete denture consists of two component parts: (1) a base material and (2) denture teeth. The typical denture base material is composed of acrylic and appears as a very faint radiopacity on a dental image or, in some cases, may not be seen at all. Denture teeth may be composed of porcelain or acrylic and vary in appearance. Porcelain denture teeth appear radiopaque and resemble the radiodensity of dentin. Anterior porcelain denture teeth include one or two metal retention pins, or diatorics. On a dental image, diatorics appear as tiny, dense radiopacities superimposed over the radiopaque porcelain denture teeth (Fig. 32-33). Posterior porcelain denture teeth

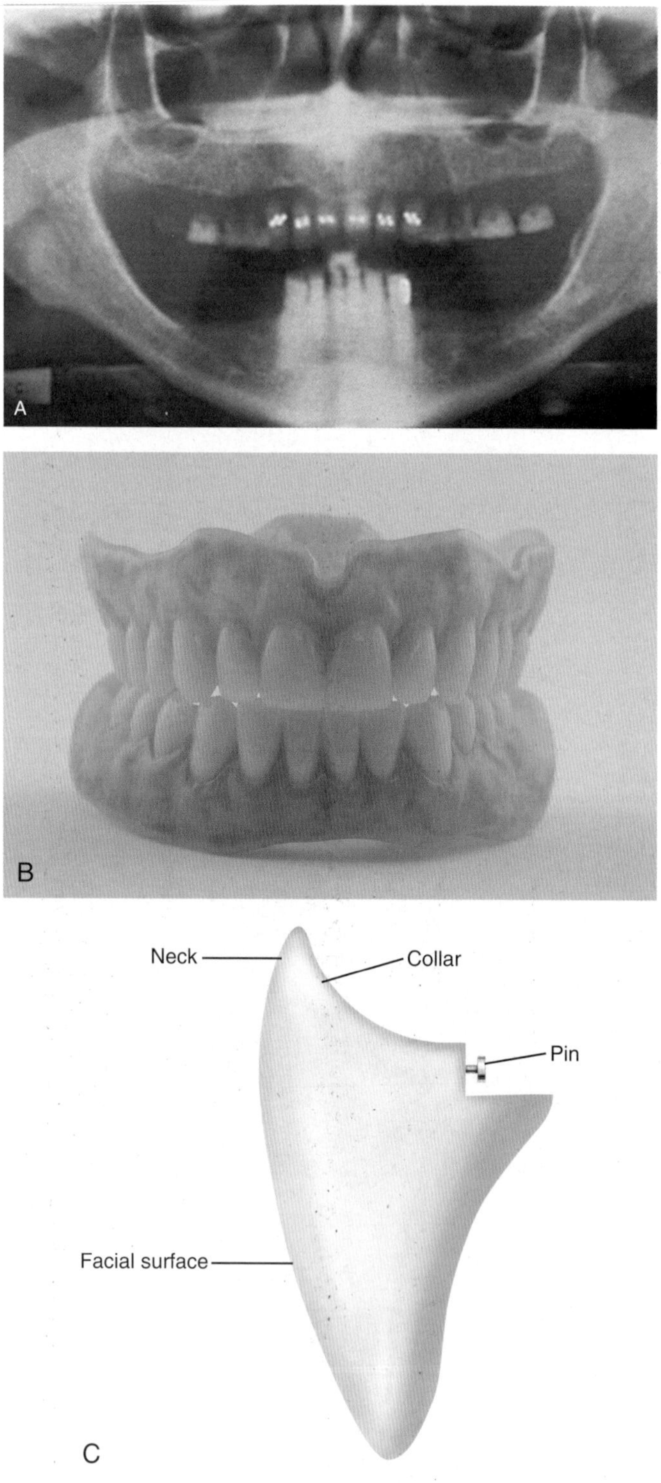

Fig 32-33 A, Diatorics seen on the teeth of the maxillary denture. B, Complete dentures. (Copyright Alexshor/iStock.com.) C, Diagram of denture tooth with retention pin (diatoric).

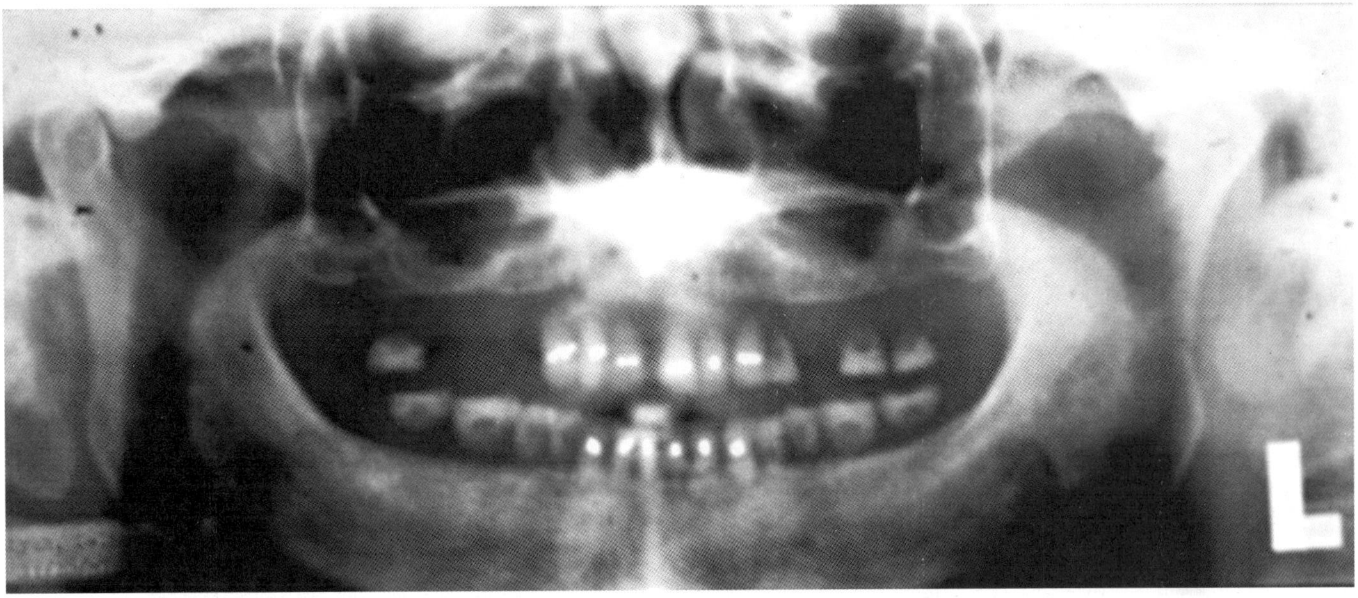

Fig 32-34 Maxillary and mandibular denture teeth appear to be "floating" in this panoramic image.

also appear radiopaque but do not contain diatorics. Acrylic (plastic) denture teeth lack density and appear faintly radiopaque or radiolucent on a dental image.

A complete denture that is not removed before the exposure of a dental image gives the illusion of rootless, or "floating," teeth (Fig. 32-34).

Removable Partial Dentures. A removable partial denture can be constructed from a variety of base materials, including cast metal, a combination of cast metal and acrylic, and all acrylic. The removable partial denture constructed of cast metal appears radiopaque on a dental image. The size and shape of the radiopacity depend on the design of the metal framework of the partial denture. A removable partial denture constructed of a metal base with acrylic saddles appears densely radiopaque where metal is present and slightly radiopaque in the areas of acrylic. A removable partial denture base constructed totally of acrylic is usually seen with wrought-metal clasps. The acrylic base appears slightly radiopaque on a dental image. The metal clasps appear radiopaque and are seen resting on abutment teeth.

Teeth in a removable partial denture may be composed of acrylic or porcelain. Porcelain teeth appear radiopaque and resemble the radiodensity of dentin. Acrylic teeth appear faintly radiopaque (Fig. 32-35).

Materials Used in Orthodontics

Orthodontic bands, brackets, and wires may be observed on dental images. Each of these orthodontic materials has a characteristic radiopaque appearance (Figures 32-36, 32-37, and 32-38). Fixed orthodontic retainers may also be observed on dental images and have an equally characteristic appearance (Figure 32-39).

Materials Used in Oral Surgery

Implants. Implants are being used in oral surgery with increased frequency. The appearances of the numerous endosteal implants that are currently used vary, depending on their shapes and designs. The endosteal implant is made of a metallic material and appears radiopaque on a dental image (Figures 32-40 through 32-43).

Bone Grafts. As dental implant placement becomes more popular and commonplace in dentistry, bone augmentation procedures have also been increasing. Not all patients present with the required bone level for a solid foundation to hold implants properly. Bone augmentation or grafting procedures include ways to add bone material to areas that were deficient in quantity of hard tissue. For implants to be successful over time, not only does the volume of bone need to be sufficient to hold the implant in place, but the grafting material must also encourage osseointegration while withstanding occlusal forces (Figures 32-44 and 32-45).

Fracture Stabilization Materials. Suture wires, metal splints and plates, bone screws, and stabilizing arches are used in oral surgery to stabilize fractures of the maxilla and the mandible. Suture wires appear as thin radiopaque lines. Metal splints, plates, screws, and stabilizing arches also appear radiopaque; their characteristic shapes and sizes may vary (Figures 32-46 and 32-47).

IDENTIFICATION OF OBJECTS

A number of miscellaneous objects, including earrings, necklaces, nose jewelry, eyeglasses, napkin chains, hearing aids, and shrapnel, can be viewed on dental images. Such objects may obscure important diagnostic information. Some miscellaneous objects may be seen on intraoral images; others may be noted on extraoral images.

To avoid nondiagnostic images, patients should be instructed to remove all earrings, necklaces, nose jewelry, eyeglasses, napkin chains, and hearing aids (if possible) before exposure of extraoral images. In the case of intraoral images, patients should be instructed to remove eyeglasses and nose jewelry, if necessary.

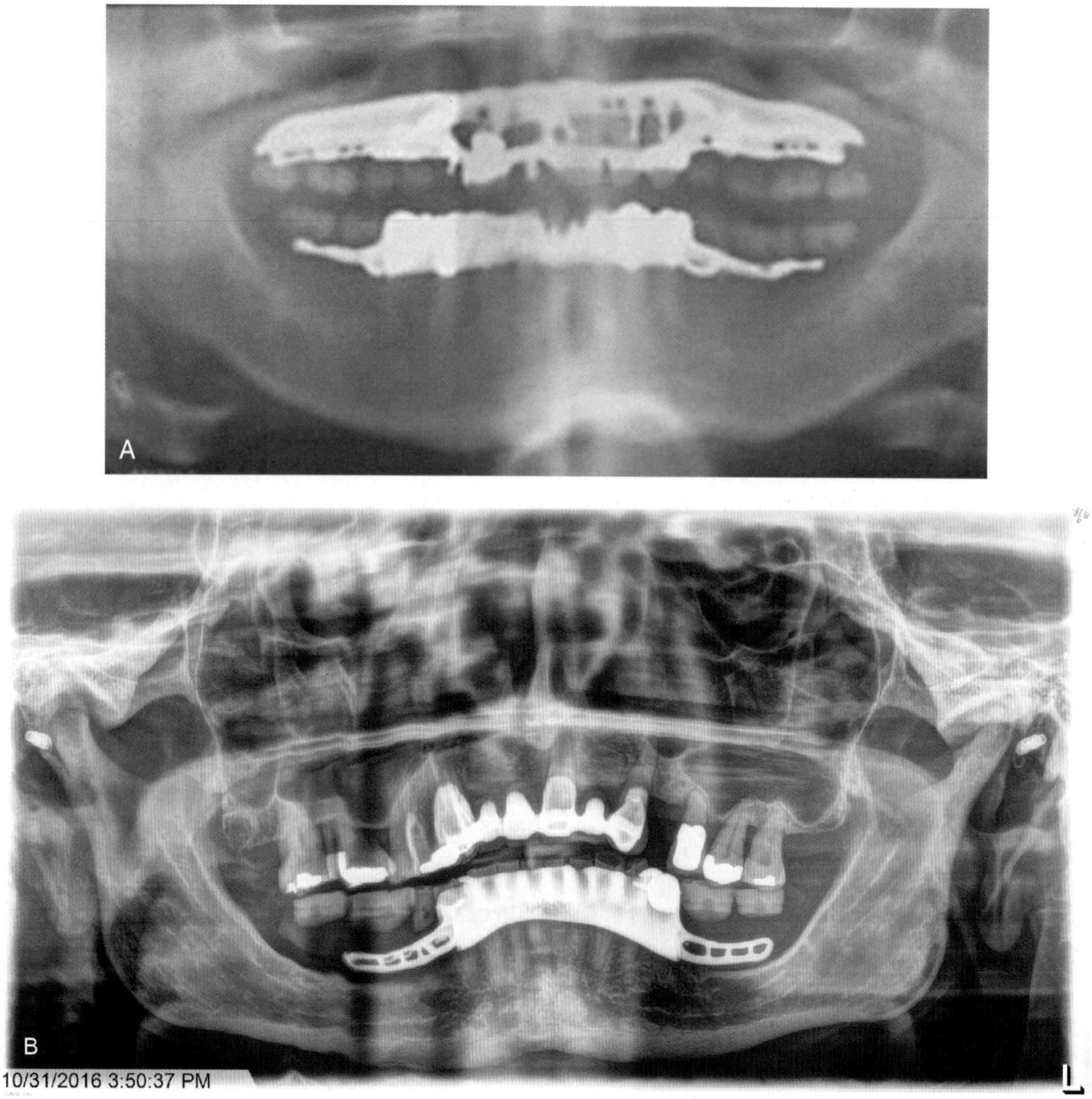

Fig 32-35 A, Metal framework of both partial dentures and porcelain teeth in the posterior quadrants of both arches is visible in this panoramic image. **B,** This panoramic image was exposed with the patient wearing a removable mandibular partial denture.

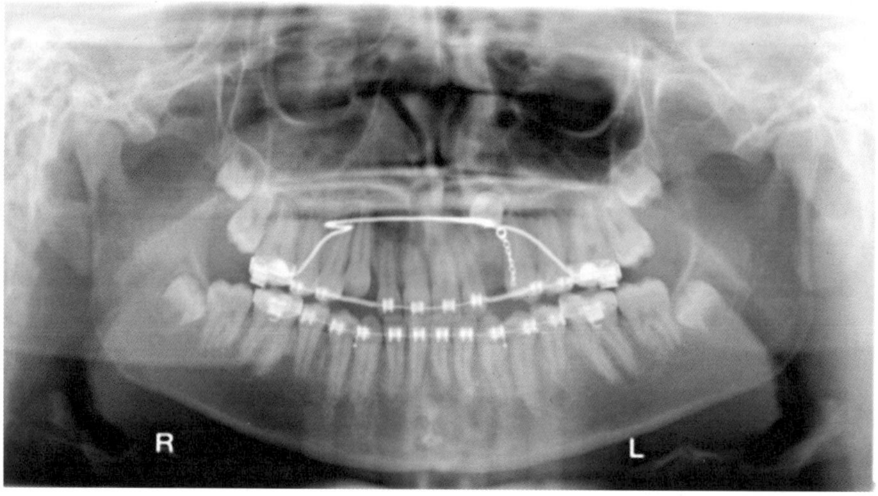

Fig 32-36 Orthodontic appliances that aid in the proper eruption of the maxillary canines.

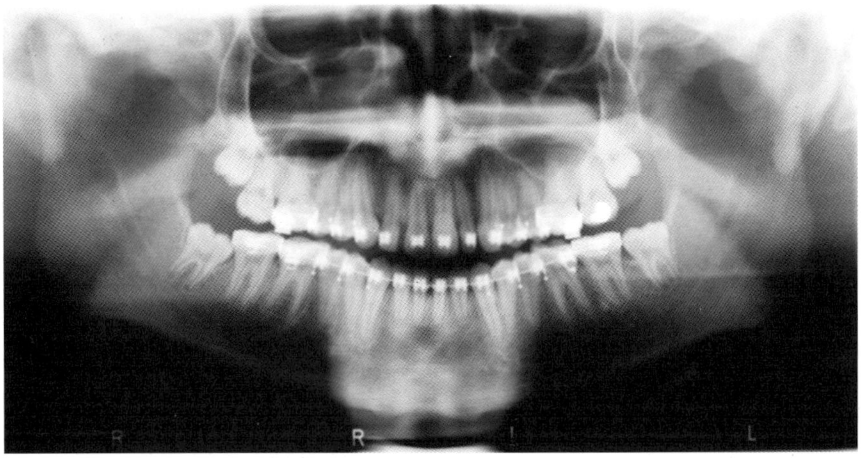

Fig 32-37 Orthodontic bands are recognizable on a panoramic image.

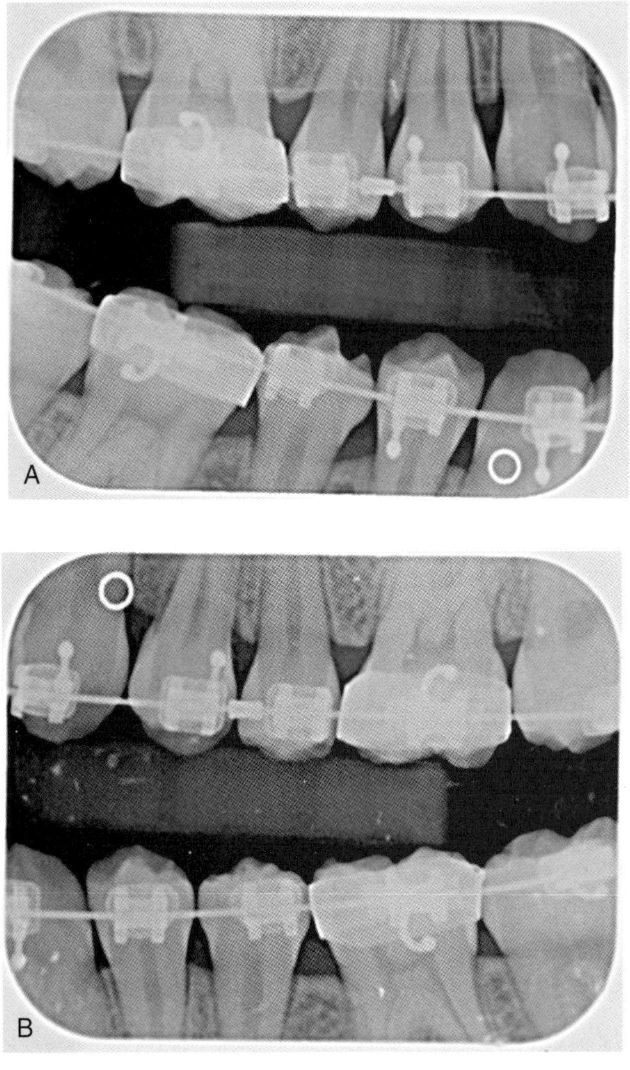

Fig 32-38 A, B, Orthodontic appliances are recognizable on bite-wing images. (Courtesy Cary Pediatric Dentistry, Cary, NC.)

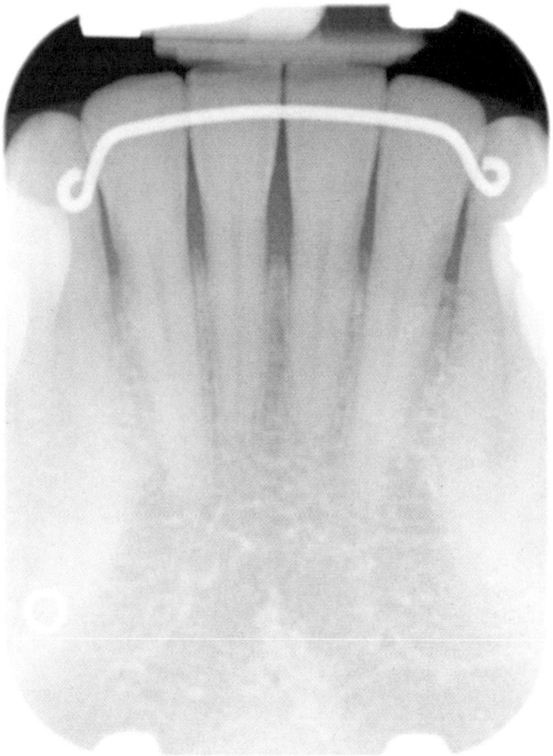

Fig 32-39 Fixed orthodontic retainer seen in the mandibular anterior region.

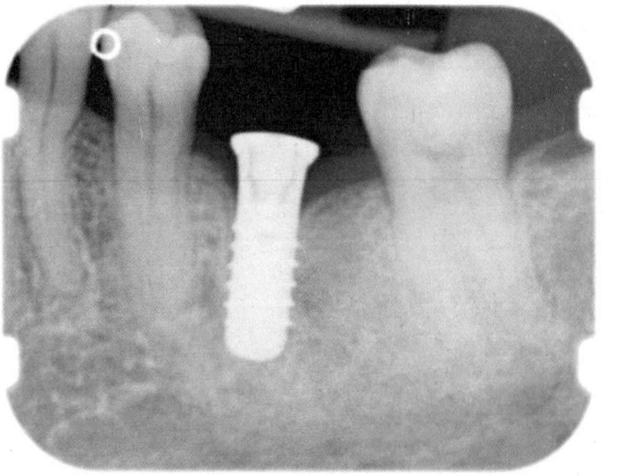

Fig 32-40 A dental implant is placed in the area of the mandibular left first molar.

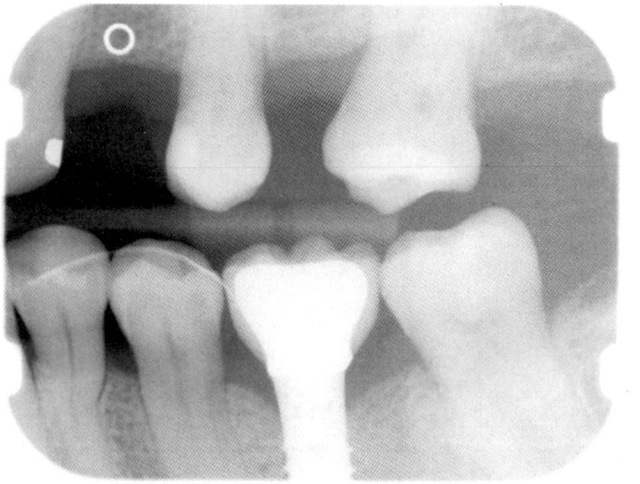

Fig 32-42 A dental implant is placed in the area of the mandibular left first molar.

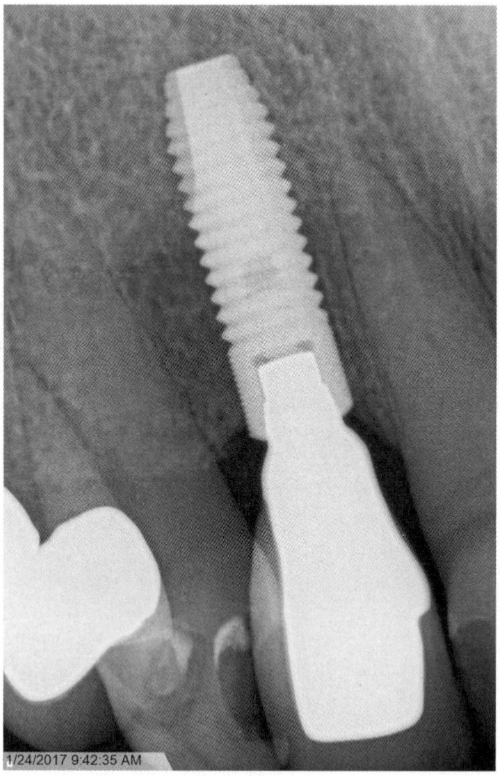

Fig 32-41 A dental implant is placed in the area of the maxillary lateral incisor.

Jewelry

Earrings. Earrings most often appear on extraoral images. Metal earrings appear as dense radiopacities on a dental image; the size and shape of the radiopacity correspond to the size and shape of the earring (Figures 32-48 and 32-49). Plastic earrings with metallic posts and backings or metal clips can also be seen on dental images; the metallic portions appear as radiopacities. A radiodense object, such as a metal earring, causes an artifact, known as a ghost image, on panoramic images (see Chapter 25). Ghost images can obscure important information about teeth and bones and render the image nondiagnostic.

Necklace. A necklace may also appear on an extraoral image as a radiopacity that corresponds in shape and size to the jewelry (Figure 32-50).

Nose Jewelry. Nose jewelry (small studs or hoop earrings worn on the nose) may be seen on extraoral as well as intraoral images (e.g., maxillary anterior periapical images). This type of jewelry appears as a radiopacity on a dental image and corresponds in size and shape to the object it represents (Figure 32-51).

Oral Piercings. Piercings of the tongue, lip, or cheek may be encountered during radiographic procedures. As with other metallic appliances, it is recommended to remove jewelry if possible prior to exposures. Similar to nose jewelry, oral piercings appear radiopaque and resemble the size and shape of the metal they represent (Figure 32-52).

Eyeglasses

Eyeglasses may be seen on extraoral and intraoral images. Most eyeglasses have some metal components in their frames. The metal portion of the frames appears as a radiopacity on a dental image (Figure 32-53).

Miscellaneous Objects

Napkin Chain. The napkin chain, similar to a necklace, may be seen on an extraoral image. If the napkin chain is in the path of the x-ray beam, a radiopacity resembling the napkin chain will be seen on the image.

Hearing Aids. A hearing aid is a small device that fits in or on the ear and is worn by a person who has impaired hearing to amplify

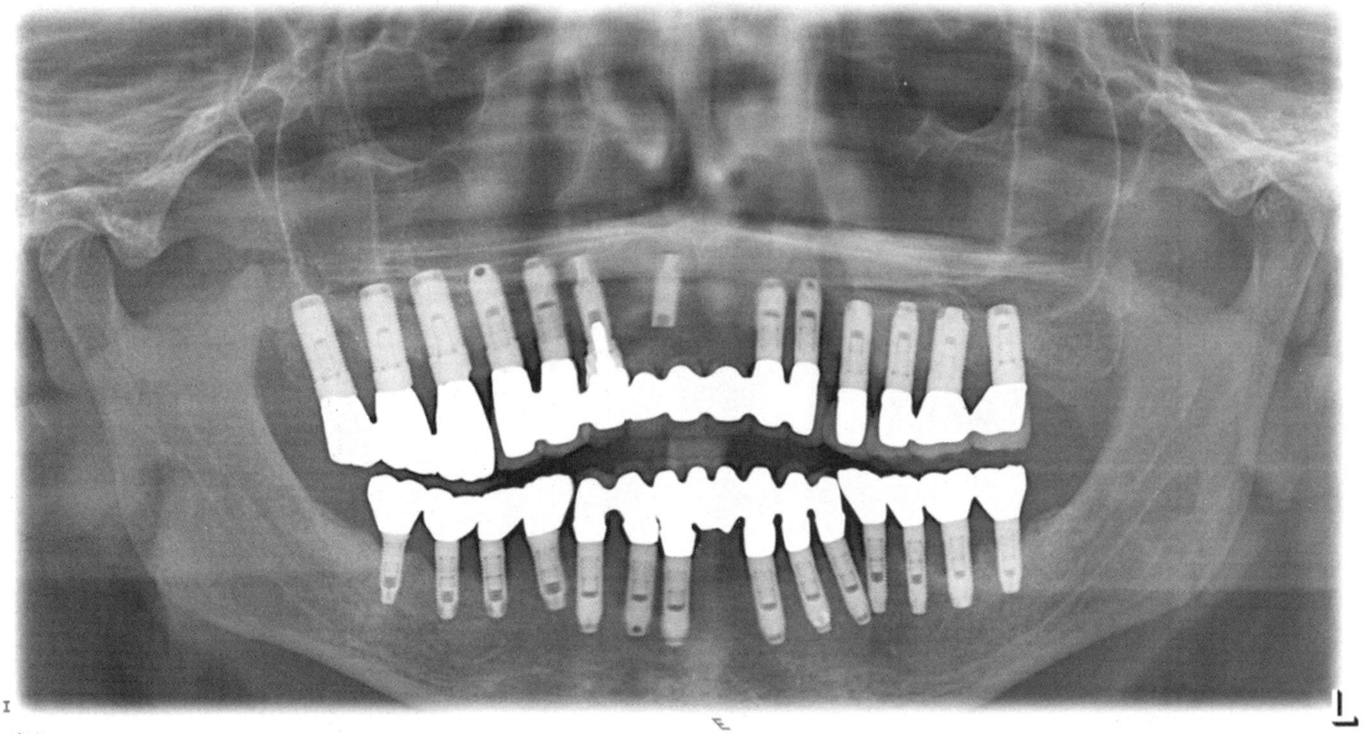

Fig 32-43 Dental implants are seen in both maxillary and mandibular arches, replacing all natural teeth. (Courtesy Timothy W. Godsey, DDS, MS, Chapel Hill Periodontics and Implants, Chapel Hill, NC.)

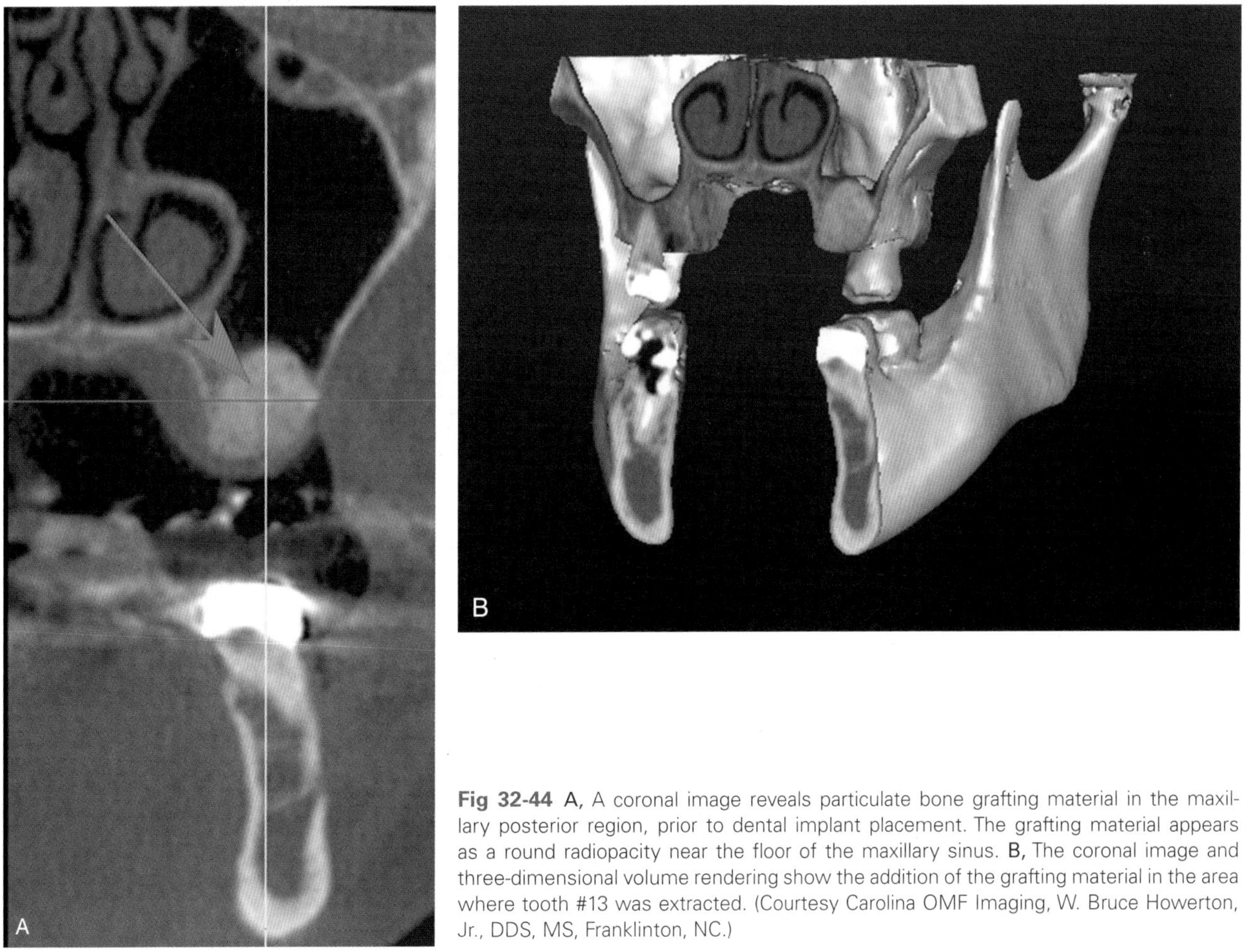

Fig 32-44 A, A coronal image reveals particulate bone grafting material in the maxillary posterior region, prior to dental implant placement. The grafting material appears as a round radiopacity near the floor of the maxillary sinus. B, The coronal image and three-dimensional volume rendering show the addition of the grafting material in the area where tooth #13 was extracted. (Courtesy Carolina OMF Imaging, W. Bruce Howerton, Jr., DDS, MS, Franklinton, NC.)

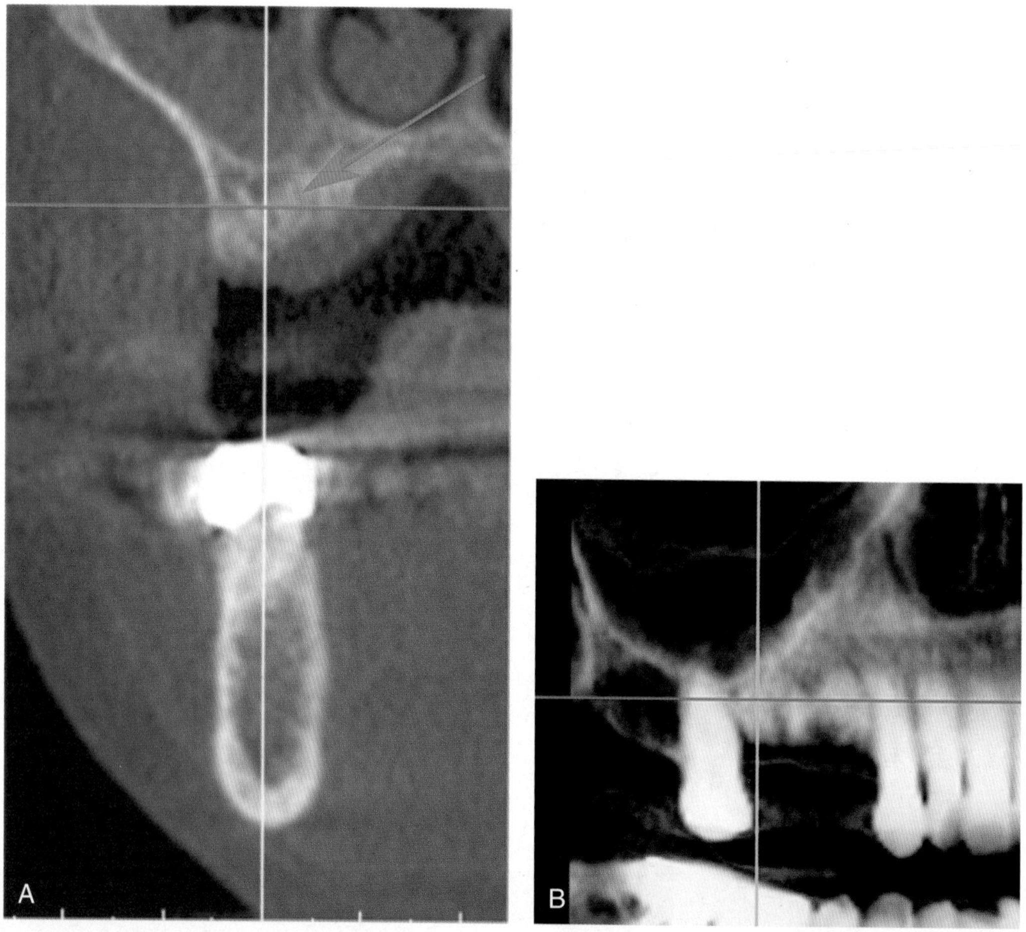

Fig 32-45 A, A coronal view reveals bone grafting material placed in the maxillary right quadrant prior to implant placement. B, A section of a panoramic image reveals the radiopaque grafting material in the areas where teeth #4 and #5 were extracted. (Courtesy Carolina OMF Imaging, W. Bruce Howerton, Jr., DDS, MS, Franklinton, NC.)

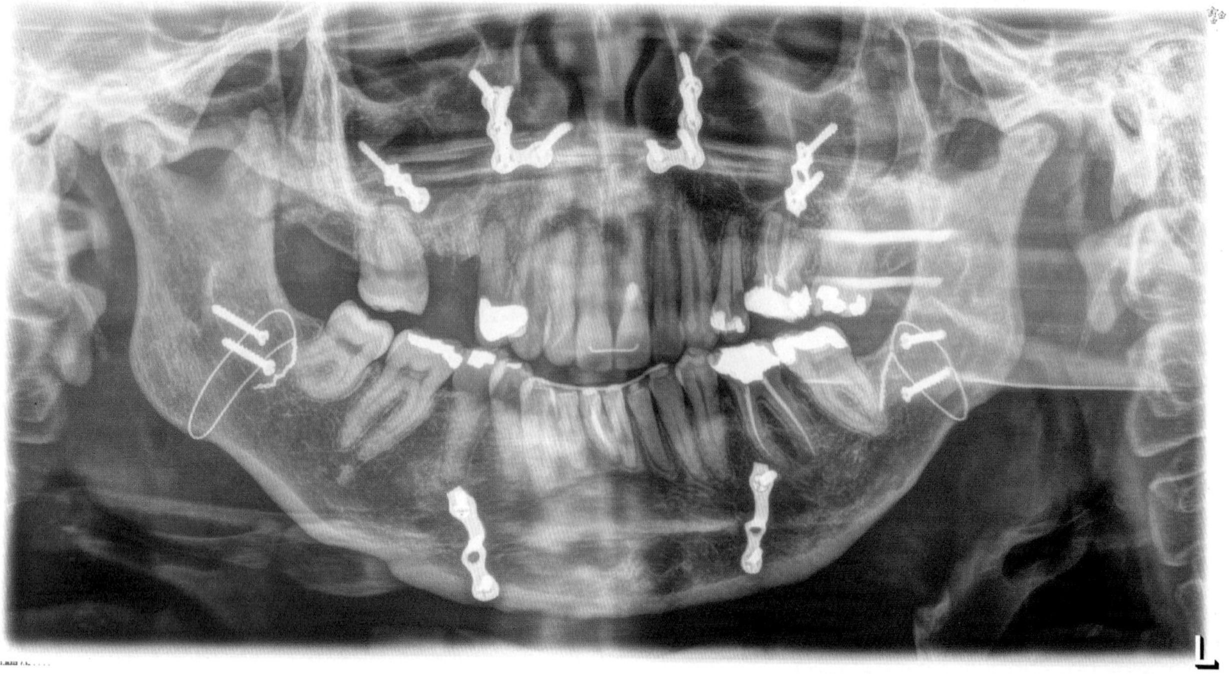

Fig 32-46 Suture wires, screws, and stabilizing metal plates seen on a panoramic image.

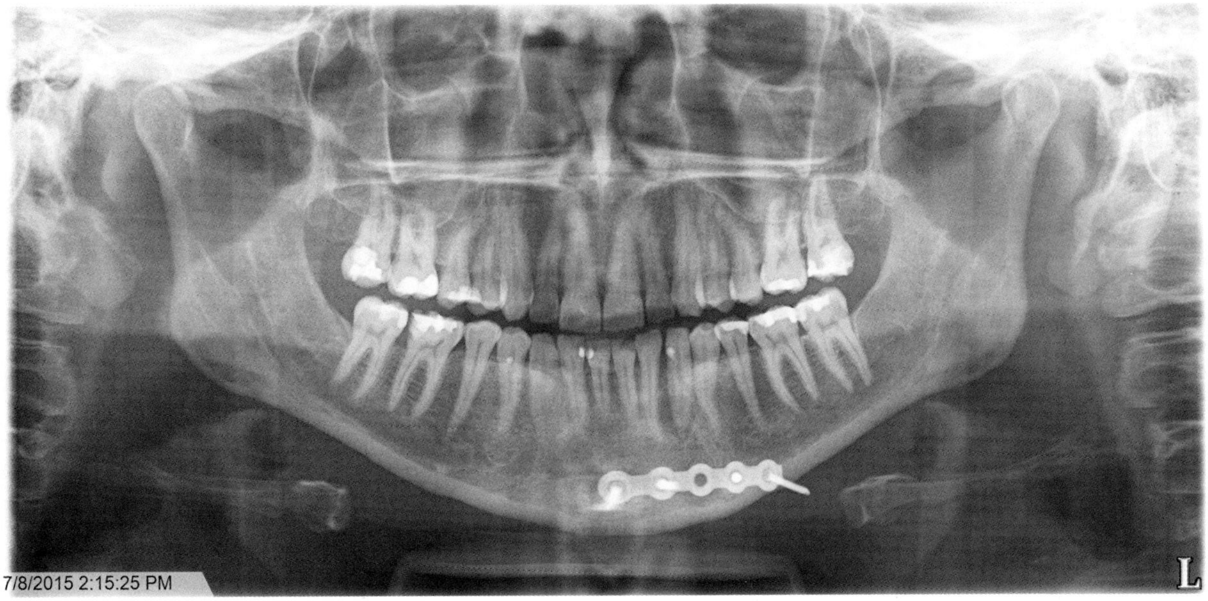

Fig 32-47 Metal plate and screws seen on a panoramic image.

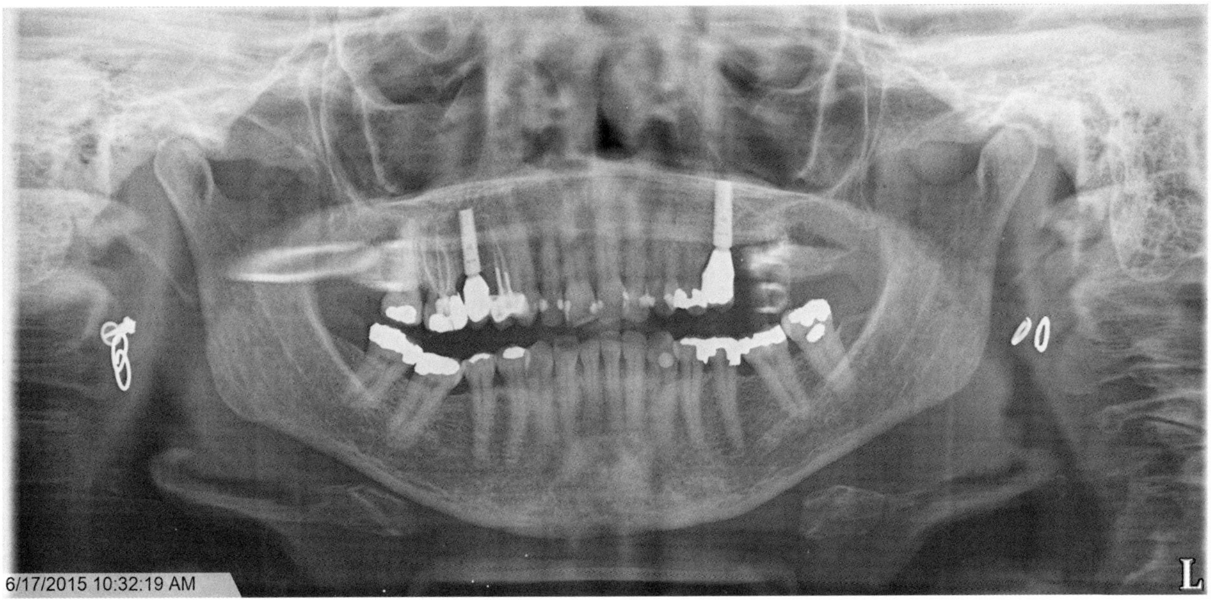

Fig 32-48 Earrings and ghost images seen on a panoramic image.

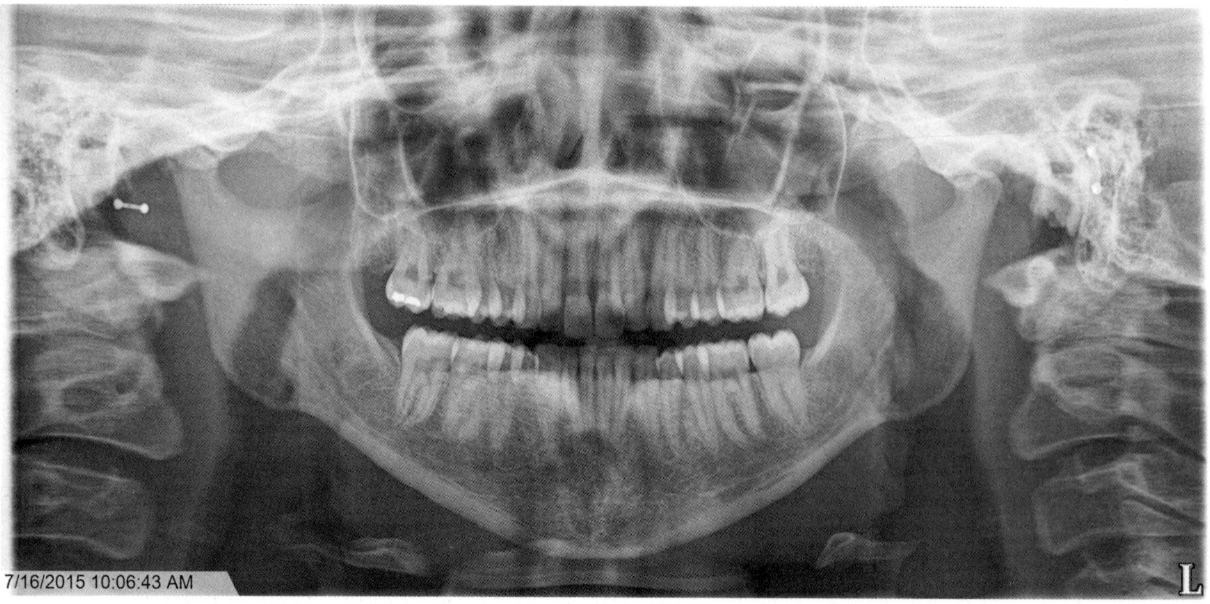

Fig 32-49 Tragus piercings and ghost images seen on a panoramic image.

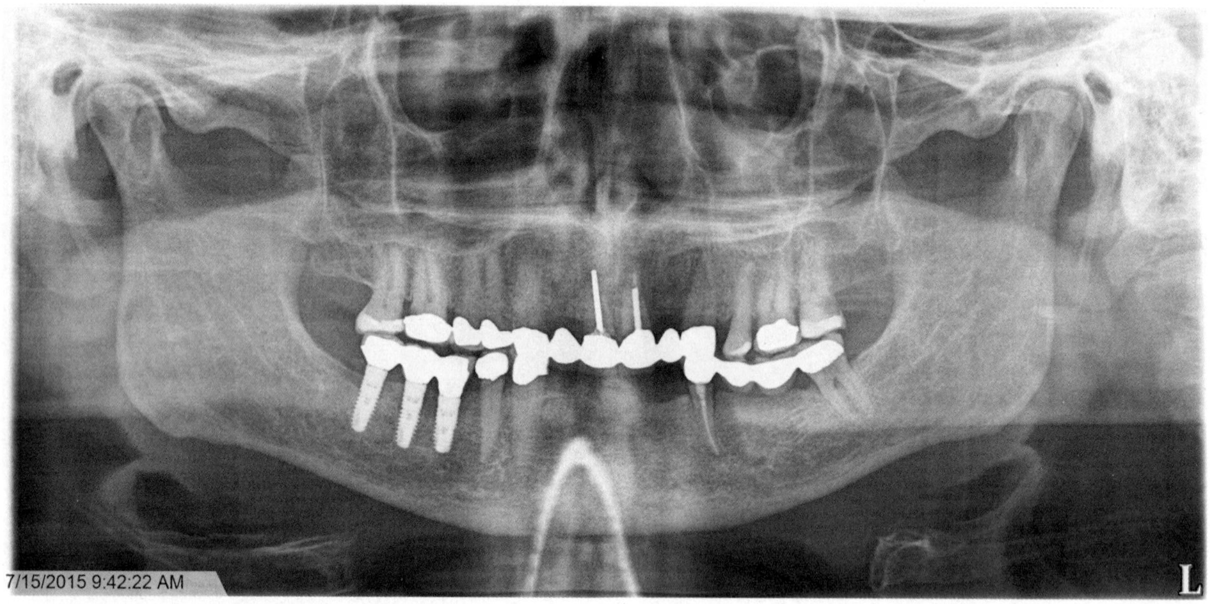

Fig 32-50 A metallic necklace appearing as a radiopaque loop in the region of the mandible.

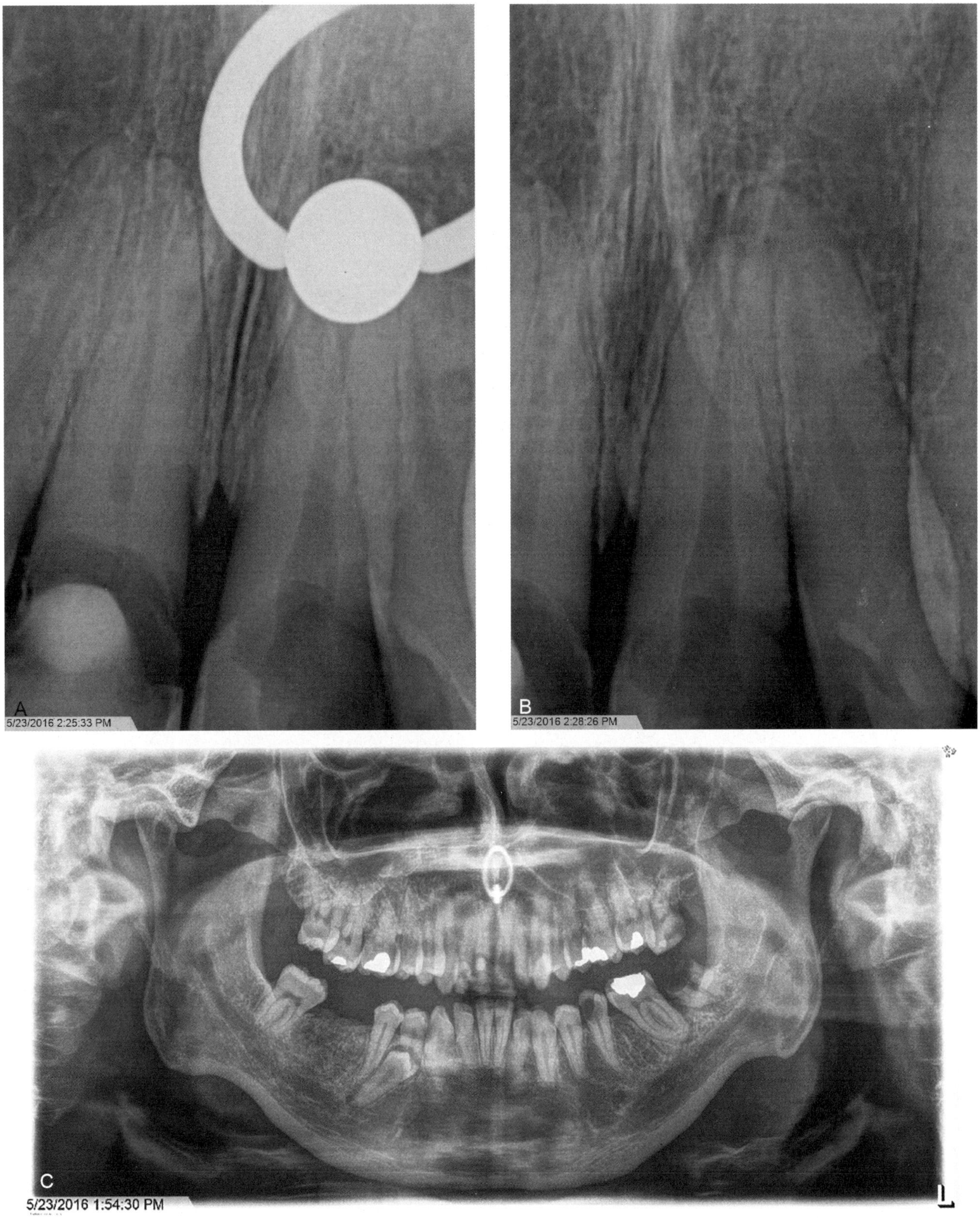

Fig 32-51 **A,** A maxillary anterior periapical image exposed with nose jewelry in place. **B,** The same exposure with the jewelry removed. **C,** A panoramic image of nose jewelry.

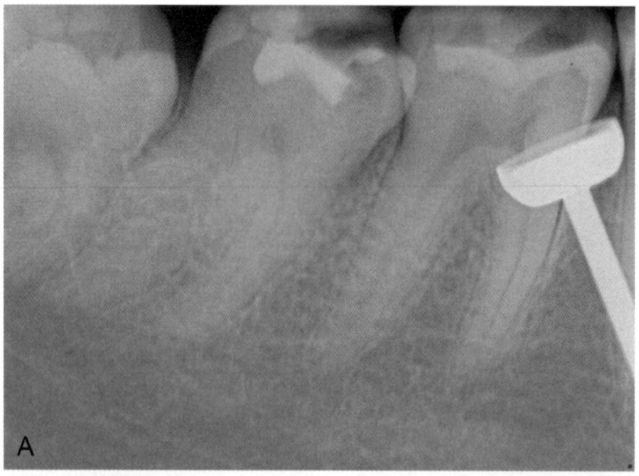

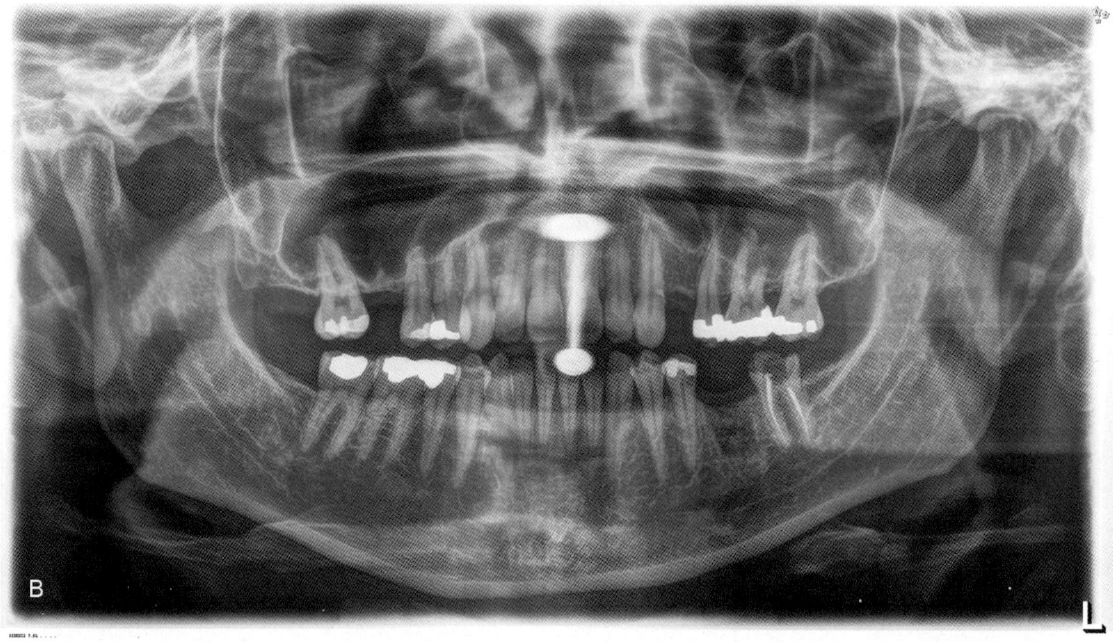

Fig 32-52 A, A mandibular posterior periapical image revealing an oral piercing. B, A panoramic image of tongue jewelry.

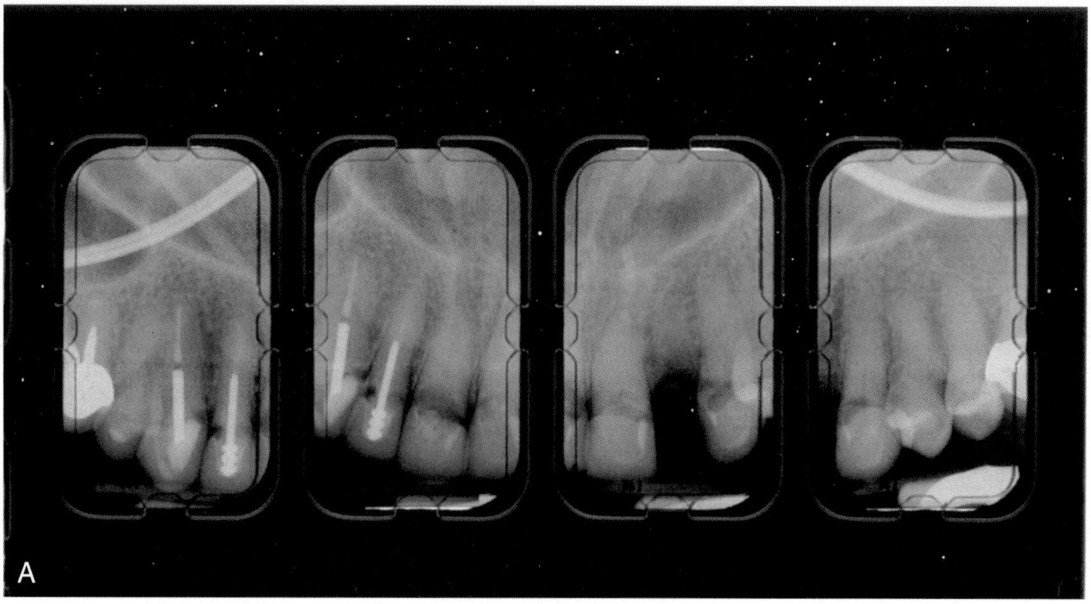

Fig 32-53 A, The rim of eyeglasses appear on both maxillary canine periapical images. B, The metal framework of the sides of eyeglasses seen on a panoramic image.

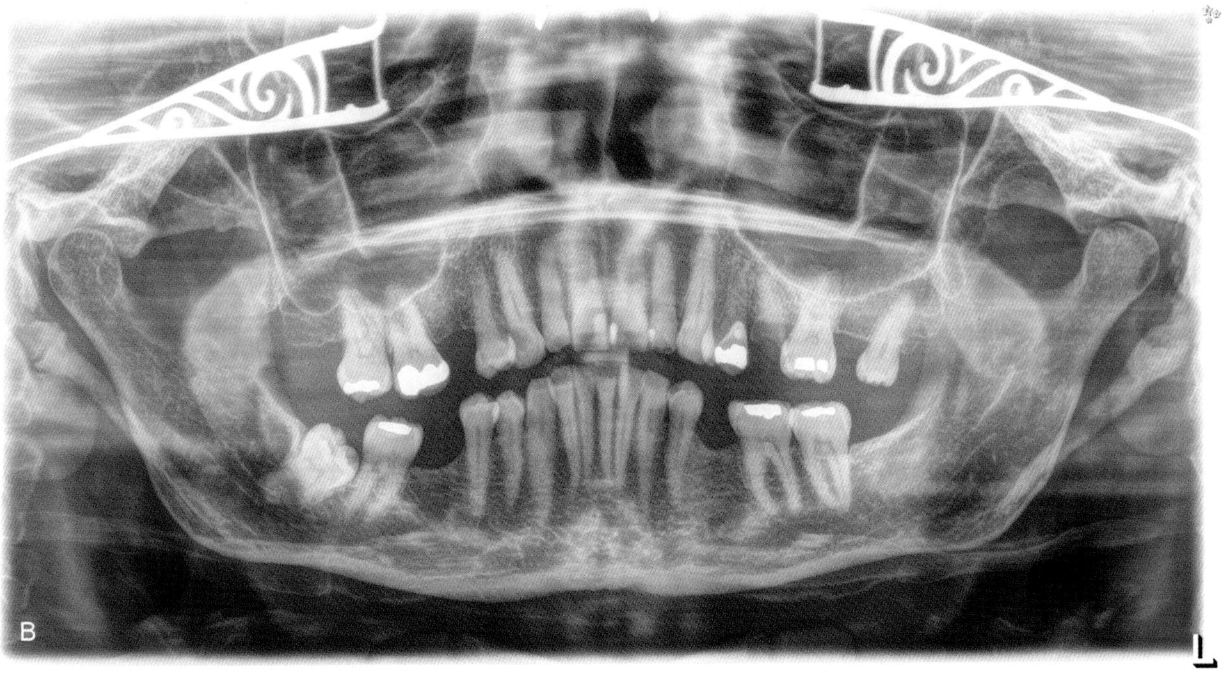

Fig 32-53 (Continued).

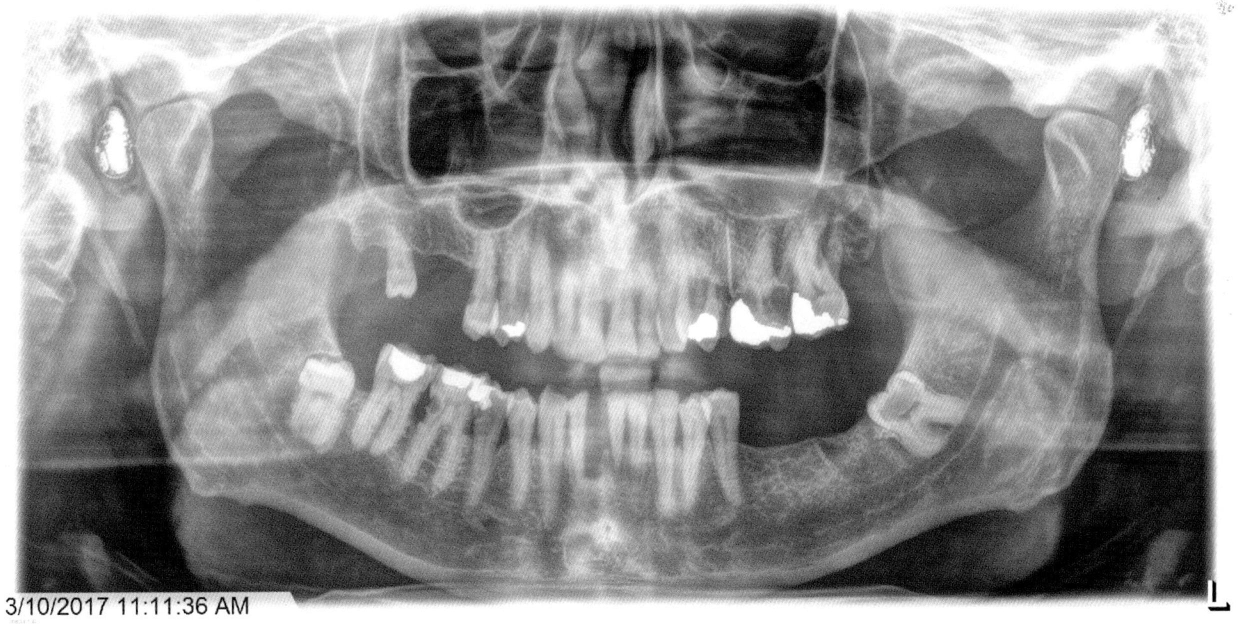

Fig 32-54 Panoramic image of a patient who did not remove hearing aids during exposure.

sound. If the hearing aid has any metal components, it should be removed prior to the exposure of extraoral images. The dental radiographer should provide imaging instructions to the patient while the hearing aid is in place, and then ask the patient to remove the hearing aid for the exposure. Figure 32-54 is a panoramic image of a patient whose hearing aids were left in during exposure.

Shrapnel. Although not seen often, shrapnel or small metal fragments that scatter outward from an exploding device may be viewed on dental images. Figure 32-55 reveals a patient who sustained a gunshot injury that resulted in embedded metal fragments in the oral and maxillofacial region. These fragments became embedded in both hard and soft tissue and, because the shrapnel is composed of metal, appear radiopaque.

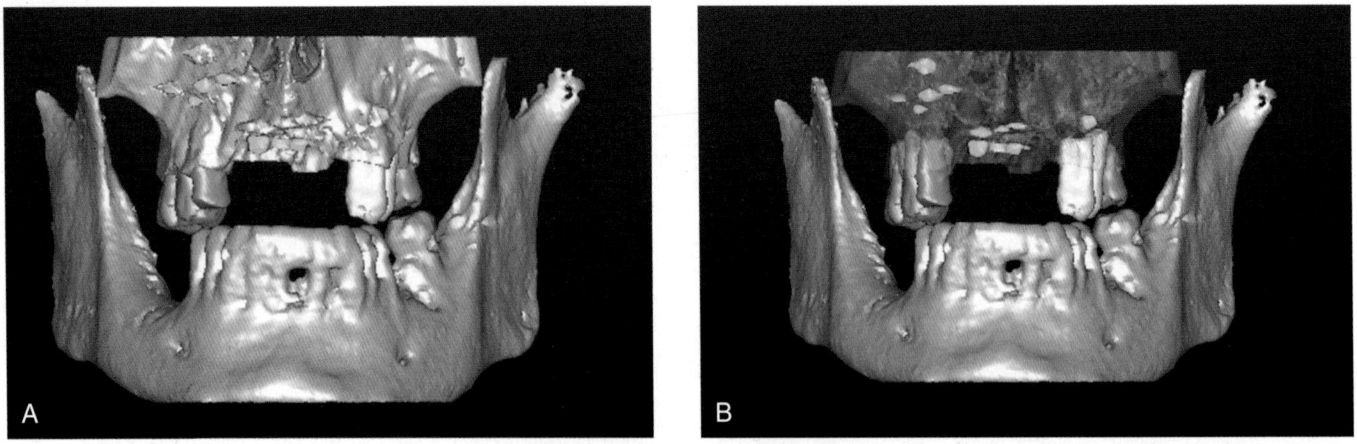

Fig 32-55 **A,** Shrapnel as indicated in green is seen scattered throughout the hard and soft tissues of a maxilla on this three-dimensional volume rendering. **B,** The same patient with a transparent maxilla. (Courtesy Carolina OMF Imaging, W. Bruce Howerton, Jr., DDS, MS, Franklinton, NC.)

SUMMARY

- Dental restorations, dental materials, and miscellaneous objects can be seen and evaluated on extraoral and intraoral images.
- The appearances of restorations, materials, and miscellaneous objects vary, depending on material composition, density, and thickness. The appearances of restorations and materials can range from radiopaque to radiolucent.
- Some restorations and objects are easily identified on dental images; others may require additional clinical information. Dental images play an important role in the evaluation of dental restorations, materials, and objects.
- It is important that the dental professional interpret dental images with the patient present. Without the patient present, important clinical information is not available.
- With the patient present, if a question arises about what is seen on a dental image, a clinical examination can provide additional information or verify what is seen.

BIBLIOGRAPHY

Frommer HH, Stabulas-Savage JJ: Film mounting and radiographic anatomy. In Radiology for the dental professional, ed 9, St Louis, 2011, Mosby.

Heymann HO, Swift EJ, Ritter AV: Sturdevant's art and science of operative dentistry, ed 6, St Louis, 2013, Mosby.

Langlais RP: Exercises in oral radiology and interpretation, ed 4, St Louis, 2004, Saunders.

Mallya SM, Lam EWN: Radiographic anatomy. In White and Pharoah's Oral radiology: principles and interpretation, ed 8, St. Louis, 2019, Elsevier.

White SC, Pharoah MJ: Implants. In Oral radiology: principles and interpretation, ed 7, St Louis, 2014, Mosby.

QUIZ QUESTIONS

Identification

1. Identify the restorative material used in the pulp canal of the maxillary first molar (Figure 32-56).

____

____

2. Identify the restorative material seen in each tooth of this dental image (Figure 32-57).

____

____

3. Identify the restorative material used to fabricate this bridge (Figure 32-58).

____

____

4. Identify the restorative material used in the maxillary anterior region (Figure 32-59).

____

____

5. Identify the restoration present in the area of the mandibular first molar (Figure 32-60).

____

____

6. Identify the large radiopacity seen in the posterior mandible (Figure 32-61).

____

____

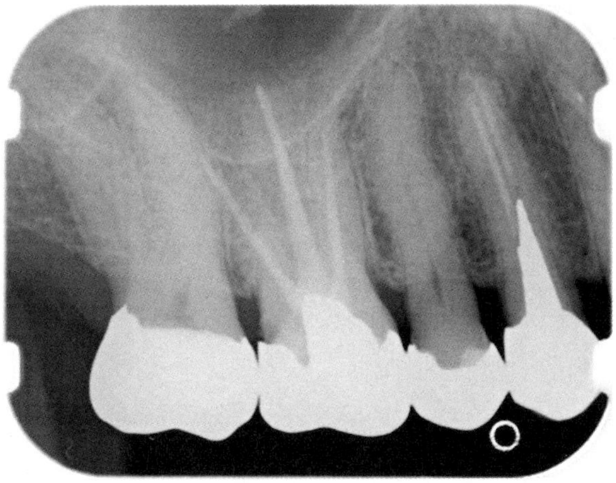

Fig 32-56

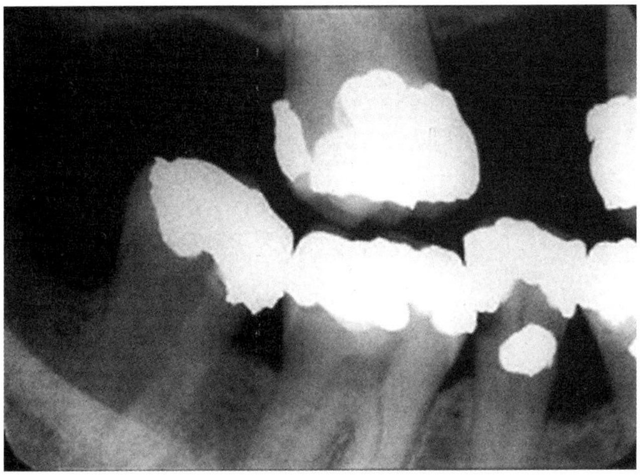

Fig 32-57

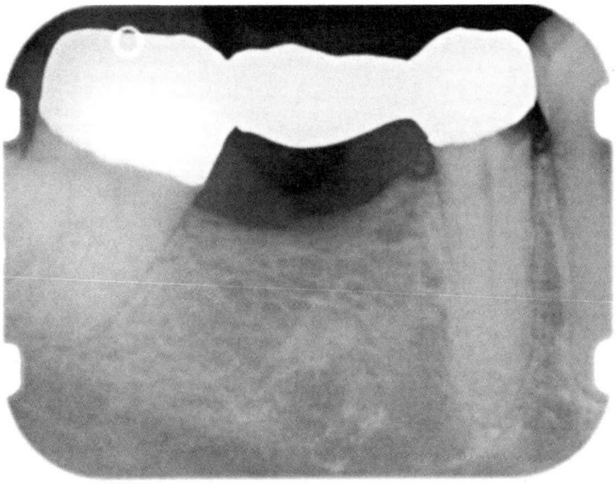

Fig 32-58

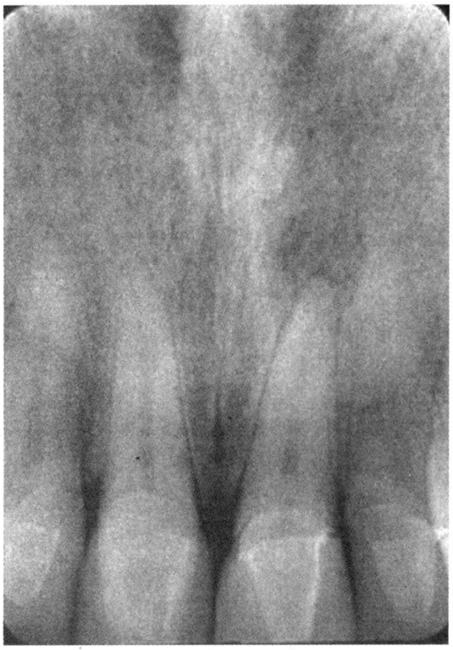

Fig 32-59

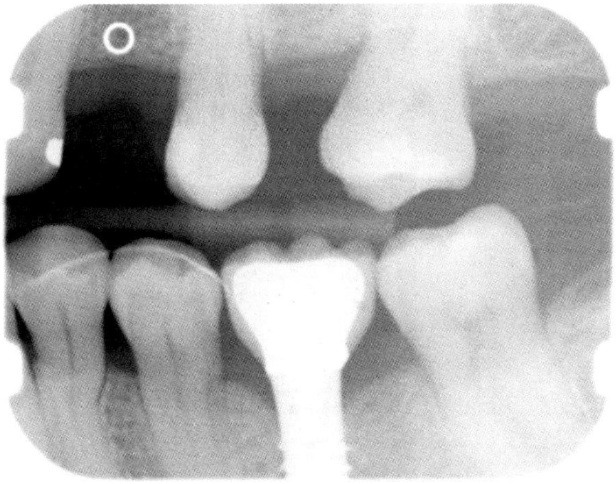

Fig 32-60

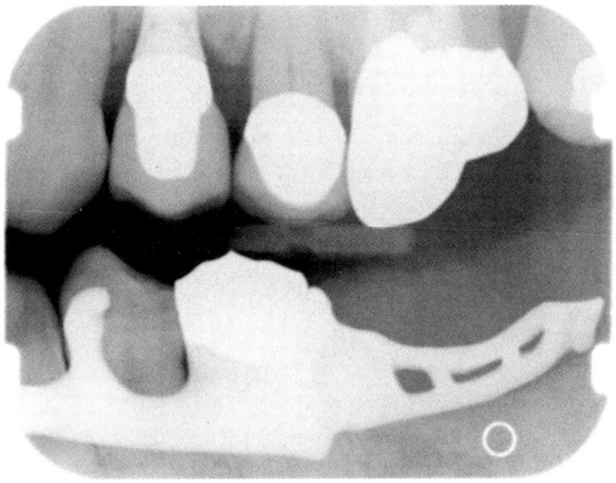

Fig 32-61

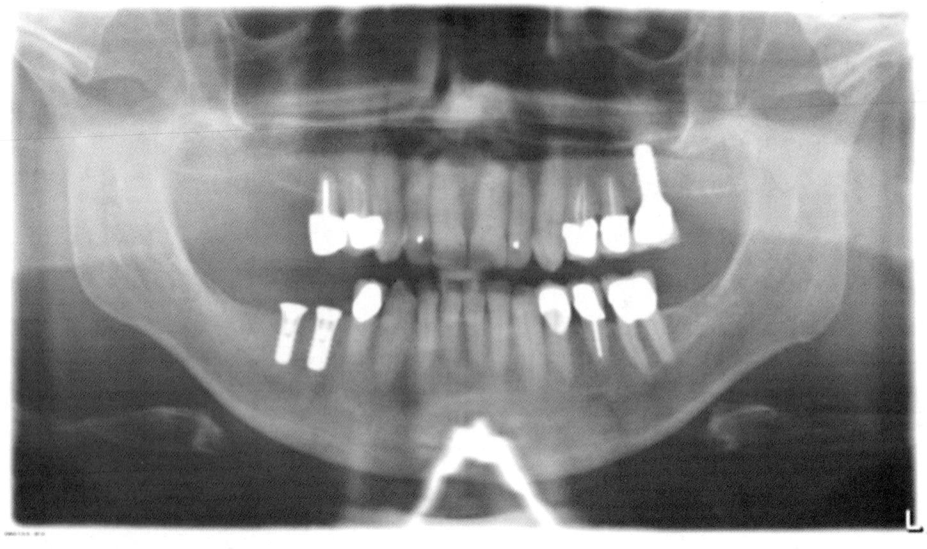

Fig 32-62

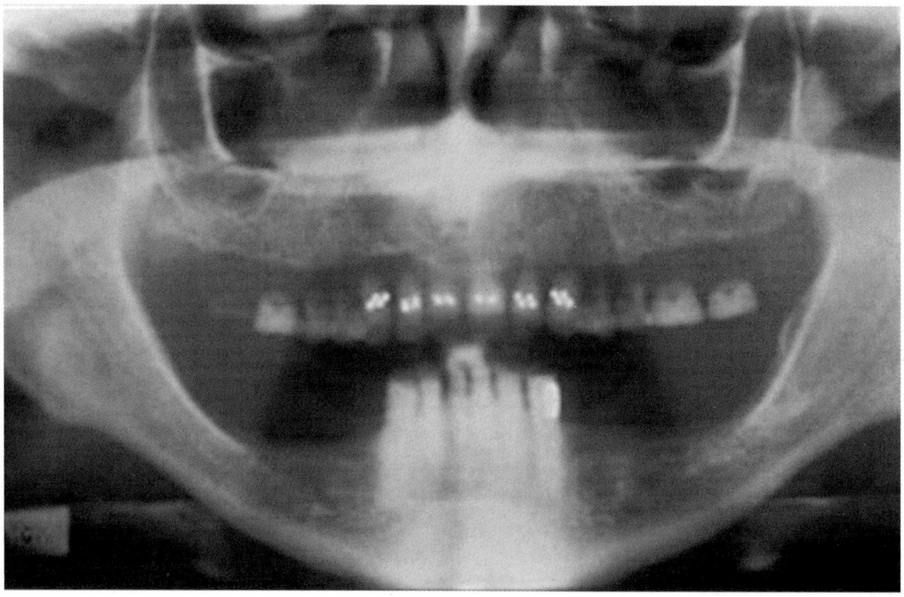

Fig 32-63

7. Identify the radiopacity seen in the middle of this panoramic image obscuring the border of the mandible (Figure 32-62).

____

____

8. Explain why the maxillary teeth in this dental image appear to be "floating" (Figure 32-63).
9. Identify at least six different types of restorative materials seen in this panoramic image (Figure 32-64).
10. Identify the dental materials seen in the maxilla; identify the radiopaque framework material seen on the mandible on this panoramic image (Figure 32-65).

____ **11.** Rank the following restorative materials from most radiopaque (1) to least radiopaque or radiolucent (4).

____ gutta percha

____ acrylic restorations

____ amalgam

____ stainless steel crown

Multiple Choice

____ **12.** Which restorative materials appear equally radiopaque on a dental image?

a. gold crowns and amalgam

b. gold crowns and porcelain crowns

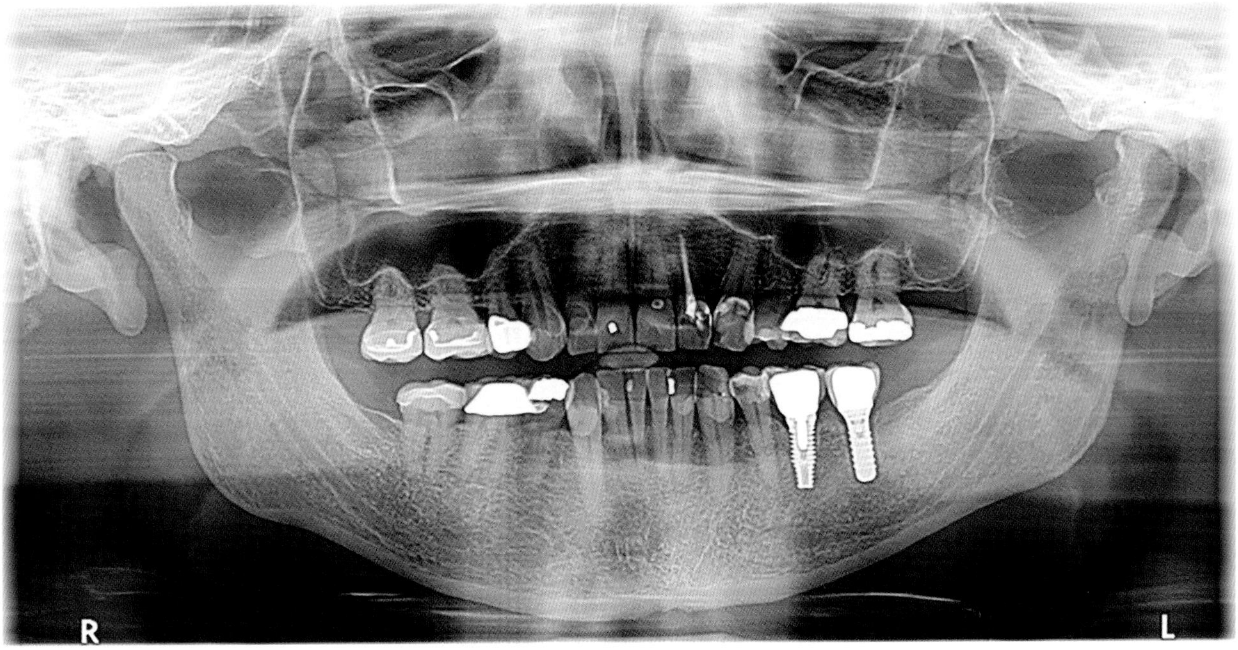

Fig 32-64 (Courtesy Carolina OMF Imaging, W. Bruce Howerton, Jr., DDS, MS, Franklinton, NC.)

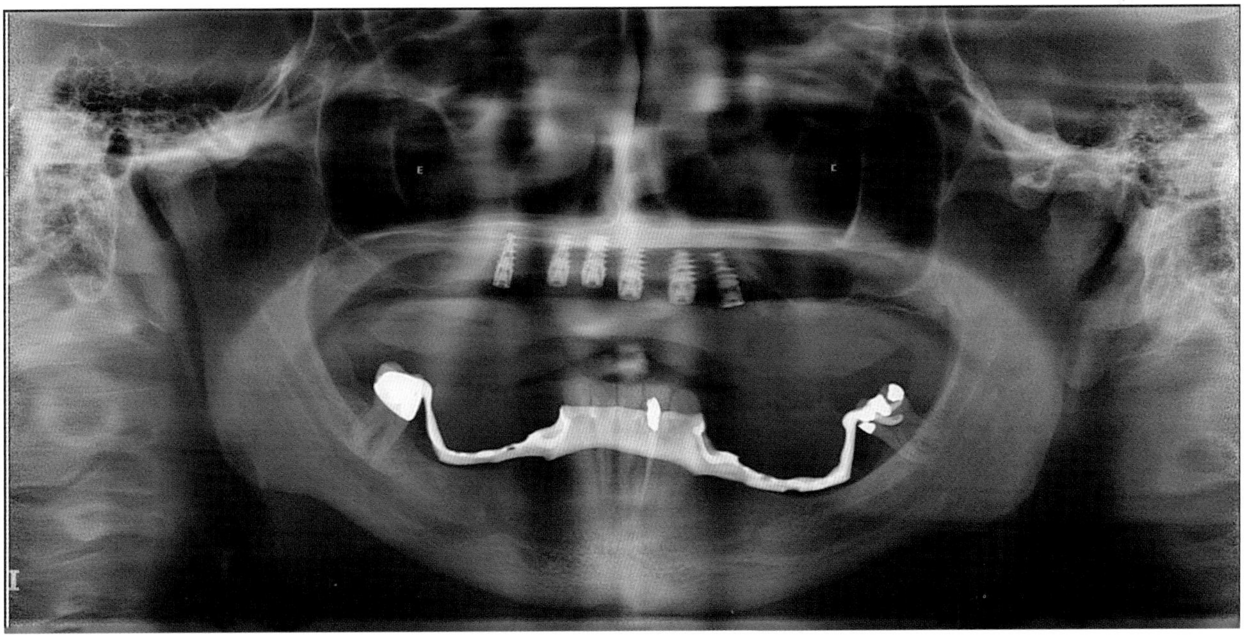

Fig 32-65

c. gutta percha and silver points
d. gold crowns and stainless steel crowns

____ 13. Which restorative material is most radiopaque?
a. amalgam
b. porcelain
c. composite
d. acrylic

____ 14. Which restorative material is least radiopaque?
a. amalgam
b. porcelain
c. stainless steel
d. acrylic

____ 15. Which describes how gold can be distinguished from amalgam on a dental image?
a. Gold appears more radiopaque than amalgam.
b. Gold appears more radiolucent than amalgam.
c. Gold margins are smooth and regular.
d. Amalgam margins are smooth and regular.

SHORT ANSWER

16. Describe the difference between a gold crown and a stainless steel crown as viewed on a dental image.

____

____

17. Describe the difference between gutta percha and silver points as viewed on a dental image.

____

____

18. Discuss the importance of interpreting dental images with the patient present.

____

____

33

Interpretation of Dental Caries

LEARNING OBJECTIVES

After completion of this chapter, the student will be able to do the following:

1. Define the key terms associated with the interpretation of dental caries.
2. Describe dental caries.
3. In relation to the detection of dental caries:
   - Explain why caries appears radiolucent on a dental image.
   - Discuss the importance of dental caries in relation to the clinical examination.
   - Discuss the importance of dental caries in relation to the dental image examination.
4. Discuss interpretation tips for evaluating caries on a dental image.
5. Discuss the factors that may influence the image interpretation of dental caries.
6. In relation to classifying caries on dental images:
   - Detail the classification of caries on dental images.
   - On a dental image, identify and describe the appearance of the following: incipient, moderate, advanced, and severe interproximal caries.
   - On a dental image, identify and describe the appearance of the following: incipient, moderate, and severe occlusal caries.
   - On a dental image, identify and describe the appearance of the following: buccal, lingual, root surface, recurrent, and rampant caries.
7. On a dental image, identify conditions that may be confused with dental caries including cervical burnout, restorative materials, attrition, and abrasion.

In the practice of dentistry, caries is one of the most frequent reasons for prescribing and exposing dental images. The dental radiographer must be confident about the identification and recognition of caries as viewed on a dental image. An overview of the interpretation of caries is presented in this chapter. Detailed information about dental caries, however, is beyond the scope of this text. The purpose of this chapter is to describe dental caries and its detection. In addition, interpretation tips and factors that influence caries interpretation are presented, and an introduction to the classification of caries on dental images is included.

DESCRIPTION OF CARIES

Dental caries, or tooth decay, is the localized destruction of teeth by microorganisms. Normal mineralized tooth structure (enamel, dentin, cementum) is altered and destroyed by dental caries. The term *caries* comes from the Latin *cariosus,* which means "rottenness" and literally refers to the "rotting of the teeth." A carious lesion, or an area of tooth decay, is often referred to as a cavity. In dentistry, the term *cavity* refers to a cavitation, or hole, in a tooth that is the result of the caries process (Figure 33-1).

DETECTION OF CARIES

To detect dental caries, both a careful clinical examination and interpretation are necessary. A dental examination for caries cannot be considered complete without dental images. Dental images enable the dental professional to identify carious lesions that are not visible clinically. In addition, dental images allow the dental professional to evaluate the extent and severity of carious lesions.

Clinical Examination

Some carious lesions can be detected by simply looking into the mouth, and some cannot. All teeth must be examined clinically for dental caries using a mirror and an explorer. The mirror can be used to reflect light, to allow indirect vision, and to retract the tongue. The explorer can be used as a tactile device to detect the presence of any changes in consistency (e.g., "catches" or "tug-back") in the pits, grooves, and fissures of teeth. Air is also helpful to dry tooth surfaces to allow a careful examination of the teeth.

A number of color changes may be seen in teeth with dental caries. Occlusal surfaces may show dark staining in the fissures, pits, and grooves or may show an obvious cavitation. Smooth surfaces may exhibit a chalky white spot, or opacity, indicating demineralization. An interproximal ridge overlying a carious lesion may also appear discolored.

Although some teeth with dental caries exhibit a discolored area or a cavitation (Figure 33-2), others have no visible changes. In addition, caries that occurs between teeth may be difficult or impossible to detect clinically. In such cases, dental images play an important role. It is important to remember that a clinical examination alone is not adequate to detect dental caries; the clinical examination must be used in conjunction with the exposure of dental images.

Dental Image Examination

Dental images are useful in the detection of caries because of the nature of the caries disease process. Demineralization and destruction of hard tooth structures result in loss of tooth density in the area of the lesion. Decreased density allows greater penetration of x-rays in the carious area, so the carious lesion appears radiolucent (dark or black) on a dental image. Dental caries is the most frequently encountered radiolucent lesion identified on dental images.

The bite-wing is the image of choice for the evaluation of caries because it provides the dental professional with diagnostic information that cannot be obtained from any other source. A periapical image using the paralleling technique can also be used for the evaluation of dental caries (Figure 33-3).

INTERPRETATION OF CARIES ON DENTAL IMAGES

To recognize caries on a dental image, the dental professional must be confident in the use of interpretation methods and must be able to identify factors that influence the interpretation of caries.

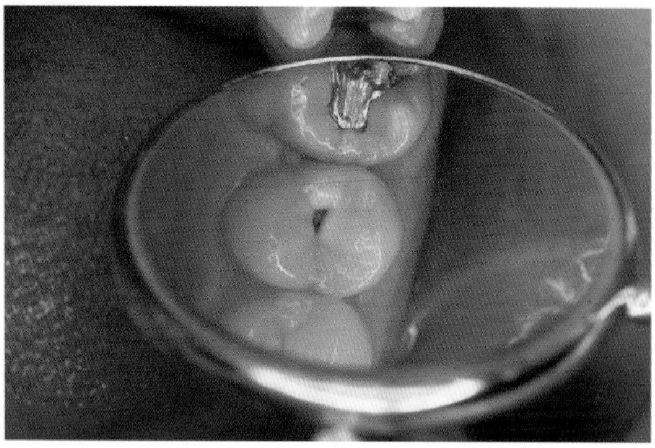

Fig 33-1 A cavitation is a hole in the tooth that results from the carious process.

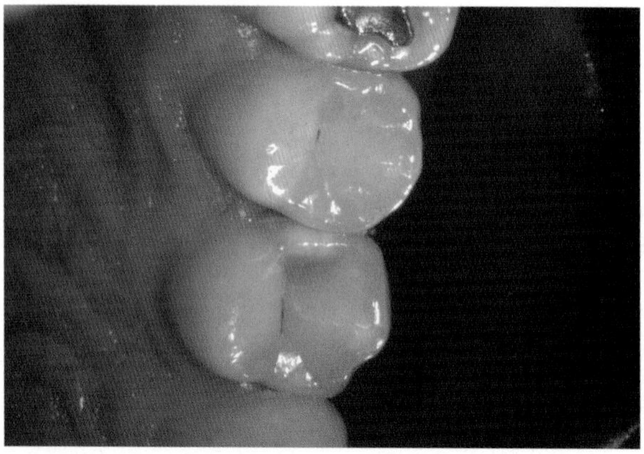

Fig 33-2 Discoloration on the mesial of the maxillary second premolar represents dental caries.

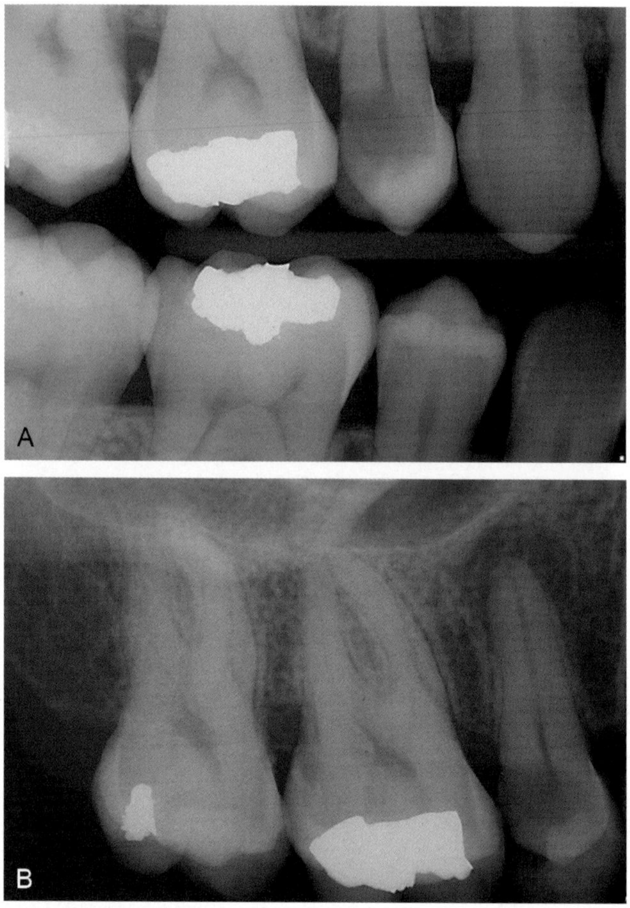

Fig 33-3 Dental caries appears on the distal surface of tooth #5 in both the (A) horizontal bite-wing and (B) periapical images.

Interpretation Tips

As reviewed in Chapter 11, proper mounting and viewing techniques are essential in the interpretation of dental images, especially the evaluation of dental caries. With digital images, all exposures should be properly displayed on the computer monitor before interpretation. Individual images may be enlarged to full screen to view in detail and determine the presence or absence of dental caries.

With film, all radiographs must be properly mounted before image interpretation. Mounted films should be viewed in a room with subdued lighting that is free of distractions. An illuminator or viewbox is required for accurate viewing and interpretation of images. If the screen of the viewbox is not completely covered by the mounted radiographs, the harsh light around must be masked to reduce glare and intensify the detail and contrast of the radiographic images. The use of a pocket-sized magnifying glass is helpful in evaluating the radiographic appearance of dental caries and can be used to detect slight changes in density and contrast in radiographic images. As discussed in Chapter 11, all dental images should be viewed in the presence of the patient.

Factors Influencing Caries Interpretation

A number of factors can influence the interpretation of dental caries on dental images. Images must be of diagnostic quality to allow accurate evaluation of dental caries. As described in Chapter 22, errors in technique may result in nondiagnostic images. For example, a bite-wing image used to detect dental caries must exhibit open contacts. Improper horizontal angulation causes overlapped contact areas and makes it impossible to identify dental caries in the interproximal regions.

As discussed in Chapter 22, errors in exposure may also result in nondiagnostic images. For example, a dental image used to detect dental caries must have proper contrast and density. Incorrect exposure factors result in images that are too dark or too light and thus useless in the detection of caries.

CLASSIFICATION OF CARIES ON DENTAL IMAGES

The appearance of caries on dental images can be classified according to the location of the caries on the tooth. Caries that involves interproximal, occlusal, buccal, lingual, or root surfaces may be seen on a dental image. In addition, recurrent and rampant caries may also be viewed on dental images.

Interproximal Caries

The term **interproximal** means "between two adjacent surfaces." Caries found between two teeth is termed **interproximal caries** (Figure 33-4). On a dental image, interproximal caries is typically seen at or just below (apical to) the contact point (Figure 33-5). This area is difficult, if not impossible, to examine clinically with an explorer.

As the caries progresses inward through the enamel of the tooth, it assumes a triangular configuration; the apex (or point) of the triangle

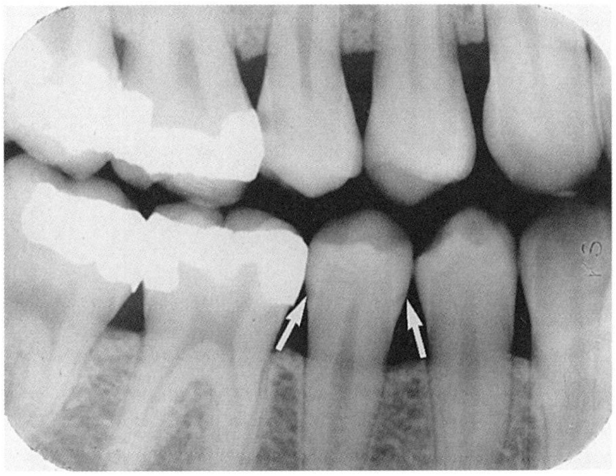

Fig 33-4 Interproximal caries found at or just below the contact area. From Haring JI, Lind LJ: Radiographic interpretation for the dental hygienist, Philadelphia, 1993, Saunders.

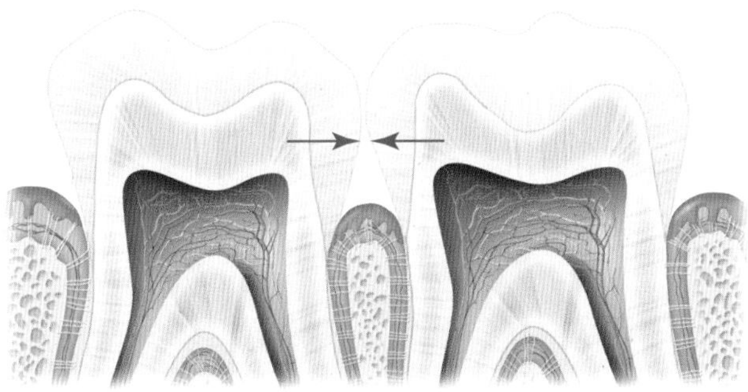

Fig 33-5 Caries found at or just below the contact area.

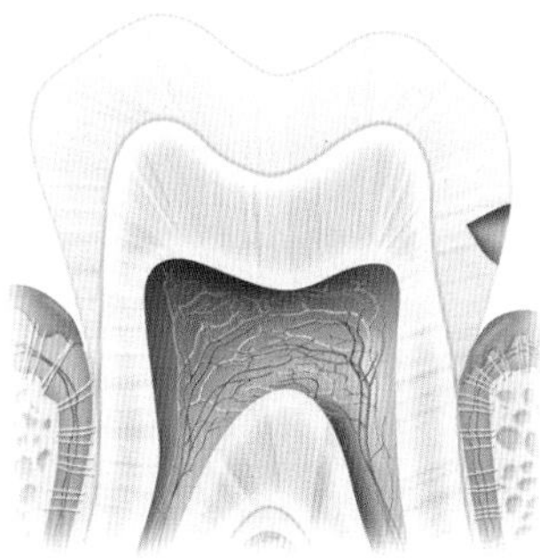

Fig 33-6 Caries confined to enamel, exhibiting a triangular configuration.

is seen at the dentino-enamel junction (DEJ) (Figure 33-6). As the caries reaches the DEJ, it spreads laterally and continues into dentin. Another triangular configuration is seen in dentin; this time the base of the triangle is along the DEJ, and the apex is pointed toward the pulp chamber (Figure 33-7).

Interproximal caries can be classified according to the depth of penetration of the lesion through enamel and dentin. Interproximal carious lesions can be classified as incipient, moderate, advanced, and severe.

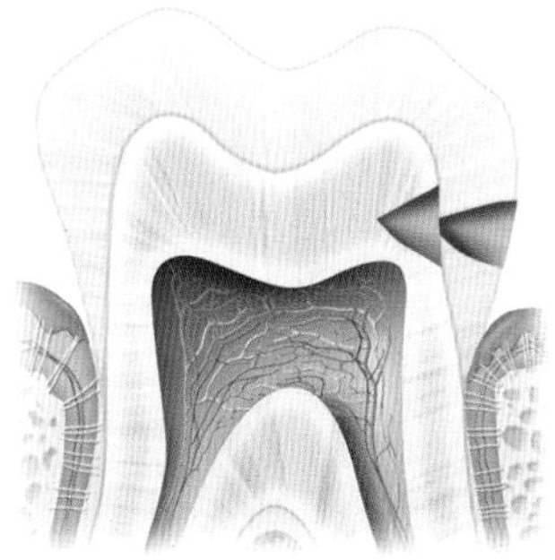

Fig 33-7 Caries that has reached the dentino-enamel junction (DEJ) and has spread along the DEJ, resulting in another triangular configuration.

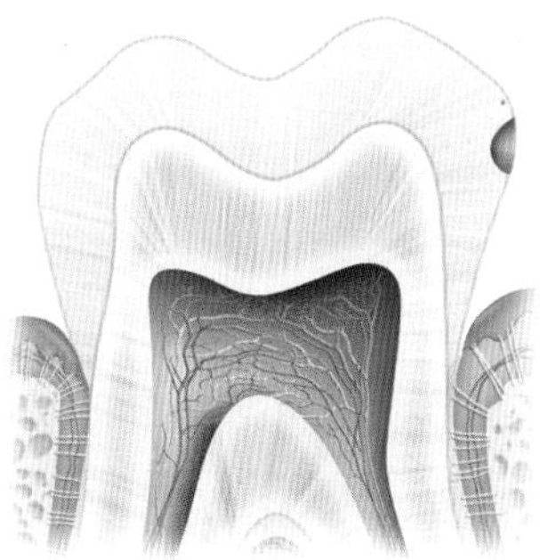

Fig 33-8 An incipient carious lesion, which extends less than halfway through enamel.

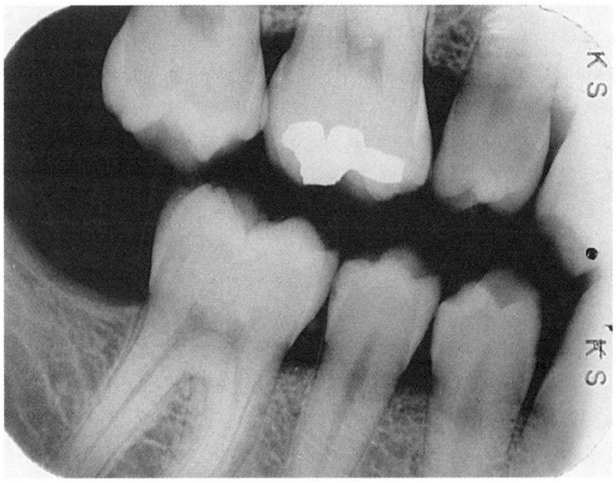

Fig 33-9 An incipient carious lesion on the distal surface of the mandibular second premolar. From Haring JI, Lind LJ: Radiographic interpretation for the dental hygienist, Philadelphia, 1993, Saunders.

Incipient Interproximal Caries. Incipient interproximal caries extends less than halfway through the thickness of enamel (Figures 33-8 and 33-9). The term incipient means "beginning to exist or appear." An incipient, or class I, lesion is seen *only* in enamel.

Moderate Interproximal Caries. Moderate interproximal caries extends more than halfway through the thickness of enamel but does not involve the DEJ (Figures 33-10 and 33-11). A moderate, or class II, lesion is seen *only* in enamel.

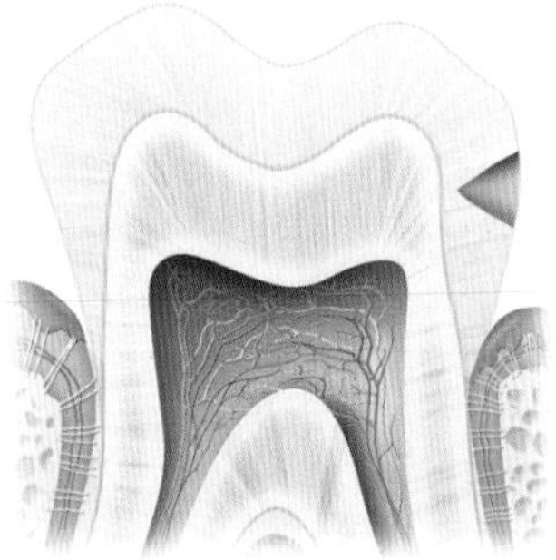

Fig 33-10 A moderate carious lesion, which extends more than halfway through enamel but does not involve the dentino-enamel junction (DEJ).

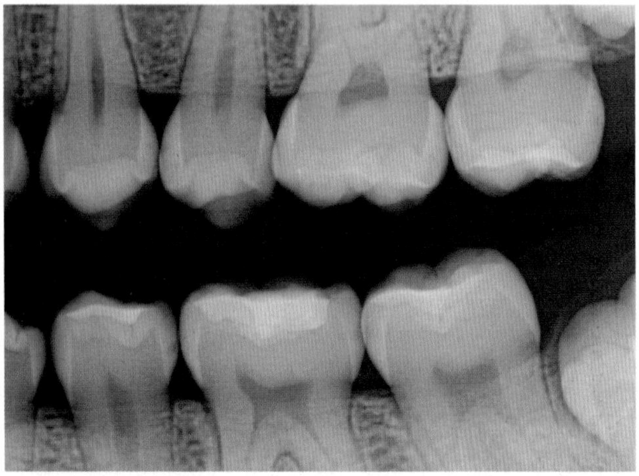

Fig 33-11 A moderate carious lesion on the distal surface of the mandibular second premolar.

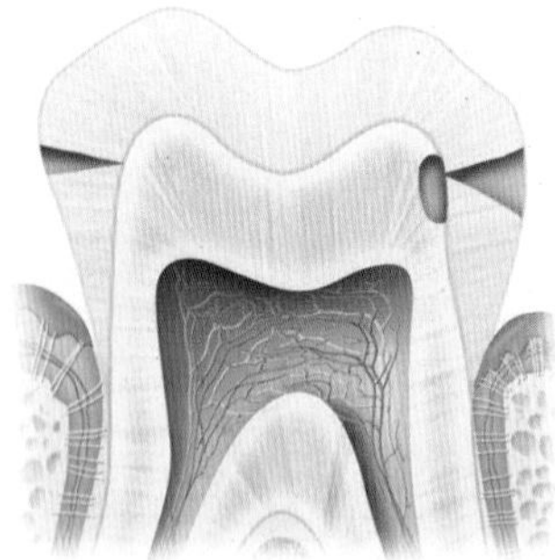

Fig 33-12 An advanced carious lesion, which extends through enamel and to or through the dentino-enamel junction (DEJ) but does not extend through dentin more than half the distance to the pulp chamber.

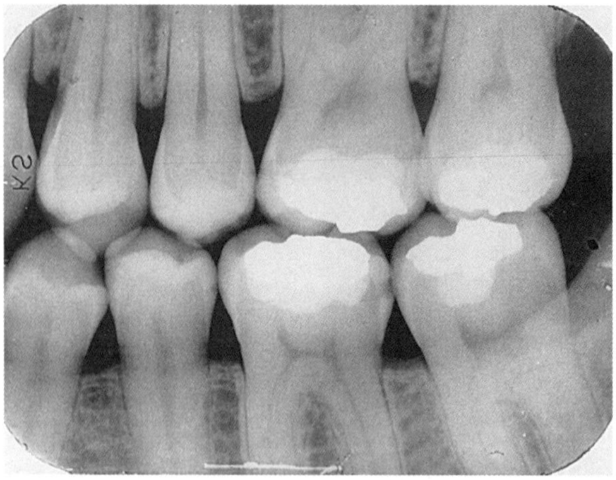

Fig 33-13 An advanced carious lesion, which extends through the dentino-enamel junction (DEJ) and into dentin, seen on the distal surface of the mandibular first molar. (From Haring JI, Lind LJ: Radiographic interpretation for the dental hygienist, Philadelphia, 1993, Saunders.)

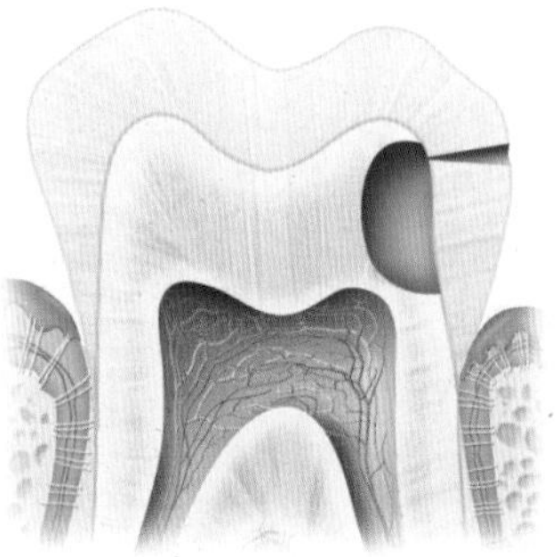

Fig 33-14 A severe carious lesion, which extends through enamel and dentin more than half the distance to the pulp chamber.

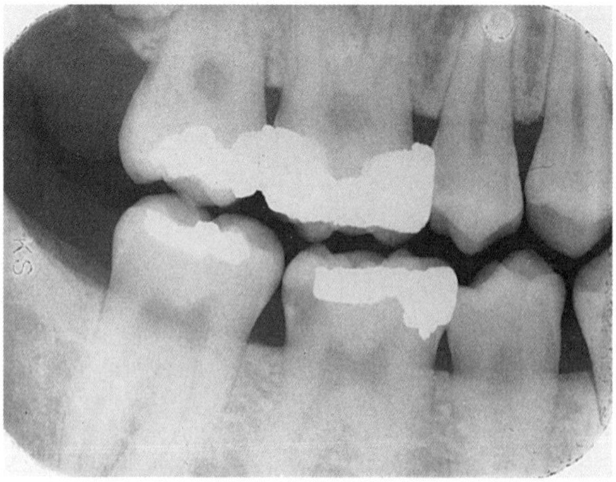

Fig 33-15 A severe carious lesion on the distal surface of the mandibular first molar. (From Haring JI, Lind LJ: Radiographic interpretation for the dental hygienist, Philadelphia, 1993, Saunders.)

Advanced Interproximal Caries. **Advanced interproximal caries** extends to or through the DEJ and into dentin but does not extend through dentin more than half the distance toward the pulp (Figures 33-12 and 33-13). An advanced, or class III, lesion affects *both* enamel and dentin.

Severe Interproximal Caries. **Severe interproximal caries** extends through enamel, through dentin, and more than half the distance toward the pulp (Figures 33-14 and 33-15). A severe, or class IV, lesion involves *both* enamel and dentin and may appear clinically as a cavitation in the tooth.

Occlusal Caries

The term occlusal refers to the chewing surfaces of teeth. Caries that involves the chewing surfaces of posterior teeth is termed occlusal caries. A thorough clinical examination with the mirror, explorer, and light is the method of choice for the detection of occlusal caries. Because of the superimposition of the dense buccal and lingual enamel cusps, early occlusal caries is difficult to see on a dental image. Consequently, occlusal caries is not seen on a dental image until involvement of the DEJ occurs. Occlusal carious lesions can be classified as incipient, moderate, or severe.

Incipient Occlusal Caries. Incipient occlusal caries cannot be seen on a dental image and must be detected clinically with an explorer.

Moderate Occlusal Caries. Moderate occlusal caries extends into dentin and appears as a very thin radiolucent line (Figures 33-16 and 33-17). The radiolucency is located under the enamel of the occlusal surface of the tooth. On a dental image, little, if any, change is noted in enamel.

Severe Occlusal Caries. Severe occlusal caries extends into dentin and appears as a large radiolucency (Figures 33-18 and 33-19). The radiolucency extends under the enamel of the occlusal surface of the tooth. Severe occlusal caries is apparent clinically and appears as a cavitation in the tooth.

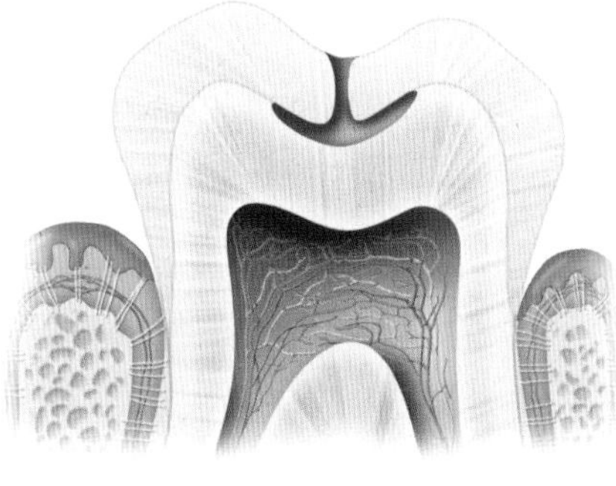

Fig 33-16 A moderate occlusal carious lesion, which extends through enamel and into dentin along the dentino-enamel junction (DEJ).

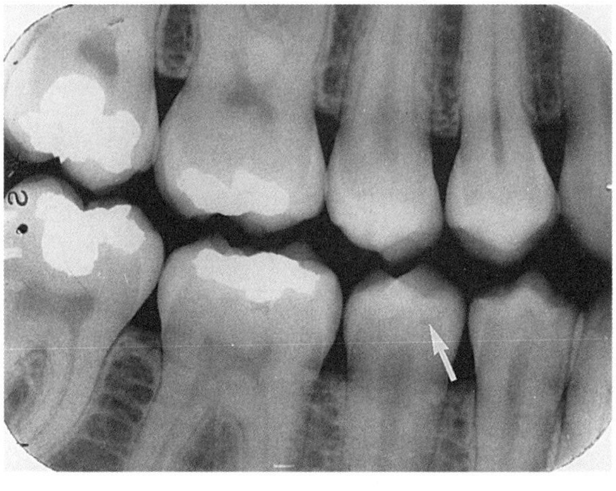

Fig 33-17 Occlusal caries, which appears as a tiny radiolucency just below the dentino-enamel junction (DEJ) on the mandibular second premolar. (From Haring JI, Lind LJ: Radiographic interpretation for the dental hygienist, Philadelphia, 1993, Saunders.)

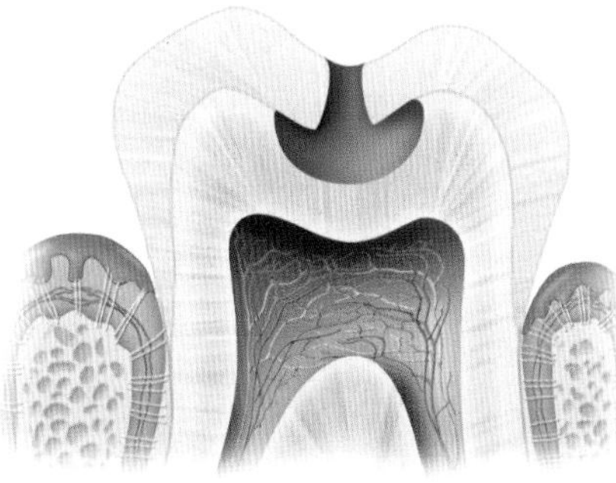

Fig 33-18 Severe occlusal caries, which extends through enamel and into dentin beyond the dentino-enamel junction (DEJ).

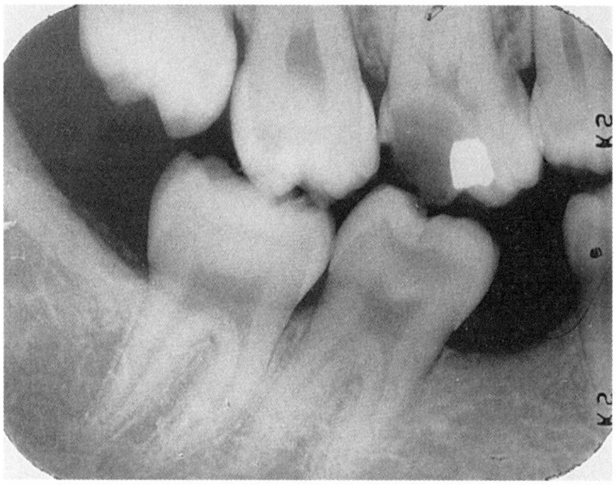

Fig 33-19 A severe occlusal carious lesion seen as a large radiolucency in dentin on the mandibular first molar. (From Haring JI, Lind LJ: Radiographic interpretation for the dental hygienist, Philadelphia, 1993, Saunders.)

Buccal and Lingual Caries

As the names suggest, buccal caries involves the buccal tooth surface, whereas lingual caries involves the lingual tooth surface. Because of the superimposition of the densities of normal tooth structure, buccal and lingual caries are difficult to detect on a dental image and are best detected clinically. When viewed on a dental image, caries that involves the buccal or lingual surface appears as a small, circular radiolucent area (Figures 33-20 and 33-21). To determine the location of the lesion, clinical examination with an explorer is necessary.

Root Surface Caries

Root surface caries involves only the roots of teeth. The cementum and dentin located just below the cervical region of the tooth are involved (Figures 33-22 and 33-23). No involvement of enamel occurs. Bone loss and corresponding gingival recession precede the caries process and result in exposed root surfaces.

Clinically, root surface caries is easily detected on exposed root surfaces. The most common locations include the exposed roots of mandibular premolar and molar areas. On a dental image, root surface caries appears as a cupped-out or crater-shaped radiolucency just below the cemento-enamel junction (CEJ). Early lesions may be difficult to detect on a dental image.

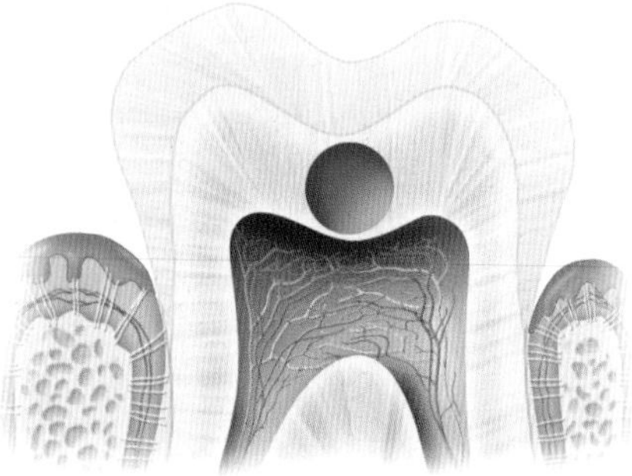

Fig 33-20 Buccal or lingual caries seen as a round radiolucency on molars.

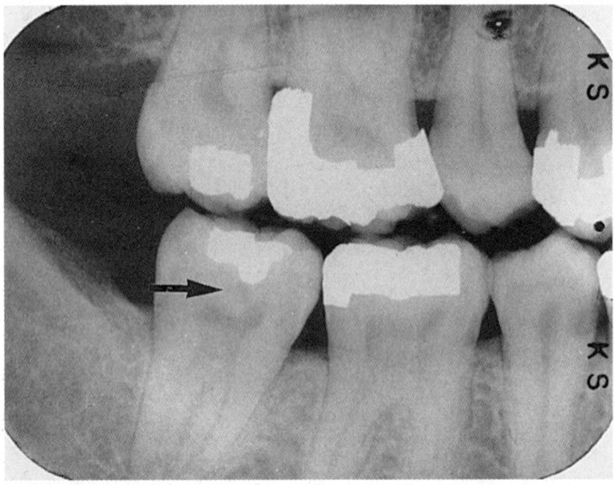

Fig 33-21 Buccal caries seen as a small, circular radiolucency on the mandibular second molar. (From Haring JI, Lind LJ: Radiographic interpretation for the dental hygienist, Philadelphia, 1993, Saunders.)

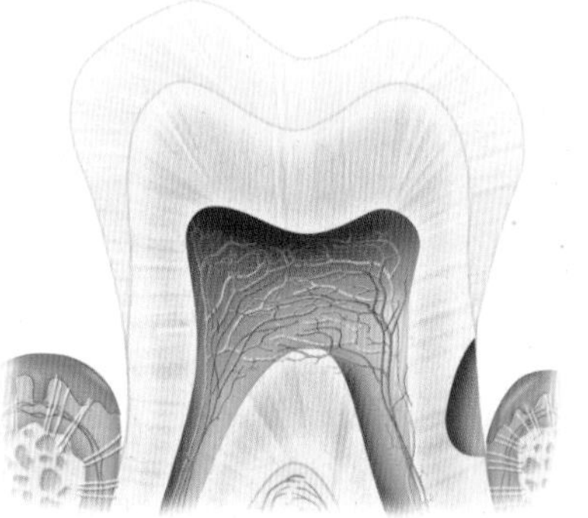

Fig 33-22 Root caries involving only cementum and dentin, not enamel.

Recurrent Caries

Secondary caries, or recurrent caries, occurs adjacent to a pre-existing restoration. Caries occurs in this region because of inadequate cavity preparation, defective margins, or incomplete removal of caries before placement of the restoration material. On a dental image, recurrent caries appears as a radiolucent area just beneath a restoration (Figure 33-24). Recurrent caries occurs most often beneath the interproximal margins of a restoration.

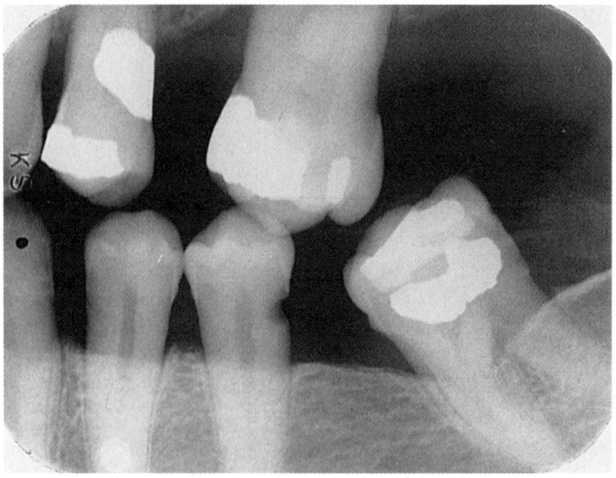

Fig 33-23 Root caries appearing as a crater-shaped radiolucency just below the cemento-enamel junction (CEJ) on the mandibular second premolar. (From Haring JI, Lind LJ: Radiographic interpretation for the dental hygienist, Philadelphia, 1993, Saunders.)

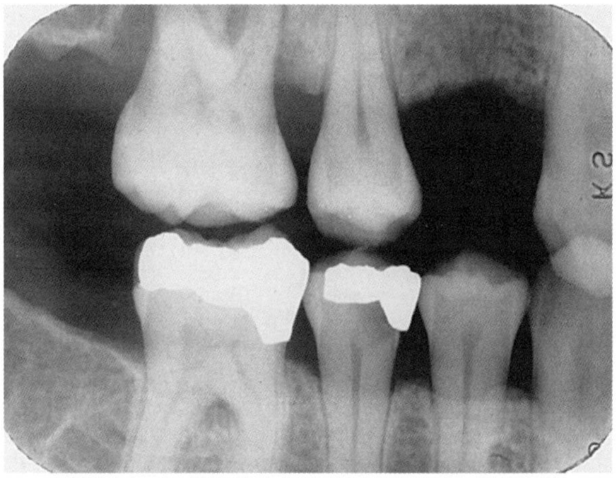

Fig 33-24 Recurrent caries seen as a radiolucency below a two-surface amalgam restoration on the mandibular second premolar. (From Haring JI, Lind LJ: Radiographic interpretation for the dental hygienist, Philadelphia, 1993, Saunders.)

Rampant Caries

The term rampant means "growing or spreading unchecked." Rampant caries is advanced and severe caries that affects numerous teeth (Figure 33-25). Rampant caries is typically seen in children with poor dietary habits or in adults with decreased salivary flow.

CONDITIONS RESEMBLING CARIES

A number of radiolucencies involve the crowns and roots of teeth and may be confused with caries. On a dental image, conditions that may be confused with caries include cervical burnout, restorative materials, attrition and abrasion. The dental professional must remember that the dentist establishes the final diagnosis of caries only after the clinical and image findings are corroborated.

Cervical Burnout

Cervical burnout, a radiolucent artifact seen on dental images, may be confused with caries. Cervical burnout appears as a collar-shaped or

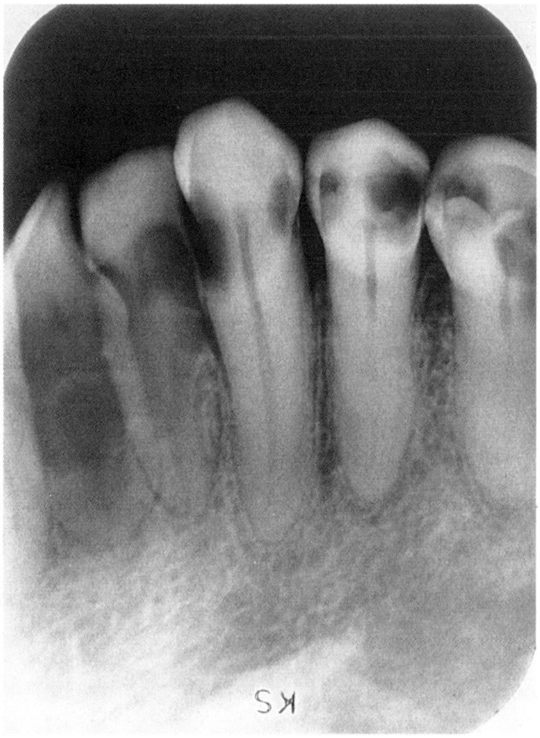

Fig 33-25 Rampant caries. (From Haring JI, Lind LJ: Radiographic interpretation for the dental hygienist, Philadelphia, 1993, Saunders.)

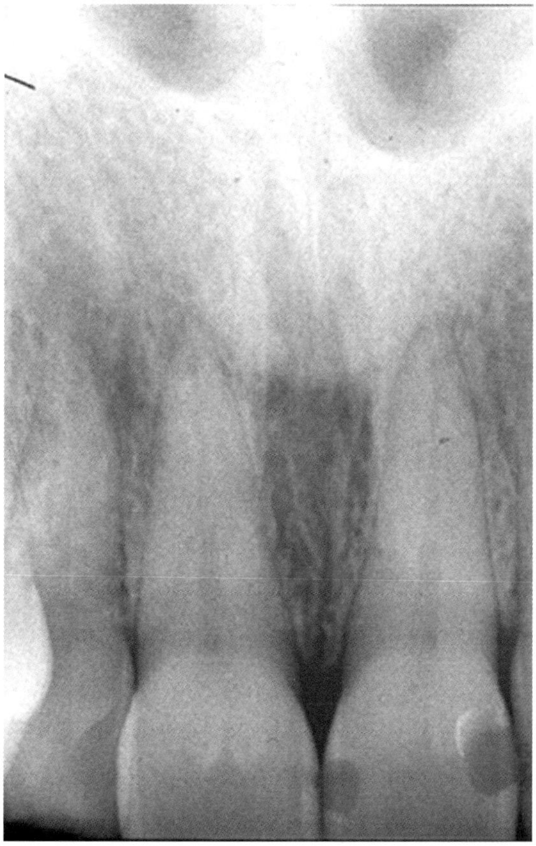

Fig 33-26 Collar-shaped cervical burnout seen on anterior teeth. (From Haring JI, Lind LJ: Radiographic interpretation for the dental hygienist, Philadelphia, 1993, Saunders.)

wedge-shaped area between the CEJ and alveolar bone. When collar-shaped, this radiolucent artifact is seen in anterior teeth because of the difference in densities of adjacent tissues. The tissue at the CEJ is less dense than the regions above and below it. Above the CEJ, enamel covers the crown, and below the CEJ, bone covers the root (Figure 33-26).

Cervical burnout may also appear as an ill-defined wedge-shaped radiolucency on the mesial or distal root surfaces near the CEJ of posterior teeth, because of the anatomic root concavities found in this area (Figure 33-27).

Restorative Materials

Restorative materials, such as composites, silicates, and acrylics, may appear radiolucent and resemble caries on a dental image. The appearance of an anterior cavity preparation restored with these materials differs from the appearance of interproximal caries and can be identified by the well-defined, smooth outline (Figure 33-28). In addition, a careful clinical exam helps the dental professional determine the difference between a restorative material and dental caries.

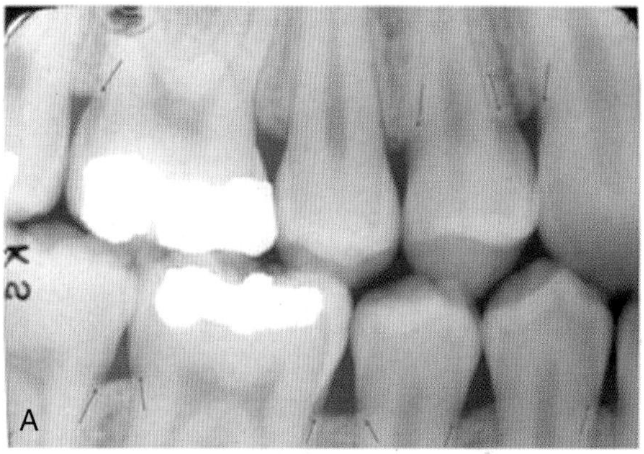

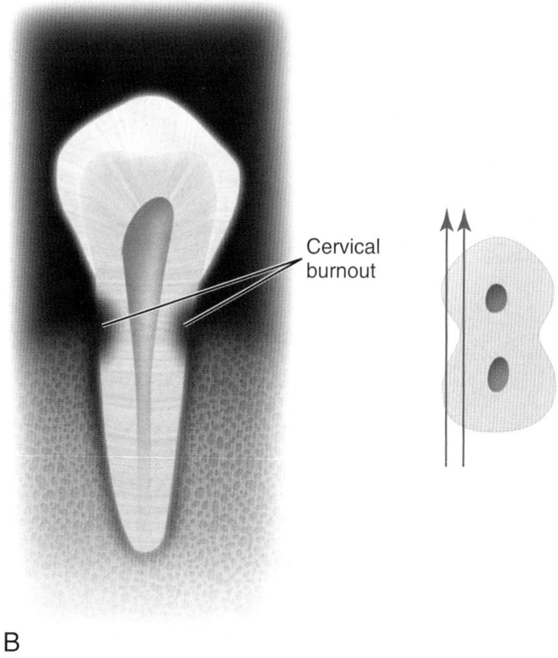

Fig 33-27 A, Wedge-shaped cervical burnout seen on posterior teeth. (From Haring JI, Lind LJ: Radiographic interpretation for the dental hygienist, Philadelphia, 1993, Saunders.) B, Invagination of the proximal root surfaces allow more x-rays to pass through this area, resulting in a more radiolucent appearance known as *cervical burnout.*

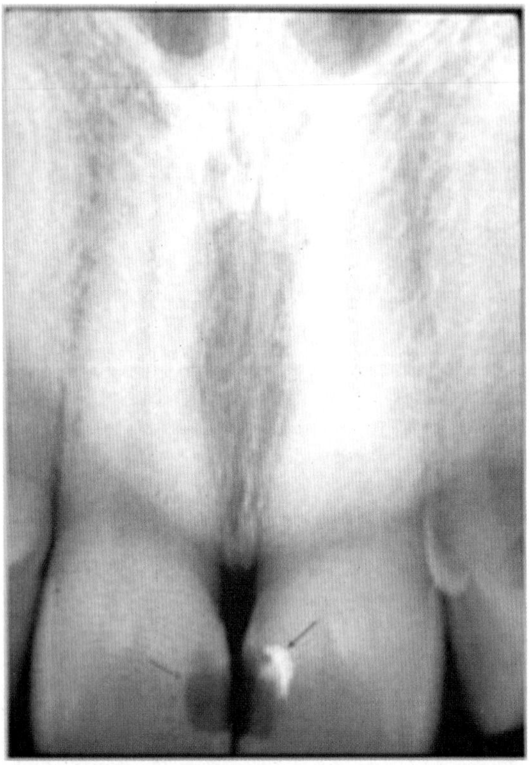

Fig 33-28 Composite restorations, when radiolucent, may be confused with caries. (From Haring JI, Lind LJ: Radiographic interpretation for the dental hygienist, Philadelphia, 1993, Saunders.)

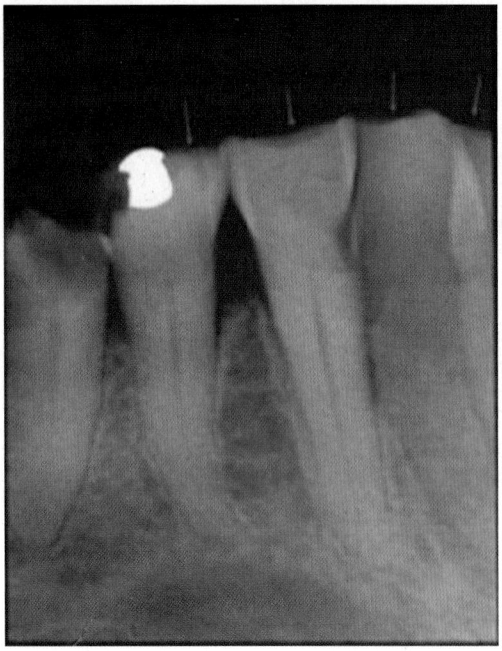

Fig 33-29 Attrition. (From Haring JI, Lind LJ: Radiographic interpretation for the dental hygienist, Philadelphia, 1993, Saunders.)

Attrition

Attrition, or the mechanical wearing down of teeth, may be mistaken for caries on a dental image. Attrition may be seen on the incisal or occlusal surfaces of deciduous or permanent teeth. When the incisal or occlusal enamel is worn away, the underlying dentin wears away rapidly, and shallow concavities may form (Figure 33-29). These concavities may resemble occlusal or incisal caries on a dental image. Clinical examination enables the dental professional to distinguish attrition from caries.

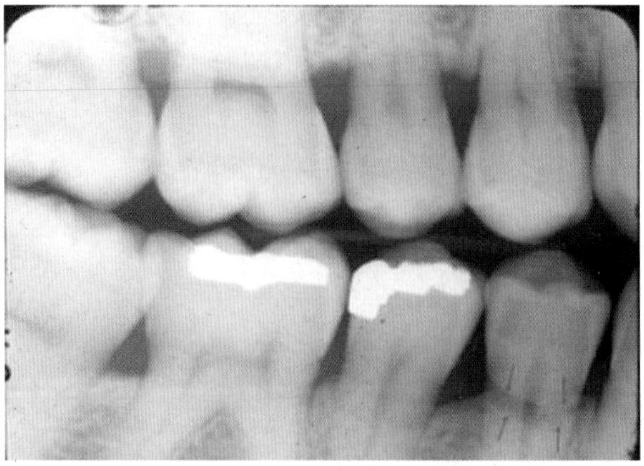

Fig 33-30 Abrasion. (From Haring JI, Lind LJ: Radiographic interpretation for the dental hygienist, Philadelphia, 1993, Saunders.)

Abrasion

Abrasion refers to the wearing away of tooth structure from the friction of a foreign object. The surface of the tooth affected depends on the causative factor. The most frequent type of abrasion is caused by improper toothbrushing and is seen at the cervical margin of the teeth. Toothbrush abrasion affects the root surface of a tooth and may be confused with root surface caries. On a dental image, toothbrush abrasion appears as a well-defined horizontal radiolucency along the cervical region of a tooth. Clinically, the areas affected by abrasion appear as hard, highly polished defects in dentin and should not be confused with root caries that appears brown and leathery (Figure 33-30).

SUMMARY

- Dental caries is a destructive process that causes decalcification of enamel, destruction of enamel and dentin, and cavitation of teeth.
- To detect dental caries, careful clinical examination and interpretation are necessary.
- Dental images allow the dental professional to identify carious lesions that are not visible clinically.
- Caries appears radiolucent on a dental image. Of all the radiolucent lesions that can be seen on a dental image, dental caries is seen most frequently.
- The dental professional must be confident in the use of interpretation methods to identify dental caries and to recognize factors that influence caries interpretation (e.g., errors in technique and exposure).
- Dental caries may involve any surface of the tooth crown or root. The appearance of dental caries can be classified according to the location of the caries on the tooth. Caries involving interproximal, occlusal, buccal, lingual, or root surfaces may be seen on dental images.
- On a dental image, the appearance of interproximal caries can be classified as incipient, moderate, advanced, or severe, depending on the amount of enamel and dentin involved in the caries process.
- On a dental image, the appearance of occlusal caries can be classified as incipient, moderate, or severe, depending on the amount of enamel and dentin involved in the caries process.

- Buccal and lingual carious lesions are difficult to detect on dental images because of the superimposition of normal tooth structure. Instead, these lesions are best detected clinically.
- Root surface caries involves cementum and dentin and is easily detected clinically. On a dental image, root surface caries appears as a cupped-out radiolucency below the cemento-enamel junction.
- On a dental image, other appearances of dental caries include recurrent caries, which appears as a radiolucency adjacent to an existing restoration, and rampant caries, which affects numerous teeth.
- On a dental image, conditions that may be confused with dental caries include cervical burnout, restorative materials, attrition, and abrasion.

BIBLIOGRAPHY

Frommer HH, Stabulas-Savage JJ: Caries and periodontal disease. In Radiology for the dental professional, ed 9, St. Louis, 2011, Mosby.

Haring JI, Lind LJ: Dental caries. In Radiographic interpretation for the dental hygienist, Philadelphia, 1993, Saunders.

Johnson ON: Preliminary interpretation of the radiographs. In Essentials of dental radiography for dental assistants and hygienists, ed 9, Upper Saddle River, NJ, 2011, Prentice Hall.

Mallya SM, Lam EWN: Dental caries. In White and Pharoah's Oral radiology: principles and interpretation, ed 8, St. Louis, 2019, Elsevier.

Miles DA, Van Dis ML, Jensen CW, et al: Interpretation: normal versus abnormal and common radiographic presentation of lesions. In Radiographic imaging for the dental team, ed 4, Philadelphia, 2009, Saunders.

QUIZ QUESTIONS

Identification

For questions 1 to 5, refer to Figures 33-31 through 33-35. On each dental image, identify the classification of the carious lesion shown.

1. ______________________________

2. ______________________________

3. ______________________________

4. ______________________________

5. ______________________________

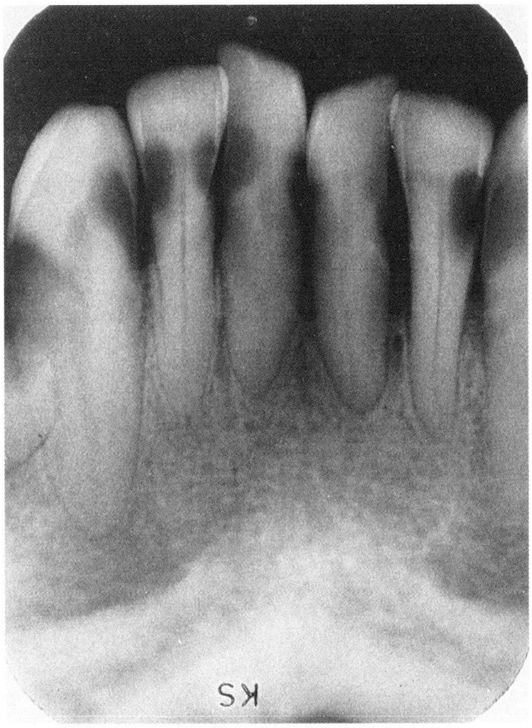

Fig 33-31 (From Haring JI, Lind LJ: Radiographic interpretation for the dental hygienist, Philadelphia, 1993, Saunders.)

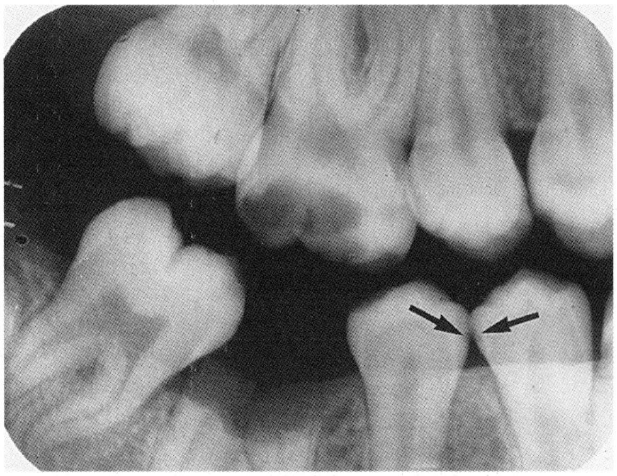

Fig 33-32 (From Haring JI, Lind LJ: Radiographic interpretation for the dental hygienist, Philadelphia, 1993, Saunders.)

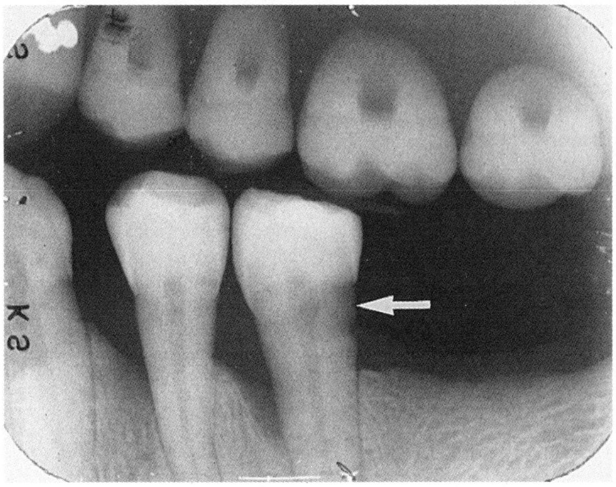

Fig 33-33 (From Haring JI, Lind LJ: Radiographic interpretation for the dental hygienist, Philadelphia, 1993, Saunders.)

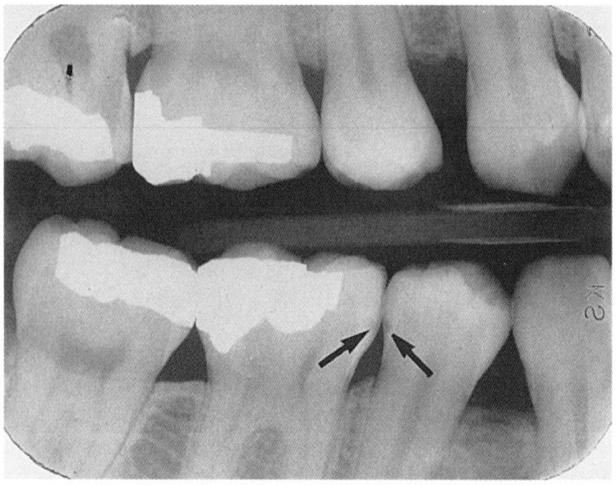

Fig 33-34 (From Haring JI, Lind LJ: Radiographic interpretation for the dental hygienist, Philadelphia, 1993, Saunders.)

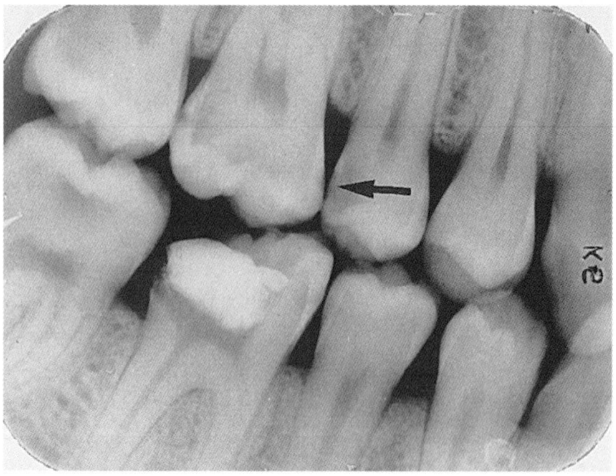

Fig 33-35 (From Haring JI, Lind LJ: Radiographic interpretation for the dental hygienist, Philadelphia, 1993, Saunders.)

Matching

For questions 6 to 12, match the classification of caries with the appropriate description.

a. Caries that extends more than halfway through enamel but does not involve the dentino-enamel junction (DEJ)
b. Caries that extends to or through the DEJ but does not extend more than half the distance to the pulp
c. Caries that cannot be seen on an image
d. Caries that extends through enamel, through dentin, and more than half the distance to the pulp
e. Caries that extends less than halfway through enamel
f. Caries seen as a large radiolucency in dentin under the enamel of the chewing surfaces of teeth
g. Caries seen as a thin radiolucent line in dentin under the enamel of the chewing surfaces of teeth
h. None of the above

_____ 6. Incipient interproximal
_____ 7. Moderate interproximal
_____ 8. Advanced interproximal
_____ 9. Severe interproximal
_____ 10. Incipient occlusal
_____ 11. Moderate occlusal
_____ 12. Severe occlusal

SHORT ANSWER

13. Describe dental caries.
14. Explain why caries appears radiolucent on a dental image.
15. List the classifications of interproximal caries on a dental image.
16. List the classifications of occlusal caries on a dental image.
17. Describe the appearance of root caries on a dental image.
18. Describe the appearance of recurrent caries on a dental image.
19. Describe the appearance of rampant caries on a dental image.
20. In Figure 33-36, examine the mesial and distal interproximal surfaces of each tooth. Describe each area of caries as incipient, moderate, advanced, or severe.

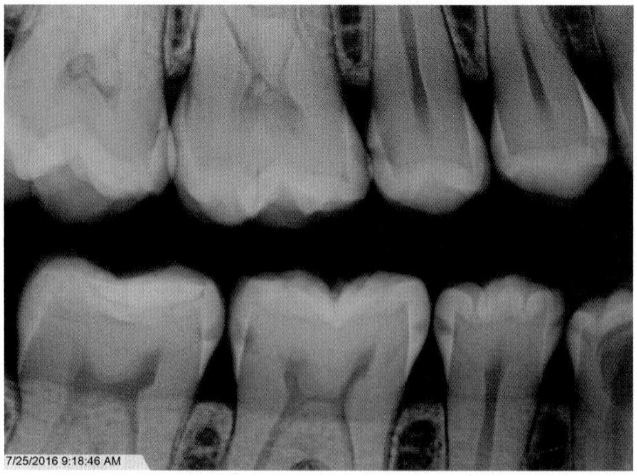

Fig 33-36

34

Interpretation of Periodontal Disease

LEARNING OBJECTIVES

After completion of this chapter, the student will be able to do the following:

1. Define the key terms associated with interpreting periodontal disease.
2. Describe the healthy periodontium.
3. Briefly describe periodontal disease and the progression to disease.
4. In relation to the detection of periodontal disease:
   - Discuss the importance of the clinical examination.
   - Discuss the importance of dental image examination, including different techniques used.
   - Describe the limitations of dental images in the detection of periodontal disease.
   - Describe the type of dental images that should be used to document periodontal disease and the preferred exposure technique.
5. In relation to the interpretation of periodontal disease on dental images:
   - State the difference between horizontal bone loss and vertical bone loss.
   - State the difference between localized bone loss and generalized bone loss.
   - State the differences among mild, moderate, and severe bone loss.
6. Discuss the characteristics described in the 2018 Classification of Periodontal and Peri-implant Diseases that pertain to the interpretation of dental images.
7. List predisposing factors for periodontal disease and recognize and describe the appearance of calculus on dental images.

Dental images play an integral role in the assessment of periodontal disease. An examination of dental images is essential for diagnostic purposes because it enables the dental professional to obtain vital information about supporting bone, as this information cannot be obtained clinically. Detailed information about the clinical aspects of periodontal disease is beyond the scope of this text. The purpose of this chapter is to introduce the dental radiographer to the description and detection of periodontal disease. The interpretation of periodontal disease as viewed on dental images, with an emphasis on a description of bone loss, and identification of predisposing factors, is also presented.

DESCRIPTION OF THE PERIODONTIUM

The term periodontium refers to tissues that invest and support teeth, such as the gingiva and alveolar bone. As described in Chapter 28, the normal anatomic landmarks of alveolar bone include the *lamina dura, alveolar crest*, and *periodontal ligament space*. The appearance of healthy alveolar bone on a dental image can be described as follows:

Lamina dura: In health, the lamina dura of teeth appears as a dense radiopaque line around the roots. The lamina dura represents the thin, smooth cortical bone of the tooth socket (Figure 34-1). On a dental image, the lamina dura is continuous with the cortical bone of the interdental septa.

Alveolar crest: The alveolar crest appears as a smooth, intact surface between adjacent teeth. The normal healthy alveolar crest is located approximately 1.5 to 2.0 mm apical to the cemento-enamel junctions (CEJs) of adjacent teeth (see Figure 34-1). The shape and density of the alveolar crest vary between the anterior and posterior regions of the mouth. The contour of the alveolar crest is an indicator of periodontal health. In the anterior regions, the alveolar crest appears pointed and sharp and is normally very radiopaque (Figure 34-2). In the posterior regions, the alveolar crest appears rounded or flat, and parallel to a line between adjacent CEJs (Figure 34-3). The alveolar crest in the posterior regions appears slightly less radiopaque than that in the anterior regions.

Periodontal ligament space: The normal periodontal ligament space appears as a thin radiolucent line between the root of the tooth and the lamina dura. In health, the periodontal ligament space is continuous around the root structure and is of uniform thickness (see Figure 34-1). On a dental image, a widening of the periodontal ligament space may be seen when resorption of the mesial or distal areas of the alveolar crest exists. This results in a triangular or funnel pattern of the remaining crestal bone, often referred to as *triangulation* or *funneling*. Also visible on a dental image is the uniform widening of the periodontal ligament space seen around the entire root, frequently indicating tooth mobility.

DESCRIPTION OF PERIODONTAL DISEASE

The term periodontal literally means "around a tooth." Periodontal disease refers to a group of diseases that affect the tissues around teeth. Periodontal disease may range from a superficial inflammation of the gingiva to the destruction of supporting bone and the periodontal ligament. With periodontal disease, the gingiva exhibits varying degrees of inflammation. Gingival tissues affected by periodontal disease may not appear stippled, pink, and firm. Instead, the gingiva may appear swollen, red, and bleeding, and formation of soft tissue pockets is seen.

As discussed in Chapter 28, the alveolar process is the portion of the maxilla and mandible that supports the teeth. The tooth is also supported by the periodontal ligament and cementum that covers the root surface. These structures are not static and will respond to local and systemic factors, such as the presence of plaque, infection, or other disease.

On a dental image, the appearance of alveolar bone affected by periodontal disease differs from that of healthy alveolar bone. With periodontal disease, the alveolar crest is no longer located 1.5 to 2.0 mm

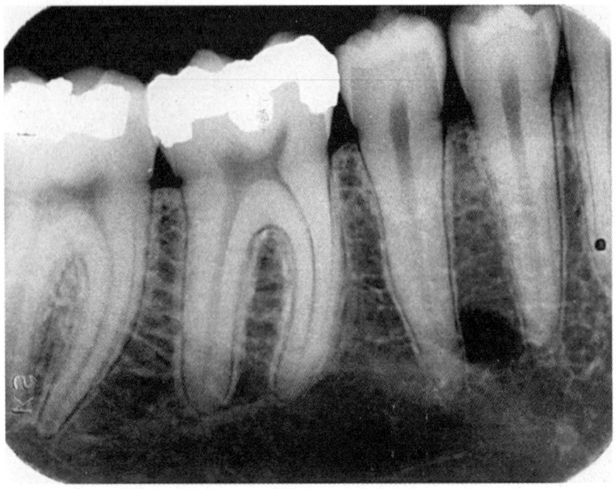

Fig 34-1 Healthy alveolar crest, normal lamina dura, and periodontal ligament space on a periapical image. (From Haring JI, Lind LJ: Radiographic interpretation for the dental hygienist, Philadelphia, 1993, Saunders.)

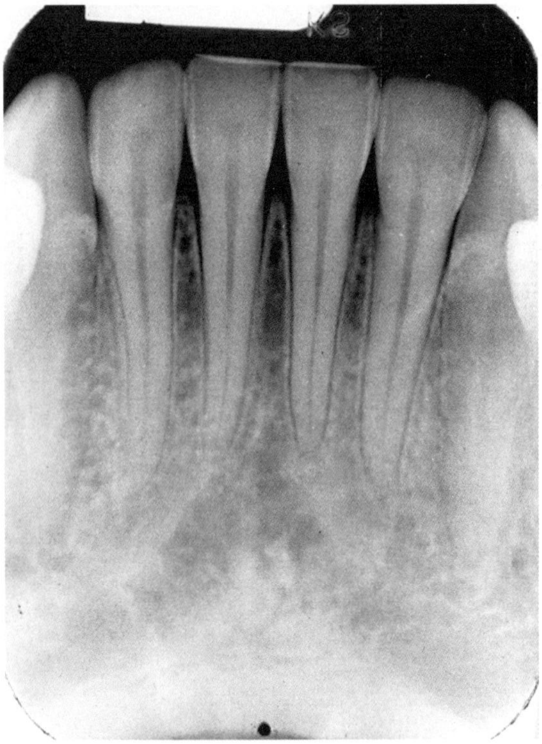

Fig 34-2 Healthy alveolar crest in the anterior region that appears pointed and highly radiopaque. (From Haring JI, Lind LJ: Radiographic interpretation for the dental hygienist, Philadelphia, 1993, Saunders.)

apical to the CEJ and no longer appears radiopaque. Instead, the alveolar crest appears indistinct, and bone loss is seen. Periodontal disease may result in severe destruction of bone and loss of teeth.

DETECTION OF PERIODONTAL DISEASE

To detect periodontal disease, both clinical examinations and interpretation of dental images are necessary. Dental images *must* be used in conjunction with a clinical examination. In general, what is seen clinically cannot be evaluated on dental images, and what is viewed on dental images cannot be evaluated clinically. Clinical examination

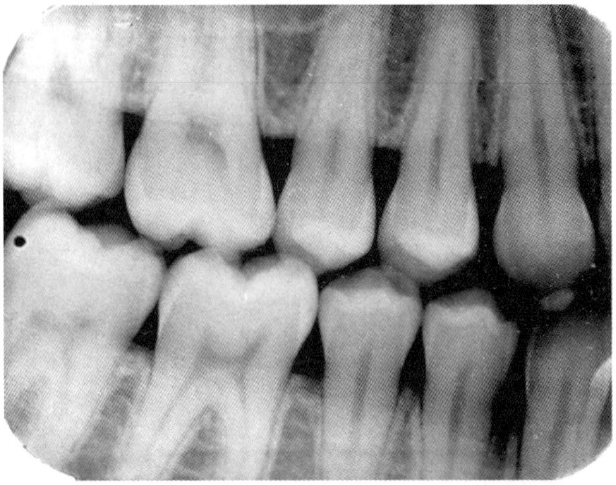

Fig 34-3 Healthy alveolar crest in the posterior region that appears flat, smooth, and radiopaque. (From Haring JI, Lind LJ: Radiographic interpretation for the dental hygienist, Philadelphia, 1993, Saunders.)

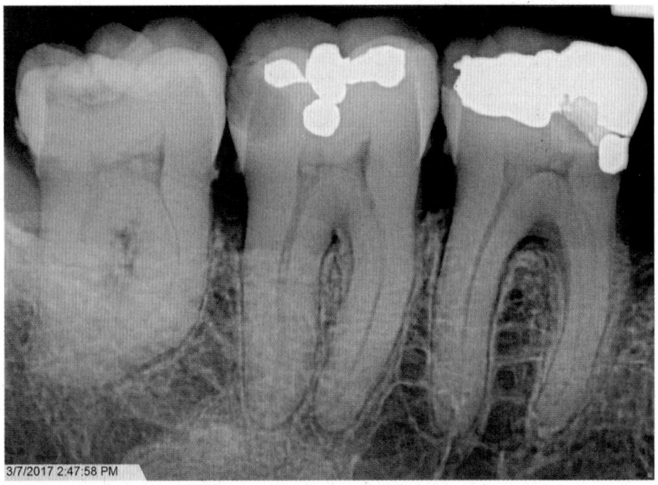

Fig 34-4 The height of crestal bone is accurately represented by the periapical image exposed with the paralleling technique.

provides information about soft tissues, whereas dental images permit evaluation of hard tissues, such as bone.

Clinical Examination

A clinical examination must be performed, including an evaluation of soft tissues (gingiva) for signs of inflammation (e.g., redness, bleeding, swelling, pus). A thorough clinical assessment includes periodontal probing. Whenever clinical evidence of periodontal disease is present, images should be exposed in order to get maximum diagnostic information.

Dental Image Examination

Dental images, along with clinical examination, enable the dental professional to determine the extent of periodontal disease. Dental images provide an overview of the amount of bone present and indicate the pattern, distribution, and severity of bone loss resulting from periodontal disease. In addition, dental images enable the dental professional to document periodontal disease at specific points in time.

The *periapical image* is recommended for the evaluation of periodontal disease (Figure 34-4). The *paralleling technique* is the preferred periapical exposure method for the demonstration of the anatomic features of periodontal disease. With the paralleling technique, the height of crestal bone is accurately recorded in relation to the tooth root. If the bisecting technique is used to expose periapical images, a dimensional distortion of bone may result from errors with vertical angulation. Therefore periapical images exposed using the bisecting technique may show more or less bone loss than is present (Figure 34-5).

The *horizontal bite-wing image* alone should not be used to document moderate to severe periodontal disease. This image has limited use in the detection of periodontal disease; severe interproximal bone loss cannot be adequately visualized on horizontal bite-wing images (Figure 34-6).

The *vertical bite-wing image* can be used to examine bone levels and is best used for post-treatment and follow-up purposes (Figure 34-7). The panoramic image has less diagnostic value in the identification of periodontal disease and is not recommended to demonstrate the anatomic features of this condition.

Dental images alone cannot be used to diagnose periodontal disease because of limitations in detecting and diagnosing the condition; images must be used in conjunction with a thorough clinical examination. For example, dental images do not provide information about the condition of soft tissues or the early bony changes seen in periodontal disease. Because dental images record two-dimensional images of three-dimensional structures, certain areas of teeth and bone are difficult, if not impossible, to examine in this manner. Buccal and lingual areas are particularly difficult to evaluate. For example, bone loss in the furcation area—the area between the roots of multirooted teeth—may not be detected on a dental image because of the superimposition of buccal and lingual bone (Figure 34-8). Although the periapical image is recommended, CBCT imaging may also be helpful in the diagnosis of bone loss in the buccal and lingual areas of teeth.

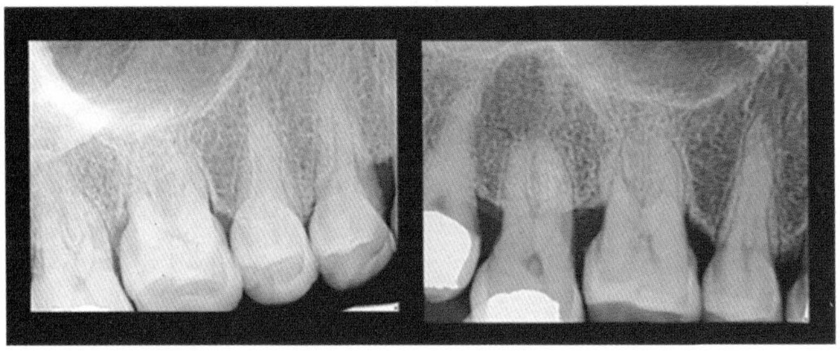

Fig 34-5 Bisecting technique distorts the level of bone present seen on an image because of the vertical angulation used. Paralleling technique is used to examine the same area. Note the difference in bone level. With the paralleling technique, the height of crestal bone is accurately recorded in relation to the tooth root.

INTERPRETATION OF PERIODONTAL DISEASE ON DENTAL IMAGES

The dental radiographer must be familiar with the appearance of periodontal disease. As viewed on dental images, early signs of periodontitis include fuzzy crestal bone, a widened periodontal ligament space near the crestal margin, and an increased radiolucent appearance of the interdental bone. All images should be evaluated for early bone changes and bone loss, and the identification of predisposing factors that may contribute to periodontal disease.

Bone Loss

A dental image allows the dental professional to view the amount of bone remaining rather than the amount of bone lost. However, in documenting bone levels, the amount of bone loss that has occurred is recorded rather than the amount of bone that remains. The amount of bone loss can be estimated as the difference between the physiologic bone level and the height of remaining bone (Figure 34-9). Bone loss can be described in terms of the pattern, distribution, and severity of loss (Figure 34-10).

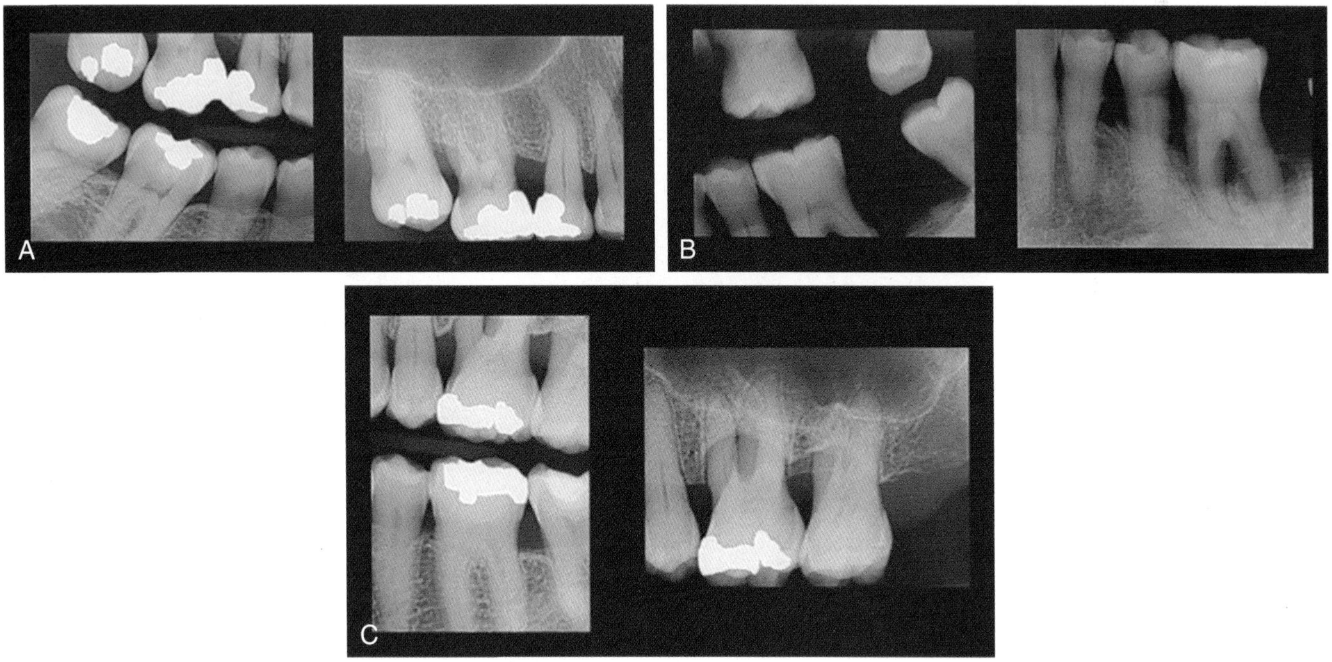

Fig 34-6 A-C With moderate to severe bone loss, a horizontal or vertical bite-wing may not adequately document the level of bone. In each of these examples, compare the bite-wing image to the corresponding periapical image for documentation of bone loss. In each case, the bite-wing image did not adequately document the bone level.

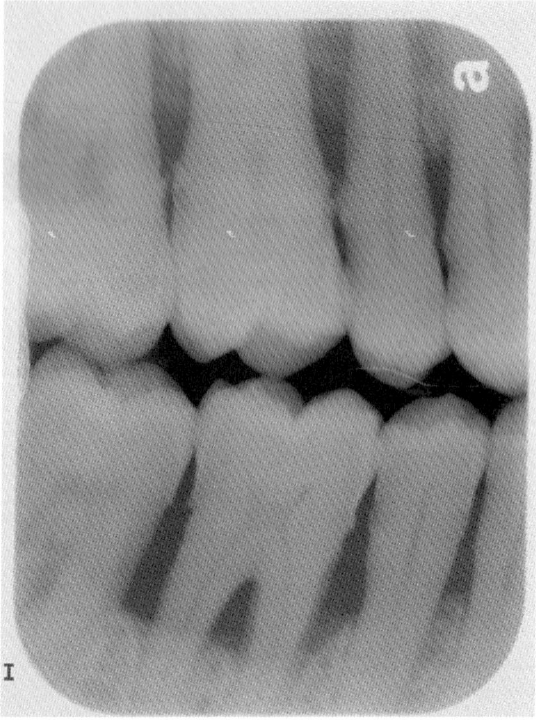

Fig 34-7 Compared with a horizontal bite-wing, the vertical bite-wing image allows for additional information about the bone loss and calculus deposits. (Courtesy Timothy W. Godsey, DDS, MS, Chapel Hill Periodontics and Implants, Chapel Hill, NC.)

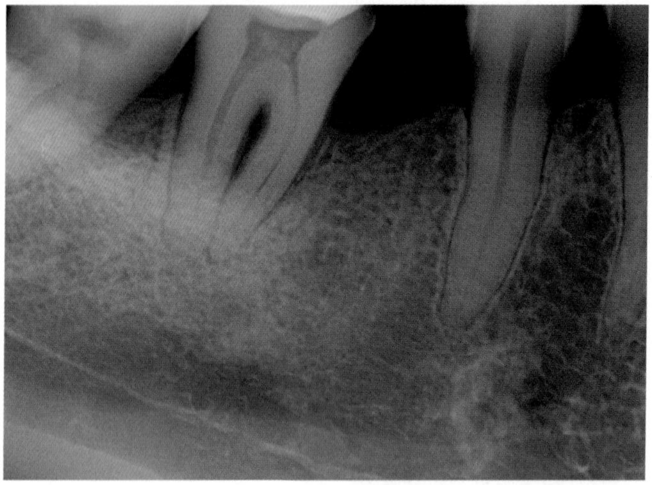

Fig 34-8 Furcation involvement.

Pattern. The pattern of bone loss viewed on a dental image can be described as horizontal or vertical. The CEJs of adjacent teeth are used as a plane of reference in determining the pattern of bone loss present. With horizontal bone loss, the bone loss occurs in a plane parallel to the CEJs of adjacent teeth (Figures 34.11 and 34-12). With vertical bone loss (also known as *angular bone loss*), the bone loss does not occur in a plane parallel to the CEJs of adjacent teeth (Figures 34-13 and 34-14).

Distribution. The distribution of bone loss seen on a dental image can be described as localized or generalized, depending on the areas involved. Localized bone loss occurs in isolated areas, with less than 30% of the sites involved (Figure 34-15). Generalized bone loss occurs

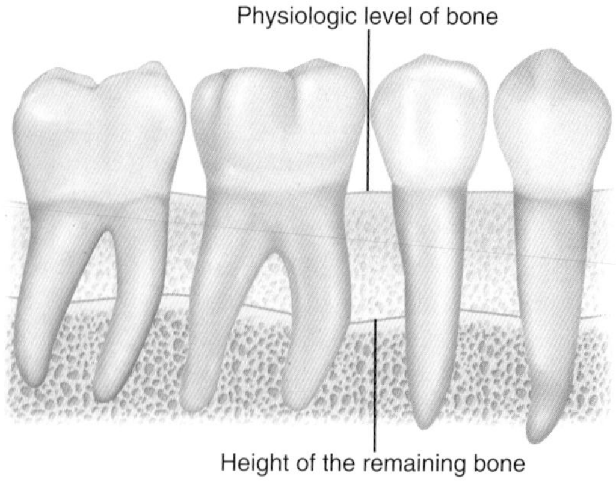

Fig 34-9 Bone loss estimated as the difference between the physiologic level of bone and the height of the remaining bone.

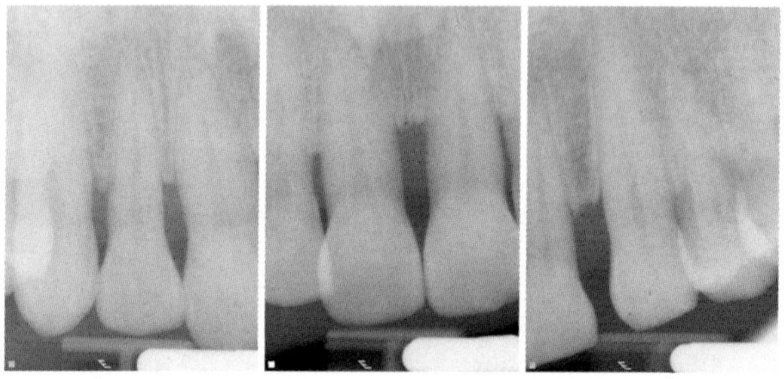

Fig 34-10 The height of the remaining bone is visualized on images of the maxillary anterior teeth. (Courtesy Timothy W. Godsey, DDS, MS, Chapel Hill Periodontics and Implants, Chapel Hill, NC.)

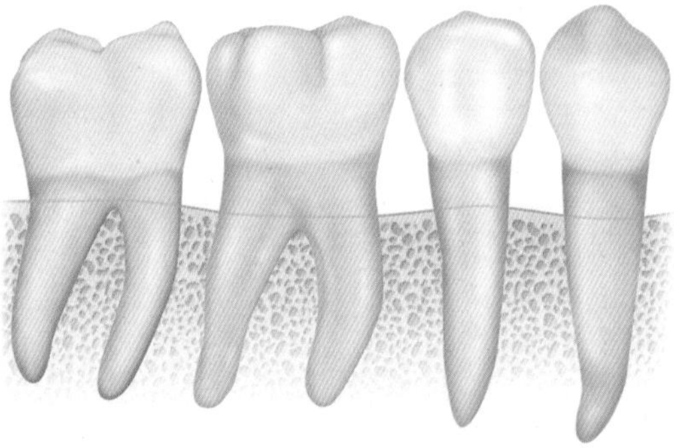

Fig 34-11 Horizontal bone loss occurs in a plane parallel to the cemento-enamel junctions (CEJs) of adjacent teeth.

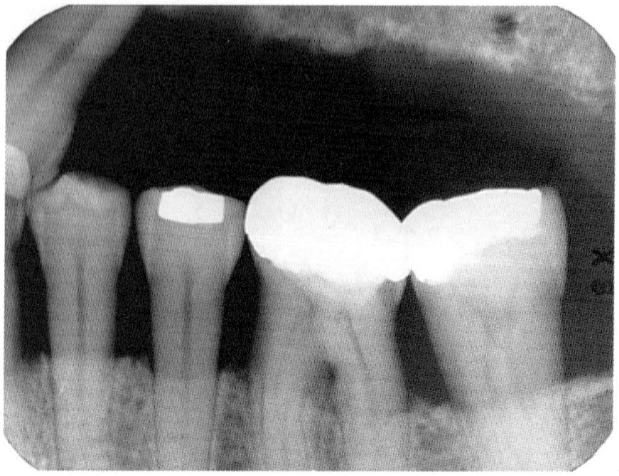

Fig 34-12 Horizontal bone loss. (From Haring JI, Lind LJ: Radiographic interpretation for the dental hygienist, Philadelphia, 1993, Saunders.)

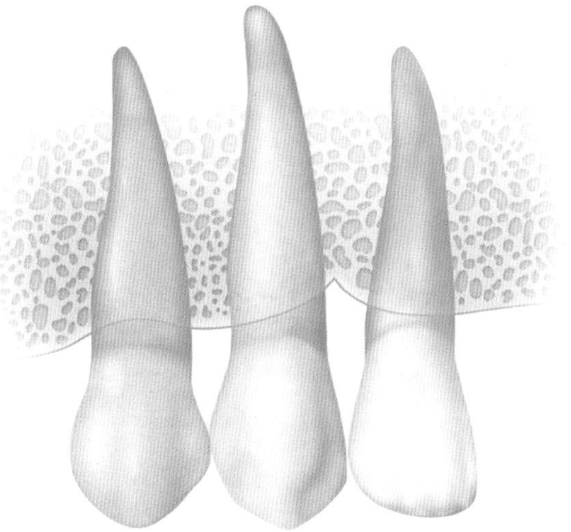

Fig 34-13 Vertical bone loss occurs in a plane not parallel to the cemento-enamel junctions (CEJs) of adjacent teeth.

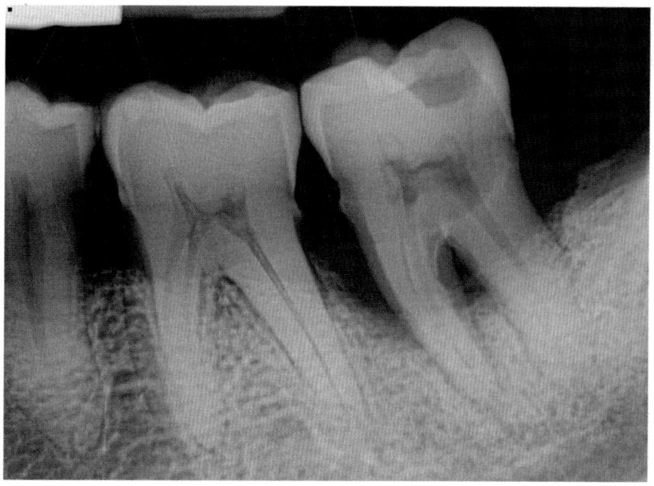

Fig 34-14 Vertical bone loss.

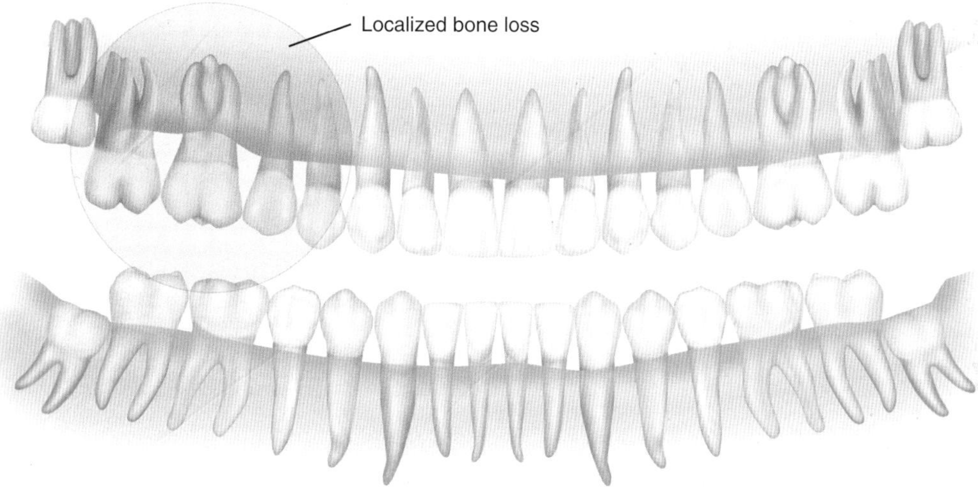

Fig 34-15 Localized bone loss occurs in isolated areas.

evenly throughout the dental arches, with more than 30% of the sites involved (Figure 34-16).

Severity. Bone loss viewed on a dental image can be classified as slight, moderate, or severe. The severity of bone loss is measured by the clinical attachment loss (CAL). The CAL is a measurement of the distance in millimeters from the CEJ to the base of the sulcus or periodontal pocket; the calibrated periodontal probe measures CAL. (*Note:* Clinical conditions, such as recession or gingival overgrowth, must be considered when determining CAL.) The severity of bone loss can be defined as follows:

- *Slight* bone loss: 1 to 2 mm
- *Moderate* bone loss: 3 to 4 mm
- *Severe* bone loss: 5 mm or greater

Classification of Periodontal Disease

Classification systems are routinely used to provide a framework to study clinical findings and for the treatment of disease. The American Academy of Periodontology (AAP) revised the classification system for periodontal disease in 1999. Clinical information regarding disease categories, including gingival disease, age-related terminology, and the pathogenesis of periodontal disease, was highlighted in this classification system. In 2017 the AAP revised the 1999 guidelines and provided an updated system for the diagnosis of periodontal disease. The motivation behind the revision was to allow periodontal disease be based on more of an individualized diagnosis for each patient. Factors taken into consideration include: the stage of severity of the disease process; the extent and distribution of the disease; the complexity, management, and response to therapies; and a grading system that relates to the progression of periodontal disease. The AAP revised the periodontal diagnosis to allow dental health care professionals to provide more patient-centered care.

Dental images are used in the classification of periodontal disease. The updated AAP guidelines classify the amount of radiographic bone loss present to determine the stage of disease. Radiographic bone loss seen in periodontal disease is categorized as follows:

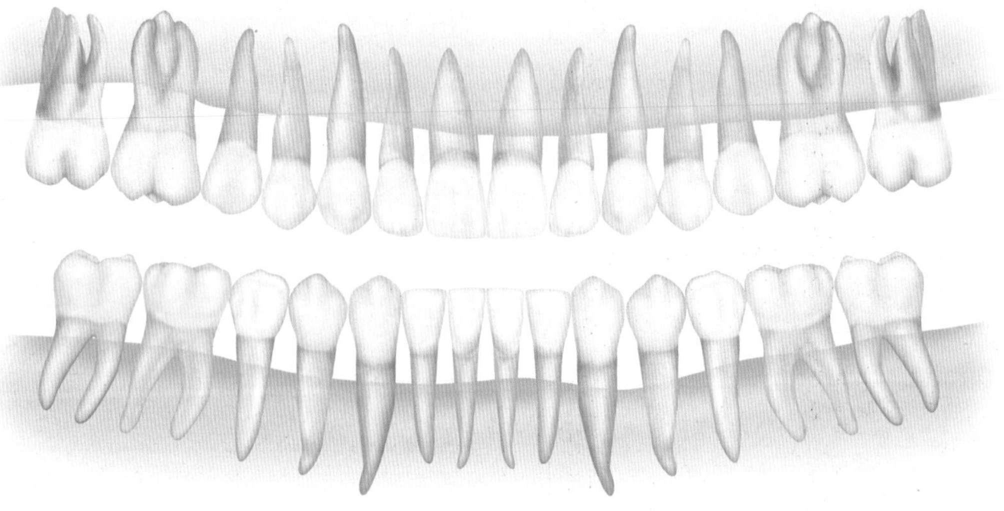

Fig 34-16 Generalized bone loss occurs throughout the dental arches.

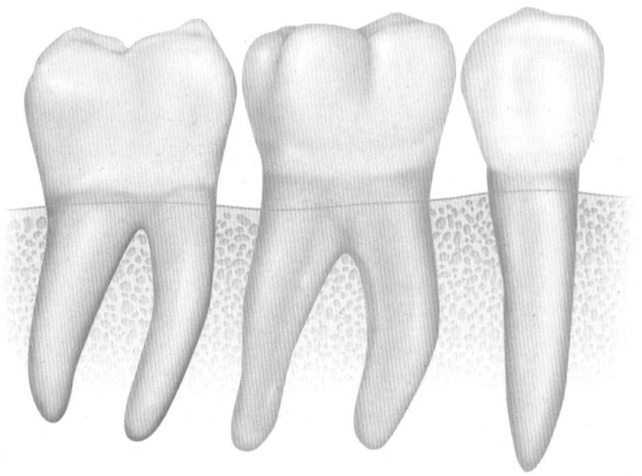

Fig 34-17 Mild bone loss.

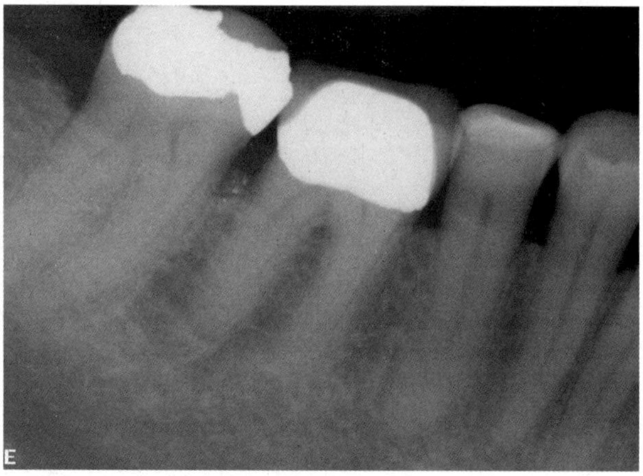

Fig 34-18 Horizontal bone loss and mild crestal changes. (Courtesy Timothy W. Godsey, DDS, MS, Chapel Hill Periodontics and Implants, Chapel Hill, NC.)

Stage I Radiographic Bone Loss in the coronal third of the root <15%.

Stage II Radiographic Bone Loss in the coronal third of the root from 15% to 33%.

Stage III Radiographic Bone Loss extending to the mid-third of the root including vertical bone loss and furcation involvement.

Stage IV Radiographic Bone Loss extending to the mid-third of the root and beyond including vertical bone loss, furcation involvement, and tooth mobility.

Each stage of disease has a specific appearance. Dental images can also be used to detect the contributing factors for periodontal disease, such as calculus and defective restorations.

THE PROGRESSION OF PERIODONTAL DISEASE

Inflammation of the gingival tissues is typically the first sign of periodontal disease. No bone loss is associated with gingivitis; therefore no change in bone is seen on the dental image. The crestal lamina dura is present, and the alveolar crest is approximately 1 to 2 mm apical to the CEJ. Clinically, bleeding on probing may be present. The inflammatory process affects only the gingival tissues in this stage of periodontal disease; no hard tissue changes are seen.

If untreated, gingival inflammation may progress to slight or mild periodontitis. The radiographic appearance reveals bone loss associated with mild crestal changes (Figures 34-17 to 34-19). The crestal lamina

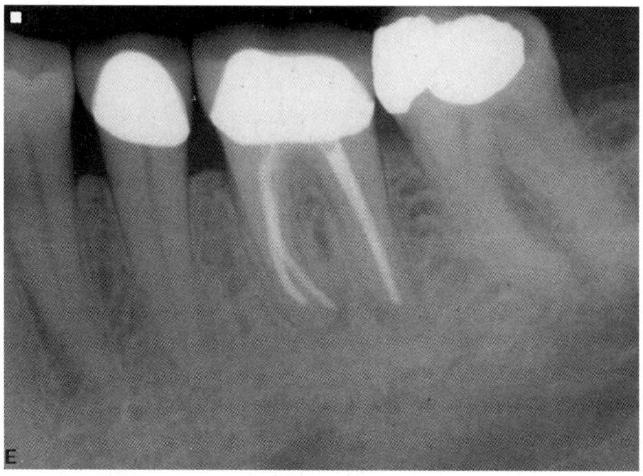

Fig 34-19 Mild crestal changes and horizontal bone loss. (Courtesy Timothy W. Godsey, DDS, MS, Chapel Hill Periodontics and Implants, Chapel Hill, NC.)

dura becomes unclear and fuzzy and no longer appears to be a continuous radiopaque line. Horizontal bone loss is seen more often in this stage of periodontal disease, with the alveolar bone level approximately 3 to 4 mm apical to the CEJ. Clinically, bleeding may occur on probing, and pocket depths resulting from attachment loss and localized areas of gingival recession may be evident.

With advancing periodontal disease, horizontal or vertical bone loss may be present; the distribution of the bone loss may be localized or generalized (Figures 34-20 to 34-23). The alveolar bone level is approximately 4 to 6 mm apical to the CEJs of adjacent teeth. Bleeding upon probing may be present. Furcation involvement, or the extension of periodontal disease between the roots of multirooted teeth, may also be seen in this stage of disease. When bone in the furcation area is destroyed, a radiolucent area is evident on the dental image (Figure 34-24). Clinically, pocket depths and attachment loss up to 6 mm are evident. Recession, furcation involvement areas, and slight mobility may also be present.

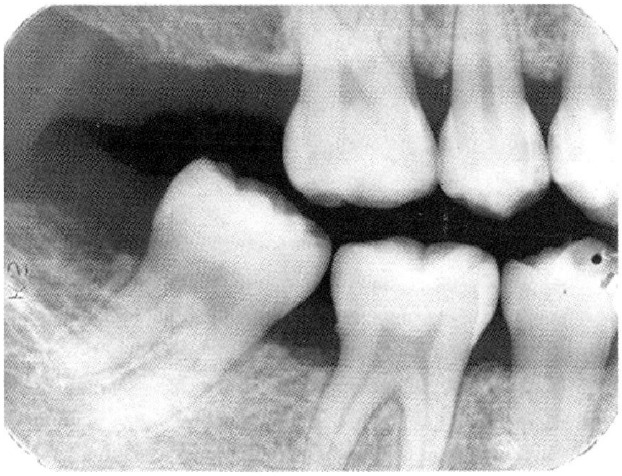

Fig 34-20 Moderate bone loss. (From Haring JI, Lind LJ: Radiographic interpretation for the dental hygienist, Philadelphia, 1993, Saunders.)

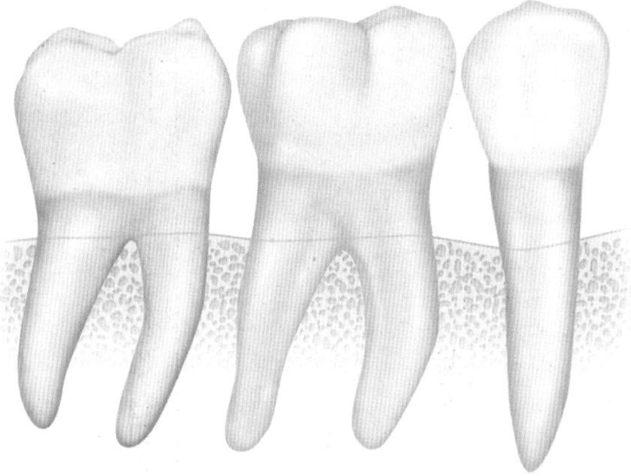

Fig 34-21 Moderate bone loss.

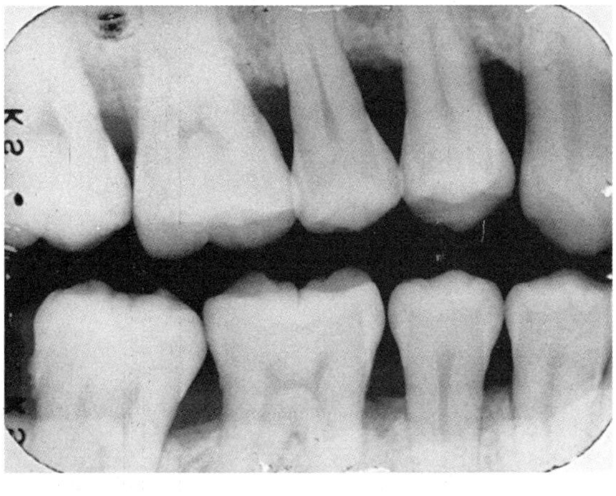

Fig 34-22 Moderate bone loss seen in the maxilla and mandible on this bite-wing image. (From Haring JI, Lind LJ: Radiographic interpretation for the dental hygienist, Philadelphia, 1993, Saunders.)

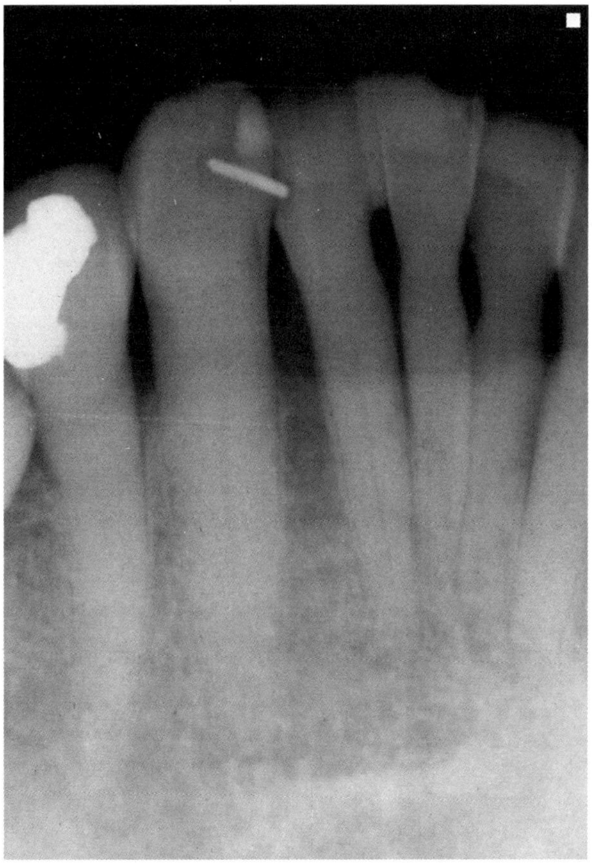

Fig 34-23 Generalized horizontal bone loss. (Courtesy Timothy W. Godsey, DDS, MS, Chapel Hill Periodontics and Implants, Chapel Hill, NC.)

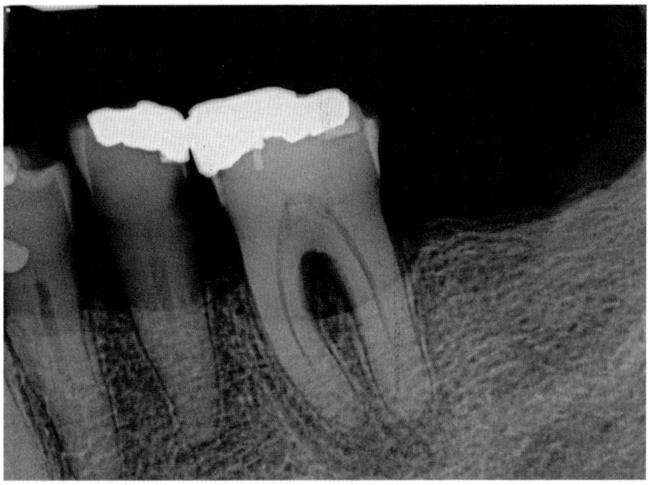

Fig 34-24 Furcation involvement and horizontal bone loss.

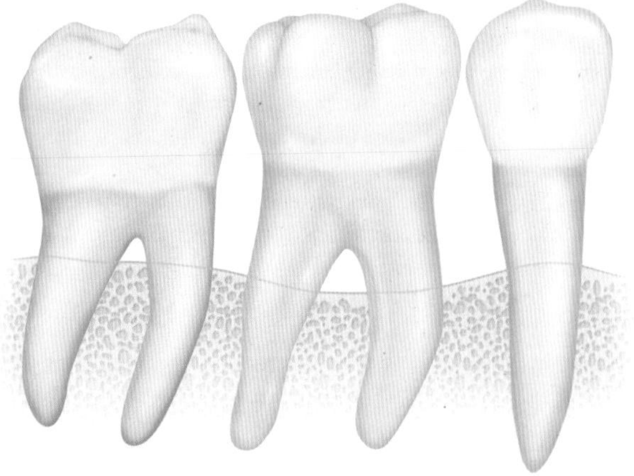

Fig 34-25 Severe bone loss.

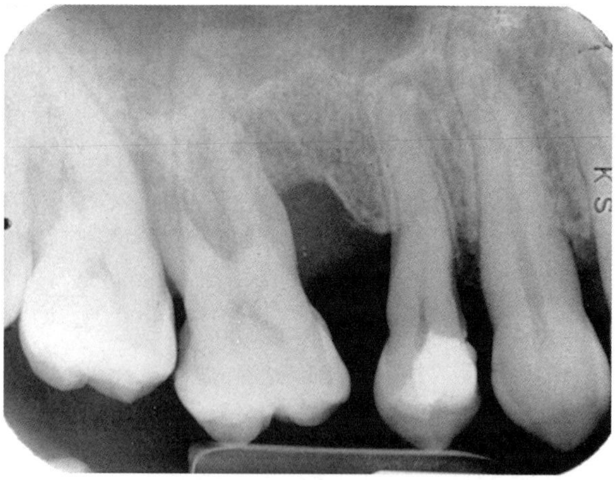

Fig 34-26 Severe horizontal and vertical bone loss.

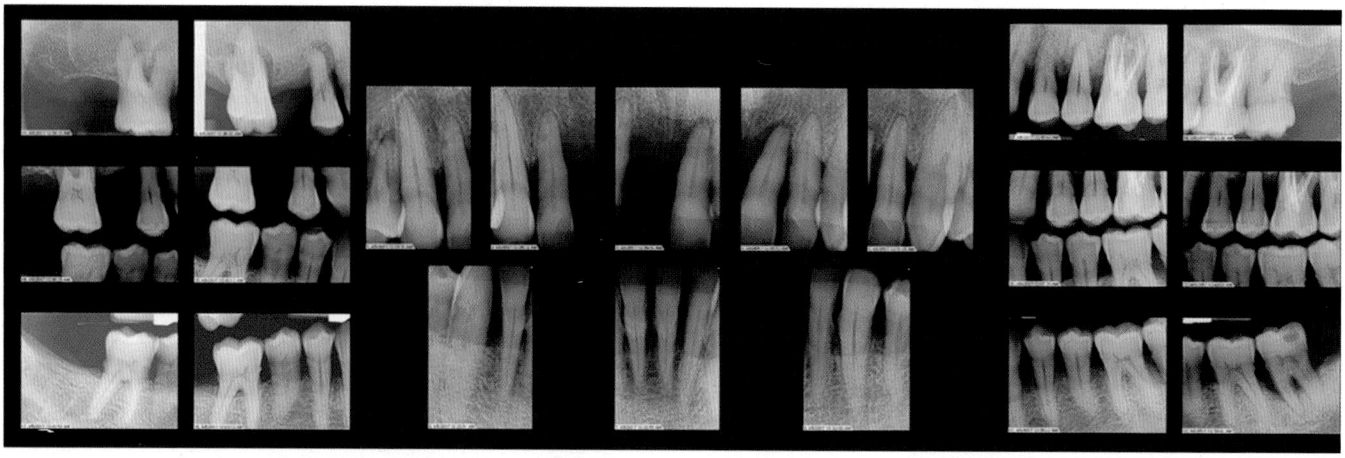

Fig 34-27 Generalized severe bone loss as viewed on a complete series of images.

The bone loss associated with advanced or severe periodontitis indicates further progression of the disease and is considered severe (Figures 34-24 to 34-27). The pattern of bone loss may be horizontal or vertical, and the alveolar bone level is 6 mm or greater from the CEJ. Furcation involvement is readily viewed on posterior images. Bleeding on probing is evident. Clinically, pocket depths and attachment loss are greater than 6 mm, and furcation involvement and mobility are more severe.

Predisposing Factors

The effects of certain medications, tobacco use, and various medical conditions are all considered risk factors for periodontal disease. A number of other factors may predispose the patient or contribute to periodontal disease. The identification, detection, and elimination of local irritants are important in the management and treatment of periodontal disease. Dental images play a major role in the detection of local irritants such as calculus and defective restorations.

Calculus. Calculus is a stonelike concretion that forms on the crowns and roots of teeth caused by the calcification of bacterial plaque. Calculus acts as a contributing or predisposing factor to the progress of

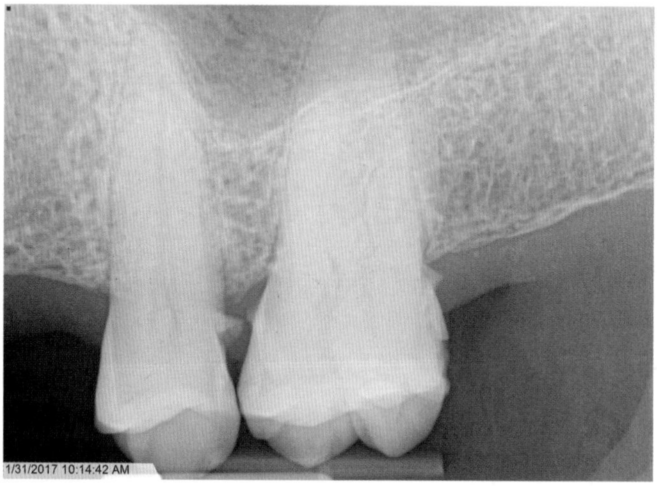

Fig 34-28 Interproximal calculus appears as irregular radiopaque projections.

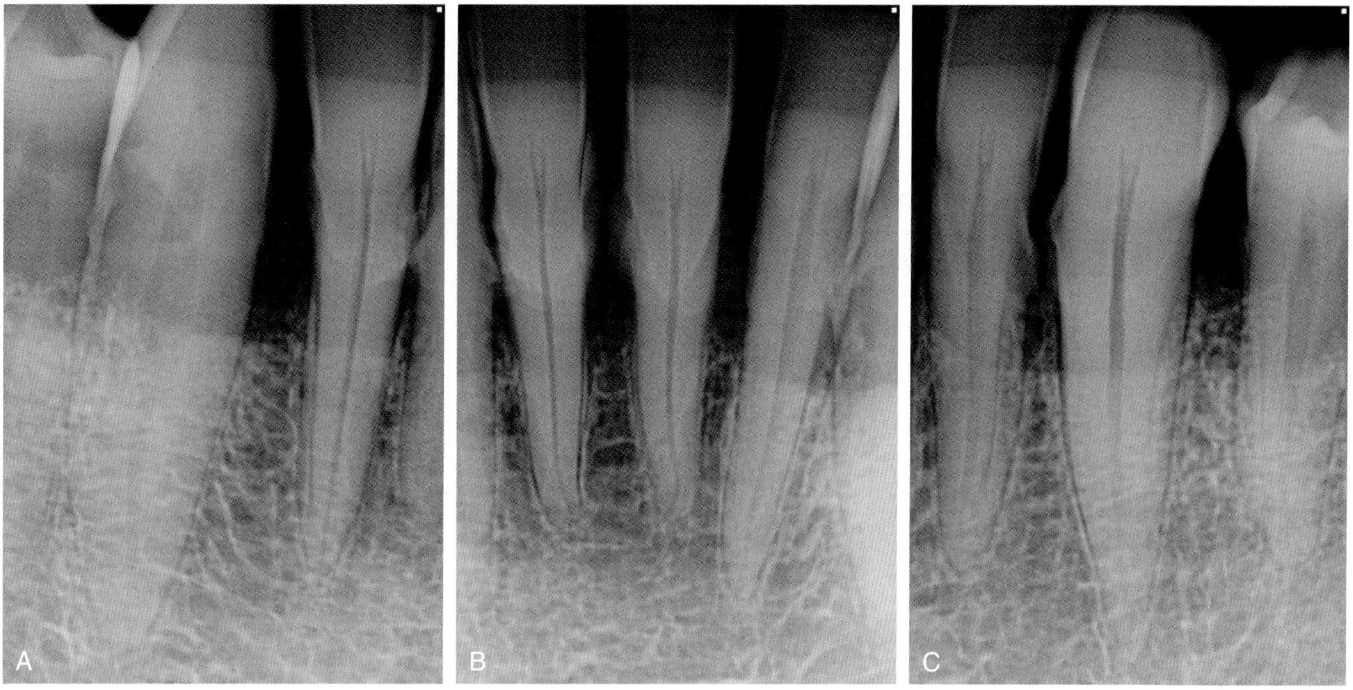

Fig 34-29 A-C, Calculus appears as radiopacities along the surfaces of mandibular anterior teeth.

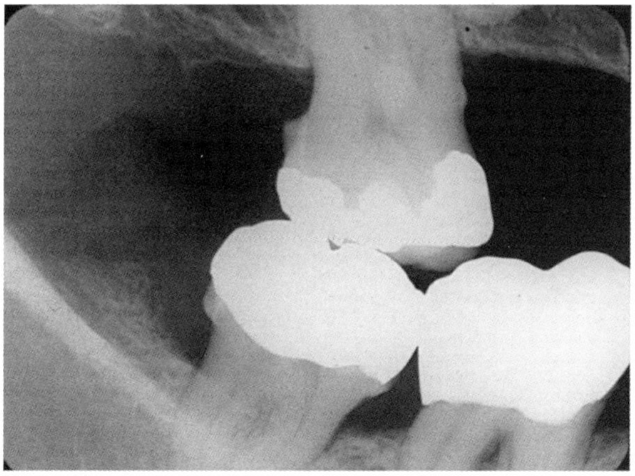

Fig 34-30 Calculus appears as a ringlike radiopacity around the cervical region of a tooth. (From Haring JI, Lind LJ: Radiographic interpretation for the dental hygienist, Philadelphia, 1993, Saunders.)

periodontal disease. Calculus appears radiopaque on a dental image (Figure 34-28). Although calculus may have a variety of appearances on dental images, it most often appears as pointed or irregular radiopaque projections extending from proximal root surfaces (Figure 34-29). Calculus may also appear as a ringlike radiopacity encircling the cervical portion of a tooth (Figure 34-30), a nodular radiopaque projection (Figure 34-31), or a smooth radiopacity on a root surface (Figure 34-32).

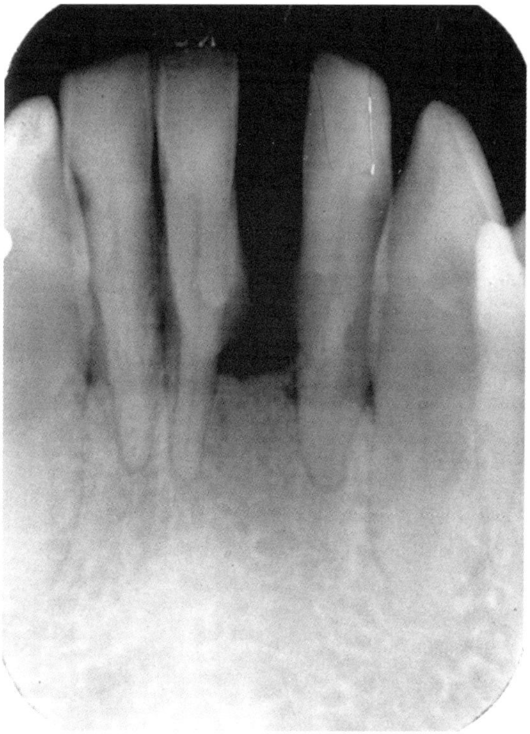

Fig 34-31 Calculus appears nodular, seen between two mandibular incisors. (From Haring JI, Lind LJ: Radiographic interpretation for the dental hygienist, Philadelphia, 1993, Saunders.)

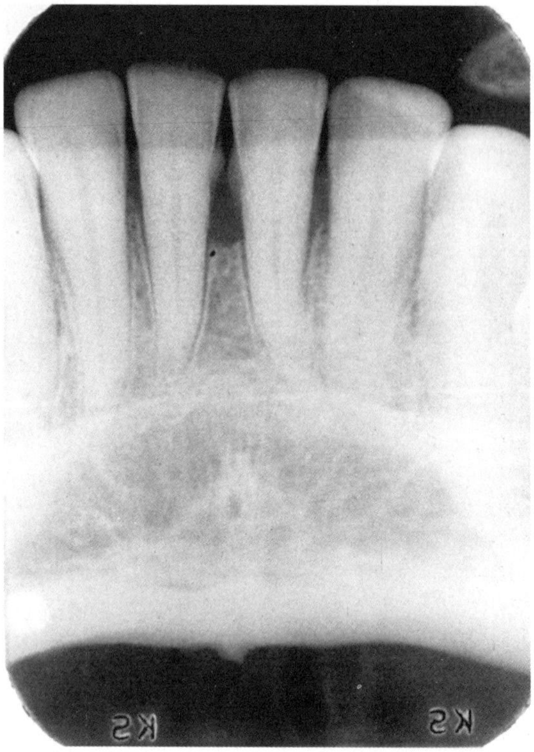

Fig 34-32 Calculus appearing as a smooth radiopacity. (From Haring JI, Lind LJ: Radiographic interpretation for the dental hygienist, Philadelphia, 1993, Saunders.)

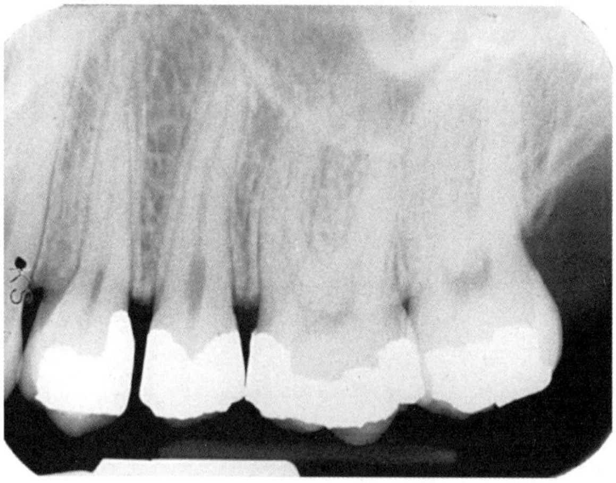

Fig 34-33 Open contact between maxillary premolars. (From Haring JI, Lind LJ: Radiographic interpretation for the dental hygienist, Philadelphia, 1993, Saunders.)

Defective Restorations. Faulty dental restorations act as potential food traps and lead to the accumulation of food debris and bacterial deposits. Defective restorations are contributing factors to periodontal disease and can be detected both clinically and on dental images. Dental images allow the dental professional to identify restorations with open or loose contacts, poor contours, uneven marginal ridges, overhangs, and inadequate margins, all of which may contribute to periodontal disease (Figures 34-33 to 34-39).

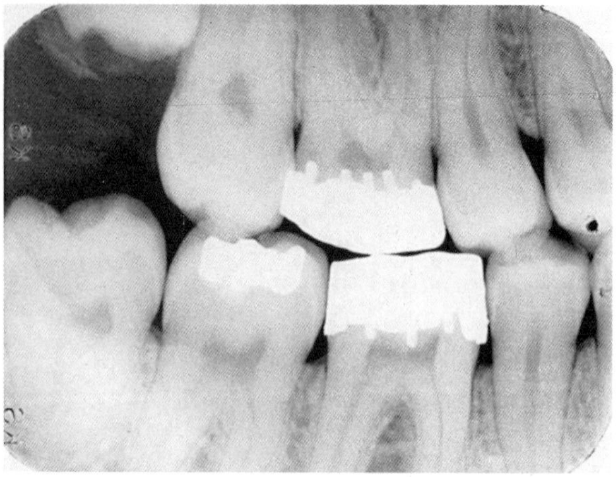

Fig 34-34 Poorly contoured crowns on maxillary and mandibular first molars. (From Haring JI, Lind LJ: Radiographic interpretation for the dental hygienist, Philadelphia, 1993, Saunders.)

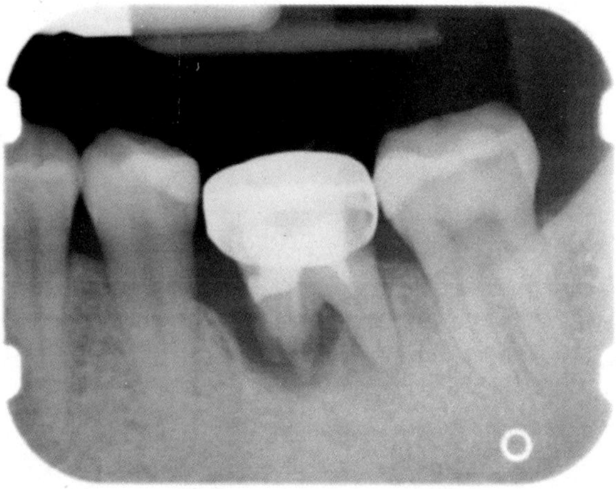

Fig 34-35 A poorly contoured stainless steel crown causing bone loss on a mandibular first molar.

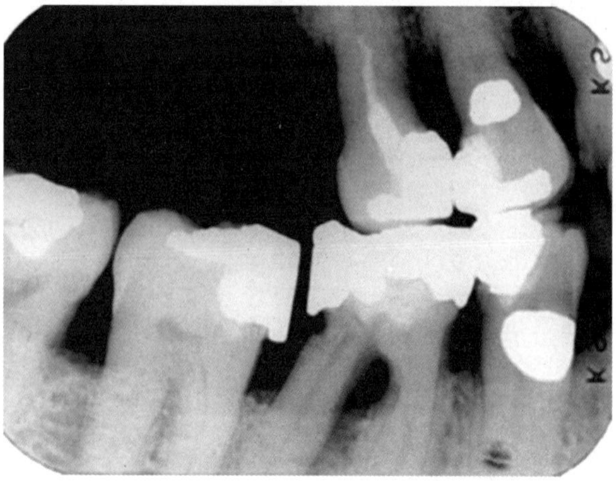

Fig 34-36 Uneven marginal ridges, open contacts, overhangs, and poorly contoured restorations on a bite-wing image. (From Haring JI, Lind LJ: Radiographic interpretation for the dental hygienist, Philadelphia, 1993, Saunders.)

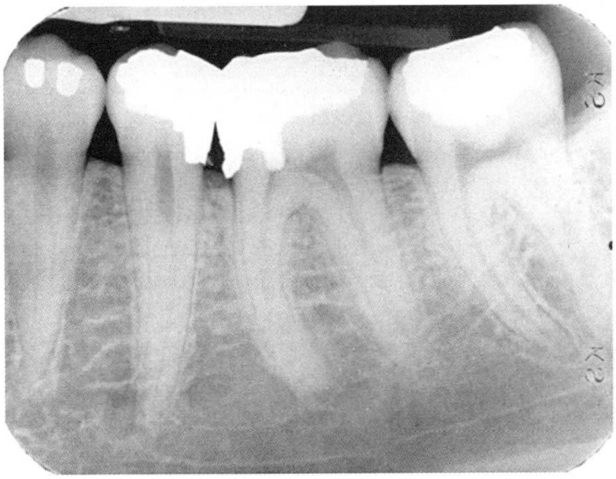

Fig 34-37 Amalgam overhang on the mesial surface of the mandibular first molar. (From Haring JI, Lind LJ: Radiographic interpretation for the dental hygienist, Philadelphia, 1993, Saunders.)

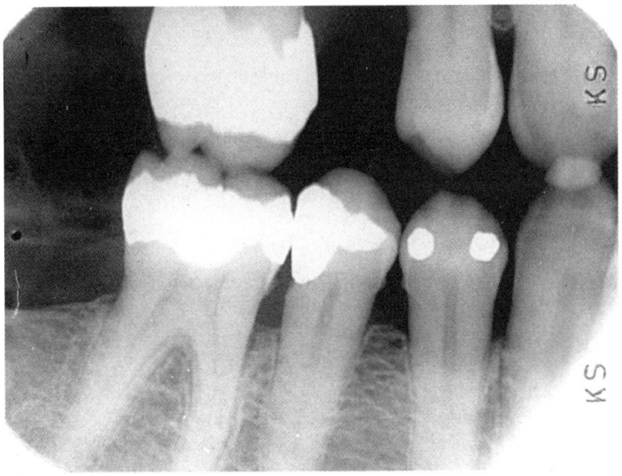

Fig 34-38 Inadequate margin on the distal surface of a mandibular second premolar. (From Haring JI, Lind LJ: Radiographic interpretation for the dental hygienist, Philadelphia, 1993, Saunders.)

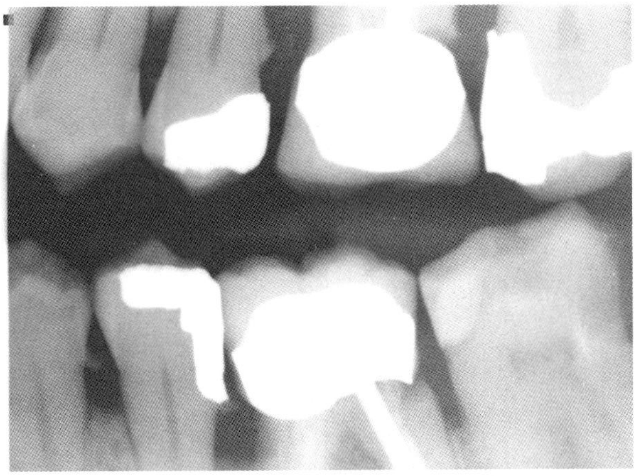

Fig 34-39 Ill-fitting restorations and open contacts between teeth contributing to the periodontal condition of this patient. (Courtesy Timothy W. Godsey, DDS, MS, Chapel Hill Periodontics and Implants, Chapel Hill, NC.)

SUMMARY

- The term *periodontal disease* refers to a group of diseases that affect the tissues around teeth.
- Thorough clinical and dental image examinations are necessary to detect, diagnose, and evaluate periodontal disease. Clinical examination provides information about soft tissues, and the dental image examination provides information about supporting bone and hard tissues.
- Dental images can be used to document periodontal disease and determine the success or failure of periodontal therapy.
- Interpretation of periodontal disease on dental images should include an evaluation of alveolar bone; bony changes can be described in terms of pattern (horizontal or vertical), distribution (localized or generalized), and severity (slight, moderate, or severe).
- In addition to the amount of bone loss viewed on images, periodontal disease is classified using clinical characteristics as described in the 2018 Classification of Periodontal and Peri-implant Diseases (Tonetti et al. J Periodontal. 2018; 89 (Supp 1):S159-S172).
- Dental images can also be used to detect local irritants, including calculus and defective restorations, which contribute to periodontal disease.

BIBLIOGRAPHY

American Academy of Periodontology: Treatment of plaque-induced gingivitis, chronic periodontitis and other clinical conditions, J Periodontol 72:1790, 2001.

American Academy of Periodontology: Proceedings from the 2017 World Workshop On The Classification Of Periodontal And Peri-Implant Diseases And Conditions. www.perio.org.

Armitage GC: Development of a classification system for periodontal diseases and conditions, Ann Periodontol 4(1), 1999.

Frommer HH, Stabulas-Savage JJ: Caries and periodontal disease. In Radiology for the dental professional, ed 9, St. Louis, 2011, Mosby.

Haring JI, Lind LJ: Periodontal disease. In Radiographic interpretation for the dental hygienist, Philadelphia, 1993, Saunders.

Mallya SM, LamEWN: Periodontal diseases. In White and Pharoah's Oral radiology: principles and interpretation, ed 8, St. Louis, 2019, Elsevier.

Miles DA, Van Dis ML, Jensen CW, et al: Basics of interpretation: normal versus abnormal and common radiographic presentation of lesions. In Radiographic imaging for the dental team, ed 4, Philadelphia, 2009, Saunders.

Newman MG, Takei H, Carranza FA: Classification of diseases and conditions affecting the periodontium. In Carranza's clinical periodontology, ed 10, Philadelphia, 2006, Saunders.

Tonetti MS, Greenwell H, Kornman KS: Staging and grading of periodontitis: Framework and proposal of a new classification and case definition, J Periodontol 89(Suppl 1):S159–S172, 2018.

QUIZ QUESTIONS

Identification

For questions 1 to 11, identify the pattern of and severity of bone loss represented by each dental image in Figures 34-40 to 34-50.

1. ______
2. ______
3. ______
4. ______
5. ______
6. ______
7. ______
8. ______
9. ______
10. ______
11. ______

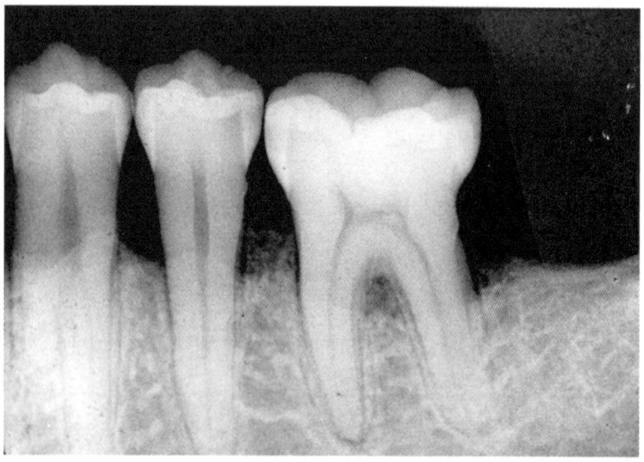

Fig 34-40 (From Haring JI, Lind LJ: Radiographic interpretation for the dental hygienist, Philadelphia, 1993, Saunders.)

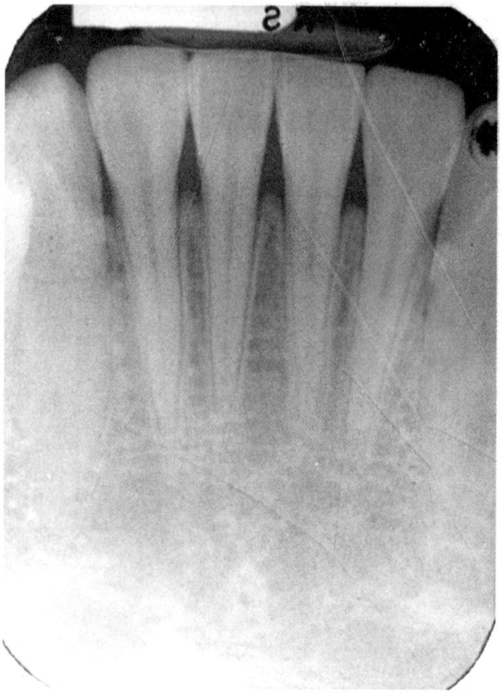

Fig 34-41 (From Haring JI, Lind LJ: Radiographic interpretation for the dental hygienist, Philadelphia, 1993, Saunders.)

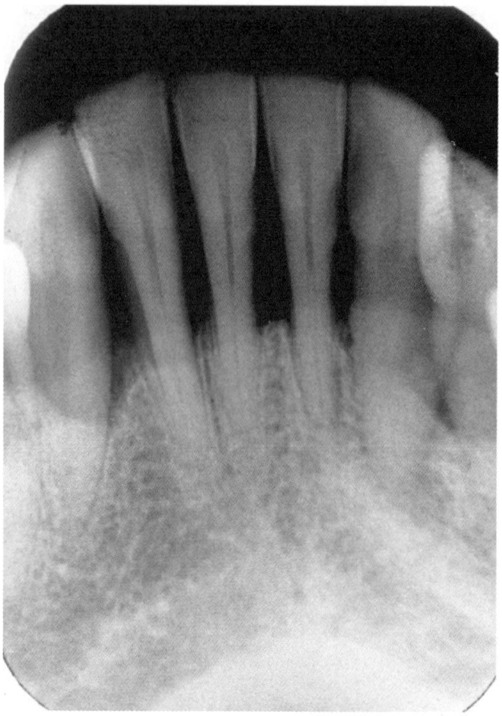

Fig 34-42 (From Haring JI, Lind LJ: Radiographic interpretation for the dental hygienist, Philadelphia, 1993, Saunders.)

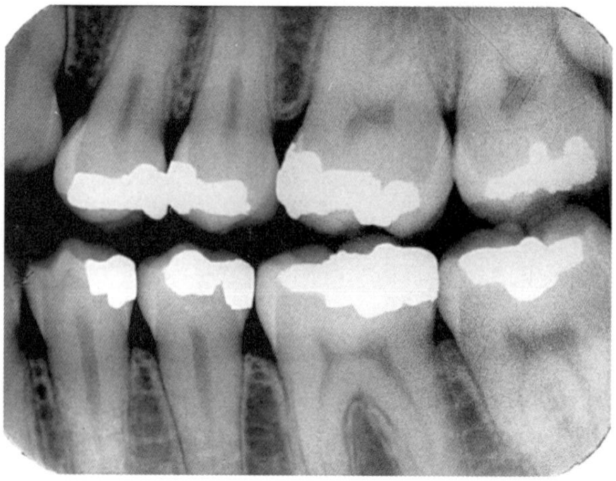

Fig 34-43 (From Haring JI, Lind LJ: Radiographic interpretation for the dental hygienist, Philadelphia, 1993, Saunders.)

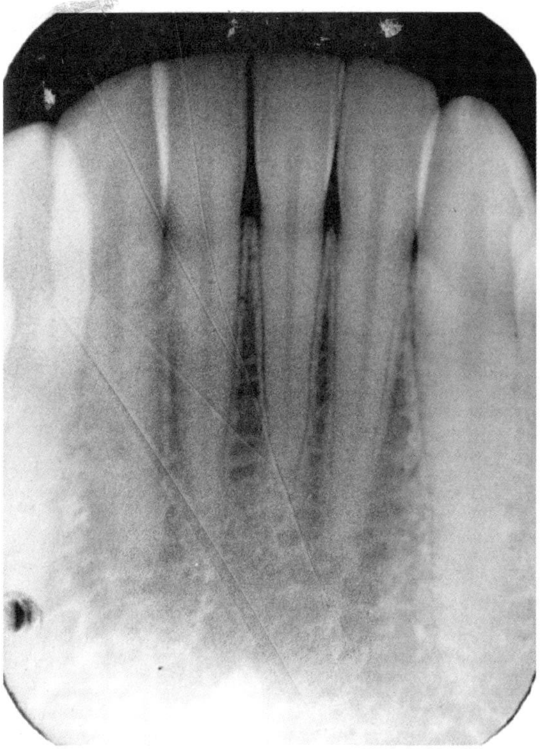

Fig 34-44 (From Haring JI, Lind LJ: Radiographic interpretation for the dental hygienist, Philadelphia, 1993, Saunders.)

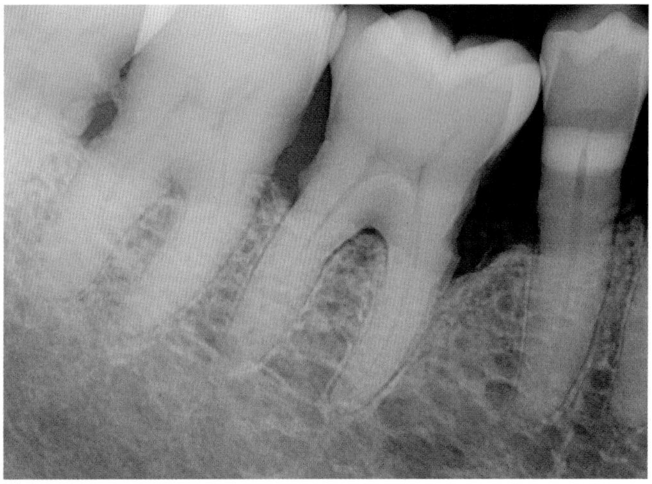

Fig 34-46

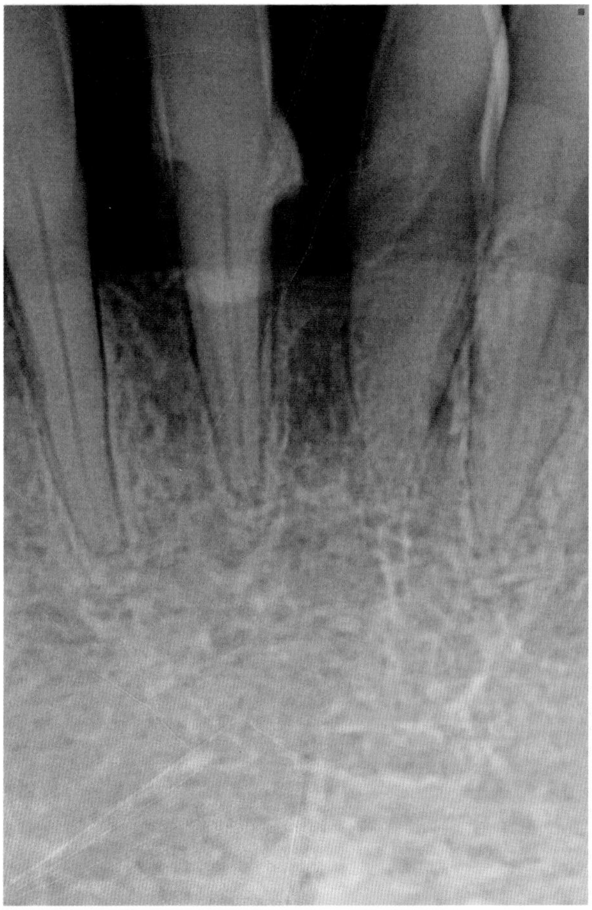

Fig 34-45

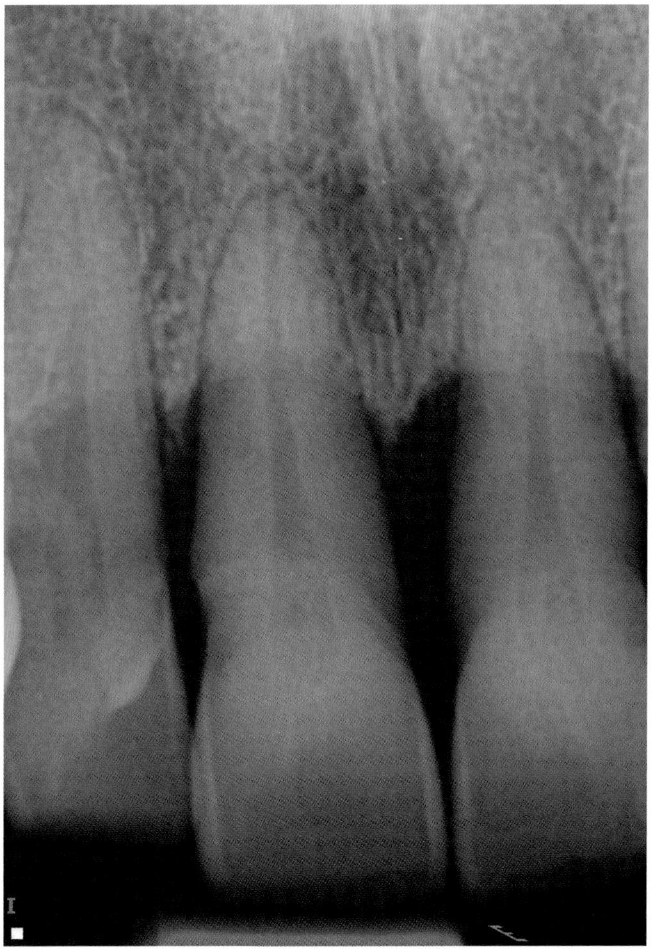

Fig 34-47

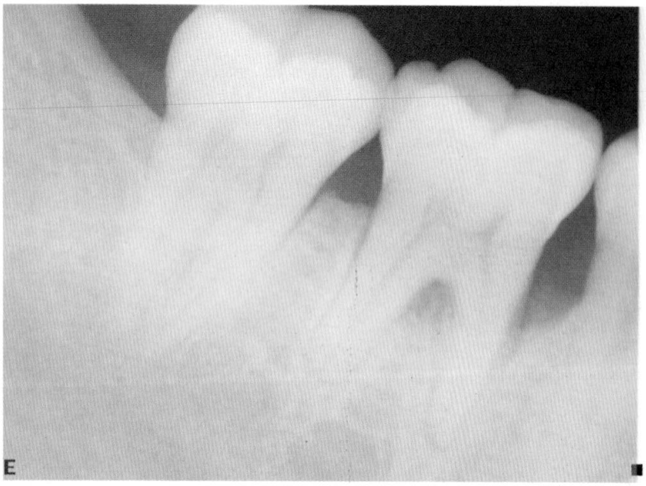

Fig 34-48

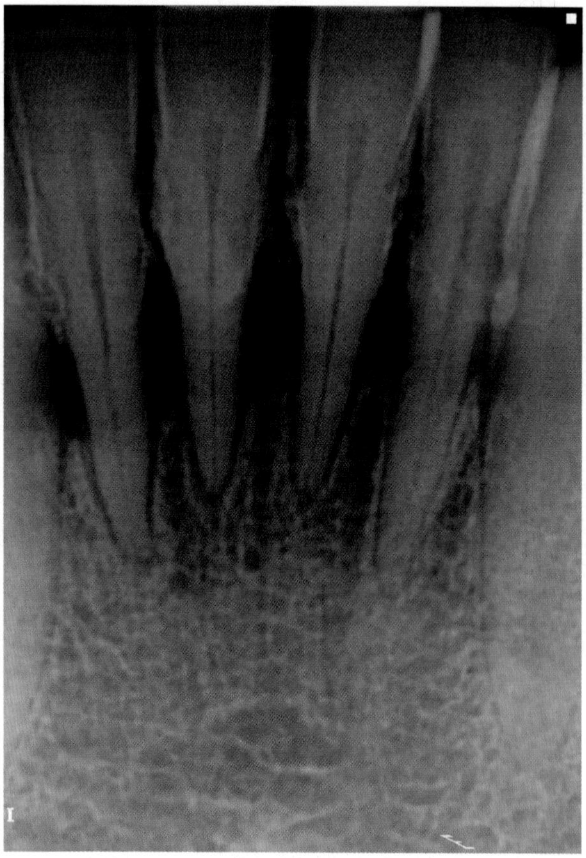

Fig 34-49

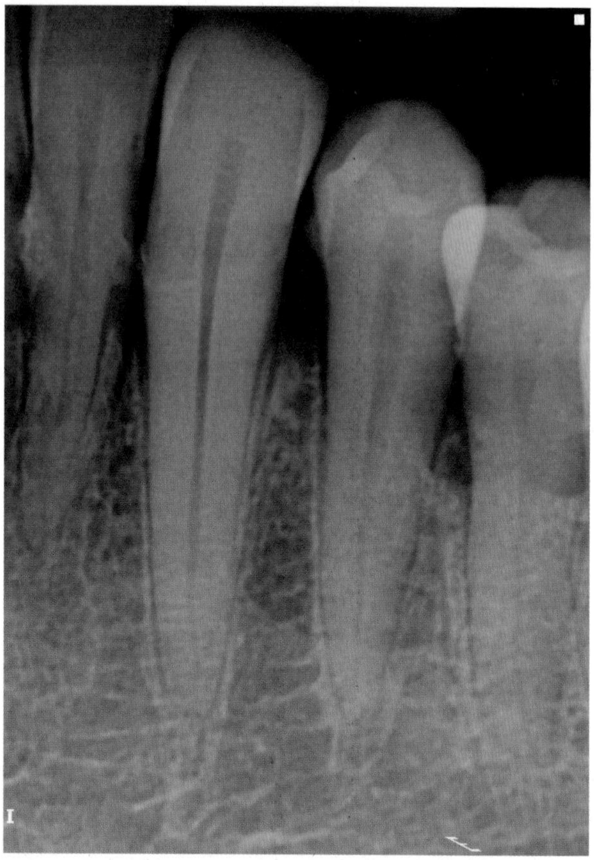

Fig 34-50

Short Answer

12. Tissues that invest and support teeth.__________
13. A term that refers to "around a tooth."__________
14. The area between the roots of multirooted teeth.__________
15. The image of choice for the evaluation of periodontal disease.__________
16. The preferred method of intraoral exposure for receptors documenting periodontal disease.__________
17. Bone loss that occurs in a plane parallel to the CEJs of adjacent teeth.__________
18. Bone loss that does not occur in a plane parallel to the CEJs of adjacent teeth.__________
19. A group of diseases that affect the tissues found around teeth.__________
20. Bone loss that occurs in isolated areas.__________
21. Bone loss that occurs evenly throughout the arches.__________
22. A stonelike concretion that forms on the crowns and roots of teeth as a result of the calcification of plaque.__________

35

Interpretation of Trauma, Pulpal Lesions, and Periapical Lesions

LEARNING OBJECTIVES

After completion of this chapter, the student will be able to do the following:

1. Define the key terms associated with the interpretation of trauma, resorption, and pulpal and periapical lesions as viewed on a dental image.
2. Describe and identify the appearance of crown, root, and jaw fractures as viewed on a dental image.
3. Describe and identify the appearance of a luxation and an avulsed tooth as viewed on a dental image.
4. Describe and identify the appearance of external and internal resorption as viewed on a dental image.
5. Describe and identify the appearance of pulpal sclerosis, pulp canal obliteration, and pulp stones as viewed on a dental image.
6. Discuss periapical radiolucencies and describe the appearance of periapical granuloma, cyst, and abscess as viewed on a dental image, and explain what is necessary to establish a definitive diagnosis.
7. Discuss periapical radiopacities and describe and identify the appearance of condensing osteitis, sclerotic bone, and hypercementosis as viewed on a dental image.

Changes associated with trauma, resorption, and pulpal and periapical lesions can all be viewed on dental images. Dental images allow for the evaluation of areas that cannot be examined clinically, such as the roots, pulp chambers, and periapical regions of teeth. Detailed information about trauma, resorption, and pulpal and periapical lesions is beyond the scope of this text. For more information on these topics, the dental radiographer should refer to additional interpretation resources.

The purpose of this chapter is to provide a brief overview of the common features of trauma, resorption, and pulpal and periapical lesions as viewed on dental images.

TRAUMA VIEWED ON DENTAL IMAGES

Trauma can be defined as an injury produced by an external force. Trauma may affect the crowns and roots of teeth, as well as the alveolar bone. Trauma may result in fractures of the jaws and teeth, as well as the displacement of teeth.

Fractures

A **fracture** can be defined as the breaking of a part. The maxilla, mandible, and teeth may all exhibit fractures. Whenever a fracture is evident or suspected, dental imaging of the injured area is indicated.

Crown Fractures

Description. A crown fracture may involve enamel only, or may include all tissues of the teeth (Figure 35-1). A crown fracture most often involves anterior teeth.

Cause. Most crown fractures result from a fall or a motor vehicle accident.

Image findings. The missing part of a crown caused by a fracture is evident on a dental image (Figure 35-2). The image allows for evaluation of the fracture location in relationship to the pulp cavity.

Root Fractures

Description. A root fracture may occur at any level along the root (Figure 35-3). A root fracture occurs most often in the maxillary central incisor region.

Cause. Most root fractures result from an accident or a traumatic blow.

Image findings. On a periapical image, if the x-ray beam is parallel with the plane of the fracture, the root fracture appears as a sharp radiolucent line (Figure 35-4). If the x-ray beam is not parallel with the fracture, adjacent areas of the tooth structure obscure the fracture site; as a result, the fracture cannot be identified on the dental image. Over time, a root fracture may enlarge because of displacement of root fragments, hemorrhage, or edema. Consequently, a root fracture that was not initially identified on a dental image may be identified on subsequent images.

Jaw Fractures

Description. A fracture of the maxilla most often involves the anterior alveolar bone and may or may not involve the tooth socket (Figure 35-5). A fracture of the lower jaw most often involves the condyle, angle, and body regions of the mandible.

Cause. A fracture of the maxilla may result from a fall or motor vehicle crash. A fracture of the mandible is seen as the result of assaults, accidents, and sports injuries.

Image findings. On a panoramic image, a mandibular fracture appears as a radiolucent line at the site where the bone has separated (Figure 35-6). The panoramic image and images produced with cone-beam computed tomography are recommended for the evaluation of a mandibular fracture.

Injuries

In addition to fractures, trauma may result in the displacement of teeth. Dental images allow for the evaluation of structures after tooth displacement. Tooth displacement includes luxation (intrusion or extrusion) and avulsion.

Luxation

Description. **Luxation**, the abnormal displacement of teeth, can be categorized as either intrusion or extrusion. **Intrusion** refers to the abnormal displacement of a tooth *into* bone (Figure 35-7). **Extrusion** refers to the abnormal displacement of a tooth *out of* bone (Figure 35-8).

Cause. Most displaced teeth result from trauma associated with assault or an accidental fall.

Image findings. A periapical image is used to evaluate a displaced tooth for root and adjacent alveolar bone fractures, damage to the

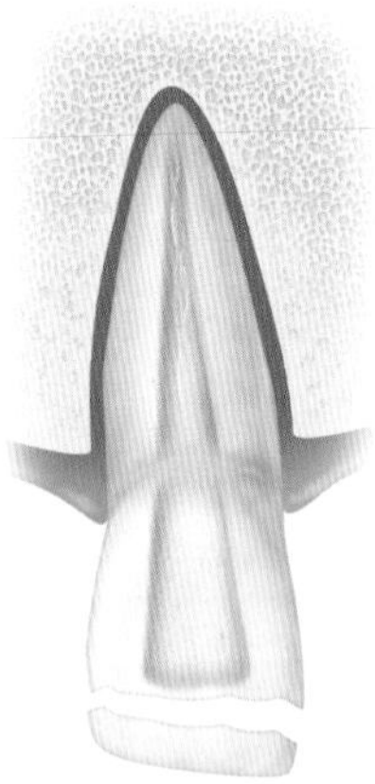

Fig 35-1 A crown fracture.

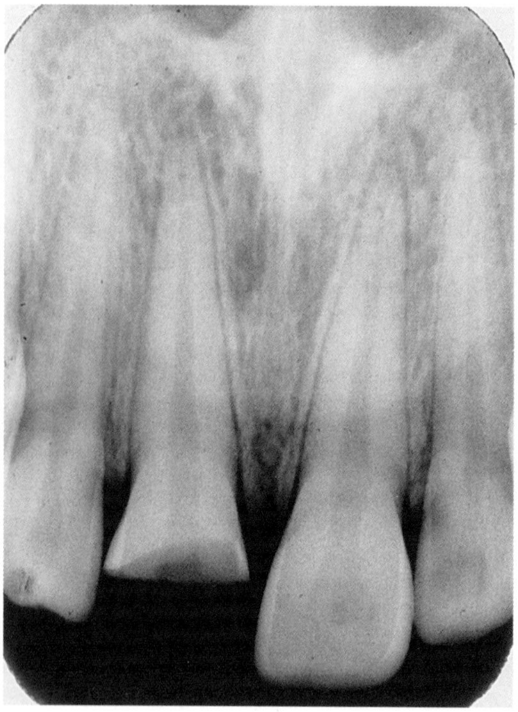

Fig 35-2 A fractured central incisor. (From Haring JI, Lind LJ: Radiographic interpretation for the dental hygienist, Philadelphia, 1993, Saunders.)

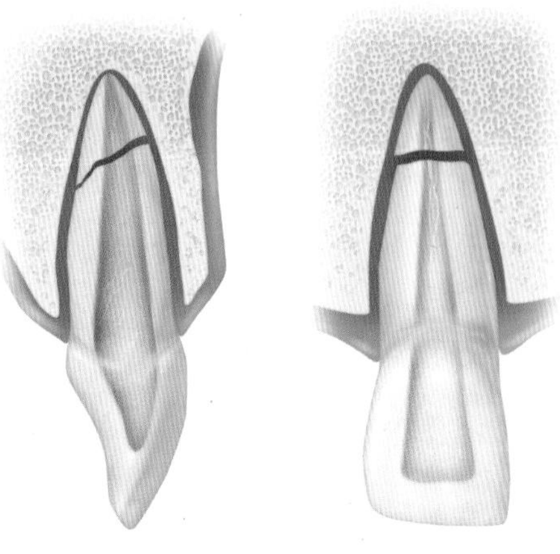

Fig 35-3 A root fracture.

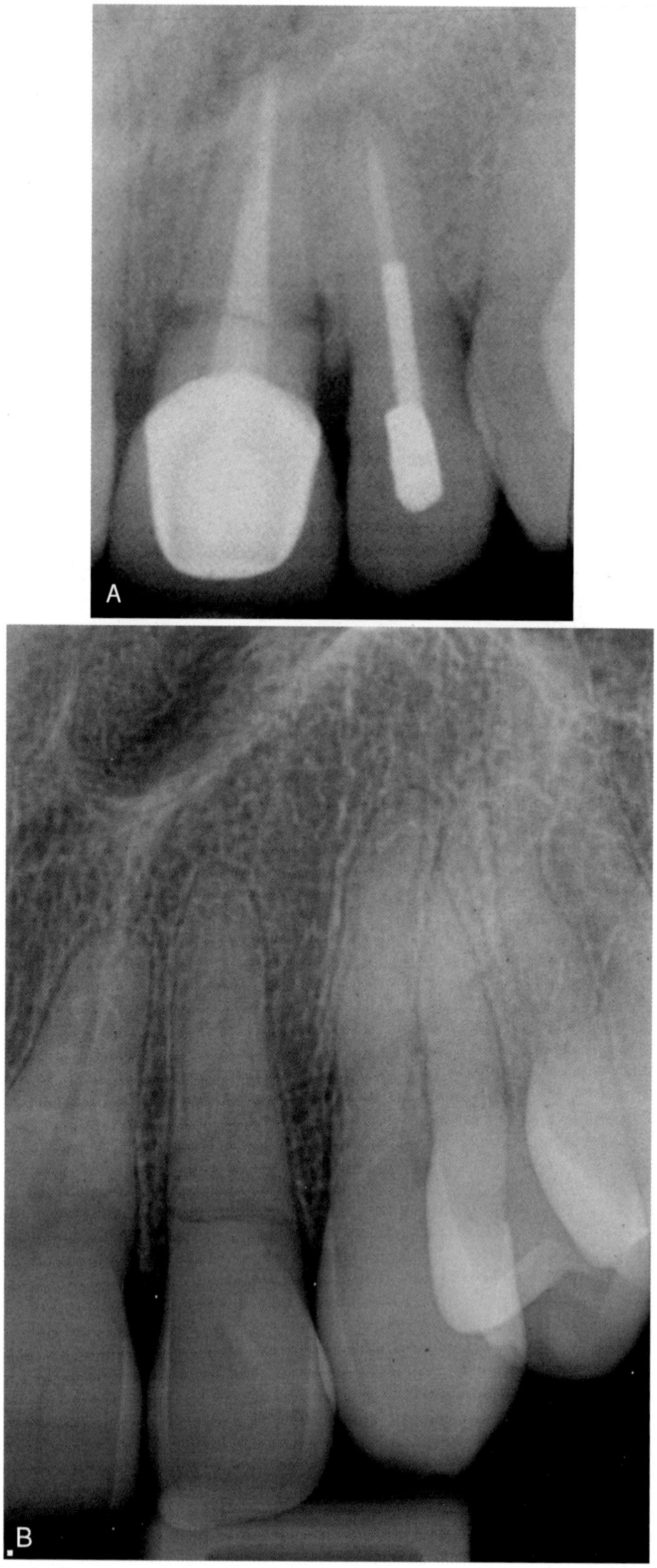

Fig 35-4 A, A root fracture on a maxillary central incisor. B, A root fracture on a maxillary lateral incisor.

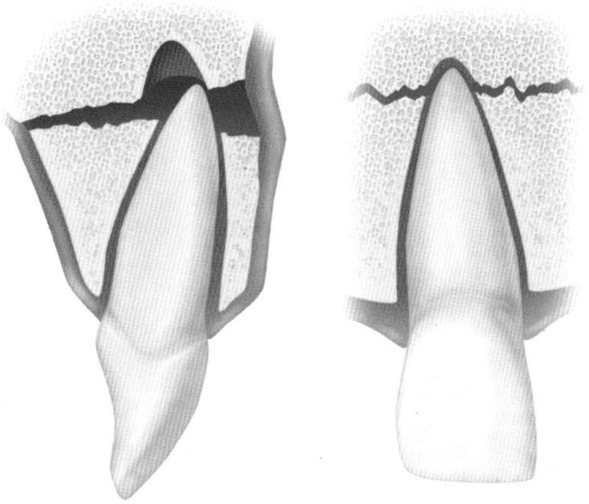

Fig 35-5 A fracture of alveolar bone.

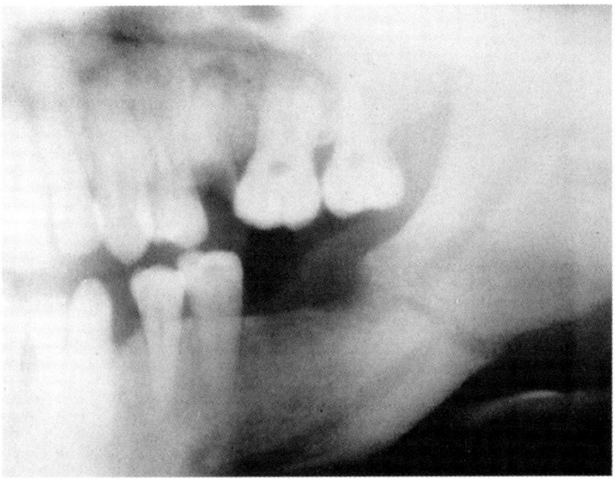

Fig 35-6 A mandibular fracture. (From Haring JI, Lind LJ: Radiographic interpretation for the dental hygienist, Philadelphia, 1993, Saunders.)

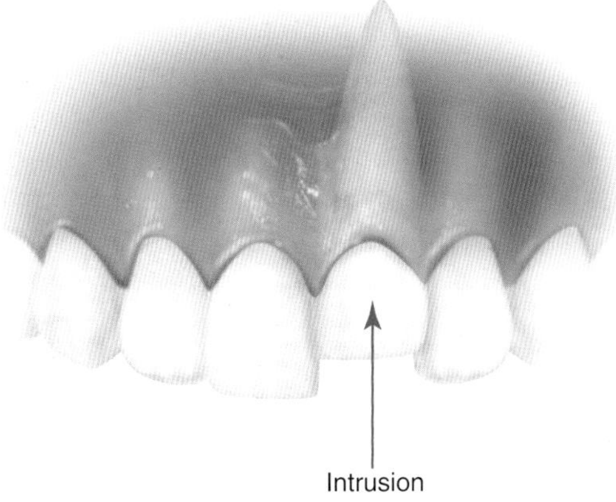

Fig 35-7 An intruded crown.

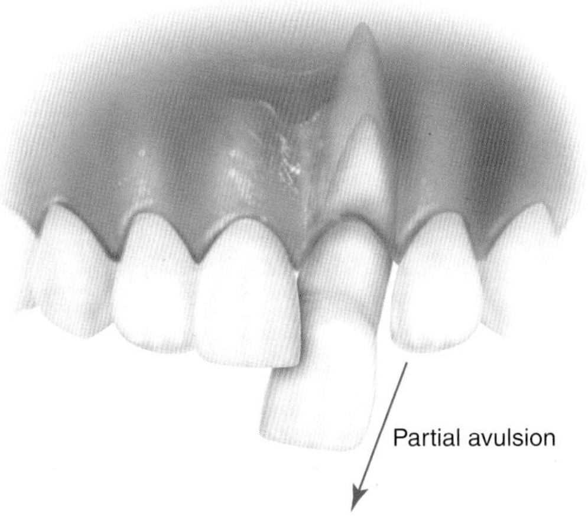

Fig 35-8 A partial avulsion (extruded crown).

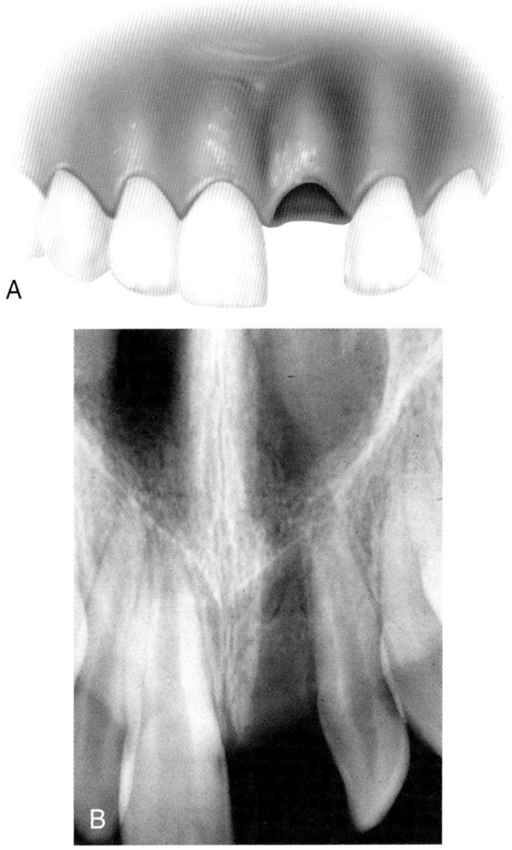

Fig 35-9 A, An avulsed tooth results in an empty tooth socket. B, Image showing socket without a tooth. (From Dean, JA, Avery DR, and McDonald RE: McDonald and Avery's Dentistry for the child and adolescent, ed 9, St. Louis, 2011, Mosby.)

periodontal ligament, and pulpal problems. Depending on the extent and severity of the injury and the treatment provided, displaced teeth often require follow-up images and evaluation for a period of years.

Dental Avulsion

Description. **Dental avulsion** is the complete displacement of a tooth from alveolar bone.

Cause. Most avulsed teeth result from trauma associated with assault or an accidental fall.

Image findings. An avulsed tooth is not seen on a dental image; instead, a periapical image reveals a tooth socket without a tooth (Figure 35-9). Dental images are important in the evaluation of the socket area and should be used to examine the region for splintered bone.

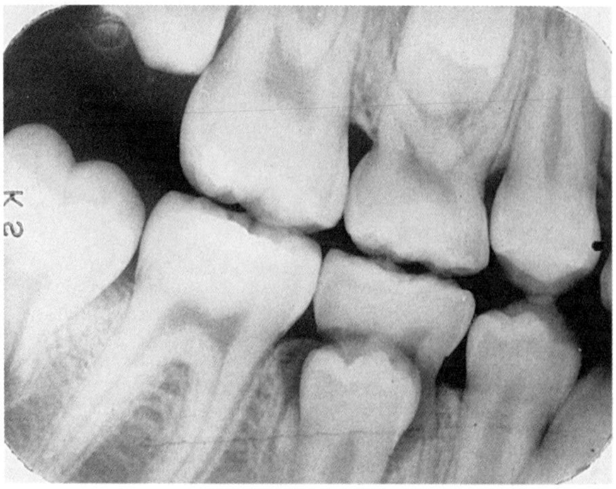

Fig 35-10 Physiologic resorption of a mandibular deciduous second molar. (From Haring JI, Lind LJ: Radiographic interpretation for the dental hygienist, Philadelphia, 1993, Saunders.)

RESORPTION VIEWED ON DENTAL IMAGES

Two types of resorption are associated with teeth: physiologic and pathologic. Physiologic resorption is a process that is seen with the normal shedding of primary teeth. The roots of a primary tooth are resorbed as the permanent successor moves in an occlusal direction; the primary tooth is shed when resorption of the roots is complete (Figure 35-10). Pathologic resorption is a regressive alteration of tooth structure that is observed when a tooth is subjected to abnormal stimuli. The pathologic resorption of teeth can be described as external or internal, depending on the location of the resorption process.

External Resorption

Description. External resorption is the destruction of root structure along the periphery of the root surface. The apical region is most often involved.

Cause. External resorption is often associated with reimplanted teeth, abnormal mechanical forces, trauma, chronic inflammation, tumors and cysts, impacted teeth, or idiopathic causes.

Image findings. On a dental image, the apical region appears blunted and the length of the root appears shorter than normal (Figure 35-11). Both the lamina dura and the bone around the blunted apex appear normal.

Clinical findings. External resorption is not associated with any signs or symptoms and is not detected clinically. A tooth with external resorption is *not* mobile.

Treatment. Currently, no effective treatment is available for external resorption.

Internal Resorption

Description. Internal resorption is the destruction of dentin around the pulp cavity within the crown or root of a tooth.

Cause. Precipitating factors such as trauma, pulp capping, and pulp polyps are believed to stimulate the internal resorption process. These factors serve as irritants and cause a chronic inflammation of the pulp that in turn destroys the surrounding dentin.

Image findings. On a dental image, internal resorption appears as a round-to-ovoid radiolucency in the mid-crown or mid-root portion of a tooth (Figures 35-12 and 35-13). It involves the pulp chamber, pulp canals, and surrounding dentin.

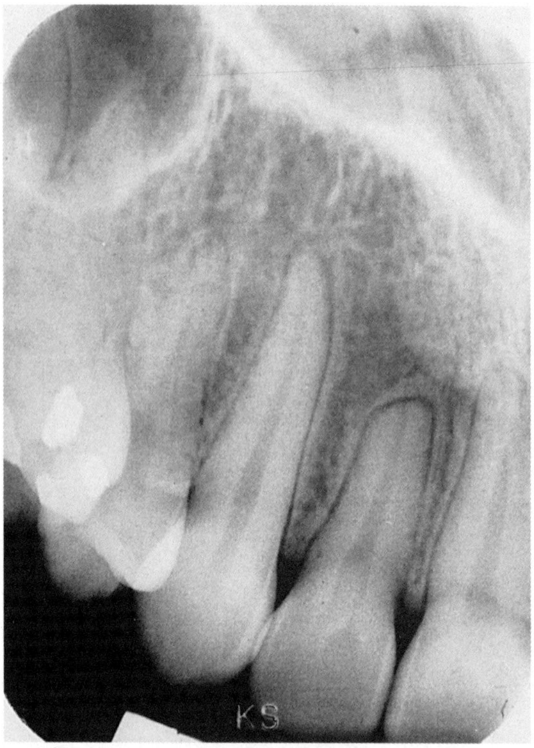

Fig 35-11 External resorption of the apical region of a maxillary lateral incisor. (From Haring JI, Lind LJ: Radiographic interpretation for the dental hygienist, Philadelphia, 1993, Saunders.)

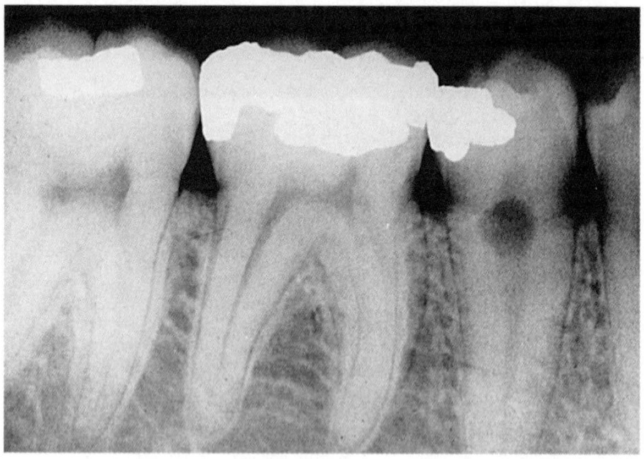

Fig 35-12 Internal resorption seen as a round radiolucency in the cervical region of a mandibular second premolar. (From Haring JI, Lind LJ: Radiographic interpretation for the dental hygienist, Philadelphia, 1993, Saunders.)

Clinical findings. Internal resorption is generally asymptomatic. The incisors are most often affected.

Treatment. Treatment is variable; endodontic therapy may be used if the resorptive process has not physically weakened the tooth. Extraction is recommended if the tooth is weakened by the resorptive process, or if a root perforation exists.

PULPAL LESIONS VIEWED ON DENTAL IMAGES

Many dental procedures require information about the size and location of the pulp cavity before treatment begins. Without dental images, examination of pulp chambers and canals is impossible. Pulpal

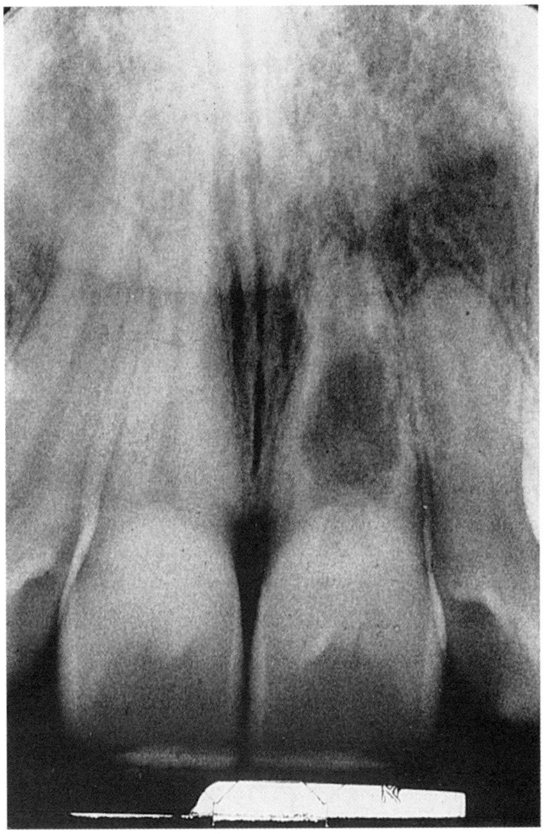

Fig 35-13 Internal resorption seen as a radiolucency in the root of a maxillary central incisor. (From Haring JI, Lind LJ: Radiographic interpretation for the dental hygienist, Philadelphia, 1993, Saunders.)

sclerosis, pulp canal obliteration, and pulp stones are common conditions of the pulp cavity that can be seen on dental images.

Pulpal Sclerosis

Description. Pulpal sclerosis is a diffuse calcification of the pulp chamber and pulp canals.

Cause. For unknown reasons, pulpal sclerosis is associated with aging.

Image findings. On a dental image, a pulp cavity of decreased size with very thin pulp canals is seen (Figure 35-14).

Clinical findings. No clinical features are associated with pulpal sclerosis; it is considered an incidental finding and has little clinical significance unless endodontic therapy is indicated.

Pulp Canal Obliteration

Description. Pulp canal obliteration is the calcification, or deposition of hard tissue, within the pulp cavity.

Cause. Conditions such as attrition, abrasion, caries, dental restorations, trauma, and abnormal mechanical forces may act as pulpal irritants and stimulate the production of secondary dentin that results in obliteration of the pulp cavity.

Image findings. On a dental image, a tooth with pulp canal obliteration has no visible pulp chamber and/or pulp canals (Figure 35-15).

Clinical findings. A tooth that exhibits pulp canal obliteration is nonvital and clinically may appear discolored (Figure 35-16).

Pulp Stones

Description. Pulp stones are dystrophic calcifications found in the pulp chamber or pulp canals of teeth.

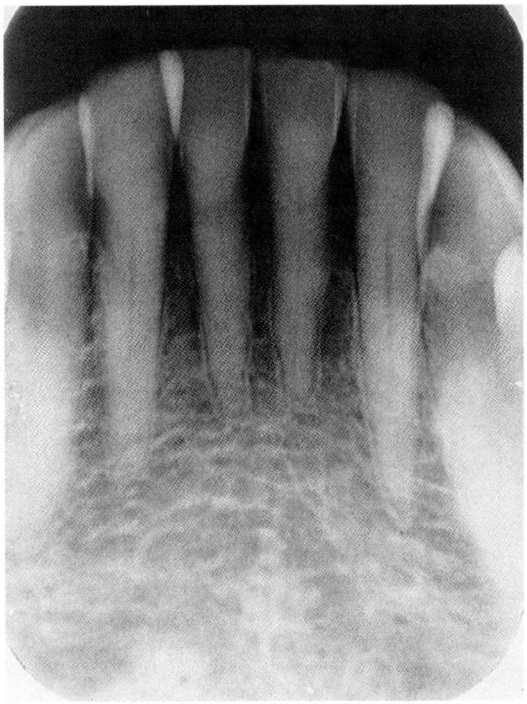

Fig 35-14 Thin atrophic pulp chambers in mandibular incisors. (From Haring JI, Lind LJ: Radiographic interpretation for the dental hygienist, Philadelphia, 1993, Saunders.)

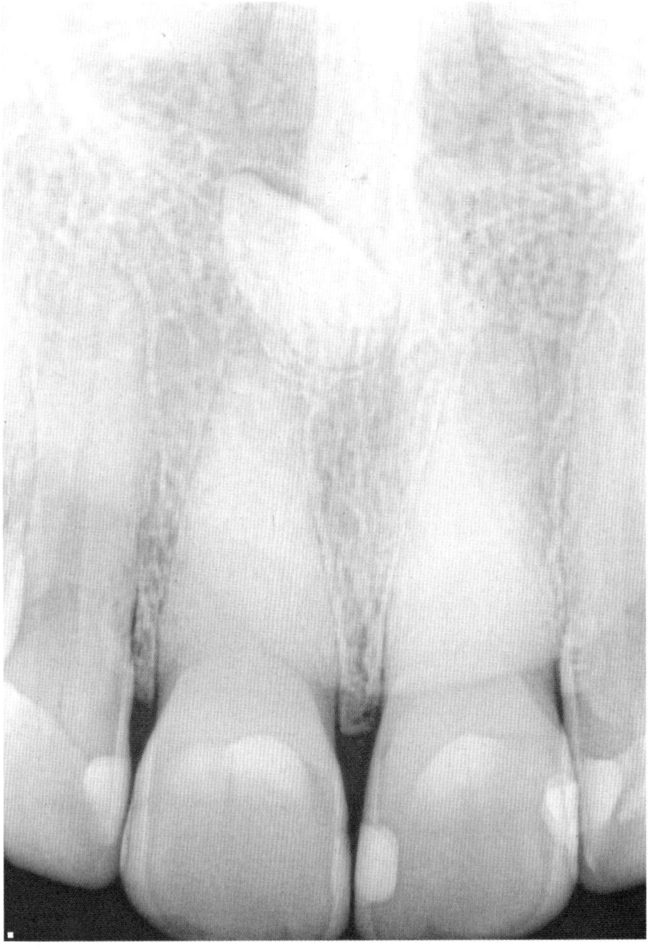

Fig 35-15 Pulp canal obliteration in both maxillary central incisors.

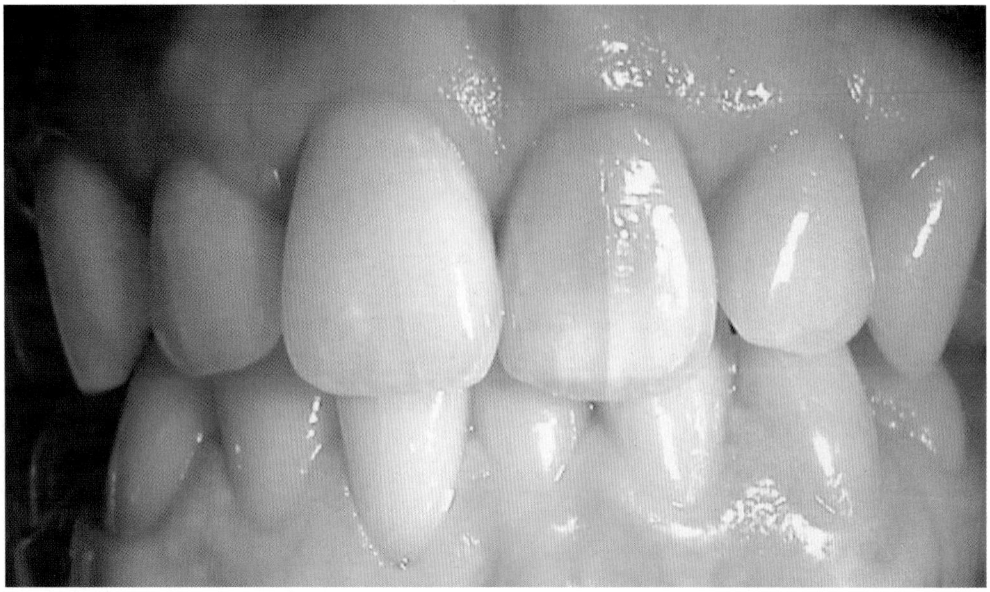

Fig 35-16 A nonvital tooth often appears discolored, as seen in this maxillary central incisor. (From Wilson N, Millar B: Principles and practice of esthetic dentistry: essentials of esthetic dentistry, London, 2015, Elsevier.)

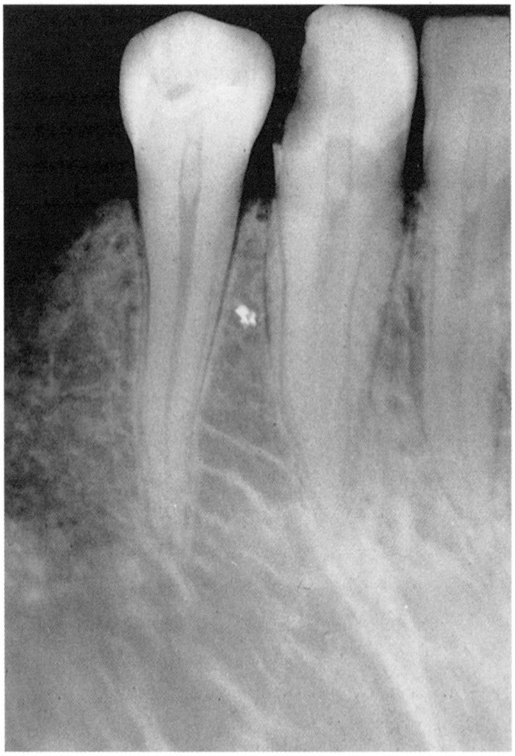

Fig 35-17 Cylindrical pulp stones in the mandibular canine and premolar. (From Haring JI, Lind LJ: Radiographic interpretation for the dental hygienist, Philadelphia, 1993, Saunders.)

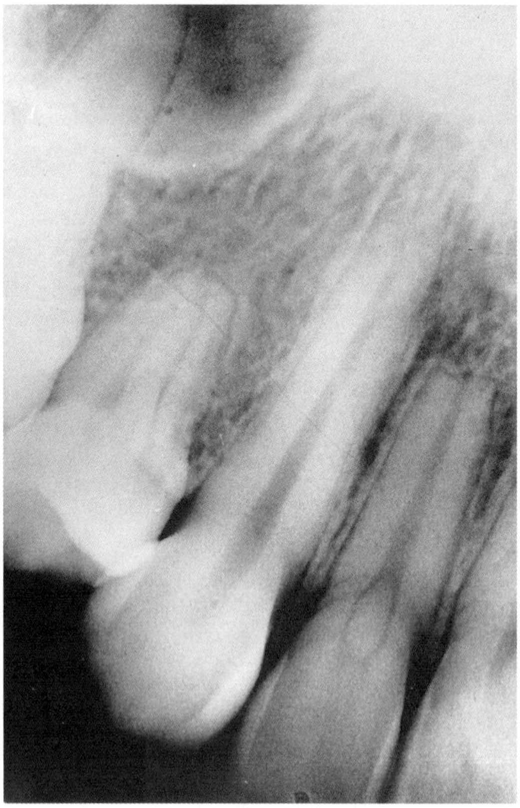

Fig 35-18 An ovoid pulp stone in a maxillary lateral incisor. (From Haring JI, Lind LJ: Radiographic interpretation for the dental hygienist, Philadelphia, 1993, Saunders.)

Cause. The cause of pulp stones is unknown.

Image findings. On a dental image, pulp stones appear as round, ovoid, or cylindrical radiopacities; some pulp stones may conform to the shape of the pulp chamber or canal (Figures 35-17 and 35-18). Pulp stones may vary in size and number.

Clinical findings. No clinical features are associated with pulp stones. Pulp stones are considered an incidental finding with little clinical significance unless endodontic therapy is indicated.

PERIAPICAL LESIONS VIEWED ON DENTAL IMAGES

A **periapical lesion** is located around the apex (tip of the root) of a tooth. The use of dental imaging is particularly important in the identification of periapical lesions. On dental images, periapical lesions may appear either *radiolucent* or *radiopaque*.

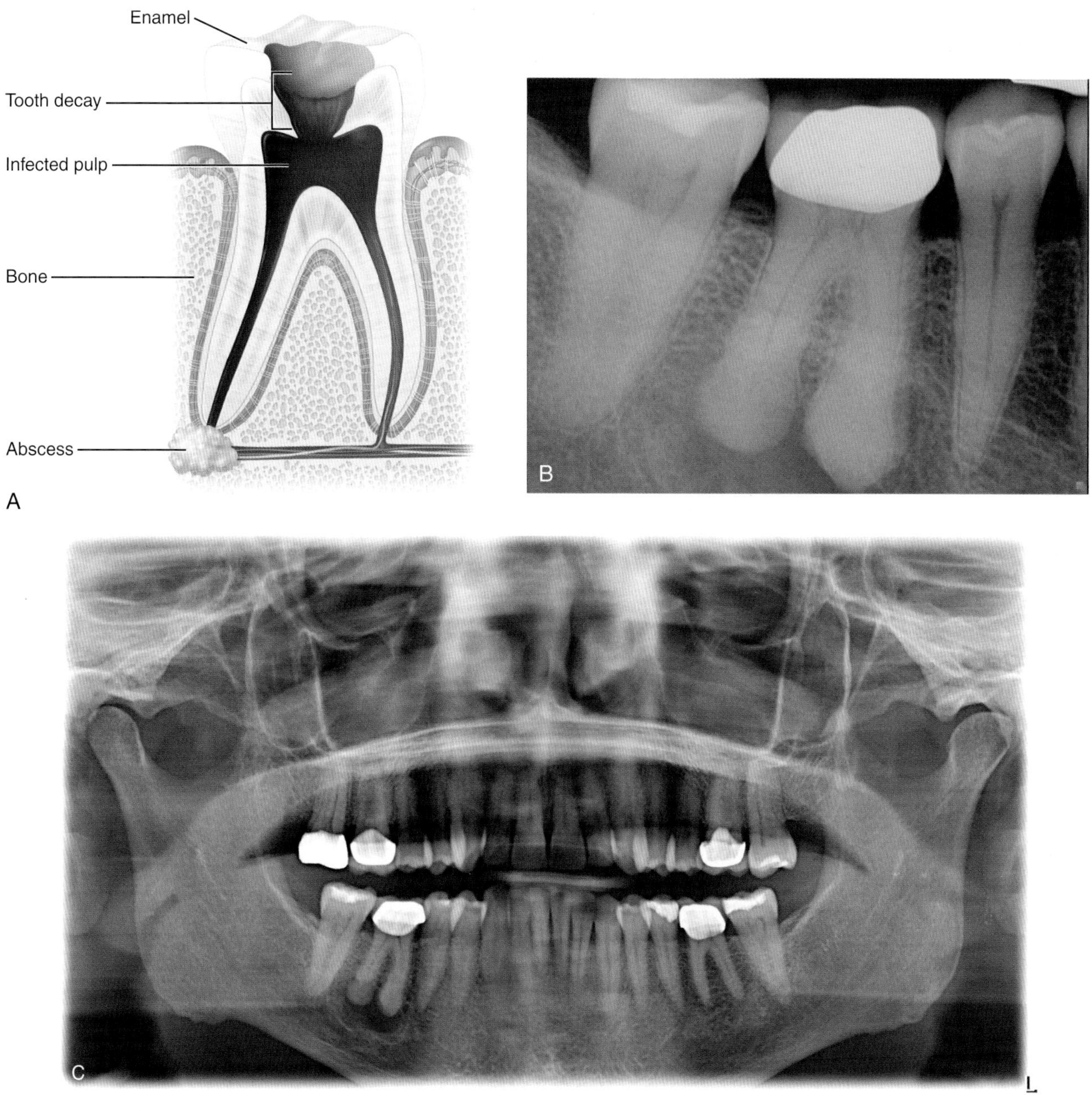

Fig 35-19 **A,** Infection of the pulp results in necrosis. A periapical granuloma, cyst, or abscess forms at the apex. **B,** Periapical image shows infection of the pulp of tooth #30. **C,** Panoramic image of the same patient.

Periapical Radiolucencies

A periapical radiolucent lesion results from pulpal death and necrosis. The most frequent cause of pulpal death and necrosis is dental caries. Trauma may also be a cause. With pulpal necrosis, an inflammatory process is seen that extends from the pulp chamber and canals to the periapical region of the affected tooth (Figure 35-19). The lesion that results may be a periapical granuloma, periapical cyst, or periapical abscess.

A periapical radiolucency viewed on a dental image may represent a periapical granuloma, cyst, or abscess. On a dental image, no distinctive differences between these three lesions are evident. A periapical granuloma, cyst, or abscess **cannot** be identified from a dental image. A definitive diagnosis can be established only with microscopic examination. Whenever a periapical radiolucency is seen on a dental image, it is best to document the finding as a "periapical radiolucency." The terms *periapical granuloma, cyst,* and *abscess* imply a specific diagnosis and should not be used to describe what is seen on a dental image.

Periapical Granuloma.

Description. A periapical granuloma is a localized mass of chronically inflamed granulation tissue at the apex of a nonvital tooth.

Cause. A periapical granuloma results from pulpal death and necrosis and is the most common sequela of *pulpitis* (inflammation of the pulp).

Image findings. On a dental image, a periapical granuloma may appear initially as a widened periodontal ligament space at the root apex (Figure 35-20). With time, the widened periodontal ligament space enlarges and appears as a round or ovoid radiolucency (Figure 35-21). The lamina dura is *not* visible between the root apex and the apical lesion.

Clinical findings. A tooth with a periapical granuloma is nonvital. It is typically asymptomatic but has a previous history of prolonged sensitivity to heat or cold.

Diagnosis. A periapical granuloma cannot be diagnosed from a dental image; a definitive diagnosis is possible only with microscopic examination.

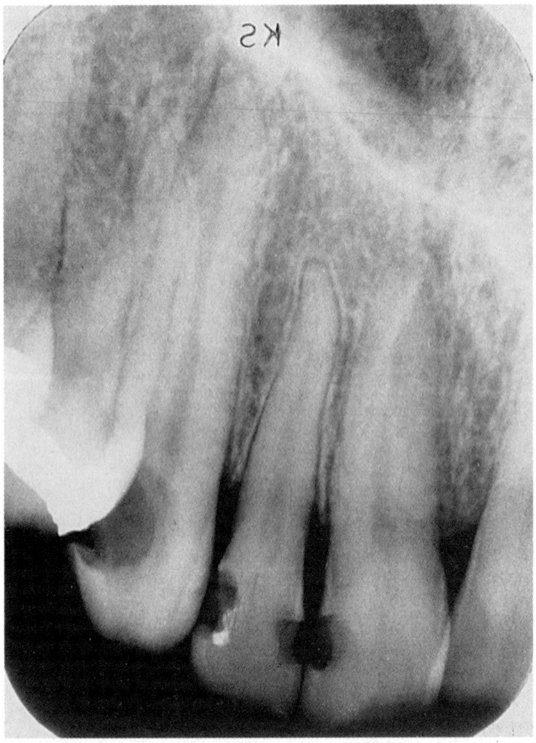

Fig 35-20 A widened periodontal ligament space at the apex of a maxillary lateral incisor. (From Haring JI, Lind LJ: Radiographic interpretation for the dental hygienist, Philadelphia, 1993, Saunders.)

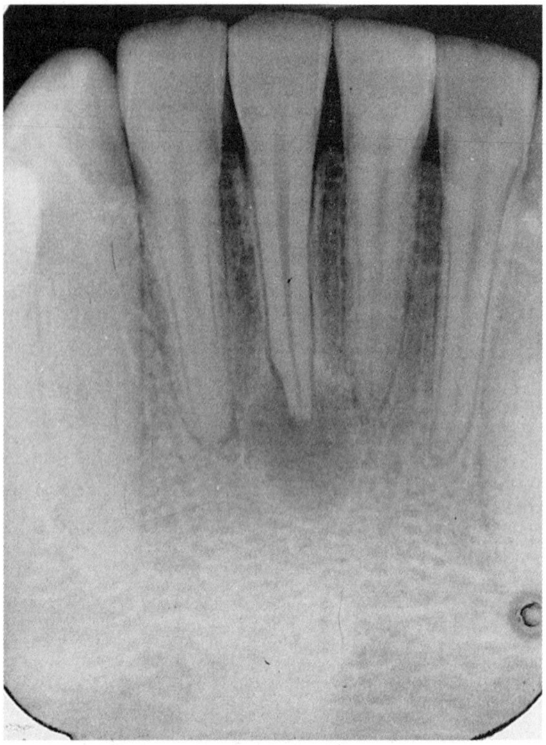

Fig 35-22 A well-defined round radiolucency seen at the apex of a mandibular central incisor. (From Haring JI, Lind LJ: Radiographic interpretation for the dental hygienist, Philadelphia, 1993, Saunders.)

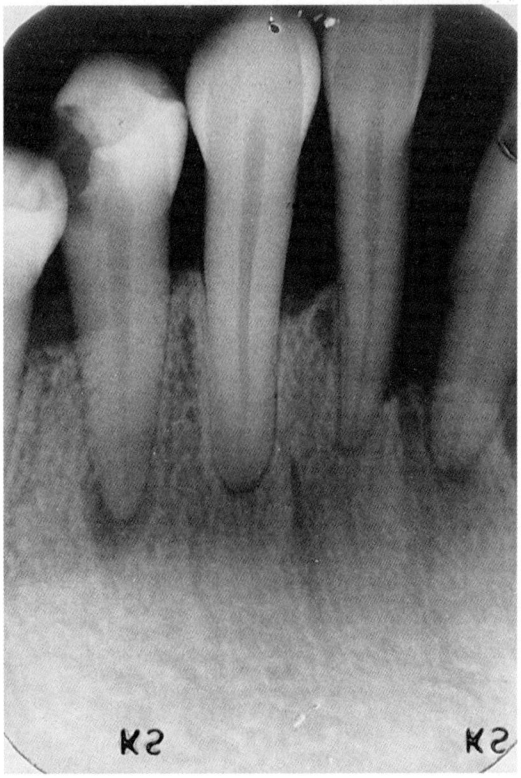

Fig 35-21 A periapical radiolucency associated with a mandibular premolar. (Note that the lamina dura is not visible.) (From Haring JI, Lind LJ: Radiographic interpretation for the dental hygienist, Philadelphia, 1993, Saunders.)

Treatment. Treatment for a periapical granuloma may include endodontic therapy or removal of the tooth with curettage of the apical region.

Periapical Cyst

Description. A **periapical cyst** (also known as a *radicular cyst*) is a lesion with an epithelial lining located at the apex of a nonvital tooth.

Cause. The periapical cyst results from pulpal death and necrosis and is formed over a prolonged period after cystic degeneration within a periapical granuloma. Most periapical cysts originate from preexisting granulomas.

Image findings. On a dental image, the typical periapical cyst may appear as a round or ovoid radiolucency (Figure 35-22). The lamina dura is *not* visible between the root apex and the apical lesion.

Clinical findings. A tooth with a periapical cyst is nonvital. The periapical cyst is typically asymptomatic. The periapical cyst is the most common of all tooth-related cysts and accounts for 50% to 70% of all cysts identified in the oral region.

Diagnosis. A periapical cyst cannot be diagnosed from a dental image; a definitive diagnosis is possible only with microscopic examination.

Treatment. Treatment may include endodontic therapy or extraction of the tooth and curettage of the apical region. If left untreated, a periapical cyst may slowly enlarge, expand cortical plates, and destroy the surrounding bone (Figure 35-23).

Periapical Abscess. A **periapical abscess** is a localized collection of pus around the apex of a nonvital tooth. It results from pulpal death. A periapical abscess may be *acute* or *chronic*.

Description. An *acute* periapical abscess is a localized collection of pus around the apex of a nonvital tooth that has features of an acute

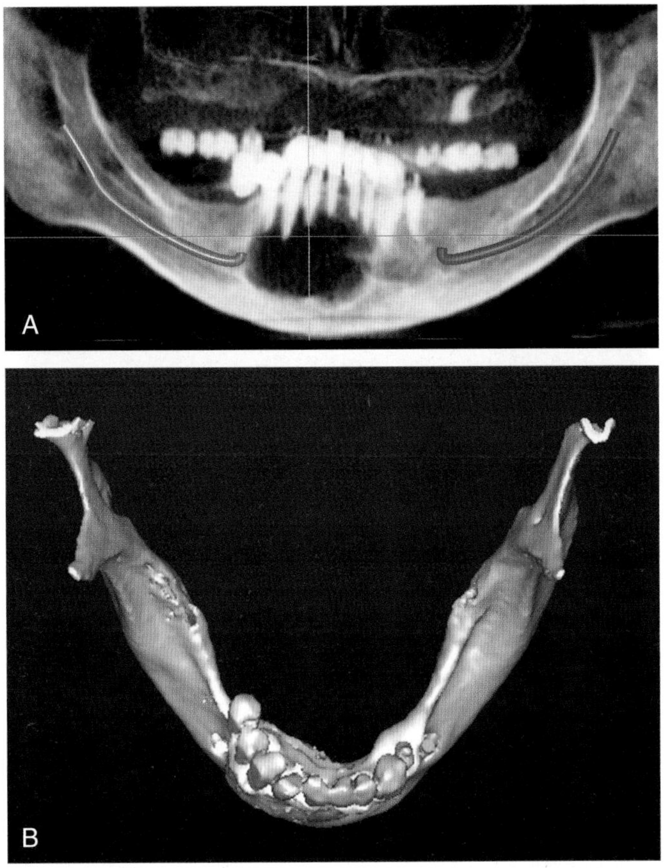

Fig 35-23 **A,** A large periapical radiolucent region appears on this panoramic image in the anterior mandible. **B,** A three-dimensional volume rendering reveals the expanded facial and lingual cortical borders of the mandible where thinning has occurred. (Courtesy Carolina OMF Imaging, W. Bruce Howerton, Jr., DDS, MS, Franklinton, NC.)

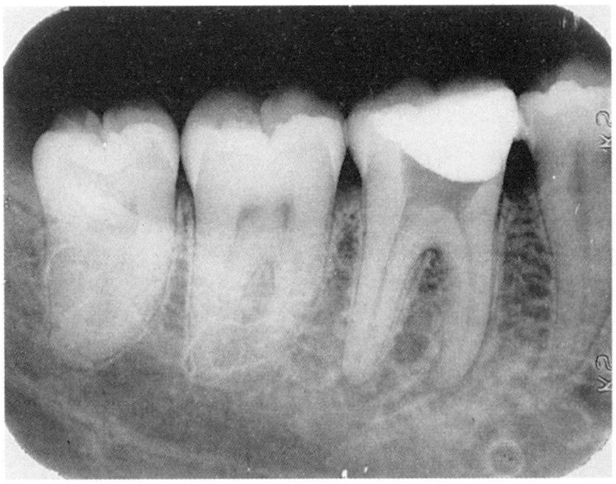

Fig 35-24 An increased widening of the periodontal ligament space seen in the periapical region of the mandibular first molar. (From Haring JI, Lind LJ: Radiographic interpretation for the dental hygienist, Philadelphia, 1993, Saunders.)

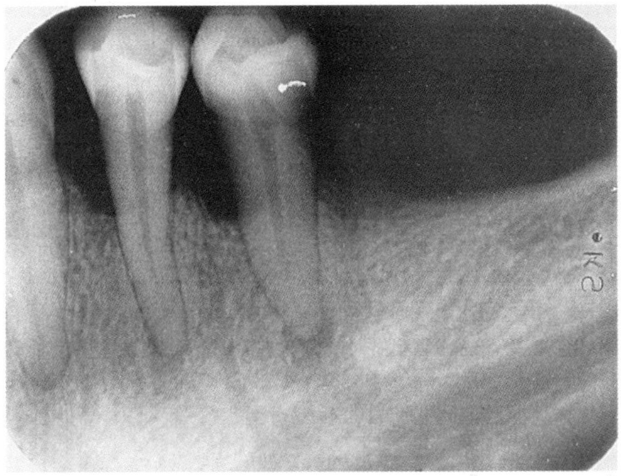

Fig 35-25 Periapical radiolucencies associated with mandibular premolars. (From Haring JI, Lind LJ: Radiographic interpretation for the dental hygienist, Philadelphia, 1993, Saunders.)

pus-producing process. A *chronic* periapical abscess is a localized collection of pus around the apex of a nonvital tooth that has features of a long-standing, low-grade, pus-producing process.

Cause. Whether acute or chronic, a periapical abscess results from pulpal death and necrosis.

Image findings. On a dental image, an *acute* periapical abscess may exhibit no change at the apex, or a slight increased widening of the periodontal ligament space may be seen (Figure 35-24). A *chronic* periapical abscess may appear as a round or ovoid apical radiolucency with poorly defined margins (Figure 35-25). The lamina dura is *not* visible between the root apex and the apical lesion.

Clinical findings. Whether acute or chronic, a tooth with a periapical abscess is nonvital. An *acute* periapical abscess is painful; the pain may be intense, throbbing, and constant. The tooth is sensitive to pressure, percussion, and heat. A *chronic* periapical abscess is usually asymptomatic because the pus drains through bone or the periodontal ligament space. Clinically, a *gum boil* (parulis) may be seen in the apical region of the tooth at the site of drainage.

Diagnosis. A periapical abscess (acute or chronic) cannot be diagnosed from a dental image; a definitive diagnosis is possible only with microscopic examination.

Treatment. Whether acute or chronic, treatment of a periapical abscess includes drainage and endodontic therapy or extraction of the tooth with curettage of the apical region.

Periodontal Abscess. It is important to note the difference between a periapical abscess and a periodontal abscess. One infection originates within the tooth, while the other originates in the periodontal structures surrounding the tooth. The *periapical abscess* is a collection of pus that results from a *necrotic pulp* (within the tooth); a periodontal abscess is a collection of pus that results from *infection within the periodontal tissues* (surrounding the tooth).

Description. The periodontal abscess is an acute destructive process resulting from a bacterial infection within the walls of periodontal tissues.

Cause. The periodontal abscess occurs as a complication of advanced periodontal disease. It occurs when the opening of a periodontal pocket becomes obstructed.

Image findings. A periodontal abscess appears as a radiolucent area along the lateral aspect of the root. The lamina dura is *not* visible. With extensive bone loss, the tooth may appear to be floating (Figure 35-26).

Clinical findings. The most common symptom of a periodontal abscess is deep and throbbing pain. As the pus forms, the pressure and pain increases until it spontaneously drains via a periodontal pocket. As the lesion drains, a bad taste is noted. Mobility may be present, depending on the amount of bone destruction.

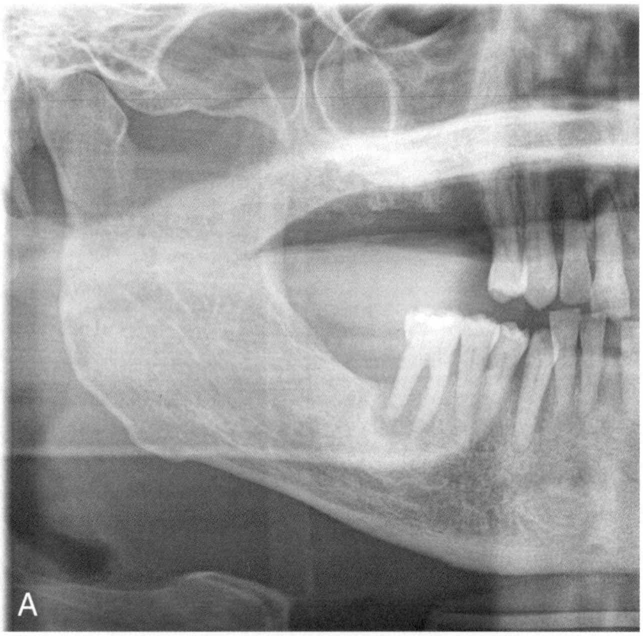

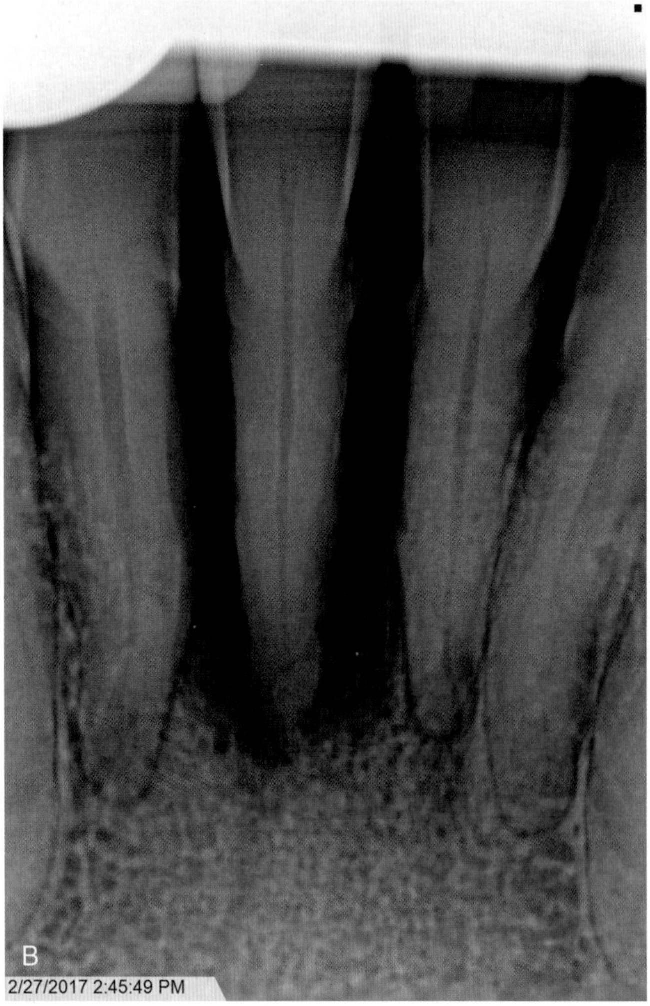

Fig 35-26 A, A periodontal abscess surrounds the roots of tooth #30. B, A periodontal abscess surrounds the root of tooth #25.

Treatment. Therapy includes drainage, subgingival scaling, and debridement of periodontal tissues. The prognosis depends on the remaining periodontal support, the amount of bone loss, and mobility.

Periapical Radiopacities

Condensing osteitis, sclerotic bone, and hypercementosis are some common radiopacities seen on dental images. Any one of these radiopacities found near a tooth apex may be diagnosed based on the characteristic dental image findings and corroborating clinical information.

Condensing Osteitis

Description. Condensing osteitis (also known as *chronic focal sclerosing osteomyelitis*) is a well-defined radiopacity seen below the apex of a nonvital tooth (Figure 35-27).

Cause. The opacity represents a proliferation of bone that results from a low-grade inflammation or mild irritation caused by pulpal necrosis.

Image findings. On a dental image, this radiopacity may vary in size and shape and is not attached to the tooth root. Condensing osteitis does not involve the periodontal ligament space.

Clinical findings. A tooth associated with condensing osteitis is nonvital. It typically has a large carious lesion or a large restoration with a history of long-standing pulpitis. The tooth most frequently involved is the mandibular first molar. Condensing osteitis is the most common periapical radiopacity observed in adults.

Treatment. Because condensing osteitis is believed to represent a physiologic reaction of bone to inflammation, no treatment is necessary. Treatment of the nonvital tooth requires endodontic therapy or extraction.

Sclerotic Bone

Description. Sclerotic bone (also known as *osteosclerosis* or *idiopathic periapical osteosclerosis*) is a well-defined radiopacity that is seen below the apex of a vital, noncarious tooth (Figure 35-28).

Cause. The cause of sclerotic bone is unknown; however, it is *not* believed to be associated with inflammation.

Image findings. On a dental image, this radiopacity is not attached to a tooth root. It varies in size and shape, and the margins may appear smooth or irregular and diffuse. The borders are continuous with adjacent normal bone, and no radiolucent outline is seen.

Clinical findings. Sclerotic bone is asymptomatic.

Treatment. No treatment is required.

Hypercementosis

Description. Hypercementosis, or the excessive deposition of cementum, appears as a radiopaque band along all or part of a root surface (Figure 35-29).

Cause. Hypercementosis may result from supra-eruption, inflammation, or trauma. In some cases, no obvious cause exists.

Image findings. On a dental image, hypercementosis appears as a radiopaque band along the root surface. It most often affects the apical area of the root, giving it an enlarged and bulbous appearance. Hypercementosis seen along the root surface is clearly separated from the periapical bone by a normal-appearing periodontal ligament space and surrounding lamina dura.

Clinical findings. A tooth affected by hypercementosis is vital. No signs or symptoms are associated with hypercementosis.

Treatment. No treatment is required.

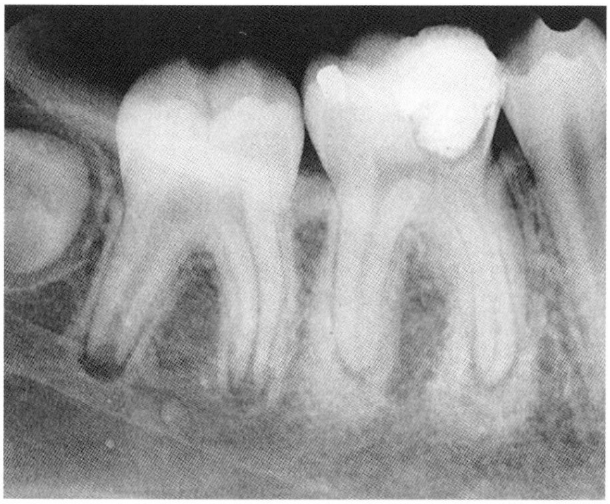

Fig 35-27 A radiopacity seen along the roots of a mandibular first molar. (From Haring JI, Lind LJ: Radiographic interpretation for the dental hygienist, Philadelphia, 1993, Saunders.)

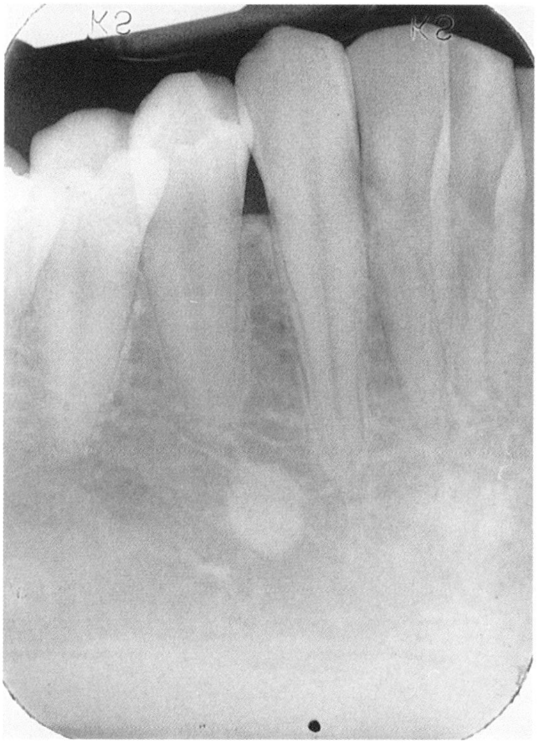

Fig 35-28 A well-defined radiopacity below the apex of a mandibular premolar. (From Haring JI, Lind LJ: Radiographic interpretation for the dental hygienist, Philadelphia, 1993, Saunders.)

SUMMARY

- Changes associated with trauma, resorption, and pulpal and periapical lesions can be viewed on dental images.

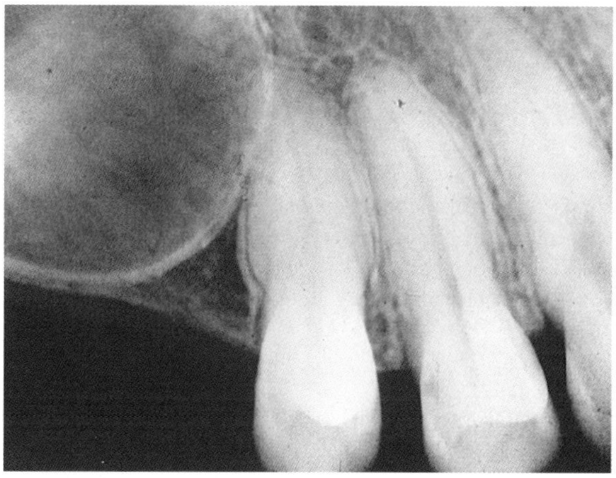

Fig 35-29 Hypercementosis of a maxillary premolar. (From Haring JI, Lind LJ: Radiographic interpretation for the dental hygienist, Philadelphia, 1993, Saunders.)

- Dental imaging allows the dental professional to evaluate the roots, pulp cavities, and periapical regions of teeth, all of which are areas that cannot be examined clinically.
- Dental imaging is important in the evaluation of trauma and injury and can be used for diagnostic, treatment, and post-treatment purposes.
- Dental imaging is useful in the evaluation of tooth and jaw fractures and of tooth injuries, including intrusion, extrusion, and avulsion.
- Dental imaging is useful in identifying regressive alterations of teeth, such as external and internal resorption. These alterations are usually asymptomatic and discovered only through dental imaging.
- Dental imaging is also useful in examining and in obtaining information about the pulp cavity. Pulpal sclerosis, pulp canal obliteration, and pulp stones are common conditions that can be viewed on dental images.
- Periapical lesions cannot be examined without the aid of dental images. Examples include periapical granulomas, periapical cysts, periapical abscesses, condensing osteitis, sclerotic bone, and hypercementosis.

BIBLIOGRAPHY

Frommer HH, Stabulas-Savage JJ: Pulpal and periapical lesions. In Radiology for the dental professional, ed 9, St. Louis, 2011, Mosby.

Haring JI, Lind LJ: Trauma, pulpal and periapical lesions. In Radiographic interpretation for the dental hygienist, Philadelphia, 1993, Saunders.

Herrera D, Roldçn S, Sanz M: The periodontal abscess: a review, J Clin Periodontol 27(6):377, 2000.

Johnson ON: Preliminary interpretation of the radiographs. In Essentials of dental radiography for dental assistants and hygienists, ed 9, Upper Saddle River, NJ, 2011, Prentice Hall.

Mallya SM, Lam EWN: Trauma. In White and Pharoah's Oral radiology: principles and interpretation, ed 8, St. Louis, 2019, Elsevier.

Manson-Hing LR: Interpretation and value of radiographs. In Fundamentals of dental radiography, ed 3, Philadelphia, 1990, Lea & Febiger.

Miles DA, Van Dis ML, Jensen CW, et al: Basics of interpretation: normal versus abnormal and common radiographic presentation. In Radiographic imaging for the dental team, ed 4, Philadelphia, 2009, Saunders.

QUIZ QUESTIONS

Matching

For questions 1 to 6, match each term with the appropriate definition.

a. Abnormal displacement of teeth
b. An injury produced by an external force
c. Complete displacement of a tooth from alveolar bone
d. Abnormal displacement of teeth out of bone
e. The breaking of a part
f. Abnormal displacement of teeth into bone

_____ 1. Trauma
_____ 2. Fracture
_____ 3. Luxation
_____ 4. Intrusion
_____ 5. Extrusion
_____ 6. Avulsion

Identification

For questions 7 to 16, refer to Figures 35-30 to 35-39. Identify or describe the periapical and pulpal lesions shown in each image.

7. ______________________________

8. ______________________________

9. ______________________________

10. ______________________________

11. ______________________________

12. ______________________________

13. ______________________________

14. ______________________________

15. ______________________________

16. ______________________________

Identification

For questions 17 and 18, refer to Figures 35-40 and 35-41. Identify or describe the trauma shown in each image.

17. ______________________________

18. ______________________________

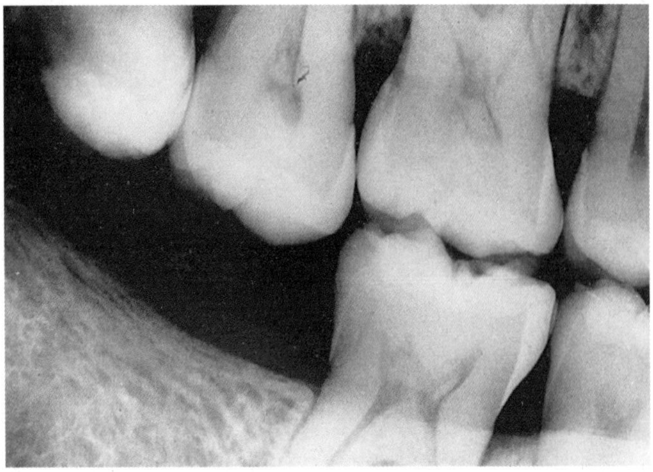

Fig 35-30 (From Haring JI, Lind LJ: Radiographic interpretation for the dental hygienist, Philadelphia, 1993, Saunders.)

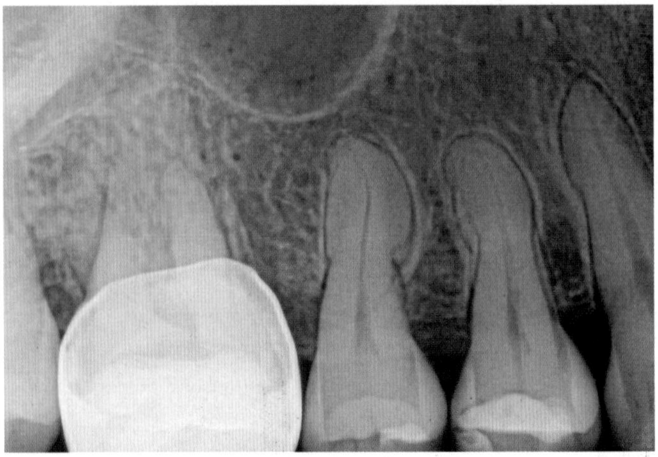

Fig 35-31

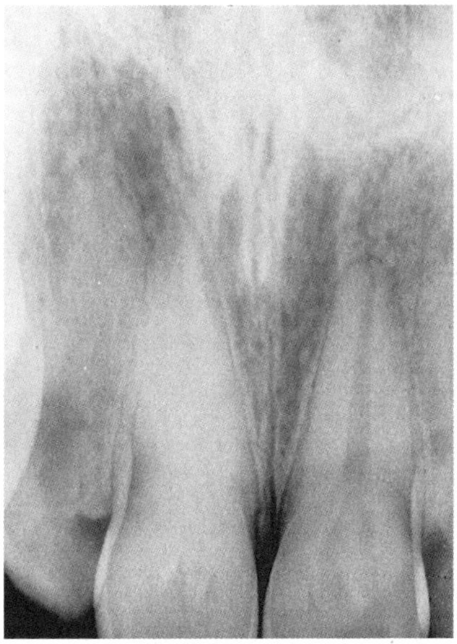

Fig 35-32 (From Haring JI, Lind LJ: Radiographic interpretation for the dental hygienist, Philadelphia, 1993, Saunders.)

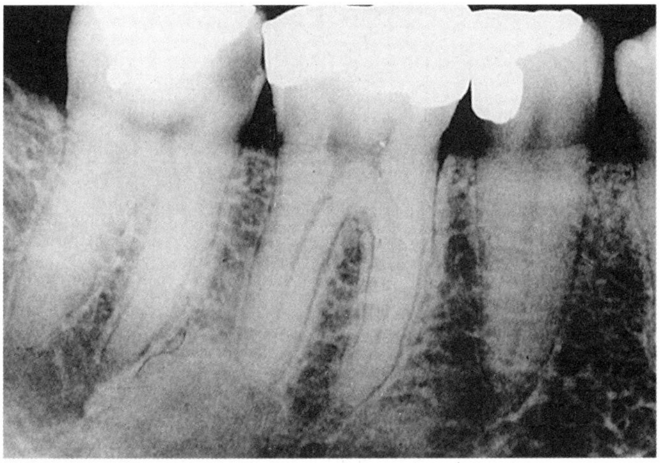

Fig 35-33 (From Haring JI, Lind LJ: Radiographic interpretation for the dental hygienist, Philadelphia, 1993, Saunders.)

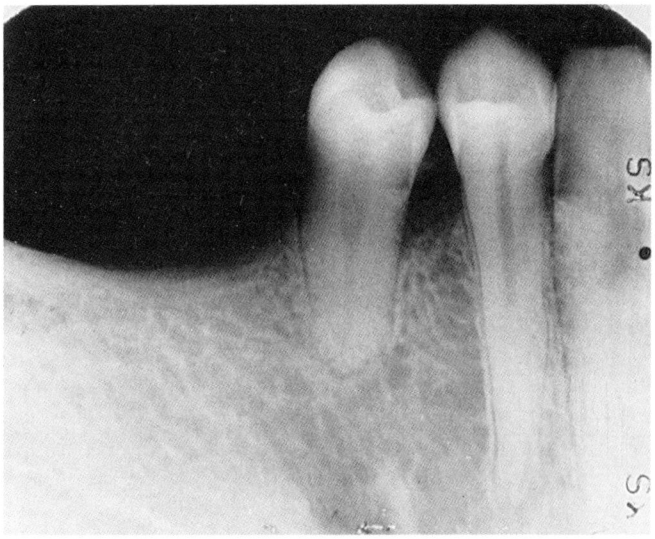

Fig 35-34 (From Haring JI, Lind LJ: Radiographic interpretation for the dental hygienist, Philadelphia, 1993, Saunders.)

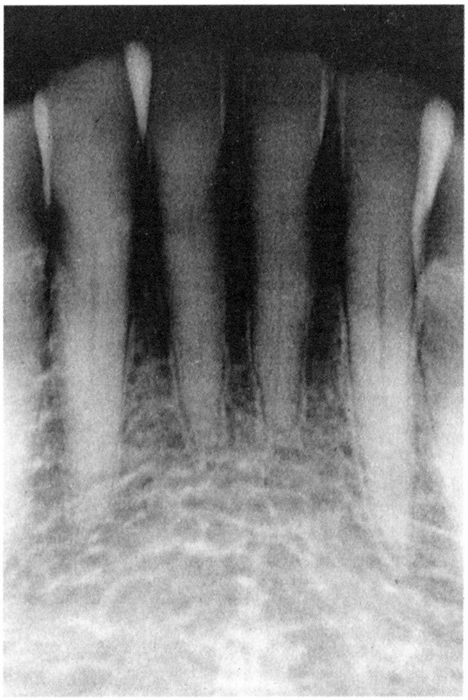

Fig 35-35 (From Haring JI, Lind LJ: Radiographic interpretation for the dental hygienist, Philadelphia, 1993, Saunders.)

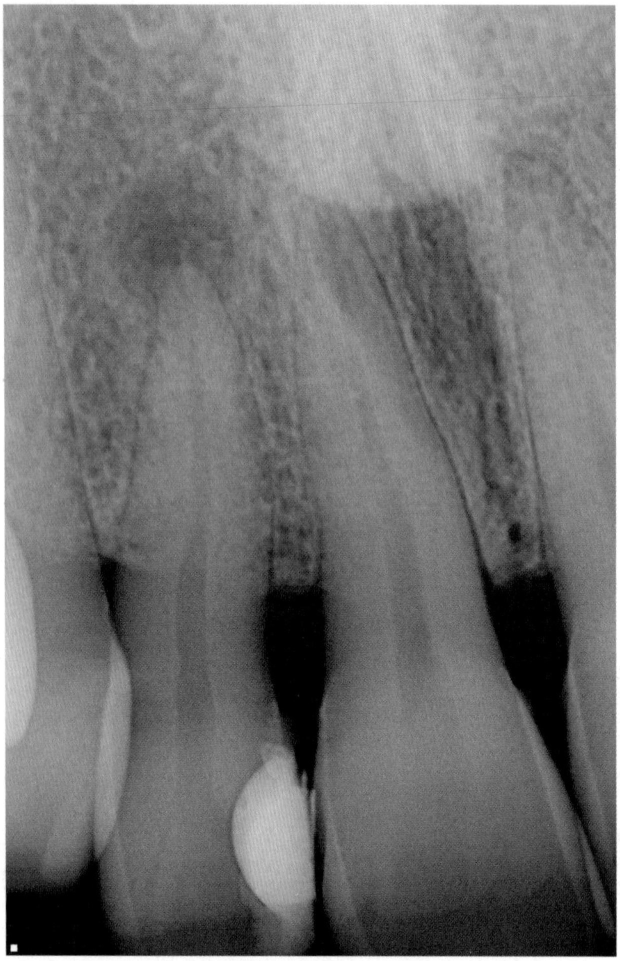

Fig 35-36

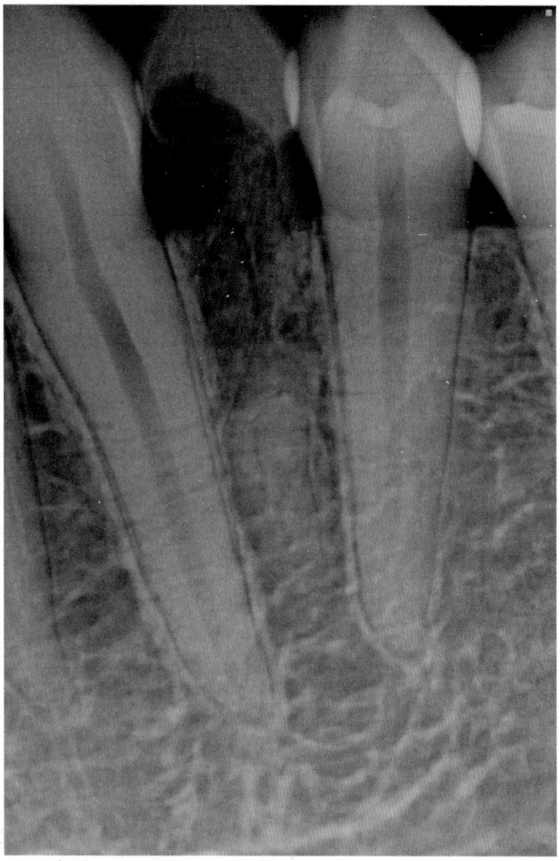

Fig 35-38

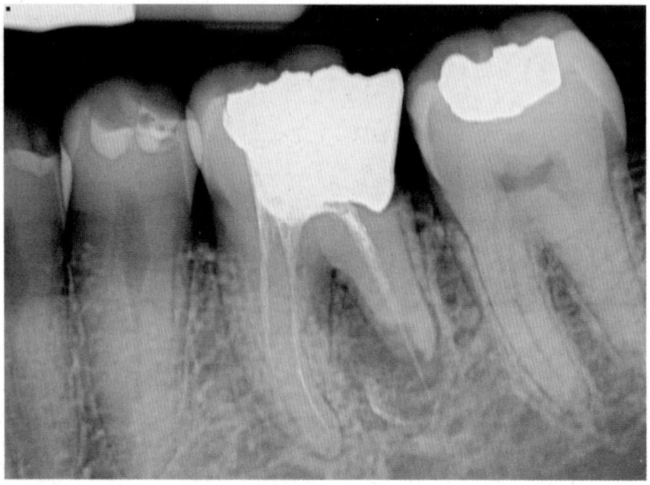

Fig 35-37

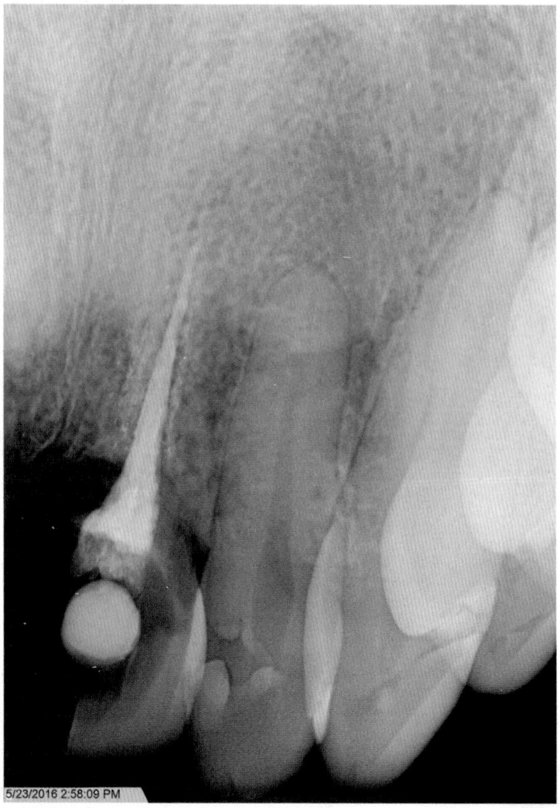

Fig 35-39

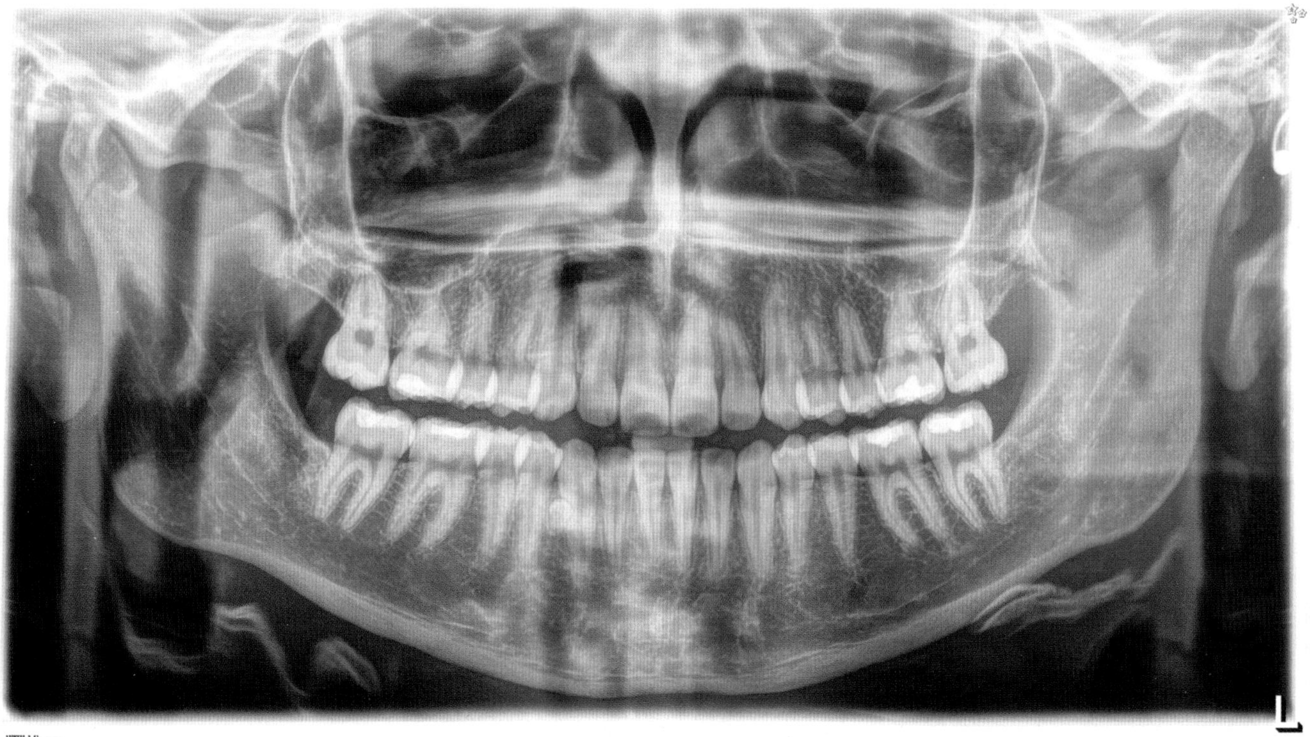

Fig 35-40

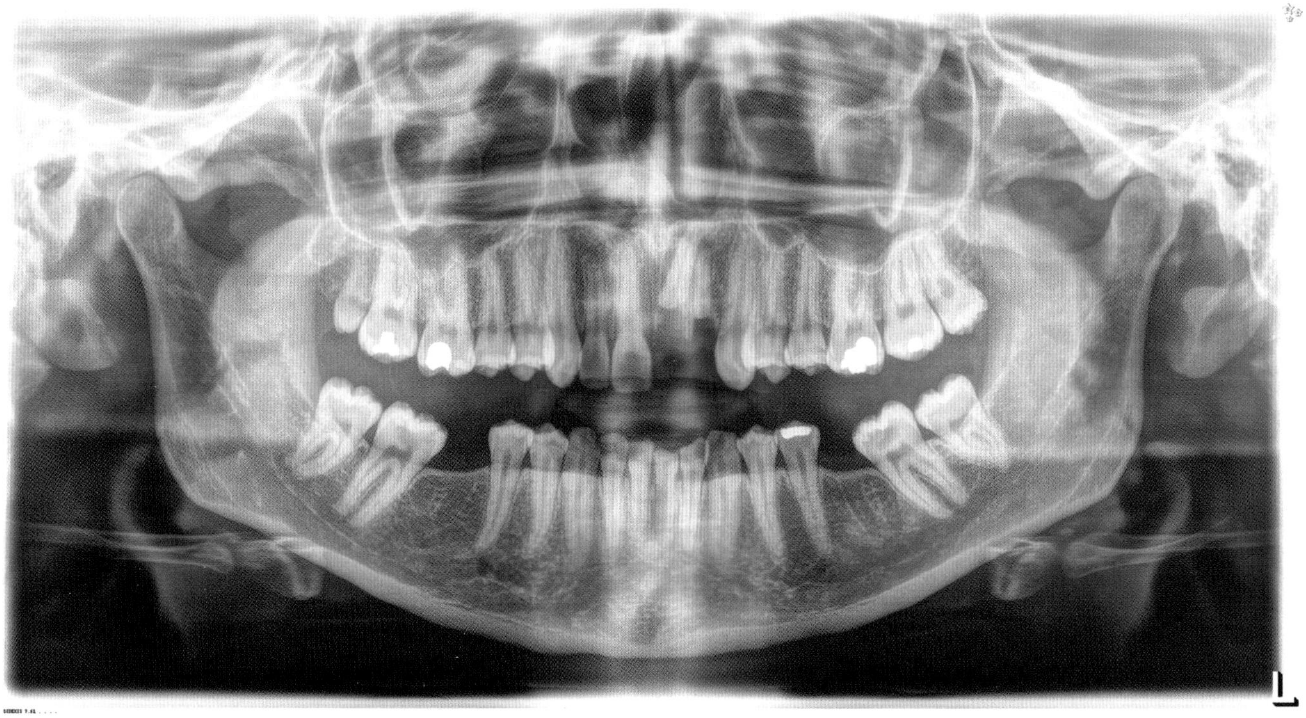

Fig 35-41

Periodontal and Peri-Implant Diseases

2018 **Classification of Periodontal and Peri-Implant Diseases**

Periodontal Health, Gingivitis & Gingival Conditions	Periodontitis	Other Conditions Affecting the Periodontium	Peri-Implant Diseases & Conditions
Periodontal Health & Gingival Health	Necrotizing Periodontal Diseases	Systemic Diseases or Conditions affecting periodontal supporting structures	Peri-Implant Health
Gingivitis: Biofilm Induced	Periodontitis as a manifestation of systemic diseases	Periodontal Abscesses & Endodontic-Periodontal Lesions	Peri-Implant Mucositis
Gingival diseases: Non-Biofilm Induced	Periodontitis	Mucogingival Deformities & Conditions	Peri-Implantitis
		Traumatic Occlusal Forces	Peri-Implant soft & hard tissue deficiencies
		Tooth & Prostheses-related factors	

Adapted from *Caton et al. J Periodontol 2018.*

(*2018 Classification of Periodontal and Peri-Implant Diseases* From The Procter & Gamble Company, Cincinnati, Ohio)

Health

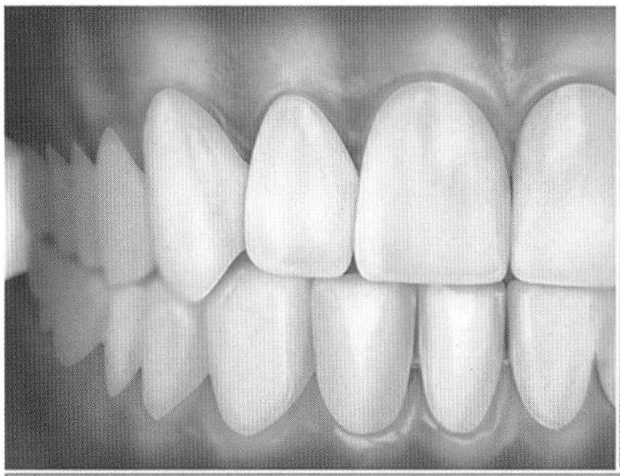

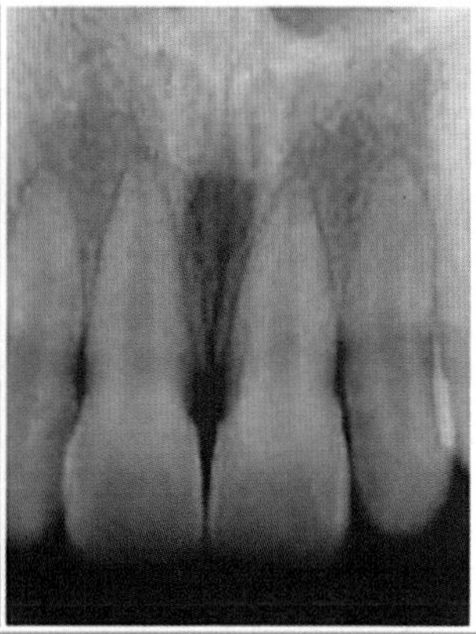

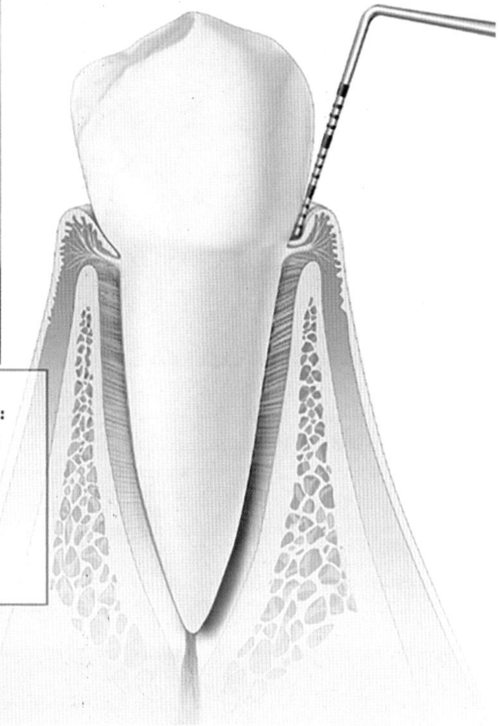

Clinical Gingival Health on an Intact Periodontium

Clinical Characteristics

BOP <10%
PD ≤3mm
Probing Attachment Loss – no
RBL – no

Clinical Gingival Health on a Reduced Periodontium:
Stable Periodontitis Patient

BOP <10%
PD ≤ 4mm
(no site ≥4mm with BOP)
Probing Attachment Loss – yes
RBL – yes

Clinical Gingival Health on a Reduced Periodontium:
Non-Periodontitis Patient (ie. recession; crown lengthening etc.)

BOP <10%
PD ≤3mm
Probing Attachment Loss – yes
RBL – possible

Gingivitis

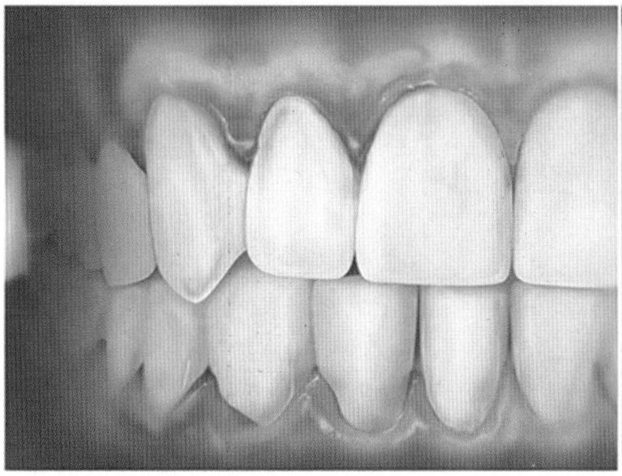

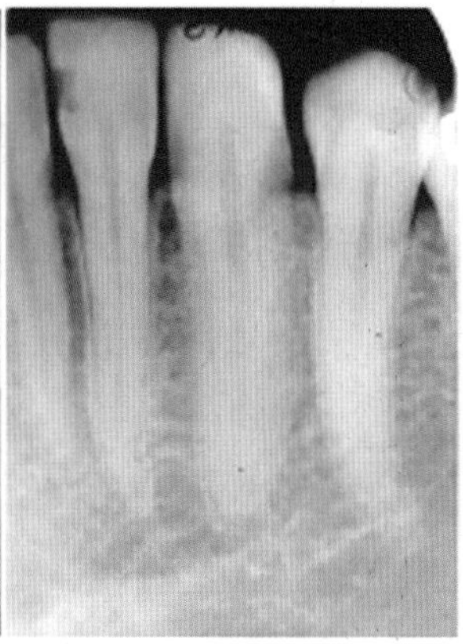

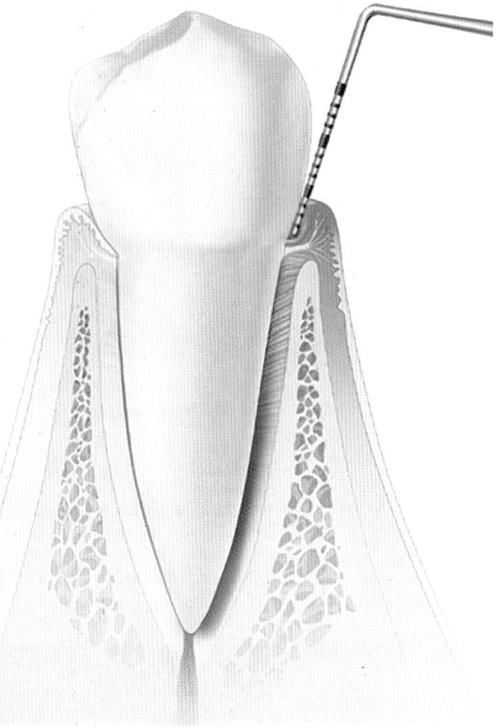

Gingivitis Intact Periodontium

Clinical Characteristics

BOP ≥ 10%
PD 0-3 mm
CAL – none
RBL – none

Gingivitis with Reduced Periodontium
Stable Periodontitis Patient

BOP ≥10%
PD ≤ 3mm
CAL – yes
RBL – yes

Gingivitis with Reduced Periodontium
Non-Periodontitis Patient
ie. recession; crown lengthening, etc)

BOP ≥10%
PD ≤ 3mm
CAL – yes
RBL – possible

(*2018 Classification of Periodontal and Peri-Implant Diseases* From The Procter & Gamble Company, Cincinnati, Ohio)

Periodontitis **Stage I - Grade B***

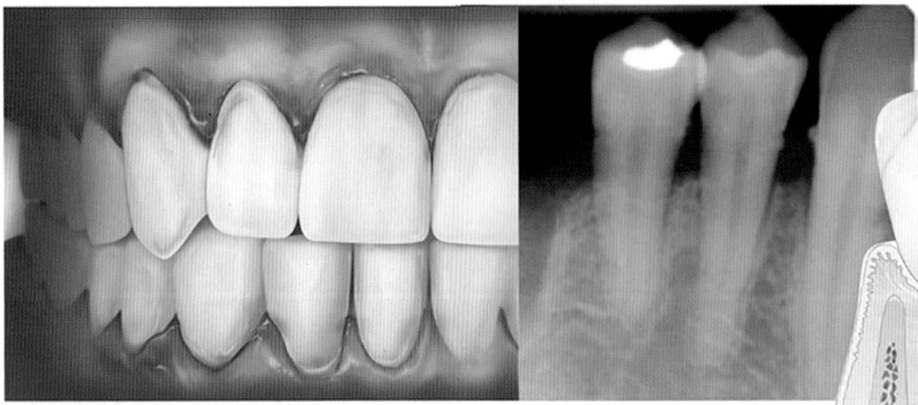

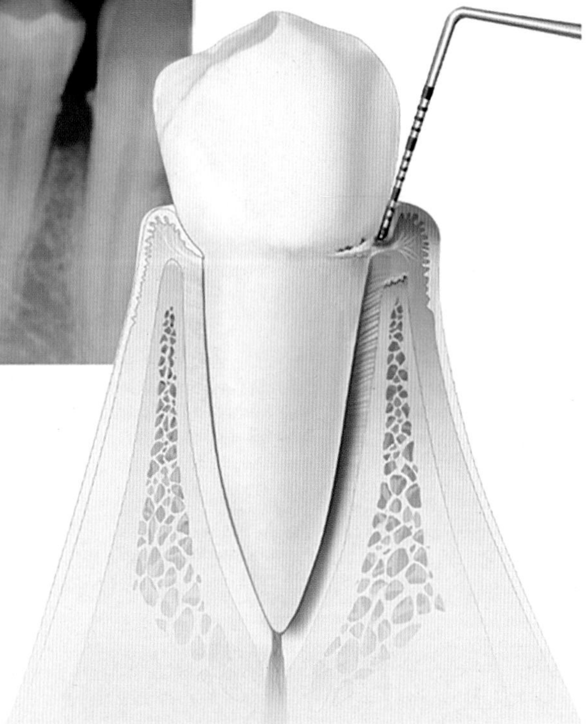

Clinical Characteristics

BOP – yes (>10%)	No tooth loss due to periodontitis
PD ≤4 mm	Moderate rate of progression
CAL 1-2 mm	If Smoker < 10 cigs/day
RBL < 15% & generally horizontal	If Diabetic HbA1c < 7.0%
Biofilm – slight - heavy	

* Grade is determined by rate of progression

Periodontitis **Stage II - Grade B***

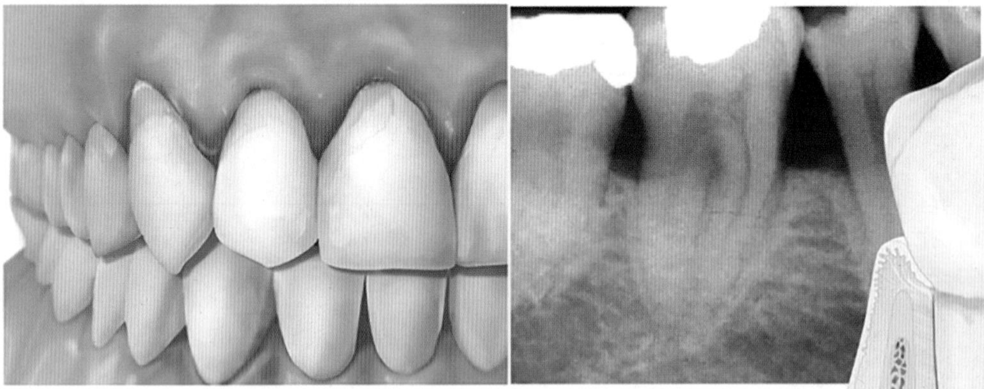

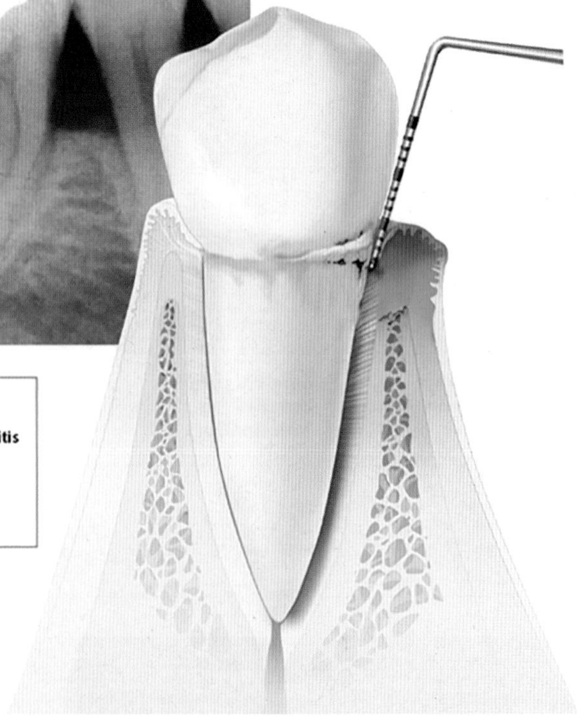

Clinical Characteristics

BOP – yes	No tooth loss due to periodontitis
PD ≤5 mm	Moderate rate of progression
CAL 3-4 mm	If Smoker < 10 cigs/day
RBL – 15%-33% & mostly horizontal	If Diabetic HbA1c < 7.0%
Biofilm – slight - heavy	

* Grade is determined by rate of progression

(*2018 Classification of Periodontal and Peri-Implant Diseases* From The Procter & Gamble Company, Cincinnati, Ohio)

Periodontitis **Stage III - Grade B***

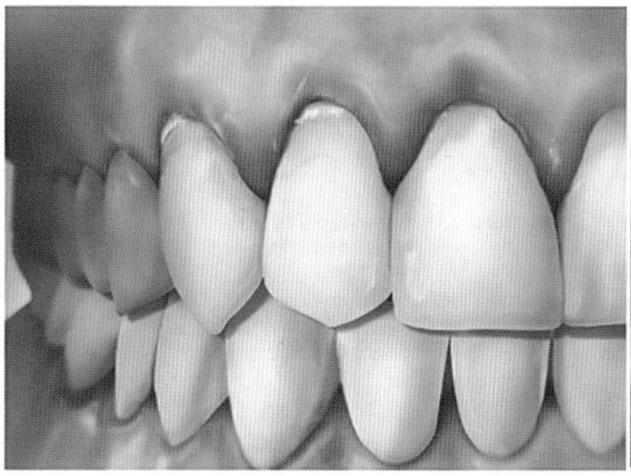
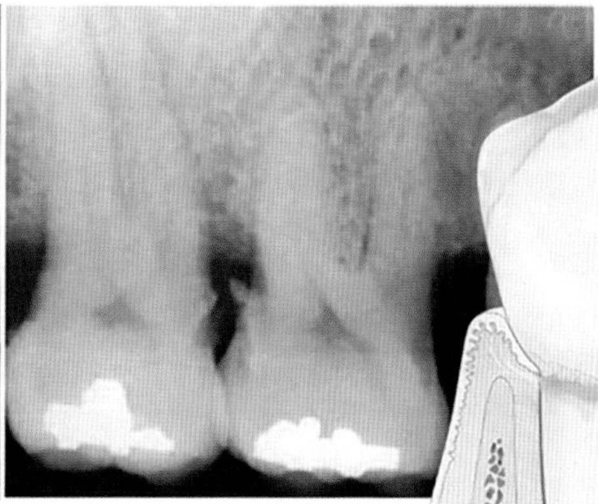
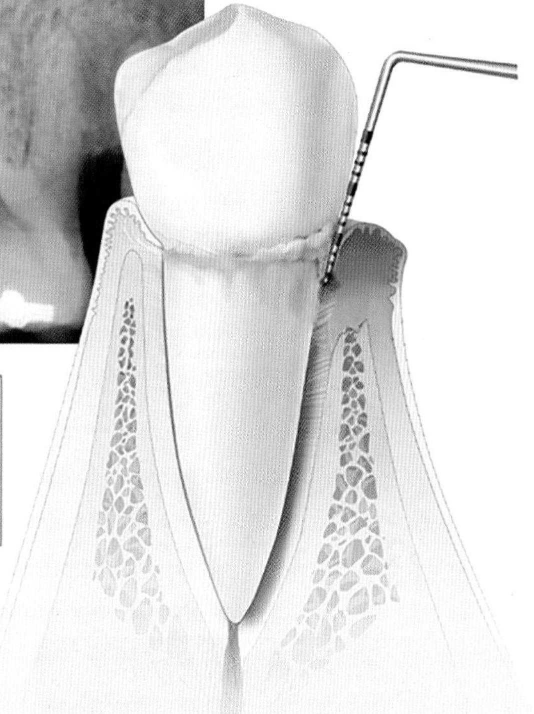

Clinical Characteristics

- BOP – yes
- PD ≥ 6 mm
- CAL ≥5 mm
- RBL ≥50% horizontal≥ 3mm vertical
- Biofilm – slight - heavy
- Tooth loss due to periodontitis ≤ 4 teeth
- Furcation involvement – Class II or III
- Moderate ridge defect
- If Smoker < 10 cigs/day
- If Diabetic HbA1c < 7.0%

* Grade is determined by rate of progression

Periodontitis **Stage IV - Grade B*** and **Stage IV - Grade C***

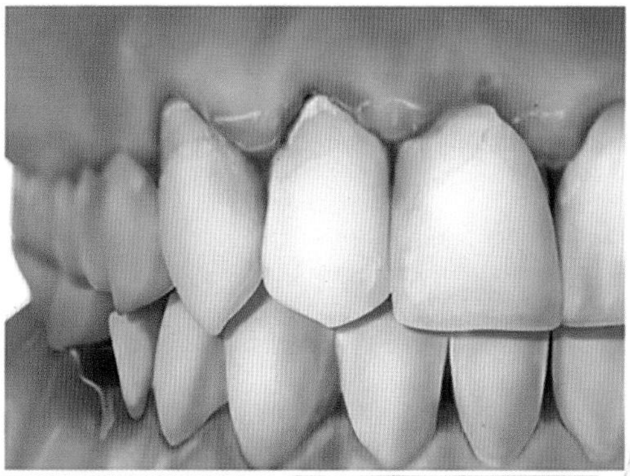
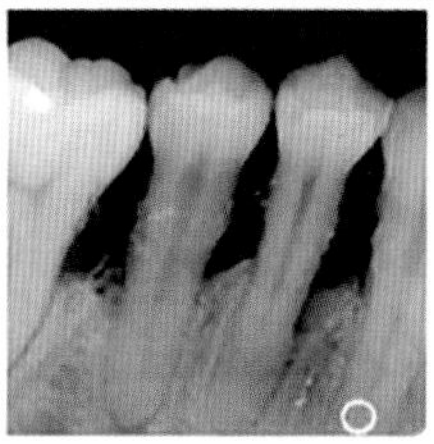
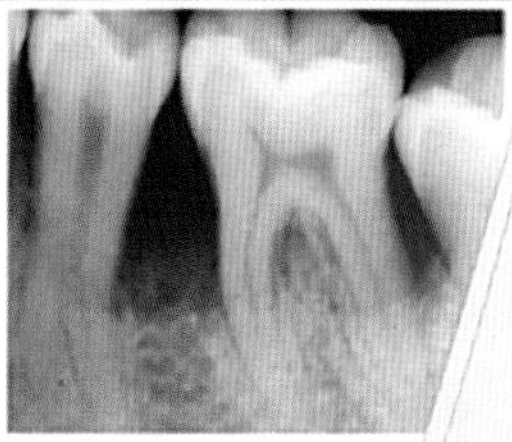
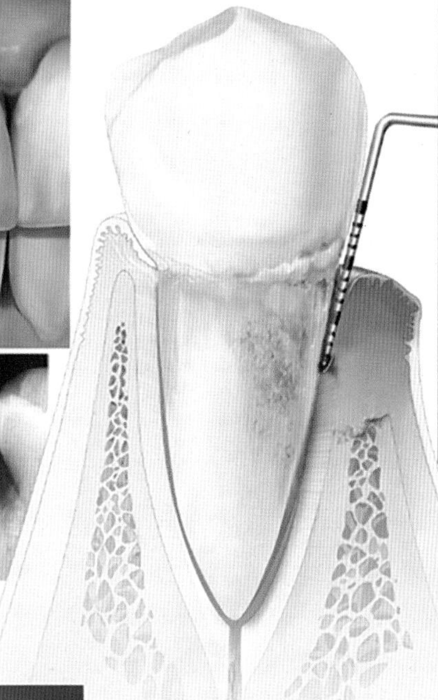

Stage IV Grade B*

Clinical Characteristics

- BOP – yes
- PD ≥ 6 mm
- CAL ≥5 mm
- RBL ≥50% horizontal ≥ 3mm vertical
- Biofilm – slight - heavy
- Tooth loss due to periodontitis ≥ 5 teeth
- Furcation involvement= Class II or III
- Moderate ridge defect
- If Smoker < 10 cigs/day
- If Diabetic HbA1c < 7.0%
- Need for complex rehabilitation

Stage IV Grade C*

Clinical Characteristics

- BOP – yes
- PD ≥ 6 mm
- CAL ≥5 mm
- RBL ≥50% horizontal ≥ 3mm vertical
- Biofilm – slight - heavy
- Tooth loss due to periodontitis ≥ 5 teeth
- Furcation involvement= Class II or III
- Moderate ridge defect
- Bone loss exceeds expectations given biofilm
- If Smoker ≥ 10 cigs/day
- If Diabetic HbA1c ≥7.0%
- Need for complex rehabilitation

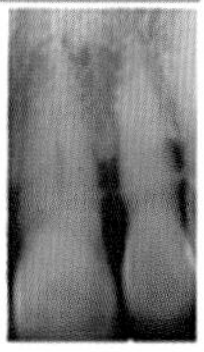

* Grade is determined by rate of progression

(*2018 Classification of Periodontal and Peri-Implant Diseases* From The Procter & Gamble Company, Cincinnati, Ohio)

Periodontitis **Staging**

Periodontitis	Stage I	Stage II	Stage III	Stage IV
Severity				
Interdental CAL at site of greatest loss	1-2mm	3-4mm	≥5mm	≥5mm
Radiographic Bone Loss	Coronal third (<15%)	Coronal third (15%-33%)	Extending to mid-third of root and beyond	Extending to mid-third of root and beyond
Tooth Loss	No tooth loss due to Periodontitis	No tooth loss due to Periodontitis	Tooth loss due to Periodontitis of ≤4 teeth	Tooth loss due to Periodontitis of ≥5 teeth
Complexity				
Local	• Maximum Probing Depth ≤ 4mm • Mostly horizontal bone loss	• Maximum Probing Depth ≤ 5mm • Mostly horizontal bone loss	*In addition to Stage II complexity:* • Probing depth ≥ 6mm • Vertical bone loss ≥3mm • Furcation involvement (Class II or III) • Moderate ridge defect	*In addition to Stage III complexity:* Need for complex rehabilitation due to: • Masticatory dysfunction • Secondary occlusal trauma (tooth mobility degree ≥2) • Severe ridge defect • Bite collapse, drifting, flaring • Less than 20 remaining teeth (10 opposing pairs)
Extent and distribution	*For each stage, describe extent as localized (<30% teeth involved), generalized, or molar/incisor pattern*			

Adapted from Tonetti et al. J Periodontal. 2018;89(Supp 1):S159-S172)

Periodontitis **Grading**

Periodontitis		Grade A Slow rate of progression	Grade B Moderate rate of progression	Grade C Rapid rate of progression
Primary Criteria				
Direct Evidence of Progression	Longitudinal data (Radiographic bone loss or CAL)	Evidence of no RBL or CAL loss over 5 years	< 2mm over 5 years	≥2mm over 5 years
Indirect Evidence of Progression	% Bone Loss/age	<0.25	.25 - 1.0	>1.0
	Case Phenotype	Heavy biofilm deposits with low levels of destruction	Destruction commensurate with biofilm deposits	• Destruction exceeds expectation given biofilm deposits • Specific clinical patterns suggestive of periods of rapid progression and/or early-onset disease (eg. molar/incisor pattern; lack of expected response to standard bacterial control therapies)
Grade Modifiers				
Risk Factors	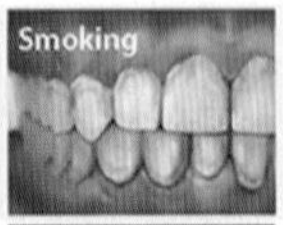	Non-smoker	Smoker <10 cigarettes/day	Smoker ≥10 cigarettes/day
	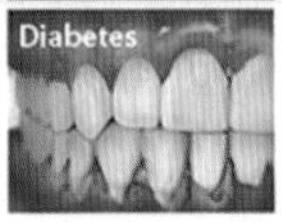	Normoglycemic/ no diagnosis of diabetes	HbA1c<7.0%	HbA1c ≥7.0% in patients with diabetes

Adapted from Papapanou et al. J Clin Periodontal. 2018;45(Supp 20):S162-S170)

(*2018 Classification of Periodontal and Peri-Implant Diseases* From The Procter & Gamble Company, Cincinnati, Ohio)

GLOSSARY

A

Absorption The total transfer of energy from the x-ray photon to the atoms of matter through which the x-ray beam passes. Absorption depends on the energy of the x-ray beam and the composition of the absorbing matter or tissues.

Accelerator One of the basic ingredients of the developer solution; sodium carbonate activates and provides an alkaline environment for the developing agents and softens the film emulsion.

Acetic acid See Acidifier.

Acidifier One of the basic ingredients of the fixer solution (e.g., acetic acid or sulfuric acid); the acidifier neutralizes the alkaline developer and stops further action of the developer.

Adhesive layer A thin layer of adhesive material that covers both sides of the film base and attaches the emulsion to the base.

Air bubbles A film handling error; white spots appear on a film as a result of trapped air that remains on the film surface after the film has been placed in the processing solution.

ALARA concept A concept of radiation protection that states that all exposure to radiation must be kept to a minimum, or "as low as reasonably achievable."

Alpha particles A type of particulate radiation emitted from the nuclei of heavy metals; alpha particles contain two protons and two neutrons and are positively charged.

Aluminum disks Disks or sheets of aluminum, usually 0.5 mm thick, that are placed in the path of the x-ray beam; filter out the nonpenetrating, longer-wavelength x-rays.

Alveolar bone Bone of the maxilla and the mandible that supports and encases the roots of teeth; appears radiopaque.

Alveolar bone loss A loss of bone that surrounds and supports teeth in the maxilla or the mandible.

Alveolar crest The most coronal portion of alveolar bone found between teeth; composed of cortical bone; appears radiopaque (also known as *crestal bone*).

Alveolar process Portion of the maxilla or mandible that encases and supports teeth.

Amalgam Most common restorative material used in dentistry.

Ammonium thiosulfate A chemical found in the fixing agent that clears the unexposed, undeveloped silver halide crystals from the film emulsion.

Amperage The number of electrons that pass through a conductor; the strength of an electrical current.

Ampere (A) The unit of measure used to describe the number of electrons passing through a conductor (electrical current strength); the intensity of an electric current produced by 1 volt acting through a resistance of 1 ohm.

Analog image An image produced on conventional film that looks like (is "analogous to") the thing it represents.

Anatomic order The order in which teeth are arranged within the dental arches.

Angle In geometry, a figure formed by two lines diverging from a common point.

Angle, right In geometry, an angle of 90 degrees formed by two lines perpendicular to each other.

Angle of mandible Area of the mandible where the body meets the ramus; the corner portion formed by the junction of the posterior and lower borders or the ramus.

Angulation The alignment of the central x-ray beam in the horizontal and vertical planes.

Angulation, horizontal The positioning of the position-indicating device (PID) in a horizontal, or side-to-side, plane.

Angulation, negative vertical The positioning of the position-indicating device (PID) below the occlusal plane that directs the central ray upward.

Angulation, positive vertical The positioning of the position-indicating device (PID) above the occlusal plane that directs the central ray downward.

Angulation, vertical The positioning of the position-indicating device (PID) in a vertical, or up and down, plane.

Anode The positive electrode in the x-ray tube; consists of a wafer-thin tungsten plate embedded in a solid copper rod; converts electrons into x-ray photons.

Anterior nasal spine A sharp projection of the maxilla located at the anteroinferior portion of the nasal cavity; appears radiopaque.

Antiseptic A substance that inhibits the growth of bacteria.

Articular eminence A rounded projection of the temporal bone located anterior to the glenoid fossa; appears radiopaque.

Asepsis The absence of pathogens or disease-causing microorganisms.

Atom A tiny, invisible particle that is the fundamental unit of matter; the smallest part of an element that has the properties of that element.

Atom, neutral An atom that contains an equal number of protons (positive charges) and electrons (negative charges).

Atomic number The total number of protons in the nucleus, which is also equal to the number of electrons outside of the nucleus.

Atomic weight The total number of protons and neutrons in the nucleus of an atom (also known as *mass number*).

Attrition The mechanical wearing of tooth structure.

Autotransformer A voltage compensator that corrects for minor fluctuations in the current flowing through the x-ray machine.

Avulsion, dental The complete displacement of a tooth from alveolar bone.

B

Barrier sleeve A plastic shield that protects an intraoral receptor from saliva and is used to minimize contamination.

Beam alignment device A device used to align the position-indicating device (PID) in relation to tooth and receptor; positions the intraoral receptor in the mouth and retains the receptor in position during exposure; helps stabilize the receptor in the mouth and reduces the chances of movement, thus reducing the patient's exposure to x-radiation.

Beta particles Fast-moving electrons emitted from the nucleus of radioactive atoms.

Binding energy The attraction between the positive nucleus and the negative electrons that maintains electrons in their orbits; determined by the distance between the nucleus and electrons (also known as *electrostatic force* or *binding force*).

Bisect To divide into two equal parts.

Bisecting technique An intraoral imaging technique used to expose periapical receptors: the receptor is placed along lingual surface of the tooth; the central ray of x-ray beam is directed perpendicular to the imaginary bisector formed by the receptor and the long axis of the tooth; receptor holder is used to stabilize the receptor.

Bisector, imaginary An imaginary plane that divides in half the angle formed by the receptor and the long axis of the tooth; creates two equal angles and provides a common side for the two imaginary equal triangles.

Bit-depth image The number of possible gray-scale combinations for each pixel.

Bite-wing, horizontal The bite-wing receptor is placed in the mouth with the long portion of the receptor in a horizontal direction.

Bite-wing, vertical The bite-wing receptor is placed in the mouth with the long portion of the receptor in a vertical direction.

Bite-wing tab A heavy paperboard tab or loop fitted around an intraoral receptor and used to stabilize the receptor during the exposure (also known as *bite loop* or *bite tab*).

Bite-wing technique An intraoral imaging technique in which the interproximal surfaces of teeth are examined (also known as *interproximal technique).*

Bloodborne pathogens Microorganisms present in blood that cause disease in humans.

Body of mandible The U-shaped horizontal portion of the mandible that extends from ramus to ramus.

Bone loss, angular See Bone loss, vertical.

Bone loss, generalized Bone loss that occurs evenly throughout the dental arches.

Bone loss, horizontal Bone loss that occurs in a plane parallel to the cemento-enamel junctions of adjacent teeth.

Bone loss, localized Bone loss that occurs in isolated areas.

Bone loss, vertical Bone loss that does not occur in a plane parallel to the cemento-enamel junctions of adjacent teeth (also known as *angular bone loss*).

Bremsstrahlung See Radiation, general.

Buccal object rule Used to illustrate the orientation of structures portrayed in two images exposed at different angulations; used to determine the buccal–lingual relationship of an object.

C

Calculus A stone like concretion that forms on the crowns and roots of teeth as a result of the calcification of bacterial plaque; appears radiopaque.

Canal A tubelike passageway through bone that houses nerves and blood vessels; appears radiolucent with radiopaque borders.

Cancellous Refers to a lattice like structure; the soft, spongy bone located between two layers of dense cortical bone; appears radiolucent (also known as *trabecular bone*).

Caries Tooth decay caused by microorganisms; appears radiolucent.

Caries, buccal Caries located on the buccal tooth surface.

Caries, interproximal Caries located between two adjacent teeth.

Caries, interproximal advanced Caries located between two teeth that extends to the dentino-enamel junction (DEJ) or through the DEJ and into dentin but does not extend through the dentin more than half the distance toward the pulp.

Caries, interproximal incipient Caries located between two teeth that extends less than halfway through the thickness of enamel.

Caries, interproximal moderate Caries located between two teeth that extends more than halfway through the thickness of enamel but does not involve the dentino-enamel junction (DEJ).

Caries, interproximal severe Caries located between two teeth that extend through enamel, through dentin, and more than half the distance toward the pulp.

Caries, lingual Caries located on the lingual tooth surface.

Caries, occlusal Caries located on the chewing surface of posterior teeth.

Caries, occlusal incipient Caries located on the chewing surface of posterior teeth; cannot be seen on a dental image.

Caries, occlusal moderate Caries located on the chewing surface of posterior teeth that extends into dentin; appears as a thin radiolucent line.

Caries, occlusal severe Caries located on the chewing surface of posterior teeth that extends into dentin; appears as a large radiolucency.

Caries, rampant Caries that affects numerous teeth in the dentition.

Caries, recurrent Caries located adjacent to a pre-existing restoration (also known as *secondary caries*).

Caries, root surface Caries located on the roots of teeth.

Cassette A light-tight device used in extraoral imaging to hold the film and intensifying screens.

Cathode The negative electrode in the x-ray tube; consists of a tungsten wire filament in a molybdenum cup; supplies the electrons necessary to generate x-rays.

Cathode ray A stream of high-speed electrons that originates from the cathode in an x-ray tube.

Cavitation A hole in a tooth that results from the caries process; appears radiolucent (also known as a *cavity*).

Cavity See Cavitation.

Cell The basic structural unit of living organisms.

Cell differentiation Individual characteristics of a cell that determine the response of the cell to radiation exposure (e.g., cells that are immature [not highly specialized] are more sensitive to radiation).

Cell metabolism The physical and chemical processes of a cell that determine the response of the cell to radiation exposure (e.g., cells with a high metabolic rate are more sensitive to radiation).

Central ray The central portion of the primary beam of x-radiation, abbreviated CR.

Cephalostat In extraoral imaging, a device that includes a receptor holder and head positioner that allow the dental radiographer to position both receptor and patient easily.

Cervical burnout A radiolucent artifact seen on dental images between the cemento-enamel junction (CEJ) and alveolar bone.

Chairside manner The manner in which a dental professional conducts himself or herself at the chairside of a patient.

Charge-coupled device (CCD) A solid-state silicon chip detector that converts light or x-ray photons into an electrical charge or signal; a CCD is found in the intraoral sensor.

Circuit A path of electrical current.

Circuit, filament The circuit that regulates the flow of electrical current to the filament of the x-ray tube; controlled by the milliampere settings (also known as *low-voltage circuit*).

Circuit, high-voltage The circuit that provides the high voltage required to accelerate electrons and to generate x-rays in the x-ray tube; controlled by the kilovoltage settings.

Circuit, low-voltage See Circuit, filament.

Clinical attachment loss (CAL) The measurement in millimeters of the distance between the cemento-enamel junction (CEJ) and the base of the sulcus or periodontal pocket.

Coherent scatter One of the interactions of x-radiation with matter in which the path of an low-energy x-ray photon interacts with an outer-shell electron. No change in the atom occurs, and an x-ray photon of scattered radiation is produced (also known as *unmodified scatter*).

Collimating device See Collimator.

Collimation The restriction of the size and shape of the x-ray beam in order to reduce patient exposure.

Collimator A diaphragm, usually made of lead, used to restrict the size and shape of the x-ray beam.

Communication The process by which information is exchanged between two or more persons.

Compartment, developer A component part of the automatic processor that holds the developer solution.

Compartment, fixer A component part of the automatic processor that holds the fixer solution.

Compartment, water A component part of the automatic processor that holds circulating water.

Complementary metal oxide semiconductor—active pixel sensor (CMOS-APS) Silicon-based detector used in digital imaging; differs from the charge-coupled device (CCD) detector in the way that the pixels are read.

Complete mouth series (CMS) An intraoral series of dental images that show all the tooth-bearing areas of the upper and lower jaws (also known as *full mouth series or complete series*).

Compton electron An outer-shell electron that is ejected from its orbit during Compton scatter; this electron carries a negative charge.

Compton scatter One of the interactions of x-radiation with matter in which the x-ray photon collides with a loosely bound, outer-shell electron and gives up part of its energy to eject the electron from its orbit. The x-ray photon loses energy and continues in a different direction at a lower energy level.

Condensing osteitis A well-defined radiopacity seen below the apex of a nonvital tooth that has a history of long-standing pulpitis (also known as *chronic focal sclerosing osteomyelitis*); appears radiopaque.

Cone beam computed tomography (CBCT) Computer-assisted digital imaging in dentistry; this imaging technique uses a cone-shaped x-ray beam to acquire information and present it in three dimensions.

Cone beam volume tomography (CBVT) Computer-assisted digital imaging in dentistry; used interchangeably with *cone beam volume imaging* (CBVI); terms used to differentiate this procedure from medical computed tomography (CT).

Cone-cut A clear, unexposed area on a dental image that occurs when the position-indicating device (PID) is misaligned and the x-ray beam is not centered over the receptor.

Confidential Private; in dental imaging, all information contained in the dental record is confidential.

Contact areas The area where adjacent tooth surfaces contact each other.

Contacts, open On a dental image, open contacts appear as a thin radiolucent line between adjacent tooth surfaces.

Contacts, overlapped On a dental image, the area where the contact area of one tooth is superimposed over the contact area of an adjacent tooth.

Contrast How sharply dark and light areas are differentiated or separated on an image; the difference in the degrees of blackness (densities) between adjacent areas on a dental image.

Contrast, film The characteristics of the film that influence contrast.

Contrast, high A term describing an image with many very dark areas and very light areas and few shades of gray.

Contrast, long-scale A term describing an image with many densities, or many shades of gray; long-scale contrast results from the use of a higher kilovoltage range.

Contrast, low A term describing an image with many shades of gray and few areas of black and white.

Contrast, scale of The range of useful densities seen on a dental image.
Contrast, short-scale A term describing an image with predominantly areas of black and white; short-scale contrast results from the use of a lower kilovoltage range.
Contrast, subject The characteristics of the subject (patient) that influence contrast; characteristics include the size and thickness of the patient.
Control devices The components of the control panel of the x-ray machine that regulate the x-ray beam; includes the timer, kilovoltage, and milliamperage selectors.
Control panel A part of the dental x-ray machine that contains an on-off switch and an indicator light, an exposure button and indicator light, and control devices to regulate the x-ray beam.
Copper stem A portion of the anode that dissipates heat away from the tungsten target.
Coronavirus A type of virus that has caused a worldwide pandemic of respiratory illness; it is spread from person to person and demonstrates symptoms which include cough, fever, chills shortness of breath, muscle aches, sore throat, loss of taste or smell, fatigue, and vomiting (also known as *COVID-19*).
Coronoid process A marked prominence of bone located on the anterior ramus of the mandible; appears radiopaque.
Cortical The dense outer layer of bone; appears radiopaque; (also known as *compact bone).*
Cough etiquette See Respiratory hygiene
Coulomb (C) A unit of electrical charge; the quantity of electrical charge transferred by 1 ampere in 1 second.
Critical organ An organ that, if damaged, diminishes the quality of an individual's life (e.g., in dentistry, the skin, thyroid gland, lens of the eye, bone marrow).
Cumulative effects The additive effects of repeated radiation exposure.
Cumulative occupational dose For occupationally exposed workers, the accumulated lifetime radiation dose.
Current, alternating (AC) A current in which electrons flow in opposite directions.
Current, direct (DC) A current in which electrons flow in one direction.
Curve of Spee The anterior-posterior anatomic curvature of the occlusal surfaces of the teeth.

D

Darkroom A completely darkened room where x-ray film is handled and processed.
Darkroom plumbing Plumbing in the darkroom that includes hot and cold water and mixing valves to adjust water temperature.
Darkroom storage space An area in the darkroom used to store chemical processing solutions, film cassettes, and other miscellaneous supplies.
Darkroom work space A clean counter area where films can be unwrapped before processing.
Daylight loader A light-shielded compartment on an automatic film processor; films can be unwrapped in a daylight loader in a room with white light.
Density The overall darkness or blackness of an image.
Dentin The tooth layer found beneath the enamel and surrounding the pulp cavity; appears radiopaque.
Dentino-enamel junction (DEJ) The junction between the dentin and enamel of a tooth.
Dentulous With teeth; areas that exhibit teeth.
Developer cutoff A film-handling error; a straight white border appears on a film as a result of using too low a level of developer solution during manual processing; represents an undeveloped portion of the film.
Developer solution A chemical solution used in film processing that distinguishes between the exposed and unexposed silver halide crystals and makes the latent image visible.
Developer spots A chemical contamination error; dark spots appear on the film because the developer solution has come in contact with the film before processing.
Developing agent One of the four basic ingredients of the developer solution; contains two chemicals, hydroquinone and elon, which reduce halides in the film emulsion to black metallic silver.
Development The first step in film processing; the developer solution reduces the halides in the film emulsion to black metallic silver and softens the film emulsion.
Diagnosis Identification of a disease by examination or analysis; the dentist is responsible for establishing a diagnosis.
Diatorics Metal retention pins that are included in anterior porcelain denture teeth.
DICOM Data The universal format for handling, storing and transmitting three-dimensional images; the acronym refers to *Digital Imaging and Communications in Medicine.*
Digital image An image composed of pixels.
Digital imaging A filmless imaging system; a method of capturing an image using a sensor, breaking it into electronic pieces, and presenting and storing the image using a computer.
Digital imaging, three-dimensional An image that demonstrates structures in three dimensions.
Digital subtraction One of the features of digital imaging; a method of reversing the gray scale as an image is viewed; radiolucent images (normally black) appear white and radiopaque images (normally white) appear black.
Digitize In digital imaging, to convert an image into digital form that, in turn, can be processed by a computer.
Direct digital imaging A method of obtaining a digital image in which an intraoral sensor is exposed to x-radiation to capture an image that can be viewed on a computer monitor.
Direct theory A theory that suggests that cell damage results when ionizing radiation hits critical areas directly within the cell.
Disability A physical or mental impairment that substantially limits one or more of an individual's major life activities.
Disability, developmental A substantial impairment of mental or physical functioning that occurs before age 22 and is of indefinite duration.
Disability, physical A physical impairment involving vision, hearing, or mobility.
Disclosure In dental imaging, the process of informing a patient about the particulars of exposing dental images.
Disinfect To inhibit or destroy disease-causing microorganisms through use of a chemical or physical procedure.
Disinfectant, high-level Chemicals classified by the U.S. Environmental Protection Agency (EPA) as "sterilants–disinfectants"; used to disinfect heat-sensitive, semicritical dental instruments.
Disinfectant, intermediate-level Chemical germicides classified by the U.S. Environmental Protection Agency (EPA)- as both "hospital disinfectants" and "tuberculocidals"; recommended for all surfaces that have been contaminated.
Disinfectant, low-level Chemical germicides classified by the U.S. Environmental Protection Agency (EPA)- as "hospital disinfectants"; recommended for general housekeeping purposes.
Disinfection The act of disinfecting; see Disinfect.
Distance, object-receptor The distance from the object being imaged (tooth) to the receptor influences image magnification; less image magnification results when the tooth and the receptor are as close as possible, and, more magnification results when the tooth and receptor are far apart.
Distance, target-object The distance from the source of x-rays (tungsten target in anode) to the object being imaged (tooth).
Distance, target-receptor The distance from the source of x-rays (tungsten target in the anode) to the receptor. Influences image magnification; less image magnification results when a longer position-indicating device (PID) is used, and more magnification results when a shorter PID is used.
Distance, target-surface The distance from the source of x-rays (tungsten target in anode) to the surface of the patient's skin.
Distortion A geometric characteristic that refers to a variation in the true size and shape of the object being imaged; distortion (e.g., elongation and foreshortening) is influenced by object-receptor alignment and the vertical angulation of the x-ray beam.
Dose The amount of energy absorbed by a tissue.
Dose, total The quantity of radiation received, or the total amount of radiation energy absorbed.
Dose equivalent A measurement used to compare the biologic effects of different types of radiation.
Dose rate Rate at which exposure to radiation occurs and absorption takes place (dose rate = dose/time).
Dose–response curve A curve that can be used to correlate the "response," or damage, of tissues with the "dose," or amount, of radiation received.
Drying chamber A component part of the automatic processor in which heated air is used to dry the wet films.

E

Ear Anatomic structure composed of cartilage with a thin covering of connective tissue and skin; on a panoramic image, appears as a radiopaque shadow projecting anteriorly and inferiorly from the mastoid process.

Edentulous Without teeth; an area where teeth are no longer present.

Edentulous patient A patient without teeth.

Edentulous zone An area where teeth are no longer present.

Electrical current The flow of electrons through a conductor; an electrical current is used to produce x-rays.

Electricity Electrical current used as a source of power; the energy used to make x-rays.

Electromagnetic radiation Propagation of wavelike energy (without mass) through space or matter.

Electromagnetic spectrum The entire range of wavelengths of electromagnetic radiations; extends from gamma rays (with the shortest wavelengths) to radio waves (with the longest wavelengths).

Electron A tiny negatively charged particle found outside of the nucleus in the atom.

Electron volt The unit of measurement for the binding energies of orbital electrons.

Electrostatic force The attraction between the positive nucleus and the negative electrons that maintains electrons in their orbits; determined by the distance between the nucleus and electrons (also known as *binding energy* or *binding force*).

Element Substances made up of only one type of atom.

Elon A chemical found in the developing agent that generates the many shades of gray of the radiographic image.

Elongated image An image of a tooth that appears long and distorted; see Elongation.

Elongation A term used in imaging to describe the image of a tooth that appears longer than the actual tooth; elongation is the result of flat or insufficient vertical angulation.

Enamel The densest structure found in the human body; the outermost radiopaque layer of the crown of a tooth.

Endodontic Within a tooth.

Endodontic patient A patient who has undergone root canal therapy.

Endodontics A branch of dentistry dealing with the diagnosis and treatment of diseases of the dental pulp.

Energy What occurs when matter is altered.

Erg A unit of energy equivalent to 1.0×10^{-7} joules or 2.4×10^{-8} calories.

Expansile Capable of expansion.

Exposure A measure of ionization produced in air by x-radiation or gamma radiation.

Exposure, occupational Contact with blood or other infectious materials involving the skin, eye, or mucous membranes that results from procedures performed by the dental professional.

Exposure, parenteral Contact with blood or other infectious materials that results from piercing or puncturing the skin barrier.

Exposure button A component of the dental x-ray machine control panel; activates the dental x-ray machine to produce x-rays.

Exposure factors Factors that influence the density of an image (e.g., milliamperage, kilovoltage, exposure time).

Exposure incident A specific incident involving contact with blood or other potentially infectious materials that results from procedures performed by the dental professional.

Exposure light A component of the dental x-ray machine control panel; provides a visible signal when x-rays are produced.

Exposure sequence A defined order to place and expose intraoral receptors.

Exposure time The interval during which x-rays are produced.

Extension arm A part of the dental x-ray machine; suspends the x-ray tubehead and houses electrical wires that extend from the control panel to the tubehead.

External auditory meatus A hole or opening in the temporal bone located superior and anterior to the mastoid process (also known as the *external acoustic meatus).*

External oblique ridge A linear prominence of bone located on the external surface of the body of the mandible; appears radiopaque (also known as *external oblique line*).

Extraoral Outside the mouth.

Extraoral imaging An inspection of large areas of the skull or jaws; requires the use of extraoral imaging receptors.

Extrusion The abnormal displacement of teeth out of bone.

F

Facilitation skills Interpersonal skills used to ease communication and to develop a trusting relationship between the dental professional and the patient.

Field of view (FOV) The area that can be captured when performing imaging procedures; With CBCT imaging, region of interest of the patient anatomy.

Filament circuit Uses 3 to 5 volts; regulates the flow of electrical current to the filament of the x-ray tube, and is controlled by the milliampere settings.

Film, cleaning An extraoral-size film used to clean the rollers of the automatic processor.

Film, D-speed The slowest intraoral film; the letter D identifies the film speed.

Film, duplicating A special type of photographic film used to make an identical copy (duplicate) of an intraoral or extraoral radiograph; this film is not exposed to x-radiation.

Film, extraoral Film placed outside the mouth to examine large areas of the skull or jaws.

Film, F-speed The fastest intraoral film available; the letter F identifies the film speed; also called *InSight.*

Film, fast A type of dental x-ray film that requires less radiation for exposure.

Film, fogged A processing error; fogged film appears gray and lacks detail and contrast; results from improper safelighting or light leaks in the darkroom.

Film, green-sensitive An extraoral film that requires the use of a screen for exposure and is sensitive to green fluorescent light; this film must be paired with screens that produce green light.

Film, intraoral Film placed inside the mouth during x-ray exposure; used to examine teeth and supporting structures.

Film, nonscreen An extraoral film that does not require the use of a screen for exposure.

Film, occlusal A film used to examine large areas of the maxilla or the mandible; the patient "occludes" or bites on the entire film.

Film, overdeveloped A processing error; appears dark and results from excessive development time, inaccurate timer, hot developer solution, inaccurate thermometer, or concentrated developer solution.

Film, overlapped A film handling error; white or dark areas appear on films where overlap has occurred, results when two films come into contact with each other during processing.

Film, periapical An intraoral film used to examine the entire tooth (crown and root) and supporting bone.

Film, scratched A film handling error; white lines appear on films; results from the emulsion having been removed from the film base by a sharp object (e.g., a film clip or hanger).

Film, screen An extraoral film that requires the use of a screen for exposure; this film is sensitive to the light emitted from intensifying screens.

Film, standard A size 2 film.

Film, underdeveloped A processing error; an underdeveloped film appears light; results from inadequate development time, inaccurate timer, cool developer temperature, inaccurate thermometer, or depleted or contaminated developer solution.

Film, x-ray An image receptor that consists of a film base, adhesive layer, film emulsion, and protective layer; three types of x-ray film may be used in dental radiography: (1) intraoral film, (2) extraoral film, and (3) duplicating film.

Film, yellow-brown A processing error; film appears yellow-brown; results from exhausted developer or fixer, insufficient fixation time, or insufficient rinsing.

Film base A flexible piece of plastic that is constructed to withstand heat, moisture, and chemical exposure and provides strength and stable support for the film emulsion.

Film duplicator A light source used to expose duplicating film.

Film emulsion A coating attached to both sides of the film base by the adhesive layer to give the film greater sensitivity to x-radiation; homogenous mixture of gelatin and silver halide crystals.

Film feed slot An opening on the outside of the automatic processor housing; used to insert unwrapped films into the automatic processor.

Film hangers A stainless steel device equipped with clips; used to hold films during manual processing.

Film mount A cardboard, plastic, or vinyl holder used to support and arrange dental radiographs in anatomic order.

Film mounting The placement of radiographs in a supporting structure or holder.
Film recovery slot An opening on the outside of the automatic processor housing where dry, processed radiographs emerge.
Film speed The amount of radiation required to produce a radiograph of standard density.
Film viewing The examining of dental radiographs on a light source.
Filtration The use of absorbing materials (e.g., aluminum) for removing the low-energy x-rays from the primary beam.
Filtration, added Aluminum disks inserted in the dental x-ray machine between the x-ray tubehead seal and collimator; removes low-energy x-rays.
Filtration, inherent Portions of the x-ray tubehead that serve to filter low-energy x-rays; includes the glass window of the x-ray tube, the insulating oil, and the tubehead seal.
Filtration, total The combination of the inherent filtration and added filtration in an x-ray machine.
Fingernail artifact A film handling error; film appears with a black, crescent-shaped mark it was damaged by the operator's fingernail during rough handling.
Fingerprint artifact A film handling error; a black fingerprint appears on a film where the film has been touched by fingers contaminated with fluoride or developer.
Fixer cutoff A film handling error; a straight black border appears on a film as a result of using too low a level of fixer solution during manual processing; represents an unfixed portion of the film.
Fixer solution A chemical solution used in film processing; removes the unexposed silver halide crystals and creates white or clear areas on the film.
Fixer spots A chemical contamination error; white spots appear on a film as a result of fixer solution contacting the film before processing.
Fixing One of the steps in film processing; A chemical solution known as *the fixer* removes the unexposed, unenergized silver halide crystals from the film emulsion.
Fixing agent One of the four basic ingredients of the fixer solution; contains hypo (sodium thiosulfate or ammonium thiosulfate), which removes or clears all unexposed and undeveloped silver halide crystals from the film emulsion (also known as *clearing agent*).
Floor of nasal cavity A bony plate formed by the palatal processes of the maxilla and the horizontal portions of the palatine bones; appears radiopaque.
Fluoresce To emit visible light in the blue or green spectrum.
Fluorescence The emission of a glowing light by certain substances when struck by a particular wavelength.
Focal opacity A term used to describe a well-defined, localized radiopaque lesion viewed on a dental image.
Focal spot The tungsten target of the anode; converts bombarding electrons into x-ray photons, concentrating the electrons and creating an enormous amount of heat.
Focal spot size The size of the tungsten target of the anode; ranges from 0.6 mm^2 to 1.0 mm^2 and is determined by the manufacturer of the x-ray machine.
Focal trough A three-dimensional curved zone in which structures are clearly demonstrated on a panoramic image; in panoramic imaging, a patient must be positioned so that the dental arches are located within the focal trough area (also called *image layer*).
Foramen An opening or hole in bone that permits the passage of nerves and blood vessels; appears radiolucent.
Foreshortened image An image of a tooth that appears short and distorted; see Foreshortening.
Foreshortening A term describing the image of a tooth that appears shorter than the actual tooth; foreshortening is the result of steep or excessive vertical angulation.
Fossa A broad, shallow, scooped-out or depressed area of bone; appears radiolucent.
Fracture The breaking of a part; appears as a thin radiolucent line.
Frankfort plane The imaginary plane that intersects the orbital rim of the eye and the opening of the ear.
Free radical An uncharged, neutral atom or molecule that exists with a single, unpaired electron in its outermost shell.
Frequency The number of wavelengths that pass a given point in a certain amount of time; frequency indicates the energy of a radiation (e.g., high-frequency radiations have more energy than do low-frequency radiations).
Full mouth series (FMS or FMX) See Complete mouth series (CMS).
Furcation area The area between the roots of multi-rooted teeth.

G

Gag reflex Retching that is elicited by stimulation of the sensitive tissues of the soft palate region (also known as *pharyngeal reflex*).
Gagging The strong involuntary effort to vomit (also known as *retching*).
Gelatin A component of the film emulsion that suspends and disperses silver halide crystals over the film base.
Genetic cells Cells that contain genes; reproductive cells (e.g., ova, sperm).
Genetic effects Effects of radiation that are not seen in the person irradiated but are passed on to future generations through genetic cells.
Genial tubercles Tiny bumps of bone located on the lingual surface of the anterior mandible; serve as attachment sites for the genioglossus and geniohyoid muscles; appear radiopaque.
Ghost image An artifact on a dental image produced when a radiodense object (e.g., earring) is penetrated twice by the x-ray beam; appears radiopaque.
Glenoid fossa A concave, depressed area of the temporal bone where the mandibular condyle rests.
Glossopharyngeal air space Refers to airspace of the pharynx (*pharyngeal*) located posterior to the tongue (*glosso*) and oral cavity; on a panoramic image, appears as a vertical radiolucent band superimposed over the ramus of the mandible.
Gray (Gy) A unit for measuring absorbed dose; the SI unit equivalent to the rad; 1 gray = 100 rad.
Grid In extraoral imaging, a device used to prevent scatter radiation from reaching the film during exposure.
Ground glass appearance A term used to describe a radiopacity viewed on a dental image that resembles pulverized glass (also known as an *orange-peel appearance*).
Gutta percha Rubberlike material used in endodontic therapy to fill the pulp canals and pulp chamber.

H

Half-value layer (HVL) The thickness of material that, when placed in the path of the x-ray beam, reduces the exposure rate by one-half.
Halide A chemical compound that is sensitive to radiation or light; in dental film, a halide, such as silver bromide, is suspended in the gelatin of the emulsion.
Hamulus A small, hooklike projection of bone that extends from the medial pterygoid plate of the sphenoid bone; appears radiopaque (also known as the *hamular process*).
Hardening agent One of the four basic ingredients of the fixer solution; contains the chemical potassium alum, which hardens and shrinks the gelatin in the film emulsion.
Head positioner One of the component parts of a panoramic unit that is used to position and stabilize the patient's head; includes a chin rest, notched bite-block, forehead rest, and lateral head supports.
Herringbone pattern The pattern seen on a dental radiograph when the film has been placed in the mouth backward and exposed (also known as *tire-track pattern*).
High-voltage circuit Uses 65,000 to 100,000 volts; provides the high voltage required to accelerate electrons and to generate x-rays in the x-ray tube, and is controlled by the kilovoltage settings.
Humidity level The amount of moisture in the air.
Hydroquinone A chemical found in the developing agent that generates the black tones and sharp contrast of the radiographic image.
Hyoid bone A horseshoe-shaped bone that lies below the mandible, between the chin and thyroid cartilage; viewed on a panoramic image and appears radiopaque.
Hypercementosis The excess deposition of cementum on the root surfaces of teeth; appears radiopaque.
Hypo Sodium thiosulfate or ammonium thiosulfate; a common name for these chemicals found in the fixing agent.
Hypotenuse In geometry, the side of a right triangle opposite the right angle.

I

Identification dot A small raised bump that appears in one corner of an intraoral film; used to determine film orientation.
Image A picture or likeness of an object.
Image, bite-wing Intraoral image that is used to examine the interproximal surfaces of teeth.

Image, dental A two-dimensional representation of a three-dimensional object produced by the passage of x-rays through teeth and supporting structures.

Image, diagnostic A dental image that allows for the identifying and monitoring diseases or injuries.

Image, double An exposure error that occurs when a film or PSP receptor is exposed twice in the patient's mouth; appears dark as the result of two superimposed images.

Image, extraoral An image that results when a receptor is placed outside the mouth and exposed to x-rays; extraoral receptors are used to examine large areas of the skull or jaws.

Image, intraoral An image that results when a receptor is placed inside the mouth and exposed to x-rays; intraoral receptors are used to examine teeth.

Image, overexposed An exposure error that results in a dark image; results from excessive exposure time, kilovoltage, or milliamperage or a combination of these factors.

Image, panoramic An image that shows the wide view of the maxilla and the mandible and surrounding structures.

Image, periapical Intraoral image that is used to examine the crowns and roots of teeth.

Image, real In panoramic imaging, the image that is recorded when a structure is located between the receptor and moving rotation center.

Image receptor A recording medium; examples include x-ray film, PSP plate or digital sensors.

Image, underexposed An exposure error that results in a light image; results from inadequate exposure time, kilovoltage, or milliamperage or a combination of these factors.

Imaging, dental The creation of digital, print or film representations of anatomic structures for the purpose of diagnosis.

Impulse In dental imaging, a measure of exposure time; 60 impulses occur in 1 second.

Incipient Small; beginning to exist or appear.

Incisive canal A passageway through bone that extends from the superior foramina of the incisive canal to the incisive foramen (also known as the *nasopalatine canal*).

Incisive foramen An opening or hole in bone located at the midline of the anterior hard palate directly posterior to the maxillary central incisors; appears radiolucent.

Indicator light A component of the dental x-ray machine control panel; when illuminated, indicates that the dental x-ray machine is turned on.

Indirect digital imaging A method of obtaining a digital image from a sensor after exposure to x-rays by using a scanner to convert information into a digital form so that it can be viewed on a computer monitor.

Indirect theory A theory suggesting that cell damage results indirectly; x-ray photons are absorbed with the cell, causing the formation of toxins; toxins, in turn, damage the cell.

Infection prevention Procedures used to prevent the transmission of infectious diseases

Infectious waste Waste that consists of blood, blood products, contaminated sharps, or other microbiologic products.

Inferior border of mandible A linear prominence of cortical bone that defines the lower border of the mandible; appears radiopaque.

Inferior nasal conchae Wafer-thin, curved plates of bone that extend from the lateral walls of the nasal cavity; appear radiopaque.

Informed consent Consent given by a patient after complete disclosure about the particulars of a procedure.

Infraorbital foramen A hole or opening in bone found inferior to the border of the orbit; viewed on a panoramic image and appears radiolucent.

Instrument, critical Instruments that are used to penetrate soft tissue or bone; must be sterilized after each use.

Instrument, noncritical Instruments that do not come in contact with mucous membranes.

Instrument, Rinn XCP A type of beam alignment device that is used with the paralleling technique; includes plastic bite-blocks, plastic aiming rings, and metal indicator arms.

Instrument, semicritical Instruments that contact but do not penetrate soft tissue or bone; must be sterilized after each use.

Insulating oil Oil that surrounds the x-ray tube and transformers inside the tubehead.

Intensity The total energy of the x-ray beam; the product of the quantity (number of x-ray photons) and quality (energy of each photon) per unit of area per time of exposure.

Internal oblique ridge A linear prominence of bone located on the internal surface of the mandible that extends downward and forward from the ramus; appears radiopaque.

Interpersonal skills Skills that promote good relationships between individuals.

Interpret To offer an explanation.

Interpretation An explanation.

Interpretation, image An explanation of what is viewed on a dental image; the ability to read what is revealed by a dental image.

Interproximal Between two adjacent surfaces.

Interproximal examination An intraoral inspection used to examine the crowns of both maxillary and mandibular teeth on a single image.

Inter-radicular Between the roots of adjacent teeth.

Intersecting Cutting across or through.

Intraoral Inside the mouth.

Intraoral imaging examination A dental imaging inspection of teeth and intraoral adjacent structures.

Intrusion The abnormal displacement of teeth into bone.

Inverse square law A rule that states that "the intensity of radiation is inversely proportional to the square of the distance from the source of radiation;" as distance is increased, the radiation intensity at the object is decreased, and vice versa.

Inverted Y A landmark viewed on dental images above the maxillary canine; represents the intersection of the anterior border of the maxillary sinus and the lateral wall of the nasal fossa; appears radiopaque.

Ion An electrically unbalanced particle; an atom that gains or loses an electron.

Ion pair A pair of ions, one positive and one negative, that results when an electron is removed from an atom in the ionization process. The atom becomes the positive ion, and the ejected electron becomes the negative ion.

Ionization The production of ions; the process of converting an atom into an ion, resulting in the formation of a positive atom and a dislodged negative electron.

Ionizing radiation Radiation that is capable of producing ions by removing or adding an electron to an atom. It can be classified into two groups: (1) particulate radiation and (2) electromagnetic radiation.

Isometry Equality of measurement.

Isometry, rule of A geometric principle that states that "two triangles are equal if they have two equal angles and share a common side."

J

Joule (J) The SI unit of measurement equivalent to the work done by the force of 1 newton acting over the distance of 1 meter.

K

Kiloelectron volt (keV) 1000 electron volts; the unit of measurement for the binding energies of orbital electrons.

Kilogram (kg) 1000 grams; a unit equivalent to 2.205 pounds.

Kilovolt (kV) 1000 volts; unit of measure for voltage.

Kilovoltage In dental imaging, the x-ray tube peak voltage used during an exposure; measured in kilovolts.

Kinetic energy Energy of motion.

L

Label side The side of the x-ray film packet that is color-coded and contains printed information; the label side of the film faces the tongue.

Labial mounting A film mounting method in which radiographs are placed in the film mount with the raised side of the identification dot facing the viewer; the dental radiographer then views the radiographs from the labial aspect.

Lamina dura The wall of the tooth socket that surrounds the root of a tooth; appears radiopaque.

Latent image The pattern of stored energy on the exposed film; the invisible image produced when the film is exposed to x-rays and that remains invisible until the film is processed.

Latent image centers Aggregates of neutral silver atoms on exposed crystals that collectively become the latent image on the emulsion of the film.

Latent period The amount of time that elapses between exposure to ionizing radiation and the appearance of observable clinical signs.

Lateral cephalometric projection An extraoral image that is used to determine facial growth and development, trauma, disease, and developmental abnormalities.

Lateral fossa A smooth, depressed area of the maxilla located just inferior and medial to the infraorbital foramen between the maxillary canine and lateral incisor; appears radiolucent.

Lateral jaw projection—body of mandible An extraoral projection used to evaluate the posterior body of the mandible; used to evaluate impacted teeth, fractures, and lesions located in the body of the mandible.

Lateral jaw projection—ramus of mandible An extraoral projection used to image the ramus of the mandible; used to evaluate impacted third molars, large lesions, and fractures that extend into the ramus of the mandible.

Lateral pterygoid plate A wing-shaped bony projection of the sphenoid bone located distal to the maxillary tuberosity region; viewed on a panoramic image and appears radiopaque.

Lead apron A flexible lead shield used to protect the patient's reproductive and blood-forming tissues from scatter radiation.

Lead collimator A lead diaphragm used to restrict the size and shape of the x-ray beam.

Lead foil sheet One of the four components of the dental x-ray film packet; a single piece of embossed lead foil placed behind the film to shield the film from scattered radiation.

Leaded-glass housing Portion of the glass housing of the x-ray tube that includes lead that prevents x-rays from escaping in all directions.

Liability Legal accountability.

Liable Accountable; legally obligated.

Light leak (1) In the darkroom setting, any white light that is seen when all the lights are turned off and the door is closed; (2) an exposure error; a black area with a fuzzy border that is seen on a radiograph as a result of exposure of the film to white light.

Light-tight A term used to describe the darkroom, a room that is completely dark and excludes all white light.

Line pairs/millimeter (lp/mm) A measurement used to evaluate the ability of the computer to capture the resolution (or detail) of an image.

Lingula A small, tongue-shaped projection of bone seen adjacent to the mandibular foramen; appears radiopaque.

Lingual foramen A small opening or hole in bone surrounded by the genial tubercles and located at the midline of the internal surface of the mandible; appears radiolucent.

Lingual mounting A film mounting method in which radiographs are placed in the film mount with the depressed side of the identification dot facing the viewer; the dental radiographer then views the radiographs from the lingual aspect.

Lipline An area of soft tissue seen on panoramic images formed by the positioning of the patient's lips.

Localization techniques Method used to locate the position of a tooth or object in the jaws.

Long axis (of tooth) An imaginary line that divides a tooth longitudinally into two equal halves.

Long-term effects Effects of radiation that appear years, decades, or generations after exposure; associated with small amounts of radiation absorbed repeatedly over a long period.

Luxation The abnormal displacement of teeth.

M

Magnification A geometric characteristic; refers to an image that appears larger than the actual size of the object it represents; influenced by target-receptor distance and object-receptor distance.

Malpractice Improper or negligent conduct or treatment.

Mandible The lower jaw.

Mandibular canal A tubelike passageway through bone that travels the length of the mandible; appears radiolucent with radiopaque borders.

Mandibular condyle A rounded projection of bone extending from the posterosuperior border of the ramus of the mandible; appears radiopaque.

Mandibular foramen A round or ovoid hole in bone on the lingual aspect of the ramus of the mandible; appears radiolucent.

Mandibular notch A scooped-out concavity of bone located distal to the coronoid process on the ramus of the mandible.

Mass number See Atomic weight.

Mastoid process A marked prominence of the temporal bone located posterior and inferior to the temporomandibular joint; viewed on a panoramic image and appears radiopaque.

Matter Anything that occupies space and has mass.

Maxilla The upper jaw.

Maxillary sinuses Paired cavities or compartments of bone located within the maxilla and located superior to the maxillary posterior teeth; appear radiolucent.

Maxillary tuberosity A rounded prominence of bone that extends posterior to the third molar region; appears radiopaque.

Maximum permissible dose (MPD) Maximum dose equivalent that a body is permitted to receive in a specific period. MPD is the dose of radiation that the body can endure with little or no injury.

Median palatal suture The immovable joint between the two palatine processes of the maxilla; appears radiolucent.

Mental foramen An opening or hole in bone located on the external surface of the mandible in the region of the mandibular premolars; appears radiolucent.

Mental fossa A scooped-out, depressed area of bone located on the external surface of the anterior mandible; appears radiolucent.

Mental ridge A linear prominence of cortical bone located on the external surface of the anterior portion of the mandible; appears radiopaque.

Metal housing The metal casing of the dental x-ray tubehead that houses the x-ray tube and transformers.

Metallic restoration Restorations that completely absorb x-rays; as a result, little to no radiation contacts the receptor; appears radiopaque (e.g., amalgam, gold).

Midsagittal plane An imaginary line or plane passing through the center of the body that divides it into right and left halves.

Milliamperage In dental imaging, the quantity, or number, of x-rays emitted from the tubehead; measured in milliamperes.

Milliampere (mA) 1/1000 of an ampere; a unit of measurement used to describe the intensity of an electrical current.

Mitotic activity Process of cell division; determines the response of a cell to radiation exposure (cells that divide frequently are more sensitive to radiation).

Mixed lucent–opaque A term used to describe a lesion viewed on a dental image that exhibits both radiolucent and radiopaque components.

Molecule Two or more atoms joined together by chemical bonds, or the smallest amount of a substance that possesses its characteristic properties. Molecules are formed in one of two ways: (1) by the transfer of electrons or (2) by the sharing of electrons between the outermost shells of atoms.

Molybdenum cup A portion of the cathode in the x-ray tube; focuses the electrons into a narrow beam and directs the beam across the tube toward the tungsten target in the anode.

Mount To place in an appropriate setting, as for display or study.

Movement Motion of the receptor or patient during image exposure; movement results in an image with decreased sharpness.

Multifocal confluent radiopacity A term used to describe multiple radiopacities on dental image that appear to overlap or flow together.

Multilocular A term used to describe a radiolucent lesion on a dental image that exhibits multiple compartments.

Multiplanar reconstruction (MPR) The reconstruction of raw data into images when imported into viewing software to create three anatomic planes of the body.

Mylohyoid ridge A linear prominence of bone located on the internal surface of the mandible that extends from the molar region downward and forward toward the lower border of the mandible; appears radiopaque.

N

Nanometer A measurement used for wavelength; 1 nanometer equals one-billionth (10^{-9}) of a meter.

Nasal cavity A pear-shaped compartment of bone located superior to the maxilla; appears radiolucent (also known as the *nasal fossa).*

Nasal septum A vertical bony wall or partition that divides the nasal cavity into the right and left nasal fossae; appears radiopaque.

Nasopharyngeal air space Refers to the airspace portion of the pharynx (*pharyngeal*) located posterior to the nasal cavity (*naso*); on a panoramic image, the nasopharyngeal air space appears as a diagonal radiolucency located superior to the radiopaque shadow of the soft palate and uvula.

Negligence Omission or failure to provide reasonable precaution, care, or action; occurs when the diagnosis made or the dental treatment delivered falls below the standard of care.

Neutral atom An atom that contains an equal number of protons (positive charges) and electrons (negative charges).

Neutron An electrically neutral or uncharged particle.

Nonmetallic restoration Restorations that do not completely absorb x-rays; vary in appearance from slightly radiopaque to radiolucent, depending on the density of the material (e.g., porcelain, composite, acrylic).
Nonstochastic effects Effects of radiation that have a threshold and increase in severity with increasing absorbed dose.
Normalizing device A commercially available device used to monitor developer strength and film density.
Nucleon Part of an atomic nucleus (e.g., protons, neutrons).
Nucleus The central, positively charged core of an atom; composed of *protons* and *neutrons*.
Nutrient canal(s) A tiny tubelike passageway through bone which contains blood vessels and nerves that supply teeth and interdental areas; appears radiolucent.

O

Occlusal Refers to the chewing surfaces of the teeth.
Occlusal examination A type of intraoral examination used to inspect large areas of the maxilla or the mandible on one image.
Occlusal projection, mandibular cross-sectional A type of occlusal projection used to examine the buccal and lingual aspects of the mandible and locate foreign bodies (e.g., salivary stones) in the floor of the mouth.
Occlusal projection, mandibular pediatric A type of occlusal projection used to examine the anterior teeth of the mandible; recommended for children aged 5 years or younger.
Occlusal projection, mandibular topographic A type of occlusal projection used to examine the anterior teeth of the mandible.
Occlusal projection, maxillary lateral A type of occlusal projection used to examine the palatal roots of molar teeth and locate foreign bodies or lesions in the posterior maxilla.
Occlusal projection, maxillary pediatric A type of occlusal projection used to examine the anterior teeth of the maxilla; recommended for children aged 5 years or younger.
Occlusal projection, maxillary topographic A type of occlusal projection used to examine the palate and anterior teeth of the maxilla.
Occlusal surfaces The chewing surfaces of posterior teeth.
Occlusal technique The method used to expose a receptor in occlusal examination.
On-off switch A component of the control panel on the dental x-ray machine; turns the dental x-ray machine on or off.
Operating kilovoltage See Kilovoltage.
Orbit (1) The well-defined path of an electron around the nucleus of an atom (also known as *shell*); (2) The bony cavity that contains the eyeball.
Outer package wrapping One of the four components of the dental x-ray film packet; a soft vinyl or paper wrapper that serves to protect the film from exposure to light and saliva. It has two sides: the tube side and the label side.
Oxidation A chemical reaction that occurs when processing solutions are exposed to air; the chemicals break down, resulting in a decreased concentration of solution strength.

P

Packet, film The intraoral film and its surrounding packaging.
Packet, one-film A film packet containing one film.
Packet, two-film A film packet containing two films.
Palate Roof of the mouth.
Palate, hard The bony plate that separates the nasal cavity from the oral cavity; the anterior portion of the roof of the mouth; appears radiopaque.
Palate, soft The fleshy, movable posterior portion of the roof of the mouth separating the mouth and pharynx.
Palatoglossal air space Refers to the space found between the palate (*palato*) and tongue (*glossal*); on a panoramic image, appears as a horizontal radiolucent band located superior to the apices of maxillary teeth.
Panoramic A wide view.
Panoramic imaging An extraoral technique used to examine the upper and lower jaws on a single projection (also known as *rotational panoramic imaging*).
Paper film wrapper One of the four components of the dental x-ray film packet; a black paper protective sheet covers the film and shields it from light.
Parallel Moving or lying in the same plane; always separated by the same distance and not intersecting.
Paralleling technique An intraoral imaging technique used to expose periapical receptors: the receptor is placed parallel to the long axis of the tooth; the central ray is directed perpendicular to the receptor and the long axis of tooth; a beam alignment device must be used to keep the receptor parallel to the long axis of the tooth (also known as *extension cone paralleling [XCP] technique, right-angle technique*, and *long-cone technique*).
Particulate radiations Tiny particles of matter that possess mass and travel in straight lines and at high speeds. Particulate radiations transmit kinetic energy by means of their extremely fast-moving small masses. Four types of particulate radiation are recognized.
Pathogen A microorganism capable of causing disease.
Patient relations The relationship between the patient and the dental professional.
Pediatric A term derived from the Greek word *pedia*, meaning child.
Pediatric patient A child patient.
Pediatrics, dental A branch of dentistry dealing with the diagnosis and treatment of dental diseases in children.
Penumbra The unsharpness or blurring of the edges of a structure (e.g., tooth) viewed on a dental image.
Periapical Around the apex of a tooth.
Periapical abscess A lesion characterized by a localized collection of pus around the apex of a nonvital tooth that results from pulpal death; appears radiolucent.
Periapical cyst A lesion characterized by an epithelial-lined cavity or sac located around the apex of a nonvital tooth that results from pulpal death; appears radiolucent (also known as a *radicular cyst*).
Periapical examination A type of intraoral imaging examination used to view the entire tooth (crown and root) and supporting bone.
Periapical granuloma A lesion characterized by a localized mass of granulation tissue around the apex of a nonvital tooth; appears radiolucent.
Periapical lesion A lesion located around the apex of a tooth.
Pericoronal Around the crown of a tooth.
Periodic table of the elements A chart that arranges elements in increasing atomic number.
Period of injury Occurs after the latent period following exposure to radiation; can include a variety of cellular injuries.
Periodontal Around a tooth.
Periodontal abscess A lesion that originates in a soft tissue pocket and is characterized by the accumulation of pus and destruction of bone; is often painful; appears radiolucent.
Periodontal disease A group of diseases that affects the tissues around teeth.
Periodontal ligament space (PDL space) A space that exists between the root of a tooth and the lamina dura; contains connective tissue fibers, blood vessels, and lymphatics; appears radiolucent.
Periodontium Specialized tissues that surround and support teeth, such as the gingiva, cementum, periodontal ligament and alveolar bone.
Perpendicular Intersecting at or forming right angles.
Personal protective equipment (PPE) Equipment worn by dental professionals to protect themselves from hazards; includes protective attire, gloves, mask, and eyewear.
Phosphors Minute fluorescent crystals that cover intensifying screens and fluoresce, or emit visible light, when exposed to x-rays.
Photoelectric effect One of the interactions of x-radiation with matter; the x-ray photon collides with a tightly bound, inner-shell electron and gives up all its energy to eject the electron from its orbit. All the energy of the photon is absorbed by the displaced electron in the form of kinetic energy.
Photon A bundle of energy with no mass or weight that travels as a wave at the speed of light and moves through space in a straight line.
Pixel A discrete unit of information; in digital electronic images, digital information is contained in, and presented as, discrete units of information (also known as *picture element*).
Plane, axial A horizontal plane that divides the body into superior and inferior parts; runs parallel to the ground.
Plane, coronal A vertical plane that divides the body into anterior and posterior sides; runs perpendicular to the ground.

Plane, sagittal A vertical plane that divides the body into right and left sides; runs perpendicular to the ground.

Polychromatic x-ray beam An x-ray beam containing many different wavelengths of varying intensities.

Position-indicating device (PID) An open-ended, lead-lined cylinder extending from the opening of the tubehead; aims and shapes the x-ray beam (also called the *cone*).

Posteroanterior projection An extraoral projection of the skull used to evaluate facial growth, trauma, diseases, and developmental abnormalities.

Potassium alum See Hardening agent.

Potassium bromide See Restrainer.

Preservative (1) One of the four basic ingredients of the developer solution; sodium sulfite prevents the developer solution from oxidizing in the presence of air; (2) one of the four basic ingredients of the fixer solution; sodium sulfite prevents the chemical deterioration of the fixing agent.

Primary beam See Radiation, primary.

Process A marked prominence or projection of bone; appears radiopaque.

Processing, automatic A method used to process films in which all film processing steps are automated.

Processing, film A series of steps that collectively produce a visible, permanent image on a dental radiograph.

Processing, manual A method used to process films in which all film processing steps are performed manually (also known as *hand processing or tank processing*).

Processor, automatic A machine that automates all film processing steps.

Processor housing The housing, or protective covering, of the automatic film processor; encases all the component parts of the automatic processor.

Protective barrier A barrier of radiation-absorbing material used to protect the operator from primary and scatter radiation (e.g., a wall).

Protective layer One of the four basic components of x-ray film; a thin, protective coating on top of the emulsion that protects the film from manipulation and mechanical and processing damage.

Proton A positively charged particle with a mass of one.

Pterygomaxillary fissure A narrow space or cleft that separates the lateral pterygoid plate and the maxilla; viewed on a panoramic image and appears radiolucent.

Pulp canal obliteration The calcification, or deposition, of hard tissue within the pulp cavity; no visible pulp chamber or canals visible on dental image.

Pulp cavity A cavity within a tooth that includes both the pulp chamber and the pulp canals; contains blood vessels, nerves, and lymphatics; appears radiolucent.

Pulp stones Calcifications found in the pulp chamber or pulp canals of teeth; appear radiopaque.

Pulpal sclerosis A diffuse calcification of the pulp chamber and pulp canals of teeth that results in a pulp cavity of decreased size; appears radiopaque.

Q

Quality (of x-ray beam) The mean energy or penetrating ability of the x-ray beam; the quality of the x-ray beam is controlled by kilovoltage.

Quality administration The management of the quality assurance plan in the dental office.

Quality assurance Special procedures used to assure the production of high-quality, diagnostic images.

Quality control tests Specific tests designed to maintain and monitor dental x-ray equipment, supplies, and film processing.

Quality factor (QF) A factor used for radiation protection purposes that accounts for the exposure effects of different types of radiation; for x-rays, QF = 1.

Quanta See Photon.

Quantity (of x-ray beam) The number of x-rays produced in the dental x-ray unit; the quantity of x-rays produced is controlled by milliamperage.

R

Radiation A form of energy carried by waves or a stream of particles.

Radiation, background A form of ionizing radiation that is ubiquitous in the environment; includes cosmic and terrestrial radiation.

Radiation, braking See Radiation, general.

Radiation, characteristic A form of radiation that occurs when a high-speed electron dislodges an inner-shell electron from an atom, causing excitation, or ionization, of the atom.

Radiation, electromagnetic The propagation of wavelike energy through space or matter; the propagated energy is accompanied by electric and magnetic fields, thus the term *electromagnetic;* examples include cosmic rays, gamma rays, x-rays, ultraviolet rays, visible light, infrared light, radar waves, microwaves, and radio waves.

Radiation, general A form of radiation that occurs when speeding electrons slow down because of their interactions with the tungsten target in the anode (also known as *bremsstrahlung* or *braking radiation*).

Radiation, ionizing Radiation capable of producing ions; includes particulate or electromagnetic radiation.

Radiation, leakage Any radiation, with the exception of the primary beam, that is emitted from the dental x-ray tubehead.

Radiation, particulate Tiny particles of matter that possess mass and travel in straight lines and at high speeds (e.g., electrons, β-particles, α-particles, protons, and neutrons).

Radiation, primary The penetrating x-ray beam produced at the target of the anode and exits the tubehead (also known as the *primary beam* or *useful beam*).

Radiation, scatter A form of secondary radiation; results from an x-ray beam that has been deflected from its path by the interaction with matter.

Radiation, secondary Radiation created when the primary beam interacts with matter; secondary radiation is less penetrating than primary radiation.

Radiation absorbed dose (rad) A unit for measuring absorbed dose; the traditional unit of dose equivalent to the gray (Gy); 100 erg of energy per gram of tissue; 100 rad = 1 Gy.

Radiation biology The study of the effects of ionizing radiation on living tissues.

Radiation monitoring badge A device used to measure and monitor radiation exposure; worn by persons frequently exposed to radiation.

Radioactivity The process by which certain unstable atoms or elements undergo spontaneous disintegration, or decay, in an effort to attain a more balanced nuclear state.

Radiograph An image or picture produced on a receptor by exposure to ionizing radiation.

Radiograph, dental A photographic image produced on film by the passage of x-rays through teeth and related structures.

Radiograph, duplicate An identical copy of a radiograph that is made through the process of film duplication.

Radiograph, reference A radiograph processed under ideal conditions and then used to compare the film densities of radiographs that are processed daily.

Radiographer, dental Any person who positions, exposes, and processes dental x-ray image receptors.

Radiography The art and science of making radiographs by the exposure of film to x-rays.

Radiography, dental The production of radiographs of teeth and adjacent structures by the exposure of an image receptor to x-rays.

Radiology The science or study of radiation as used in medicine; a branch of medical science that deals with the use of x-rays, radioactive substances, and other forms of radiant energy in the diagnosis and treatment of disease.

Radiolucent The portion of an image that is dark or black; a radiolucent structure readily permits the passage of the x-ray beam and allows more x-rays to reach the receptor.

Radiopacity, irregular A term used to describe a radiopacity viewed on a dental image that has irregular, ill-defined borders.

Radiopaque The portion of an image that is light or white; a radiopaque structure resists the passage of the x-ray beam and limits the amount of x-rays that reach the receptor.

Radioresistant cell A cell that is resistant to radiation (e.g., bone, muscle, and nerve cells).

Radiosensitive cell A cell that is sensitive to radiation (e.g., small lymphocytes; blood, immature reproductive, young bone, and epithelial cells).

Rampant Growing or spreading unchecked.

Ramus Vertical portion of the mandible that is found posterior to the third molar. The mandible has two rami, one on each side.

Receptor Something that responds to a stimulus; a recording medium (examples: x-ray film, PSP plates or digital sensors).

Receptor, bite-wing An intraoral receptor used to examine the crowns of both maxillary and mandibular teeth on one image.

Receptor, extraoral Receptor placed outside the mouth to examine large areas of the skull or jaws.
Receptor, intraoral A receptor placed inside the mouth during x-ray exposure; intraoral receptors are used to examine teeth and supporting structures.
Receptor, occlusal A receptor used to examine large areas of the maxilla or the mandible; the patient "occludes" or bites on the entire receptor.
Receptor, panoramic Receptor used in panoramic examination, shows a wide view of the maxilla and the mandible.
Receptor, periapical An intraoral receptor used to examine the entire tooth (crown and root) and supporting bone.
Receptor holder Device used to hold an intraoral receptor in the mouth; used to stabilize the receptor's position during the exposure.
Receptor placement The specific area where the receptor must be positioned before exposure.
Recoil electron See Compton electron.
Recovery period The period during which cellular damage caused by radiation is followed by repair.
Rectification The conversion of alternating current to direct current.
Reduction A chemical reaction during film processing in which the halide portion of the exposed energized silver halide crystal is removed.
Reduction, selective A chemical reaction during film processing in which the energized exposed silver halide crystals are changed into black metallic silver, while the unenergized unexposed silver halide crystals are removed from the film.
Replenisher A superconcentrated solution added to a processing solution to compensate for the loss of volume and strength that results from oxidation.
Replenisher pump A component part of the automatic film processor; automatically maintains proper concentrations and levels of solutions.
Replenisher solutions See Replenisher.
Resolution, contrast The number of gray scale colors available to be chosen for each pixel in the image.
Resolution, spatial A measurement of pixel size in multiplanar reconstruction.
Resorption, external A regressive alteration of root structure that occurs along the periphery of the root surface.
Resorption, internal The destruction of dentin around the pulp cavity within the crown or root of a tooth; appears as a radiolucency.
Resorption, pathologic Resorption of a tooth *not* associated with the normal shedding of deciduous teeth.
Resorption, physiologic Resorption of the teeth associated with the normal shedding of deciduous teeth.
Respirator, N95 filtering facepiece An air-purifying respirator which filters at least 95% of airborne particles; this mask protects against airborne particle transmission and liquids that could contaminate the face.
Respiratory hygiene An infection prevention measure designed to limit the transmission of disease spread by respiratory pathogens via droplet or airborne routes (also known as *cough etiquette*).
Restrainer One of the four basic ingredients of the developer solution; potassium bromide is used to prevent the development of unexposed silver halide crystals; also prevents film fogging.
Reticulation of emulsion A temperature error; a film has a cracked appearance as a result of being subjected to sudden temperature changes between the developer solution and the water bath.
Reverse Towne projection An extraoral projection used to identify fractures of the condylar neck and ramus area.
Ridge A linear prominence of bone; appears radiopaque.
Right-angle technique A localization technique in which the orientation of structures can be seen in two images (one periapical and one occlusal).
Rinn Snap-A-Ray Holder A simple intraoral receptor holder used to stabilize a receptor during exposure.
Rinsing One of the steps in film processing; a water bath is used to rinse the developer from the film and stop the development process.
Risk The likelihood of adverse effects or death resulting from exposure to a hazard.
Risk management The policies and procedures that the dental professional should follow to reduce the chance that a patient will take legal action against the dental professional or the supervising dentist.
Roentgen (R) The traditional unit of exposure for x-rays; the quantity of x-radiation or gamma radiation that produces an electrical charge of 2.58×10^{-4} coulombs in 1 kilogram of air at standard pressure and temperature conditions.
Roentgen equivalent (in) man (rem) The traditional unit of the dose equivalent; the product of absorbed dose (rad) and a quality factor (QF) specific for the type of radiation; 100 rems = 1 sievert (Sv).
Roller film transporter A component part of the automatic film processor; a system of rollers is used to move the film rapidly through the developer, fixer, water, and the drying compartments.
Room lighting One of the two essential types of lighting in a darkroom; room lighting provides adequate illumination for the size of the room to perform tasks such as cleaning, stocking of materials, and mixing of chemicals.
Rotation center In panoramic imaging, the axis or pivotal point on which the receptor and x-ray tubehead rotate around the patient.

S

Safelight filter A filter placed over the safelight that is designed to remove the short wavelengths in the blue-green portion of the visible light spectrum that are responsible for exposing and damaging x-ray film.
Safelighting One of the two essential types of lighting in a darkroom; a low-intensity light composed of long wavelengths in the red-orange portion of the visible light spectrum; safelighting provides sufficient illumination in the darkroom to carry out processing activities without exposing or damaging the film.
Sclerotic bone A term used to describe a well-defined radiopacity viewed on a dental image located below the apices of vital, noncarious teeth (also known as *osteosclerosis* or *idiopathic periapical osteosclerosis*).
Screen, calcium tungstate A type of intensifying screen used in extraoral imaging; contains phosphors that emit blue light.
Screen, intensifying A device used in extraoral imaging that converts x-ray energy into visible light; the light, in turn, exposes the screen film.
Screen, rare earth A type of intensifying screen used in extraoral imaging; contains phosphors not usually found in the earth that emit green light.
Self-determination The legal rights of an individual to make choices about the care he or she receives, including the opportunity to consent to or refuse treatment.
Sensitivity speck An irregularity within the lattice structure of the exposed silver halide crystals that attracts the silver atoms.
Sensor In digital imaging, a receptor that is used to capture an intraoral or extraoral image.
Septum Bony wall or partition that divides a cavity into separate areas; appears radiopaque (plural: septa).
Sharp Any object that can penetrate skin, including, but not limited to, needles and scalpels.
Sharpness Refers to the capability of the receptor to reproduce the distinct outlines of an object; influenced by focal spot size, film composition, and movement.
Shell See Orbit.
Short-term effects Effects of radiation that appear within minutes, days, or weeks; associated with large amounts of radiation absorbed in a short time.
Sievert (Sv) A unit of measurement for dose equivalent; the SI unit of measurement equivalent to the rem; 1 Sv = 100 rems.
Sigmoid notch A curved depression located between the mandibular condyle and the coronoid process of the mandible (also known as the *mandibular notch*).
Silver halide crystals Crystals that are suspended in the emulsion of the dental x-ray film (e.g., silver bromide, silver iodide); function to absorb radiation during x-ray exposure and store energy from the radiation.
Sinus A hollow space, cavity, or recess in bone; appears radiolucent.
Sodium carbonate See Accelerator.
Sodium sulfite See Preservative.
Sodium thiosulfate See Fixing agent.
Soft tissue opacity A term used to describe a well-defined radiopacity viewed on a dental image that is located in soft tissue.
Somatic cells All the cells in the body, with the exception of the reproductive cells.
Somatic effects Radiation injuries that produce changes in somatic cells and produce poor

health in the irradiated individual (e.g., the induction of cancer, leukemia, or cataracts).

Spine A sharp, thornlike projection of bone; appears radiopaque.

Stabe Biteblock A disposable Styrofoam device that can be used to hold a receptor during exposure.

Standard of care In dentistry, the quality of care that is provided by dental practitioners in a similar locality under the same or similar conditions.

Standard precautions Measures that include a standard of care designed to protect health care personnel and patients from pathogens that can be spread by blood or any other body fluid, excretion, or secretion.

Static electricity A film handling error; thin, black, branching lines on a film that result from static that occurs when opening a film packet too quickly.

Statute of limitations A period during which a patient may bring a malpractice action against a dentist or an auxiliary.

Stepwedge A device constructed of uniform-layered thicknesses of an x-ray absorbing material, usually aluminum; different steps absorb varying amounts of x-rays and are used to demonstrate film densities and contrast scales.

Sterilization The act of sterilizing; see Sterilize.

Sterilize The use of a physical or chemical procedure to destroy all pathogens, including highly resistant bacterial and fungal spores.

Stimuli, psychogenic Stimuli originating in the mind.

Stimuli, tactile Stimuli originating from touch.

Stirring paddle A device used in manual processing; agitates the developer and fixer solutions and equalizes the temperature of the solutions before processing.

Stirring rod See Stirring paddle.

Stochastic effects Biologic effects from radiation that occur as a direct function of dose; the probability of occurrence increases with increasing absorbed dose; however, the severity of effects does not depend on the magnitude of the absorbed dose.

Storage phosphor imaging An indirect method of obtaining a digital image in which the image is recorded on phosphor-coated plates and then placed into an electronic processor, where a laser scans the plate and produces an image on a computer screen.

Styloid process A long, pointed, and sharp projection of bone that extends downward from the inferior surface of the temporal bone; located anterior to the mastoid process; viewed on a panoramic image and appears radiopaque.

Subject thickness The thickness of soft tissue and bone in a patient.

Submandibular fossa A depressed area of bone located on the internal surface of the mandible inferior to the mylohyoid ridge; appears radiolucent (also known as *mandibular fossa*).

Submentovertex projection An extraoral projection used to identify the position of the condyles, demonstrate the base of the skull, and evaluate fractures of the zygomatic arch.

Sulfuric acid See Acidifier.

Superior foramina of the incisive canal Two tiny openings or holes in bone that are located on the floor of the nasal cavity; appear radiolucent.

Suture An immovable joint that represents a line of union between adjoining bones of the skull; appears radiolucent.

T

Tank, insert In manual processing, a component part of the processing tank; two removable insert tanks are placed in the master tank and hold the developer and fixer solutions.

Tank, master In manual processing, a component part of the processing tank; the master tank is filled with circulating water that surrounds and suspends the two insert tanks.

Tank, processing A tank used in manual processing; divided into compartments for the developer solution, water bath, and fixer solution; a processing tank has two insert tanks and one master tank.

Target lesion A term used to describe a well-defined, localized radiopacity viewed on a dental image that is surrounded by a uniform radiolucent halo.

Teeth, anterior Incisors and canines.

Teeth, posterior Premolars and molars.

Temporomandibular joint (TMJ) The jaw joint; includes the temporal bone (glenoid fossa and articular eminence), the mandible (condyle) and the articular disc between the two bones.

Temporomandibular joint tomography An extraoral imaging technique used to examine the temporomandibular joint (TMJ).

Thermionic emission The release of electrons from the tungsten filament when the electrical current passes through it and heats the filament.

Thermometer A device used to measure temperature.

Three-dimensional volume rendering A three-dimensional shape that is created from two-dimensional images.

Thyroid collar A flexible lead shield used to protect the thyroid gland from scatter radiation.

Timer A mechanical device used to measure time intervals.

Tomogram An extraoral image used to examine the bony components of the temporomandibular joint (TMJ).

Tomography Imaging technique that allows the examination of one layer or section of the body while blurring images from structures in other planes.

Tongue A movable muscular organ attached to the floor of the mouth.

Tooth-bearing areas Regions of the maxilla and mandible in which the 32 teeth of the human dentition are normally located.

Torus A bony growth in the oral cavity (plural, *tori*).

Torus, mandibular A bony growth seen along the lingual aspect of the mandible (also known as *torus mandibularis*).

Torus, maxillary A nodular mass of bone along the midline of the hard palate (also known as *torus palatinus*).

Total dose Quantity of radiation received, or the total amount of radiation energy absorbed.

Transcranial projection An extraoral projection used to evaluate the superior surface of the condyle and the articular eminence; also used to evaluate the movement of the condyle when the mouth is opened and to compare the joint spaces.

Transformer A device used to increase or decrease the voltage of incoming electricity.

Transformer, step-down In dental imaging, a device used to decrease the incoming voltage from 110 or 220 volts to the low voltage required, usually 3 to 5 volts.

Transformer, step-up In dental imaging, a device used to increase the incoming line voltage from 110 or 220 volts to the high voltage required, usually 65,000 to 100,000 volts.

Trauma Injury produced by an external force.

Triangle In geometry, a figure formed by connecting three points not in a straight line by three straight-line segments; the figure has three angles.

Triangle, equilateral In geometry, a triangle with three equal sides.

Triangle, right In geometry, a triangle with one 90-degree angle (right angle).

Triangles, congruent In geometry, triangles that are identical and correspond exactly when superimposed.

Tube side The outer side of the x-ray film packet that is solid white and exhibits a raised bump in one corner; the tube side of the film faces the teeth and tubehead.

Tubehead The tightly sealed heavy metal housing that contains the dental x-ray tube; includes the metal housing, insulating oil, tubehead seal, x-ray tube, transformers, aluminum disks, lead collimator, and position-indicating device (PID); contains a filament used to produce electrons and a target used to produce x-rays.

Tubehead seal The aluminum or leaded-glass covering of the tubehead that seals the oil in the tubehead and filters the x-ray beam.

Tubercle A small bump or nodule of bone; appears radiopaque.

Tuberosity A rounded prominence of bone; appears radiopaque.

Tungsten filament A portion of the cathode in the x-ray tube; a coiled wire of tungsten that produces electrons when heated.

Tungsten target A portion of the anode in the x-ray tube; serves as a focal spot and converts bombarding electrons into x-ray photons.

U

Unilocular corticated A term used to describe a radiolucency on a dental image that exhibits one compartment with a well-defined outer border.

Unilocular noncorticated A term used to describe a radiolucency on a dental image that exhibits one compartment without a well-defined outer border.

Unmodified scatter See Coherent scatter.

Useful beam See Radiation, primary.

Uvula A small, fleshy extension located on the free edge of the soft palate at the midline.

V

Vacuum tube A sealed glass tube from which most of the air has been evacuated.

Valve, mixing In manual processing, a device that mixes the incoming hot and cold water to produce a water bath of optimum temperature (68°F).

Velocity Speed; in dental imaging, the speed of a wave.

Viewbox A light source used to view dental radiographs (also called the *illuminator*).

Viewing Examining or inspecting; see Film viewing.

Volt (V) Unit of measure for voltage.

Voltage In dental imaging, measurement of force that refers to the potential difference between two electrical charges.

Voxel The smallest element of a three-dimensional image; also referred to as *volume element* or *three-dimensional pixel.*

W

Washing A step in film processing; water is used to wash a film after fixing; removes excess chemicals from the emulsion.

Waters projection An extraoral projection used to evaluate the maxillary sinus area.

Wavelength The distance between the crest of one wave to the crest of the next wave; determines the energy and penetrating power of the radiation; the shorter the wavelength, the higher the energy.

X

X-radiation A high-energy radiation produced by the collision of a beam of electrons with a metal target in an x-ray tube; see X-ray(s).

X-ray(s) A beam of energy that has the power to penetrate substances and record image shadows on receptors (photographic film or digital sensors).

X-ray beam angulation One of the influencing factors for image distortion; refers to the direction of the x-ray beam; less image distortion results when the x-ray beam is directed perpendicular to the tooth and receptor.

X-ray tube A component part of the x-ray tubehead that generates x-rays; includes a leaded-glass vacuum tube, cathode, and anode.

Z

Zygoma The cheekbone; articulates with the zygomatic process of the maxilla and appears as a diffuse radiopaque band posterior to the zygomatic process of the maxilla (also call *zygomatic bone* or *malar bone*).

Zygomatic process of maxilla A bony projection of the maxilla that articulates with the zygoma; appears as a J-shaped or U-shaped radiopacity on a maxillary molar periapical image.

INDEX

Page numbers followed by "*f*" indicate figures, "*b*" indicate boxes, and "*t*" indicate tables.